THE CANADIAN MEDICAL ASSOCIATION

HOME MEDICAL ENCYCLOPEDIA

VOLUME ONE · A – H

MEDICAL EDITOR

Peter Morgan, M.D.

Reader's Digest

The Reader's Digest Association (Canada) Ltd.
Montreal

A Dorling Kindersley book

Published in Canada in 1992 by
The Reader's Digest Association (Canada) Ltd.
215 Redfern Avenue
Westmount, Que. H3Z 2V9

The Canadian Medical Association Home Medical Encyclopedia provides information on a wide range of health and medical topics. The encyclopedia is not a substitute for medical diagnosis, however, and you are advised always to consult your physician for specific information on personal health matters. The naming of any organization, product, or alternative therapy in this encyclopedia does not imply CMA endorsement; the omission of any such names does not indicate CMA disapproval.

Canadian Cataloguing in Publication Data
Main entry under title:
The Canadian Medical Association home medical encyclopedia

1st Canadian ed.
Includes index.
ISBN 0-88850-186-2 (set)
ISBN 0-88850-184-6 (v. 1)
ISBN 0-88850-185-4 (v. 2)

  I. Medicine, Popular – Dictionaries. I. Morgan, Peter, 1927 –   . II. Canadian Medical Association. III. Reader's Digest Association (Canada). IV. Title: Home medical encyclopedia.

RC81.A2C36 1991   610.3   C91-090378-6

Computerset by MFK Typesetting Limited, England
Reproduction by Mandarin Offset Limited, Hong Kong
Printed and bound in the U.S.A.

92 93 94 95 96 / 5 4 3 2 1

PREFACE

Good health is a most precious asset and Canadians are especially fortunate in having one of the most modern and efficient health care systems in the world. But there is more to health care than access to competent physicians, modern diagnostic technology, and well-equipped hospitals. Both the public and the medical profession increasingly believe that people must become active in promoting and protecting their own health.

The public's concern is evident in the questions of patients and their families: How good are the health promotion programs being touted? How do physicians make a diagnosis and decide to treat—or not to treat—a problem? What diseases can be prevented and how? When should some of the spectacular new technologies be used, and when are the older methods better? How can I get the right kind of care for my problem? How common is this disease? Should I see a specialist? Will this drug make me feel sick? What questions should I ask the physician next time?

Information in the popular press about health and disease is often fragmentary and sometimes inaccurate. Our schools teach little about the workings of the human body and the effects of disability and disease. Many manuals and books available in bookstores offer limited information or present a biased point of view. Although health care professionals have increased their efforts to educate and inform the public and their patients, it is impossible in an office visit to explain the workings of the human body or the causes and mechanisms of a patient's disease "from the ground up."

The Canadian Medical Association believes there is a pressing need for a medical encyclopedia to help people make informed decisions about their health and to share these decisions with their physicians. Indeed, the success of any course of medical diagnosis and treatment largely depends on mutual understanding—on knowledge shared between the physician and the patient.

THE CANADIAN MEDICAL ASSOCIATION HOME MEDICAL ENCYCLOPEDIA is by far the most authoritative source of health information available to the Canadian public. Its contents have been reviewed extensively by several groups of medical experts. It contains thousands of clear answers to questions people are asking every day. It describes the symptoms and signs of both common and rare diseases, shows—in words and illustrations—the anatomy and function of all parts of the body, and gives current information on nutrition, safety, and other good health practices for all age groups. It also presents Canadian statistical information on many important diseases, a glossary of Canadian drugs, a compendium of Canadian self-help organizations, and all the essential facts about the Canadian health care system. The encyclopedic format allows rapid access to all this information.

The Canadian Medical Association is proud to present THE CANADIAN MEDICAL ASSOCIATION HOME MEDICAL ENCYCLOPEDIA as evidence of its commitment to better medical care and as a contribution to the better health of Canadians.

Léo-Paul Landry

Léo-Paul Landry, M.D.
Secretary General
Canadian Medical Association

CANADIAN MEDICAL ASSOCIATION

Carole Guzman, *President*
Léo-Paul Landry, *Secretary General*
Susan Stockwell, *Director, Department of Publications*
Bruce P. Squires, *Editor in chief*
Leesa D. Bruce, *Managing Editor*
Deborah A. Rupert, *Editorial Assistant*

EDITORIAL TEAM

Peter Morgan, M.D., Medical Editor; Bruce P. Squires, M.D., Ph.D.; Martha Plaine, Researcher;
Gene Krysak, Ph.M., Pharmaceutical consultant

CONSULTANTS

Lynne Cohen, Garth Dickinson, M.D., Theresa Gyorkos, Ph.D., Eike-Henner Kluge, Ph.D.,
Robert E. Lee, Eleanor Paulsen, Gerald Rotenberg, B.Sc.Phm., F.A.C.A.

ACKNOWLEDGMENTS

Canadian Centre for Occupational Health and Safety, Canadian Chiropractic Association, Canadian College of Family Physicians, Canadian National Institute for the Blind, Canadian Nurses Association, Canadian Pharmaceutical Association, Canadian Red Cross, Health and Welfare Canada, National Cancer Institute of Canada, St. John's Ambulance, Statistics Canada, The Association of Local Official Health Agencies, University of Ottawa Heart Institute

Medical reviewers and contributors to the work on which *The Canadian Medical Association Home Medical Encyclopedia* is based are:

MEDICAL REVIEWERS

Mr. John Ballantyne, C.B.E., F.R.C.S.
Professor Arnold E. Bender, D.Sc., Ph.D.
Dr. Brendan M. Buckley, D.Phil., F.R.C.P.(I)
Professor James Calnan, F.R.C.S., F.R.C.P.
Dr. Dewi Davies, M.D., F.R.C.P.
Dr. A.K. Dixon, M.D., F.R.C.R.
Dr. James Owen Drife, M.D., F.R.C.S.(Ed)
Mr. Edgar Gordon, M.Sc., D.D.S.

Professor Terry J. Hamblin, D.M., F.R.C.P.
Dr. Anthony John Holland, M.Phil., M.R.C.P.
Dr. Helen M. Kingston, M.D., M.R.C.P.
Professor W.R. Lee, M.D., F.R.C.P.
Dr. E.B. Lewis, M.B., F.F.A.R.C.S.
Mr. C.D.R. Lightowler, F.R.C.S.
Dr. G. Keith Morris, M.D., F.R.C.P.
Dr. Graham Peter Mulley, D.M., F.R.C.P.
Dr. R.T.D. Oliver, M.D., F.R.C.P.

Dr. Alex Paton, M.D., F.R.C.P.
Dr. T. Richards, M.R.C.P, M.R.C.G.P.
Dr. J.A. Savin, M.D., F.R.C.P.
Dr. Leonard Sinclair, F.R.C.P., D.C.H.
Dr. R.N.T. Thin, M.D., F.R.C.P.
Mr. Patrick D. Trevor-Roper, M.D., F.R.C.S.
Mr. Robert H. Whitaker, M.D., F.R.C.S.
Dr. George Bernard Wyatt, F.R.C.P., D.C.H.

CONTRIBUTORS

Vivienne Owen Ankrett, M.R.C.G.P., D.R.C.O.G.
Igor Anrep, L.R.C.P., M.R.C.S.
Ann Ashworth, Ph.D.
Alan Bailey, M.B., M.R.C.P.
Julian Barth, M.B., M.R.C.P.
Margaret A. Barrie, F.R.C.P., D.R.C.O.G.
R.J. Berry, F.R.C.P., F.R.C.R.
A.K. Bhalla, M.D., M.R.C.P.
Charles Eric Blank, Ph.D., M.B.
Geoffrey Blundell
Susan Bosanko
Arthur William Boylston, M.D., M.R.C.Path.
Amanda Bridges
Peter Bromwich, M.B., M.R.C.O.G.
W.B.J. Broom, M.B.
N.F. Burnett Hodd, F.B.C.O., D.C.L.P.
E.P. Cameron, M.Ch., F.R.C.S.

Rosalind Carr, M.B., D.R.C.O.G.
Nicola Jane Carroll
N.R. Carroll, B.D.S., L.D.S.R.C.S.
Simon StC. Carter, M.B., F.R.C.S.
Michael D. Chard, M.B., M.R.C.P.
Lyn Cheater
Julian Chomet, M.Sc.
Neil Citron, M.Chir., F.R.C.S.
A.M. de Lacy Costello, M.B., M.R.C.P.
Richard Dawood, F.R.C.R., D.T.M. & H.
J.J. Dawson, M.S., F.R.C.S.
Johnathan H. Dean
Jane Deverson
John H. Dubois
Andrew Duncombe, M.B., M.R.C.P.
Patrick Durston, F.A.S.I., R.E.M.T.
Adrian Eddleston, D.M., F.R.C.P.

Martin Brian Edwards, B.D.S., F.D.S.R.C.S.
Anne Eldred, M.B., M.R.C.G.P.
Christopher John Ellis, F.R.C.P., D.T.M. & H.
M.G. Falcon, F.R.C.S., F.C.Ophth.
Ivor L. Felstein, M.B.
P.H. Fentem, M.B., M.R.C.P.
Colin Fergusson, M.B., F.R.C.S.
Loraine Fergusson
Richard E. Field, F.R.C.S.E.
Michael W. Flowers, M.B., F.R.C.S.
Michael D. Flynn, M.B., M.R.C.P.
John Foley, M.D., F.R.C.P.
T.J. Fowler, D.M., F.R.C.P.
Roger Gabriel, M.B., F.R.C.P.
Ruth Garland
Michael Glasspool, F.R.C.S., D.O.
Max Glatt, F.R.C.P., F.R.C.Psych.

READER'S DIGEST

Editor Alice Philomena Rutherford • **Researchers** Wadad Bashour (Chief), Penelope Body,
Gladys Pollack, Aleli Balagtas, Françoise Giovannangeli, Catherine Korman
Copy preparation Joseph Marchetti • **Production** Holger Lorenzen
Coordinators Marilyn Ghadirian, Susan Wong • **Indexer** Jane Broderick

DORLING KINDERSLEY LIMITED

Managing Editor Ruth Midgley
Editors Andrea Bagg, Dr. Stephen Carroll, Robert Dinwiddie, Gail Lawther, Mary Lindsay,
Richenda Milton-Thompson, Ricki Ostrov, Martyn Page, Jillian Somerscales, Tony Whitehorn,
Dr. Frances Williams • **Additional editorial assistance from** Maria Adams, Simon Adams, Donald Berwick,
Deirdre Clark, Jean Cooke, Mike Darton, Elizabeth Galfalvi, Ann Kramer, Cathy Meeus, Terence Monaighan,
Theodore Rowland-Entwistle, Ruth Swan, Rena Taylor, Kay Wright, Pat White
Editorial Director Amy Carroll

Managing Art Editors Chez Picthall, Denise Brown
Art Editors Melissa Gray, Caroline Murray • **Designers** Sandra Archer, Peter Cross, Tina Hill, Gail Jones,
Sarah Ponder, Tracy Timson, Lydia Umney, Bryn Walls • **Additional design assistance from** Peter Blake,
Carol Briggs, Thomas Keenes, Anne Renel, Chris Scollens
Illustrators Tony Graham, Karen Cochran, Peter Cooper, Sandra Doyle, Simone End, Will Giles, Brian Hewson,
Chris Jenkins, Kevin Jones, Kevin Marks, Janos Marffy, Coral Mula, Frazer Newman, Nick Oxloby,
Lynda Payne, Sandra Pond, Patricia Sempron, Mark Surridge, John Woodcock
Picture research Sandra Schneider • **Production** Eunice Paterson

EMERGENCY FIRST AID TECHNIQUES

Use this quick-reference list to find illustrated first aid boxes containing step-by-step instructions for performing emergency techniques.

SYMPTOM CHARTS

Use this quick-reference list to find question-and-answer flow charts that indicate the possible causes and significance of many common symptoms.

CONTENTS

HOW TO USE THE ENCYCLOPEDIA

This highly illustrated encyclopedia is an informative and authoritative guide to all aspects of health and medical care. For swift and easy reference, entries within the main part of the encyclopedia are arranged alphabetically, and longer entries are subdivided into sections, each with a descriptive subheading. Information within entries is presented in clear, concise language, and technical or unfamiliar medical terms are generally explained as they appear.

The main body of the encyclopedia, the **A to Z of Health and Medicine**, contains some 5,000 entries covering a vast range of health, medical,

and medically related topics. In any manageable compendium it is obviously impossible to provide separate entries for every single medical term, but many additional terms and topics are discussed within relevant entries.

The encyclopedia also contains a full-color introductory section, **Health and Medicine Today**, which describes the latest advances in diagnosis and treatment. At the back of the book, additional information on generic-name and brand-name drugs is contained in the **Drug Glossary**. There are also addresses and phone numbers of **Self-help Organizations** and a comprehensive **Index**.

HOW TO FIND THE INFORMATION YOU WANT

All entries in the **A to Z of Health and Medicine** and in the **Index** are arranged alphabetically using the "letter-by-letter" system. In this system, any spaces or punctuation in the entry titles are ignored. Thus, *Sick building syndrome* is followed by *Sickle cell anemia* and then by *Sick sinus syndrome*: the fifth letter gives you the order.

When the name of a topic consists of more than one word, begin by looking up what seems to be the key word. Thus, for information on general anesthesia you will find what you want under the heading *Anesthesia, general*. If the key word is not obvious, you may find it easier to turn first to the **Index**, although many alternative

topic names and common abbreviations are included as short cross-reference entries within the main part of the book. You will also find cross-references within entries. These are indicated by italic type and take several forms. Examples of the different forms are shown and explained in the annotated illustration below.

Standard subheadings
Standard subheadings are used to tell you what each part of the entry is about.

Subordinate subheadings
A second level of subheading is sometimes used. In such cases, the text continues on the same line.

"See" cross-references
Italicized "see" cross-references within parentheses refer you to other entries for more detailed information.

Cross-references
Italicized cross-references within sentences refer you to other entries for more detailed information.

"See also" cross-references
At the end of some entries, "see also" cross-references direct you to related entries that may be of interest to you.

Technical terms
Medical and other technical terms are explained briefly in parentheses.

Names of organisms
Scientific names of organisms are printed in italic small capital letters.

10

HOW TO FIND INFORMATION ON SYMPTOMS

The **A to Z of Health and Medicine** contains individual entries on the whole range of physical and psychological symptoms. In general, you will find the main description of a particular symptom under its common name, if it has one. Thus, for example, *Vomiting* is the main entry and *Emesis*, the medical term for vomiting, is a short cross-reference entry. Alternative names for symptoms also appear in the **Index**.

Symptom charts

The question-and-answer symptom charts will help you understand the significance of common symptoms that have no obvious cause. Each chart singles out possible causes of the symptom, refers you to relevant entries in the encyclopedia, and suggests appropriate action, if any. Start at the top of the chart and answer "yes" or "no" to the series of carefully selected questions until you reach the box that advises you on your particular problem. For the page numbers of all symptom charts, consult page 8.

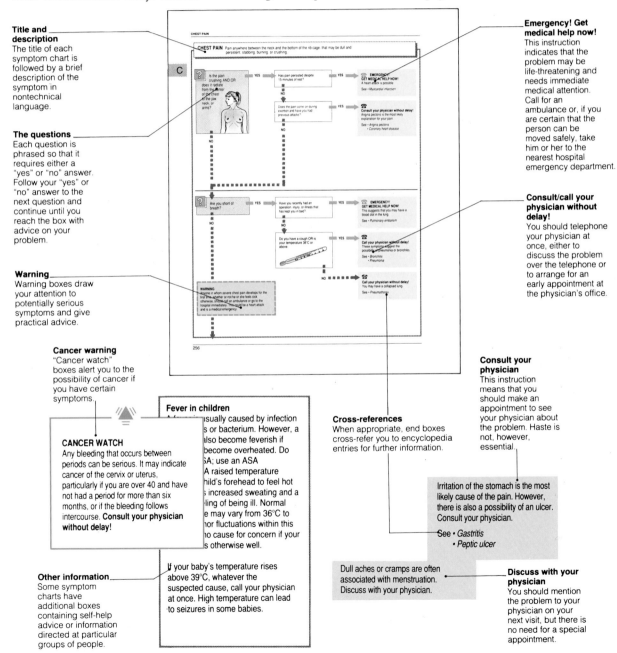

Title and description
The title of each symptom chart is followed by a brief description of the symptom in nontechnical language.

The questions
Each question is phrased so that it requires either a "yes" or "no" answer. Follow your "yes" or "no" answer to the next question and continue until you reach the box with advice on your problem.

Warning
Warning boxes draw your attention to potentially serious symptoms and give practical advice.

Cancer warning
"Cancer watch" boxes alert you to the possibility of cancer if you have certain symptoms.

CANCER WATCH
Any bleeding that occurs between periods can be serious. It may indicate cancer of the cervix or uterus, particularly if you are over 40 and have not had a period for more than six months, or if the bleeding follows intercourse. **Consult your physician without delay!**

Other information
Some symptom charts have additional boxes containing self-help advice or information directed at particular groups of people.

Fever in children
A fever is usually caused by infection ...s or bacterium. However, a ...lso become feverish if ...become overheated. Do ...A; use an ASA
A raised temperature ...ild's forehead to feel hot ...s increased sweating and a ...ling of being ill. Normal ...e may vary from 36°C to ...or fluctuations within this ...o cause for concern if your ...s otherwise well.

If your baby's temperature rises above 39°C, whatever the suspected cause, call your physician at once. High temperature can lead to seizures in some babies.

Emergency! Get medical help now!
This instruction indicates that the problem may be life-threatening and needs immediate medical attention. Call for an ambulance or, if you are certain that the person can be moved safely, take him or her to the nearest hospital emergency department.

Consult/call your physician without delay!
You should telephone your physician at once, either to discuss the problem over the telephone or to arrange for an early appointment at the physician's office.

Consult your physician
This instruction means that you should make an appointment to see your physician about the problem. Haste is not, however, essential.

Cross-references
When appropriate, end boxes cross-refer you to encyclopedia entries for further information.

Irritation of the stomach is the most likely cause of the pain. However, there is also a possibility of an ulcer. Consult your physician.
See • *Gastritis*
     • *Peptic ulcer*

Dull aches or cramps are often associated with menstruation. Discuss with your physician.

Discuss with your physician
You should mention the problem to your physician on your next visit, but there is no need for a special appointment.

HOW TO FIND INFORMATION ON DISORDERS

The **A to Z of Health and Medicine** has individual entries on all major and many minor disorders. There are also general entries on groups of disorders, such as *Genetic disorders*, or disorders that affect different parts of the body in different ways, such as *Cancer*. These group entries provide an overview and explain the basic disease processes; specific forms, such as *Hemophilia* or *Breast cancer*, are covered in separate entries. Group entries contain cross-references to more specific entries. If you look up certain group entries in the **Index**, you will find references to disorders in those groups.

Consult the **Index**, too, if you fail to find an entry on a specific disorder within the **A to Z of Health and Medicine**. You may find that the disorder has an alternative name. For example, if you look up *Decubitus ulcer* in the **Index** you will be directed to the encyclopedia entry on *Bedsores*; decubitus ulcer and bedsore are alternative names for the same condition. In other cases, the **Index** will show you that a specific disorder is covered in a more general entry. For example, conductive deafness is included in the *Deafness* entry.

Disorder boxes

Entries on the main organs and body parts are accompanied by boxed summaries of the various disorders that may affect them. These disorder boxes help you see at a glance the types of problems most often associated with a particular organ or body part. These boxes also cross-refer you to entries on specific disorders and investigation techniques.

Cross-references
Italicized cross-references direct you to entries on specific disorders for more information.

Subheadings
Different disorders are grouped under standard subheadings, allowing you to see at a glance the problems most likely to affect a particular body part.

Illustrations
Some disorder boxes have an annotated illustration showing areas most likely to be affected by different disorders.

Investigation box
A summary of investigation techniques is given here, including italicized cross-references to entries on diagnostic procedures.

HOW TO FIND INFORMATION ON ANATOMY AND PHYSIOLOGY

All body systems (e.g., *Biliary system*) and major organs and body parts (e.g., *Brain* and *Coccyx*) have individual entries in the **A to Z of Health and Medicine**. There are also entries on the senses (e.g., *Vision*) and on other body processes (e.g., *Breathing* and *Blood clotting*). Anatomy and physiology entries explain how the healthy body works and provide a background for understanding medical disorders.

Most anatomy and physiology entries are accompanied by illustrated boxes. Annotated illustrations show the main structural features of body parts, the location of different body parts in relation to each other, and, for physiology entries, the main stages in important body processes.

Medical images
Pictures obtained by specialized imaging techniques, such as X rays or scans, are used in many cases.

Location diagrams
Most anatomy boxes include a diagram showing the part's position within the body.

Anatomical drawings
Detailed drawings, often with cutaway sections, show the structure of body parts.

Entire body systems
Large illustrations show the structure and relative position of organs within different body systems.

How body systems work
Clearly written captions give detailed descriptions of the different stages in physiological processes.

HOW TO FIND INFORMATION ON MEDICAL TESTS

Many different tests for diagnosing or monitoring medical conditions have individual entries within the **A to Z of Health and Medicine**. Many of these entries are illustrated by step-by-step diagrams.

More general information on tests is given in the entry headed *Tests, medical*. This entry is accompanied by a table that shows the tests used to investigate different parts of the body and directs you to individual entries within the encyclopedia. You can also find out the various types of tests used to investigate a major body organ by consulting the investigation section of the disorder box for that particular organ.

Entries on specific disorders in the **A to Z of Health and Medicine** cross-refer you to entries on the tests used to diagnose and monitor them.

Illustrations showing techniques
Clear illustrations show a test's most important stages, including, for example, where a needle is inserted in the body or how samples are prepared for testing.

Step-by-step text
Concise captions describe the various stages in each test, including what happens to the patient and how test samples are analyzed in the laboratory.

Test results
Diagrams, photographs, and captions explain the results of the test.

PREGNANCY TEST KIT
Just one of the many types of pregnancy test kit is shown. No kit is 100 percent accurate. Whether a test indicates pregnancy or gives a negative result despite a missed period, it is wise to consult a physician for confirmation.

Indicator stick
Dropper with test solution
Test tube
Stopper

Components of test kit
The kit has three main parts—a dropper tube containing a test solution, a test tube with stopper, and an indicator stick.

1 The end of the dropper tube is squeezed gently to introduce the test solution into the test tube, which is held upright in a stand provided.

2 The lid of the test kit is used to collect a urine sample early in the morning. Some urine is drawn up into the dropper tube by squeezing and releasing.

Negative
Positive

3 Five drops of urine are added to the solution in the test tube. The stopper is put in the test tube, the contents are shaken, and the stopper is removed.

4 The indicator stick is placed in the test tube. The result can be read after 30 minutes. If the end of the stick changes color, it signifies a pregnancy.

HOW TO FIND INFORMATION ON SURGICAL PROCEDURES

Surgical procedures are described either in individual entries or in the treatment section of disorder entries. In many cases, entries are accompanied by illustrated boxes.

Individual entries on surgical procedures are included under their generally accepted medical names. In many cases, these names are self-explanatory—*Heart-lung transplant* or *Hernia repair*, for example.

If you do not know the name of a particular procedure, look up the encyclopedia entry on the disorder for which it is a treatment, where you will find a description of, or a cross-reference to, the appropriate procedure. Alternatively, consult the **Index**, which lists some popular names. For example, if you look up "Stomach removal," you will be referred to the encyclopedia entry on *Gastrectomy*.

Surgery in progress
True-to-life drawings show surgical procedures in progress and provide an accurate representation of current surgical practice.

Incision sites
A red line superimposed on a photograph of the relevant part of the body shows the position and shape of the surgeon's incision.

HEART-LUNG TRANSPLANT
In this procedure, both the heart and lungs of a patient are removed and replaced with organs taken from a brain-dead donor. The removed heart can sometimes be given to another patient.

HOW IT IS DONE
Heart and lungs must be removed from both donor and patient; the donor organs are then inserted into the patient.

1 The donor heart and lungs must be healthy, and the lungs must match the size of the patient's chest, as measured by chest X rays.

2 In both donor and patient, the heart and lungs are reached via an incision made in the sternum, and the chest is opened up.

Site of incision

Equipment
Detailed illustrations show the workings of special equipment, such as a heart-lung machine.

3 The patient is connected to a heart-lung machine. It takes over the function of heart and lungs, oxygenating blood taken from the venae cavae and pumping it back to the body via the aorta.

Trachea
Aorta
Right atrium/Vena cava

4 In both patient and donor, heart and lungs are removed through cuts in the trachea, aorta, and where the heart connects to the venae cavae. The blood vessels linking donor heart and lungs are left intact.

Tracheal reconnection
Aortic reconnection
Right atrium/Vena cava reconnection

Step-by-step text and illustrations
Explanatory captions and anatomically correct illustrations take you through the most important stages of surgical procedures. Large numbers show the sequence of events and help you follow the different stages.

WHY IT IS DONE
Subject to availability of a donor, a heart-lung transplant can offer hope to someone who is dying of a terminally chronic lung disease, whether or not he or she is also suffering from heart disease. Diseases treated include *emphysema, cystic fibrosis, sarcoidosis,* or *interstitial pulmonary fibrosis.* The heart-lung transplant operation has a better success record than that of lung transplant alone.

5 Insertion of the donor organs into the patient is, in some respects, easier than in the heart transplant, since fewer reconnections have to be made. The main reconnections are between the patient's and donor's tracheas and aortas and between the right atrium of the donor heart and the patient's venae cavae.

Reasons for surgery
Different medical images—such as photographs, X rays, or scans—of diseased tissue show why operations are necessary.

These sections were taken from a healthy lung (left) and an emphysematous

lung; transplantation of heart and lungs may give an emphysema patient new hope.

HOW TO FIND INFORMATION ON DRUGS

The **A to Z of Health and Medicine** contains entries on all major drug groups (from *ACE inhibitor drugs* to *Vasodilator drugs*) and on the most important generic drugs (from *Acebutolol* to *Zidovudine*). Other information on drugs can be found in general entries, such as *Drug, Drug dependence,* and *Drug poisoning.*

The **Drug Glossary** gives concise information on some 1,300 generic-name and brand-name drugs, showing the generic equivalents of brand-name drugs, and identifying the drug groups to which individual drugs belong. Each glossary entry cross-refers you to appropriate entries in the **A to Z of Health and Medicine**.

Drug charts
Selected entries on individual drugs are accompanied by an illustrated chart that summarizes important information about the drug.

Group to which the drug belongs

Forms in which the drug is available

Availability on prescription or over-the-counter

Generic name

Injection

Intravenous infusion

Suppository or pessary

Inhaler

Drops

Applicable symbols are printed in red

Transdermal patch

Digitoxin

DIGITALIS

Tablet   Liquid   Injection

Prescription needed

Tablet

Capsule

Liquid

Powder

Cream or ointment

Drug group charts
Most drug group entries are accompanied by a chart showing examples of common drugs within the group.

Group name

Division within the main drug group

Generic-name examples

Antirheumatic drugs

COMMON DRUGS
Corticosteroid drugs *Dexamethasone Prednisolone*
Immunosuppressant drugs *Azathioprine Chlorambucil*
Others *Auranofin Chloroquine Gold Penicillamine*

WARNING
Sudden withdrawal of corticosteroid drugs may cause serious illness or death. Always inform a physician if you are taking or have recently taken corticosteroids.

Drug warning
Warning boxes draw your attention to the possible dangers associated with taking particular types of drugs.

HOW TO USE THE ENCYCLOPEDIA IN AN EMERGENCY

EMERGENCY FIRST-AID TECHNIQUES

Turn to page 8 for the page numbers of emergency first-aid boxes.

Lifesaving and other, less urgent, first aid techniques are explained in easy-to-follow first aid boxes. These boxes accompany relevant entries in the **A to Z of Health and Medicine**. All first aid boxes have a distinctive red border and a special heading. A list of first aid boxes describing emergency techniques, with their page numbers, is given on page 8.

Distinctive appearance
Bold red borders and special headings make first aid boxes easy to find.

WARNING
Warning boxes contain essential advice and indicate when professional help should be sought.

WARNING
Frostbite is often accompanied by hypothermia, which must be treated first. Proper medical attention should be sought promptly, but first aid should be given immediately.

DO NOT
■ rub the affected parts
■ attempt to burst blisters
■ warm the affected area with direct heat
■ allow the victim to walk on a frostbitten foot

DO NOT
These boxes tell you what not to do when treating an injured person.

Step-by-step
First aid techniques are clearly described in numbered sequences of text and illustrations.

Close-ups
More detailed illustrations show you exactly what to do.

FIRST AID: CHOKING

CONSCIOUS VICTIM
1 A person clutching the throat may be choking. Encourage the victim to cough up the obstruction. If this fails, and the victim can no longer speak or cough, use the method below.

UNCONSCIOUS VICTIM
1 Straddle the victim. Place the heel of one hand on the victim's abdomen, slightly above the navel; place your other hand on top, fingers interlaced. With elbows straight, press in with a quick upward thrust. Repeat 6 to 10 times.

2 Clasp the victim, placing one clenched fist just under the sternum (breastbone) and grasping the fist with the other hand. Then make a quick, hard, thrusting movement inward and upward

2 If this fails, try to remove the obstruction with your index finger. If the victim is still unconscious, summon emergency help. If breathing has stopped, start artificial respiration

HEALTH AND MEDICINE TODAY

KEEPING HEALTHY

An individual's health is determined partly by inheritance and partly by external factors. Health and longevity tend to run in families, so a person whose grandparents lived beyond the age of 80 is likely to do the same. However, this is not always the case. Even the intrinsically healthiest body can be damaged by neglect or by external factors, especially by the unwise use of drugs, including tobacco and alcohol. With AIDS still spreading, adherence to safe sex practices and programs to stop users of illicit intravenous drugs from sharing needles are essential.

Good health requires lifelong maintenance of the body. A health-promoting life-style in youth not only reduces the chances of premature death from heart disease or cancer but also slows the natural process of aging. Researchers have been able to identify certain factors that speed up the decline of the vital organs—of which the most important are alcohol and tobacco. It has also been possible to identify various factors that slow down the aging process—of which the most important are the taking of regular vigorous exercise and the maintenance of body weight within recommended limits.

A positive approach to health is fundamental to any personal health-care program. The fact that you can control many of the different factors that affect your health means that you can exert a major influence on your own well-being.

There is no need for a personal health-care program to be unpleasant—it is perfectly possible to combine health promotion with enjoyment.

Exercise and your heart
Running is a good way of maintaining cardiovascular fitness and reducing the risk of heart disease.

SIX WAYS OF KEEPING HEALTHY

By paying attention to each of the following six aspects of personal health care, you can make an important start toward improving or maintaining your individual levels of general health and physical fitness.

Eat sensibly
Eating a balanced diet is a key feature of any personal health-care plan.

Take exercise
Regular exercise can improve or maintain physical and mental fitness.

Limit alcohol
Keeping alcohol consumption within safe limits is vital for health.

Watch weight
People who are very overweight or underweight tend to die prematurely.

Don't smoke
The link between tobacco-smoking and killer diseases has been proved.

Visit the doctor
Seek medical advice as soon as you suspect a health problem.

Diet and nutrition

Although there are many different views on healthy eating, experts generally agree that diets should be varied and should contain adequate but not excessive amounts of protein, carbohydrates, fats, minerals, and vitamins. You can combine pleasure with health promotion by eating a healthy mix of foods that appeals to your palate.

Alcohol consumption

Excessive alcohol consumption is a major health hazard. Alcohol not only contributes to problems at home and at work, to accidents, and to violent crime, it can also cause irreversible damage to the heart, liver, brain, and nervous system. Limiting alcohol consumption is essential for long-term health.

Tobacco smoking

Giving up smoking is the single most important measure that any tobacco smoker can take to improve his or her own health. The life expectancy of nonsmokers is significantly higher than that of smokers. Smoking is a major cause of lung cancer, heart disease, and chronic bronchitis.

Exercise and fitness

Regular exercise benefits every part of your body, enhancing both physical and mental well-being. Different types of exercise vary in the extent to which they improve the three main aspects of health and fitness: heart and lung efficiency, joint suppleness, and muscle power. The best exercises for improving general fitness are aerobic exercises, such as jogging, swimming, and cycling. Most people should be able to select a sport or activity that they find interesting and stimulating as well as beneficial to their health.

Weight control

People who are significantly overweight or underweight tend to die younger than people who are of normal weight. Maintaining a healthy weight involves paying attention to what you eat and drink, and making sure that you take adequate exercise.

Stress control

A certain amount of stress is natural in any demanding or difficult situation, but if feelings of anxiety become persistent, they can become the cause of psychological and physical symptoms. Being able to cope with stress is an important aspect of keeping healthy. Often you can alleviate stress, even avoid it altogether, by modifying your behavior—in

Ensuring nutritional balance
This selection of protein sources, fruits, and vegetables shows the variety possible even within the food groups (see box, following page). Milk and milk products, breads, and cereals are other essentials of a nutritionally balanced diet.

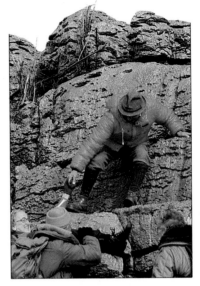

Exercise for life
As you grow older, taking regular exercise will help you maintain the normal functioning of your bones, joints, muscles, tendons, and ligaments. Your joints will stay mobile and your muscle strength, coordination, and confidence will be retained.

effect changing your response to stressful situations. Reacting with anger or aggression, or seeking escape through drugs or alcohol almost invariably compound stress without resolving the underlying problem. Conversely, it is nearly always helpful to talk problems through with family, friends, employers, or professionals. Relaxation techniques can often help relieve tension caused by stress.

Safety measures

Accidents and injury are a major cause of death and disability, especially in young people. Paying attention to basic standards of safety in the home, at work, near water, and particularly on the roads can considerably reduce the risk of accidents. Keeping healthy also depends on keeping safe.

Medical help

People used to believe that medical help was necessary only when they became ill. It is now widely recognized that preventive medicine is important in maintaining health. Immunization can prevent a range of formerly common infectious diseases, and screening tests make it possible to detect certain types of medical problem at an early stage when they can be treated more easily.

EATING WELL

If you eat a balanced diet, you are already well on the way to good health. The function of food is to provide your body with appropriate amounts of the necessary nutrients—fats, protein, carbohydrates, vitamins, minerals, fiber, and water—ideally in as pleasant a form as possible. Many people in developed countries, however, consume too much fat, salt, sugar, alcohol, and refined food. A diet of this type contributes to numerous health problems, such as diabetes, heart disease, dental decay, liver disease, and some cancers.

THE FOUR FOOD GROUPS
There are four main food groups; a balanced diet should include several servings from each group per day. The "meat" group also contains fish, nuts, and eggs.

Milk group
Servings required per day: two (adults); two to four (children)

Typical servings

Milk	250 ml
Yogurt, plain	150-175 ml
Hard cheese	45 g
Cottage cheese	125 ml

Meat group
Servings required per day: two

Typical servings

Meat, lean	60–90 g
Fish	60–90 g
Eggs	2
Peanut butter	4 tablespoons

Fruit and vegetable group
Servings required per day: four to five

Typical servings

Vegetables	½ cup
Apple	1 medium
Potato	1 medium
Grapefruit	½ cup

Bread and cereal group
Servings required per day: three to five

Typical servings

Bread	1 slice
Pasta	½ to ¾ cup
Rice	½ to ¾ cup
Breakfast cereal	¾ cup

Fats

Fats provide energy, and are a structural component of body cells. Fats fall into two main types: saturated and unsaturated.

Saturated fats include most animal fats, such as those found in whole milk, butter, cheese, pork, beef, lamb, and eggs; some vegetable oils are also saturated. Unsaturated fats include most of the fats found in fish and poultry, and in soya, sunflower, and corn oils. A high intake of saturated fats tends to increase the blood levels of cholesterol, which in turn can increase the risk of atherosclerosis and heart disease.

To keep your diet as healthy as possible, reduce your overall intake of fats, and choose unsaturated fats instead of saturated ones whenever possible.

Protein

Protein is needed regularly by the body for growth, and also for the repair and replacement of cells. The main sources of dietary protein are meat, fish, eggs, some dairy products, grains, and legumes.

AN UNHEALTHY MEAL
Although it looks tempting, the meal shown below is high in calories and very high in saturated fats. It contains some protein, but very little fiber and few vitamins.

Eggs
Although they are a good source of protein, eggs are high in cholesterol. Here they have been fried, which has increased their fat and calorie levels substantially.

Potatoes
Potatoes are high in fibre and healthy carbohydrate, but cutting them up small and frying them has drastically boosted their calorie and fat levels.

Parsley
The sprig of parsley used as garnish is the only fresh, uncooked vegetable.

Meat
These fried hamburgers are packed with saturated fats, and may contain unsuspected ingredients—for example, rusk, soya, sugar, monosodium glutamate, salt, water, colorings, preservative, and meat flavorings—as well as meat.

For a healthy diet, choose fish and poultry instead of red meats. Grains and legumes are other good sources of protein.

Carbohydrates

Carbohydrates are the body's main source of energy, and are necessary for cell metabolism. There are two main groups of carbohydrates: starches and sugars. Starches are found in large amounts in foods such as flour, grains, pasta, bread, and legumes; sugars occur in large amounts in fruits and some vegetables, and in foods such as jams, cakes, and soft drinks.

A high intake of carbohydrates, especially in the form of refined sugar, contributes to obesity and dental decay; obesity in turn can contribute to heart disease, diabetes, and arthritis.

Make your diet healthier by avoiding high-sugar products. As far as possible, obtain your dietary carbohydrates from rela-

---

FOOD HYGIENE

In recent years the incidence of food poisoning—particularly involving bacterial contamination—has risen substantially. You can minimize the risk by following the simple guidelines set out below.

1 Buy the freshest produce you can, and never eat food after its "best before" or expiry date. If food smells bad, throw it away, even if it hasn't reached its "best before" date.

2 Store food properly. All food should be covered, wrapped with foil or plastic wrap or kept in an airtight container. Perishable food should be refrigerated at 2.2°C to 4.5°C or frozen at -17.8°C. Fresh fruit and vegetables should be kept in the crisper or stored loosely in moisture-resistant paper.

3 Wash your hands thoroughly before handling food, immediately after handling raw meat, and between prepared meat and preparing other foods. Wash fruit and vegetables in clean water before eating or preparing them.

4 Ensure that kitchen surfaces, cutting boards, and cooking utensils are thoroughly clean before use; keep pets away from food, work surfaces and utensils.

5 Thaw frozen meats (especially poultry, pork, and seafood) thoroughly before cooking. Don't keep food warm for extended periods; if reheating is necessary, do so quickly but thoroughly on a high heat.

---

tively low-calorie, high-fiber foods, such as bread, potatoes, and whole-grain cereals.

Fiber

Fiber is an indigestible substance found in plants. Although it does not provide the body with any nutrients, fiber is essential for the healthy functioning of the digestive system.

Diets that are low in fiber contribute to constipation, diverticular disease, and some bowel cancers; high-fiber foods provide dietary bulk without excess calories.

Foods that are particularly high in fiber include whole-grain breads and cereals, legumes, dried fruits, and nuts. Fiber is also found in all fruit and vegetables.

Vitamins

Vitamins help to ensure that all the body's cells and organs are functioning well. A balanced diet should provide all the vitamins you need; healthy people do not need vitamin tablets. Fresh fruit and vegetables are very good sources of vitamins.

Minerals

Many different minerals, such as calcium, sodium, potassium, iron, zinc, and iodine, are necessary to keep the organs, bones, and muscles functioning properly. A balanced diet usually provides all the necessary minerals.

Water

Water is essential to sustain life. Although most foods contain substantial amounts of water, it is sensible also to drink several glasses of pure water each day.

A HEALTHY MEAL
As this meal shows, healthy eating does not have to be just cottage cheese and carrots. The meal below provides a good variety of taste and texture, but is low in fat and relatively low in calories.

Fish
Grilled, non-oily fish provides a low-calorie nutritious "meat" serving that is also low in fat.

Lemon
Juice from a lemon wedge gives the food extra taste without the fat and sugar of thick, high-calorie dressings.

Vegetables
A mixture of fresh, uncooked salad vegetables provides vitamins, minerals, and fibre without too many calories or any fat content.

EXERCISE AND HEALTH

Regular exercise is an important means of improving health. Exercise keeps the muscles and bones in good health, and also slows down the aging process; it improves fitness levels and increases muscle tone and flexibility, producing a general sense of well-being.

Also, if you exercise regularly and vigorously several times a week you will improve the efficiency of your heart and lungs, and significantly reduce your risk of developing coronary artery disease or of having a myocardial infarction (heart attack).

Types of exercise

There are many different types of exercise, which can be performed to fulfil different functions. For instance, certain exercises may be chosen to improve the efficiency of the heart and lungs, others may be used to improve flexibility, and others to increase muscular strength or physical endurance. A well-balanced exercise program will contain activities that provide a combination of benefits.

Aerobic exercise is activity that requires the lungs to take in additional oxygen to meet the requirements of the muscles—the kind of exercise that makes you breathless. Activities such as jogging, cycling, squash, and swimming fall into this category. Aerobic exercise is the best kind of exercise for improving cardiovascular fitness, and also usually improves the strength and flexibility of certain muscle groups at the same time. For example, jogging improves and strengthens the leg muscles as well as increasing cardiovascular fitness.

Isometric exercise is exercise without movement, in which one group of muscles exerts pressure against an immovable object (a wall, for example) or against an opposing group of muscles. Isometric exercises improve muscle strength, but they do not have any effect on cardiovascular fitness or on flexibility.

Isotonic exercise is a form of exercise in which the body works against its own weight or against an external weight. Weight lifting and calisthenics (repetitive exercises that have been designed to stretch and strengthen particular muscle groups) are examples of isotonic exercises.

Isokinetic exercise combines elements of isometric and isotonic exercise. This is the kind of exercise usually performed on the sophisticated fitness training equipment found in sports centers and gymnasiums.

Improving health

Exercise improves the blood flow to muscles, providing them with nutrients and removing waste products. Muscles are strengthened and so are the ligaments that attach them to the bones, thus improving the strength and mobility of the joints. The muscle tone is improved and, because the muscles require more energy, fat stored in the body is broken down and utilized, which can lead to a reduction in weight. Specific exercises of the right

FITNESS VALUE OF SELECTED ACTIVITIES

Different physical activities and exercises benefit different aspects of fitness to varying degrees. The table below illustrates the ways in which six common activities benefit three major elements of overall fitness.

Key
★ ★ ★ ★ Excellent ★ ★ ★ Good ★ ★ Fair ★ Minimal

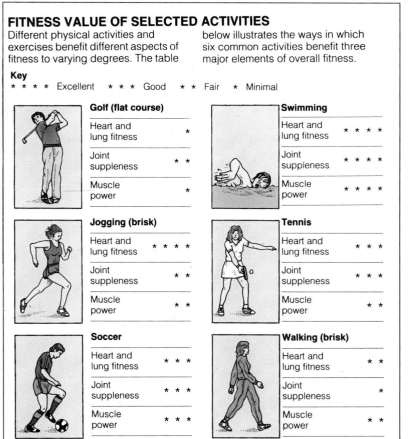

Golf (flat course)	
Heart and lung fitness	★
Joint suppleness	★ ★
Muscle power	★

Swimming	
Heart and lung fitness	★ ★ ★ ★
Joint suppleness	★ ★ ★ ★
Muscle power	★ ★ ★ ★

Jogging (brisk)	
Heart and lung fitness	★ ★ ★ ★
Joint suppleness	★ ★
Muscle power	★ ★

Tennis	
Heart and lung fitness	★ ★ ★
Joint suppleness	★ ★ ★
Muscle power	★ ★

Soccer	
Heart and lung fitness	★ ★ ★
Joint suppleness	★ ★ ★
Muscle power	★ ★ ★

Walking (brisk)	
Heart and lung fitness	★ ★
Joint suppleness	★
Muscle power	★ ★

ENERGY EXPENDITURE

The table below gives the approximate amount of energy expended during 30 minutes of various activities. The figures are based on levels of exertion likely to be kept up by typical amateurs.

Activity	Energy used
Easy walking	90 cal
Light gardening	135 cal
Golf	135 cal
Housework	135 cal
Brisk walking	150 cal
Badminton	170 cal
Heavy gardening	210 cal
Gymnastics	210 cal
Tennis	240 cal
Hockey	270 cal
Rugby	270 cal
Soccer	270 cal
Squash	300 cal
Brisk jogging	315 cal
Cycling	330 cal
Swimming	360 cal

THE BODY DURING EXERCISE

During vigorous aerobic activity many of the body's systems are exercised. The illustration shows the effects of strenuous exercise on different parts of the body.

Lungs
The rate and depth of breathing increases, which improves the oxygenation of the blood; this leads to an increased feeling of fitness and well-being.

Heart and circulation
The heart beats faster and stronger, so the speed at which blood flows through the circulation is increased. Regular aerobic exercise usually leads to a fall in the resting blood pressure.

Body weight
When the blood's immediate supply of energy has been exhausted, stored body fat is mobilized and converted to energy to feed the muscles, helping to control weight.

Bones and joints
The blood flow to bones increases, which helps to maintain the density of the bones and protect them against injury. Joints are kept flexible and mobile by exercise.

Muscles
The blood flow to the muscles is increased and the muscles are strengthened and toned up.

kind can restore mobility to damaged joints and can ease some kinds of back pain.

Avoiding heart disease

Regular aerobic exercise has been shown to reduce the likelihood of coronary artery disease. During aerobic exercise the heart beats more rapidly and more powerfully. This strengthens the heart muscle and improves its efficiency; the blood pressure while at rest is also usually reduced. Aerobic exercise is also thought to help protect the body against the development of atherosclerosis (the accumulation of fatty deposits in the arteries), which can lead to a myocardial infarction.

Exercise in later life

Because mobility and energy tend to decrease in later life, an elderly person's joints may become stiff and weak while his or her bones may become more liable to fracture.

Regular, gentle exercise will maintain joint mobility and help to strengthen the muscles, joints, and bones. This in turn will help maintain mobility and independence into old age.

EXERCISE WARNING

Stop exercising and seek medical advice if you suffer from any of the following symptoms.

- Chest pain
- Pain in neck or left arm
- Palpitations
- Severe breathlessness
- Feeling faint

SMOKING AND DRINKING

Smoking and drinking are two of the greatest enemies of a healthy life-style. In recent years, tobacco smoking and alcohol consumption have both been convincingly implicated in a wide range of health problems. Numerous working days are lost each year through disorders related to smoking or drinking, and both activities increase the risk of cancer and heart disease, and therefore of premature death. Women who smoke or drink during pregnancy risk causing damage to the health of their unborn children.

Both alcohol and nicotine are addictive drugs; people who begin smoking or drinking socially often find themselves, several years later, unable to give up the habit.

The effects of tobacco

The harmful effects of tobacco on the body are mainly due to three constituents of its smoke: nicotine, carbon monoxide, and tar.

Nicotine is a tranquilizer, and is also addictive; it is the absence of nicotine that causes the physical and psychological withdrawal symptoms that may occur when a regular smoker suddenly stops. The presence of carbon monoxide in the blood decreases the amount of oxygen reaching the tissues, and in the long term can lead to atherosclerosis (the accumulation of fatty deposits in the arteries). Tar causes chronic irritation of the respiratory tract, and contains carcinogens (cancer-causing agents).

Smoking and cancer

The link between smoking and lung cancer is well known; 90 percent of lung cancer deaths can be attributed to smoking. Lung cancer is, however, only one of the malignant tumors that can be caused by, or aggravated by, tobacco smoking. Other smoking-related tumors include cancers of the mouth, throat, lip, cervix, and bladder.

Pipe and cigar smokers inhale less smoke than most cigarette smokers and they are therefore somewhat less likely to develop lung cancer; they are, however, more prone to cancers of the mouth and throat.

Other risks of smoking

Many people do not realize that smoking also contributes significantly to numerous other diseases and disorders.

The irritant effect of tobacco smoke causes the respiratory tract to produce excessive sputum (phlegm), leading to the classic "smoker's cough." Tobacco smoke also causes the alveoli (tiny air sacs in the lungs) to lose their elasticity and eventually become fused; this makes them less efficient, and ultimately leads to emphysema. Many heavy smok-

Cigarette-smoking comparisons
Campaigns to reduce smoking have had some success. In 1965, 53 percent of Canadian men and 32 percent of Canadian women smoked cigarettes regularly. In 1990, only 30 percent of men and 25 percent of women smoked. The smaller decline in women is a concern for health educators, since most women start smoking in their teens. Only about 5 percent of Canadian physicians smoke.

ers die from respiratory failure caused by chronic bronchitis and/or emphysema.

People who smoke also face a great risk of premature death from coronary artery disease. Smokers have been found to suffer more commonly than nonsmokers from angina (chest pain due to inadequate blood supply to heart muscle), and also from the kind of myocardial infarction (heart attack) that does not produce symptoms.

Arterial disease makes smokers more likely than nonsmokers to have a stroke. They are also more likely to develop gastric and duodenal ulcers.

A little exercise does your heart good.

Step 1. Step 2. Step 3.

Look after your HEART!

Health education poster
Antismoking posters, such as the one shown here, have a major part to play in persuading people not to smoke. The link between smoking and heart disease is less well known than the link between smoking and cancer but is no less serious. For example, the risk of coronary artery disease in a young man who smokes 20 cigarettes a day is about three times that of a nonsmoker.

Cirrhosis of the liver
The two photomicrographs above show healthy liver tissue (left), and liver tissue damaged by alcoholic cirrhosis (right). In the healthy liver, the cells are arranged regularly; in the cirrhotic liver, healthy cells have been destroyed by alcohol and replaced by scar tissue (colored blue). Eventually the cirrhotic liver loses normal function.

Reducing the risk

If you give up smoking, you immediately reduce your chances of developing smoking-related diseases; the more years you subsequently go without smoking, the lower is your risk.

Alcohol and disease

The dangers of drink are not confined to people who are considered to be alcoholics; many people who drink regularly or heavily are at risk of developing alcohol-related disorders.

Liver disorders are common among heavy drinkers, who have an increased incidence of fatty

DEATHS FROM CIRRHOSIS

As the population in a given country drinks more, so the death rate from cirrhosis of the liver rises. This graph shows death rates from cirrhosis and other chronic liver disease in four countries in 1987.

As the graph shows, the death rates for Canada are slightly lower than for the US. In France and Italy, however, where heavy drinking is more common, the death rate is very much higher.

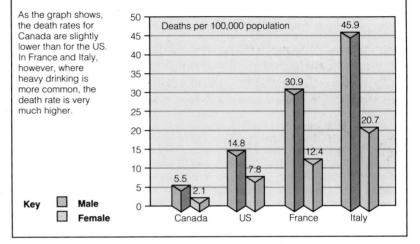

Deaths per 100,000 population

	Male	Female
Canada	5.5	2.1
US	14.8	7.8
France	30.9	12.4
Italy	45.9	20.7

Key: Male / Female

liver, alcoholic hepatitis, cirrhosis of the liver (in which healthy cells are replaced by scar tissue), and liver cancer. There is also an increased risk of cardiovascular diseases, such as hypertension (high blood pressure), coronary artery disease, and stroke.

Heavy drinkers often suffer from disorders of the digestive tract, partly because of the constant irritant effect of the alcohol. Gastritis, pancreatitis, peptic ul-

cer, and cancers of the mouth, tongue, pharynx, larynx, esophagus, and stomach are all more common than average in heavy drinkers. People who drink heavily tend not to eat a balanced diet, and may therefore suffer from nutritional disorders.

Long-term overindulgence in alcohol leads to impairment of brain function, affecting intellectual abilities and movement.

Women who drink regularly or heavily during pregnancy are likely to damage the physical and mental development of their unborn children to a greater or lesser degree.

Social problems

Alcohol is implicated in a wide range of social problems; it is a significant factor in absenteeism, traffic accidents, drowning, domestic violence, marital breakdown, child abuse, sexual assault, and other violent crimes. Also, there is strong evidence that young people who drink heavily are more likely to experiment with other addictive drugs. For your own sake and for the sake of others, it is sensible to stick to safe drinking limits.

HOW MUCH IS TOO MUCH?

First count how many units of alcohol you drink in a week. Each of the following is one unit:
- half a pint of ordinary beer or lager;
- a glass of wine;
- a single whisky, a vermouth, or a small glass of sherry.

Then check your rating against the table below. Remember that cider and strong beers account for more units of alcohol per half pint than ordinary beers. Remember, too, that home and party measures are usually larger than measures in a bar.

Men: 21 units or under per week
Women: 14 units or under per week
Your drinking is within generally safe limits; try not to increase the amount of alcohol you drink. Remember, though, not to drink and drive.

Men: 22-35 units per week
Women: 15-21 units per week
Your drinking level is probably not doing lasting damage if it is spread out evenly through the week, but if it is in two or three binges you could be damaging your health. Try to drink less.

Men: 36-49 units per week
Women: 22-35 units per week
Your drinking is at a level which is likely to do long-term damage to your health. Examine your drinking habits and work out ways in which you can cut down.

Men: 50 units or more per week
Women: 36 units or more per week
Your drinking is almost certainly causing serious damage to your health, and you may well be dependent on alcohol. Cut down your drinking drastically, and seek help if you have trouble doing this.

THE VALUE OF SCREENING

"If only we'd caught this earlier." All too commonly, it is necessary for a physician to explain that the disease responsible for a patient's symptoms is too far advanced for a cure to be possible. In many cases, however, modern diagnostic tests could have detected the disease months or even years before the appearance of symptoms or any upset to health. The detection of early signs of a disease in its hidden, presymptomatic stage allows treatment to be more effective—and often curative; this detection process is known as screening. In recent years, more and more general practices, health centers, and clinics have begun to offer screening programs for different groups of people.

Screening tests

Screening tests may be suitable for the whole population or for subgroups at special risk (such as people over a certain age, people belonging to particular racial groups, people with relatives who have a particular disorder, or people who are employed in hazardous occupations).

Most screening tests need to be performed by physicians or nurses, but it is possible to carry out some types of screening tests yourself—self-examination of the testes or breasts, for example.

Criteria for screening

A good screening test is both sensitive and specific. A test is sensitive if it detects all, or almost all, of the people with the disorder (i.e., there are few false negatives). A test is specific if it does not cause many false alarms (i.e., there are few false positives).

The condition being tested for should be reasonably common (for example, there is not much point screening Canadians for leprosy). Another criterion for screening is the availability of an effective treatment for the condition at the stage at which it can be detected by the test. Also, there should be good evidence that early diagnosis by screening substantially improves the chance of a cure or of prolonged freedom from symptoms.

These criteria for screening are now fulfilled by a whole range of tests, starting immediately after birth and continuing into old age.

Common screening tests

Newborn infants are examined by a pediatrician, who looks for various conditions, such as heart defects, and disorders of the brain and nervous system. Blood is taken from newborn infants to test for phenylketonuria (a chemical disorder) and hypothyroidism (a hormonal disorder), which, if undetected, may cause serious illness later in childhood. Infants and children are tested regularly to monitor growth, and to assess mental and physical development (including vision and hearing).

In early adult life, everyone should have his or her blood pressure measured; this test should then be repeated every three to five years throughout life. Early detection of raised blood pressure

TAKING THE BLOOD PRESSURE
Blood pressure is measured by using a sphygmomanometer (an inflatable cuff attached to a pressure gauge) and a stethoscope to listen for sounds of blood flow. Two pressure readings are recorded: the higher (systolic) pressure and the lower (diastolic) pressure. Blood pressure measurements are conventionally expressed in millimetres of mercury (mm Hg).

During the procedure
With the cuff on one arm, the patient sits with the arm on a firm surface and with the inside of the elbow turned up.

Placing the stethoscope
The physician positions the end of the stethoscope over the patient's brachial artery at the elbow, just below the cuff.

Reading the gauge
The pressure dial of the sphygmomanometer allows the physician to read the systolic and diastolic blood pressure levels.

The stethoscope
The stethoscope allows the physician to hear changes in the flow of blood which relate to blood pressure levels.

is the most useful screening test available, and is both safe and simple. Also important is regular personal measurement of weight.

Screening for cancer

Screening tests for cancer fall into two groups: those appropriate for the whole population, and those for high-risk groups.

All men should learn how to examine their testes regularly for signs of cancer. Cancer of the testis is the most common cancer in men under the age of 40, and is easily curable if detected early.

All women should learn how to examine their breasts, and should begin regular mammographic screening for cancer at the age of 50.

All women who have ever had sexual intercourse should have a cervical smear test done every three to five years (or more often if they have had a viral infection of the genital region).

After the age of 50, anyone with a family history of intestinal cancer should have an annual test for blood in the feces. Workers in some industries are more likely to develop some forms of cancer and may therefore benefit from screening; current and past workers in certain chemical industries, for example, should have regular urine tests to check for cancer of the bladder.

Other screening tests

Regular eye tests are important, particularly after the age of 40. Vision should be checked, and the

Cervical smear tests
These photomicrographs show the results of a normal smear (above left) and an abnormal smear (above right). The normal smear shows red-stained healthy cells with small nuclei; the abnormal smear shows numerous abnormal blue-stained cells with large, dark nuclei.

interior of the eye examined. Anyone with a family history of glaucoma should have the fluid pressure in their eyes measured at two-yearly intervals from the age of 40 onward.

Despite all the recent publicity about cholesterol tests, present medical advice is that these tests are unnecessary for most people. Physicians currently recommend the measurement of blood cholesterol only for people with relatives who have had a heart attack before the age of 50, or for people with other high-risk factors—such as a combination of raised blood pressure and heavy smoking.

Dental health has improved dramatically following many years' use of fluoride toothpaste and fluoridated water. Regular checkups by a dentist are, however, still essential, and are recommended every six months until the age of 21, and every one to two years thereafter.

Heel-prick blood test
This blood test is performed eight to 14 days after birth. The baby's heel is pricked and a few drops of blood are collected and sent to the laboratory to be tested for phenylketonuria, an inherited chemical disorder, and for hypothyroidism (thyroid deficiency).

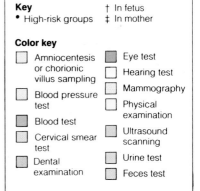

TYPES OF SCREENING TESTS
The table lists tests that can be used to screen people for different conditions.

Prenatal screening tests

| Chromosomal abnormalities |
| Sickle cell disorders |
| Genetic disorders (e.g., muscular dystrophy) |
| Hemophilia; thalassemia |
| Anemia |
| Blood group (including Rh) |
| Hepatitis B; HIV infection |
| Rubella; syphilis |
| Spina bifida (and other malformations) |

Infant and child screening tests

| Hypothyroidism; phenylketonuria |
| Sickle cell; thalassemia |
| Dental caries |
| Cataracts; squint; visual defects |
| Deafness |
| Heart disease, congenital |
| Hip dislocation; talipes |
| Testes, ectopic or undescended |

Adult screening tests

| Hypertension |
| Hyperlipidemia |
| Cervical cancer |
| Glaucoma; visual defects |
| Breast cancer |
| Testicular cancer |
| Bladder cancer |
| Intestinal cancer |

Key
• High-risk groups
† In fetus
‡ In mother

Color key

Amniocentesis or chorionic villus sampling	Eye test
Blood pressure test	Hearing test
Blood test	Mammography
Cervical smear test	Physical examination
Dental examination	Ultrasound scanning
	Urine test
	Feces test

IMMUNIZATION AGAINST DISEASE

A range of dangerous diseases can now be avoided thanks to immunization—the artificial creation of immunity against infection. Smallpox, a former killer-disease, has already been successfully eliminated, and the World Health Organization hopes that several more infectious diseases will be eradicated from developed countries by the year 2000.

Immunization protects most children completely, but in the rare cases in which an immunized child does catch the disease, the illness is much milder than if the child had not been immunized. No child should be denied immunization without very good reason—not only for the child's sake, but also for that of the community at large.

How immunization works

When an infecting microorganism enters the body, the immune system attacks the invader and produces blood proteins called antibodies, which help to destroy the organism. The immune system is able to "remember" this destruction process, so that if the invader returns, a repeat attack can be mounted faster. This phenomenon is called immunity.

Immunization is the process of creating immunity artificially. This can be done either by passive or by active immunization.

In passive immunization, a person is injected with a preparation of ready-made human antibodies, taken from general blood donors or from people recovering from specific infections. Passive immunization gives immediate protection, but this protection lasts only for a few weeks.

In active immunization, a person is given a vaccine that may contain living, weakened organisms (e.g., measles vaccine), dead organisms (e.g., pertussis vaccine), or weakened forms of bacterial poisons (e.g., diphtheria vaccine). The vaccine stimulates the immune system to produce its own particular antibodies, which provide longer-lasting immunity.

Immunization schedules

For protection against some diseases, only one dose of vaccine is necessary; for other diseases, an initial course followed by booster doses is required.

Your physician will probably discuss immunization when your baby is very small, and you will be reminded when the immunizations are due. Premature babies are at greater than average risk from infectious diseases, so every effort should be made to have them vaccinated at the recommended schedule dates. Your child can be immunized by your family physician or at a public health clinic. Most immunizations are given by injection into the upper arm or thigh. Polio vaccines, however, are now given orally in all provinces.

TYPICAL IMMUNIZATION SCHEDULE

Vaccine	3 months	5 months	9 months	15 months	4–5 years	10–14 years (girls only)	13 years	15–19 years
Diphtheria	Yes*	Yes*	Yes*		Booster†			
Pertussis (whooping cough)	Yes*	Yes*	Yes*					
Tetanus	Yes*	Yes*	Yes*		Booster†			Booster
Poliomyelitis	Yes‡	Yes‡	Yes‡		Booster‡			Booster‡
Measles				Yes§				
Mumps				Yes§				
Rubella (German measles)				Yes§		Yes		
Tuberculosis							Yes	

Key
*Combined diphtheria, pertussis, and tetanus (DPT) vaccine
†Combined diphtheria and tetanus vaccine
‡Oral vaccine
§Combined measles, mumps, and rubella (MMR) vaccine

Immunization side effects

All vaccines are extensively tested for safety and effectiveness. When side effects do occur, they are usually mild. The risk of harmful side effects is very small, and for any vaccine this is always less than the risk of serious effects from the disease itself.

Immunization or not?

There are very few genuine reasons why a child should not be immunized; the physician will discuss these with you. Vaccination should be postponed if the child is suffering from a feverish illness, but does not need to be put off if he or she simply has a snuffly nose.

If the child has had a severe reaction to a previous dose, or a serious allergic reaction to egg, certain vaccines will not be given. There is no reason why a child with asthma, eczema, or hay fever, or who is older than the scheduled age, should not be immunized.

Live vaccines are generally not given to pregnant women, because of the theoretical risk of harm to the developing fetus; to people suffering from certain forms of cancer or immune system disorders; or to people receiving any treatment that suppresses the immune system.

Travel immunization

Various immunizations are necessary or recommended for people of any age who plan to travel to certain countries where there is a risk of contracting particular infections. You should check your immunization requirements with your physician, travel agent, or local medical officer of health at least two months before traveling.

TRAVEL PROTECTION

If you travel abroad you may be exposed to potentially serious infections to which you are not immune. Always check the immunizations recommended for your destination, and obtain immunization for the diseases against which you have no current protection.

Disease	Duration of immunity
Cholera	6 months
Hepatitis A	5–6 months
Meningococcal meningitis	3–5 years
Poliomyelitis	10 years
Rabies	2–3 years
Tetanus	10 years
Tuberculosis	15 years (minimum)
Typhoid fever	3 years
Yellow fever	10 years

PROTECTING YOUR CHILD

For most children, the benefits of immunization far outweigh any slight risks that might be involved. The consequences of catching these avoidable diseases can be very serious, as shown below.

Visual defects
Measles can damage the optic nerve. Visual defects due to brain damage can follow measles, pertussis, mumps, and rubella.

Brain damage
Measles, pertussis, mumps, and rubella can all cause brain inflammation, sometimes leading to permanent brain damage.

Heart and lung damage
Diphtheria attacks the heart and affects breathing. Pertussis and measles may cause pneumonia, bronchitis, and permanent lung damage. Tuberculosis can cause permanent lung damage.

Hearing loss
Permanent hearing loss may result from nerve damage due to mumps, from ear infections due to measles, or from brain damage due to mumps, measles, pertussis, or rubella.

Muscle problems
Poliomyelitis and diphtheria attack the nervous system and may cause muscle paralysis. Tetanus causes painful muscle spasms.

AN ACCEPTABLE RISK

Despite some public fears about the safety of pertussis vaccine, the risks of immunization are much lower than the risks of the disease itself. This graph compares the risk of death or brain damage from pertussis in unvaccinated children with the risk of pertussis vaccination.

% of children who die or suffer brain damage

2.4%

0.0003%

☐ Not vaccinated against pertussis
◼ Vaccinated against pertussis

DIAGNOSING DISEASE

Diagnosis is the identification by a physician of a disease process that is causing a person's ill health or other complaint. Without knowing the identity of a disorder, a physician is able only to relieve symptoms, such as pain or fever. Once the physician has made a diagnosis, however, it becomes possible to make a prognosis—an estimate of the outcome of a certain disorder—and to begin appropriate treatment.

Diagnosis and prognosis

The concepts of diagnosis and prognosis go back to the fifth century B.C., when the Greek physician Hippocrates (c. 460–c. 377 B.C.) attempted to identify diseases rather than symptoms, and to describe the sequence of events that occurred in individual diseases. These concepts led to a system of medical training based

on pattern recognition that continues to the present day. Physicians are taught to recognize and distinguish diseases by history taking—during which the physician asks a series of questions and listens to the patient's own account of the events of the illness—and by performing a physical examination, which may be either general or local depending on the patient's symptoms.

Anatomy and pathology

Diagnosis remained mostly guesswork until the 17th century, when anatomists and pathologists began to make use of dissection to study the structure of the human body, and to investigate the changes that disease causes in body tissues and organs.

The process of diagnosis was also aided by the development in the 17th century of the single-lens microscope, which led to a greater understanding of the structure and function of the body and of the effects of disease.

The 19th century brought another major advance in the history of diagnosis, with the discovery that microorganisms, such as bacteria and fungi, can cause disease. This discovery led to the development of the germ theory of disease by, among others, the French microbiologist and chemist Louis Pasteur (1822-1895) and the German bacteriologist Robert Koch (1843-1910). The germ theory of disease is generally regarded as being one of the most important achievements of medical and biological science.

Muscular and skeletal systems
Muscles Muscle biopsy; EMG.
Bones Biopsy; imaging techniques (X ray, CT, MRI, diskography, radionuclide scanning); arthroscopy; densitometry; blood tests

Reproductive system
Men Biochemical analysis of blood and semen; biopsy; culture
Women Endoscopy (laparoscopy, colposcopy, fetoscopy); imaging techniques (mammography, ultrasound, hysterosalpingography); cytology; culture; biopsy; blood tests; amniocentesis; chorionic villus sampling

Respiratory system
Pulmonary function tests; bronchoscopy; culture; biopsy; blood tests; imaging techniques (X ray, CT, MRI, lung tomography)

Modern diagnostic techniques

Today, physicians still rely heavily on history taking and physical examination in order to arrive at a diagnosis. However, the speed and accuracy with which diagnoses are made have been greatly increased by the numerous different investigative procedures that can now be performed.

As recently as 50 years ago, the diagnosis of many diseases became certain only after an affected person had died, when his or her body could be fully examined by a pathologist. Nowadays, equal certainty in diagnosis is possible early in the course of a disease, either because it is possible to remove samples of the diseased organs for examination or because diagnostic testing provides a precise, accurate picture of the interior of the body.

The development of these diagnostic methods has led to hospitals being equipped with an enormous range of biochemical, immunological, and microbiological tests on body fluids and tissues. The past 20 years has also seen a revolution in the scale and accuracy of imaging techniques, such as endoscopy, ultrasound, CT scanning, MRI, and PET scanning, which have made it possible to obtain detailed, accurate information about the structure and function of internal organs. Modern diagnostic techniques are able to provide valuable information for physicians, while involving only minimal risk and discomfort to patients.

Some of the most common diagnostic techniques that can be used to investigate disorders affecting the different body systems are listed with the illustrations on these two pages.

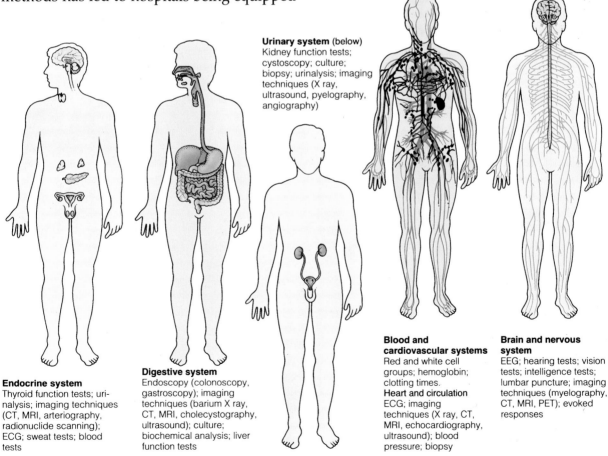

Urinary system (below)
Kidney function tests; cystoscopy; culture; biopsy; urinalysis; imaging techniques (X ray, ultrasound, pyelography, angiography)

Endocrine system
Thyroid function tests; urinalysis; imaging techniques (CT, MRI, arteriography, radionuclide scanning); ECG; sweat tests; blood tests

Digestive system
Endoscopy (colonoscopy, gastroscopy); imaging techniques (barium X ray, CT, MRI, cholecystography, ultrasound); culture; biochemical analysis; liver function tests

Blood and cardiovascular systems
Red and white cell groups; hemoglobin; clotting times.
Heart and circulation
ECG; imaging techniques (X ray, CT, MRI, echocardiography, ultrasound); blood pressure; biopsy

Brain and nervous system
EEG; hearing tests; vision tests; intelligence tests; lumbar puncture; imaging techniques (myelography, CT, MRI, PET); evoked responses

YOU AND YOUR PHYSICIAN

Your physician is trained to diagnose and treat many diseases and disorders. When you consult your physician about a particular problem, you will find that the consultation typically consists of two main parts. First of these is history taking, in which the physician asks carefully selected questions designed to build a picture of your problem; second is a physical examination, which confirms or corrects your physician's first impressions. These two procedures are among the physician's most important tools.

Before your visit

Before you visit your physician, check in your own mind just why it is that you want an appointment, and what questions you want to ask. Be totally honest from the outset; for instance, if your specific symptom is that you have an upset stomach, but you also know that you have been feeling run-down, tell your physician about both symptoms—this will enable your physician to get to the root of the problem more quickly.

If your mind tends to go blank as soon as you get to the office, write down your symptoms before you go, and either present the list to the physician or use it yourself to check that you have not missed anything out. Your physician is likely to begin by asking you a few questions about your general health—so take a little time before your visit to think over how you have been feeling lately,

Talking to your physician
Your physician will be able to help you most easily if you give him or her a full description of your problem. Always feel free to tell the physician about anything that is bothering you. He or she will ask you a series of questions designed to help build up a full picture of your problem

whether you have noticed any change in your eating habits, bowel habits, or sleeping pattern, and whether you have any particular worries.

Taking the history

The first thing your physician will want to know is why you have asked for an appointment. Relate your symptoms as simply and clearly as possible, and be as specific as you can. The more clues you can give, the easier the diagnosis will be.

While you are relating your symptoms, the physician will be seeing whether your appearance

Eye examination
The physician is using an ophthalmoscope, which uses a deflecting prism to illuminate the inside of the eye.

Throat examination
Here the physician is using a tongue depressor to hold the tongue down, and a flashlight to illuminate the throat.

Listening to the chest
A stethoscope is here being used by the physician to listen for abnormal sounds from the heart or lungs.

gives any clues to your state of health—for example, whether you look generally fit and relaxed, or seem pale, tired, or worried; whether your skin, eyes, hair, and teeth look healthy; and whether you are noticeably overweight or underweight.

Your physician will make notes on the symptoms you describe, and will then ask you questions to supplement this information: for instance, if you mention that you have a pain in your abdomen, the physician might ask you about the frequency of your bowel movements. The physician will also ask you questions about your previous health record and about the medical history of members of your family.

Once your physician is satisfied that a good picture of your specific symptoms has been built up, he or she might ask you more general questions about your everyday health and life-style.

Physical examination

Your physician may then perform a physical examination. The part or parts of the body that are to be examined will depend on the symptoms that you have described; for instance, if it seems likely that you have a broken arm, the physician will probably just do

URINE TEST
Urinalysis involves testing a sample of urine to see whether its constituents are abnormal, or present in abnormal quantities. Here, urine is being tested for the presence of protein. A test stick has been dipped in the urine, and has changed color; the color is being compared against a chart of possible results.

a careful examination of the damaged arm, but if you are feeling under the weather or run-down, he or she is likely to do a thorough general examination to see if your main body systems are functioning properly.

Examination techniques that your physician might use include visual examinations of the ears, eyes, nose, throat, and skin; listening to the chest through a stethoscope; palpating (feeling) body parts such as the abdomen or armpit to detect tenderness or swelling; testing reflexes; and percussion (tapping the chest or abdomen with the fingers to

see from the vibrations whether the different internal organs appear to be normal).

Your physician may take your temperature to see whether you have a fever, and may also measure your blood pressure, take your pulse, and weigh you. If you are a woman and your symptoms seem to suggest a gynecological condition, the physician may perform a pelvic examination, in which the vagina is examined visually and manually to see if the reproductive organs seem to be healthy.

What happens next?

In some cases, your physician may tell you that further tests are necessary before a diagnosis can be made or confirmed. He or she may ask you to provide a sample of urine, or may take a blood sample or a throat swab, which will then be sent to a laboratory for various types of analysis. In some cases, your physician will refer you to a hospital for further examinations and tests.

Once your condition has been diagnosed, an appropriate course of treatment can be recommended. In most cases, treatment will be supervised by your own physician, but in some cases you will be placed under the care of a hospital physician.

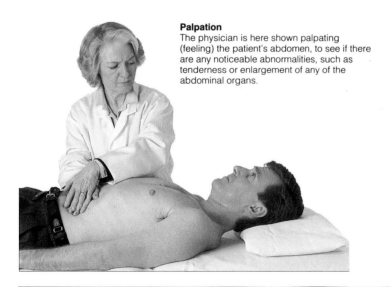

Palpation
The physician is here shown palpating (feeling) the patient's abdomen, to see if there are any noticeable abnormalities, such as tenderness or enlargement of any of the abdominal organs.

DIAGNOSTIC TECHNIQUES 1

Physicians today can make use of a variety of sophisticated techniques to help them reach an accurate diagnosis. Major advances have been the development of new imaging techniques that provide detailed pictures of internal organs, and fiber-optic endoscopes that enable physicians to look directly into many parts of the body without any need for open surgery. Also of great value in diagnosis are numerous biochemical, immunological, and microbiological tests, as well as techniques of genetic analysis.

X rays

Following their discovery by Wilhelm Roentgen in 1895, X rays soon became an important aid to medical diagnosis. Despite the development of newer techniques, X-ray imaging continues to be a widely used and extremely valuable means of seeing inside the body.

X rays are a form of electromagnetic radiation of extremely short wavelength. They are invisible but blacken photographic film—a property that is used to produce X-ray images. When a beam of X rays is directed at a part of the body, such as the chest, the rays are absorbed more by dense structures, such as the ribs or heart muscle, than by less dense structures, such as the skin or lungs.

This causes shadows of variable intensity to be cast onto photographic film placed behind the patient. The result is the classic X-ray picture, in which dense tissues appear white, and softer tissues appear as shades of gray.

X rays cause no sensation when passed through body tissues, but large or frequent radiation doses may damage the skin and internal organs, and may cause cancer in later life. Today, the risk involved in having an X ray is extremely small, because radiation doses are kept to a minimum.

Contrast X rays

The development of contrast X-ray imaging techniques has extended the usefulness of X rays. Fluid-filled or hollow parts of

A chest X ray
The lungs, which are full of air, appear as dark areas on X-ray film; denser structures, such as the heart and skeleton, appear white.

the body that would not show up well on conventional X rays can be seen clearly on X rays if they are first filled with a contrast medium (substance opaque to X rays).

Commonly used examples of contrast X-ray techniques are urography, which is performed to obtain X-ray pictures of the urinary system, and barium X-ray examinations, which are used to investigate the digestive tract. Angiography, an imaging technique which requires contrast medium to be injected into blood vessels, is used to investigate diseases that alter the appearance of the blood vessels.

Digital subtraction angiography

The technique of digital subtraction angiography uses computers to process images obtained before and after the injection of contrast medium into the bloodstream. The computer subtracts (i.e.,

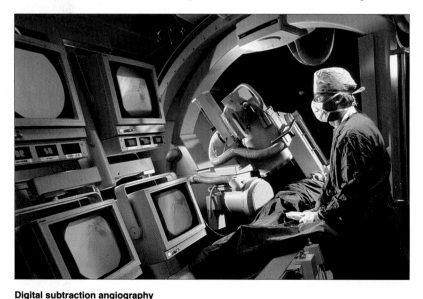

Digital subtraction angiography
This technique is a form of contrast X-ray imaging that uses computers to improve the image. Physicians monitor the introduction of a contrast medium into the patient's bloodstream, thus obtaining a clear image of the arteries.

CT SCANNING

CT scanning can be used to obtain images of virtually any part of the body. This technique combines the use of X rays with computer technology to produce a two- or three-dimensional image of an area. The CT scan included here shows a cross section through the trunk along the plane shown, at the level of the kidneys. The image has been artificially colored by computer to make the internal structures (the most important of which have been labeled) more clearly visible.

Plane of scan

Intestine (gas-filled)

Rib

Rib

Fat around kidney

Liver

Left kidney

Right kidney

Vertebral canal (containing spinal cord)

Thoracic vertebra

Paravertebral muscles

A radionuclide bone scan
This radionuclide bone scan shows a front view of the complete skeleton of a healthy person. Bone scanning is an essential step in assessing treatment for some types of cancer, such as breast cancer, because it can reveal whether or not the cancer has spread beyond its primary site and developed secondary growths in the bones. Cancerous areas appear as bright "hot spots" on scans.

removes) unwanted background detail, leaving a clear image of the blood vessels.

CT scanning

Conventional X rays are essentially shadow photographs, but CT (computed tomography) scanning uses X rays in a completely different way. Multiple beams of X rays are passed through the body, and their degree of absorption is recorded by sensors. The scanner moves around the patient, emitting and recording X-ray beams from every point. The resulting data are then analyzed by a computer, which uses the variations in absorption of the X rays to construct cross-sectional "slices" through the body.

CT images are more detailed than those produced by conventional X-ray techniques. A further advantage of CT scanning is that images can be manipulated by the computer to obtain a better view of the area under study, or to produce a three-dimensional image. CT scanning was first used, in the early 1970s, for studying the brain. The technique quickly

became a first-line test in the investigation not only of brain disorders but also of symptoms affecting virtually every other part of the body.

Radionuclide scanning

Images obtained by conventional X-ray techniques or by CT scanning depend on physical differences (notably in density) among body structures. Imaging by radionuclide scanning utilizes another approach. In this technique, radioactive chemicals are either swallowed by the patient or injected into the bloodstream. These chemicals are taken up by certain organs or tissues, which then give off radiation that can be detected and analyzed by a gamma camera.

The amount of radiation emitted by a part of the body depends mainly on the level of metabolic activity of its constituent cells. Thus, cells that are dividing rapidly (such as cancer cells) show up in some cases as "hot spots" on radionuclide scans.

The substances used in radionuclide scanning are usually

either radioactive forms of elements that are normally found in the body, such as iodine, or synthetic radioactive elements, such as technetium. The levels of radiation to which the body is exposed in radionuclide scanning are very low, usually considerably lower than in conventional X rays.

DIAGNOSTIC TECHNIQUES 2

MRI

Unlike X-ray imaging, CT scanning, and radionuclide imaging, MRI (magnetic resonance imaging) does not use potentially harmful ionizing radiation. Instead, it exploits the natural behavior of the protons (nuclei) of hydrogen atoms when they are subjected to a very strong magnetic field and radio waves.

For MRI, the patient lies inside a large, hollow, cylindrical magnet in which the body is exposed to a magnetic field many thousands of times more powerful than that of the Earth. Under the influence of the scanner's magnetic field, the protons in the body, which normally point randomly in different directions, line up parallel to each other. A strong pulse of radio waves is then used to knock the protons out of alignment. As the protons realign themselves, they produce detectable radio signals, which are picked up by radio receiver coils in the scanner. A computer then converts these radio signals into a two-dimen-

MRI chest scans
These scans show cross-sectional views through a normal chest (above) and through the chest of a patient with a lung tumor (above right). The lungs appear as black areas in the middle and the ribs as yellow-red crescents. The tumor is indicated by the increased blue area and by the affected lung's small size.

sional or a three-dimensional image based on the strength and location of the signals.

The most abundant sources of protons in the body are the hydrogen atoms in water molecules; an MRI scan thus reflects differences in the water content of tissues.

Superficially, MRI scans look like CT scans. However, MRI scans give a much more detailed picture of the structure of soft tissues because of the differences in water content within these tissues. MRI scans are particularly useful for studying the brain and spinal cord. They are also useful for imaging other soft tissues.

A newer application of MRI, known as magnetic resonance spectroscopy, relies on the detection of other chemical elements, such as phosphorus and calcium. Magnetic resonance spectroscopy can provide useful information on organ function.

Ultrasound scanning

The diagnostic use of ultrasound is based on the principle of naval sonar, in which sound waves are used to locate underwater objects

MRI SCAN OF HEAD
This MRI scan shows a longitudinal section through the middle of the head and upper neck. The image has been colored to differentiate the internal structures according to differences in water content. MRI scanning is very useful for studying the brain because it allows the detailed structure of the soft brain tissues to be clearly imaged.

- Skull
- Cerebrospinal fluid between meninges
- Cerebrum
- Ventricle
- Corpus callosum
- Pituitary gland
- Midbrain
- Pons
- Medulla oblongata
- Brainstem
- Cerebellum
- Spinal cord
- Vertebrae in neck

by their echoes. Ultrasound scanning causes no discomfort and is thought to be completely safe.

In ultrasound scanning, a device called a transducer is placed on the skin and transmits inaudible high-frequency sound waves into the body, where they are reflected by the internal structures. The transducer detects these echoes, which are converted to numerical data and then displayed directly on a screen or analyzed by computer to produce an image of the structures.

The technique is especially useful in obstetrics because it enables the obstetrician to examine the fetus at no known risk to either the pregnant woman or her developing child. Ultrasound waves are converted into an image of the fetus and enable the obstetrician to identify multiple pregnancies, to measure the size of the fetus (so that its age can be assessed), and to detect various defects.

Another ultrasound procedure, known as echocardiography, provides information about the heart, including the structure and flexibility of heart valves, the condition of the heart muscle, and the flow of blood within the heart.

A modification of the basic ultrasound technique makes use of the Doppler effect (the change in pitch that occurs when a sound source is moving relative to the detector) to give information about the rate of blood flow through the heart and blood vessels. This procedure enables the physician to detect narrowing of blood vessels or turbulence in the flow of blood.

PET scanning

PET (positron emission tomography) scanning is a development of radionuclide scanning. Both techniques use a radioactive substance to produce an image that reflects the level of metabolic activity of cells within the tissues. However, PET scanning, unlike radionuclide scanning, allows a cross-sectional image to be built up.

In PET scanning, a substance that takes part in normal metabolic processes is radioactively labeled (i.e., replaced with a radioactive form of the substance) and then injected into the bloodstream. The radioactive substance is taken up by the most metabolically active areas of tissue, where it emits positrons. The positrons, in turn, release photons, which are then detected by an array of sensors around the patient. The sensors are linked to a computer, which calculates the origins of the photons to construct an image of the distribution of the substance within the tissues.

PET scanning is currently being used for investigating brain tumors, for locating the origin of epileptic activity, and for study-

PET scan of brain
This PET scan shows a section through a normal brain. Methionine (an essential amino acid) has been used to show levels of protein synthesis within the brain; different levels of metabolic activity show up as different colors in the scan. Other brain functions can be imaged by using different substances, such as the use of a radioactive form of glucose to show different levels of carbohydrate metabolism.

ing the brain function in various mental illnesses. It is also being used for investigating the heart, and it is expected to be useful for studying other organs.

Biochemical analysis

A physician may arrange for biochemical tests on samples of blood, urine, and other body fluids such as spinal fluid, saliva, or sweat. These tests may be part of a diagnostic investigation in which the chemical constituents of body fluids are checked primarily to confirm the physician's diagnosis. Biochemical tests may also be used to assess the function of a particular organ, such as the liver or kidneys.

Fetal ultrasound
The photograph (above) shows the ultrasound transducer being passed over the pregnant woman's abdomen, and the ultrasound images being displayed on computer screens. The ultrasound scan (right) shows a 12-week-old fetus, whose body parts are annotated in the accompanying diagram (far right).

Arm
Head
Leg
Body
Uterine wall

Biopsy

Biopsy is the removal of a sample of tissue or cells from a living patient. Such samples are then examined under a microscope and may be subjected to a variety of biochemical tests. Biopsy thus provides a valuable aid in establishing a precise diagnosis.

Samples of some types of tissue may be removed by passing a hollow needle through the skin and into the target organ or tissue. Other samples may be removed surgically or endoscopically.

Biopsy is useful in the investigation of tumors or cysts in organs such as the breast, ovary, testis, or thyroid. This procedure provides physicians with an important means of determining whether a tumor is benign or malignant, thus allowing appropriate treatment to be carried out. Biopsy can also be used to determine the cause of other disorders, such as unexplained inflammation or degeneration of the liver, kidneys, muscle, or skin.

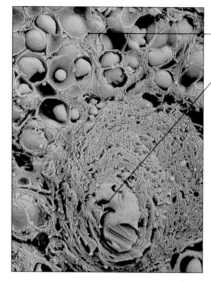

Normal ovarian tissue

Malignant teratoma

Ovarian biopsy sample
The development of biopsy—in which samples of tissue are removed from the body for microscopic analysis—has proved very useful in the diagnosis of a great many disorders. Biopsy samples may be examined in the laboratory under a light microscope or, occasionally, under a scanning electron microscope. This example of a scanning electron micrograph shows a sample of ovarian tissue in which a malignant teratoma (a type of ovarian cancer) can be seen invading the normal ovarian tissue.

Endoscopy

Endoscopy is an investigative procedure that enables a physician to look directly into a patient's body by means of a viewing instrument known as an endoscope.

Early endoscopes were rigid or partially rigid tubes, sometimes with complex lens systems and interior lighting. The application of fiber optics to endoscopy in the 1950s allowed the development of flexible endoscopes and made the technique more versatile.

Today, many specialized endoscopes, both rigid and flexible, are available, enabling physicians to view virtually any structure in the body, including the digestive tract, nasal sinuses, lungs, bladder, abdominal cavity, and joints. Many types of endoscope can be fitted with attachments for the removal of biopsy samples.

Fetoscopy

Fetoscopy is a procedure for directly observing a fetus inside the uterus by means of a fetoscope, a type of endoscope. The fetoscope is passed into the woman's uterus through a small incision in the abdomen.

Fetoscopy may be performed if the obstetrician suspects that a fetus may have a physical malformation, such as spina bifida or a cleft lip or palate. Attachments on the fetoscope also make it possible to remove samples of skin or blood from the fetus so that tests may be performed to identify certain genetic or other disorders.

ENDOSCOPY OF COLON
The colon can be viewed through a flexible endoscope known as a colonoscope. The technique of colonoscopy is useful in the diagnosis of such disorders as intestinal polyps, inflammatory bowel disorders, and cancer of the large intestine. The inset photograph shows normal intestinal lining as seen through a colonoscope.

A view through an endoscope showing a healthy colon wall

Physician

Endoscope

Patient

Key

☐ Cytosine

☐ Guanine

☐ Adenine

☐ Thymine

☐ Sugar-phosphate side chain

Structure of DNA
DNA is a large, double-helix-shaped molecule, as shown in the computer-generated model (left). The DNA molecule consists of two sugar-phosphate side chains linked by the nucleotide bases cytosine, guanine, adenine, and thymine, as shown in the diagram (above). The DNA within each cell carries the 50,000-plus genes that control cellular activities; thus a defective gene may disrupt cellular activity and lead to a genetic disorder, such as cystic fibrosis or hemophilia.

Amniocentesis

Amniocentesis is the removal and testing of a sample of the amniotic fluid that surrounds the fetus in the uterus. Tests on the cells and fluid removed can be used to diagnose certain fetal abnormalities early enough in pregnancy for elective abortion to remain a feasible option. However, because amniocentesis carries a small risk of causing miscarriage, this procedure is recommended only in some cases.

Amniocentesis is not usually performed before about the 16th to 18th week of pregnancy because there is not enough amniotic fluid before this time. Results from an amniocentesis cannot usually be obtained until the 18th to 20th week of pregnancy.

The sample of amniotic fluid contains fetal cells, which are cultured to provide chromosomes for analysis. Analysis of chromosomes makes it possible to identify chromosomal abnormalities, such as Down's syndrome. Amniocentesis also allows the measurement of various substances in the amniotic fluid. Abnormal levels of such substances may indicate other, non-chromosomal disorders of the fetus. For example, raised levels of alpha-fetoprotein may indicate spina bifida.

Chorionic villus sampling

Chorionic villus sampling is another method of diagnosing fetal abnormalities. The sample can be taken as early as eight to nine weeks into pregnancy, and testing can usually begin at once. This technique thus gives earlier results than amniocentesis.

Chorionic villus sampling is performed by removing a small sample of tissue from the fetal side of the placenta, and then analyzing this sample in the laboratory. The cells in the tissue sample are genetically identical to those of the fetus, and analysis of this sample shows whether the fetus has certain types of chromosomal or genetic disorders.

Genetic analysis

Genetic analysis may be performed in high-risk pregnancies (i.e., when there is a family history of a genetic disorder or when a couple has had a child with such a disorder) to investigate whether a fetus has a disorder of this type, such as hemophilia or cystic fibrosis. Cell samples for genetic analysis during pregnancy are obtained by amniocentesis or by chorionic villus sampling.

Genetic analysis may also be used to determine whether a person with a family history of a genetic disorder is affected by the disorder, or is a carrier of the disorder and is thus at risk of having affected children.

An important technique in genetic analysis involves the use of genetic probes. A genetic probe is a specific fragment of DNA (the genetic material contained in the chromosomes of all cells) that can be used in laboratory tests to determine whether a particular gene defect is present.

Geneticists are currently building up a complete picture of how human DNA is arranged, showing the position of individual genes in each chromosome. This information is invaluable in the identification of genetic disorders. In many cases, it is not yet possible to detect a defective gene itself. However, for certain gene defects, researchers have identified markers (sections of DNA with a specific base sequence) that very commonly occur on particular chromosomes in association with the defect. The presence of a marker thus provides strong evidence that the associated gene defect is also present.

Sickle cell anemia
Beta-thalassemia
Methemoglobinemia
Polycythemia vera

Acute intermittent porphyria

Gene map of chromosome 11
This gene map shows the location of gene defects responsible for various inherited blood disorders, and for the metabolic disorder acute intermittent porphyria. Other gene defects have been located on other chromosomes.

TREATING DISEASE

Most illnesses and injuries are not serious, and most sufferers recover completely within a few days without ever having to see a physician. In other cases, however, a medical consultation will be necessary, so that a physician can diagnose the disorder and prescribe suitable treatment. Sometimes a physician will need to refer patients to a consultant for specialist treatment.

Self-treatment

For treating many disorders, simple self-help measures are all that is needed. Most self-treatments—such as resting in bed, drinking plenty of fluids, or taking over-the-counter medications—are intended to relieve symptoms and to help you feel more comfortable until your illness has run its natural course. Cold remedies, for example, will help relieve the symptoms of nasal congestion, fever, and aches, but will not attack the virus that has caused the cold.

Seeing your physician

If your symptoms persist, or get worse, you may need to consult a physician so that your problem can be diagnosed and treated.

If specific treatment is available, the physician will arrange this. For example, he or she may insert stitches to treat a cut, or may prescribe antihypertensive drugs to treat raised blood pressure. If no specific treatment is available, as in the case of many viral infections, the physician will provide or advise treatment that will relieve symptoms and help make you feel more comfortable while the disease runs its course.

If your problem needs further investigation, or some form of specialist treatment, you will usually be referred by your physician to a hospital-based consultant. Specialist treatment may involve taking medication, undergoing surgery, or receiving some other form of treatment.

Drug treatment

Until well into this century, physicians had few effective drugs with which to work, and as a result were unable to cure or even to slow down the progress of many diseases. Traditionally, many of the drugs that have proved useful, such as morphine and digitalis, were derived from plants.

The situation changed dramatically in the 1930s, with the introduction of antibacterial drugs, advances in the production of synthetic drugs, and the development of drugs that act on the body's metabolic processes. Since then, progress has been rapid, with the development of an even wider range of effective drugs, and with developments in drug production, such as the application of genetic engineering techniques.

Although immunization began in 1796, when Edward Jenner gave the first smallpox inoculation, it was not until this century that

Bed rest
Simply resting in bed may be all that is needed for recovery.

vaccines against other potentially lethal human diseases were developed. Today, vaccines are available against measles, mumps, diphtheria, poliomyelitis, tetanus, pertussis, rubella, tuberculosis, and various other, less common, diseases such as hepatitis, typhoid, rabies, cholera, and yellow fever.

Before any new substance can be marketed as a drug, it must be thoroughly tested for effectiveness and safety and approved by the Health Promotion Branch of Health and Welfare Canada. The form in which a drug is produced may depend on the nature of the drug itself, the dosage in which it needs to be taken, and the length of time over which it will act.

Surgical treatment

Considerable advances in surgery in the 19th and early 20th centuries—the introduction of general anesthesia in the 1840s, antiseptic procedures in the 1870s, and blood transfusions in the early 1900s—paved the way for many new surgical techniques.

Nevertheless, until about the 1940s, most surgery involved the cutting out of diseased, damaged, or deformed tissues or structures.

Drug remedies
Over-the-counter drugs or drugs obtained on a physician's prescription are an important aspect of treatment for many disorders.

The primary exception was orthopedic surgery, in which surgeons were attempting to encourage the healing of bones by employing rods, pins, and immobilization.

Since then, however, surgery has been transformed by technological advances, such as the operating microscope, the laser scalpel, and the endoscope. Today, many operations emphasize repair or replacement rather than excision, and there have been exciting developments in the fields of implant surgery and transplant surgery.

Other treatments

Drug treatment and surgery are still the primary divisions of medical care, but technological advances have led to the development of other forms of treatment. Radiation therapy plays a central part in the treatment of many forms of cancer, and modern medicine increasingly employs recently developed procedures, such as endoscopy, lithotripsy, and laser treatment, that avoid the need for open surgery. Some new areas of treatment, such as intensive care or neonatology, have become so specialized in recent years that they have developed into separate branches of medicine.

Surgery
Surgical procedures are necessary for the treatment of a wide variety of disorders. Operations may be performed under general anesthesia (as here) or under local anesthesia.

HOME NURSING

The nature and amount of home nursing that an ill person requires depends on the effects and duration of the illness and on how much help the patient needs to perform daily activities, such as eating and washing. A child who has chickenpox obviously needs very different home nursing from an old person who is suffering from the effects of a severe stroke. In all cases, however, the overall aim when looking after an ill person at home should be to keep the patient as comfortable and cheerful as possible.

Patient care

Whenever you are nursing someone at home, you will probably find it useful to establish a daily routine for tending to his or her basic needs. Although you may have to provide help with many activities, you can help pre-serve your patient's self-esteem by letting him or her attend to personal needs as far as possible.

When preparing food for a sick person, try to make it look as appetizing as possible. Most people prefer to feed themselves if possible, but you may have to pro-vide help with feeding in some cases. Make sure that the patient sits upright and is well supported by pillows before he or she starts to eat. If you have to help with feeding, do not rush the patient; allow plenty of time between mouthfuls for food to be chewed and swallowed.

In some cases, you may need to help your patient visit the bathroom or toilet. A bedridden patient will have to be bathed and helped with a bedpan. You may also need to learn how to turn a patient regularly to prevent bed-sores, how to change a bed with the patient in it, or how to sit the patient up in bed. Sometimes, two people will be needed for these tasks. A visiting nurse will often be able to provide valuable advice and practical assistance. Health care in your province or community may include professional home-care nursing.

CHANGING A BED
Two people are needed to change a bed with the patient in it. Before you begin, tell the patient exactly what you are going to do.

1 Remove the covers except for one blanket. Roll the patient to one side of the bed, and support his or her back and thigh. Your helper should then roll the dirty bottom sheet toward the patient.

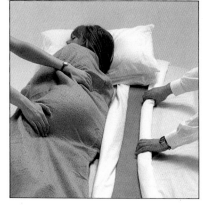

2 Continue to support the patient's back and thigh while your helper tucks in the new bottom sheet and unrolls it, as shown above, toward the patient's back. The clean sheet should be rolled over the bed until it meets the rolled dirty sheet.

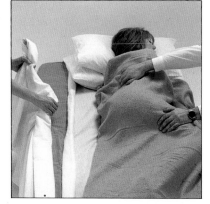

3 You and your helper can then roll the patient over the ridge formed by the two rolled sheets onto the newly laid clean sheet. Your helper should then support the patient while you remove the dirty sheet and tuck in the clean sheet.

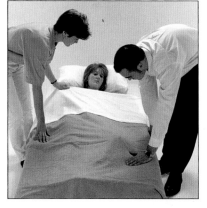

4 Raise the patient's head and shoulders while you replace the pillowcase. Unfold the clean top sheet over the blanket covering the patient. Remove the blanket, tuck in the sheet, and then replace the blanket and other covers over the sheet.

The sickroom

The ideal sickroom should be cheerful in appearance, close to a bathroom, reasonably quiet, maintained at a comfortable temperature, adequately lit, well ventilated, and kept as clean as possible. In many cases, a person's own bedroom will be suitable and preferable.

Many patients will benefit from the stimulation and entertainment provided by reading materials, radio, audio equipment, television, or videotapes.

Some people will want certain items within easy reach, such as drinking water, tissues, a telephone, or a bell to call for assistance. Do not leave medications within reach of children or patients who are confused.

Your patient may be more comfortable if he or she is given extra supports for sitting up in bed, such as a backrest or triangular pillows. Orthopedic bed boards can be placed under ordinary soft mattresses for use by people with back problems.

Blinds
These are useful for controlling glare and giving privacy.

Window
An easily opened window allows the room to be ventilated.

Washbasin
It is very useful to have a washbasin close at hand.

Heating devices
A hot-water bottle or electric blanket can provide comfort and extra warmth.

A WELL-PLANNED SICKROOM
This illustration shows various features and equipment that can help to make a sickroom more comfortable and convenient for patient and carer.

Curtains
Well-fitting curtains help to stop draughts.

Angled light
An angled light clamped to the bedhead is easy to use.

New bedding
It is a good idea to keep clean sheets and extra blankets in the sickroom.

TV and video
Remote-controlled TV and video can provide hours of entertainment.

Bedside table
This should be of a height that can be easily reached by the patient.

Flowers
These add colour and help cheer up the patient.

Bed-tray
A bed-tray provides a firm surface for meals, writing paper, and games.

Chairs
Comfortable chairs are useful for patient and visitors.

The bed
This should have a firm mattress, and should allow access on both sides for easy changing.

METHODS OF TREATMENT 1

This century has seen major advances in the treatment of disease. Large numbers of new drugs have been discovered and developed. Many lives are now saved by new intensive-care methods and by techniques such as dialysis and radiation therapy. Surgical advances—including developments in transplant surgery, implant surgery, and microsurgery—have increased the surgeon's range. For some disorders, surgery has been superseded by less invasive techniques, such as lithotripsy and laser treatment.

Drug treatment

The value of drugs in the treatment of disorders has been known for many thousands of years, and the use of drugs is still an extremely important aspect of medical treatment.

Some drugs, such as ASA, can be bought over the counter without a physician's prescription. Other drugs, such as penicillin, can be obtained only on presentation of a prescription to a pharmacist in a drugstore or hospital pharmacy. Certain drugs, such as the anticancer drug cisplatin, are normally administered only by physicians or nurses in a hospital.

Drugs are available in many different forms, including tablets, capsules, liquids, sprays and inhalers, ointments and creams, suppositories and pessaries, drops, powders, injections, and transdermal patches.

Drug sources

For many centuries, drugs were obtained from diverse natural sources, including many species of plants and animals, and various minerals. More recently, advances in drug production have helped pharmacologists and biochemists to develop an immense range of new drugs. In many cases, these drugs are manufactured synthetically by various chemical processes, or are produced by the newer technique of genetic engineering.

Natural drugs

Drugs that continue to be obtained from natural sources include digoxin, obtained from

Culture of *PENICILLIUM NOTATUM*
This species of mold was an early source of the antibiotic penicillin. Today, synthetic forms of the drug are usually used.

the foxglove; vinblastine and vincristine, obtained from the periwinkle; and phenoxymethylpenicillin, obtained from a type of penicillin mold.

Other drugs, such as atropine, caffeine, and streptomycin, are still sometimes obtained from natural sources but are now more often prepared synthetically.

Drugs from plant sources were originally obtained directly from various parts of the plant. For example, drug preparations could be obtained by grinding a plant's roots or seeds, or by making an infusion of its dried leaves.

Today, most drugs derived from plant sources are obtained in purer form by extracting the active ingredient in the laboratory. For example, morphine and codeine are commercially refined from opium, which is a substance obtained from the unripe seed pods of the opium poppy.

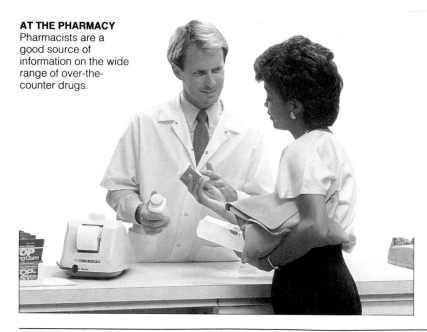

AT THE PHARMACY
Pharmacists are a good source of information on the wide range of over-the-counter drugs.

Genetically engineered drugs

Genetic engineering is a recently developed technique for modifying the genetic structure of living organisms. To date, the principal medical use of genetic engineering has been to produce hormones and other natural body chemicals for use as drugs.

Although technically difficult to achieve, producing a human hormone or other body chemical by genetic engineering is simple in theory. The gene that instructs human cells to produce the hormone is identified, isolated, and inserted into the genetic material of a microorganism such as a bacterium or yeast. The microorganism is then cultured in large vats so that it multiplies and produces large amounts of the hormone for commercial purposes.

Genetic engineering has been applied to the production of human insulin, anistreplase (a tissue-plasminogen activator), factor VIII (used in the treatment of hemophilia), erythropoietin (used to treat some forms of anemia), human growth hormone, and hepatitis B vaccine.

SOURCES OF DRUGS

Drugs can be placed in one of three categories according to whether they are naturally occurring, synthetically produced, or genetically engineered. At present, most are synthetically produced.

Sources	Drug names	Disorders treated
Natural drugs	Digoxin	Cardiac arrhythmias
	Phenoxymethylpenicillin	Infections
	Vinblastine	Cancers
Synthetic drugs	Cimetidine	Peptic ulcer
	Diazepam	Anxiety
	Acetaminophen	Pain
	Propanolol	Hypertension
Genetically engineered drugs	Anistreplase	Coronary thrombosis
	Factor VIII	Hemophilia
	Growth hormone	Growth hormone deficiency
	Human insulin	Diabetes mellitus

Synthetic drugs

The active ingredients of many drugs that were originally derived from natural sources are now produced synthetically from chemicals. Synthetic production ensures that drugs are of consistent potency and that they are available in sufficient quantities when required.

Furthermore, recent advances in our understanding of the functioning of the body have made it possible to "tailor-make" drugs for specific purposes, rather than relying solely on synthetic equivalents of natural substances. For example, propranolol was developed specifically to block the action of the natural hormones epinephrine and norepinephrine on the heart and blood vessels; this blocking effect is useful in treating some cases of high blood pressure, angina, or abnormal heart rhythms. Cimetidine was tailor-made to treat ulcers by reducing the stomach's acid-secreting response to histamine.

Drugs may also be synthesized to supplement hormones or other body chemicals that are produced in insufficient amounts due to disease. One example is the synthetic drug levodopa, which is given to counteract the deficiency of the natural chemical dopamine that occurs in Parkinson's disease. Drugs developed in this purposeful way to meet particular needs may be further modified chemically to increase their potency and duration of action, or to reduce possible adverse effects.

Photomicrograph of epinephrine
Epinephrine (shown here in a polarized light photomicrograph) is an example of the many different drugs that can now be produced synthetically. Naturally occurring epinephrine is a hormone secreted by the adrenal gland. Synthetically produced epinephrine is used to treat cardiac arrest and to control bleeding in surgery.

METHODS OF TREATMENT 2

Intensive care

The intensive care of seriously ill patients is an important aspect of modern medical treatment. The provision of such care has become so specialized in recent years that intensive care is now commonly considered to be a separate branch of medicine. All major hospitals have an intensive-care unit staffed by specially trained medical and nursing staff.

An intensive-care unit contains all the equipment needed to provide continuous monitoring of vital body functions (heart rate, breathing rate, blood pressure, etc.), and to maintain a stable condition in the patient. Careful monitoring of patients allows any worsening of their condition to be detected and treated at once.

Patients in an intensive-care unit are usually given fluids intravenously through a drip, and nutrients and drugs may also be administered in this way. Many intensive-care patients also need artificial ventilation.

A coronary care unit is a type of intensive-care unit designed to provide care for patients who have had, or are suspected of having had, a myocardial infarction (heart attack).

Neonatal care

Advances in neonatal care have greatly increased the survival rate of newborn babies, especially babies who are born prematurely. The internal organs of premature babies may not be mature enough to cope independently, and many physiological functions, such as those that regulate body temperature, may not be sufficiently well developed.

Intensive-care equipment in a neonatal unit can support the vital functions of a premature or severely ill baby. For example, an incubator may be used to provide an external environment in which the temperature, humidity, and oxygen levels can be carefully controlled, and in which the baby can be closely monitored.

Many babies in a neonatal unit will also require other support measures, such as the use of a ventilator to maintain breathing, and the use of an intravenous drip or a nasogastric tube for feeding.

Dialysis

A person whose kidneys fail will die within a few days unless the impurities that accumulate in his or her blood can be removed. Removal of impurities from the blood can be achieved artificially by the procedure of dialysis. There are two methods: hemodialysis and peritoneal dialysis.

In hemodialysis, a dialysis machine removes impurities by filtering the patient's blood through a semipermeable membrane immersed in a special dialysis solution. The procedure takes a few hours and is usually necessary several times a week.

In peritoneal dialysis, the patient's abdominal cavity lining is used to filter impurities from the blood into the dialysis solution, which is passed into and out of the abdomen through a tube.

Dialysis may be necessary for only a few days if kidney failure is temporary, but it is also effective as a long-term treatment for permanent kidney failure. In

Neonatal intensive care
This photograph, taken in a neonatal intensive-care unit, shows a premature baby being examined after undergoing surgery. The baby is being artificially ventilated to assist breathing and is being given fluids intravenously. The heater above the baby's cot maintains the environment at a controlled temperature.

most cases of permanent kidney failure, however, the best remedy for the patient's condition is a kidney transplant.

Lithotripsy

Extracorporeal lithotripsy is a nonsurgical procedure that uses ultrasound to pulverize calculi (stones) in the body. This technique seems likely to replace surgery as the usual treatment for certain types of kidney stones, and is currently under investigation in the treatment of gallstones.

In lithotripsy, repeated pulses of high-energy ultrasound waves are focused on a stone to break it down into tiny particles; the particles can then be passed out of the body via the urine (in the case of kidney stones) or via the feces (in the case of gallstones).

Psychiatric treatment

People with mental disorders were formerly incarcerated in remote mental asylums. Today, most sufferers are treated in units within general hospitals or in community settings.

Lithotripsy
This technique involves focusing ultrasound shock waves on a stone until it breaks into tiny fragments that can be passed out of the body. The patient lies on a couch or in a water bath. The physician uses ultrasound or X-ray imaging to locate the stone, and then positions the patient and the shock-wave emitter for treatment. Shock-wave pulses are then applied until the stone is pulverized.

Arm for positioning shock-wave emitter
Ultrasound shock-wave emitter
Location display screen
Control unit
Movable couch
Ultrasound location transducer

The development of antipsychotic drugs and other drugs to treat psychiatric problems has transformed the outlook for many patients with severe mental disorders, such as schizophrenia or manic-depressive illness. Drug therapy enables many people to resume varying degrees of activity within the community.

Psychotherapy may be useful in the treatment of people with neuroses, personality disorders, or forms of abnormal behavior, such as alcohol dependence or drug addiction. Psychotherapy may take the form of psychoanalysis, group therapy, or counseling.

Radiation therapy

The use of X rays and implants of radium (a naturally radioactive substance) to treat cancers dates from the turn of this century. Today, X rays are still used in radiation therapy, but the range of treatment has been greatly expanded to include other forms or sources of radiation (e.g., neutron beams or radioactive varieties of substances such as iodine or yttrium). Damage to surrounding healthy tissue was a significant drawback of early radiation treatment, but with modern technology it is now possible to focus radiation beams more accurately, thereby concentrating them on the tumor and minimizing damage to normal tissue.

Radiation therapy may be used alone to treat some tumors—such as basal cell carcinomas and certain tumors of the pituitary gland—but it is more often used in combination with surgery, chemotherapy, or both of these.

Preparing for radiation therapy
The metal platform between the radiation source and the patient protects against excessive radiation. The illuminated pattern shows the areas to be irradiated.

METHODS OF TREATMENT 3

Surgical treatment

Surgery is the main form of treatment for a great variety of disorders. Common procedures include the removal of diseased tissue or organs, the relief of blockages, the repositioning of displaced structures, the implantation of mechanical or electronic devices, and the transplantation of tissues or organs.

Surgical implants

There are four main problems in replacing a part of the body with an artificial implant. First, the implant must be made of a material that does not provoke the immune system to reject it. Second, it must be tough enough to last for many years, so that the operation does not have to be repeated. Third, a reliable means must be found to secure the implant firmly in position. Fourth, implant surgery requires scrupulous operative techniques

Bone marrow transplant
This photograph shows healthy bone marrow being removed via a syringe from a donor's hip bone. This marrow will be injected into the recipient's bloodstream after the recipient's own diseased marrow has first been destroyed by radiation. Immunosuppressant drugs are needed after the operation.

in order to prevent infection of the surrounding tissues.

Today, these problems have largely been solved, and most implants are successful; hip-joint replacements last for 10 years or more in 70 percent of cases. Furthermore, a wide range of implants is now available: knee and finger joints as well as hip joints; heart valves; artificial lenses for the eyes; sections of blood vessels; and replacements for parts of the skull.

Transplant surgery

In the early days of transplant surgery, the only transplants that were possible without rejection were corneal transplants (which are not subject to rejection because there is no blood supply to the cornea), and those between identical twins; this inevitably limited the number of operations that could be done.

Soon, however, physicians began to treat transplant patients with immunosuppressant drugs to prevent rejection of the new organ. Because drugs that prevent rejection also suppress the immune system, they reduce resistance to infection. Consequently, many early transplant recipients survived the operation to replace a diseased organ, but died later as a result of infection.

Gradually, the technical problems were overcome, first with kidney transplants and later with heart and liver transplants.

Improved immunosuppressant drugs were then developed, notably cyclosporine. As a result, the success rates for transplants are now generally high.

The primary problem today is the lack of available donor organs. Many transplants are performed using organs from dead donors, but transplants of kidneys can be

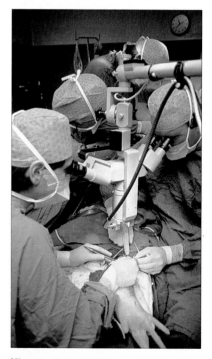

Microsurgical operation
The two surgeons in this photograph are shown performing a delicate microsurgical operation. Each is looking through a binocular eyepiece of an operating microscope, which magnifies the structures being operated on and allows the surgeons to achieve extreme precision.

Hip replacement
This colored X ray shows a patient's artificial hip joint. The replacement of a damaged hip joint by an artificial substitute is one of the most successful types of implant surgery. Hip-joint replacement is most commonly performed on joints that have been damaged by arthritis.

done from a live donor (usually, but not always, related to the recipient); bone marrow transplants are always done from live donors. Occasionally, tissue from animals is used, for instance the transplantation of heart valves from pigs to humans. The use of fetal tissue and organs for transplantation poses technical and ethical problems that are currently a subject of debate.

Microsurgery

In microsurgery, surgeons use a specially designed microscope, delicate instruments, and fine sutures (stitches) to perform operations on minute structures, such as small nerves or blood vessels. One of the major advantages of microsurgery is that more of the tiny blood vessels and nerves can be preserved, minimizing damage to the tissues being repaired and thus reducing the amount of scar tissue formed.

Today, microsurgical techniques are used in many operations on the eye and ear. These techniques are also used in operations that involve the joining of blood vessels, such as in reconstructive surgery during which the tiny arteries and veins in skin flaps are sewn together.

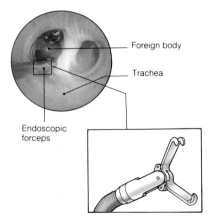

Endoscopic removal of an object
This circular view through an endoscope shows forceps removing an inhaled object from the trachea.

LASER TREATMENT
Lasers are effective at removing certain skin blemishes, such as birthmarks caused by excessive growth of blood vessels in the skin. In such treatment (shown right), the physician and patient both wear goggles to protect their eyes. Lasers can also be used to remove unwanted tattoos.

- Protective goggles
- Fibre-optic cable from laser source
- Laser beam

Microsurgery has also enabled surgeons to reattach severed fingers, toes, and complete limbs, and to rejoin the two sections of a vas deferens separated in a vasectomy operation.

Laser surgery

A laser produces a narrow beam of intense energy that surgeons can use as a "light knife" to cut through tissue, usually without causing damage beyond the target area. As it cuts, the laser simultaneously cauterizes blood vessels, thus sealing them and stemming blood flow.

Lasers are widely used in ophthalmology, especially for operations on the retina. Ophthalmic uses include the repair of retinal tears and the destruction of small retinal tumors. Uses in other branches of surgery include the sealing of bleeding arteries in peptic ulcers; the destruction of abnormal cells in various parts of the body, such as the cervix; the treatment of endometriosis; and the removal of some skin blemishes.

Endoscopic surgery

Endoscopes are used not only for diagnosis, but also for performing certain surgical procedures. Special attachments, such as scissors or a wire loop, may be fitted to remove tumors, and sharp-toothed forceps may be used to grasp and remove foreign bodies.

Other operations for which endoscopes are used include the removal of stones from the urinary tract, and the repair of damaged joint cartilage.

Endoscopic surgery is generally safer and easier to perform than conventional surgical techniques. Surgery performed using an endoscope also causes less tissue damage, producing less discomfort and a quicker recovery for the patient.

USES OF ENDOSCOPY
Listed here are some uses for various types of endoscopy; all these procedures formerly required open surgery.

Endoscope	Possible uses
Arthroscopy	Repair of damaged joint cartilage
Bronchoscopy	Removal of foreign bodies from bronchi
Colonoscopy	Removal of intestinal polyps
Cystoscopy	Removal of bladder calculi (stones)
Fetoscopy	Correction of fetal urinary tract defects
Gastroscopy	Treatment of bleeding peptic ulcers
Laparoscopy	Female sterilization

NEW DISEASES

Advances in medical science have made it possible to diagnose and treat many diseases that were previously unknown. Recent decades have seen the identification of several important diseases that had not formerly been found in humans. Only a few of these, such as AIDS, are thought to be completely new. Far more common are diseases, such as legionnaires' disease, for which the causes have only recently been recognized although the diseases themselves are thought to have existed for some time.

AIDS

The first cases of AIDS were recognized in 1981 among young homosexual men in the US. By the end of the 1980s, approximately 50,000 men, women, and children in the US had died from AIDS. By the same time, there had been around 2,600 deaths in Canada and perhaps 100,000 worldwide.

AIDS is caused by infection with HIV (human immunodeficiency virus). Transmission of the virus can occur through sexual contact, through blood-to-blood contact, or from a pregnant woman to her unborn child. HIV infection follows an unpredictable course. Some of those infected develop full-blown AIDS and soon die; others remain in apparently good health for many years. There is still no cure for AIDS, but certain antiviral drugs, such as zidovudine, have been found to slow the progression of HIV infection.

Legionnaires' disease

Although legionnaires' disease was identified only after an outbreak among delegates at a 1976 American Legion convention, it is in fact much older. Once the causative bacterium was identified, research showed that outbreaks had occurred over the past 40 years. Legionnaires' disease now accounts for 10 percent of pneumonia cases outside hospitals.

Legionella
This photograph shows LEGIONELLA PNEUMOPHILA, one of the bacteria that cause legionnaires' disease. This recently discovered disease is a form of pneumonia that was identified after an outbreak among delegates at an American Legion convention.

Listeriosis

The microorganism LISTERIA MONOCYTOGENES has been known for many years as a rare cause of meningitis, but in the 1980s there was growing awareness that Listeria could cause food poisoning. Listeriosis may be serious in the elderly and in anyone with impaired immunity. In pregnant women it may cause miscarriages and stillbirths; newborn babies may be seriously affected. Most cases are associated with poorly refrigerated soft cheeses and precooked frozen meals.

Lyme disease

Lyme disease is a bacterial infection spread by ticks that causes skin disorders and arthritis. This disease was first recognized in 1975 in Lyme, Conn., but is now thought to have been in existence before that time; some cases have been confirmed in Canada.

Hepatitis C

In 1989 the cause of many cases of non-A non-B hepatitis was found to be a newly identified virus, which has been given the name of hepatitis C virus.

The AIDS virus
This photomicrograph shows the human immunodeficiency virus (HIV), the virus that causes AIDS. The virus (here colored orange) can be seen budding from an infected lymphocyte (here colored blue). HIV infection may last for years without causing symptoms; it is not yet known whether full-blown AIDS develops in all infected people.

THE A TO Z
OF MEDICINE

A

Abdomen

The region of the body between the chest and the hips. The abdominal cavity is bounded by the ribs and the diaphragm above, and by the muscles and bones of the pelvis below, with the spine and the abdominal muscles forming the back, side, and front walls. The abdominal cavity contains the liver, stomach, intestines, spleen, pancreas, and kidneys. In the lower part of the abdomen, enclosed by the pelvis, are the bladder, rectum, and, in women, the uterus and ovaries.

STRUCTURE

The spine, pelvis, and ribs provide attachments for the layers of muscle that make up the abdominal walls. There is a layer of fat between the muscles and the skin; in obese people this layer may be several centimetres thick. The inner surface of the abdominal muscles is covered by a thin membrane, the peritoneum, which also covers the organs, such as the pancreas and kidneys, that are fixed to the back wall. Folds of peritoneum also cover the mobile organs, such as the stomach and intestines.

Abdomen, acute

The medical term for persistent, severe abdominal pain of sudden onset, usually associated with spasm of the abdominal muscles, vomiting, and fever. These symptoms suggest inflammation of one or more organs in the abdomen and indicate that urgent medical investigation is needed. Such an investigation usually includes detailed questioning, a physical examination, laboratory tests, and imaging procedures, such as X rays and ultrasound scanning. A *laparotomy* (surgical exploration of the abdomen) or a *laparoscopy* (internal examination using a viewing instrument) may be necessary in some cases.

CAUSES AND TREATMENT

The most common cause of an acute abdomen is *peritonitis* (inflammation of the membrane that lines the abdomen). Inflammation of any structure in the abdomen may lead to peritonitis—for example, *salpingitis* (inflammation of the fallopian tubes); intestinal disorders, such as *appendicitis*, *Crohn's disease*, or *diverticulitis*; or a perforated *peptic ulcer*. Abdominal injury may also be the cause.

Other possible causes of acute abdomen include urinary tract disorders, such as a stone in the ureter (see *Calculus, urinary tract*), a stone in the duct that drains the gallbladder (see *Gallstones*), or a disorder that stretches the covering of the liver, such as *hepatitis*, or of the kidneys.

In their early stages, these conditions produce similar symptoms, and the physician will often make observations at regular intervals over several hours before reaching a final diagnosis. Abdominal pain often begins as a vague pain in the center but then commonly becomes localized to a particular region (such as on the right side in appendicitis). If peritonitis spreads, the abdominal muscles become rigid and the pain generalized.

Treatment depends on the underlying cause, but if the diagnosis is prompt and accurate, the outlook is generally good.

Abdominal pain

Discomfort in the abdominal cavity. Accompanying symptoms may include belching, nausea, vomiting, rumbling and gurgling noises, and flatulence (wind).

CAUSES

Minor degrees of abdominal pain are experienced by everybody at some time, and often the cause is easily recognized—for example, eating unwisely, or an attack of *diarrhea*.

Many women experience pelvic or lower abdominal pain during part of their menstrual cycle. The pain may occur before or during a period, or around the time of ovulation. Occasionally, the pain is due to a gynecological disorder, such as *endometriosis* (in which fragments of uterine lining are present in abnormal sites within the abdomen).

A common cause of pain very low in the abdomen is *cystitis* (inflammation of the bladder). Distention of the bladder due to urinary obstruction may also cause pain.

Abdominal colic is the term used for pain that occurs every few minutes as one of the internal organs goes into muscular spasm. Waves of colicky pain may originate in the intestines, bile ducts, ureters, or uterus. Colic is an attempt by the body to overcome an obstruction, partial or total, that may be due to a stone, a tumor, or an area of inflammation. The attacks of colic may become more severe and associated with vomiting—giving the features of an ''acute abdomen'' (see *Abdomen, acute*).

LOCATION OF THE ABDOMEN

The abdomen is bounded by the lower ribs at the top and the pelvis below. The illustration shows the position of the abdominal organs in an adult woman.

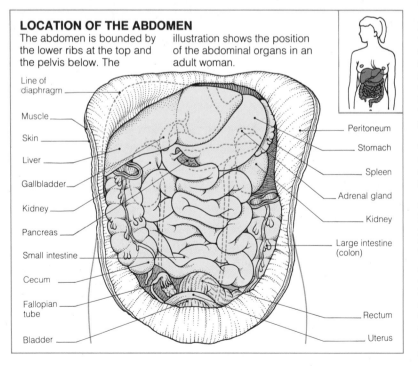

Line of diaphragm
Muscle
Skin
Liver
Gallbladder
Kidney
Pancreas
Small intestine
Cecum
Fallopian tube
Bladder

Peritoneum
Stomach
Spleen
Adrenal gland
Kidney
Large intestine (colon)
Rectum
Uterus

A

ABDOMINAL PAIN General or localized pain between the bottom of the rib cage and the groin that has occurred within the last 24 hours. See also Recurrent abdominal pain chart.

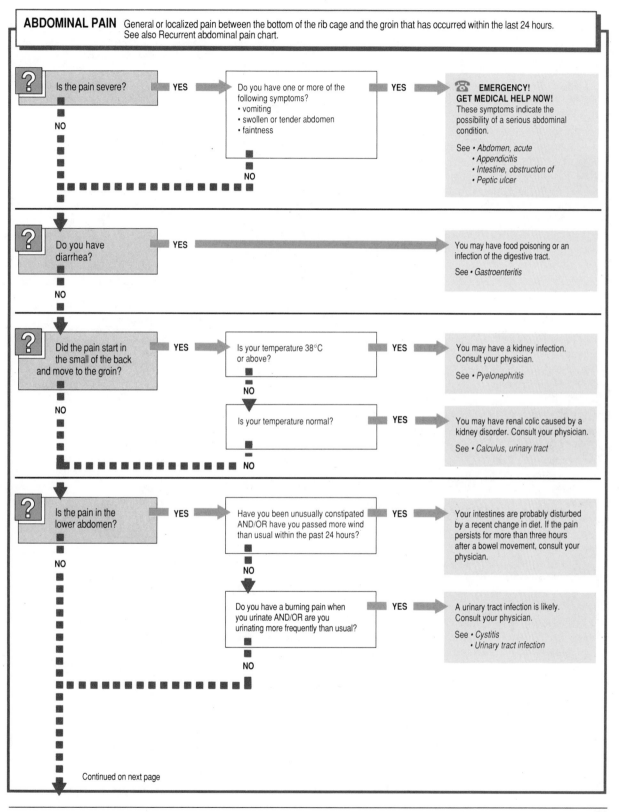

Is the pain severe?

YES → Do you have one or more of the following symptoms?
• vomiting
• swollen or tender abdomen
• faintness

YES → ☎ **EMERGENCY!**
GET MEDICAL HELP NOW!
These symptoms indicate the possibility of a serious abdominal condition.

See • *Abdomen, acute*
 • *Appendicitis*
 • *Intestine, obstruction of*
 • *Peptic ulcer*

NO

NO

Do you have diarrhea?

YES → You may have food poisoning or an infection of the digestive tract.

See • *Gastroenteritis*

NO

Did the pain start in the small of the back and move to the groin?

YES → Is your temperature 38°C or above?

YES → You may have a kidney infection. Consult your physician.

See • *Pyelonephritis*

NO

Is your temperature normal?

YES → You may have renal colic caused by a kidney disorder. Consult your physician.

See • *Calculus, urinary tract*

NO

NO

Is the pain in the lower abdomen?

YES → Have you been unusually constipated AND/OR have you passed more wind than usual within the past 24 hours?

YES → Your intestines are probably disturbed by a recent change in diet. If the pain persists for more than three hours after a bowel movement, consult your physician.

NO

Do you have a burning pain when you urinate AND/OR are you urinating more frequently than usual?

YES → A urinary tract infection is likely. Consult your physician.

See • *Cystitis*
 • *Urinary tract infection*

NO

NO

Continued on next page

A

? Is the pain mainly just below the ribs on the right side and have you been vomiting?

YES → You may have a gallbladder disorder. Consult your physician.

See • *Cholecystitis*
• *Gallstones*

NO ↓

WARNING
Severe abdominal pain
Severe and continuous abdominal pain requires immediate medical attention in the following cases:
• if it persists for more than four hours
• if it is accompanied by vomiting
• if the abdomen is swollen and tender
• if it is accompanied by faintness, drowsiness, or confusion

Waiting for medical attention
While waiting for medical help to arrive, do not eat or drink anything in case you need to undergo surgery immediately. Do not take ASA or drink alcohol to relieve the pain; they can further inflame an irritated stomach and, in some circumstances, can cause dangerous internal bleeding.

? Do you have a burning pain on one side only AND does your skin feel sensitive along the site of the pain?

YES → You may be developing a nerve infection. Consult your physician.

See • *Herpes zoster*

NO ↓

? Did the pain follow excessive eating or a bout of heavy drinking?

YES → Overeating or tension is a likely cause of abdominal pain, especially if it occurs soon after a meal. The lining of your stomach may be inflamed.

See • *Gastritis*
• *Indigestion*

NO ↓

? Is the pain in the center of the upper abdomen?

YES → Is it a dull cramping pain that extends up your chest or down your arms?

YES → ☎ **EMERGENCY!**
GET MEDICAL HELP NOW!

These symptoms may indicate a heart disorder.

See • *Angina pectoris*
• *Chest pain*
• *Myocardial infarction*

NO ■■■■■■■■■■■ **NO** ↓

NO ↓

? Are you a woman and do you have intermittent lower abdominal cramping pains?

YES → Are you having a menstrual period?

YES → Dull aches or cramps are often associated with menstruation. Discuss with your physician.

NO ↓

Could you be in the first three months of pregnancy AND/OR have you noticed any vaginal bleeding?

YES → ☎
Consult your physician without delay!
A serious complication, such as a threatened miscarriage or ectopic pregnancy (pregnancy outside the womb), is a possibility.

See • *Ectopic pregnancy*
• *Miscarriage*

NO ↓

NO ↓

Continued on next page

Continued on next page, column 2

A

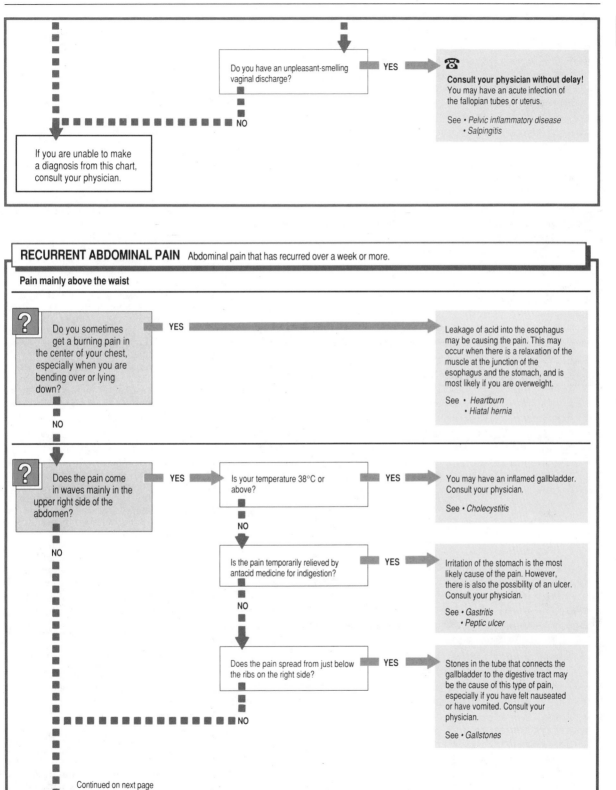

Do you have an unpleasant-smelling vaginal discharge?

YES

☎

Consult your physician without delay!
You may have an acute infection of the fallopian tubes or uterus.

See • *Pelvic inflammatory disease*
• *Salpingitis*

NO

If you are unable to make a diagnosis from this chart, consult your physician.

RECURRENT ABDOMINAL PAIN Abdominal pain that has recurred over a week or more.

Pain mainly above the waist

? Do you sometimes get a burning pain in the center of your chest, especially when you are bending over or lying down?

YES

Leakage of acid into the esophagus may be causing the pain. This may occur when there is a relaxation of the muscle at the junction of the esophagus and the stomach, and is most likely if you are overweight.

See • *Heartburn*
• *Hiatal hernia*

NO

? Does the pain come in waves mainly in the upper right side of the abdomen?

YES

Is your temperature 38°C or above?

YES

You may have an inflamed gallbladder. Consult your physician.

See • *Cholecystitis*

NO

NO

Is the pain temporarily relieved by antacid medicine for indigestion?

YES

Irritation of the stomach is the most likely cause of the pain. However, there is also the possibility of an ulcer. Consult your physician.

See • *Gastritis*
• *Peptic ulcer*

NO

Does the pain spread from just below the ribs on the right side?

YES

Stones in the tube that connects the gallbladder to the digestive tract may be the cause of this type of pain, especially if you have felt nauseated or have vomited. Consult your physician.

See • *Gallstones*

NO

Continued on next page

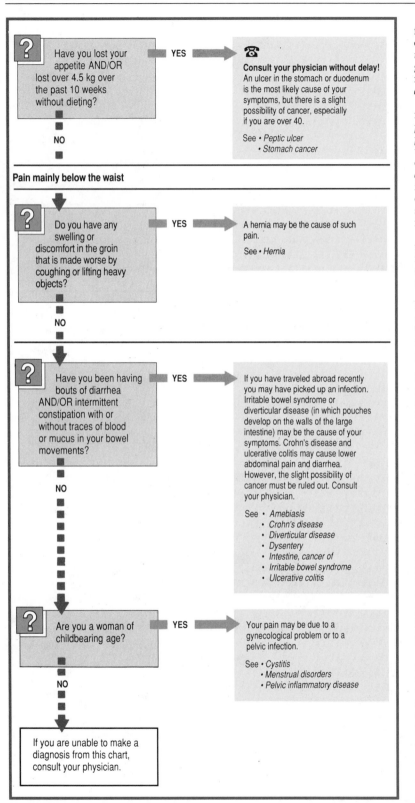

Have you lost your appetite AND/OR lost over 4.5 kg over the past 10 weeks without dieting?

YES →

☎ **Consult your physician without delay!**
An ulcer in the stomach or duodenum is the most likely cause of your symptoms, but there is a slight possibility of cancer, especially if you are over 40.

See • *Peptic ulcer*
• *Stomach cancer*

NO

Pain mainly below the waist

Do you have any swelling or discomfort in the groin that is made worse by coughing or lifting heavy objects?

YES →

A hernia may be the cause of such pain.

See • *Hernia*

NO

Have you been having bouts of diarrhea AND/OR intermittent constipation with or without traces of blood or mucus in your bowel movements?

YES →

If you have traveled abroad recently you may have picked up an infection. Irritable bowel syndrome or diverticular disease (in which pouches develop on the walls of the large intestine) may be the cause of your symptoms. Crohn's disease and ulcerative colitis may cause lower abdominal pain and diarrhea. However, the slight possibility of cancer must be ruled out. Consult your physician.

See • *Amebiasis*
• *Crohn's disease*
• *Diverticular disease*
• *Dysentery*
• *Intestine, cancer of*
• *Irritable bowel syndrome*
• *Ulcerative colitis*

NO

Are you a woman of childbearing age?

YES →

Your pain may be due to a gynecological problem or to a pelvic infection.

See • *Cystitis*
• *Menstrual disorders*
• *Pelvic inflammatory disease*

NO

If you are unable to make a diagnosis from this chart, consult your physician.

An increase in the amount of acid formed in the stomach may be associated with the development of a *peptic ulcer*, which produces a recurrent gnawing pain that is temporarily relieved by food, milk, or by taking *antacid drugs.*

Another possible cause of abdominal pain is infection, such as *pyelonephritis* (infection of the kidneys) or *pelvic inflammatory disease* (infection of the female internal reproductive organs). Pain may also be due to *ischemia* (lack of blood supply), as occurs, for instance, when a *volvulus* (twisting of the intestine) obstructs blood vessels or when a clot forms in one of the intestinal blood vessels.

Tumors affecting any of the abdominal organs can cause pain by stretching the lining of the organ, by pressing on surrounding structures, or by ulcerating or rupturing.

In rare cases, disorders of organs outside the abdomen can cause abdominal pain. For example, pneumonia of the right lower lobe of the lung may produce pain in the upper right part of the abdomen.

Abdominal pain can have a psychological origin. For example, it may result from anxiety, such as that felt by a child starting a new school or an adult changing jobs.

TREATMENT

Many people have recurrent attacks of mild abdominal pain that they learn to recognize as transient. In such circumstances, self-treatment with simple measures is often effective—a milky drink, a hot-water bottle, or simply a night's sleep. Any unusual pain, or pain that is not relieved by vomiting, or that persists for more than six hours, or that is associated with sweating or faintness should be reported to a physician without delay. Urgent attention is also necessary if the abdominal pain is accompanied by persistent vomiting, by vomiting of blood (which may appear brown), or by the passing of bloodstained or black feces.

Abdominal pain that is accompanied by weight loss without dieting, or by a change in bowel habits—sudden constipation or attacks of diarrhea—should also be investigated by a physician.

INVESTIGATION

The physician will make a diagnosis based on the patient's detailed description of the pain and its relationship to eating, passing urine, and bowel movements, along with a thorough physical examination.

DIAGNOSING ABDOMINAL PAIN

The physician conducts a physical examination and listens to the patient's description of the pain. More investigations, such as blood tests or X rays, may be carried out. If the diagnosis is still in doubt, gastroscopy, colonoscopy or laparoscopy may be performed.

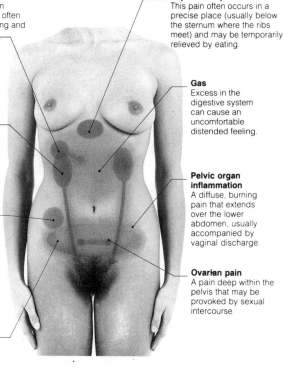

Gallbladder pain
A crampy or steady pain under the right ribs and often accompanied by vomiting and fever.

Kidney pain
An intermittent pain that may begin in the flank and radiate to the groin.

Appendicitis pain
This pain starts around the navel and settles in the body's lower right side.

Menstrual pain
Cramping pain occurring at the beginning of a monthly period; it usually begins during the teenage years.

Peptic ulcer pain
This pain often occurs in a precise place (usually below the sternum where the ribs meet) and may be temporarily relieved by eating.

Gas
Excess in the digestive system can cause an uncomfortable distended feeling.

Pelvic organ inflammation
A diffuse, burning pain that extends over the lower abdomen, usually accompanied by vaginal discharge.

Ovarian pain
A pain deep within the pelvis that may be provoked by sexual intercourse.

If there is any doubt about the diagnosis, further investigations may be carried out. The investigations may include a urine test, blood tests, X rays, and *ultrasound scanning*.

If the cause still cannot be diagnosed after such tests, endoscopic examination (looking into a body cavity with a viewing tube) may be necessary. This may take the form of *gastroscopy* (inspecting the stomach and duodenum), *colonoscopy* (inspecting the large intestine), or *laparoscopy* (inspecting the contents of the abdominal cavity). In some cases, the diagnosis can be confirmed only by an exploratory operation on the abdomen, known as a *laparotomy*.

Abdominal swelling

Distention of the abdomen, which may be due to any of a number of causes. It is the natural result of *obesity* and of enlargement of the uterus during pregnancy, generally noticeable after about 12 weeks.

Some causes of abdominal swelling are harmless. Gas in the stomach or intestine may cause uncomfortable, bloating distention of the whole abdomen. Many women experience lower abdominal distention due to temporary water retention just before a menstrual period.

Other causes of abdominal swelling may be more serious. For instance, *ascites* (accumulation of fluid in the abdomen) may be a symptom of underlying cancer, heart disease, kidney disease, or liver disease; the swelling may also be caused by an *intestinal obstruction* or an *ovarian cyst*.

INVESTIGATION AND TREATMENT
Diagnosis of the underlying cause may involve abdominal X rays or *ultrasound scanning* to look for abnormalities in the size or shape of the internal organs or for signs of intestinal obstruction. If ascites is present, some of the fluid may be drained for examination. Occasionally, a *laparotomy* (surgical exploration of the abdomen)

or *laparoscopy* (internal examination of the abdomen using a flexible viewing tube) may also be necessary. (See also *Abdominal swelling* symptom chart.)

Abdominal X ray

An X-ray examination of the abdominal contents. An abdominal X ray is often one of the first steps in the investigation of acute abdominal disease (after the physician has taken a careful medical history and performed a physical examination).

X rays do not reveal the internal structure of organs but do show their outlines. Thus a radiologist can see whether any organ is enlarged and is able to spot swallowed foreign bodies within the digestive tract. Useful information is also gained by studying patterns of fluid and gas. Distended loops of bowel containing collections of fluid often indicate an obstruction (see *Intestine, obstruction of*); gas outside the intestine (in most cases under the diaphragm) indicates intestinal *perforation*.

Calcium, which is opaque to X rays, is present in most kidney stones (see *Calculus, urinary tract*) and a small proportion of *gallstones*; these can sometimes be detected on an abdominal X ray. Some aortic *aneurysms* contain calcium and therefore are visible.

Abdominal X rays often need to be followed by other procedures that give more detailed information, such as *endoscopy*, *ultrasound scanning*, *CT scanning*, *barium X-ray examinations*, or intravenous *pyelography*.

Abducent nerve

The sixth *cranial nerve*. The abducent nerve supplies only one muscle of each eye, the lateral rectus muscle, which is responsible for moving the eyeball outward. The abducent nerve originates in the pons (part of the *brain stem*) and extends along the base of the skull, eventually entering the back of the eye socket through a gap between the skull bones.

As a result of its long path inside the skull, the abducent nerve is often damaged in fractures of the base of the skull, or by a disorder, such as a tumor, that distorts the brain. Such damage may give rise to *double vision* or a *squint*.

Abduction

Movement of a limb away from the central line of the body, or of a digit away from the axis of a limb. Muscles that carry out this movement are called abductors. (See also *Adduction*.)

A

ABDOMINAL SWELLING
Generalized swelling over the whole abdomen between the bottom of the rib cage and the groin that is not due to simply being overweight.

Of sudden onset – within 24 hours

? Have you had severe abdominal pain for more than an hour?

YES → Do you have one or both of the following symptoms?
- vomiting
- no relief of pain by passing gas

YES → ☎ **EMERGENCY GET MEDICAL HELP NOW!** These symptoms may indicate a dangerous abdominal condition.

See • *Abdomen, acute*
• *Intestine, obstruction of*

NO → See • *Abdominal pain*

NO

Sudden abdominal swelling that is not accompanied by severe and continuous pain is most likely to be the result of gas in the bowel.

Of gradual onset/long-standing duration

? Are your ankles puffy AND/OR do they pit when you press them with your finger?

YES → Are you short of breath, particularly at night?

YES → You may have fluid retention as a result of a heart, liver, or kidney disorder. Consult your physician.

See • *Heart failure*

NO ↓

Are you passing less urine than usual?

YES → You may have a kidney disorder. Consult your physician.

See • *Glomerulonephritis*
• *Nephrotic syndrome*

NO

NO

? Does the swelling reduce slightly when you pass urine?

YES → ☎

Consult your physician without delay! Retention of urine in the bladder may cause such swelling, which in men may be the result of enlargement of the prostate gland.

See • *Prostate gland*

NO

? Does your skin or do the whites of your eyes look yellow?

YES → ☎

Consult your physician without delay! This suggests a liver disorder.

See • *Cirrhosis*

NO

Continued on next page

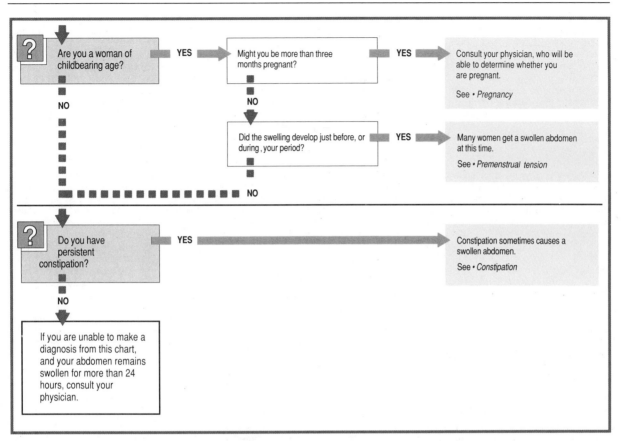

Are you a woman of childbearing age? — **YES** → Might you be more than three months pregnant? — **YES** → Consult your physician, who will be able to determine whether you are pregnant.

See • *Pregnancy*

NO (from "Might you be more than three months pregnant?") → Did the swelling develop just before, or during, your period? — **YES** → Many women get a swollen abdomen at this time.

See • *Premenstrual tension*

NO

Do you have persistent constipation? — **YES** → Constipation sometimes causes a swollen abdomen.

See • *Constipation*

NO

If you are unable to make a diagnosis from this chart, and your abdomen remains swollen for more than 24 hours, consult your physician.

Ablation

The removal of dead or diseased tissue by excision (cutting away with a sharp instrument), *cryosurgery* (freezing), *radiotherapy*, *diathermy* (burning), or *laser treatment*. Ablation of the thyroid gland is achieved with radioactive iodine isotopes.

Abnormality

A physical deformity or malformation, a behavioral or mental problem, or a variation from what is considered normal in the structure or function of a cell, tissue, or organ.

Abortifacient

An agent that causes *abortion*. Various substances have been claimed to cause abortion, such as large amounts of castor oil or gin, but such folk remedies are generally ineffective. In medical practice, *prostaglandin drugs* are used to induce abortion; they cause softening and widening of the cervix (neck of the uterus) and muscular contractions of the uterus. These drugs are usually administered in the form of suppositories that are placed high in the vagina.

Abortion

In medical terminology, a word denoting either spontaneous abortion (see *Miscarriage*) or medically induced termination of pregnancy.

Abortion, induced

Intentional termination of pregnancy by any means.

Canada has had no legislation governing abortion since 1988, when the Supreme Court ruled that the legislation of the day violated a woman's constitutional right to security of the person. The House of Commons later approved a bill making abortion a criminal offense punishable by up to two years' imprisonment, unless a physician had determined that the pregnancy would endanger the mother's physical, mental, or psychological health. But the bill, defeated in the Senate in January 1991, never became law.

MEDICAL REASONS FOR ABORTION

A physician may recommend an abortion for conditions affecting either the woman or the fetus. In the woman, examples of conditions that may worsen during pregnancy and possibly become life-threatening include severe heart disease, chronic kidney disease, and cancer, especially of the breast or cervix.

Fetal conditions, revealed by *ultrasound scanning*, *amniocentesis*, or *chorionic villus sampling*, include severe developmental defects incompatible with normal life (such as *anencephaly*) and serious *chromosomal abnormalities* (such as *Down's syndrome*). Termination may also be recommended if the woman contracts *rubella* (German measles) during the early stages of pregnancy; this virus can severely damage the baby, especially his or her eyes, ears, and heart. Certain other infections in the woman may also damage the fetus. Termination is recommended if the mother has been infected by the *AIDS* virus as this virus can be transmitted to the baby.

HOW IT IS DONE

EARLY ABORTION Vacuum suction techniques are the simplest and safest means of terminating an early pregnancy. When this is done within two weeks of a missed period, before pregnancy has been confirmed, it is termed *menstrual extraction* (which is performed as an outpatient suction procedure). More commonly, vacuum suction curettage is performed between the 7th and 12th week of pregnancy, as either an outpatient or an inpatient procedure.

The procedure may be performed under either a general or a local anesthetic. If local anesthesia (paracervical block) is used, it may be supplemented by an intravenous narcotic or a tranquilizer. The cervix is dilated with curved metal rods, and a narrow plastic tube is then inserted into the uterus. The outer end of the tube is connected to a suction machine, which sucks out the fetal and placental tissue into a vacuum bottle. After this procedure, which usually takes less than 10 minutes, the physician scrapes the lining of the uterus with a curet (a spoonlike instrument) to make sure that no placental tissue has been left behind. The tissue may be analyzed in a laboratory to confirm that a pregnancy existed and that the tissue appears complete. This is done because an *ectopic pregnancy* (development of an embryo outside the uterus) would require more surgery. In most cases, the operator knows from his or her examination that there has been a pregnancy and that the uterus has been emptied completely.

Recovery is fast, although strenuous activity should be avoided for several days. There is usually some bleeding, and occasionally mild cramps, for up to a week. A normal period starts four to six weeks after the termination. Sexual intercourse can be resumed after two to three weeks.

LATE ABORTION Between the 12th and 15th week of pregnancy, either the suction procedure used in early abortion or the evacuation procedure described below may be recommended, depending on the facilities available. After the 15th week, it is normally considered safer to perform an abortion by causing the uterus to contract so that the fetus is expelled, as in natural labor. Contractions are induced by introducing a *prostaglandin* hormone into the uterus. This may be done either by injection directly through the woman's abdomen into the amniotic fluid or by infusion, via the cervix, into the gap between the amniotic sac (the membrane that surrounds the fetus) and the uterine wall. Alternatively, a pessary containing prostaglandin may be placed high in the vagina.

It usually takes about 12 to 24 hours for the fetus to be expelled, during which time the woman is given analgesic drugs (painkillers). She remains in hospital for 24 to 48 hours after completion of the termination to be monitored for complications.

COMPLICATIONS

If termination is performed in a well-equipped clinic or hospital by a qualified gynecologist, complications are rare. Infection, resulting in a condition called septic abortion, or serious bleeding occurs in fewer than 1 percent of cases.

Mortality is less than one per 100,000 when abortion is performed before the 13th week, rising to three per 100,000 after the 13th week. (For comparison, maternal mortality for full-term pregnancy is nine per 100,000.) Repeated terminations may increase the risk of miscarriage in subsequent pregnancies, although there is little evidence that a single termination affects future fertility.

Nonmedical abortions, by nonphysicians for reasons other than the woman's health, are still common in many parts of the world. Not surprisingly, they carry a high risk of complications. Infertility or death often results.

Abrasion, dental

The wearing away of tooth enamel, often accompanied by the wearing away of dentin (the layer beneath the enamel) and cementum (the bonelike tissue that covers the tooth root), usually through too vigorous brushing. The areas most commonly affected are the root surface and the front surfaces of the canine and premolar teeth where they emerge from the gum.

The depressions produced by abrasion are often sensitive to very cold or hot food or drink, and may require the use of a desensitizing toothpaste and perhaps protection with a *bonding* agent or *filling*.

Abreaction

The process of becoming consciously aware of repressed thoughts and feelings. In Freudian theory, abreaction ideally occurs via *catharsis*, the open expression of emotions associated with forgotten memories. The term abreaction is sometimes used interchangeably with catharsis but, in its strictest sense, is the result of catharsis. Abreaction is an important part of some forms of *psychotherapy* and is more easily achieved when a recent, specific traumatic event is the source of the patient's symptoms.

Abscess

A collection of pus formed as a result of infection by microorganisms, usually bacteria. The pus is formed from destroyed tissue cells, from leukocytes (white blood cells) that have been carried to the area to fight infection, and from dead and live microorganisms. Usually, a lining (pyogenic membrane) gradually forms around the abscess.

TYPES

Abscesses may develop in any organ and in the soft tissues beneath the skin in any area. Common sites include the breast (see *Breast abscess*) and gums (see *Abscess, dental*). Rarer sites include the liver (see *Liver abscess*) and the brain (see *Brain abscess*).

Common sites for abscesses under the skin include the axilla (armpit) and the groin; these two areas have a large number of lymph glands that are responsible for fighting infection. A collar-stud abscess is one in which a small abscess cavity under the skin connects via a sinus (channel) to a much larger one in deeper tissues.

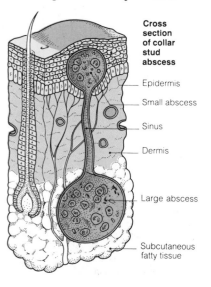

Cross section of collar stud abscess

Epidermis
Small abscess
Sinus
Dermis
Large abscess
Subcutaneous fatty tissue

CAUSES

Common bacteria, such as staphylococci, are the usual cause, although the bacillus responsible for tuberculosis is an important abscess-forming type. Fungal infections sometimes cause abscesses, while amebae (single-celled animal parasites) are an important cause of liver abscesses (see *Amebiasis*). Infectious organisms usually reach internal organs via the bloodstream or penetrate to tissues under the skin by way of an infected wound or bite.

A

SYMPTOMS AND SIGNS

Symptoms of discomfort or pain depend mainly on the site of the abscess, but most larger abscesses, because they are a source of infection within the body, cause fever (sometimes with chills), sweating, and malaise. Abscesses may produce a sensation of intense pressure and those close to the skin usually cause inflammation with redness, increased skin temperature, and tenderness. Tuberculous abscesses are the exception; hence their description as cold abscesses.

DIAGNOSIS

An abscess within an organ may be apparent from symptoms and signs. Occasionally, the diagnosis is confirmed by imaging techniques, such as *CT scanning*, *MRI*, or *radionuclide scanning* (using radioactively labeled white blood cells or the element gallium, which concentrates in areas where pus has recently formed).

TREATMENT

Antibiotics are usually prescribed to treat bacterial infections, antifungal drugs to treat fungi, and antiamebic drugs to treat *amebiasis*. However, the lining of the abscess cavity tends to reduce the amount of drug that can penetrate to the source of infection from the bloodstream. The cavity itself therefore needs to be drained by making a cut in the lining and providing an escape route for the pus, either through a drainage tube (see *Drain, surgical*) or by leaving the cavity open to the skin. Most abscesses require surgical drainage.

OUTLOOK

Many abscesses subside after drainage alone. Others subside after drainage and drug treatment. Some abscesses burst and drain spontaneously through the skin. Occasionally, the presence of an abscess within a vital organ, such as the liver or brain, damages enough surrounding tissue to cause some permanent loss of normal function, or even death.

Abscess, dental

A pus-filled sac in the tissue around the root of a tooth.

CAUSE

An abscess may occur when bacteria invade the pulp (the nerves and blood vessels that fill the central cavity of the tooth), causing the pulp to die. This most commonly happens as a result of dental *caries*, which destroys the tooth's enamel and dentin, allowing bacteria to reach the pulp. Bacteria can also gain access to the pulp when a tooth is injured. Bacteria enter either directly through a fracture or along damaged blood vessels. The infection in the pulp spreads into the surrounding tissue to form an abscess.

Abscesses can also result from *periodontal disease*, in which bacteria accumulate in the deep pockets that form between the teeth and gums.

SYMPTOMS AND SIGNS

The affected tooth aches or throbs, and biting or chewing is usually extremely painful. The gum around the tooth is tender and may be red and swollen. An untreated abscess eventually erodes a sinus (small channel) through the jawbone to the gum surface, where it forms a gumboil (swelling). The gumboil may burst, discharging foul-tasting pus into the mouth, which usually lessens the pain. As the abscess spreads through surrounding tissues and bone, the glands in the neck and the side of the face may become swollen. Eventually, symptoms of infection, such as headache and fever, may develop.

TREATMENT

The dentist will usually try, if possible, to save the tooth by endodontic treatment. To do this, the abscess is drained by drilling through the crown of the tooth and into the pulp cavity to allow the pus to escape. The pulp cavity is then carefully cleaned and disinfected. An antibiotic may be prescribed if the infection has spread beyond the tooth. When the infection has cleared up, the cavity is filled with dental cement (see *Root-canal treatment*), sealed, and crowned.

When an abscess is caused by diseased pulp and the infection cannot be cleared up with endodontic treatment, it is necessary to extract the tooth. *Extraction* removes the source of infection and drains the abscess. Antibiotics are usually prescribed to clear up any residual infection.

An abscess in a periodontal pocket can usually be treated by the dentist passing a probe into the pocket and gently scraping away infected material; sometimes it is necessary to make a small incision in the pocket to reach the abscess. If there is loss of bony support and periodontal ligament attachment due to severe periodontal disease, a dental extraction may need to be performed.

Absence

In medical terminology, a temporary loss or impairment of consciousness that occurs in some forms of *epilepsy*, typically petit mal seizures.

Acanthosis nigricans

A rare, untreatable condition characterized by thickened dark patches of skin in the groin, armpits, neck, and other skin folds. It may occur in young people as a genetic (inherited) disorder, or as the result of an endocrine disorder, such as *Cushing's syndrome*. It also occurs in people with carcinomas (malignant tumors) of the lung and other organs. The affected skin is thickened, rough, may itch, and is gray to black in color.

Pseudoacanthosis nigricans is a much more common condition, usually seen in dark-complexioned people who are overweight. In this form, the skin in fold areas, such as the groin, armpits, or neck, is both thicker and darker than the surrounding skin, and there is usually excessive sweating in affected areas. The condition may improve with dieting.

Accessory nerve

The 11th *cranial nerve*. The accessory nerve differs from the other cranial nerves in that only a small part of it originates from the brain; most of the nerve comes from the spinal cord.

The part of the nerve originating from the brain supplies many muscles of the palate, pharynx (throat), and larynx (voice box). Damage to this part of the nerve may give rise to dysphonia (difficulty in speaking) and dysphagia (difficulty in swallowing).

The spinal part of the nerve supplies some large muscles of the neck and back, notably the sternomastoid (which runs from the breastbone to the side of the skull) and the trapezius (a large, triangular muscle of the upper back, shoulder, and neck). Damage to the spinal fibers of the nerve paralyzes these muscles. Such damage usually occurs as a result of surgery for cancer in which lymph nodes in the neck are removed.

Access to care

One of five federal criteria for measuring provincial health care programs. All Canadian residents are entitled to necessary medical and hospital care. The provinces are responsible for providing this care, which is partly financed (about 43 percent) by the federal government. To qualify for federal aid, the provinces must meet federally set standards of accessibility, universality, comprehensiveness, portability and public administration.

The Canada Health Act (1984) defines accessibility as reasonable access to insured health care for all

ACCIDENTAL DEATH

Every year thousands of Canadians die needlessly in automobiles or as a result of falls or drownings. Many of these are young people; in traffic accidents, the big killer, males under 34 years are the most likely victims. The annual toll is evident from this table, which highlights another tragic aspect of preventable deaths, potential years of life lost, a term for the years lost if a person dies before age 75.

* Potential years of life lost (PYLL) are the years lost if one dies before reaching age 75. For example, there are 40 PYLL when a 35-year-old dies; there are also 40 PYLL when four 65-year-olds die.

ACCIDENTAL DEATHS AND POTENTIAL YEARS OF LIFE LOST* BY LEADING CAUSES IN A TYPICAL YEAR

	← Number of deaths (000's)				Potential years of life lost (000's) →						
	3	2	1	0	20	40	60	80	100	120
Motor vehicle accidents										
Drownings										
Fire and flames										
Falls										
Poisonings										
Suffocation										

Male Female

Canadians, on uniform terms and conditions. This allows for some variations in the services available to areas with vastly different populations. For example, remote areas cannot expect the same range of specialized and intensive care services as exist in heavily populated areas.

Accidental death

Death from an accidental or unintended injury. Accidents are the leading cause of death for those under the age of 45, and fourth (after cardiovascular disease, cancer, and respiratory diseases) for all ages combined. The six leading causes of accidental death overall are motor vehicle accidents, falls, fires, suffocation, drownings, and poisonings. Men are twice as likely as women to die in accidents, and they are much more likely than women to die by drowning, which accounts for more than 8 percent of accidental male deaths.

The bright side of course is that accidental deaths have been decreasing steadily for many years. Even motor vehicle fatalities have declined, probably because of compulsory seat belt laws, better road construction, improved safety engineering of cars, and a number of programs to reduce drinking and driving.

Alcohol continues to be a factor in many accidents, however: about 60 percent of fatally injured drivers have some alcohol in their blood, and 35 percent have twice the legal limit.

Motor vehicle accidents are by far the commonest cause of accidental death until age 65, when falls take the lead. Because the majority of those killed on the roads are young, the toll in terms of potential years of life lost is much greater than from any other accidental death. (See table above.)

Off the roads, the home—perhaps because people spend more time there than anywhere else—is the most dangerous place. Children and the elderly are most often the victims: fires, suffocation, poisonings and falls are the leading causes of death. Up to the age of 1 year, choking on food or an object in the mouth is the commonest cause of accidental death. Smothering on bedclothes, plastic bags or other materials is also a major home hazard for infants.

Accidents at work, including farm accidents, comprise less than 2 percent of all non-traffic-related deaths.

Accommodation

Adjustment, especially the process by which the eye adjusts itself to focus on near objects. At rest, the eye is focused for distant vision, when its

THE MECHANISM OF ACCOMMODATION

In a normal, healthy eye, light reflected from a near object is brought into focus on the retina by a process called accommodation. Focusing is achieved by an automatic change in lens shape.

Focusing on a near subject
To bring a near object into sharp focus, the ciliary muscles contract and the lens becomes more convex in shape.

Focusing on a distant object
The lens focused on a distant object is thin, flat, and completely relaxed.

Ciliary muscle

Near object Lens

Distant object

Ciliary muscle

Lens

lens is relatively thin and flat. To make it possible to focus on a nearer object, the ciliary muscle of the eye contracts, reducing the pull on the outer rim of the lens, so permitting it to become thicker and more convex.

With age, the lens loses its elasticity and, as a result, accommodation becomes increasingly difficult. This results in a form of farsightedness called *presbyopia*.

Accreditation

A national program that develops standards for hospitals, long-term care centers, nursing homes, rehabilitation centers and psychiatric facilities. The institutions are inspected and accreditation certificates are given to those that meet the standards.

Acebutolol

A *beta-blocker drug* commonly used in the treatment of *hypertension* (high blood pressure), *angina pectoris* (chest pain due to impaired blood supply to heart muscle), and certain types of *arrhythmia* (abnormal heart rhythm) in which the heart beats too rapidly. It is safer than other beta-blockers for people with lung problems.

ACE inhibitor drugs

COMMON DRUGS

Captopril Enalapril

A group of *vasodilator drugs* introduced in 1981. ACE inhibitors (*angiotensin*-converting enzyme inhibitors) are used to treat *hypertension* (high blood pressure) and *heart failure* (reduced pumping efficiency). They are often prescribed with other drugs, for example, *diuretic drugs* or *beta-blocker drugs*.

HOW THEY WORK

ACE inhibitor drugs block the action of the enzyme that converts angiotensin (a protein present in the blood) from an inactive form, angiotensin I, to an active form, angiotensin II, which constricts (narrows) blood vessels. By reducing production of angiotensin II, ACE inhibitors reduce constriction of blood vessels, which makes it easier for the blood to flow through them, and thus reduces blood pressure.

POSSIBLE ADVERSE EFFECTS

These include nausea, loss of taste, headache, dizziness, and a dry cough. The first dose may reduce blood pressure so dramatically that the patient collapses; treatment is therefore often started in hospital.

Acetaminophen

ANALGESIC

Tablet Liquid

Available over-the-counter

An *analgesic drug* (painkiller). Acetaminophen is used to treat mild pain (for example, from headache or toothache) and to reduce fever. It has been widely used since 1955.

Unlike ASA, acetaminophen does not cause stomach irritation or bleeding and so is particularly useful as a painkiller for people who suffer from *peptic ulcer* or who cannot tolerate ASA. Acetaminophen may be used with safety to treat children, for whom it is available as a syrup. Acetaminophen does not have an anti-inflammatory effect, however, and so is less effective than ASA, as a treatment for injury to soft tissues such as muscles and ligaments.

POSSIBLE ADVERSE EFFECTS

Taken in normal doses, acetaminophen may rarely cause nausea or rash. An overdose may cause permanent liver damage and can be fatal.

Acetazolamide

A type of *diuretic drug* known as a carbonic anhydrase inhibitor. Acetazolamide is used in the treatment of *glaucoma* (raised pressure in the eyeball) and, occasionally, to prevent or treat symptoms of *mountain sickness* (headache, weakness, or other symptoms occurring at high altitudes).

During treatment with acetazolamide, adverse effects may include lethargy, nausea, diarrhea, weight loss, and impotence.

Acetic acid

The colorless, pungent, organic acid that gives vinegar its characteristic sour taste. In medicine, acetic acid is an ingredient of antiseptic jellies that are used to restore the normal acidity of the vagina in certain types of vaginal infections.

Acetylcholine

A type of *neurotransmitter* (a chemical that transmits messages between nerve cells or between nerve and muscle cells). Acetylcholine (sometimes abbreviated to ACh) is the neurotransmitter at all nerve-muscle junctions as well as at many other sites in the nervous system. The actions of acetylcholine are called cholinergic actions and are blocked by *anticholinergic drugs*.

Acetylcysteine

A drug used as an antidote for *acetaminophen* overdose. It is also a *mucolytic drug* used in the treatment of chronic *bronchitis* and *emphysema*.

HOW IT WORKS

To be effective as an antidote to acetaminophen poisoning, acetylcysteine must be given by injection within a few hours of the overdose; it works by reducing the amount of toxic substances produced during the breakdown of acetaminophen, thus reducing the risk of liver damage. Taken by mouth, acetylcysteine makes the mucus in sputum less sticky and therefore easier to cough up. Usually this drug is administered as a nebulized (fine) spray.

POSSIBLE ADVERSE EFFECTS

In rare cases, vomiting, rash, or breathing difficulty may occur when acetylcysteine is taken in large doses.

Acetylsalicylic acid (ASA)

ANALGESIC (NONNARCOTIC)

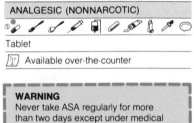

Tablet

Available over-the-counter

WARNING
Never take ASA regularly for more than two days except under medical supervision; it may mask the symptoms of a serious disorder.

An *analgesic drug* (painkiller) that has been used for more than 80 years to treat disorders such as headache, menstrual pain, and muscle discomfort. Because ASA has an anti-inflammatory action, it is particularly useful in treating joint pain and stiffness caused by types of *arthritis*. ASA also reduces fever and is therefore included in some *cold remedies*.

In small doses ASA reduces the stickiness of platelets (blood particles involved in clotting). This has led to its use in preventing *thrombosis* (abnormal blood clots) in some individuals at risk of having a *stroke* or *myocardial infarction* (heart attack).

ASA reduces the production of certain *prostaglandins* (hormonelike chemicals) that can be responsible for inflammation, pain, fever, or clumping of platelets.

POSSIBLE ADVERSE EFFECTS

In children there is a slight risk of *Reye's syndrome* (a rare brain and liver disorder). ASA should not be given to children except under close medical supervision; *acetaminophen* should be used instead in most circumstances.

ASA may cause irritation of the stomach lining, resulting in indigestion or nausea. These side effects may be reduced by taking the drug with food or by taking a coated tablet that does not release the drug until it reaches the intestine. Prolonged use of this medication may cause bleeding from the stomach due to *gastric erosion* (disruption of the surface lining of the stomach) or *peptic ulcer* (a deeper penetration of the wall of the stomach or duodenum).

Achalasia

A condition in which the muscles at the lower end of the *esophagus* and the sphincter (valve) between the esophagus and the stomach fail to relax enough to let food into the stomach after swallowing.

Food normally stimulates the muscles in the wall of the esophagus to begin a series of contractions that push food toward the stomach in waves. In achalasia, the sphincter does not relax to allow food to pass from the esophagus to the stomach, and the lowest part of the esophagus becomes narrowed, distorted, and blocked with food while the part above widens.

This rare condition can occur at any age, but is unusual before age 15. The underlying cause is unknown.

SYMPTOMS AND SIGNS
Symptoms include difficulty and pain with swallowing and pain in the lower chest and upper abdomen. Regurgitated food that may have been swallowed a day or two earlier may cause a foul taste and bad breath. The patient's ability to swallow gradually deteriorates even more until he or she has difficulty swallowing liquids as well as solids.

DIAGNOSIS
A barium swallow (a type of *barium X-ray examination*) will show abnormal, ineffective movement of the esophageal wall and varying degrees of dilatation (widening) of the esophagus, as well as narrowing at the lowest end of the esophagus and failure of the sphincter to open after swallowing. *Gastroscopy*, in which a narrow viewing tube is passed down the esophagus, is used to check the narrowing and to rule out cancer.

In achalasia, the pressure in the area of the lower sphincter is markedly raised; pressure recordings reveal that the sphincter is incompletely relaxed after swallowing.

TREATMENT
Drug treatment is rarely successful. It is possible to widen the esophagus for prolonged periods by passing a slender rubber bag down it and filling the bag with air or water to stretch the muscles (see *Esophageal dilatation*). There is also a surgical procedure that cuts some of the muscles at the stomach entrance to widen the passageway for food.

Achilles tendon

The tendon that pulls up the back of the heel. It is formed from the calf muscles (the gastrocnemius, soleus, and plantar muscles) and is attached to the *calcaneus* (heel bone). The tendon is named after the legendary Greek hero Achilles, who was vulnerable only in the heel.

Minor injuries to the tendon are common. They are usually due to too much exercise, faulty running technique, or wearing incorrect footwear. All of these can cause inflammation of the tendon (*tendinitis*) and tearing of the tendon fibers. In most cases, these conditions clear up with rest and physiotherapy.

Violent stretching of the Achilles tendon can cause it to rupture. In such cases, surgical repair of the tendon may be necessary.

Achlorhydria

Absence of stomach acid secretions. This may be due to chronic atrophic *gastritis* or to an absence or malfunction of acid-producing parietal cells in the lining of the stomach.

About one in every 20 normal people has achlorhydria without symptoms. Achlorhydria in itself is no cause for concern. However, the condition is present in some people with stomach cancer, and is also a feature of pernicious anemia, a blood disorder caused by defective absorption of vitamin B_{12} from the stomach (see *Anemia, megaloblastic*).

Achondroplasia

A rare disorder of bone growth, present from birth and leading to *short stature* (once called dwarfism). The affected bones are mainly the long bones of the arms and legs. The cartilage that links each bone to its epiphysis (the growing area at its tip) is converted to bone too early, thus preventing further limb growth. Most other bones are able to grow normally.

Individuals who are affected by achondroplasia have short, strong limbs, a well-developed trunk, and a

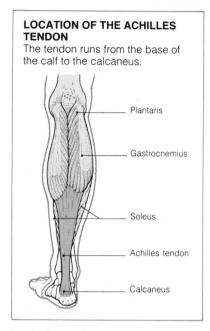

LOCATION OF THE ACHILLES TENDON
The tendon runs from the base of the calf to the calcaneus.

- Plantaris
- Gastrocnemius
- Soleus
- Achilles tendon
- Calcaneus

head of normal size except for a somewhat protruding forehead.

INCIDENCE AND CAUSES
The condition is caused by a gene defect of the dominant variety (see *Genetic disorders*), although exactly how the gene defect leads to the disorder of bone growth is not known.

The parents of most achondroplastics are of normal stature. In these cases, the abnormality has arisen from a gene *mutation* (new gene defect). However, the children of achondroplastics have a 50 percent chance of inheriting the defective gene and of being achondroplastic.

SYMPTOMS AND OUTLOOK
Achondroplasia is usually obvious at birth or during the first year of life, when there is already a noticeable stunting of the limbs relative to the size of the head. Growth of the limb bones slows and stops during childhood, and no treatment is available to alter the outlook. Intelligence and sexual development are not affected, and lifespan is close to normal.

Acid

A substance defined as a donor of hydrogen ions (atoms of hydrogen with positive electrical charges). When mixed with, or dissolved in, water, acid molecules dissociate (split up) to release their constituent ions; all acids release hydrogen as the positive ion (positively charged ions are called cations, negatively charged ones are called anions).

A wide variety of substances are acids. Examples of acids within the body include hydrochloric acid, which is a corrosive mineral acid produced by the stomach lining, and many organic acids, such as lactic acid, carbonic acid, ascorbic acid (vitamin C), and pyruvic acid. (See also *Acid-base balance; Alkali.*)

Acid-base balance
A combination of mechanisms that ensures that the body's fluids are neither too *acid* nor too alkaline (*alkalis* are also called bases). The body functions healthily only when its fluids are close to chemical neutrality.

In body metabolism, sugars and fats are broken down and energy is released. This breakdown involves the use of oxygen, and the production of carbon dioxide (which forms carbonic acid when dissolved in water) and organic acids, such as pyruvic acid. Thus, the body's metabolic processes cause fluctuations in the acidity and alkalinity of the blood as well as in other body fluids.

The body has three mechanisms for the maintenance of normal acid-base balance: buffers, breathing, and the activities of the kidneys. Buffers are substances in the blood that tend to neutralize acid or alkaline wastes. Rapid breathing increases the rate at which carbon dioxide is eliminated from the blood, thereby making it less acidic; conversely, slow breathing allows the blood to become more acidic. The kidneys help maintain a constant acidity level in the blood by regulating the amounts of acid or alkaline wastes in the urine.

Disturbances of the body's acid-base balance result in either *acidosis* (excessive blood acidity) or *alkalosis* (excessive blood alkalinity).

Acidosis
A disturbance of the body's *acid-base balance* in which there is an accumulation of acid or a loss of alkali (base). There are two types of acidosis: metabolic and respiratory.

CAUSES
In metabolic acidosis, an increased amount of acid is produced by metabolic processes. Ketoacidosis, a form of metabolic acidosis, occurs in uncontroled *diabetes mellitus* and, to a lesser degree, in starvation. Metabolic acidosis may also be caused by loss of bicarbonate (an alkali) through severe diarrhea. In kidney failure there is insufficient excretion of acid in the urine. One unusual cause of acidosis

is an overdose of ASA, which may cause an increase in acids produced by cell metabolism.

Respiratory acidosis occurs when breathing fails to remove enough carbon dioxide from the lungs. This causes increased acidity of the blood because the excess carbon dioxide remains in the blood, where it dissolves to form carbonic acid. Impaired breathing leading to respiratory acidosis may be due to conditions such as *bronchitis*, bronchial *asthma*, or *airway obstruction*.

Acid reflux
Regurgitation of acidic fluid from the stomach into the *esophagus* (the tube connecting the throat to the stomach). Acid reflux is associated with heartburn (a burning pain in the chest) and often leads to *esophagitis*.

Mild acid reflux is common and of no serious significance. It may occur in pregnancy and often affects people who are overweight.

Acid reflux is attributed to inefficiency of the muscular valve at the lower end of the esophagus, which permits regurgitation of the acidic fluid. Repeated episodes of discomfort may indicate the presence of a *hiatal hernia* (a weakness in the diaphragm that permits part of the stomach to protrude into the chest).

Acne
A chronic skin disorder caused by inflammation of the hair follicles and the sebaceous glands in the skin.

TYPES
The most common type of acne is acne vulgaris, which mainly affects adolescents. Tropical acne typically affects young white people on unaccustomed exposure to hot, humid environments. Infantile acne, a rare condition affecting male infants, is associated with subsequent severe acne vulgaris in adolescence. Chemical acne is caused by exposure to certain chemicals and oils, and results in acne in unusual sites, such as on the legs. Chloracne is a form of acne caused by exposure to chlorinated hydrocarbon chemicals; many cases occurred following a severe explosion at a chemical factory in Seveso, Italy, in 1976.

INCIDENCE
Acne vulgaris almost always begins during puberty, although it may develop later in life; most adolescent boys and many girls have some acne.

CAUSE
Acne spots are caused by the obstruction of hair follicles by sebum (the oily

substance secreted by the sebaceous glands). When a plug of sebum becomes trapped in a follicle, bacteria multiply and the follicle becomes inflamed. The cause of the change in sebum secretion at puberty is uncertain but it seems to be linked with increased levels of *androgen hormones* (male sex hormones). There may also be a genetic factor, since acne can run in families.

Some drugs may bring on or aggravate existing acne (e.g., corticosteroids and androgens, which increase oil production in the skin). Other drugs that can aggravate acne include barbiturates, isoniazid, rifampin, bromides, and iodides.

Oil and grease may also cause acne. The natural oil from the scalp may cause acne around the hairline. Regular contact with mineral or cooking oils, as may occur in restaurant kitchens, can make the condition worse. Cosmetics with oily bases are also associated with an increased tendency to develop acne.

SYMPTOMS
Acne occurs in areas that have a high concentration of sebaceous glands, mainly the face, center of the chest, upper back, shoulders, and around the neck. The most common acne spots are comedones (blackheads), milia (whiteheads), pustules, nodules (firm swellings below the skin), and cysts (larger, fluid-filled swellings in the skin). As spots heal, others tend to appear. Healing spots often fade to a pink mark that eventually disappears, although some spots, particularly cystic spots, may leave scars. Acne scars often appear as small, depressed pits. Occasionally keloids (overgrowths of scar tissue) may form.

PREVENTION
There are many myths about the prevention of acne, particularly relating to diet. There is no evidence that diet plays any part in causing acne. For example, there is little point in avoiding chocolate. Although washing affected areas does not prevent acne, it may keep it from spreading. The skin should be washed twice daily; more frequent washing is unnecessary, since washing simply removes surface oil.

TREATMENT
There is no instant cure for acne, although many treatments are available to relieve it. Topical (applied to the skin) treatments act by unblocking the pores and removing sebum. They also help to promote healing. Topical applications that are most often used

Severe acne
An example of cystic acne, with widespread scarring across the back. Few cases are as extensive as this.

include benzoyl peroxide, retinoic acid, antibiotic lotions, and sulfur-containing creams.

Ultraviolet light is often beneficial in treating acne. Moderate exposure to natural sunlight is helpful in most instances, and artificial ultraviolet light may be used to treat severe cases. The spots should not be picked or squeezed; this kind of interference can worsen the condition and can lead to scarring.

If acne is severe and does not respond to topical treatment, long-term therapy with oral antibiotics often helps. The antibiotics are prescribed regularly for up to six months at a time. They not only have an effect on the bacteria in the skin but also may have a direct anti-inflammatory effect on cells in acne spots; because of this, such antibiotics may discourage sebum production.

A recent development in the treatment of acne is the use of retinoid drugs. These drugs are prescribed only for severe acne when antibiotics and other measures have not helped. Retinoid drugs reduce oil production and have a drying effect on the skin, but must be taken cautiously because they may cause liver damage and other serious problems.

Acne cysts can often be treated by intralesional therapy (direct injection of a drug into the acne spots), which also helps to reduce scarring. In cases of severe and extensive scarring, *dermabrasion* (removal of the top layer of affected skin by high-speed sanding) can also improve appearance.

OUTLOOK
Acne improves slowly over a period of time, often clearing up by the end of the teenage years. With modern treatment, nobody should have severe, scarring acne.

Acoustic nerve
Also called the auditory nerve, the acoustic nerve is the part of the *vestibulocochlear nerve* (the eighth *cranial nerve*) concerned with hearing.

Acoustic neuroma
A rare, benign tumor arising from supporting cells that surround the eighth cranial (auditory or acoustic) nerve, usually within the internal auditory meatus (the canal in the skull through which the nerve passes from the inner ear to the brain).

INCIDENCE AND CAUSES
Acoustic neuromas constitute about 5 to 7 percent of primary *brain tumors*. Acoustic neuromas most commonly occur in people between the ages of 40 and 60 and are slightly more common in women than in men.

Usually the cause of acoustic neuromas is unknown. In some cases, however, tumors simultaneously affect the nerves on both sides of the head and may be part of a widespread *neurofibromatosis*, a disease characterized by changes in the nervous system, skin, and bones.

SYMPTOMS AND DIAGNOSIS
Acoustic neuroma can cause *deafness, tinnitus* (noises in the ear), loss of balance, and pain in the affected ear. As the tumor enlarges, it may compress the brain stem and cerebellum, causing *ataxia* (loss of coordination). As it expands, the tumor presses on the trigeminal nerve (fifth cranial nerve), causing pain in the face, or on the *abducent nerve* (sixth cranial nerve), causing double vision.

Diagnosis is made by *hearing tests* and tests of balance, such as the *caloric test* or *electronystagmography*, followed by X rays or *CT scanning* to visualize the internal auditory meatus.

TREATMENT
The tumor is treated by surgical removal. Before the operation, CT scanning or *MRI* (magnetic resonance imaging) is used to show the location of the tumor and its approximate size, so that the surgeon can decide on the best route for removal.

The results of surgery depend on the size of the tumor; in many cases, there is no residual damage to the acoustic nerve and hearing is preserved. Occasionally, however, numbness and weakness of part of the face result from unavoidable damage to neighboring nerves.

Acrocyanosis
A condition in which the hands and feet turn blue, may become cold, and sweat excessively. Acrocyanosis is caused by spasm of the small blood vessels and is usually aggravated by cold weather.

Acrocyanosis is related to another circulatory disorder, *Raynaud's disease*, in which the skin of the fingers and toes may be damaged by reduced blood flow.

Acrodermatitis enteropathica
A rare, inherited disorder in which areas of the skin (most commonly the fingers, toes, scalp, and the areas around the mouth and anus) are reddened, ulcerated, and covered with pustules (pus-containing spots).

Acrodermatitis enteropathica is caused by an inability to absorb enough zinc from food, and addition of zinc supplements to the diet usually produces a rapid improvement in a person's condition.

Acromegaly
A rare disease characterized externally by abnormal enlargement of the skull, jaw, hands, and feet.

Appearance of acromegaly
The woman in profile at left shows many of the typical features of acromegaly—including lengthening of the face, enlargement of the jaw and nose, and general coarsening of the facial features.

CAUSE AND SYMPTOMS
Acromegaly is caused by excessive secretion of *growth hormone* from the anterior pituitary gland at the base of the brain and is the result of a benign *pituitary tumor*.

If such a tumor develops within the first 10 years of life, the result is *gigantism* (in which growth is accelerated) and not acromegaly. More commonly, the tumor develops after growth in the long bones of the limbs has stopped. This leads to acromegaly, although it may take several years before the symptoms and signs of the condition appear.

Symptoms and signs of acromegaly include enlargement of the hands and feet, coarsening of the facial features, enlargement of the ears and nose, a jutting jaw, and a long face. Sufferers may notice a gradual increase in ring, shoe, glove, and hat size, and deepening or huskiness of the voice. Other possible symptoms are those common to any tumor in the brain, such as headache and visual disturbances.

DIAGNOSIS AND TREATMENT

If a person appears to be developing acromegaly, the level of growth hormone in the blood is measured before and after a quantity of glucose has been administered. Glucose usually suppresses growth hormone secretion; if it has no effect on the blood level of the hormone, this confirms uncontrolled secretion of the hormone by the pituitary gland. *CT scanning* or *MRI* may reveal a tumor or overgrowth of the pituitary gland.

In some cases, the drug bromocriptine may cause the pituitary tumor to regress. Alternatively, the tumor may be removed surgically or treated by *radiation therapy*.

Acromioclavicular joint

The joint between the outer end of the clavicle (collarbone) and the acromion (the bony prominence at the top of the shoulder blade).

INJURIES TO THE JOINT

Injuries to the joint are rare. They are usually due to a fall on the shoulder and may result in subluxation (partial dislocation with the bones still in contact) or, rarely, dislocation (complete displacement of the bones).

In subluxation, the synovium (joint lining) and the ligaments around it are stretched and bruised, the joint is swollen, and the bones are felt to be slightly out of alignment. In dislocation, the ligaments are torn, the swelling is greater, and the bone deformity is pronounced. In both subluxation and dislocation, the joint is painful and tender, and movement of the shoulder is restricted.

Subluxation is treated by resting the arm and shoulder in a sling. If the pain and tenderness persist, injection of a corticosteroid and a local anesthetic into the joint often helps.

Dislocation requires a strapping around the clavicle and elbow to pull the outer end of the clavicle back into position. The strapping is usually left on for three weeks. Occasionally, an operation may be needed.

Osteoarthritis (degeneration of the joint), which makes shoulder movement painful, can develop if the joint suffers repeated injuries.

Acroparesthesia

A medical term used to describe tingling in the fingers or toes (see *Pins and needles*).

ACTH

The commonly used abbreviation for adrenocorticotropic hormone (also called corticotropin), which is produced by the anterior part of the *pituitary gland* and stimulates the adrenal cortex (outer layer of the *adrenal glands*) to release various *corticosteroid hormones*. ACTH is also necessary for the maintenance and growth of the cells of the adrenal cortex.

ACTIONS

ACTH stimulates the adrenal cortex to increase production of the hormones *hydrocortisone* (cortisol), *aldosterone*, and *androgen hormones*. Most important of these is its stimulation of hydrocortisone production.

ACTH production is partly controlled by the *hypothalamus* (an area in the center of the brain) and partly by the level of hydrocortisone in the blood. When ACTH levels are high, the production of hydrocortisone is increased; this, in turn, suppresses the release of ACTH from the pituitary gland. If ACTH levels are low, hydrocortisone production falls and the hypothalamus releases factors that stimulate the pituitary gland to increase ACTH production.

ACTH levels increase in response to stress, emotion, injury, infection, burns, surgery, and a decrease in blood pressure. The level of ACTH naturally fluctuates in a diurnal (24-hour) pattern.

DISORDERS

A tumor of the pituitary gland can cause excessive ACTH production which, in turn, leads to overproduction of hydrocortisone by the adrenal cortex, resulting in *Cushing's syndrome*. Insufficient ACTH production due, for example, to hypopituitarism (underactivity of the pituitary gland), is rare. When it does occur, it causes *adrenal failure*.

MEDICAL USES

ACTH is used very rarely to treat inflammatory disorders, such as *arthritis*, *ulcerative colitis*, and some types of *hepatitis*. It has also been employed to induce remissions in *multiple sclerosis* but its efficacy in this respect is uncertain. ACTH is also used to diagnose disorders of the adrenal glands.

Acting out

Impulsive actions which may reflect unconscious wishes. The term is most often used by psychotherapists to describe behavior during analysis when the patient "acts out" rather than reports fantasies, wishes, or beliefs. Acting out can also occur outside psychoanalysis as a reaction to frustrations encountered in everyday life. In this case it usually takes the form of antisocial, aggressive behavior that may be directed toward oneself (e.g., wrist-cutting) or others.

Actinic

Pertaining to changes caused by the ultraviolet rays in sunlight, as in actinic *dermatitis* (inflammation of the skin) and actinic *keratosis* (roughness and thickening of the skin). Both are caused by overexposure to solar radiation, which is especially likely to occur near the sea in summer and from the snow in winter.

Actinomycosis

An infection caused by *ACTINOMYCES ISRAELII* or related actinomycete bacteria. These bacteria resemble fungi and cause diseases of the mouth and jaw, pelvis, and chest.

TYPES

The most common form of actinomycosis affects the jaw area. A painful swelling appears, usually under the jaw, and small openings develop in the skin. Pus and characteristic yellow granules discharge through the openings. Poor oral hygiene may contribute to this form of the infection.

Another form of actinomycosis, affecting the pelvis, occurs in women

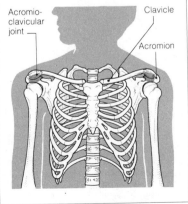

LOCATION OF THE ACROMIOCLAVICULAR JOINT
The joint lies at the junction of the outer end of the clavicle and the acromion.

Acromioclavicular joint

Clavicle

Acromion

A

and may cause lower abdominal pain, fever, and bleeding between menstrual periods. This form of actinomycosis has been associated with the use of *IUDs* that do not contain copper. Rare forms of actinomycosis affect the appendix or lung.

DIAGNOSIS AND TREATMENT

A diagnosis of actinomycosis is usually confirmed by finding the typical granules and by identifying the causative bacteria in a culture.

The infection can usually be treated successfully with large doses of a penicillin drug.

Acuity, visual

See *Visual acuity*.

Acupressure

A derivative of *acupuncture* in which pressure instead of a needle is applied.

Acupuncture

A branch of Chinese medicine in which needles are inserted into a patient's skin as therapy for various disorders or to induce anesthesia.

Traditional Chinese medicine holds that the chi (life-force) flows through the body along 14 meridians (channels), which affect particular parts of the body. A blockage in one or more of these meridians is believed to cause ill health. Acupuncturists aim to restore health by inserting needles at appropriate sites, known as acupuncture points, on the affected meridians.

A cautious view is taken of acupuncture by orthodox medical practitioners, but some use it to complement other treatments. In Canada acupuncturists in some provinces must be licensed physicians; in others, they are licensed as nonmedical practitioners; in still others, no licensing is required.

HOW IT WORKS

Research suggests that acupuncture causes the release within the central nervous system of *endorphins* (substances resembling morphine), which act as natural analgesics (painkillers). It has also been suggested that acupuncture may work by inducing a form of hypnosis, or that insertion of the acupuncture needles stimulates the peripheral nerves, acting as a distraction from, or a counter-irritant to, the original pain.

WHY IT IS DONE

Acupuncture has been used successfully as an anesthetic for dental procedures and surgical operations, and also during labor and delivery (includ-

ing cesarean sections). Some practitioners use acupuncture to reduce pain after operations and also to relieve chronically painful conditions, such as arthritis, that are not responding to standard treatments.

Acupuncture is claimed to be particularly effective for conditions that affect muscles, bones, joints, eyes, heart, and the digestive, respiratory, and nervous systems; it is also claimed to help in the treatment of addiction, depression, and anxiety.

HOW IT IS DONE

The traditional Chinese physician recognizes that accurate diagnosis is essential so that the acupuncturist knows which acupuncture points to use. Diagnosis in traditional Chinese medicine is made by examination of the patient's 12 pulses (six in each wrist). Each pulse is believed to give information about the health of a particular body region.

The precise disorder being treated, or the degree of anesthesia required, determines the temperature of the needle used, the angle of insertion, whether needles are twisted or vibrated while inserted, the speed of insertion and withdrawal, and the length of time the needles remain in position. Some practitioners pass a mild current through the needle to act as a stimulant in unblocking the meridian; others inject homeopathic remedies into the acupuncture point.

RISKS

Infection is a possible risk but good practitioners avoid this by using scrupulous sterilization techniques. It is rare for a blood vessel, body cavity, or organ to be punctured.

Some people find that they experience a temporary exacerbation of their symptoms immediately following acupuncture treatment. Others experience light-headedness, drowsiness, or exhilaration, although these feelings disappear soon after the treatment session has ended.

Acute

A term often used to describe a disorder or symptom that comes on suddenly. Acute conditions may or may not be severe, and they are usually of short duration. (See also *Chronic*.)

Acyclovir

ANTIVIRAL				
Tablet	Liquid	Injection	Cream	Eye ointment

Prescription needed

An antiviral drug introduced in 1982 and used in the treatment of *herpes simplex* infections. Acyclovir is also used in the treatment of *herpes zoster* (shingles). Acyclovir also has some effect against *cytomegalovirus* and *Epstein-Barr virus* infections. To be effective, acyclovir must be prescribed soon after infection; however, it does not provide a cure, nor does it always prevent attacks from recurring, but it does reduce their severity.

POSSIBLE ADVERSE EFFECTS

Adverse effects are uncommon. Acyclovir ointment may cause skin irritation or a rash. When taken by mouth, acyclovir may cause headache, dizziness, nausea, or vomiting. In rare cases, acyclovir injections can cause kidney damage.

Adam's apple

A projection at the front of the neck, just beneath the skin, that is formed by a prominence on the thyroid cartilage, part of the *larynx* (voice box). It enlarges in males at puberty.

LOCATION OF THE ADAM'S APPLE
This projection at the front of the neck, beneath the skin, is formed by a prominence on the thyroid cartilage.

Trachea — — Thyroid cartilage

Addiction

A dependence on, and craving for, a particular drug, such as alcohol, diazepam (a tranquilizer), or heroin. Reducing or stopping intake of the drug may lead to characteristic physiological or psychological symptoms (see *Withdrawal syndrome*), such as tremor or anxiety. (See also *Alcohol dependence; Drug dependence*.)

Addison's disease

A rare disorder in which symptoms are caused by a deficiency of the corticosteroid hormones *hydrocortisone* and *aldosterone*, normally produced by the adrenal cortex (outer part of the adrenal glands). The disease is named after the English physician Thomas Addison (1793-1860). It was invariably fatal before hormone treatment became available in the 1950s.

CAUSES

Addison's disease can be caused by any disease process that destroys the adrenal cortices. The most common cause is an *autoimmune disorder*, in which a person's immune system produces antibodies that attack the adrenal glands. *Tuberculosis* of the adrenal glands, once the main cause, is now extremely rare.

In addition to the deficient production of aldosterone and hydrocortisone by the adrenal glands, excessive amounts of *ACTH* and other hormones are secreted by the pituitary gland. One of these hormones (called melanocyte-stimulating hormone, or MSH) increases the synthesis of melanin pigment in the skin.

SYMPTOMS AND DIAGNOSIS

Addison's disease generally has a slow onset and chronic course, with symptoms developing gradually over months or years. However, acute episodes, called Addisonian crises, can also occur; they are brought on by infection, injury, or other stresses. The crises occur because the adrenal glands cannot increase their production of aldosterone and hydrocortisone, which normally help the body to cope with stress.

The symptoms of Addisonian crises are mainly due to aldosterone deficiency, which leads to excessive loss of sodium and water in the urine, extreme muscle weakness, dehydration, *hypotension* (low blood pressure), confusion, and coma. Deficiency of hydrocortisone leads to *hypoglycemia* (low blood sugar).

Symptoms of the chronic form of Addison's disease include tiredness, weakness, vague abdominal pain, and weight loss. A more specific symptom of the condition is darkening of the skin in the creases of the palms and pressure areas of the body, and particularly in the mouth. The darkening is caused by the excessive production of MSH.

Diagnosis is generally made if the patient fails to respond to an injection of ACTH, which normally stimulates the secretion of hydrocortisone.

TREATMENT

Treatment of acute Addisonian crises involves monitoring blood pressure and heart rate during the rapid infusion of saline and glucose, and supplementary doses of hydrocortisone and fludrocortisone to correct the sodium deficiency and dehydration. Lifelong treatment will include *corticosteroid drugs*.

Because patients with Addison's disease cannot increase their output of corticosteroid hormones in response to stress, they are at risk during stressful situations, such as infection, surgery, or injury. Their physicians must instruct them in the use of increased doses of corticosteroid drugs at such times so that the body mechanisms that fight infection and promote healing are not impaired.

Adduction

Movement of a limb toward the central line of the body, or of a digit toward the axis of a limb. Muscles that carry out this movement are often called adductors. The opposite movement is called *abduction*.

Adenitis

Inflammation of lymph nodes. Cervical adenitis (swollen, tender lymph nodes in the neck) occurs in certain infections, such as those caused by streptococcal bacteria (especially *tonsillitis*) and infectious *mononucleosis* (glandular fever). In the past, adenitis was often due to scrofula (tuberculous infection of the cervical lymph nodes).

Mesenteric lymphadenitis is inflammation of the lymph nodes in the peritoneum (the membrane that encloses the intestines) caused by a viral infection. Symptoms of mesenteric lymphadenitis—abdominal pain and tenderness—may mimic those of acute appendicitis and may require an operation to confirm a diagnosis.

Treatment of adenitis may include analgesic drugs (painkillers), hot compresses or a heating pad, and, if a bacterial infection is suspected, antibiotic drugs. The inflammation usually subsides within a few days.

Adenocarcinoma

The technical name for a *cancer* of a gland or glandular tissue, or for a cancer in which the cells form glandlike structures. An adenocarcinoma arises from epithelium (the layer of cells that lines the inside of organs).

Cancers of the colon (the main part of the large intestine), breast, pancreas, and kidney are usually adeno-carcinomas, as are a proportion of cancers of the cervix, esophagus, salivary glands, and many other organs. (See also *Intestine, cancer of; Kidney cancer; Pancreas, cancer of.*)

Adenoidectomy

Surgical removal of the *adenoids*, usually performed on a child with abnormally large adenoids that are causing recurrent infections of the middle ear or air sinuses. The operation is often performed together with *tonsillectomy*.

Adenoidectomy is generally an operation with minimal after effects. The patient can usually begin to eat normally the following day.

Adenoids

A midline swelling at the back of the nose, above the tonsils, made up of *lymph nodes* (tissues that contain lymphocytes, which are white cells that help fight infection). These nodes form part of the body's defenses against upper respiratory tract infections; they tend to enlarge during early childhood, a time when such infections are common.

DISORDERS

In most children, adenoids shrink after the age of about 5 years, disappearing altogether by puberty. In some children, however, they become even larger and obstruct the passage from the nose to the throat, causing snoring, breathing through the

---

LOCATION OF THE ADENOIDS
These two glandular swellings are found at the back of the nasal passage above the tonsils. Enlarged adenoids are sometimes implicated in *sleep apnea*.

Nasal cavity

Tongue

Tonsil   Trachea

Adenoids

mouth, and a characteristically nasal voice. They can also block the eustachian tube (which connects the middle ear to the throat), causing infection and deafness.

Obstruction to the flow of secretions behind the nose can result in *rhinitis* (inflammation of the nose), which can spread to the middle ear (see *Otitis media*) and to the air sinuses behind the nose (see *Sinusitis*).

DIAGNOSIS AND TREATMENT To discover whether ear, nose, and throat infections are being caused by abnormally enlarged adenoids, the physician usually inspects the back of the throat using a mirror with a light attached. Sometimes an X ray may be taken.

Infections usually respond to antibiotic drugs; however, if infections recur frequently, *adenoidectomy* (surgical removal of the adenoids) may be recommended.

Adenoma

A benign (noncancerous) tumor or cyst that resembles glandular tissue and arises from the epithelium (the layer of cells that lines the inside of most body organs).

Adenomas of *endocrine glands*, such as the pituitary gland, thyroid gland, adrenal glands, and pancreas, can cause excessive hormone production, leading to disease. Pituitary adenomas, for example, can result in *acromegaly* or *Cushing's syndrome*.

Adenomatosis

An abnormal condition of glands in which they are affected either by *hyperplasia* (overgrowth) or by the development of numerous *adenomas* (benign tumors).

Adenomatosis may simultaneously affect two or more different endocrine glands, such as the adrenal glands, parathyroid glands, pituitary gland, and pancreas.

ADH

The abbreviation for antidiuretic hormone (also called vasopressin), which is released from the posterior part of the *pituitary gland* and acts on the kidneys to increase their reabsorption of water into the blood.

ACTIONS
ADH reduces the amount of water lost in the urine and helps control the body's overall water balance. Water is continually being taken into the body in food and drink and is also produced by the chemical reactions in cells. Conversely, water is also continually being lost in urine, sweat, feces, and

in the breath as water vapor. ADH helps maintain the optimum amount of water in the body.

ADH production is controlled by the *hypothalamus* (an area in the center of the brain), which detects changes in the concentration and volume of the blood. If the blood concentration increases (i.e., the blood contains less water), the hypothalamus stimulates the pituitary to release more ADH. If the blood is too dilute, less ADH is produced; as a result, more water is lost from the body in the urine.

DISORDERS
Various factors can affect ADH production and thus disturb the body's water balance. For example, alcohol reduces ADH production by direct action on the brain, resulting in a temporary increase in the production of urine. Urine production is also increased in *diabetes insipidus*, a disorder in which there is either insufficient production of ADH in the pituitary gland or, rarely, failure of the kidneys to respond to ADH.

The reverse effect, water retention, may result from temporarily increased ADH production after a major operation or serious accident. Water retention may also be caused by the secretion of ADH by some tumors, especially of the lung.

DRUG THERAPY
Synthetic ADH is given via the nose or by injection to treat diabetes insipidus. High intravenous doses cause narrowing of blood vessels and may stop bleeding from *esophageal varices*. Adverse effects include abdominal cramps, nausea, headache, drowsiness, and confusion.

Adhesion

Joining of normally unconnected body parts by bands of fibrous tissue. Adhesions are sometimes present from birth, but most develop as a result of scarring after inflammation.

Adhesions are most common in the abdomen, where they often form after *peritonitis* (inflammation of the abdominal lining) or after surgery. Sometimes, loops of intestine are bound together by adhesions, resulting in *intestinal obstruction*. In such cases, an operation is usually required to cut the bands of fibrous tissue and free the intestinal loops.

Adipose tissue

A layer of fat just beneath the skin and around various internal organs. After puberty, the distribution of superficial adipose tissue differs in males and

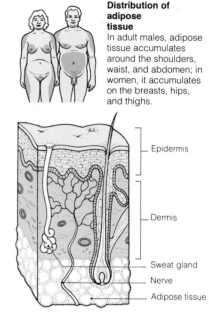

Distribution of adipose tissue
In adult males, adipose tissue accumulates around the shoulders, waist, and abdomen; in women, it accumulates on the breasts, hips, and thighs.

Epidermis

Dermis

Sweat gland
Nerve
Adipose tissue

females. Adipose tissue makes up a larger proportion of the total body weight of women than of men.

FUNCTIONS AND DISORDERS
Adipose tissue is built up from fat deposited as a result of excess food intake, thus acting as an energy store; excessive amounts of adipose tissue produce *obesity*. The tissue acts as an insulator against loss of body heat, particularly in babies. Adipose tissue helps absorb shock in areas subject to sudden or frequent pressure, such as the buttocks and feet. Adipose tissue also surrounds and cushions the heart, kidneys, and various other internal organs.

Adjuvant

A substance that enhances the action of another substance in the body. The term is usually used to describe an ingredient added to a *vaccine* to increase the production of antibodies by the immune system, therefore enhancing the vaccine's efficiency in conferring immunity. Adjuvant chemotherapy is the use of anticancer drugs in addition to surgical removal of a tumor.

Adlerian theory

The psychoanalytical ideas set forth by the Austrian psychiatrist Alfred Adler (1870-1937). Also known as individual psychology, Adler's theories were based on the central idea that everyone is born with natural feelings of inferiority. Life is seen as a constant struggle to overcome these feelings; failure to do so leads to symptoms of neurosis. (See also *Psychoanalytic theory*.)

Adolescence

The period between childhood and adulthood. Broadly speaking, adolescence corresponds to the teenage years. A complex stage of personality development and psychological upheaval, adolescence commences and overlaps with, but is not the same as, *puberty*. Puberty is the period of hormonally regulated development when the secondary sexual characteristics appear, marking the onset of physical and sexual maturity.

FEATURES

Adolescence is a time of much change for the individual and for the adolescent's family. The adolescent must come to terms with the body's physical changes and with the fact that family and society no longer expect or tolerate childish behavior. During adolescence, the adult's self-identity is formed. This involves achieving reorientation of emotional ties with parents; understanding and developing control and direction of adult sexual and other drives; occupation and career orientation; and eventually developing a mature set of values with responsible self-direction. Adolescence is also a time of forming attitudes and opinions.

Adolescents would like to be independent but many must still rely on adults for emotional and financial support. Family conflicts may arise when adolescents demand increased independence before their parents consider them ready for it.

During the process of achieving an adult identity, the adolescent ceases to define himself or herself only in terms of the adults who are at home and at school. He or she may seek other figures (such as singers or sports personalities) as role models, and may rebel against parental standards and family. Adolescents experiment with views and opinions, with allegiances to peer groups and gangs, and with political movements. They may adopt outrageous fashions of dress, appearance, and behavior.

Sexual experimentation occurs in fantasy and in reality, alone and with others. Gender identity may be questioned; this may be the time that a person first realizes that he or she is homosexual. Often during adolescence, homosexual behavior occurs temporarily. Coming to terms with

sexual drives may be influenced by the adolescent's perception of his or her parents' relationship.

PROBLEMS

Problems may have physiological, psychological, and/or social origins. Common patterns of adolescent behavior include moodiness, loss of interest in school, fluctuating school performance, and truancy. Adolescents may worry about their physical appearance, their changing body shape, and whether they are physically attractive. They may feel nervous, may become painfully shy and lacking in confidence. Often they feel very unsure of their personal identity, suffering a so-called "identity crisis." There may be a strong sense of alienation from parents, who may feel they can no longer talk to their children.

Some adolescents are overassertive and strive prematurely for independence. Rebellion against parents is often exaggerated in adolescents who were overdependent on, or overprotected by, their parents during childhood. Childhood deprivation that has resulted in poor *bonding* between child and parents can also lead to rebelliousness. On the other hand, a teenager who remains too dependent may remain stuck in adolescence and not develop sufficiently to make his or her own decisions or to form new relationships outside the family.

Aggressive drives that are not controlled and used constructively can lead to outbursts of temper or other undesirable behavior. Delinquency is usually a transient phase and may be dealt with by a mixture of firmness and understanding.

Adolescents (and younger children) may become involved in drug or solvent abuse. Youngsters who take drugs to relieve anxiety or depression are more likely to become dependent than others who experiment because of peer-group pressure.

A high proportion of adolescents with serious or prolonged psychological and behavioral problems, particularly delinquency and *drug dependence*, come from disturbed or deprived home environments, where there is poverty, marital disharmony, alcoholism, violence, or psychiatric disturbance in the parents.

Adolescents are often referred for specialist advice because parents or teachers are worried about their behavior. Only a small percentage of those referred need psychiatric treatment; most have temporary problems that resolve on their own. Family

problems or difficulties with relationships may provoke suicide attempts in disturbed adolescents.

Maintaining communication between parents and their offspring is important but not always easy. Parents should give advice on practical problems, such as acne and diet, but should never laugh off or underestimate seemingly minor problems; to do so may undermine the adolescent's confidence. The most valuable support a parent can give an adolescent is to encourage self-confidence and responsibility and thus prepare him or her to cope with adult life.

ADP

Abbreviation for adenosine diphosphate, the chemical that takes up energy released during biochemical reactions to form *ATP* (adenosine triphosphate), the main energy-carrying chemical in the body. When ATP releases its energy, ADP is reconstituted. (See also *Metabolism*.)

Adrenal failure

Insufficient production of hormones by the adrenal cortex (outer part of the *adrenal glands*). It can be acute (of sudden onset) or chronic (of more gradual onset). Adrenal failure may be due to a disorder of the adrenal glands, in which case it is called *Addison's disease*. Alternatively, it may be due to reduced stimulation of the adrenal cortex by *ACTH*, a hormone produced by the pituitary gland (see *Adrenal glands* disorders box).

Adrenal glands

A pair of small, triangular *endocrine glands* (glands that secrete hormones directly into the bloodstream) located above the kidneys. Each adrenal gland can be divided, anatomically and functionally, into two distinct parts: the outer adrenal cortex and the smaller, inner adrenal medulla.

THE ADRENAL CORTEX

This part of the gland secretes a group of hormones called *corticosteroid hormones*, which have a variety of important effects on the body. The adrenal cortex is made up of three zones that can be distinguished under a microscope. The outermost zone secretes the hormone *aldosterone*, which, by inhibiting the amount of sodium excreted in the urine, helps maintain blood volume and blood pressure.

The inner and middle zones together secrete the hormones *hydrocortisone* (also called cortisol) and corticosterone, as well as small amounts of

A

ANATOMY OF THE ADRENAL GLANDS

Also sometimes called the suprarenal glands, the adrenal glands are situated on top of the kidneys. Each one is divided into two regions: the adrenal cortex (which secretes hormones that affect the metabolism) and the adrenal medulla (which is part of the sympathetic nervous system).

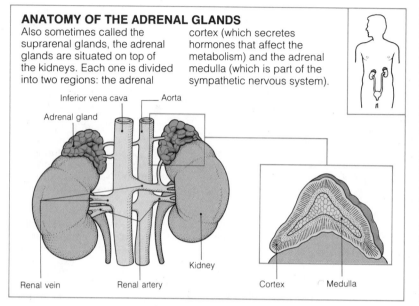

Inferior vena cava — Aorta
Adrenal gland
Kidney
Renal vein — Renal artery
Cortex — Medulla

androgen hormones (hormones that stimulate the development of male sex characteristics). Hydrocortisone is the most important human corticosteroid, controlling the body's use of fats, proteins, and carbohydrates. Hydrocorti-sone and corticosterone also have the effect of suppressing inflammatory reactions in the body and, to a limited extent, inhibiting the activities of the *immune system*.

Production of hormones by the adrenal cortex is governed by other hormones made in the *hypothalamus* and *pituitary gland*. The rate of hydrocortisone secretion is controlled by the release of *ACTH* (adrenocorticotropic hormone) by the pituitary gland, and normally varies during a 24-hour cycle, being minimal at midnight, rising to a peak at around 6 a.m., and then falling slowly during the course of the day.

Emotion, stress, and injury are potent stimulators of ACTH and hydrocortisone release; without hydrocortisone, the body is unable to recover properly from stress.

THE ADRENAL MEDULLA

The adrenal medulla is part of the sympathetic division of the *autonomic nervous system*, which is the body's first line of defense against physical and emotional stresses. The adrenal medulla is closely related to nervous tissue and secretes the hormones *epinephrine* and *norepinephrine* in response to stimulation by sympathetic nerves. These nerves are most active during times of stress.

The release of these hormones into the circulation produces effects similar to sympathetic nerve stimulation. The heart rate and also the force of contraction of the heart muscle increase so that more blood can be pumped around the body, and the airways of the lungs are widened to make breathing easier. The hormones constrict blood vessels in the intestines, kidneys, and liver, and widen blood vessels supplying the skeletal muscles. Consequently, more blood is supplied to the active muscles and less to the internal organs.

Adrenal hyperplasia, congenital

An uncommon disorder, also called adrenogenital syndrome or virilizing adrenal hyperplasia. The condition is present (although not always apparent) from birth. It results from inheritance of a recessive genetic defect (see *Genetic disorders*). The gene defect causes variable *enzyme* defects and blocks the production of the hormones *hydrocortisone* and *aldosterone* by the adrenal glands.

CAUSES AND SYMPTOMS

The enzyme block results in the production of progestogens, which are converted to *androgens* (male hormones) that accumulate in the fetus. In girls, these androgens virilize the genital tract, causing enlargement of the clitoris and some fusion of the labia majora (outer lips of the vulva),

FEEDBACK MECHANISM

The rate at which many glands produce hormones is influenced by other hormones, especially those secreted by the pituitary gland and the hypothalamus. If the amount of hormone produced is increased, negative feedback mechanisms act on the hypothalamus and pituitary so that they produce less of their stimulating hormones, thus reducing the target gland's activity. If the amount of hormone produced is decreased, the feedback weakens, swelling production of stimulating hormones.

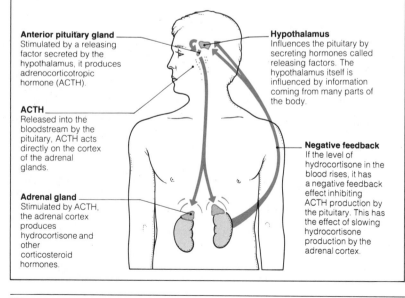

Anterior pituitary gland
Stimulated by a releasing factor secreted by the hypothalamus, it produces adrenocorticotropic hormone (ACTH).

ACTH
Released into the bloodstream by the pituitary, ACTH acts directly on the cortex of the adrenal glands.

Adrenal gland
Stimulated by ACTH, the adrenal cortex produces hydrocortisone and other corticosteroid hormones.

Hypothalamus
Influences the pituitary by secreting hormones called releasing factors. The hypothalamus itself is influenced by information coming from many parts of the body.

Negative feedback
If the level of hydrocortisone in the blood rises, it has a negative feedback effect inhibiting ACTH production by the pituitary. This has the effect of slowing hydrocortisone production by the adrenal cortex.

resulting in ambiguity of the genitals (see *Sex determination*). About half of the affected males have an enlarged penis, which may be evident at birth or develop later.

Another result of the enzyme defect is that the body is unable to retain salt and water. This in turn may cause dehydration, weight loss, and low blood pressure, and may lead to shock. There may also be hypoglycemia (low blood sugar).

Normally, hydrocortisone suppresses secretion by the pituitary gland of *ACTH* (adrenocorticotropic hormone), the hormone that stimu-lates the adrenal glands. An affected person's adrenal glands produce insufficient hydrocortisone, leading to excessive secretion of ACTH. This causes hyperplasia (enlargement) of the adrenal glands.

The excessive secretion of ACTH and another hormone, called melano-cyte-stimulating hormone, causes excessive skin pigmentation, with dark skin creases and dark nipples.

In severe cases, the condition becomes apparent in the first weeks of life. In milder cases, features of the disorder appear later, sometimes pro-ducing premature puberty in boys, and delayed menstruation, hirsutism, and potential infertility in girls. These more mildly affected individuals do not usually have problems with salt regulation.

DIAGNOSIS AND TREATMENT

The diagnosis is suggested by the signs and symptoms at birth or later in childhood or adolescence. Congenital adrenal hyperplasia is confirmed by the measurement of corticosteroid hormones in the blood and urine. *Ultrasound scanning* shows the adrenal glands to be enlarged but with no tumor present. Treatment consists of replacing the missing hormones. If

DISORDERS OF THE ADRENAL GLANDS

Excessive or deficient production of hormones by the adrenal glands can occur in a variety of ways. These disorders are uncommon, but may be serious. Disturbed hormone production by the adrenal cortex is more common than disturbance of the adrenal medulla.

CONGENITAL DEFECTS

Congenital *adrenal hyperplasia* affects about one newborn in 10,000. The adrenal cortex is unable to synthesize sufficient hydrocortisone and (sometimes) aldosterone, and the baby is ill or fails to thrive. As a side effect of the reduced hydrocortisone production, the glands are stimulated to produce androgens (male sex hormones) in excess; this can cause masculinization of female babies.

TUMORS

Growths in the adrenal glands are rare and generally lead to excess hormone production. Excess secretion of aldosterone causes *aldosteronism* (also known as Conn's syndrome), a condition characterized by thirst and high blood pressure. Excess secretion of hydrocortisone causes *Cushing's syndrome*, which has various features including muscle-wasting and obesity of the trunk. Androgens may also be produced to excess, causing masculinization in females.

Tumors of the adrenal medulla include *pheochromocytoma* and *neuroblastoma*. Excess epinephrine and norepinephrine are secreted.

AUTOIMMUNE DISORDERS

Deficient production of hormones by the adrenal cortex is called *adrenal failure*; if due to disease of the adrenal glands themselves, it is called *Addison's disease*. The most common cause of Addison's disease is an autoimmune process (in which the body's immune system attacks its own tissues). Addison's disease can take a chronic course, characterized by weakness, weight loss, and skin darkening, or an acute form (Addisonian crisis or acute adrenal failure), in which the patient may become confused and comatose.

INFECTION

Destruction of the adrenal glands by *tuberculosis* was once a major cause of Addison's disease but is now uncommon. The onset of an infection or other acute illness in someone with Addison's disease can precipitate acute adrenal failure.

IMPAIRED BLOOD SUPPLY

Loss or obstruction of the blood supply to the adrenals, sometimes as a result of arterial disease, is another possible cause of Addison's disease or acute adrenal failure.

OTHER DISORDERS

In many cases disturbed activity of the adrenals is caused not by disease of the glands themselves, but by an increase or decrease in the blood level of hormones that influence the activity of the glands.

Hydrocortisone production by the adrenal cortex is controlled by the secretion of *ACTH* (adrenocortico-tropic hormone) by the pituitary gland. A tumor or other disorder of the pituitary, or tumors in the lung, breast, and elsewhere, can cause excess ACTH secretion, leading to too much hydrocortisone being produced by the adrenals and, hence, to Cushing's syndrome. Pituitary disease is, in fact, the most common cause of Cushing's syndrome.

Destruction or removal of the pituitary stops ACTH secretion, which prevents stimulation of the adrenal cortex, and leads to adrenal failure.

INVESTIGATION

Suspected disturbance of adrenal function is investigated by serial measurement of the levels of hormones such as hydrocortisone, aldosterone, epinephrine, and ACTH in the blood and/or urine. Tests may also be carried out to measure the effects of an injected substance that would normally modify the production of a hormone. Such tests can help localize the underlying cause of the disorder—for example, to distinguish Cushing's syndrome due to an adrenal tumor from that due to pituitary disease.

If disease of the adrenal glands is suspected, the glands may be imaged by such techniques as an *X ray* (perhaps after first introducing air around the glands), *CT scanning*, *arteriography*, *radionuclide scanning*, or intravenous *pyelography* (to detect distortion of the kidney by an adrenal gland tumor). A tumor or gland overgrowth is usually detectable by one of these techniques.

the condition is recognized and treatment started early, normal sexual development and fertility usually follow. Plastic surgery needs to be undertaken in most affected females. (See also *Hermaphroditism; Sex determination.*)

Adrenaline
See *Epinephrine.*

Adrenal tumors
Rare malignant or benign tumors within the *adrenal glands*, usually causing excess secretion of hormones.

Tumors of the adrenal cortex may secrete aldosterone, causing primary *aldosteronism* (also called Conn's syndrome), or hydrocortisone, causing *Cushing's syndrome.*

Tumors of the adrenal medulla may cause excess secretion of epinephrine and norepinephrine. There are two types of tumor affecting the adrenal medulla: *neuroblastoma* and *pheochromocytoma.* These tumors cause intermittent *hypertension* (high blood pressure) and sweating attacks.

Surgical removal of a tumor, or even a whole adrenal gland, often cures the conditions caused by the excess hormone secretion. (See also *Adrenal glands* disorders box.)

Adrenocorticotropic hormone
See *ACTH.*

Adrenogenital syndrome
See *Adrenal hyperplasia, congenital.*

Aerobic
Requiring oxygen to live, function, and grow. Humans and almost all other forms of life are dependent on oxygen for "burning" foods to produce energy (see *Metabolism*). Because of this dependence, they are described as obligate aerobes. In contrast, many bacteria have fundamentally different metabolisms and thrive without oxygen (some of them are even killed by it); such microorganisms are described as *anaerobic.* There are also some bacteria and yeasts (called facultative aerobes) that flourish in oxygen but can also live without it. (See also *Aerobics.*)

Aerobics
Exercises that allow muscles to work at a steady rate with a constant, adequate supply of oxygen-carrying blood. Oxygen is necessary to release energy from the body's stores of fat, glycogen (a starchy storage material), and sugars.

During aerobic exercises, such as swimming, jogging, and cycling, the muscles' increased demand for oxygen is met continuously as the rate at which oxygen reaches the muscles keeps pace with the rate at which it is used up. Because of this continual replenishment, the activity can be sustained for long periods.

To fuel aerobic exercise, the muscles use fatty acid rather than glucose, burning it completely to produce energy, carbon dioxide, and water. By contrast, anaerobic exercise relies on a different series of biochemical reactions to obtain energy from the stores of sugar and fat in muscle. The waste products of anaerobic exercise are acidic and, as they accumulate in the muscles, cause muscle fatigue. High-intensity exercises are anaerobic and can be performed for only relatively short periods.

Unexercised muscle

Unhealthy muscle   Fat deposits

Exercised muscle

Healthy muscle
Good flow of oxygen

Benefits of aerobic exercise
Regular aerobic exercise improves the condition of the muscles. The supply of blood carrying oxygen to the muscles is increased and the cells' capacity to use oxygen is consequently enhanced.

BENEFITS OF AEROBIC EXERCISE
To benefit your health, aerobic exercises should involve the large muscles of the trunk and limbs. In addition, the exercises need to be performed continuously for 20 minutes at least three times a week.

When performed regularly, aerobic exercises improve stamina and endurance. They encourage the growth of capillaries (small blood vessels),

thus improving the supply of blood to the cells. Aerobic exercises also increase the size and number of mitochondria (energy-producing organelles) within muscle cells, thus improving the cells' capacity to use oxygen and increasing the amount that the body can use in a given time.

The condition of the heart also improves as the body becomes fitter. The heart rate becomes slower, both at rest and during exercise; the heart muscle becomes thicker and stronger; and the stroke volume (the amount of blood pumped with each beat) increases. The overall result of these changes is that the heart needs to do less work to achieve the same level of efficiency in pumping blood around the body.

For all-round fitness, which includes strength and suppleness, other types of exercise should be performed as well as aerobics. (See also *Exercise; Fitness.*)

Aerodontalgia
Sudden pain in a tooth brought on by a change in surrounding air pressure. Flying at a high altitude in a lowered atmospheric pressure can cause a pocket of air within the dental pulp chamber to expand and irritate the nerve in the root. Common sources of aerodontalgia are improperly fitting fillings, poorly filled root canals, and inflammation of the pulp.

Aerophagia
Excessive swallowing of air. It may occur during rapid eating or drinking or be caused by anxiety. Aerophagia may also be a deliberate action to relieve indigestion by belching. After *laryngectomy* (surgical removal of the larynx), voluntary aerophagia is used to produce esophageal speech.

Affect
A term used to describe a person's mood. The two extremes of affect are elation and depression. A person who experiences extreme moods or changes in moods may have an *affective disorder.* A person whose responses to events seem flat—so that nothing excites, nothing angers—is said to have a shallow, flattened, or reduced affect; this characteristic may be a sign of *schizophrenia* or of an organic *brain syndrome.*

Affective disorders
Mental illnesses characterized predominantly by marked changes in *affect* (mood). Mood may vary over time between *mania* (extreme elation)

and severe *depression*. The disorders may be psychotic or neurotic. (See also *Manic-depressive illness*.)

Affinity

A term used to describe the attraction between chemicals that causes them to bind together, as, for example, between an antigen and an antibody (see *Immune response*). In microbiology, affinity describes the physical similarity between organisms (for example, viruses). In psychology, the term affinity describes an attraction between two people.

Aflatoxin

A poisonous substance produced by *ASPERGILLUS FLAVUS* molds, which contaminate stored foods, especially grains, peanuts, and cassava. Aflatoxin has been found to cause liver cancer in laboratory animals and is believed to be one of the factors responsible for the high incidence of this cancer in tropical Africa.

Afterbirth

The common name for the tissues that are expelled from the uterus after delivery of a baby. The afterbirth includes the *placenta* and the membranes that surrounded the fetus.

Afterpains

Contractions of the uterus that continue after childbirth. Afterpains are normal and indicate that the uterus is shrinking as it should. They are experienced by many women, especially after a second or subsequent delivery. The pains typically occur during the first few days after delivery and are particularly painful during breast-feeding. Afterpains disappear after a few days but may require analgesic drugs (painkillers).

Agar

An extract of certain seaweeds with properties similar to those of gelatin. Its full name is agar-agar. It is taken to soften and give bulk to feces in cases of constipation, and to relieve indigestion and heartburn because of its bland, soothing properties. Another use of agar is as a gelling agent in media for growing bacterial *cultures*.

Age

Of medical significance in diagnosis and in determining treatment, age is usually measured chronologically (in terms of the period of time since birth). However, age can also be measured in terms of physical, mental, or developmental maturity.

PHYSICAL AGE

Physical age can be measured even before birth. The age of a fetus is measured in terms of gestational age. Estimation of gestational age is important in neonatal pediatrics for identifying those babies who are too small for their gestational age and who may have problems because of their low birth weight. Gestational age can be assessed from the date of the woman's last menstrual period and by the size of her pregnant uterus. More accurate determination is made by measuring the size of the fetus by *ultrasound scanning*. The gestational age of a newborn baby can be estimated to within about two weeks by physical examination.

Children vary greatly in the rate at which they develop and grow, but their physical age is a measure of maturity that provides a common scale of development that can be used throughout the period of growth. In adults, physical age is difficult to assess other than through physical appearance. Physical age can be estimated after death by the state of certain organs, particularly by the amount of atheroma (fatty deposits) lining the arteries.

The most useful measure of physical development in children is bone age. Bone age measures how much the bones of a body area have matured, as seen on an X ray. Measures such as height and weight are less useful as age standards because they vary greatly among individuals of the same chronological age. In contrast, all healthy individuals reach the same adult level of skeletal maturity and each bone passes through the same sequence of changes of shape as it grows.

Assessment of bone age is particularly useful in investigating delayed *puberty* or *short stature* in children. A prediction of the final adult height can be made if the chronological age, bone age, and current height are known.

Dental age is another, though less useful, measure of physical maturity. It can be assessed by counting the number of teeth that have erupted (see *Eruption of teeth*), and by comparing the amount of dental calcification (as seen on X rays) with standard values in much the same way as bone age is measured.

MENTAL AND DEVELOPMENTAL AGE

Mental age is assessed by comparing scores achieved in intelligence or achievement tests with standard scores for different chronological ages (see *Intelligence tests*).

A young child's age can be expressed in terms of developmental level. Patterns of normal development have been described for children from birth to the age of 5 years in the fields of speech, vision, hearing, and motor skills (principally walking and delicate hand-eye coordination). Specific tasks in these fields are achieved at certain ages (see *Child development*).

Agenesis

The complete absence at birth of an organ or component of the body, caused by failure of development in the embryo.

Agent

Any substance or force capable of bringing about a biological, chemical, or physical change. An agent can also be a person acting on behalf of someone else. (See also *Reagent*.)

Agent Orange

A herbicide which the major constituent (50 percent by volume) is the phenoxy acid herbicide 2,4,5-T. That substance may be contaminated with the highly toxic poison TCDD, commonly known as dioxin, a by-product in the herbicide's manufacture (see *Defoliant poisoning*).

Age spots

Blemishes that appear on the skin with increasing age. Most common are seborrheic *keratoses*, which are brown or yellow, slightly raised spots that can occur at any site and sometimes get caught on clothing. Also common in the elderly are freckles, solar keratoses (small, blemishes caused by overexposure to the sun), and *De Morgan's spots*, which are red, pinpoint blemishes on the trunk.

Treatment is usually unnecessary for any of these age spots apart from solar keratoses, which may progress to skin cancer. Freezing the keratoses with liquid nitrogen is the usual treatment; they may also be removed surgically under a local anesthetic.

Most spots are harmless but any unexplained blemish, or one that grows rapidly or bleeds, should be seen by your doctor because of the possibility of skin cancer.

Ageusia

Lack or impairment of the sense of taste (see *Taste, loss of*).

A

Aggregation, platelet

The clumping together of platelets (small, sticky blood particles). Platelet aggregation takes place when a blood vessel is damaged, forming the first stage of *blood clotting* and thus helping to plug the injured vessel. Aggregation can also have adverse effects. It contributes to the formation of atheroma (the fatty substance that accumulates inside arteries and causes *atherosclerosis*) and thrombi (blood clots), which can cause *thrombosis*.

In the treatment of disorders in which thrombosis plays a part—*coronary artery disease*, for example—drugs such as ASA, dipyridamole, or sulfinpyrazone may be prescribed to reduce aggregation.

Aggression

A general term for a wide variety of acts of hostility, some of which may be outside the range of normal social behavior.

CAUSES

Among animals, aggression serves to protect the individual by way of self-defense and in defense of food, territory, and the young. In humans, there seem to be other factors, perhaps based on the needs of prehistoric survival. Some people believe aggression results from frustration, lack of affection, and the attitudes of parents.

EEG studies show changes in brain-wave patterns in people who are continuously aggressive. Aggression centers (for example, the amygdaloid area in the brain) have been described. Brain disease (such as a tumor) or head injury may sometimes result in aggressive behavior. Even so, such outbursts do seem to be related to events; the person does not start fights for no reason at all, but rather overreacts aggressively to problems.

Androgen hormones, the male sex hormones, seem to promote aggression, whereas *estrogen hormones*, the female sex hormones, actively suppress it. Age is another factor, because aggression is more common in adolescence and the early 20s, but becomes increasingly rare the older people get.

Psychiatric conditions associated with aggressive outbursts are *schizophrenia* (especially the catatonic and paranoid types), *antisocial personality disorder*, *mania*, and abuse of amphetamines or alcohol. *Temporal lobe epilepsy*, *hypoglycemia*, and *confusion* due to physical illnesses are other, less common, medical causes. *Dementia*, whether associated with *Alzheimer's*

disease or *alcohol dependence*, may remove control of aggression.

Aging

The physical and mental changes that occur with the passing of time. The aging process is sometimes seen as bringing with it only frailty and increased vulnerability to disease and injury, but many societies value their old people for their wisdom and experience and recognize other virtues that often come with age (e.g., patience and acceptance).

BIOLOGICAL AGING

All animals have a finite life span, and the maximum for humans seems to have changed little since biblical times. Very few people live beyond 100 years, and the average life span in the absence of disease seems to be about 85 years.

Gerontologists have yet to agree on the biological processes that underlie aging. Among the many theories are the "worn template" concept—that every time cells divide, the copying mechanism is more likely to introduce errors; the accumulated toxins theory, according to which the body is gradually poisoned by the accumulation of chemicals it cannot excrete; and the immune surveillance theory, which postulates that there is a progressive decline in the immune system's ability to detect and destroy microorganisms and developing tumors.

Aging is associated with degenerative changes in various organs and tissues, such as the skin, bones, joints, blood vessels, and nervous tissue (see chart). These changes may be accelerated by factors such as smoking, excessive alcohol consumption, poor diet, insufficient exercise, and excessive exposure of the skin to strong sunlight.

Nevertheless, the evidence of 90-year-olds who have smoked and drunk alcohol all their lives shows that an important factor determining life expectancy is genetic. Just as a person's height is determined by the interaction of diet and environment with the genetic potential inherited from the parents, so life span depends to a large extent on heredity.

NORMAL CHANGES

As people age, they discover that their physical performance declines, although not by as much as is often believed. A 60-year-old who has always exercised regularly may retain some 80 percent of the physical strength and stamina that he or she had at the age of 25. However, the

natural decline in lung function limits exertion past the age of about 60. Wound healing and resistance to infection also decline.

Sexual activity past the age of 60 is variable. Prolonged abstinence tends to lead to loss of libido and potency, whereas those who have remained sexually active often find little, if any, decline in their sex life.

As with physical performance, certain of our mental abilities inevitably deteriorate with increasing age. Most people over 60 experience some degree of "benign forgetfulness," finding it more difficult, for example, to recall names or telephone numbers that were once familiar. However, *dementia* (a general decline in all areas of mental ability) occurs in fewer than 20 percent of people older than 80.

AGING AND SOCIETY

In the 20th century there have been dramatic changes in the age structure of developed societies because infant and childhood mortality have declined markedly. Today, few adults under the age of 50 die from natural causes (accidental death is now much more frequent in young adults than death from disease). The result has been a substantial increase in the proportion of people living beyond the age of 65; the proportion living to beyond 75 continues to increase. However, about one third of the people over 75 who are living today have some disability that in some way restricts their everyday activities; improvements in preventive medicine are likely to reduce this proportion in the future.

Agitation

Restless inability to keep still, usually due to underlying anxiety or tension. Agitated people may pace up and down, pluck at clothes or sheets, wring their hands, and start tasks without completing them. Because they cannot relax or concentrate, agitated people constantly repeat such aimless activities.

Agitation is usually caused by worry over a particular situation—a father anxiously awaiting the birth of his child, for example. Persistent agitation is also seen in *anxiety disorders*, especially when there is an underlying physical cause such as alcohol withdrawal. Depressive illness (see *Depression*) in older people is usually accompanied by severe agitation. The restlessness that is sometimes caused by certain drugs, such as the *phenothiazines*, can mimic agitation.

THE PRACTICAL EFFECTS OF AGING

In the body, aging is associated with loss of elasticity in the skin, blood vessels, and tendons. There is also progressive decline in the functioning of organs such as the lungs, kidneys, and liver. Mechanical wear and tear causes cumulative damage to certain organ systems. Brain cells, specialized kidney units, and many other body structures are never replaced after they have reached maturity.

EFFECTS OF AGING

Organ or tissue	Natural effects	Accelerated by
Skin	Loss of elastic tissue causes skin to sag and wrinkle. Weakened blood capillaries cause skin to bruise more easily.	Exposure to sun; smoking.
Brain and nervous system	Loss of nerve cells leads to reduction in ability to memorize or to learn new skills. Reaction time of nerves increases, making responses slower.	Excessive consumption of alcohol and other drugs; repeated head trauma (for example, from boxing).
Senses	Some loss of acuity in all senses, mainly due to loss of nerve cells.	Loud noise (hearing); smoking (smell/taste).
Lungs	Loss of elasticity with age, so that breathing is less efficient.	Air pollution; smoking; lack of exercise.
Heart	Becomes less efficient at pumping, causing reduced tolerance to exercise.	Excessive use of alcohol and cigarettes; a fatty diet.
Circulation	Arteries harden, causing poor blood circulation and higher blood pressure.	Lack of exercise; smoking; poor diet.
Joints	Pressure on intervertebral disks causes height loss; wear on hip and knee joints reduces mobility.	Athletic injuries; being overweight.
Muscles	Loss of muscle bulk and strength.	Lack of exercise; starvation.
Liver	Becomes less efficient in processing toxic substances in the blood.	Damage from alcohol consumption and virus infections.

Hip joint in young person
The X ray shows the rounded head of the thighbone (femur) separated by cartilage from the surrounding hip socket.

Hip joint in elderly person
This X ray of an osteoarthritic hip shows almost complete degeneration and disappearance of the cartilage in the joint.

Young skin
The outer skin layer has an appreciable thickness. The deeper layers contain numerous collagen fibers, which give the skin elasticity.

Older skin
The outer layer has become thinned, wrinkled, and prone to injury. There are fewer elastic fibers in the deeper layers.

Agnosia

An inability to recognize objects despite adequate sensory information about them reaching the brain via the eyes or ears or through touch. For an object to be recognized, the sensory information about it must be interpreted, which involves recall of memorized information about similar objects. Agnosia is caused by damage to areas of the brain involved in these interpretative and recall functions. The most common causes of such damage are *stroke* and *head injury*.

TYPES AND SYMPTOMS

Agnosia is usually associated with just one of the sensations of vision, hearing, or touch. For example, an object may be recognizable by hearing and sight but not by touch. Some people, after a stroke that damages the right cerebral hemisphere, may seem unaware of any disability in their affected left limbs. This is called anosognosia or sensory inattention.

TACTILE AGNOSIA is an inability to recognize by touch alone objects that are placed in the hands, despite adequate sensation in the fingers.

VISUAL AGNOSIA is an inability to recognize and name objects despite normal vision. Affected people may be able to describe the color, shape, and size of an object but cannot name what they see or indicate its use.

AUDITORY AGNOSIA is an inability to recognize familiar sounds despite normal hearing.

OUTLOOK

There is no specific treatment for agnosia but some of the lost interpretative ability may return eventually.

Agoraphobia

Fear of going into open spaces and of entering shops, restaurants, or other public places. The condition often overlaps with *claustrophobia* (fear of enclosed spaces), another *phobia*.

The thought of visiting a public place or of mixing with many other people fills sufferers with such dread that they make up any number of excuses to remain at home. If they do venture out, they may have a *panic attack*, which leads to further restriction of activities. Eventually, people suffering from agoraphobia become completely housebound.

People afflicted with the condition seek psychiatric treatment more often than for any other phobia. Treatment by *behavior therapy* is usually successful; *antidepressant drugs* are occasionally needed.

Agraphia

Loss of, or impaired, ability to write, despite normal functioning of the hand and arm muscles, caused by damage to the parts of the cerebrum (the main mass of the brain) that are concerned with writing.

CAUSES

Writing depends on a complex sequence of mental processes, including the selection of words, recall from memory of how these words are spelled, formulation and execution of the hand movements required, and visual checking that written words match their representation in the brain. These processes probably take place in a number of connected regions of the brain. Agraphia may be caused by damage to various parts of these regions (usually within the left cerebral hemisphere) and can be of different types and degrees of severity. The most common reasons for such damage are *head injury*, *stroke*, and *brain tumors*.

Agraphia rarely occurs on its own. Often this condition is accompanied by *alexia* (loss of the ability to read) or may be part of an expressive *aphasia* (general disturbance in the expression of language).

TREATMENT AND OUTLOOK

There is no specific treatment for agraphia. However, some of the lost writing skills may return as time passes after brain injury that is due to a stroke or other event.

Ague

An outdated term for malaria or other diseases causing fever in which the sufferer alternately feels excessively hot and shiveringly cold.

AIDS

A deficiency of the *immune system* due to infection with *HIV* (human immunodeficiency virus). In its present form, AIDS (acquired immune deficiency syndrome) appears to be new to the human population. As yet, there is no curative treatment and no vaccine for AIDS, but the symptoms and complications variably respond to *antibiotic drugs*, *antiviral drugs*, *anticancer drugs*, and *radiation therapy*.

INCIDENCE

AIDS is not present in all individuals who are infected with HIV. The proportion of those infected whose condition progresses to AIDS has varied widely in different countries and in different risk groups. Every year, AIDS will develop in between 1 and 5 percent of people infected with HIV, but there is some evidence that in a few infected people (less than 1 percent) both the virus and the antibodies eventually disappear from the blood, suggesting that the body has fought off the infection.

Once AIDS has been diagnosed, the condition is considered fatal. By the end of the 1980s, nearly 100,000 men, women, and children in the United States had been diagnosed as having AIDS and about half of them had died. In the same period, Canada had reported more than 3,500 cases: 60 percent of the patients died. The number of reported cases is doubling every 21 months.

The main risk groups are homosexual or bisexual men and people who inject themselves with drugs using unsterile needles and syringes. Other risk categories include heterosexual contacts of individuals infected with the disease and children born to infected women. Many people with *hemophilia* became infected in the early 1980s as a result of receiving infected blood products, but this route of infection has now been closed by better screening of blood.

HISTORY

In 1981, the Centers for Disease Control (CDC) in Atlanta, Georgia, was alerted to reports of cases of a rare lung infection in previously healthy homosexual men in Los Angeles and then in New York. Infection was found to be with *PNEUMOCYSTIS CARINII*, a protozoan organism that had previously caused pneumonia only in patients whose immune defenses were suppressed.

Later, cases of a rare tumor (*Kaposi's sarcoma*) were reported in young homosexual men. Kaposi's sarcoma was recognized as a slow-growing skin tumor previously seen mainly in Africa. In people with AIDS, the tumor behaved much more aggressively and was found in parts of the body other than the skin.

Soon it appeared that there was a rapidly increasing epidemic of conditions associated with depression of the immune system. Several other infections were reported—most of them being the so-called *opportunistic* *infections* (i.e., infections that do not ordinarily affect individuals with efficient immune defenses).

These conditions were observed not only in male homosexuals, but also in intravenous drug users and hemophiliacs, suggesting that transmission was related to blood as well as to sexual activity. An infective cause seemed likely and, in 1984, French and American researchers identified the virus responsible. It was named LAV (lymphadenopathy-associated virus) by the French, and HTLV III (human T-cell lymphotropic virus, type III) by the Americans. In 1986, the virus was renamed HIV.

THE EFFECTS OF THE VIRUS

The virus infects a type of white blood cell known as the T4, CD4, or T-helper lymphocyte, which is crucial for the regulation of the immune mechanisms. The infected cell may die or the virus may remain dormant in the cell, with the possibility of later reactivation. Many infected individuals have no sign of disease; they are "asymptomatic carriers." Or they have vague complaints, such as weight loss, fevers, sweats, or unexplained diarrhea. People in this group have been referred to as having AIDS-related complex (ARC).

In its most severe form (i.e., AIDS), HIV infection interferes with the immune system to make the individual susceptible to a variety of infections and cancers, such as Kaposi's sarcoma and *lymphomas*.

METHODS OF TRANSMISSION

HIV has been isolated from blood, semen, saliva, tears, nervous system tissue, breast milk, and female genital tract secretions. However, only semen and blood have been proved to transmit infection. Transmission is by sexual contact (penis to anus, vagina, or mouth), blood to blood (through transfusions or needle sharing in drug users), and from woman to fetus. Other rare methods are through accidental needle injury, artificial insemination by donated semen, and kidney transplants.

"Casual" or household spread does not occur. The infection is not spread by touching or hugging, by breathing the same air, or by sharing cutlery or crockery. Heterosexual transmission does occur. By early 1990, this mode of transmission accounted for approximately 7 percent of all known cases in Canada. In Africa, AIDS affects men and women equally; heterosexual transmission plays a more important role for many reasons, including an increased rate of transmission in people also infected with sexually transmitted diseases.

SYMPTOMS AND SIGNS

Individuals infected with the virus may have no symptoms; others experience a short-lived illness, which sometimes resembles infectious *mononucleosis*, when they first become infected. Medical examination of patients without symptoms may reveal abnormalities, most commonly lymph gland enlargement.

Minor features of HIV infection include skin disorders such as seborrheic *dermatitis* (skin inflammation particularly affecting the face). More severe features include marked weight loss, diarrhea, fever, and oral *candidiasis* (thrush).

Other infections that are more common or more severe in HIV-infected patients include *herpes simplex* infections, *shingles, tuberculosis*, salmonellosis, and shigellosis. HIV may also affect the brain, causing a variety of neurological disorders, including *dementia*.

The features of full-blown AIDS include cancers (such as Kaposi's sarcoma and lymphoma of the brain), autoimmune diseases (especially *thrombocytopenia*), and various infections (such as *pneumocystis pneumonia*, severe *cytomegalovirus* infection, *toxoplasmosis*, diarrhea caused by CRYPTOSPORIDIUM or ISOSPORA, candidiasis, disseminated *strongyloidiasis, cryptococcosis*, and chronic or persistent herpes simplex).

DIAGNOSIS

HIV infection may be suspected in someone with lymph gland enlargement or unexplained weight loss if the person is in a high-risk group. Confirmation of HIV infection involves testing a blood sample for antibodies to HIV; testing for the virus itself is more difficult. A positive HIV antibody test result indicates exposure to the virus; most antibody-positive individuals are virus carriers. Positive test results are always checked by a confirmatory test. A negative test result may occur in someone who has only recently come into contact with the virus; for this reason a negative result should be followed by repeated testing after six months if the individual concerned is in a high-risk group.

HOW AIDS HAS BEEN CONTRACTED IN CANADA

Cases (percentage of patients, adults and children, diagnosed as having AIDS)

%	Category
79.2%	**Male homosexual or bisexual activity** — This has accounted for most cases to date
5.4%	**Receiving infected blood or blood-product transfusions** — Most of this group consists of hemophiliacs who were infected before the risk was recognized. Since 1985 all Canada's blood supplies have been tested for AIDS
1.0%	**Needle-sharing by drug abusers** — The number of cases is increasing in this group
3.3%	**Male-to-female sexual transmission** — In Canada, this has accounted for relatively few cases, but the percentage is increasing
3.7%	**Female-to-male sexual transmission** — Again, this has accounted for relatively few cases, but the percentage is increasing
1.2%	**Mother-to-child via placenta** — A baby born to a woman who has AIDS or is HIV-positive has a risk of being infected
3.0%	**Multiple risk factors** — This group consists of people with more than one risk factor—mainly homosexual males who have also shared needles
3.2%	**Other/unknown** — This group consists of people who contracted AIDS by another means (e.g., accidental injury with an infected needle), or by unknown means

---

NO-RISK ACTIVITIES

Touching
AIDS virus cannot be transmitted by social contact such as shaking hands.

"Dry" kissing
Kissing without exchange of saliva poses no risk of virus transmission.

Embracing
There is no risk of transmitting the virus by embracing or cuddling.

Sharing utensils
The virus cannot be transmitted by sharing a glass or cutlery.

Giving blood
Only sterile needles are used for taking blood from donors in Canada.

Other contact
The virus cannot be caught from toilet seats or other objects.

A

CAUSES AND PREVENTION OF AIDS

AIDS is caused by the human immunodeficiency virus (HIV) (right), which consists of some nucleic acid (genetic material) inside two protective shells and an outer envelope. Full-blown AIDS develops in only some people infected with HIV.

Surface proteins

Outer envelope

Outer shell

Inner shell

Nucleic acid

HIV (the AIDS virus)

The electron micrograph at left shows a human immunodeficiency virus (HIV) particle erupting from an infected human lymphocyte (cell of the immune system).

HOW HIV (THE AIDS VIRUS) AFFECTS THE IMMUNE SYSTEM

In a person with a healthy immune system, various types of lymphocytes combat disease organisms.

In a person infected with HIV, the immune system is weakened; in some cases, this may lead to AIDS.

NORMAL IMMUNE SYSTEM

T4-lymphocytes

Disease organisms

1 Disease organisms entering the body alert T4-lymphocytes and other immune system components.

T4-lymphocytes

Other lymphocytes

2 The T4-lymphocytes help regulate the response of other lymphocytes (cells of the immune system).

Other lymphocytes

Disease organisms

3 These lymphocytes then counterattack and destroy the disease organisms by various mechanisms.

IMMUNE SYSTEM IN AIDS VICTIM

HIV

T4-lymphocytes

1 HIV (the AIDS virus) multiplies within, and ultimately may destroy, the body's T4-lymphocytes.

Disease organisms

Destroyed T4-lymphocytes

2 When disease organisms invade, immune responses may fail, due to absence of the vital T4-lymphocytes.

Disease organisms

3 The disease organisms may then overwhelm the immune system and lead to the features of AIDS.

RECOMMENDATIONS FOR PREVENTING THE SPREAD OF AIDS

- Do not have sexual intercourse with persons known or suspected of having AIDS, with many people, or with people who have had many partners.

- Do not use intravenous (IV) drugs. If you use IV drugs, do not share needles or syringes.

- Do not have sex with people who use IV drugs.

- People with AIDS or who have had positive HIV antibody test results may pass the disease on to others and should not donate blood, plasma, body organs, other tissues, or sperm. They should not exchange body fluids during sexual activity.

- There is a risk of infecting (or being infected by) others through sexual intercourse, sharing needles, and, possibly, exposure of others to saliva through oral-genital contact or "wet" kissing. The effectiveness of condoms in preventing infection with HIV is not proved, but their consistent use may reduce transmission, since exchange of body fluids is known to increase risk.

- Toothbrushes, razors, or other implements that could become contaminated with blood should not be shared.

Diagnosis of full-blown AIDS is based on positive results to tests for HIV, along with the characteristic infections and tumors.

PREVENTION OF INFECTION

Until a cure or vaccine is found, prevention is the most important measure against contacting the AIDS virus. The risk of infection can be reduced by practicing *safe sex*.

Anyone who feels that he or she may have been exposed to the virus may request a blood test, although it is wise to obtain counseling first on the advisability of the test and on the implications of a positive result. A person who knows that he or she has been infected should alter his or her sexual life-style to avoid transmitting the virus. An uninfected person should also adopt safe-sex procedures to avoid becoming infected.

Safe-sex techniques involve reducing the number of sex partners; ideally, sex should be restricted to partners whose sexual histories are known. Unprotected anal and vaginal intercourse should be avoided. Hugging, touching, mutual masturbation, and dry kissing are safe.

Saliva may contain the virus but is unlikely to be important in transmission; the risk of wet kissing with saliva exchange is unknown. If penile penetration takes place, a condom should be worn. Spermicidal jellies seem to inactivate the virus and should also be used. The risk of oral sex is not fully known, but ejaculation into the mouth should be avoided.

Intravenous drug users should not share needles, so as to prevent the spread of infection; their sexual partners may also be at risk. (Needle-exchange programs have been introduced in some communities.)

In Africa, prostitutes show a high rate of infection. Although rates are very much lower in Canada, prostitutes are a potential means of spread. They should be encouraged to require use of condoms to protect themselves and their clients.

There is a small risk to hospital and other health workers when handling infected blood products or needles. The risk of transmission by needles in hospitals has, however, been lower than expected; it is minimized if care is taken with all procedures involving sharp instruments.

People in risk groups should not donate blood, semen, or organs. All donated blood, semen, and organs are screened for HIV antibodies; blood products are also heat-treated.

TREATMENT

There is no cure for AIDS. Supportive treatment is available only for its complications. Pneumocystis pneumonia is treated with antibiotic drugs (such as pentamidine or co-trimoxazole), but troublesome side effects often occur and the infection commonly recurs. Treatment of Kaposi's sarcoma by radiation therapy or anticancer drugs is rarely curative.

Several antiviral drugs, such as *zidovudine* (AZT) and *acyclovir*, are being used to treat patients with HIV infection. Zidovudine has serious side effects and is not curative, but it does slow the progression of HIV infection. Full assessment of its value will come only after many more patients have been treated for long periods.

OUTLOOK

Research is continuing into other methods of attacking the virus or halting its effects. In laboratory tests, several drugs have inhibited an enzyme essential for viral multiplication. In practice, however, these drugs have failed in clinical trials or their use has been drastically limited because of severe side effects.

While research into drug treatment for AIDS continues, the failure of medical science to achieve curative treatment for other viral infections makes anything approaching a cure unlikely in the near future.

Medical prevention is possible if a vaccine against HIV can be developed. A successful vaccine has been developed against feline leukemia virus, which bears similarities to HIV, an encouraging sign that research is advancing.

AIDS-related complex

A combination of weight loss, fever, and enlarged lymph nodes in a person who has been infected with *HIV* (the *AIDS* virus), but does not actually have AIDS itself. Many people with AIDS-related complex (ARC) will eventually have the features of AIDS.

Air

The colorless, odorless mixture of gases that forms the Earth's atmosphere. Air consists of 78 percent *nitrogen*, 21 percent *oxygen*, small quantities of *carbon dioxide* and other gases, and some water vapor.

The balance among the various atmospheric gases is maintained largely by the mutual needs of animals and plants. Animals use oxygen and produce carbon dioxide as a waste product; plants use carbon dioxide and release oxygen in a process called photosynthesis. The level of carbon dioxide in the atmosphere is gradually increasing as a result of extensive deforestation and the large-scale burning of fossil fuels. This disturbance of the atmospheric balance is causing concern among scientists because the raised carbon dioxide levels may lead to significant global warming (the greenhouse effect), which could have potentially disastrous consequences for all life on this planet. (See also *Pollution*.)

Air conditioning

Any system that controls the purity, humidity, and temperature of the air in a building. Air conditioning is important in maintaining comfort and hygienic conditions in hospitals, hotels, offices, and other buildings.

WHY IT IS USED

Air conditioning helps to provide comfortable living and working conditions by acting on air that is already inside rooms and on air that is drawn in from outside. It works by filtering out dust, pollen, smoke, and bad smells, by adding or removing moisture as necessary, and by either cooling or heating the air to keep it at a comfortable temperature. By bringing in outside air that has been filtered and exposed to the antiseptic effect of ultraviolet light, air conditioning may also reduce the risk of airborne infections and allergies.

Hospital sterile units, used for nursing high-risk patients, have air-conditioning units fitted with special bacterial filters that minimize the risk of spreading infection.

DISORDERS

Despite its generally beneficial effects, air conditioning may be responsible for certain disorders. For example, some outbreaks of *Legionnaires' disease* (a type of pneumonia) have been linked to contaminated air-conditioning systems; and humidifier fever (a lung disease that causes fever, coughing, and breathing difficulty) is thought to be caused by the spread of infectious microorganisms (usually fungi) by air conditioning. Air conditioning has also been blamed for some cases of *sick building syndrome*, which is attributed to the physical working environment and produces headache, irritability, and loss of energy.

Air embolism

Blockage of a small artery by an air bubble carried in the blood. Air embolism is rare. In most cases, it is a result of air entering the circulation by way of a vein, either because of an injury or during surgery. Very occasionally, a scuba diver or a person in an aircraft suffers an air embolism as a result of a pressure accident in which lung tissues rupture and air bubbles escape into the bloodstream.

Air pollution
See *Pollution*.

Air swallowing
See *Aerophagia*.

Airway
A collective term for the passages through which air enters and leaves the lungs. The airway is made up of the nasal passages, oral cavity, upper part of the pharynx (throat), larynx (voice box), trachea (windpipe), bronchi (main air passages in the lungs), and bronchioles (smaller air passages off the bronchi that end with air sacs known as alveoli).

The term airway is also applied to a tube which is inserted into the mouth to hold the tongue forward and allow breathing in an unconscious patient. Preservation of the airway can also be achieved by the insertion of an *endotracheal tube* into the trachea in such a patient, either through the mouth or through an incision in the neck, as in a *tracheostomy* operation. (See also *Respiratory system*.)

Airway obstruction
Narrowing or blockage of the respiratory passages. The obstruction may be due to a foreign body, such as a piece of food, that becomes lodged in part of the upper airway and may result in *choking*. Certain diseases or disorders, such as *diphtheria* and *lung cancer*, affect the airway and can cause obstruction. Additionally, a spasm of the muscular walls of the airway, as occurs in *bronchospasm* (a feature of *asthma* and *bronchitis*), results in *breathing difficulty*. (See also *Artificial respiration*; *Lung* disorders box.)

Akathisia
An inability to sit still, occurring occasionally as a side effect of an *antipsychotic drug* used to treat mental disorders such as schizophrenia and depression. Less commonly, akathisia occurs as a complication of *Parkinson's disease*.

Akinesia
Complete or almost complete loss of movement. It may be due to loss of power in a group of muscles (e.g., as a result of damage to part of the brain by a *stroke*). Akinesia may also occur when muscle power is normal but when the muscles are abnormally rigid (e.g., in *Parkinson's disease*).

Albinism
A *genetic disorder* characterized by a lack of the pigment *melanin* that gives color to the skin, hair, and eyes. Although rare, albinism occurs in all races. Affected individuals (albinos) suffer visual problems and a tendency to have *skin cancers*.

TYPES
In oculocutaneous albinism (the most common type), the hair, skin, and eyes are all affected. In a severe form of oculocutaneous albinism, the skin and hair are snowy white throughout life (although the tips of the hairs may turn slightly yellow with age). In a less severe form, the skin and hair are white and the irises are almost transparent at birth, but all darken slightly with age and numerous freckles develop on parts of the skin exposed to the sun. In both forms, the eyes are affected by *photophobia* (intolerance to bright light), *nystagmus* (abnormal flickering movements), and, commonly, also by *squint* and *myopia* (nearsightedness).

Other rare types of albinism affect only the skin and hair or the eyes.

CAUSES AND INCIDENCE
The genetic defect results in deficiency of a specific *enzyme*; this deficiency interferes with melanin production in affected tissues. Oculocutaneous albinism shows an autosomal recessive pattern of inheritance, in which there is a one in four chance of a child being affected if both parents have normal skin coloring but carry the gene defect.

The overall prevalence of oculocutaneous albinism is low in Europe and North America—fewer than 5 people per 100,000 are affected. The prevalence varies in different ethnic groups (e.g., it is higher in the Ibo population in Nigeria).

COMPLICATIONS AND TREATMENT
SKIN The most serious complication of oculocutaneous albinism results from the lack of melanin, which normally protects the skin against harmful radiation in sunlight. The skin cannot tan, ages prematurely, and is liable to develop cancers on areas exposed to the sun. Albinos in sunny climates should therefore wear suitable protective clothing.

EYES The visual problems of albinos,

Appearance of albinism
The condition is caused by lack of melanin pigment in the skin, hair, and eyes.

Albinism in an African boy
Albinism is found in people of all races, although it occurs only rarely.

such as photophobia and nystagmus, can cause great difficulties, particularly with reading. Expert assessment and treatment should be sought at an early age; in most cases, glasses are needed, preferably tinted to help reduce photophobia.

Albumin
The most abundant protein in the *blood* plasma. Albumin is made in the liver from amino acids that have been absorbed from digested protein.

Albumin has several important functions. It helps retain substances (such as calcium, some hormones, and certain drugs) in the circulation by binding to them and thereby preventing their being filtered out by the kidneys and excreted in the urine. Albumin is also important in regulating the movement of water between tissues and the bloodstream by *osmosis* (the attraction of water to an area with a higher concentration of salts or proteins). (See also *Albuminuria*.)

Albuminuria
The presence of the protein *albumin* in the urine; a type of *proteinuria*. Normally, the glomeruli (filtering units of the kidneys) do not allow

albumin to pass through them and into the urine. Albuminuria therefore usually indicates a failure of the kidneys' filtering mechanisms. Such a failure may be due to a kidney disorder, such as *glomerulonephritis* or *nephrotic syndrome*, or it may be a sign that the kidneys have been damaged by *hypertension*.

Albuminuria can be detected by a simple test on the urine; this test is commonly included in routine medical examinations.

Alcohol

A colorless liquid produced from the fermentation of carbohydrates by yeast. Also known as ethanol or ethyl alcohol, alcohol is the active constituent of alcoholic drinks such as beer, wine, and spirits. In medicine, alcohol is used as an antiseptic and a solvent. *Methanol*, also known as methyl alcohol or wood alcohol, is a related, highly poisonous substance.

Any society where alcohol is freely used is invariably afflicted by the problems of acute *alcohol intoxication* (drunkenness), *alcohol dependence* (habitual, compulsive, long-term heavy drinking), and *alcohol-related disorders* such as liver disorders, heart disease, *hypertension*, *neuropathy*, and *Wernicke-Korsakoff syndrome* (a form of *dementia*). Alcohol is also an important factor in road traffic and industrial accidents, domestic violence, marriage breakdown, rowdyism, child abuse, physical assault, and other crimes.

EFFECTS

The effect of alcohol on the *central nervous system* (the brain and spinal cord) is as a depressant, decreasing its activity and thereby reducing anxiety, tension, and inhibitions. Taken in moderate amounts, alcohol gives the drinker a feeling of relaxation and confidence that may enable him or her to socialize more easily. However, any feeling of heightened mental and physical efficiency is illusory.

Tests have shown that even a low level of alcohol in the blood slows reactions. The more alcohol that is drunk, the greater is the impairment of concentration and judgment. At the same time, the drinker's confidence is increased—a potentially lethal combination while driving. If excessive amounts of alcohol are drunk, poisoning or intoxication results, with effects ranging from feelings of euphoria to unconsciousness.

In addition to significantly altering mood and behavior, alcohol has various physical effects on the body.

As a result of peripheral *vasodilation* (widening of the small blood vessels), the face becomes flushed and the drinker feels warm, although in fact a greater amount of body heat is lost. Small amounts of alcohol increase the flow of gastric juices and therefore stimulate the appetite; however, large amounts over a long period can cause erosive *gastritis* (inflammation and superficial ulceration of the drinker's stomach lining) and hematemesis (vomiting blood).

Urine production increases because of the inhibitory effect of alcohol on the secretion of *ADH* (antidiuretic hormone). Heavy drinkers thus often become dehydrated; great thirst, a dry tongue, and a hangover may be associated with the effects of alcohol.

The effects of alcohol on sexual behavior were aptly summarized by William Shakespeare when he wrote: "It provokes the desire but it takes away the performance."

Regular intake of alcohol adds significantly to the energy content of the diet; pure alcohol provides 700 calories per 100 g. This explains why habitual drinkers of beer or wine are commonly overweight.

TOLERANCE

Habitual drinkers acquire a tolerance to alcohol. This means that they must drink gradually increasing amounts of alcohol to obtain the same effects. The liver breaks down alcohol at a faster rate, necessitating a greater intake to achieve the same level in the blood.

At the same time, nerve cells in the brain become less and less responsive to a given amount of alcohol. Paradoxically, however, after years of drinking, many alcoholics experience a reduced tolerance.

Alcohol dependence

An illness characterized by habitual, compulsive, long-term, heavy consumption of alcohol and the development of withdrawal symptoms when drinking is suddenly stopped. The description "alcohol dependence" is generally preferred medically to "alcoholism," but the terms are often used synonymously.

INCIDENCE

The incidence of alcohol dependence has been rising throughout the world for many years. Statistics on the extent of the problem are difficult to quote with any certainty. In Canada approximately 397,000 men and 189,000 women are alcohol dependent. Among men, alcoholism is second only to schizophrenia as a cause of mental hospital admissions.

CAUSES

There is no single cause of alcohol dependence. Three causative factors interact in the development of the illness: personality, environment, and the addictive nature of alcohol. Thus, if all other factors (such as the availability of alcohol) are equal, then inadequate, insecure, or immature personalities are more at risk than more emotionally mature individuals.

ALCOHOL AND PREGNANCY

The damage that alcohol can cause a fetus has been recognized only recently. Drinking more than two alcoholic drinks per day (e.g., two shots of whisky, two glasses of wine, or two bottles of beer) increases the chance of *fetal alcohol syndrome*. This disorder consists of facial abnormalities such as *cleft lip and palate*, heart defects, abnormal limb development, and lower-than-average intelligence. This level of drinking also increases the risk of miscarriage. Occasional binge drinking may cause the same effects even if the mother drinks little otherwise. Because a proportion of the alcohol from any drink reaches the baby, there is a risk that drinking even small amounts may disrupt normal development (causing, for example, low birth weight).

Fetal alcohol syndrome
An affected baby is abnormally short, has small eyes and a small jaw, and may have heart defects or a cleft lip and palate. He or she may suck poorly, sleep badly, and be irritable.

A

ALCOHOL AND THE BODY

Alcohol is a drug and, even in small amounts, its effects on the body are noticeable. Problems arise when people fail to take into account the effects of alcohol on tasks requiring coordination (such as driving) when they become intoxicated or when they become dependent on the drug. Alcohol dependence can cause early death and is a major factor in crime, marital breakdown, child abuse, accidents, and absenteeism. Prolonged heavy drinking that stops short of dependence may cause diseases such as *cirrhosis* of the liver and *cardiomyopathy*.

Alcohol in blood (milligrams per 100 millilitres)

Maximum legal driving limit

100 — 80 — 60 — 40

Time 12 2 p.m. 4 p.m. 6 p.m. 8 p.m. 10 p.m.

Cumulative effects of alcohol
It takes time for the body to eliminate even small amounts of alcohol. For instance, if you have two drinks at lunchtime and then one or two more early in the evening, by then your cumulative blood alcohol level could be over the legal limit for driving (80 mg of alcohol per 100 ml of blood; 0.08 on a breathalyzer).

EFFECTS OF INCREASING BLOOD ALCOHOL LEVELS

Concentration (milligrams per 100 millilitres)	Observable effects
30–50 / 150–200	Flushed face, euphoria, talkativeness, increased social confidence
50–150 / 200–350	Disturbed thinking and coordination, irritability, reduced self-control, irresponsible talk and behavior
150–250 / 350–500	Marked confusion, unsteady gait, slurred speech, unpredictable shows of emotion and aggression
250–400 / 500–700	Extreme confusion and disorientation, difficulty remaining upright, drowsiness, delayed or incoherent reaction to questions progressing to coma (a state of deep unconsciousness from which the person cannot be aroused)
400–500 / 700+	Risk of death due to arrest of breathing (although habitual drinkers may survive even such high levels)

☐ Occasional social drinker

▨ Alcoholic/problem drinker

Alcohol levels in different drinks
Alcoholic drinks come in many forms and contain varying levels of pure alcohol. It can be very difficult to estimate alcohol intake because the strengths of drinks vary. The measures shown here contain approximately equal amounts of pure alcohol.

355 ml of beer (5 percent by volume) = **178 ml of wine** (10 percent by volume) = **90 ml of sherry** (20 percent by volume) = **45 ml of whisky** (40 percent by volume)

LONG-TERM EFFECTS ON THE BODY

Persistent heavy drinking eventually damages body tissues; the main effects are shown below.

Liver
The liver is the main organ responsible for metabolizing alcohol from the blood; it manifests many of the long-term effects of heavy drinking. These effects include fatty liver, hepatitis, cirrhosis, and liver cancer.

Cirrhotic liver
In this condition, commonly caused by heavy drinking, bands of scar tissue form in the liver, impairing its function.

Brain and nervous system
Alcohol depresses the central nervous system. Prolonged alcohol abuse permanently impairs brain and nerve function.

Skin
Alcohol causes facial flushing, which becomes constant in heavy drinkers.

Heart and circulation
Prolonged heavy drinking can cause coronary heart disease, hypertension, heart failure, and stroke.

Digestive system
Irritation from large amounts of alcohol can cause gastritis and ulcers.

Urinary system
Alcohol acts as a diuretic, increasing urine output. Prolonged heavy drinking can cause renal failure.

Reproductive system
Alcohol increases sexual confidence, but high levels cause impotence.

Inherited, genetic factors probably play a part in causing dependence in some cases, but it is now widely believed that any person, irrespective of environment, genetic background, or personality, can become alcoholic if he or she drinks heavily for a prolonged period.

Environmental factors are important, especially the ready availability, affordability, and widespread social acceptance of alcohol in the individual's national culture and among the people he or she associates with. Thus alcoholism is much more common in certain countries, occupations, and social groups than others.

Stress is another important factor. Many formerly moderate drinkers begin to drink excessively at times of bereavement. Women may turn to drink when their adolescent children leave home.

Once social and/or psychological factors have induced heavy drinking, the discovery that taking alcohol in the morning relieves the withdrawal symptoms induced by the previous night's drinking tends to accelerate the development of dependence.

DEVELOPMENT OF DEPENDENCE

The development of alcohol dependence can be divided into four main stages, which merge imperceptibly. The time scale of these changes may be from 5 to 25 years, although the average is about 10 years.

In the first phase, tolerance (being able to drink more alcohol before experiencing its effects) develops in the heavy social drinker. Entering the second phase, the drinker experiences memory lapses relating to events occurring during the drinking episodes. In the third phase, there is loss, or lack, of control over alcohol; the drinker can no longer be certain of discontinuing drinking whenever he or she wants to. The final phase is characterized by prolonged binges of intoxication and by observable mental or physical complications.

Some people halt their consumption, temporarily or permanently, during one of the first three phases.

SYMPTOMS AND EFFECTS

BEHAVIORAL SYMPTOMS are varied and can include any combination of the following: furtive behavior (such as hiding bottles); aggressive or grandiose behavior; personality changes (such as irritability, jealousy, uncontrolled anger, selfishness); frequent changes of job; constant promises to oneself and others to give up drinking; changes in drinking pattern (e.g.,

switching to early-morning drinking, or changing from beer to spirits); neglect of food intake and personal appearance; and lengthy periods of intoxication.

PHYSICAL SYMPTOMS can also be varied. The drinker may exhibit any of the following: nausea, vomiting, or shaking in the morning; abdominal pain; cramps; numbness or tingling; weakness in the legs and hands; irregular pulse; redness and enlarged capillaries (small blood vessels) in the face; unsteadiness; confusion; lapses of memory; and incontinence. After sudden withdrawal of alcohol, the dependent person may experience *delirium tremens* (severe shakes, hallucinations, and convulsions).

In addition, alcohol-dependent persons are more susceptible than others to a wide variety of specific physical and mental diseases and disorders (see *Alcohol-related disorders*).

Physical and psychological problems may cause difficulties at home and at work. The person's marriage often suffers and there may be financial problems. Suicide threats and attempts may occur.

PREVENTION

Steps for avoiding the development of alcohol dependence include the following: keep to safe limits of alcohol intake as recommended by medical authorities; drink slowly instead of gulping; do not drink on an empty stomach; never drink to relieve anxiety, tension, or depression.

Nobody should ever feel (or be made to feel) embarrassed about refusing an alcoholic drink.

TREATMENT

Many alcoholics require detoxification (medical help in getting over their physical withdrawal symptoms when they stop drinking). Detoxification is followed by long-term treatment. Different methods of treatment—psychological, social and physical—are appropriate for different people, and may be combined.

PSYCHOLOGICAL TREATMENTS involve *psychotherapy* and are commonly carried out in groups. There are various types of *group therapy*.

SOCIAL TREATMENTS include help with problems at work and, in particular, the inclusion of family members in the treatment process.

PHYSICAL TREATMENT is needed only by some alcoholics. It generally includes the use of disulfiram, a drug that sensitizes the drinker to alcohol so that he or she is afraid to drink because of unpleasant side effects.

Alcoholics are strongly advised to use the self-help fellowship of organizations, such as *Alcoholics Anonymous*, where the alcoholic greatly benefits from meeting fellow sufferers who share their experiences.

Alcoholics Anonymous

A worldwide fellowship of people who readily admit to being alcoholics and who help each other stay sober. Alcoholics Anonymous (AA) was started in 1935 in the United States and now consists of an estimated 67,000 local groups and more than 1.5 million members in 92 countries. In Canada there are several groups in each large city and there is at least one group in all but the smallest towns. Contact addresses can be found in telephone directories.

Membership is open to anyone who has a drinking problem and has a desire to become and/or to continue to stay sober. There is no membership fee; the organization relies on voluntary contributions from members. Members are of all races, nationalities, and occupations, and range from people whose health, careers, and relationships were totally destroyed by alcoholism to those who sought help at a much earlier stage of the illness. AA is not affiliated with any sect, political party, institution, or other organization. It has a policy of cooperation with other organizations that fight alcoholism.

Local AA meetings are of two types. At open meetings, which anyone (including members' families) can attend, speakers describe their lives as alcoholics and the effect AA has had in helping them refrain from drinking. At closed meetings, which only members can attend, new members are invited to describe their drinking problems and their difficulties in abstaining. Other members who have had the same experiences suggest methods of staying sober and ways in which other problems can be surmounted. A program of recovery is suggested. Many members find that helping other alcoholics is the best way to remain sober themselves.

Members of AA do not reveal the names of other members to people outside AA. The fellowship does not keep membership records, monitor or attempt to control its members, engage or sponsor research on alcoholism, dispense drugs or psychiatric treatment, or provide detoxification, nursing, social services, or vocational counseling.

A

Alcohol intoxication

The condition, also known as drunkenness, that results from drinking an excessive amount of alcohol, often over a relatively short period (usually about 30 minutes to several hours). Alcohol causes acute poisoning if taken in sufficiently large amounts. It depresses the activity of the central nervous system (the brain and spinal cord), leading to loss of normal mental and physical control.

In extreme cases, a person who drinks a large amount of alcohol over a short period may lose consciousness and even die.

SYMPTOMS

The effects of a large alcohol intake depend on many factors, including physical and mental state, body size, social situation, and acquired tolerance (see *Alcohol*). Thus, a person may become "jocose, lachrymose, bellicose, or comatose" (cheerful, tearful, argumentative, or unconscious). There are wide individual variations. The important factor, however, is the blood alcohol level (see *Alcohol* and the body chart).

TREATMENT

For intoxication that stops short of coma, no treatment is required. Recovery takes place naturally as the alcohol in the person's body is gradually broken down in the liver.

If a drinker lapses into a coma, medical attention should be sought, particularly if the person is known or suspected to be diabetic or to have been taking another drug, whether prescribed by a physician (such as a sedative) or illicit (such as cocaine), in addition to alcohol. The person's clothing should be loosened and the mouth and back of the throat checked to make sure there is no obstruction to breathing. No attempt should be made to make the person drink water or to make him or her vomit. If breathing stops, *artificial respiration* should be carried out until breathing restarts or medical help arrives.

For a description of the chronic mental, physical, and social effects of long-term heavy drinking, see *Alcohol dependence* and *Alcohol-related disorders*.

Alcoholism

See *Alcohol dependence*.

Alcohol-related disorders

In addition to the many health and social problems that may result from *alcohol dependence*, and the high accident rate associated with *alcohol intoxication*, people who consume large quantities of alcohol on a regular basis are susceptible to a wide variety of physical and mental disorders.

Alcohol consumption can lead to tissue damage and disease by any, or a combination, of three main mechanisms. First of all, alcohol is a drug, and it or its breakdown products from metabolism can have a direct toxic or irritant effect on body cells and tissues.

Second, many alcoholics eat little or no nutritious food. Alcohol satisfies their calorie requirements and at the same time reduces appetite through an irritant effect on the stomach. However, alcohol provides no protein, vitamins, or minerals. Consequently, chronic alcoholics are prone

ALCOHOL-RELATED DISORDERS

Cancer	High alcohol consumption increases the risk of cancers of the mouth, tongue, pharynx (back of the throat), larynx (voice box), and esophagus, probably due to irritant action. In each of these cancers, alcohol	consumption along with smoking produces a much higher total risk of cancer than the sum of their separate risks. The risk of *liver cancer*, along with most types of liver disease, is also higher among alcoholics.
Liver damage and disease	Liver diseases caused by a high alcohol consumption include fatty liver, alcoholic *hepatitis*, *cirrhosis*, and liver cancer. They develop in sequence over a period of years. It is thought that a breakdown product of alcohol (acetaldehyde) has a toxic effect on liver cells and is the main cause of these diseases, although nutritional deficiency may also play some part.	The risk of alcoholic hepatitis and cirrhosis developing increases in proportion to the amount of alcohol consumed and the number of years of high consumption; liver cancer develops in about 1 in 5 sufferers of cirrhosis. However, about one third of heavy drinkers never get liver disease and in another third, only a fatty liver develops.
Nervous system disorders	Thiamine (vitamin B$_1$) deficiency, also known as *beriberi* (which disturbs nerve functioning), may develop in alcoholics. The effect of severe deficiency on the brain produces Wernicke's encephalopathy, with symptoms such as confusion, disturbances of speech and gait, and eventual coma. Korsakoff's psychosis may also occur (see	*Wernicke-Korsakoff syndrome*). The effect on the peripheral nervous system (nerve pathways outside the brain and spinal cord) produces polyneuropathy, with symptoms such as pain, cramps, numbness, tingling, and weakness in the legs and hands. Injections of thiamine and resumption of a normal diet can produce a dramatic cure.
Heart and circulatory disorders	Severe thiamine deficiency in alcoholics can cause *heart failure* (reduced pumping efficiency of the heart), usually combined with edema (fluid collection in the tissues). A high alcohol consumption also	increases the risk of coronary heart disease, of *hypertension* (high blood pressure) and of suffering a *stroke*. Heavy drinkers of certain beers risk *cardiomyopathy*.
Other physical disorders	Other physical diseases and disorders associated with a high alcohol consumption include *gastritis*, *pancreatitis*, and *peptic ulcer*, all probably linked	to an irritant action of alcohol. Heavy drinking during pregnancy carries a risk of the baby being born with *fetal alcohol syndrome*.
Psychiatric illnesses	Alcoholics are more likely than others to suffer from *anxiety* and *depression* (frequently related to financial, work, or family problems) and from paranoia. They are also more likely to	develop *dementia* (irreversible mental deterioration). The incidence of *suicide* attempts and actual suicide is also higher among alcoholics.

to diseases caused by nutritional deficiency, particularly deficiency of thiamine (see *Vitamin B complex*).

Third, a continual high level of alcohol in the blood and tissues can cause wide-ranging disturbances in body chemistry. These disturbances can lead to *hypoglycemia* (reduced glucose in the blood) and *hyperlipidemia* (increased fat in the blood), which may contribute to malfunction and disease of the blood vessels and such organs as the heart and liver. Irreversible damage can be done to the heart, liver, and brain, and this may result in premature death.

Aldosterone

A hormone secreted by the adrenal cortex (the outer part of the *adrenal glands*). Aldosterone plays an important role in the control of blood pressure, and in the regulation of sodium and potassium concentrations in the blood and tissues.

Aldosterone acts on the kidneys to decrease the amount of sodium lost in the urine; the sodium is reabsorbed from urine before it leaves the kidneys and is replaced in the urine by potassium. The sodium draws water back into the blood with it, thereby increasing the blood volume and raising the blood pressure.

The production of aldosterone is stimulated mainly by the action of *angiotensin* II, a chemical produced by a complex series of reactions that involves the enzymes *renin* (released by the kidneys) and converting enzyme. Aldosterone production is also stimulated by the action of *ACTH*, produced by the pituitary gland.

Aldosteronism

A disorder that results from the excessive production of the hormone *aldosterone* from one or both *adrenal glands*. Aldosteronism caused by an *adrenal tumor* is known as Conn's syndrome. Aldosteronism may also be caused by disorders, such as *heart failure* or liver damage, that reduce the flow of blood through the kidneys. Reduced blood flow through the kidneys leads to overproduction of *renin* and of *angiotensin*, which, in turn, leads to excessive aldosterone production.

SYMPTOMS

Symptoms are directly related to the actions of aldosterone. Too much sodium is retained in the body, leading to a rise in blood pressure; at the same time, excess potassium is lost in the urine. The low potassium level causes tiredness and muscle weakness and impairs kidney function, leading to overproduction of urine, and thirst due to fluid loss.

DIAGNOSIS AND TREATMENT

The diagnosis is suggested by a combination of *hypertension* (high blood pressure), a raised level of sodium in the blood, and a low level of potassium. Further tests may be needed to confirm the diagnosis.

Treatment in all cases includes restriction of salt in the diet and use of the diuretic drug *spironolactone*. This drug blocks the action of aldosterone on the kidneys, leading to increased loss of sodium from the body, lowered blood pressure, and reduced loss of potassium. If the cause of aldosteronism is an adrenal tumor, this may be surgically removed.

Alexander technique

A therapy that aims to improve health by teaching people to stand and move more efficiently.

Developed in the 1920s by F. Matthias Alexander, the technique is based on the belief that bad patterns of body movement interfere with the proper functioning of the body and thus contribute to the development of disease.

The Alexander technique does not claim to take the place of medicine but, by releasing unnecessary muscle tensions, it aims to eliminate or reduce the severity of a wide range of disorders, including back pain, asthma, and stuttering.

Training is carried out in one-to-one sessions with a qualified teacher.

Alexia

Word blindness; the inability to recognize and name written words, thus severely disrupting the reading ability of a person who was previously literate. The disability is caused by damage (e.g., by a *stroke*) to part of the cerebrum (the main mass of the brain) and is a much more severe reading disability than *dyslexia*.

Alienation

Feeling like a stranger, even when among familiar people or places, and being unable to identify with a culture, family, or peer group. Alienation is common in adolescents. It also occurs in people with financial problems or who are isolated by cultural or language differences.

In some people, alienation may be an early symptom of *schizophrenia* or part of a *personality disorder*. Feelings of alienation are also thought to be a contributing cause of suicide, attempted suicide, and inner-city violence.

Alignment, dental

The movement of teeth by either fixed or removable *orthodontic appliances* (braces) to correct *malocclusion* (incorrect bite).

Alimentary tract

The tubelike structure that extends from the mouth to the anus (see *Digestive system*). It is also known as the alimentary canal.

Alkali

Also known as a base, an alkali is chemically defined as a donor of hydroxyl ions (each of which comprises an atom of hydrogen linked to an atom of oxygen and has an overall negative electrical charge).

Examples of alkalis include *antacid drugs*, such as sodium bicarbonate (bicarbonate of soda) and aluminium hydroxide. Some alkalis, such as caustic soda (sodium hydroxide), are corrosive and cause *burns*. (See also *Acid*; *Acid-base balance*.)

Alkaloids

A group of nitrogen-containing substances obtained from plants. *Morphine*, *codeine*, *nicotine*, and *strychnine* are examples.

Alkalosis

A disturbance of the body's *acid-base balance* in which there is an accumulation of alkali (base) or a loss of acid.

There are two types of alkalosis: metabolic and respiratory. In metabolic alkalosis, the increase in alkalinity may be caused by taking too much of an *antacid drug* or by losing a large amount of stomach acid as a result of severe vomiting.

Respiratory alkalosis is caused by a reduction in the level of carbonic acid (derived from carbon dioxide) in the blood. This reduction is a consequence of *hyperventilation* (overbreathing), which may occur during a panic attack or at high altitudes due to lack of oxygen. (See also *Acidosis*.)

Allergy

A collection of conditions caused by inappropiate or exaggerated reactions of the *immune system* to a variety of substances. Many common illnesses, such as *asthma* and allergic *rhinitis* (hay fever), are caused by allergic reactions to substances that in the majority of people cause no symptoms.

A

ALLERGY AND THE BODY

An allergy is an inappropriate response (causing troublesome symptoms) to substances that, in most people, cause no response. The response is mainly to harmless substances that come in contact with the skin, respiratory airways, or the eye's surface. In diagnosing an allergy, the individual's medical history is important. The physician needs to know whether the symptoms vary according to the time of the day or the season, and whether there are any pets or other likely sources of allergens in the victim's home.

THE MOST COMMON ALLERGENS

Airborne		Foods	
	Grass pollens		Dairy products
	Tree pollens		Eggs
	Spores from molds		Strawberries
	House-dust mites		Fish and shellfish
	Animal dander		Cereals

Pollen
Airborne pollen from plants (especially from grasses and trees) may trigger an allergic reaction; symptoms appear during the warmer months. The most common reaction is allergic rhinitis (hay fever), which occurs when pollen is breathed in and irritates the nasal lining.

Animal dander
It is often assumed that allergy results from contact with animal hair. In fact, allergy is caused by flakes of dead skin (dander).

Feathers
Bedding containing feathers may produce an allergic reaction. Instead, use pillows and quilts containing synthetic stuffing.

Mites in house dust
Fragments of mites and their feces in house dust may cause an allergic reaction. Keeping the house dust-free helps.

DIAGNOSING SKIN ALLERGY

Tests are performed to identify specific reactions to allergens. Small amounts of various substances are applied to the skin. A wheal indicates sensitivity to a particular allergen.

Conducting a patch test
Three different allergens are put on a patch and taped to the skin.

Results are (left to right); no reaction; mild inflammation; severe contact dermatitis.

THE ORIGIN OF AN ALLERGY

The immune system is sensitized when it is exposed to an allergen (steps 1 to 3). Symptoms occur when allergens are met again (step 4).

Lymphocyte

Allergen

1 Allergens enter the body and are recognized by lymphocytes (blood cells that form part of the body's immune system).

Antibody

2 A few days to weeks later, the lymphocytes produce antibodies specific to the allergens.

Mast cell

3 The antibodies attach to cells in the tissues called mast cells, which contain packets of histamine.

Allergens

Histamine

4 Binding of allergens to antibodies on the surface of mast cells leads to the release of histamine and to the symptoms of allergy.

In susceptible people, allergies may result from exposure of the skin to a chemical, of the respiratory system to inhaled particles of dust or pollen, or of the stomach and intestines to a particular food. Allergic reactions occur only on second or subsequent exposures to the offending agent, after the first contact has sensitized the body.

TYPES AND CAUSES

The function of the immune system is to recognize *antigens* (foreign proteins) on the surfaces of microorganisms and to form *antibodies* (also called immunoglobulins) and sensitized *lymphocytes* (white blood cells). When the immune system next encounters the same antigens, the antibodies and sensitized lymphocytes interact with them, leading to destruction of the microorganisms.

In allergies, a similar immune response occurs, except that the immune system forms antibodies or sensitized lymphocytes against harmless substances—because these allergens (as they are called) are misidentified as potentially harmful antigens.

The inappropriate or exaggerated reactions seen in allergies are termed *hypersensitivity* reactions and can have any of four different mechanisms (termed Types I to IV hypersensitivity reactions). Most well-known allergies are caused by the Type I variety (also known as anaphylactic or immediate hypersensitivity).

TYPE I HYPERSENSITIVITY REACTIONS Common allergens that can cause Type I reactions include flower, grass, and tree pollens, animal dander (tiny particles of skin and hair), house dust, house-dust mites, yeasts, certain drugs and foods, and constituents of bee and wasp venom. Foods that contain substances that commonly provoke allergic reactions include milk, eggs, shellfish, dried fruits, and nuts.

These allergens cause immediate symptoms by provoking the immune system to produce specific antibodies, belonging to a type called immunoglobulin E (IgE), which coat cells (called mast cells or basophils) present in the skin and the lining of the stomach, lungs, and upper respiratory airways. When the allergen is encountered for the second time, it binds to the IgE antibodies and causes the granules in mast cells to release various chemicals, which are responsible for the symptoms of the allergy.

Among the chemicals released is histamine, which causes blood vessels to widen, fluids to leak into tissues,

and muscles to go into spasm. Symptoms may be restricted to the skin (itchy swelling or rash), upper airways (inflammation or mucus secretion, sneezing in hay fever, and spasm and narrowing of the airways in asthma), eyes (inflammation), or stomach and intestines (vomiting and diarrhea). Sometimes the symptoms affect several organs, especially when the allergies are to injected drugs, insect venom, or some foods. Particular conditions associated with Type I reactions include asthma, hay fever, *urticaria* (nettle rash), *angioedema*, *anaphylactic shock* (a severe, generalized allergic reaction), possibly atopic *eczema*, and many food allergies.

TYPES II TO IV HYPERSENSITIVITY REACTIONS These reactions have different mechanisms from Type I reactions (see *Hypersensitivity*) and are less often implicated in allergies. However, Type II reactions are responsible for autoimmune hemolytic *anemia* and *Goodpasture's syndrome*. Type III reactions are responsible for a type of lung disease called allergic *alveolitis* (which includes *farmer's lung*) and for the skin swellings that occur after booster vaccinations. Type IV reactions are responsible for contact *dermatitis*.

It is not known why certain individuals and not others get allergies, although about one person in eight seems to have an inherited predisposition to allergies (see *Atopy*).

TREATMENT

Whenever possible, the most effective treatment for allergy of any kind is avoidance of the relevant allergen. For example, anyone with an allergy to eggs should avoid eating eggs or any dishes containing eggs as an ingredient, and should check the recipes of dishes consumed in restaurants or at parties. If pollen is the allergen, it may be harder to avoid; measures such as keeping car windows closed while driving and closing bedroom windows at night afford some protection.

Drug treatment for allergic reactions includes the use of *antihistamine drugs*, which relieve the symptoms (the itching produced by an insect bite, for example). Most available antihistamine drugs have a sedative effect, which is particularly useful in treating the itching due to eczema because they permit the sufferer to sleep more soundly. Several of the newer antihistamines do not cause drowsiness, making them more suitable for daytime use.

Other drugs, such as *sodium cromoglycate* and *corticosteroid drugs*, can be

taken regularly to prevent symptoms from developing. Creams that contain corticosteroids are useful for treating eczema, but prolonged use on the same area can damage the skin. In severe allergic diseases, such as asthma, the use of inhaled or oral corticosteroids may be necessary.

Hyposensitization can be valuable for people who suffer allergic reactions to insect venom, house-dust mites, and some pollens. Gradually increasing doses of the allergen are given to promote the formation of antibodies that will block future adverse reactions. The therapy is effective in about two thirds of cases, but usually requires two to three years of treatment.

Hyposensitization can produce mild side effects, such as itching, swelling, or rashes; occasionally, more serious side effects occur, such as bronchospasm or anaphylactic shock, and deaths have even occurred in a very few cases. Low-dosage, long-acting methods of desensitization are being researched.

Allopathy

A term that describes conventional medicine as practiced by a graduate of a medical school or university granting the degree of Doctor of Medicine. (See also *Homeopathy*.)

Allopurinol

A treatment for *gout* that works by reducing *hyperuricemia* (raised levels of uric acid in the blood). Allopurinol does not relieve pain in acute attacks but, taken long term, does reduce the frequency of attacks.

POSSIBLE ADVERSE EFFECTS

These include itching, rashes, and nausea. Occasionally, during the first few weeks of treatment, allopurinol increases the frequency of gout attacks. *Colchicine* or a *nonsteroidal antiinflammatory drug* may be prescribed to counteract this effect.

Alopecia

Loss or absence of *hair*, which is usually noticeable only on the scalp but which may occur at any hair-bearing site on the body.

TYPES

HEREDITARY ALOPECIA This includes male-pattern baldness, the most common form of alopecia. Normal hair is lost initially from the temples and crown, where it is replaced by fine, downy hair. The affected area gradually widens as the line of normal hair recedes. This pattern of hair loss is inherited; it usually affects men,

A

although young women and women who have passed the menopause are occasionally affected.

Other hereditary forms of hair loss are rare. They may be due to an absence of hair roots or to abnormalities of the hair shaft, causing it to snap under the normal effects of sun, wind, shampooing, and combing.

GENERALIZED ALOPECIA In this rare form of alopecia, the hair falls out in large amounts, leaving a nearly invisible covering over the entire scalp. Such hair loss occurs because all the hairs simultaneously enter the resting phase and then fall out about three months later. Regrowth occurs when the underlying cause is corrected.

Causes include various forms of stress, such as surgery, prolonged illness, or childbirth. Many *anticancer drugs* cause temporary alopecia.

LOCALIZED ALOPECIA This may be due to permanent damage to the skin (e.g., by burns or *radiation therapy*). Another common cause of hair loss is trauma to the hair roots. Trauma may be due to excessive pulling of the hair to produce a particular hairstyle or, rarely, to *trichotillomania* (a disorder in which sufferers pull out their hair).

Stages in male pattern baldness
In this common form of alopecia, the man loses hair first from the temples and from the crown; the bald area then gradually widens.

The most common cause is alopecia areata, which produces localized areas of hair loss in which the bald skin looks and feels normal. The cause is unknown. Usually the hair returns to normal within a few months. There is no specific treatment.

Alopecia universalis is a rare, permanent form of alopecia areata that causes all the hair on the scalp and the body to be lost, including the eyelashes and eyebrows.

Ringworm infection of the scalp (see *Tinea*) may cause localized hair loss due to breakage of weakened hair shafts. Other skin diseases, such as *lichen planus, lupus erythematosus,* and *skin tumors,* may also be responsible. The bald skin always looks abnormal in conditions such as these and hair stubble can usually be seen in the affected area.

TREATMENT
Wigs and toupees are often used to disguise alopecia affecting the scalp. *Hair transplants* are sometimes successful as a permanent method of replacing the lost hair. The antihypertensive drug *minoxidil* may cause hair regrowth in some cases.

Alpha-fetoprotein

A protein produced in the liver and gastrointestinal tract of the fetus and by some abnormal tissues in adults.

ALPHA-FETOPROTEIN IN PREGNANCY
Alpha-fetoprotein (AFP) is excreted in the fetal urine into the *amniotic fluid*; the fluid is then swallowed by the fetus, which introduces AFP into the fetal digestive system. Most of the AFP is broken down in the fetal intestine, but some passes from the fetus into the mother's circulation. AFP can be measured in the maternal blood from the latter part of the first trimester of pregnancy, and its concentration rises steadily between the 15th and 20th weeks.

Raised levels of AFP are found in some cases of fetal abnormality and occasionally when the fetus is normal. In *neural tube defects,* such as *spina bifida* or *anencephaly,* excess AFP may leak into the amniotic fluid. AFP levels are also raised in certain kidney abnormalities and can result from reduced breakdown of AFP in the intestine if the fetus cannot swallow properly due to esophageal malformation.

AFP levels are also raised in multiple pregnancy (see *Pregnancy, multiple*) and in threatened or actual *miscarriage.* They may be mistakenly thought to be raised if there has been an error in the calculation of gestation dates. AFP levels may be unusually low in pregnancies in which the fetus has *Down's syndrome.*

TESTING AFP LEVELS IN PREGNANCY Ideally, pregnant women should be offered prenatal screening by measurement of blood AFP and by *ultrasound scanning* at about 16 weeks. Scanning is performed to date the pregnancy, to detect a multiple pregnancy, and to show certain fetal abnormalities. If the blood AFP level is raised, the test is repeated one week later. If the second result is also raised, the woman may be carrying a baby with a neural tube or other defect. An ultrasound scan may strengthen or confirm the suspicion. *Amniocentesis* (removal of a small amount of the fluid surrounding the fetus) may be performed, and further measurements of AFP may be made on the sample. If the level is significantly

raised, the chances that the woman is carrying an affected baby are high; a termination of pregnancy (see *Abortion, induced*) may then be considered.

About 10 percent of cases of neural tube defect are missed during screening because AFP levels are not significantly raised in all such cases. Conversely, in about 5 cases per 1,000 in which both amniotic fluid and blood levels of AFP are raised, the fetus is normal.

AFP IN ADULTS
In adults, AFP is produced in certain abnormal tissues. Levels are commonly raised in patients with hepatoma (see *Liver cancer*) and in those with malignant *teratoma* of the testes or ovaries. Some patients with cancer of the pancreas, stomach, and lung also have raised levels. Because it is present in abnormal quantities when a person is suffering from certain cancers, AFP is known as a "tumor marker." However, AFP levels are also raised in some noncancerous conditions, including viral and alcoholic *hepatitis* and in *cirrhosis.*

AFP levels can be used to monitor the treatment of hepatomas and teratomas; increasing levels after surgery or chemotherapy are a useful indicator of tumor recurrence.

Alprazolam

A *benzodiazepine drug* used to treat *anxiety, panic attacks,* and *phobias.*

ALS

Amyotrophic lateral sclerosis (see *Motor neuron disease*).

Alternative medicine

Any medical system based on a theory of disease or method of treatment other than the orthodox science of medicine as taught in medical schools.

Every society has its *folk medicine* and traditional healers who use methods and beliefs handed down through the generations. In some cultures, such as in China (see *Chinese medicine*), textbooks of traditional medicine date back several thousands of years. Some systems, such as acupuncture, are based on theories of disease that emphasize internal balances. Many cultures have a long tradition of healing based on *herbal medicine* and some plant-based remedies, after objective analysis, have been recognized by orthodox medicine.

The early 19th century brought the development of many new alternative systems, such as *chiropractic, homeopathy,* and *naturopathy.* The popularity of alternative practices declined in the 20th century because of the successes of orthodox medicine—notably vaccines, antibiotics, diuretics, antidepressants, and advances in anesthesia and surgery. More recently, a small but increasing number of people have questioned the ability of orthodox medicine to provide all the answers. Numerous new and rediscovered disciplines, such as *aroma therapy* and naturopathy, have won a following even though there is no conclusive scientific evidence supporting them.

Many alternative practitioners are sympathetic listeners who give sensible advice backed up by treatments that are sometimes successful. The opposition by many practitioners of orthodox medicine to alternative therapies is based on the principle that the essential first step in the treatment of any disorder is accurate diagnosis, which itself requires extensive medical knowledge. Treatment of symptoms without knowing their cause is potentially disastrous if an underlying remediable but progressive condition has not been recognized. Furthermore, some herbal remedies, although based on natural ingredients, may cause adverse reactions in some people and might also be dangerous if taken at the same time as conventional medicines.

Altitude sickness
See *Mountain sickness.*

Aluminum
A light, metallic element which is abundant in bauxite and various other minerals. Aluminum compounds are found in relatively low concentrations in the human body, where they have no known useful function and are almost certainly harmful.

Sources of ingested aluminum in humans include *antacid drugs*, cooking utensils and foil, some baking powders, and food additives such as potassium alum (used to whiten flour) and aluminum calcium silicate (used to keep salt running freely). Most of the aluminum taken into the body is excreted. The remainder is stored in the lungs, brain, liver, and thyroid gland.

Aluminum chloride is a common ingredient in *antiperspirants* and aluminum acetate is used as an *astringent* skin preparation.

ADVERSE EFFECTS
Some industrial processes, such as aluminum processing and explosives manufacturing, may give off minute

droplets containing aluminum into the air. Inhalation of such droplets is occasionally associated with various lung diseases, including *fibrosis* of the lungs and *emphysema.*

Prolonged use of antacids containing aluminum hydroxide can cause weakness, tiredness, and loss of appetite. Aluminum chloride in antiperspirants can cause allergic *dermatitis* in susceptible people.

Aluminum-induced *dementia* has developed in some patients undergoing *dialysis* (artificial purification of the blood) due to the aluminum content of the water used; this problem can be prevented by adequate monitoring procedures. Most neurologists doubt any causal association between aluminum and *Alzheimer's disease.*

Alveolectomy
See *Alveoloplasty.*

Alveolitis
Inflammation and thickening of the walls of the alveoli (tiny air sacs) in the lungs. Alveolitis reduces the elasticity of the lungs during breathing and reduces the efficiency of gas transfer between the lungs and the surrounding blood vessels.

Alveolitis is most commonly caused by an allergic reaction to inhaled dust of animal or plant origin, often containing fungal spores. Such allergic alveolitis may be related to occupa-

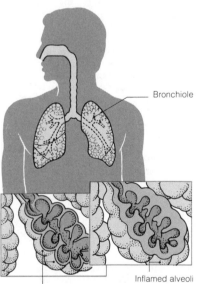

Bronchiole

Inflamed alveoli

Normal alveoli

Signs of alveolitis
The alveoli become inflamed and their walls thicken, causing the lungs to become less elastic and less efficient.

tion, as in cases of *farmer's lung* (caused by spores from moldy hay), *bagassosis* (caused by spores from moldy sugar-cane residue), and pigeon fancier's lung (caused by particles from bird droppings).

Fibrosing alveolitis may be an *autoimmune disorder* (a disorder in which the body's defense mechanisms produce antibodies that act against its own tissues). In some cases, fibrosing alveolitis occurs with other autoimmune disorders, such as systemic *lupus erythematosus* or *rheumatoid arthritis.*

Radiation alveolitis is inflammation of the alveoli caused by exposure to radiation, usually as a rare complication of *radiation therapy* treatment for lung or breast cancer.

SYMPTOMS AND DIAGNOSIS
Alveolitis usually causes a dry cough and the patient may have breathing difficulty on exertion.

A chest X ray usually shows mottled shadowing across the lungs. Blood tests may be performed to look for specific antibodies to an allergen or evidence of an autoimmune disorder. *Pulmonary function tests* show reduced lung capacity without obstruction to air flow through the bronchi. A lung *biopsy* (removal of a sample of tissue for analysis) may be the only way to make a conclusive diagnosis.

TREATMENT AND OUTLOOK
For fibrosing alveolitis, *corticosteroid drugs* may need to be taken indefinitely. For other types of alveolitis, a short course of corticosteroids may relieve symptoms.

If the cause of allergic alveolitis is recognized and avoided before lung damage occurs, there is often no permanent disability. In fibrosing alveolitis, the lung damage progresses despite treatment, causing increasing breathing difficulty and, sometimes, *respiratory failure.* The outlook for radiation alveolitis varies considerably, depending largely on the severity of the condition. (See also *Hypersensitivity; Pneumonitis.*)

Alveoloplasty
Dental surgery to remove protuberances and to smooth out other uneven areas from tooth-bearing bone in the jaw. The procedure is performed, before the fitting of dentures, on people whose alveolar ridge underlying the gums would not otherwise be even enough for dentures to be fitted easily or worn comfortably.

Minor alveoloplasty may be performed using a local anesthetic, but

A

most operations require general anesthesia (see *Anesthesia, dental*). An incision is made in the gum, which is then peeled back to expose the uneven bone. The bone is then either reshaped with large bone forceps or filed down to the required shape. Finally, the gum is drawn back over the bone and stitched together again. Some bruising and swelling of the mouth may occur, but the gum usually heals within two weeks.

Alveolus, dental
The bony cavity or socket that supports each tooth in the jaw.

Alveolus, pulmonary
One of a group of tiny, balloonlike sacs at the end of a bronchiole (one of the many small air passages in the lungs) where gases are exchanged during *respiration*. There are approximately 300 million alveoli in each lung, arranged in groups that resemble bunches of grapes.

ANATOMY OF THE ALVEOLI
These tiny sacs contain capillaries in their thin walls that allow oxygen to be absorbed into the blood.

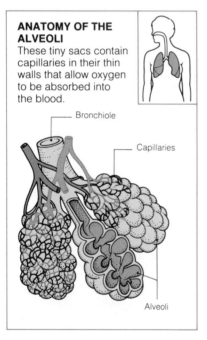

Bronchiole

Capillaries

Alveoli

Alzheimer's disease
A progressive condition in which nerve cells in the brain degenerate and the size of the brain substance shrinks. Alzheimer's disease is the single most common cause of *dementia* (a general decline in all areas of mental ability). Although originally classified as a "presenile" dementia, Alzheimer's disease is now known to be responsible for 75 percent of dementia

cases in people over 65 years old. Because of the increasing numbers of elderly people, interest in and research into the causes and treatment of Alzheimer's disease have greatly expanded in recent years. The progress of the disease (which, in most cases, means several years of intellectual and personal decline until death) cannot be arrested.

CAUSES
The cause of Alzheimer's disease is unknown, although a number of theories have been proposed, ranging from the effects of a chronic infection to those of toxic poisoning by compounds of metals such as *aluminum* (high levels of which have been found in the brains of people with Alzheimer's disease). There is also known to be a reduced level of *acetylcholine* and other brain chemicals in people with the disease. A genetic factor is another possibility; the disease is more common in people with *Down's syndrome*, and 15 percent of the victims of Alzheimer's disease have a family history of the disease.

INCIDENCE
Onset is rare before the age of 60, but thereafter increases steadily with age. Up to 30 percent of people over the age of 85 are affected.

SYMPTOMS AND SIGNS
The features of the disease vary among individuals, but there are three broad stages. At first, the patient becomes increasingly forgetful and may try to compensate by writing lists or seeking the help of others. Some deterioration in memory is a feature of normal *aging*, and this symptom alone is not evidence of dementia. Problems with memory due to Alzheimer's disease may cause the patient to feel anxious and depressed.

Forgetfulness moves almost imperceptibly into a second phase of severe memory loss, particularly for recent events. Victims may remember long-ago events, such as their schooldays and young adulthood, but they are unable to recall yesterday's visitors or what they saw on television. They also become disoriented as to time or place, losing their way even in familiar locations. Concentration and numerical ability decline and *dysphasia* (inability to find the right word) is noticeable. Anxiety increases, mood changes are unpredictable, and personality changes soon occur.

In the third stage, patients become severely disoriented and confused. They may also suffer from symptoms of *psychosis*, such as *hallucinations* and

Brain scan in Alzheimer's disease
The volume of the brain substance (gray area) has shrunk markedly. Its normal outline is shown by the dotted line.

paranoid *delusions*. Symptoms are worsened by the patient's disorientation and memory losses and are usually most severe at night. Signs of nervous system disease begin to emerge, such as abnormal *reflexes* (involuntary actions) and incontinence of urine and feces. Some patients become very demanding, unpleasant, and sometimes violent, and lose all awareness of social norms. Others become docile and helpless. They neglect personal hygiene and may wander purposelessly. Eventually the burden for caring relatives becomes impossible, and full-time hospital care and nursing are often inevitable. Once the patient is bedridden, the complications of *bedsores*, feeding problems, and *pneumonia* reduce life expectancy.

DIAGNOSIS
Alzheimer's disease is usually diagnosed from the patient's symptoms and signs. An *EEG* shows slowing of brain waves. *CT scanning* and *MRI* of the brain show evidence of reduced cerebral size. Tests of mental state indicate decreased intellectual ability.

Alzheimer's disease can be definitely diagnosed only by examination of the brain, either by *biopsy* (removal of a sample of tissue for microscopic analysis) or after death. Microscopic examination typically shows loss of nerve cells, specks of brain debris, and tangles of nerves that resemble pieces of unwound string.

Other tests should be performed to exclude other possible causes of symptoms resembling those of Alzheimer's disease. Some 10 percent of people with such symptoms have a treatable disease (such as *hypothyroidism*, *vitamin B$_{12}$* deficiency, a *brain tumor*, or a subdural *hematoma*). Other elderly people suffer from depressive pseudodementia, in which they appear to be demented but are actually suffering from the effects of *depression*, which may be treatable.

TREATMENT

The most important aspect of treatment for Alzheimer's disease is the provision of suitable nursing and social care for sufferers and their relatives. A good diet, exercise, and keeping occupied help alleviate anxiety and personal distress, especially in the earlier stages when the sufferer is still sufficiently aware of his or her condition. *Tranquilizer drugs* can often improve difficult behavior and help the patient to sleep. Counseling of sufferers' families can help prevent problems and minimize disruption of family life.

People with Alzheimer's disease are often best cared for at home. The provision of suitable day-care and short-stay facilities may reduce the burden on families and enable some people to continue living at home longer than would otherwise be possible. For advanced cases, however, inpatient care may be necessary.

Drugs, such as *tetrahydroaminoacridine*, that restore the acetylcholine content of the brain to normal are currently being tested, but results have proved disappointing. Research into drug therapy is continuing.

Amalgam, dental

A material used to fill teeth, consisting of an alloy of mercury with one or more other metals. Amalgam is soft enough to be easily workable by the dentist but sets rapidly (within two hours) into a hard, strong solid; it is therefore ideal for use as a filling, especially for back teeth (see *Filling, dental*).

Amantadine

An *antiviral drug* used in the prevention and treatment of *influenza* A. Amantadine has more recently been used to help relieve symptoms of *Parkinson's disease*.

Amaurosis fugax

Brief loss of vision, lasting for periods of seconds to minutes, usually caused by the temporary blockage of small blood vessels in the eye by tiny *emboli* (particles of solid matter such as cholesterol crystals or particles of clotted blood). These emboli are carried in the bloodstream from diseased carotid arteries in the neck or, rarely, from the heart. Sufferers typically experience a loss or dimming of vision, in one eye only, rather like a shade being pulled down or up.

Attacks may be infrequent or may occur many times a day. This symptom should never be ignored since it is a clear warning that the person has an increased risk of *stroke* or *coronary heart disease*. Medical investigation, with special attention to the state of the arteries, is urgently needed.

Ambidexterity

The ability to perform manual skills, such as writing or using cutlery, equally well with either hand because there is no definite *handedness* (preference for using one hand). Ambidexterity is an uncommon and often familial trait.

Amblyopia

A permanent defect of visual acuity in which there is usually no structural abnormality in the eye. In many cases there is a disturbance of the visual pathway between the retina and the brain. The term is also sometimes applied to toxic or nutritional causes of decreased visual acuity, as in tobacco-alcohol amblyopia.

If normal vision is to develop during infancy and childhood, it is essential that clear, corresponding visual images are formed on both retinas so that compatible nerve impulses pass from the eyes to the brain. If no images are received, normal vision cannot develop. If images from the two eyes are very different, one will be suppressed to avoid double vision, and normal vision may not develop in one of the eyes.

CAUSES

The most common cause of amblyopia is *squint* in very young children. In this condition, only one eye points at a selected object and the different image from the other eye is suppressed. Failure to form normal retinal images may also result from congenital *cataract* (opacity of the lens of the eye at birth), and severe, or unequal, focusing errors in a young child, such as when one eye is normal and the other eye has an uncorrected large degree of *astigmatism*, causing a blurred image on the retina. Toxic and nutritional amblyopia may result from damage to the retina and/or optic nerve.

TREATMENT AND OUTLOOK

It is important to treat amblyopia at an early age; after the age of 8, amblyopia usually cannot be remedied. For amblyopia due to squint, patching (covering up the good eye in order to force the deviating eye to function properly) is the usual treatment. Glasses and/or surgery to place the deviating eye in the correct position may be necessary. Glasses may also be necessary to correct severe focusing errors. Congenital cataracts may be removed surgically.

Ambulance

A vehicle for conveying sick, injured, or disabled people. An emergency ambulance takes acutely ill or severely injured people to hospital. In many parts of Canada an ambulance crew responds to 911 calls. The emergency ambulance usually contains stretchers, dressings, splints, analgesics, and oxygen and is staffed by emergency medical technicians. Some ambulances also contain intravenous fluids and equipment for diagnosing and treating *cardiac arrest*, and may be staffed by fully trained paramedical personnel. A nonemergency ambulance or Medicar is a van that takes people to and from outpatient clinics at hospitals.

Ambulatory care

A general term for care given to patients who are not in hospital.

Amebiasis

An infection caused by the ameba *ENTAMOEBA HISTOLYTICA*, a tiny single-celled animal parasite that lives in the human large intestine. The infection is characterized by recurrent moderate to severe diarrhea and, occasionally, the development of abscesses in the liver or, more rarely, in the brain or lung.

CAUSE AND INCIDENCE

Amebiasis occurs as a result of drinking water or eating food that have been contaminated by human excreta containing cysts of the ameba. Once swallowed, the walls of the cysts break down, and the amebae hatch out to parasitize the large intestine. In the intestine, the amebae multiply and develop protective capsules, forming new cysts. These cysts are passed out of the body in the feces, and can survive for long periods before the next person acquires them.

Amebiasis is prevalent in poor countries where standards of public hygiene and sanitation are low. Annual incidence in Canada has been as high as 2,100 cases. Prevalence tends to be highest among sexually promiscuous male homosexuals.

PREVENTION

Travelers to countries where sanitary standards are low can reduce their chances of acquiring amebiasis by drinking only water that has been bottled or thoroughly boiled (chlorine-releasing water-sterilization tablets are not very effective at killing amebic cysts) and by not eating uncooked vegetables (especially lettuce) or unpeeled fruit.

SYMPTOMS

Some people carry ENTAMOEBA HISTOLYTICA in their intestines and excrete cysts but have no symptoms, probably because the strain of amebae they carry is harmless.

Some strains of amebae invade and ulcerate the intestinal wall, causing diarrhea, which may vary in severity from two or more rather loose stools per day, accompanied by rumbling pains in the stomach, to full-blown dysentery, with high fever and the frequent passage of watery diarrhea accompanied by the passage of blood and mucus. Dysentery often recurs after short intermissions.

Amebae may spread via the bloodstream to the liver, where they cause abscesses. Symptoms of an amebic liver abscess include chills, fever, weight loss, and painful enlargement of the liver. Liver abscesses sometimes develop in people who are infected with amebae but who have never had digestive tract symptoms.

TREATMENT

Treatment of all forms of amebiasis is with drugs such as metronidazole or diloxanide, which effectively kill the parasite within a few weeks, leading to full recovery. Plenty of fluids should be drunk to avoid dehydration from diarrhea. Occasionally, it is necessary to drain a liver abscess.

Amebic dysentery

See Amebiasis.

Amebicides

A group of drugs used to treat amebiasis. Examples include chloroquine, diloxanide and metronidazole. They work by killing amebae in the intestine and in other body tissues.

Amelogenesis imperfecta

An inherited condition of the teeth in which the enamel is either abnormally thin or deficient in calcium. Affected teeth may be pitted and discolored (see Discolored teeth), and, depending on the type of imperfection, may be more susceptible to dental caries (tooth decay) and wear.

Amenorrhea

Absence of menstrual periods. Primary amenorrhea is defined as failure to start menstruating by the age of 16. Secondary amenorrhea is the temporary or permanent cessation of periods in a woman who has menstruated regularly in the past.

PRIMARY AMENORRHEA

The main cause of primary amenorrhea is the delayed onset of puberty. The delay is often not due to any disorder but, rarely, it may result from a disorder of the endocrine system, such as a pituitary tumor, hypothyroidism (underactivity of the thyroid gland), an adrenal tumor, or adrenal hyperplasia. Another rare cause of delayed puberty is Turner's syndrome, in which one female sex chromosome is missing.

In some cases, menstruation fails to take place because the vagina or the uterus has been absent from birth, or because there is no perforation in the hymen (the membrane across the opening of the vagina) to allow menstrual blood to escape.

SECONDARY AMENORRHEA

The most common cause of temporary secondary amenorrhea is pregnancy. Periods may also cease temporarily after a woman has stopped taking oral contraceptives; periods usually return after six to eight weeks but may not return for a year or longer in some cases. Secondary amenorrhea may also result from hormonal changes due to emotional stress, depression, anorexia nervosa, or certain drugs.

Rarely, periods may stop as a result of the same disorders of the endocrine system that can cause primary amenorrhea. Another possible cause of secondary amenorrhea is a disorder of the ovary, such as polycystic ovary or an ovarian tumor.

Amenorrhea occurs permanently after the menopause or following a hysterectomy (a surgical operation to remove the uterus).

INVESTIGATION

Investigation of amenorrhea usually includes a physical examination and blood tests to measure hormone levels. It may also involve laparoscopy to inspect the ovaries, CT scanning of the skull to exclude the possibility of a pituitary tumor, and ultrasound scanning of the abdomen and pelvis to exclude a tumor of the adrenal glands or ovaries.

TREATMENT

Some women with either primary or secondary amenorrhea may choose not to have treatment, but in every case the cause should be identified. Ovarian tumors or cysts should be removed surgically. Anorexia nervosa, too, needs treatment because of its long-term threat to health. If a woman with amenorrhea wants treatment and the cause is an endocrine disorder other than ovarian failure, ovulation can often be induced by treatment with clomiphene or gonadotropin hormones.

Ametropia

An optical defect of the eye, usually due to some distortion of the shape of the eyeball. (See Astigmatism; Hypermetropia; Myopia; Presbyopia.)

Amiloride

A potassium-sparing diuretic drug. Combined with loop or thiazide diuretic drugs, amiloride is used to treat hypertension (high blood pressure) and fluid retention due to heart failure or to cirrhosis of the liver.

Amino acids

 A group of chemical compounds that form the basic structural units of all proteins. Each amino acid molecule consists of nitrogenous amino and acidic carboxyl groups of atoms linked to a variable chain or ring of carbon atoms.

Individual amino acid molecules are linked together—by chemical bonds, called peptide bonds, between the amino and carboxyl groups—to form short chains of molecules called polypeptides. Hundreds of polypeptides are, in turn, linked together—also by peptide bonds—to form a protein molecule. What differentiates one protein from another is the sequence of the amino acids.

There are 20 different amino acids that make up all the proteins in humans. Of these, 12 can be made by the body; they are known as nonessential amino acids, because they do not need to be obtained from the diet. The other eight, known as the essential amino acids, cannot be made by the body and therefore must be obtained from the diet.

The 20 amino acids that make up proteins also occur free within cells and in body fluids. In addition, there are more than 200 other amino acids that are not found in proteins but which play an important part in chemical reactions within cells.

Aminoglutethimide

An anticancer drug that is used in the treatment of certain types of advanced breast cancer, prostate cancer, some endocrine gland tumors, and *Cushing's syndrome*, a hormonal disorder.

Aminoglycoside drugs

A group of *antibiotic drugs*. Aminoglycosides are generally reserved for the treatment of serious infections because their use can cause damage to the inner ear or kidneys. Important examples are *gentamicin*, *neomycin*, and *streptomycin*.

Aminophylline

A drug that is used to treat *asthma*, chronic *bronchitis*, and, occasionally, *heart failure*.

HOW IT WORKS

Aminophylline relieves breathing difficulty by widening the bronchi in the lungs. It also dilates (widens) blood vessels, thus improving blood flow from the heart, and increases the production of urine.

POSSIBLE ADVERSE EFFECTS

Nausea, vomiting, headache, dizziness, and palpitations may occur. During long-term treatment, blood tests may be carried out to monitor the level of aminophylline in the body.

Amiodarone

An antiarrhythmic drug used to treat various types of *arrhythmia* (irregular heartbeat). Long-term use of amiodarone may result in inflammation of the liver, thyroid problems, and damage to the eyes and lungs. Because of its possible adverse effects, amiodarone is usually given only when other drugs have not been effective.

Amitriptyline

A tricyclic *antidepressant drug* with a sedative effect. Amitriptyline is useful in the treatment of *depression* accompanied by *anxiety* or *insomnia*. Possible adverse effects include blurred vision, dizziness, and drowsiness.

Ammonia

A colorless, pungent gas that dissolves in water to form ammonium hydroxide, an alkaline solution (see *Alkali*). Ammonia consists of one nitrogen atom linked to three hydrogen atoms. Ammonia is produced in the body and plays a valuable role in maintaining the *acid-base balance*.

In severe liver damage, the capacity of the liver to convert ammonia to *urea* is diminished. This leads to a high concentration of ammonia in the blood, which is thought to be a cause of the impaired consciousness that occurs in *liver failure*.

Amnesia

Loss of the ability to memorize information and/or to recall information stored in *memory*. Amnesic conditions affect mainly long-term memory (where information is retained indefinitely) rather than short-term memory (where information is retained only for seconds or minutes).

Many people with amnesia have a memory gap that extends back for some time from the onset of the disorder. This condition, known as retrograde amnesia, is principally a deficit of recall. In most cases, the memory gap gradually shrinks over time.

Some people with amnesia are unable to store new information in the period following the onset of illness. The resultant gap in memory, known as anterograde amnesia, extends from the moment of onset of the amnesia to the time when long-term memory resumes (if at all). This memory gap is usually permanent.

CAUSES

Amnesia is caused by damage to, or disease of, brain regions concerned with memory functions. Possible causes of such damage are *head injury*, degenerative disorders (such as *Alzheimer's disease* and other forms of *dementia*), infections such as *encephalitis*, thiamine deficiency in alcoholics leading to *Wernicke-Korsakoff syndrome*, and also *brain tumors*, *strokes*, and *subarachnoid hemorrhage*. Amnesia can also occur in some forms of psychiatric illness (in which there is no apparent physical damage to the brain). Some deterioration of memory is a common feature of *aging*.

Amniocentesis

A diagnostic procedure in which a small amount of *amniotic fluid* is withdrawn from the *amniotic sac* (the membranous bag that surrounds the fetus in the uterus).

WHY IT IS DONE

The amniotic fluid contains cells and chemicals from the fetus that can be analyzed to detect fetal abnormalities, such as *Down's syndrome* and other chromosomal abnormalities. Amniocentesis can also help detect genetic disorders (such as *hemophilia*, *cystic fibrosis*, and *Tay-Sachs disease*), or developmental disorders (such as *spina bifida*). It is also used to assess fetal disorders, such as *Rhesus incompatibility*, and to check the maturity of the fetal lungs.

HOW IT IS DONE

Amniocentesis is usually performed between the 16th and 18th week of gestation. *Ultrasound scanning* is used to estimate the age and position of the fetus, the placental site, and the amount of amniotic fluid. A needle is then inserted through the abdomen and uterine wall into the amniotic sac, avoiding the fetus and placenta. A syringe is attached to the needle and about 20 to 30 ml of fluid is removed for analysis.

Anesthesia is not usually required, although occasionally a local anesthetic is used. In most cases, the woman can go home soon after the procedure but is advised to rest for about 24 hours.

RESULTS

The amniotic fluid is analyzed biochemically and fetal cells are cultured for *chromosomal analysis*. Culturing cells for chromosomal analysis may take up to four weeks and results may therefore not be available until about 20 weeks' gestation.

As well as identifying any fetal disorders that exist, chromosome analysis also reveals the sex of the fetus. A woman should therefore indicate whether or not she wishes to receive this information. Some laboratories do not report the sex of the fetus unless specifically requested to do so.

COMPLICATIONS

There is a slightly increased incidence of *miscarriage* or early rupture of the membranes after amniocentesis; recent studies show a risk of about 0.5 percent. Amniocentesis is therefore usually recommended only for women over the age of 35 (who are

Procedure for amniocentesis
A needle is introduced through the abdomen and uterine wall into the amniotic sac; a sample of amniotic fluid is then withdrawn.

more likely to have a child with Down's syndrome), or when there are other compelling medical reasons, such as a family history of a chromosomal abnormality. (See also *Chorionic villus sampling*.)

Amnion

One of the membranes that surround the *fetus* in the *uterus*. The outside of the amnion is covered by another membrane called the *chorion*.

Amnioscopy

An obstetric procedure in which an amnioscope (a tapering metal viewing tube) is inserted through the cervix toward the end of pregnancy to allow inspection of the *amniotic fluid* through the intact amniotic membrane. The amnioscope may also be inserted through the cervix during labor to allow a sample of blood to be taken from the fetal scalp, to check the condition of the fetus.

Amniotic fluid

The clear fluid (popularly called the "waters") that surrounds the fetus in the uterus throughout pregnancy. The fluid is contained within the amniotic sac (a thin membrane).

The fetus floats in the amniotic fluid and, in the early months of pregnancy, can move about freely. The amniotic fluid cushions the fetus against pressure from internal organs and protects it from any injury from the mother's movements.

The fluid is produced by the cells that line the amniotic sac and is constantly circulated. It is swallowed by the fetus, absorbed into its bloodstream, and then excreted by the fetal kidneys as urine. Amniotic fluid is 99 percent water. The remainder consists of dilute concentrations of the substances found in *blood* plasma, along with cells and *lipids* (fats) that have flaked off from the fetus.

Amniotic fluid appears during the first week after conception and gradually increases in volume until the 10th week, when the increase becomes very rapid. By 35 weeks' gestation the volume of fluid is about one litre. Thereafter it slowly declines until it is just over half a litre at term, though there is a wide variation between individuals.

In a small number of pregnancies, excessive fluid is formed; this condition is known as *polyhydramnios* or hydramnios. Less frequently, insufficient amniotic fluid is formed; this condition is called *oligohydramnios*.

Amniotic sac

The membranous bag that surrounds the *fetus* and fills with watery *amniotic fluid* as pregnancy advances. The amniotic sac is made up of two membranes; the inner *amnion* is covered by another membrane called the *chorion*.

Amniotomy

Artificial rupture of the amniotic membranes (breaking of the waters) performed for *induction of labor*.

Amoxicillin

A *penicillin drug* commonly used to treat a wide variety of infections, including *bronchitis*, *cystitis*, *gonorrhea*, and ear and skin infections.

Allergy to amoxicillin causes a blotchy rash and, rarely, fever, swelling of the mouth and tongue, itching, and breathing difficulty.

Amphetamine drugs

COMMON DRUG
Dexamphetamine

A group of *stimulant drugs* with an *appetite suppressant* effect. In the past, amphetamine drugs were commonly prescribed to treat *obesity*; this use has now been largely abandoned because of dependence problems and abuse. Amphetamines are now used mainly in the treatment of *narcolepsy* (a rare condition characterized by excessive sleepiness).

HOW THEY WORK

Amphetamine drugs stimulate the secretion of *neurotransmitters* (chemicals released by nerve endings), such as *norepinephrine*, which increase nerve activity in the brain and make a person wakeful and alert.

POSSIBLE ADVERSE EFFECTS

Taken in high doses, amphetamines can cause tremor, sweating, palpitations, anxiety, and sleeping difficulties. Delusions, hallucinations, high blood pressure, and, rarely, seizures may also occur. Prolonged use may cause *tolerance* and physical dependence (see *Drug dependence*).

ABUSE

Amphetamines are sometimes abused for their stimulant effects; for this reason, their prescription and use are regulated by the Food and Drugs Act, Part III (Controlled Drugs—General).

Amphotericin B

A drug used to treat fungal infections. Life-threatening infections, such as *cryptococcosis* and *histoplasmosis*, are treated by injection.

Adverse effects are likely only when amphotericin B is given by injection; these include vomiting, fever, headache, and, rarely, seizures.

Ampicillin

A *penicillin drug* commonly used to treat infections including *cystitis*, *bronchitis*, and ear infections. Ampicillin is also useful in the treatment of *gonorrhea*, *typhoid fever*, and infections of the *biliary system*.

Diarrhea is a common adverse effect. Some people are allergic to ampicillin and suffer from rash, fever, swelling of the mouth and tongue, itching, and breathing difficulty.

Amputation

Surgical removal of part or all of a limb. Amputation was formerly a common operation, especially in wartime, but is now rarely performed except in the treatment of severe arterial disease and cancer.

WHY IT IS DONE

Until the introduction of *antibiotic drugs* in the early 1940s, amputation was often necessary to prevent the spread of *gangrene* (tissue death) following infection of a wound.

Today, most amputations are performed on patients with *peripheral vascular disease*, in which a combination of *atherosclerosis* and *thrombosis* may completely block the blood supply to a limb, causing gangrene.

Amputation is also sometimes performed to prevent the spread of *bone cancer* or malignant *melanoma* (a type of skin cancer).

HOW IT IS DONE

Before the operation, the surgeon decides where on the limb to operate; the tissue at the amputation site must be healthy if the wound is to heal satisfactorily. Investigative techniques used at this stage include *angiography* (injection into an artery of a solution visible on X ray) and *thermography* (recordings of body-surface temperatures with a heat-sensitive camera).

During the operation, skin and muscle are cut below the level at which the bone is to be severed to create flaps that will later provide a fleshy stump. Blood vessels are tied off, the bone is sawn through, the area is washed with saline (salt solution), and the flaps of skin and muscle are stitched over the sawn end of bone to form a smooth and rounded stump.

While amputating, the surgeon tries to ensure that nerves are severed well above the stump, reducing the risk of pressure pain when a prosthesis (see *Limb, artificial*) is fitted. However, despite every precaution, a painful *neuroma* (a benign tumor of nerve tissue) sometimes develops.

In an amputation at the ankle (Syme's amputation), the tough skin of the heel pad is retained to cover the stump. The patient can then place weight on the stump without necessarily having to use a prosthesis.

Amputations below the knee are now more satisfactory than before. Newer techniques for shaping the stump make it easier to fit a prosthesis, and new prostheses, attached by suction rather than straps, are easier to put on and take off.

RECOVERY PERIOD

As the wound heals, bandaging and plaster casts are used to mold the stump to a shape suitable for accepting a prosthesis. The stump is usually swollen for about six weeks after the operation and a permanent prosthesis can be fitted only after it has settled down to a stable size. The patient with a lower limb amputation is usually fitted with a temporary prosthesis during this period to avoid becoming unaccustomed to walking.

For some time after an amputation, some patients have the unpleasant sensation that the amputated limb is still present—a phenomenon known as "phantom limb."

OUTLOOK

The prospect of a person who has had a leg amputation remaining mobile afterward depends on several factors: age, attitude, general health, the amount of limb lost, and whether the pressure of a prosthesis on the stump causes pain. Some healthy people lead almost as active lives as they did before, but many older people become confined to *wheelchairs*.

Amputation, congenital

The separation of a body part (usually a limb, finger, or toe) from the rest of the body, as a result of the part's blood supply being blocked by a band of *amnion* (fetal membrane) in the uterus. This may result in the affected part being completely separated, or showing the marks of the "amniotic band" after birth. (See *Limb defects*.)

Amputation, traumatic

Loss of a finger, toe, or limb through injury. (See also *Microsurgery*.)

Amyl nitrite

A *nitrate drug* formerly prescribed to relieve *angina pectoris* (chest pain due to impaired blood supply to the heart

muscle). Because amyl nitrite frequently causes adverse effects (including headache, hot flashes, palpitations, and restlessness) it has been superseded by other drugs.

Amyl nitrite is sometimes abused for its effect of intensifying pleasure during orgasm.

Amyloidosis

An uncommon disease in which a waxy, translucent substance called amyloid, composed of fibrous protein, accumulates in tissues and organs, including the liver, kidneys, tongue, spleen, and heart.

CAUSES

Amyloidosis may occur for no known reason, when it is called primary; more commonly, it is a complication of some other disease, when it is called secondary. Conditions that may lead to amyloidosis include *rheumatoid arthritis*, *multiple myeloma* (a cancer of bone marrow), *tuberculosis*, and some other long-standing infections, such as chronic *osteomyelitis* (bone infection). Exactly why amyloid is deposited in any of these circumstances is not known.

SYMPTOMS AND SIGNS

The symptoms and signs of amyloidosis vary, depending on which part of the body is involved.

Affected organs typically become enlarged. Accumulation of amyloid in the heart may result in *arrhythmias* (disturbances of the heartbeat) and *heart failure* (reduced pumping efficiency). If the stomach and intestines are affected, symptoms such as diarrhea may develop and the lining of these organs may become ulcerated. In some cases, the joints are affected, causing *arthritis*.

Primary amyloidosis is often characterized by deposits of amyloid in the skin. Slightly raised, waxy spots appear, usually clustered around the armpits, groin, face, and neck.

Some rare forms of amyloidosis are inherited. These forms of the disease tend to involve the nervous system. Symptoms include peripheral *neuropathy*, postural *hypotension*, urinary or fecal *incontinence*, and reduced *sweating*. Death may occur as a result of *renal failure* caused by deposits of amyloid in the kidneys.

DIAGNOSIS AND TREATMENT

Diagnosis of amyloidosis depends on microscopic and biochemical examination of a *biopsy* sample of patient tissue. Affected organs usually have a rubbery consistency and a waxy, pink or gray appearance.

There is no treatment, but secondary amyloidosis may be arrested or even reversed when the underlying disorder is treated.

Amyotrophic lateral sclerosis

See *Motor neuron disease*.

Amyotrophy

Shrinkage or wasting away of a muscle, caused by a reduction in the size of its fibers and leading to weakness. Amyotrophy is usually due to poor nutrition, reduced use of the muscle (as occurs when a limb is immobilized for a long period), or disruption of the blood or nerve supply to the muscle (as can occur in *diabetes mellitus* or *poliomyelitis*).

Anabolic steroids

See *Steroids, anabolic*.

Anaerobic

Capable of living and growing without oxygen. Many important bacteria are anaerobes and thrive in the intestinal canal or in tissue that has a poor supply of oxygenated blood. These species can cause diseases such as *food poisoning, tetanus*, and *gangrene*.

Some human body cells are capable of limited anaerobic activity. For example, when muscular exertion is so strenuous that oxygen is used faster than the blood circulation can supply it, the muscle cells can temporarily work anaerobically. When this happens, lactic acid is produced as waste (instead of the carbon dioxide from *aerobic* activity). The localized acid build up in the exercising muscle causes fatigue and pain, limiting the time for which anaerobic exercise can be tolerated. Compensation for this anaerobic activity requires oxygen to convert the lactic acid to glucose or to carbon dioxide, which explains why we need to continue to breathe rapidly after vigorous exertion. The deficit of oxygen that builds up in the muscles during exercise is known as the oxygen debt.

Anal dilatation

A procedure for enlarging the anus. Anal dilatation is used to treat conditions in which the anus becomes too tight, such as *anal stenosis* and *anal fissure*. It is also used as a treatment for *hemorrhoids*. Anal dilatation can be performed under general anesthesia by a surgeon, using fingers or an anal dilator. Minor dilatation can be performed by the patient, using a dilator and lubricating jelly.

Reflex anal dilatation, in which the anus dilates abnormally, may occur in certain disorders of the anus, in cases where there has been repeated anal penetration, and, sometimes, without any known cause.

Anal discharge

The loss of mucus, blood, or pus from the anus. *Hemorrhoids, anal fissures* (tears in the anal margin), and *proctitis* (inflammation of the rectum) can all cause anal discharge. The production of mucus from the anus tends to irritate the surrounding skin and may cause *itching* of the anus (known medically as pruritus ani).

Analeptic drugs

Drugs that stimulate breathing. Analeptic drugs, which include doxapram and nikethamide, are occasionally used in hospitals to treat *respiratory failure* in acute flare-ups of chronic bronchitis and after drug overdoses. Analeptic drugs may also be used to hasten recovery from a general anesthetic, and to treat *apnea* (absent breathing) in newborns.

Analeptics work by stimulating the respiratory center (a group of nerve endings in the brain stem that control the rate and volume of breathing).

Anal fissure

A fairly common anal disorder caused by an elongated ulcer that extends upward into the anal canal from the anal sphincter (the ring of muscle that surrounds the anal orifice). The fissure probably originates from a tear in the lining of the anus caused by the passage of hard, dry feces.

SYMPTOMS

There is usually pain during defecation and the muscles of the anus may go into spasm. There may be a small amount of bright red blood on feces or toilet paper.

TREATMENT

The tear often heals naturally in the course of a few days, although spasm of the anal muscles may delay healing. Warm sitz baths following bowel movements should bring some relief from painful spasms. Treatment of recurrent or persistent fissures usually includes *anal dilatation* (a procedure to enlarge the anus) and a high-fiber diet, including whole grain products, fruits, vegetables, and plenty of fluids, to soften the feces. Fissures usually heal within a few days after such treatment but surgery to remove the fissure is occasionally necessary. Healing occurs rapidly.

Anal fistula

An abnormal channel connecting the inside of the anal canal with the skin surrounding the anus.

An anal fistula is occasionally an indication of *Crohn's disease, colitis,* or cancer of the colon or rectum (see *Intestine, cancer of* and *Rectum, cancer of*). In most cases, an anal fistula results from an abscess that develops for unknown reasons in the anal wall. The abscess discharges pus, both into the anus and out onto the surrounding skin.

A fistula is treated surgically by opening the channel, removing the fistulous lining, and then draining the abscess of the pus it contains. The operation is performed under a general anesthetic.

Analgesia

Loss or reduction of pain sensation. Analgesia differs from *anesthesia* (loss of all sensation) in that sensitivity to touch is still preserved. (See also *Analgesic drugs.*)

Analgesic drugs

COMMON DRUGS

Nonnarcotic
Acetaminophen ASA Diflunisal Fenoprofen Ibuprofen Mefenamic acid Salsalate Sodium salicylate

Narcotic
Buprenorphine Codeine Dihydrocodeine Meperidine Morphine Pentazocine Propoxyphene

WARNING
Over-the-counter (nonnarcotic) analgesics should only be used for 48 hours before seeking medical advice. If pain persists, becomes more severe, recurs, or differs from pain previously experienced, consult your physician.

Drugs that relieve pain. The two main types are nonnarcotic and narcotic. Nonnarcotic analgesics include *acetaminophen; ASA;* and *nonsteroidal anti-inflammatory drugs* (NSAIDs) such as ibuprofen. Narcotic analgesics include *morphine* and related drugs.

WHY THEY ARE USED

Nonnarcotic analgesics are useful in the treatment of mild or moderate pain (e.g., headache or toothache). For more severe pain, a preparation combining one of the weaker narcotic analgesics (such as *codeine*) with a non-narcotic analgesic (such as ASA) is usually prescribed. In sufficient doses, the combination is more effective than either drug alone. The most potent narcotic analgesics are used only when other preparations would be ineffective.

HOW THEY WORK

When body tissues are damaged (e.g., by injury, infection, or inflammation), they produce *prostaglandins* (chemicals that trigger the transmission of pain signals to the brain). Nonnarcotic analgesics other than acetaminophen work by preventing prostaglandin production. Acetaminophen works by blocking the pain impulses in the brain itself, thereby preventing the perception of pain.

Narcotic analgesics act in a similar way to *endorphins* (substances formed within the body that relieve pain). They block pain impulses at specific sites (called opiate receptors) in the brain and spinal cord.

POSSIBLE ADVERSE EFFECTS

Adverse effects are uncommon with acetaminophen. ASA and NSAIDs may irritate the stomach lining and cause nausea, abdominal pain, and, occasionally, a *peptic ulcer.* Nausea, vomiting, drowsiness, constipation, and breathing difficulties may occur with narcotic analgesics. The stronger narcotic analgesics may also produce a feeling of euphoria.

The euphoric effects produced by some narcotic analgesics have led to their abuse. In most cases, long-term abuse causes *tolerance* and physical dependence (see *Drug dependence*). In Canada both the manufacture and the distribution of strong narcotic analgesics are controlled by the Narcotic Control Act.

Anal stenosis

A tightness of the anus, sometimes referred to as anal stricture. Anal stenosis prevents the normal passage of feces, causing constipation and pain during defecation.

The condition may be present from birth, or may be caused by a number of conditions in which scarring has occurred, such as *anal fissure, colitis,* or cancer of the anus. Anal stenosis sometimes occurs after surgery on the anus (e.g., to treat *hemorrhoids*).

Anal stenosis is treated by *anal dilatation* (a procedure to enlarge the anus), which may be performed by the patient.

Anal stricture

See *Anal stenosis.*

A

HOW ANALGESICS WORK

When tissue is damaged (for example, by injury, inflammation, or infection) the body produces prostaglandins. These substances combine with receptors (specific sites on the surface of cells in the brain and spinal cord). As a result, a signal is passed along a series of nerve cells to the brain, where the signal is interpreted as pain by brain cells. Analgesics (except for acetaminophen) work either by preventing the production of prostaglandins or by blocking pain impulses in the brain and spinal cord. Acetaminophen works by blocking the pain impulses in the brain itself. This action prevents the perception of pain.

Action of nonnarcotics
Nonnarcotic drugs block the production of prostaglandins (chemicals released in response to tissue damage). This action prevents stimulation of the nerve endings, so that no pain signal passes on to the brain. As a result, these drugs provide pain relief.

Action of narcotics
When tissue damage occurs, the body produces prostaglandins, chemicals that trigger the transmission of pain signals (above). Normally, the pain signal is transmitted between brain cells, but narcotic drugs (below) combine with opiate receptors to prevent the signals from being transmitted.

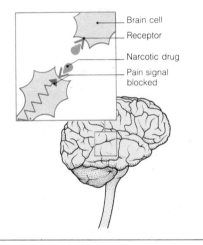

Analysis, chemical

Determination of the identity of a substance or of the individual chemical constituents of a mixture. Analysis may be qualitative, as in determining whether or not a particular substance is present, or it may be quantitative, that is, measuring the amount or concentration of one or more constituents. (See also *Assay*.)

Analysis, psychological

See *Psychoanalysis*.

Analysis scientific

See *Analysis, chemical*.

Anaphylactic shock

A rare, severe, frightening, and life-threatening allergic reaction. It is a Type I hypersensitivity reaction (see *Allergy*) that occurs rarely in people in whom an extreme sensitivity to a particular substance (allergen) has developed. The reaction occurs most commonly after an *insect sting* or as a reaction to an injected drug (e.g., penicillin, antitetanus serum, a local anesthetic, or during *hyposensitization* for an allergy). Less commonly, the reaction occurs after a particular food or drug has been taken by mouth.

Entry of the allergen into the bloodstream provokes the release of massive amounts of *histamine* and other chemicals that have effects on body tissues. The blood vessels widen, with a sudden severe lowering of blood pressure. Other symptoms include an itchy, raised rash, bronchospasm (constriction of the airways in the lungs), pain in the abdomen, swelling of the tongue or throat, and diarrhea.

FIRST AID AND TREATMENT
If a person becomes severely ill or collapses soon after an insect sting, injection, or eating a particular food, medical help should be summoned immediately. Call 911, which can send a physician or an ambulance.

The victim should be laid down and the legs raised to improve blood flow to the heart and brain. An injection of *epinephrine* is often life saving and must be given as soon as possible.

People who have suffered previous severe allergic reactions should carry a preloaded syringe of epinephrine, so that they can inject themselves (if still conscious) or can have the dose administered promptly by someone familiar with the method of injection. Otherwise, medical help should be awaited. If the person's breathing or heartbeat stops, *cardiopulmonary resuscitation* should be performed. In addition to epinephrine (injections of which may need to be repeated until the victim's condition improves), a physician may also administer *antihistamine drugs* and *corticosteroid drugs*.

Individuals who have suffered anaphylactic reactions to insect venom may respond to a course of desensitizing injections (see *Hyposensitization*, although this treatment itself carries a risk of repetition of the anaphylaxis and therefore should be carried out only by a physician with a supply of epinephrine and other emergency medications at hand.

Anastomosis

A natural or artificial communication between two tubular cavities or blood vessels that may or may not normally be joined.

A natural anastomosis usually takes the form of two blood vessels joining (see *Arteriovenous fistula*). Surgical anastomosis is used to treat various disorders. For example, if an artery is blocked by *thrombosis* (clot) or *atheroma* (fat deposits), an operation may be performed to remove the blockage and directly connect the two ends of the vessel. Alternatively, an operation to bypass the blockage may be performed by joining a synthetic substitute or a section of a .vein from the patient to the artery above and below the obstruction.

Another common use of surgical anastomosis is to treat intestinal obstruction: the obstructed section of intestine may be cut out and the healthy ends joined, or the obstruction may be bypassed by making two openings in a loop of the intestine (one either side of the defective area) and joining together the two openings. (See also *Bypass surgery*.)

Anatomy

The structure of the body of any living thing, and its scientific study. The science of human anatomy dates back to ancient Egyptian times and, together with *physiology* (the study of the functioning of the body), forms the foundation of all medical science. Dissection of human *cadavers* provides the primary source of information for anatomists today.

The ancient Greek physician Galen produced many medical treatises containing some anatomical descriptions that are still in use today, but his work is also full of gross errors. It was not until 1543 that the first accurate, comprehensive anatomical text, "De Humani Corporis Fabrica" ("On the structure of the human body"), was produced by the Flemish scientist Andreas Vesalius.

BRANCHES OF ANATOMY

Anatomy as a scientific study today is subdivided into many branches. These include comparative anatomy (the study of the differences between human and animal bodies), surgical anatomy (the practical knowledge required by surgeons, especially recognition of the surface markings of internal organs and the pattern of blood vessels within them), *embryology* (the study of structural changes that occur during the development of the embryo and fetus), systematic anatomy (the study of the structure of particular body systems, such as the urinary system), and *cytology* and *histology* (the microscopic study of, respectively, cells and tissues).

DESCRIPTIVE TERMS

In textbook descriptions of human anatomy, the body is assumed to be standing upright, with the arms hanging down and the palms facing forward. The body is divided by the median (also called the sagittal) plane into right and left halves, and by the central coronal plane into front (anterior or ventral) and rear (posterior or dorsal) halves.

Every anatomical structure is scientifically named in Latin, but today anatomists prefer to use simpler terms when they exist. For example, the main blood vessel in the thigh is usually called the femoral artery rather than the arteria femoralis.

Ancylostomiasis

See *Hookworm infestation*.

Androgen drugs

Natural or synthetic *androgen hormones* used as drugs; one of the most important of these drugs is *testosterone*.

Androgen drugs are used in the treatment of male *hypogonadism* (underactivity of the testes) to stimulate the development of sexual characteristics, such as growth of facial and pubic hair, enlargement of the genitals, and deepening of the voice. This treatment improves libido and potency but does not increase the production of sperm.

Androgen drugs are also used to stimulate production of new blood cells by the bone marrow in aplastic *anemia*. They may also occasionally be used in the treatment of certain types of *breast cancer*.

Androgen drugs are commonly used by athletes and bodybuilders wishing to increase muscle bulk and strength, but this practice is condemned by physicians due to doubts concerning the drugs' benefits and the risk of adverse effects.

POSSIBLE ADVERSE EFFECTS

Adverse effects include fluid retention, weight gain, increased levels of cholesterol in the blood, and, rarely, liver damage. When taken by women the drugs can cause deepening of the voice and other male characteristics, especially growth of facial hair. Because androgen drugs affect sexual development in babies, they are not prescribed during pregnancy or breast-feeding. They are prescribed with caution during adolescence because they may prematurely halt the growth of the long bones.

Androgen hormones

A group of hormones that cause *virilization* (development of male secondary sexual characteristics, such as the growth of facial hair, deepening of the voice, and increase in muscle bulk).

FORMATION

Androgens are produced by specialized cells in the testes in males and in the adrenal glands in both sexes. The ovaries secrete very small quantities of

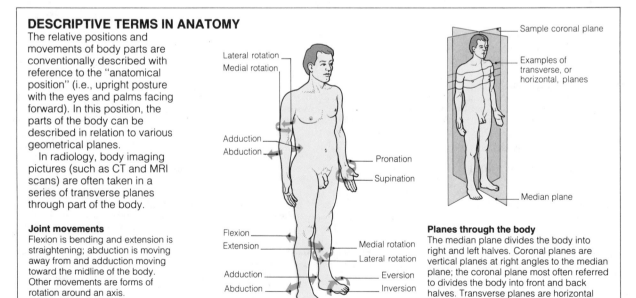

DESCRIPTIVE TERMS IN ANATOMY

The relative positions and movements of body parts are conventionally described with reference to the "anatomical position" (i.e., upright posture with the eyes and palms facing forward). In this position, the parts of the body can be described in relation to various geometrical planes.

In radiology, body imaging pictures (such as CT and MRI scans) are often taken in a series of transverse planes through part of the body.

Joint movements

Flexion is bending and extension is straightening; abduction is moving away from and adduction moving toward the midline of the body. Other movements are forms of rotation around an axis.

Lateral rotation
Medial rotation
Adduction
Abduction
Pronation
Supination
Flexion
Extension
Medial rotation
Lateral rotation
Adduction
Abduction
Eversion
Inversion

Sample coronal plane
Examples of transverse, or horizontal, planes
Median plane

Planes through the body

The median plane divides the body into right and left halves. Coronal planes are vertical planes at right angles to the median plane; the coronal plane most often referred to divides the body into front and back halves. Transverse planes are horizontal slices through the body.

androgens until the menopause. The most active androgen is *testosterone*, which is produced in the testes. Androgens produced by the adrenal glands are less active than testicular androgens, and have no significant masculinizing effects unless produced to excess.

The production of androgens by the testes is controlled by certain pituitary hormones, called *gonadotropins*. Adrenal androgens are controlled by *ACTH*, another pituitary hormone.

EFFECTS
Androgens stimulate the appearance of male secondary sexual characteristics at puberty, including enlargement of the penis and growth of facial and body hair. Androgens have what is called an anabolic effect, that is, they raise the rate of protein synthesis and lower the rate at which it is broken down. This increases muscle bulk, especially in the chest and shoulders, and accelerates growth, especially during early puberty. At the end of puberty, androgens cause the long bones to stop growing.

Androgens also promote aggression, a characteristically male trait. They stimulate sebum secretion, which, if excessive, causes *acne*. In early adult life, androgens promote male-pattern baldness. Absence of androgens protects against male-pattern baldness.

ANDROGEN DEFICIENCY
Adult males may be deficient in androgens if their *testes* are diseased or if the pituitary gland fails to secrete gonadotropins. Such men are termed "hypogonadal." The effects of androgen deficiency vary according to whether the deficiency develops before or after puberty. Typical effects include decreased body hair and beard growth, smooth skin, a high-pitched voice, reduced sexual drive and performance, underdevelopment of the genitalia, and poor muscle development.

ANDROGEN EXCESS
Overproduction of androgens may be the result of adrenal disorders (see *Adrenal hyperplasia, congenital; Adrenal tumors*), of testicular tumors (see *Testis, cancer of*), or, rarely, of androgen-secreting ovarian tumors (see *Ovary, cancer of*).

In adult males, excess androgens accentuate male physical characteristics. In boys, they cause premature sexual development. Initially they increase bone growth but adult height is reduced because they cause the long bones to stop growing.

In females, excess androgens cause virilization, that is, the development of masculine features such as increase in body hair, deepening of the voice, clitoral enlargement, and *amenorrhea* (absence of menstruation).

Anemia
A condition in which the concentration of the oxygen-carrying pigment *hemoglobin* in the blood is below normal. Hemoglobin molecules are carried inside red *blood cells* and transport oxygen from the lungs to the tissues. Under normal circumstances, stable hemoglobin concentrations in the blood are maintained by a strict balance between red cell production in the bone marrow and red cell destruction in the spleen. Anemia may result if this balance is upset.

By far the most common form of anemia worldwide is due to a deficiency of iron, an essential component of hemoglobin. However, there are numerous other causes of anemia, which is not a disease in itself but a feature of many different disorders.

TYPES AND CAUSES
Red blood cells are formed in the bone marrow over a period of about five days from less specialized cells called stem cells. During this time, the cells change their appearance and accumulate hemoglobin. The red cells released from the bone marrow into the blood are called reticulocytes. Over a few days, reticulocytes mature into adult red blood cells. The adult cells circulate in the bloodstream for about 120 days; they age and are eventually trapped in small blood vessels (mainly in the spleen) and destroyed. Some cell components, including iron, are recycled for use in new cells.

The various forms of anemia can be classified into those caused by decreased or defective production of red cells by the bone marrow (see *Anemia, aplastic; Anemia, iron-deficiency; Anemia, megaloblastic*) and those caused by decreased survival of the red cells in the blood (see *Anemia, hemolytic*). See the box on page 100.

SYMPTOMS
The symptoms common to all forms of anemia result from the reduced oxygen-carrying capacity of the blood. Their severity depends on how low the hemoglobin concentration in the blood is. Normal blood hemoglobin concentrations are in the range 13.5 to 18 g/100 ml for men and 11.5 to 16 g/100 ml for women. Concentrations below 10 g/100 ml can cause headaches, tiredness, and lethargy.

Concentrations below 8 g/100 ml can cause breathing difficulty on exercise, dizziness due to reduced oxygen reaching the brain, *angina pectoris* due to reduced oxygen supply to the heart muscle, and palpitations as the heart works harder to compensate. General signs include pallor, particularly of the skin creases, the lining of the mouth, and the inside of the eyelids, although this is not a reliable indicator of the severity of the anemia.

Symptoms also depend to some extent upon the speed of development of an anemia. The slow development of anemia is tolerated well until it becomes advanced; the sudden development of anemia causes more immediate symptoms.

Other features may occur with particular forms of anemia. For example, some degree of *jaundice* occurs in most types of hemolytic anemia, because the high rate of destruction of red cells leads to an increased level of the yellow pigment bilirubin (produced by the breakdown of the hemoglobin in red cells) in the blood.

DIAGNOSIS
Anemia is diagnosed from the patient's symptoms and by the measurement of a low level of hemoglobin in the blood. To establish the type and cause of the anemia, a sample of blood is first examined under the microscope, the numbers of different types of blood cells are counted, and their appearance is noted (see *Blood count; Blood film*). A low proportion of reticulocytes suggests that the cause is decreased production of red cells; a high proportion of reticulocytes suggests that cells are being destroyed at a high rate. The size of the red cells—whether small, normal, or large—provides further clues. With some specific forms—for example, *sickle cell anemia* (a type of hemolytic anemia)—some of the red cells have an abnormal shape.

Other investigations that may help the diagnosis include examination of cells in the bone marrow by means of a *bone marrow biopsy* and measurement of the levels of substances such as folic acid, bilirubin, and vitamin B_{12} in the blood. Sometimes, further investigations must be carried out to establish the exact cause.

Treatment is directed toward correcting, modifying, or diminishing the mechanism or process that is leading to defective red cell production or reduced red cell survival. Treatment tends to be more straightforward for anemias caused by deficiencies (iron-

TYPES AND CAUSES OF ANEMIA

Anemia results either from reduced or defective production or from an excessively high rate of destruction of oxygen-carrying red blood cells.

Four of the main types are shown below, but anemia can have many other causes (such as various forms of leukemia).

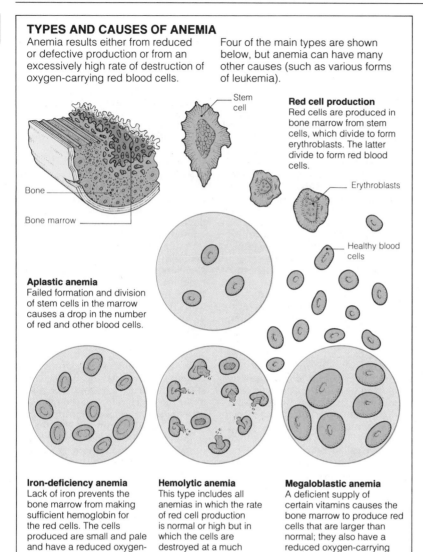

Red cell production
Red cells are produced in bone marrow from stem cells, which divide to form erythroblasts. The latter divide to form red blood cells.

Stem cell

Bone

Bone marrow

Erythroblasts

Healthy blood cells

Aplastic anemia
Failed formation and division of stem cells in the marrow causes a drop in the number of red and other blood cells.

Iron-deficiency anemia
Lack of iron prevents the bone marrow from making sufficient hemoglobin for the red cells. The cells produced are small and pale and have a reduced oxygen-carrying capacity.

Hemolytic anemia
This type includes all anemias in which the rate of red cell production is normal or high but in which the cells are destroyed at a much faster rate than normal.

Megaloblastic anemia
A deficient supply of certain vitamins causes the bone marrow to produce red cells that are larger than normal; they also have a reduced oxygen-carrying capacity.

deficiency and megaloblastic anemias) than for those caused by inherited disorders or other disease processes (*thalassemia* and many types of hemolytic anemia).

Anemia, aplastic

A rare but important type of *anemia* in which the red cells, white cells, and platelets in the blood are all reduced in number. Aplastic anemia is caused by a failure of the *bone marrow* to produce stem cells, which are the initial form of all blood cells.

CAUSES AND INCIDENCE

Treatment of cancer with *radiation therapy* or *anticancer drugs* can interfere with the bone marrow's cell-produc-

ing capacity, as can certain viral infections and other drugs. In these cases, the marrow usually recovers and resumes normal production of cells once the cause is removed.

Long-term exposure to the fumes of benzene (a constituent of gasoline) or insecticides has been implicated as a cause of more persistent aplastic anemia, and a moderate to high dose of nuclear radiation (from radioactive fallout or nuclear explosions) is another recognized cause. In about half of all cases an autoimmune process is responsible (see *Autoimmune disorders*). In other people, aplastic anemia develops for no known reason—a condition that is known as pri-

mary or idiopathic aplastic anemia. This can can occur at any age but is most common around the age of 30.

SYMPTOMS

A low level of red blood cells may result in symptoms common to all types of anemia, such as fatigue and breathlessness. Deficiency of white cells increases susceptibility to infections, while deficiency of platelets may cause a tendency to bruise easily, bleeding gums, or nosebleeds.

DIAGNOSIS

The disorder is usually suspected from the results of a blood test, particularly a *blood count*, and is confirmed by a *bone marrow biopsy*, in which a small sample of marrow is removed and examined for the presence or absence of blood-forming cells.

TREATMENT

When aplastic anemia is due to infection or treatment for cancer, transfusions of red cells and platelets are given until the marrow returns to normal. When the anemia is thought to be due to an autoimmune process, the usual first line of treatment is immunosuppression (therapy to suppress the immune system).

In persistent aplastic anemia, a *bone marrow transplant* may be carried out if a suitable donor is available. The donor must be someone (usually a brother or sister) whose tissue type closely matches that of the patient.

OUTLOOK

Recovery usually occurs from mild forms of the disease. However, without a bone marrow transplant, severe aplastic anemia is often fatal.

Anemia, hemolytic

A form of *anemia* (a reduced level of the oxygen-carrying pigment *hemoglobin* in the blood) caused by the premature destruction of red cells in the bloodstream—a process known as hemolysis. The bone marrow has the capacity to increase red cell production approximately sixfold over normal rates. Anemia results only if the shortening of the life span of red cells is sufficiently severe to overcome the marrow's reserve capacity.

TYPES AND CAUSES

Hemolytic anemias can be classified according to whether the cause of the problem is inside the red cells, in which case it is usually an inherited condition, or whether it is outside the cells, in which case it is usually acquired later in life.

RED CELL DEFECTS When hemolysis is due to a defect within the red cells, the underlying problem is an abnormal rigidity of the cell membrane (the envelope that surrounds each cell). This causes the cells to become trapped at an early stage of their life span in the smaller blood vessels (usually of the spleen) and eventually to be destroyed by macrophages (types of cell which ingest foreign and dead particles).

The abnormal rigidity may result from an inherited defect of the cell membrane (as in hereditary *spherocytosis*), from a defect of the hemoglobin within the cell (as in *sickle cell anemia*), or from a defect of one of the cell's enzymes. Only two chemical processes occurring in red cells are essential to their survival—one provides energy and one helps protect the cells from chemical damage. The last process is of great importance; a deficiency of one of the enzymes that catalyze the process, called glucose-6-phosphate dehydrogenase (see *G6PD deficiency*), is a common cause of hemolytic anemia in some countries. One variety of G6PD deficiency occurs among black people and another is common in Greece (see *Favism*).

DEFECTS OUTSIDE THE RED CELL Hemolytic anemias resulting from defects outside the red cells fall into three main groups. First are disorders in which red cells are destroyed by mechanical buffeting (e.g., when the lining of the blood vessels is abnormal, when the blood flows past artificial surfaces such as replacement heart valves, or in conditions in which a blood clot has formed inside a blood vessel). In all these conditions, the otherwise normal red cell is physically disrupted by mechanical forces.

In a second group of conditions, the red cells are destroyed by antibodies produced by the *immune system* and directed against the red cells. These immune hemolytic anemias may occur if foreign blood cells enter the bloodstream, as during an incompatible blood transfusion, or if the immune system becomes defective and fails to recognize the body's own red cells. This is a type of *autoimmune disorder*. Sometimes, the reaction is triggered by a drug such as methyldopa. In *hemolytic disease of the newborn*, the baby's red cells are destroyed by antibodies produced by the mother crossing the placenta. In most cases, however, the cause of immune hemolytic anemia is unknown.

In a third group of conditions, the red cells are destroyed by microorganisms in the blood. By far the most important cause is *malaria*.

SYMPTOMS AND DIAGNOSIS
People with hemolytic anemia may have symptoms common to all types of anemia (such as pallor, headaches, fatigue, and shortness of breath on exertion) or symptoms specifically due to the hemolysis (such as *jaundice*, caused by an excessive concentration in the blood of bile pigments formed from red cell destruction).

The diagnosis of hemolytic anemia depends on microscopic examination of the blood (see *Blood film*), which often shows a big increase in the number of immature red cells and, with some specific types, red cells that are abnormally shaped. The patient's racial background and medical history may also help establish the diagnosis.

TREATMENT
Some inherited causes of hemolytic anemia can be controlled by removing the main site of destruction of the red cells—the spleen (see *Splenectomy*). Others, such as G6PD deficiency and favism, are largely preventable by avoiding the drugs or foods that precipitate hemolysis.

Treatment of hemolysis caused by mechanical buffeting of red cells relies on reducing the disruptive forces. Those caused by immune or autoimmune processes can often be controlled by *immunosuppressant drugs*.

More specific treatments may be required in particular cases—for example, the use of antimalarial drugs in hemolysis caused by malaria. Transfusions of red blood cells, or exchange transfusions of whole blood, are sometimes required for emergency treatment of severe life-threatening anemia.

Anemia, iron-deficiency
The most common form of *anemia* (a reduced level of the oxygen-carrying pigment *hemoglobin* in the blood); it is caused by a deficiency of iron, an essential constituent of hemoglobin.

Iron-deficiency anemia develops if insufficient iron is available to the bone marrow, where hemoglobin is made and packaged into red blood cells. Anemia occurs when iron loss, along with any extra iron requirements for growth, persistently exceeds iron gained from the diet.

Small losses of hemoglobin and iron occur normally from the body through occasional minor bleeding; in women of childbearing age, these losses are much greater due to menstrual blood loss. Small amounts of iron are also shed in skin cells as they peel off from the body surface and in cells from the

lining of the bowel which are shed in the feces. Tiny amounts of iron are also lost when red blood cells are destroyed at the end of their life span (most of the mineral is efficiently repackaged into new red cells).

Because of their menstrual blood losses, women of childbearing age tend to have low, or no, built-up stores of iron and thus tend to become anemic more quickly if iron losses exceed iron intake. Pregnancy stops the menstrual losses but is replaced by an even greater drain on iron stores (from the baby); hence, pregnant women are at particular risk of iron-deficiency anemia.

CAUSES

INCREASED LOSSES The main cause of iron-deficiency anemia is loss of iron at a greater rate than normal as a result of abnormally heavy or persistent bleeding, which may be caused by disease or by particularly heavy periods (see *Menorrhagia*). The diseases most commonly responsible for persistent bleeding are those of the digestive tract, such as erosive *gastritis, peptic ulcer, stomach cancer, inflammatory bowel disease, hemorrhoids,* and bowel tumors, including cancer (see *Intestine, cancer of*). Prolonged treatment with ASA and ASA-like *nonsteroidal anti-inflammatory drugs* (NSAIDs) can cause gastrointestinal bleeding. In some countries, *hookworm infestation* of the digestive tract is an important cause of iron-deficiency anemia.

Blood lost from the lower part of the intestine and from the rectum is bright red and usually noticed when feces are passed. If the bleeding is in the stomach or upper intestine, it is invisible; when it is excessive, it usually makes the feces black.

Bleeding may also occur as a result of disorders of the urinary tract (such as *kidney tumors, bladder tumors, cystitis,* or *prostatitis*), in which case it colors the urine.

INSUFFICIENT INTAKE The second most common cause of iron deficiency is poor absorption of iron from the diet, usually as the result of surgical removal of part or all of the stomach (see *Gastrectomy*) but also sometimes due to *celiac disease*, an uncommon disorder that impairs digestion.

The third possible cause of iron deficiency, and the least common, is a diet that does not provide enough iron. Those most affected are old people who live alone and who eat a generally poor diet, children and pregnant women because of their extra needs, and slimmers who reduce their total food intake. Women should be sure to have an iron-rich diet and may be prescribed iron tablets during pregnancy.

SYMPTOMS

The symptoms are those of the underlying cause (e.g., abdominal pain and black feces in some cases of peptic ulcer), along with brittle nails and a sore mouth or tongue; and those common to all forms of anemia—fatigue and headaches, and, in severe cases, breathlessness and pain in the center of the chest.

DIAGNOSIS AND TREATMENT

The diagnosis is made from the measurement of a low level of hemoglobin in the blood and from a *blood film* that usually shows the red blood cells to be smaller and paler than normal. When the cause is not clear, investigations such as fecal analysis (for evidence of blood) and *barium X-ray examination* or *endoscopy* (to look for disorders of the digestive tract) may be carried out.

Treatment is for the underlying cause, along with a course of iron tablets or injections (or syrup for children) to build up depleted iron stores and correct the anemia.

Foods containing iron
Foods such as fruit, whole wheat bread, beans, lean meat, and green vegetables are good sources of iron that help prevent iron-deficiency anemia.

Anemia, megaloblastic

An important type of *anemia* (a reduced level of the oxygen-carrying pigment *hemoglobin* in the blood), caused by a deficiency of vitamin B_{12} or another vitamin, folic acid. Either of these deficiencies seriously interferes with the production of red blood cells in the bone marrow. An excess of cells known as megaloblasts appears in the marrow. Megaloblasts give rise to enlarged and deformed red blood cells known as macrocytes.

CAUSES

VITAMIN B_{12} DEFICIENCY Vitamin B_{12} is found only in foods of animal origin, such as meat, fish, and dairy products. It is absorbed from the small

intestine after first combining with a chemical called intrinsic factor, produced by the stomach lining. In most diets, there is much more vitamin B_{12} than the body requires; the excess is stored in the liver, where it can last for a few years. If a person on a normal diet acquires a vitamin B_{12} deficiency, it is due not to lack of the vitamin but to an inability to absorb it.

The most common cause of such a deficiency is a failure of the stomach lining to produce intrinsic factor, usually because of an *autoimmune disorder*, in which antibodies are produced that block the production of intrinsic factor. When vitamin B_{12} deficiency anemia is due to this cause it is known as pernicious anemia. This disorder has a tendency to run in families, to start in middle age, and to affect women more than men. It is sometimes associated with other disorders, such as *diabetes mellitus* or *myxedema*. Total gastrectomy (removal of the entire stomach) prevents the production of intrinsic factor by removing its source.

Other causes of defective absorption of the vitamin include removal of part of the small intestine (where vitamin B_{12} is absorbed) and the intestinal disorder *Crohn's disease*.

In a minority of cases, vitamin B_{12} deficiency is the result of a vegan diet, which excludes eggs and dairy products as well as meat and fish.

FOLIC ACID DEFICIENCY Folic acid is present to some extent in many foods, but is found mainly in green vegetables and liver. However, unlike vitamin B_{12}, it is not stored in the body in large amounts; therefore, a constant supply is needed. For this reason, the usual cause of deficiency is a poor diet. The disorder is most common in the poor and in old people living by themselves. It may also occur in people with *alcohol dependence*.

Deficiency can also be caused by anything that interferes with the absorption of folic acid from the small intestine (e.g., disorders such as *Crohn's disease* and *celiac disease* or removal of part of the small intestine).

Folic acid is required by rapidly dividing cells, as in the fetus, and the requirements during pregnancy are much higher than at other times. For this reason some physicians recommend that women should take folic acid in early pregnancy.

SYMPTOMS

Many people with mild megaloblastic anemia have no symptoms. In others, symptoms may include any or all of

Bone marrow in megaloblastic anemia
In this microscopic view, some of the large cells are abnormal red cell precursors (megaloblasts).

the following: tiredness, headaches, a sore mouth and tongue, weight loss, and *jaundice*. In severe cases there may also be instances of breathlessness, chest pain, and sometimes loss of balance and tingling in the feet due to damage to the nervous system from lack of the vitamins.

DIAGNOSIS

The anemia is usually first suspected following *blood tests* that show a low level of hemoglobin, a preponderance of large red blood cells, and low levels of either vitamin B_{12} or folic acid or both. The disease is confirmed if a *bone marrow biopsy* (removal of a small sample of marrow for analysis) reveals the presence of large numbers of megaloblasts (abnormal, immature red cells). Tests may also be carried out to discover an underlying cause in cases where this is not clear.

Pernicious anemia is sometimes diagnosed by a special test, the Schilling test, in which the absorption of vitamin B_{12} into the bloodstream is measured with the vitamin first unbound and then bound to intrinsic factor. If the vitamin is found to be absorbed only when bound to intrinsic factor, it confirms the diagnosis of pernicious anemia.

TREATMENT

When megaloblastic anemia is due to poor diet, it can be remedied by adopting a normal diet and taking a short course of vitamin B_{12} injections or folic acid tablets.

If the deficiency is due to inability to absorb vitamin B_{12}, it can sometimes be remedied by treating the underlying cause. Often the power of absorption is lost permanently however, either through digestive system surgery or because the stomach has stopped excreting intrinsic factor, which it needs to absorb vitamin B_{12}. Lifelong vitamin B_{12} injections or folic acid tablets are then required.

A

Anemia, pernicious

A type of anemia in which the underlying problem is a disorder of the stomach lining. The lining fails to produce a substance called intrinsic factor, necessary for the absorption of vitamin B_{12} from the intestines into the blood. As a result, a deficiency of vitamin B_{12} develops and without this vitamin, the bone marrow is unable to produce normal red blood cells. (See also *Anemia, megaloblastic*.)

Anencephaly

Absence at birth of the brain and cranial vault (top of the skull). Most affected infants are stillborn or survive only a few hours. Anencephaly is detectable early in pregnancy by measurement of maternal *alpha-fetoprotein*, by *ultrasound scanning*, by *amniocentesis*, or by *fetoscopy*.

CAUSES

Anencephaly is caused by a failure in development of the neural tube (the nerve tissue in the embryo that normally develops into the spinal cord and brain). Maldevelopment of the neural tube may also result in *spina bifida* and *hydrocephalus*. These abnormalities are collectively known as *neural tube defects* and seem likely to have similar causes. Anencephaly occurs in about five in every 1,000 pregnancies, but only in about one third of these does the pregnancy continue to term.

Anesthesia

Literally, the absence of all sensation; insensibility. Anesthesia can be induced artificially to abolish pain during surgical procedures and sometimes during childbirth.

HOW IT IS DONE

Two types of anesthesia are used for medical purposes: local and general. A patient given a local anesthetic (see *Anesthesia, local*) remains conscious and sensation is abolished in only part of the body. This is usually accomplished by injection of drugs that temporarily interrupt the nerve supply from the region to be anesthetized. Local anesthetics can also be given in the form of eye drops, sprays, skin creams, and suppositories. It may be possible to produce local pain relief by using *acupuncture*; this technique is widely used in China and is now being used more widely by Western practitioners.

A patient under general anesthesia (see *Anesthesia, general*) is rendered unconscious and maintained in this state with a combination of drugs that are either injected into a vein or inhaled. These drugs affect all parts of the body but have their main sites of action in the brain and spinal cord.

Damage to nerve tissues by injury or disease can produce local anesthesia. Rarely, anesthesia may be a result of extreme arousal, as in the case of boxers or soldiers who do not notice painful blows or wounds. Psychological factors may be responsible for numbness, particularly in the hand or foot (see *Conversion disorder*).

Anesthesia, dental

Loss of sensation induced in a patient to prevent pain during dental treatment. Most dental procedures are carried out using local anesthesia; general anesthesia is usually reserved for surgical procedures and people with special needs.

LOCAL ANESTHESIA

For minor restorative work, such as fillings, some patients and dentists choose no anesthesia; otherwise, a local anesthetic (e.g., lidocaine or bupivacaine) is injected into the gum at the site that is being treated. Sometimes it is not possible to inject directly into the area to be treated because the gum is painfully inflamed or because there is a risk of spreading an infection in the gum. In these cases, the anesthetic is injected into or around the nerve a short distance away from the site of operation. This procedure is known as a peripheral *nerve block*. Topical anesthetics on the surface of the gums are often used in conjunction with injected anesthetics.

SEDATION

In addition to receiving a local anesthetic, a patient who is abnormally anxious, agitated, or uncooperative may need to be calmed by sedation. To sedate the patient, an antianxiety agent is given orally or intravenously, or by inhalation. Antianxiety agents include tranquilizer drugs (such as diazepam), nitrous oxide (laughing gas), and barbiturates.

GENERAL ANESTHESIA

The most common use for general anesthesia is in surgical procedures such as periodontal (gum) surgery and multiple tooth extractions. General anesthesia is also used for young children, for people who are allergic to local anesthetics or who have extremely sensitive teeth, and for those who are unable to cooperate (e.g., because of a mental disorder or physical handicap).

For relatively short dental surgery, general anesthesia is given by an injection of a barbiturate, such as methohexitone or thiopental, into a vein. Anesthesia may then be maintained by the patient breathing a mixture of nitrous oxide, oxygen, and possibly another volatile anesthetic during surgery.

For longer or more complicated procedures, general anesthesia is carried out as for other types of surgery (see *Anesthesia, general*).

Anesthesia, general

Loss of sensation and consciousness induced to prevent pain and discomfort during surgery. The state of general anesthesia is produced and maintained by an anesthetist, who gives combinations of drugs by injection, inhalation, or both. The anesthetist is also responsible for the preanesthetic assessment and medication of patients, their safety during surgery, and their recovery during the postanesthetic period.

HISTORY

Until about the middle of the 19th century, pain relief during surgery relied on natural substances such as alcohol, opium, and cannabis. However, the relief obtained was often inadequate and short-lived. It was not until the 1840s that significant progress was made toward solving the problems of inducing unconsciousness in a manner that was safe, easily maintained for long periods, and reversible. *Ether* was first demonstrated successfully in New York in 1842 and Boston in 1846, when a tooth was extracted without pain while the patient was breathing ether. Soon after, the anesthetic properties of chloroform and nitrous oxide (laughing gas) were discovered, heralding a new era in surgery.

WHY IT IS DONE

The primary objectives of general anesthesia are to abolish pain, awareness, muscle tone, and cardiovascular reflexes in the patient and so make conditions suitable for surgery or diagnostic procedures.

HOW IT IS DONE

The principal stages in administering, maintaining, and reversing general anesthesia are shown in the illustrated box overleaf.

COMPLICATIONS

The likelihood of any complications depends on the preoperative condition of the patient, the anesthetic technique used, and the nature of the operation performed. The longer the operation, the greater the risk.

General anesthesia may cause several possible complications. These

A

TECHNIQUES FOR GENERAL ANESTHESIA

The main phases in the administration of a general anesthetic are induction (bringing on unconsciousness), maintenance, and emergence (returning the patient to consciousness). Some of the main stages are shown below. Often, to allow surgical manipulation, a muscle relaxant must be given in addition to anesthetic gases or injections. Because the relaxant temporarily paralyzes the breathing muscles, the patient's lungs must be ventilated artificially.

DRUGS USED IN GENERAL ANESTHESIA

Type	Action	Examples
Drugs given as premedication	Relax patient, abolish pain, reduce saliva and mucus formation	Diazepam, morphine, atropine
Induction agents	Induce unconsciousness	Thiopental sodium
Anesthetic gases and volatile agents	Induce and/or maintain unconsciousness	Nitrous oxide, halothane, enflurane, isoflurane
Analgesics	Abolish pain	Morphine, fentanyl
Muscle relaxants	Relax muscles	Pancuronium, vecuronium
Reversal agents	Reverse muscle relaxation	Neostigmine

1 Before the operation, the anesthetist talks to and examines the patient and assesses his or her fitness for anesthesia and surgery. He or she also answers the patient's questions.

2 Premedication may include a drug that relieves pain or anxiety and one that prevents excessive salivation.

3 The induction agent is usually given via a cannula inserted into a vein. The cannula is left in position so that other drugs can be given rapidly if needed.

4 Sometimes, anesthesia is induced or maintained with gases delivered by mask. Without muscle relaxant the patient may be able to continue breathing naturally.

5 In other cases, a breathing tube is inserted for delivery of the anesthetic gases. If a muscle relaxant is used, artificial ventilation is necessary.

Anesthetist

Assistant

Gas mask

Gas cylinder pressure meters

Pipes carrying anesthetic gas supply

6 The patient is kept at a level of anesthesia deep enough to be unaware of the operation. The gas mixture, and the patient's heart rate, breathing, blood pressure, temperature, blood oxygenation, and exhaled carbon dioxide are monitored. After surgery, anesthesia is stopped and reversal agents are given if necessary.

include such things as nausea, vomiting, *hypotension* (low blood pressure), physical injury (such as chipped teeth and muscle strains), allergic reactions, cardiac *arrhythmia* (irregular heartbeat), respiratory depression (slowed, ineffective breathing), *hypoxia, aspiration* (inhaling vomit into the lungs), and *airway obstruction*.

AWARENESS DURING ANESTHESIA It is possible (though rare with modern anesthetic techniques) for patients to remain aware of events during surgery but, because they have been given muscle-relaxant drugs, to be unable to signal this distressed state to the anesthetist. The concentrations of anesthetic agents required to produce adequate anesthesia in the majority of patients are well documented. In addition, the anesthetist can detect an inadequate level of anesthesia by noting physical signs, such as increased sweating and salivation; irregular breathing; changes in muscle tone; spontaneous eye movements; and increases in the patient's heart rate and blood pressure.

Anesthesia, local

Loss of sensation induced in a limited region of a person's body to prevent pain during examinations, diagnostic or treatment procedures, and surgical operations. Local anesthesia is produced by the administration of drugs that temporarily interrupt the action of pain-carrying nerve fibers.

HOW IT IS DONE

For minor surgical procedures, such as stitching of small wounds, local anesthesia is usually produced by direct injection into the area to be treated. When it is necessary to anesthetize a large area, or when local injection would not penetrate deeply enough into body tissues, a *nerve block* (in which nerves carrying sensation from the area to be treated are injected) may be used. Nerves can also be blocked as they branch off from the spinal cord, as in *epidural anesthesia*, which is widely used during childbirth, and spinal anesthesia (see *Spinal block*), which is used mainly for surgery of the lower limbs and lower abdomen.

Some parts of the body that are permeable to local anesthetic drugs can be anesthetized by applying an anesthetic drug directly to the area. The throat, larynx, and respiratory passages can be sprayed before *bronchoscopy*, and the urethra can be numbed with a gel before *catheterization* or *cystoscopy*. An anesthetic cream can be rubbed onto the skin prior to an injection to make it painless. Other forms of local anesthetic include anesthetic lozenges for sore throats, and ointments or rectal suppositories to relieve the discomfort of *hemorrhoids*.

For some procedures, particularly if the patient is unusually anxious, a sedative drug is given in addition to the local anesthetic.

COMPLICATIONS

Adverse reactions to an anesthetic drug may occur if the dose is too high or has been absorbed too rapidly. Such reactions include dizziness, loss of consciousness, seizures, and cardiac arrest. In rare cases, people have an allergic reaction to the drug itself. During major (epidural and spinal) blocks, blood pressure may drop, causing reduced blood flow to the brain and heart. Rarely, infections enter the body at the injection site. In a small number of susceptible patients, certain local anesthetics may cause long-term nerve damage.

Anesthetics

A term for the group of drugs that produce the state of *anesthesia* and for the medical discipline concerned with their administration.

A specialist who administers anesthetics is called an anesthetist. Before a patient goes to the operating room, the anesthetist assesses the condition of the patient's heart, lungs, and circulation. The anesthetist decides the type and amount of drugs needed to induce and maintain anesthesia, determines the patient's position on the operating table, watches for signs of trouble, and decides what actions should be taken if an emergency develops. The anesthetist is also responsible for monitoring the progress of the waking patient, and watching for and treating any complications that might develop.

Aneurysm

Abnormal dilation (ballooning) of an artery caused by the pressure of blood flowing through a weakened area. The weakening may be due to disease, injury, or a congenital defect of the arterial wall.

TYPES

Some of the common types, sites, and shapes of aneurysm are shown in the illustrated box on page 106.

A dissecting aneurysm, usually associated with *atherosclerosis*, is a condition in which a longitudinal, blood-

LOCAL ANESTHETICS

Drug	Common uses	How taken
Amethocaine	For surgery on the eye, for relief of pain during dental treatment	Eye drops, spray, cream
Benzocaine	To treat painful conditions of the mouth and throat, painful anal conditions (e.g., hemorrhoids), skin wounds; used before laryngoscopy	Lozenges, suppositories, spray, cream, ointment
Bupivacaine	As nerve block (e.g., epidural anesthesia and caudal block)	Injection
Cocaine	For surgery on the nose, throat, and larynx; formerly used in eye operations	Eye drops, spray, liquid
Lidocaine	For relief of pain during dental treatment; for spinal anesthesia, nerve blocks (e.g., epidural anesthesia), eye surgery, and before endoscopic procedures; to treat hemorrhoids	Injection, gel, spray, cream, ointment, liquid, eye drops, suppositories
Procaine	For relief of pain before surgical and dental treatment	Injection

A

filled split forms within the lining of the wall of an artery—usually the aorta —and spreads so that extensive areas of the vessel are weakened. Usually the patient suffers severe pain and the vessel may rupture. When the aneurysm is located in the aortic arch or the ascending aorta and dissects into the pericardium (membrane surrounding the heart), the pressure of the blood around the heart may be fatal because it prevents the heart from beating.

An aneurysm may sometimes develop in the heart wall due to weakening of the heart muscle as a result of a *myocardial infarction* (heart attack). Such aneurysms seldom rupture but they often interfere with the efficient pumping action of the heart.

A traumatic aneurysm is one caused by mechanical injury that weakens the blood vessel wall.

CAUSES

An aneurysm may form for several reasons. If the muscular middle layer of an artery is congenitally weak, normal blood pressure causes dilation of the blood vessel wall at the weak point. *Marfan's syndrome*, a condition in which the middle layer of the wall of the aorta is defective, is often associated with an aneurysm just above the heart. The arterial wall can also be weakened by inflammation, as occurs in *polyarteritis nodosa*.

Most aneurysms of the aorta—usually in the lower part of the vessel—are caused by atherosclerotic weakening of a segment of the wall. Aneurysm of the ascending aorta once commonly resulted from untreated *syphilis* but this is now rare. Aneurysms, known as mycotic aneurysms, may occur in smaller vessels as a result of local infection in *septicemia*. Aneurysms of arteries in the brain are often termed berry aneurysms because of their size and appearance.

SYMPTOMS AND SIGNS

Symptoms vary according to the type, size, and location of the swelling. Cerebral aneurysms may persist for many years without causing symptoms, but the close proximity of the brain makes them very dangerous. Sudden enlargement and bursting of a berry aneurysm produces obvious symptoms and signs, such as paralysis of eye movement, drooping of the lid, dilation of the pupil, rigidity of the neck, severe headache, and unconsciousness (symptoms similar to those of a *stroke*).

Pressure from an aneurysm may damage surrounding structures,

TYPES OF ANEURYSM

An aneurysm forms when pressure from the blood flow causes a weakened artery wall to distend or forces blood through a fissure.

Aneurysms can form anywhere in the body, although the most common sites are the aorta and the arteries supplying the brain.

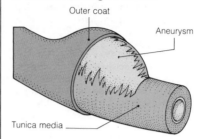

Common aneurysm
This type forms when the tunica media, the artery's middle wall, is weakened; the strong force of the blood flow distends the wall of the artery.

Dissecting aneurysm
This type occurs when there is a fissure in the internal wall of the artery; blood forced through the fissure forms a swelling.

Cerebral (or berry) aneurysm
A swelling where the arteries branch at the brain's base, often caused by congenital weakness.

Saccular aneurysm
A balloon-shaped distention of part of an artery's wall, often seen in aortic aneurysms just above the heart.

Fusiform aneurysm
A distention around an artery's circumference, tapered at both ends, often seen in lower aortic aneurysms.

especially if the aneurysm is located within the confined space of the skull.

Aneurysms may rupture, sometimes causing fatal blood loss, or, in the case of cerebral aneurysms, may cause severe damage to the brain (see *Subarachnoid hemorrhage*).

Aneurysms of the thoracic (chest) part of the aorta are usually accompanied by hoarseness (due to pressure on a nerve controlling a vocal chord), difficulty swallowing, and chest pain that may be mistaken for myocardial infarction (heart attack). Abdominal aortic aneurysm is sometimes visible as a throbbing swelling and may also cause backache.

DIAGNOSIS

X rays will sometimes reveal an aneurysm in a larger blood vessel, but

angiography provides more detailed information. In the case of cerebral aneurysms, valuable information may be obtained from *CT scanning* or *MRI*.

TREATMENT AND OUTLOOK

Treatment varies with the site of the aneurysm and the age and health of the patient.

Ruptured or enlarged aneurysms require urgent surgery (see *Arterial reconstructive surgery*). If cerebral aneurysm causes symptoms, surgery is recommended if possible. Nonurgent surgery for aortic aneurysms of the chest offers an 80 to 90 percent chance of survival.

Emergency surgery always carries a high risk, and the outlook following a ruptured aneurysm in the chest is equally poor.

A

Angel dust
One of the common names for phencyclidine, an illicit drug taken for its hallucinogenic properties. Adverse effects of the drug include slowed breathing rate, agitation, muscle rigidity, vomiting, and convulsions; several deaths have been reported.

Angiitis
See *Vasculitis*.

Angina
A term that describes a strangling or constrictive pain. Angina has become synonymous with the heart disorder *angina pectoris* (chest pain caused by lack of oxygen to the heart muscle, usually a result of poor blood supply). Other types of angina include abdominal angina (abdominal pain after eating caused by poor blood supply to the intestines) and Vincent's angina, pain caused by inflammation of the mouth (see *Vincent's disease*).

Angina pectoris
Pain in the chest due to insufficient oxygen being carried to the heart muscle in the blood. Angina pectoris usually occurs when the demand for oxygen is increased during exercise and at times of stress.

CAUSES
Inadequate blood supply to the heart is usually due to *coronary artery disease*, in which the coronary arteries are narrowed by *atherosclerosis* (fat deposits on the walls of the arteries). Other causes include coronary artery spasm, in which the blood vessels narrow suddenly for a short time but return to normal with no permanent obstruction, *aortic stenosis* (narrowing of the aortic valve in the heart), and *arrhythmias* (abnormal heart rhythms).

Rare causes of angina pectoris include severe *anemia*, which reduces the oxygen-carrying efficiency of the blood, and *polycythemia* (increased numbers of red blood cells), which thickens the blood, slowing its flow through the heart muscle. *Thyrotoxicosis* (a disorder caused by excessive production of thyroid hormones) can precipitate angina pectoris by making the heart work much faster than its blood supply will permit.

INCIDENCE
Angina pectoris is a common condition. In men, it usually starts in the 50s but may occur as early as 30; in women, it usually starts later in life.

SYMPTOMS
The chest pain varies from mild to severe and is often described as a sensation of pressure on the chest. It usually starts in the center of the chest but can spread to the throat, upper jaw, back, and arms (usually the left one) or between the shoulder blades.

The pain usually comes on when the heart is working harder and requires more oxygen—for example, during exercise, when under stress, in extremes of temperature, or during mild exercise soon after a meal. Typically the pain develops at the same stage in daily activities—for example, at the same point on a flight of stairs—and is relieved by a short rest.

Other symptoms may include nausea, sweating, dizziness, and breathing difficulty. These symptoms are usually characteristic of angina pectoris, but similar symptoms can also be caused by *esophagitis* (inflammation of the esophagus), spasm of the esophagus, arthritis in the upper spine or rib cage, even by a pulled muscle in the chest wall.

A prolonged and usually more severe attack of angina pectoris may be due to *myocardial infarction* (heart attack), in which the heart muscle is permanently damaged.

DIAGNOSIS
Angina pectoris cannot be diagnosed with certainty by a physical examination. Diagnostic tests usually include an *ECG* (measurement of the electrical activity in the heart) while the patient is at rest and a *cardiac stress test* (an ECG performed while the patient is exercising enough to cause chest pain (e.g., while walking on a treadmill). Although the resting ECG will show no signs of angina (unless an attack is actually in progress), it may show former heart damage.

Blood tests may be performed to look for an underlying cause, such as *anemia*, *polycythemia*, *thyrotoxicosis*, or *hyperlipidemia* (abnormally high levels of fat in the blood, which can cause atherosclerosis).

Coronary *angiography* (X-ray examination of the blood vessels) may also be performed.

TREATMENT
Initial treatment attempts to control the symptoms. It is important to stop smoking because nicotine and carbon monoxide contribute to the progressive development of coronary artery disease and make the symptoms worse. Overweight people should lose weight to reduce stress on the heart during exercise.

Attacks of angina pectoris may be prevented and treated by *nitrate drugs*, such as glyceryl trinitrate, which increase the flow of blood through the heart muscle and improve blood flow around the body. If nitrates are not effective, or are causing severe headaches due to an increased blood flow through the brain, other drugs may be used, including *beta-blocker drugs* and *calcium channel blockers*.

If *hypertension* (high blood pressure) is found during examination, it is treated with *antihypertensive drugs* to reduce the work load of the heart in pumping blood. Other specific causes can also be treated—for example, arrhythmias with *antiarrhythmic drugs* and hyperlipidemia with a low-fat diet and/or drugs.

Drug treatment can control the symptoms of angina pectoris for many years but it cannot cure the disorder. If attacks become more severe, more frequent, or more prolonged, despite drug treatment, and if there is angiographic evidence of advanced narrowing of vessels, then *coronary artery bypass* surgery or *angioplasty* may be performed to reestablish blood flow to the heart muscle.

OUTLOOK
The effect of angina pectoris on lifestyle depends on the severity of the underlying disease and the effectiveness of drug treatment or surgery. Some people are able to lead a normal life apart from some restriction on strenuous exercise, whereas others are severely disabled.

Angioedema
A type of reaction, also known as angioneurotic edema, caused by *allergy*. Angioedema is similar to *urticaria* (hives) and characterized by large, well-defined swellings, of sudden onset, in the skin, larynx (voice box), and other areas. These swellings may last several hours or days if they are left untreated.

INCIDENCE AND CAUSES
Angioedema primarily affects young people (especially those in their 20s) and those with a general tendency toward allergies (see *Atopy*).

The most common cause is a sudden allergic reaction to a food, such as eggs, strawberries, or seafood. Less commonly, it results from allergy to a drug (such as *penicillin*), a reaction to an insect sting or bite, or from infection, emotional stress, or exposure to animals, molds, pollens, or cold conditions. There is also a hereditary form of the disease.

SYMPTOMS
Angioedema may cause very sudden difficulty in breathing, speaking, and

swallowing, accompanied by obvious swelling of the lips, face, and neck.

Angioedema that affects the throat and the larynx is potentially life-threatening because the swelling can block the airway, causing *asphyxia* (suffocation). If the gastrointestinal tract is affected, colic, nausea, and vomiting may occur.

TREATMENT
Severe cases are treated with injections of *epinephrine* and may require intubation (passage of a breathing tube via the mouth into the windpipe) or *tracheostomy* (surgical creation of a breathing hole in the windpipe) to prevent suffocation. *Corticosteroid drugs* may also be prescribed. In less severe cases, *antihistamine drugs* often relieve symptoms.

Angiography
An imaging procedure that enables blood vessels to be seen clearly on X-ray film following the injection of a contrast medium (a substance opaque to X rays).

WHY IT IS DONE
Angiography is used to detect diseases that alter the appearance of blood vessels. These diseases include *aneurysm* (ballooning of an artery), and narrowing or blockage of blood vessels by *atherosclerosis* (fatty deposits lining artery walls) or by a *thrombus* (abnormal clot) or an *embolus* (fragment carried in the blood). Angiography is also used to detect changes in the pattern of blood vessels that supply organs which have been injured or are affected by a tumor. By noting the abnormal arrangement of blood vessels, the physician can evaluate the extent of disease and plan treatment accordingly.

Carotid angiography is sometimes performed on patients suffering from *transient ischemic attacks* (symptoms of *stroke* lasting less than 24 hours) to see whether there is a blockage or substantial narrowing in one of the carotid arteries (in the neck), which supply blood to the brain.

Cerebral angiography is used to demonstrate the presence of an aneurysm within the brain or to help pinpoint the position of a brain tumor prior to surgery.

Coronary angiography, which is often combined with cardiac *catheterization*, is carried out to identify the sites of narrowing or blockage in *coronary artery disease*.

HOW IT IS DONE
The contrast medium is usually injected into the blood vessel to be examined through a fine catheter (flexible plastic tube) that is inserted into the femoral artery at the groin, the brachial artery just over the elbow, or a carotid artery.

To insert the catheter, the skin and tissues around the artery are numbed with local anesthetic and then a hollow needle is inserted through the skin into the artery. A long, thin wire with a soft tip is inserted through the needle, the needle is removed, and the catheter is then threaded over the wire into the blood vessel. Under X-ray control, the tip of the catheter is guided further into the vessel to be examined and contrast medium is injected. A rapid sequence of X-ray pictures (or a continuous recording) is taken so that the blood flow through the vessels can be studied.

Angiography can take from as little as a few minutes to as long as two or three hours.

DIGITAL SUBTRACTION ANGIOGRAPHY
This type of angiography uses computer techniques to process images and subtract (remove) unwanted background information, leaving only an image of the blood vessels to be studied. Digital subtraction angiography requires less contrast medium than conventional angiography and is therefore safer for the patient. In some cases, digital subtraction angiography also makes it possible to avoid injecting the contrast medium directly into affected blood vessels that are not easily accessible by catheter. However, the detail provided by digital subtraction angiography is not always as good as in conventional angiography.

RISKS
Allergy to the contrast medium is a possible adverse effect, but the use of new contrast agents has reduced the risk of a severe reaction to less than one in 80,000 examinations.

Damage to blood vessels can occur at the site of injection or anywhere along the vessel during the passage of the catheter.

OUTLOOK
Angiographic techniques have, in the last few years, been adapted to allow not only diagnosis but also certain types of treatment that, in some cases, eliminate the need for surgery. For example, small balloons can be inflated at the tip of a catheter to expand a narrowed or blocked segment of artery (see *Angioplasty, balloon*), foreign material can be injected to reduce or shut off blood supply to a tumor (see *Embolization*), and medication to control bleeding or to treat tumors can be infused directly into the blood supply to individual organs. (See also *Aortography*.)

Angioma
A benign tumor made up of blood vessels (see *Hemangioma*) or lymph vessels (see *Lymphangioma*).

Angioplasty, balloon
A technique for treating narrowing or blockage of a blood vessel or heart valve by introducing a balloon into the constricted area to widen it.

WHY IT IS DONE
Balloon angioplasty is used in the treatment of *peripheral vascular disease* to increase or restore the flow of blood through a significantly narrowed artery in a limb; it is also used to treat narrowing of the coronary arteries (see *Coronary artery disease*).

COMPLICATIONS
There is a slight risk of damaging the artery or heart valve during this procedure and immediate surgery may be required. In rare cases, a *myocardial*

Angiogram of a normal kidney
Contrast medium is passed through the catheter into the kidney's arterial system and a series of X-ray pictures is taken.

Digital subtraction angiography
Here, the normal kidneys are revealed more clearly because the computer eliminates unwanted information.

PROCEDURE FOR BALLOON ANGIOPLASTY

A blockage or narrowing of a blood vessel may be treated by introducing a balloon catheter into the area and then inflating the balloon to stretch the constricted part. The balloon is then deflated and the catheter withdrawn. The procedure is carried out using a local anesthetic.

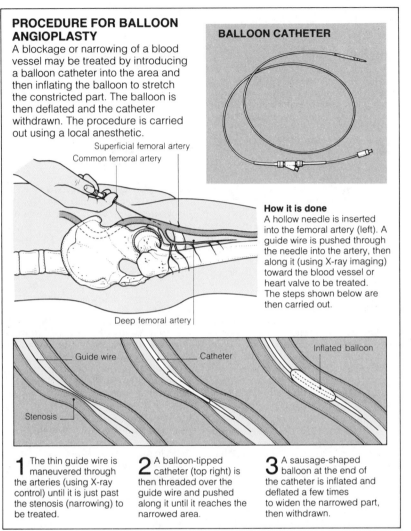

BALLOON CATHETER

Superficial femoral artery
Common femoral artery

Deep femoral artery

How it is done
A hollow needle is inserted into the femoral artery (left). A guide wire is pushed through the needle into the artery, then along it (using X-ray imaging) toward the blood vessel or heart valve to be treated. The steps shown below are then carried out.

Guide wire   Catheter   Inflated balloon

Stenosis

1 The thin guide wire is maneuvered through the arteries (using X-ray control) until it is just past the stenosis (narrowing) to be treated.

2 A balloon-tipped catheter (top right) is then threaded over the guide wire and pushed along it until it reaches the narrowed area.

3 A sausage-shaped balloon at the end of the catheter is inflated and deflated a few times to widen the narrowed part, then withdrawn.

infarction (heart attack) may be caused by prolonged interruption, by the inflated balloon, of blood supply to an area of the heart.

RESULTS

Coronary balloon angioplasty is successful in improving the condition of about two thirds of the patients who are treated in this manner. In some three quarters of these cases, the improvement continues after a year; in the remainder, stenosis, or narrowing, recurs in the affected vessel, but balloon angioplasty may be repeated successfully.

Angioplasty of peripheral vessels is most successful in treating the iliac and femoral arteries (in the legs), particularly when the affected area is small. After five years, 85 to 90 percent of iliac arteries treated by angioplasty

remain free of obstruction. For femoral arteries, the success rate is 50 to 70 percent after two years.

New techniques for angioplasty currently under investigation include devices using lasers, cutting drills, and suction to remove the atheromatous deposits blocking the arteries.

Angiotensin

The name of two related proteins involved in regulating blood pressure. The first of these, angiotensin I, is itself inactive and is converted to the second, active form, angiotensin II, by the action of a converting enzyme. Angiotensin II causes narrowing of the small blood vessels in tissues, resulting in an increase in blood pressure. It also stimulates the release from the adrenal cortex (the outer part

of each *adrenal gland*) of the hormone *aldosterone*, which also increases blood pressure. Certain kidney disorders can increase the production of angiotensin II, causing *hypertension* (high blood pressure). Whatever the cause of hypertension, it may be treated with drugs known as *ACE inhibitors* (angiotensin-converting enzyme inhibitors), which work by reducing angiotensin II formation.

Anhidrosis

Complete absence of *sweating*. (See also *Hypohidrosis*.)

Animal experimentation

The use of living animals in research and safety testing to provide information about animal biology and about human physiology or behavior. Animal experimentation is most prolific in developed countries, where medical standards are high and where there is a long-standing concern for public health and safety.

The animals most extensively used in animal experimentation are rats and mice, which are bred for laboratory research. Less than 1 percent of experiments involve cats, dogs, farm animals, nonhuman primates, frogs, fish, and birds.

LEGISLATIVE CONTROLS

Animal experimentation is controlled by law in most countries but the controls vary in their stringency. Governments must balance pressures for very tight controls against the weight of scientific opinion, which maintains that animal experiments are indispensable to public health and safety.

TYPES OF EXPERIMENTS

The experiments for which animals are used fall into several groups. One group consists of experiments to test the safety of nonmedical substances, such as pesticides, cleaning chemicals, and cosmetics, before they are released for public use.

Another group includes the many medical experiments in which a condition in an animal corresponds to a human disease. This provides the potential for testing new treatments to discover cures for the disease in the animal and therefore in humans.

Other experiments are performed to discover new drugs and medical procedures or to develop new substances for use in the environment.

ETHICAL OBJECTIONS

Campaigners for animal rights point out that animals suffer in many of these experiments. Sometimes the suffering is an implicit part of the research, as in research to study the mechanism of pain or to create models of painful conditions on which to test analgesic drugs (painkillers). Some of the conditions or effects being studied necessarily cause illness, stress, or pain, such as infecting animals with a disease or studying the irritant or poisonous effects of chemicals.

Two safety tests, often required by law, have received considerable criticism from protest groups and scientists alike. One test is the LD_{50} test, which measures acute toxicity (short-term poisonous effects) by estimating the dose that would kill 50 percent of the animals in a test group. The other test is the Draize test, which measures irritant damage of chemicals and substances to eyes and skin.

BENEFITS

Experiments on animals have contributed greatly to the advancement of science and have specifically benefited humanity by virtue of new medical and surgical treatments.

In the past 30 years alone, the incidence of poliomyelitis and other infections has been reduced enormously as a result of vaccines produced after such testing programs.

Antibiotic drugs developed using animal experiments have also prolonged and saved many lives. Drugs for the treatment of noninfectious disorders, such as arthritis, diabetes mellitus, and hypertension (high blood pressure), are also the result of animal-based research. Surgical treatments may also be developed in animals; the success of transplant operations and microsurgery techniques are notable recent advances.

ALTERNATIVES

Alternatives to animal experiments have been developed and are used whenever possible. Laboratory tests using cultured cells or tissues have replaced many experiments that once involved animals. Other alternatives involve the use of simple organisms, such as bacteria or yeasts, or the computerized or mathematical modeling of an experiment.

New techniques have also led in some cases to the replacement of animals as a source of vaccines and hormones. Cell culture techniques have now almost replaced the use of animals in vaccine production, and genetically engineered bacteria and yeasts are increasingly used to produce substances, such as insulin, that were once derived only from animals.

However, even with these newer methods, it is dangerous—and illegal—not to undertake confirmatory studies on animals before releasing a new drug or vaccine.

Anisometropia

Unequal focusing power in the two eyes, usually due to a difference in size and/or shape in the eyes. For example, one eye may be normal and the other affected by *myopia* (near-sightedness), *hyperopia* (farsightedness), or *astigmatism* (uneven curvature of the cornea).

Significant anisometropia causes visual discomfort because the image formed on one retina differs in size from that formed on the other. Glasses or contact lenses are satisfactory in most cases. In severe cases, however, it is usually better not to sharpen the image in the most affected eye because this would emphasize the difference in image size and increase visual discomfort.

Ankle joint

The hinge joint between the foot and the leg. The talus (uppermost bone in the foot) fits between the two bony protuberances formed by the lower ends of the tibia (shinbone) and the fibula (outer bone of the lower leg). Strong ligaments on each side of the ankle joint provide support and limit movement. The ankle joint allows up-and-down movements of the foot; movements, such as tilting and rotating, occur at joints in the foot itself.

DISORDERS

An ankle *sprain* is one of the most common of all injuries, and is usually

LOCATION OF THE ANKLE JOINT
This hinge joint is formed where the top of the talus fits in between the lower ends of the tibia and fibula.

Tibia

Fibula

Talus

Ligament

Calcaneus

caused by twisting the foot over onto its outside edge, which produces overstretching and bruising of the ligaments on the outside of the ankle. Very severe sprains may cause extensive tearing of the ligaments, which requires surgical repair.

Excessive or violent twisting of the ankle can cause a combined fracture and dislocation (called *Pott's fracture*), in which the fibula breaks above the ankle, and either the tibia breaks or the ligaments tear, resulting in dislocation of the ankle.

Ankylosing spondylitis

An inflammatory disease affecting joints between the vertebrae of the spine and the sacroiliac joints (joints between the spine and the pelvis).

CAUSES AND INCIDENCE

Ankylosing spondylitis is usually of unknown cause. A variant of the disorder is preceded, in some people, either by *colitis* (inflammation of the colon) or *psoriasis* (a skin disease).

Ankylosing spondylitis affects less than 1 percent of the population, is more common in men than in women, and has its onset between the ages of 20 and 40 years. The disorder also seems to run in families. A genetically determined *histocompatibility antigen* (HLA-B27) is found much more often in people with ankylosing spondylitis than in the rest of the population.

SYMPTOMS

Ankylosing spondylitis usually starts with pain and stiffness in the lower back and hips, which are worse after resting and especially noticeable in the early morning. Typically, exercise helps reduce the stiffness.

Other, less common, symptoms include pain in the chest (from the joints between the spine and the ribs), loss of appetite, tiredness, and, occasionally, redness and pain in the eyes due to *iritis* (inflammation of the iris). In about one fifth of sufferers, other joints (e.g., the hips, knees, and ankles) may be swollen and painful. Inflammation of tissues around the heel can cause pain and tenderness.

In time, the inflammation in the spine can lead to *ankylosis* (permanent stiffness and limitation of movement) and *kyphosis* (curvature of the spine). Movement is restricted and expansion of the chest is often limited.

DIAGNOSIS

A diagnosis of ankylosing spondylitis is usually made from the pattern of symptoms, backed up by blood tests and X rays. Blood tests can be used to assess inflammation and to indicate the presence of the HLA-B27 antigen on white blood cells. At the onset, X rays of the back may be normal, but later there are signs of increased bone density around the sacroiliac joints. Later still in the disease, the spine may show loss of space between joints and bony outgrowths.

TREATMENT

There is no curative treatment but symptoms may be reduced by a program of heat, massage, and supervised exercise. Regular daily exercise (such as swimming) is advisable to keep the back muscles strong. To prevent curvature of the spine, patients are taught breathing exercises and exercises to improve posture. *Antiinflammatory drugs* may be prescribed to reduce the pain and stiffness.

OUTLOOK

The inflammatory process tends to become less active with age. With treatment, most people suffer only minor deformity of the spine and are able to lead a normal life.

Ankylosis

Complete loss of movement in a joint caused by fusion of the bony surfaces. Ankylosis may be due to degeneration as a result of injury, infection, or inflammation. Ankylosis may also be produced surgically by an operation to fuse a diseased joint to correct deformity or to alleviate persistent pain (see *Arthrodesis*).

Anodontia

Failure of some or all of the teeth to develop. Anodontia may be due to absence of tooth buds at birth or may be the result of damage to developing tooth buds caused by infection or other widespread disease. Both primary and permanent teeth, or permanent teeth only, may be affected.

If only a few teeth are missing, a *bridge* can fill the gap; if all the teeth are missing, a *denture* is needed.

Anomaly

A deviation from what is accepted as normal, especially a birth defect such as a limb malformation.

Anorexia

The medical term for loss of appetite (see *Appetite, loss of*).

Anorexia nervosa

An eating disorder characterized by severe weight loss, wilful avoidance of food, and intense fear of being fat. *Amenorrhea* (absence of menstrual periods) is also typical in girls and women. Popularly known as the "slimmer's disease," anorexia nervosa is difficult to treat and is occasionally fatal.

INCIDENCE

Anorexia most often affects teenage girls and young adult women, especially from certain high-risk groups. In the population as a whole, the incidence is one in 100,000; among middle-class teenage girls and young women it is one in 100, rising to one in 20 among young female models, ballet dancers, and athletes. Males are affected only very rarely.

CAUSES

The causes of anorexia are much debated. Many sufferers seem to be part of close-knit families and to have a special relationship with one parent. Some sufferers seem to be particularly anxious to please and tend to be obsessional in their habits.

People with anorexia nervosa may see dieting as a way of controlling their lives. It seems as if they do not wish to grow up and are trying to keep their childhood shapes.

Some specialists have suggested that anorexia nervosa is a true *phobia* about putting on weight.

Other specialists believe that anorexia is a symptom rather than a disease, and that the real cause is *depression, personality disorder,* or, rarely, *schizophrenia*. However, it is frequently difficult to identify any such underlying cause.

Hormonal changes related to weight loss and absence of menstruation have led some doctors to regard anorexia nervosa as a physical illness that is caused by a disorder of the *hypothalamus* (part of the brain concerned with hunger, thirst, and sexual development).

SYMPTOMS AND SIGNS

The most obvious sign is emaciation (extreme thinness), with one third or more of the body's weight being lost. In the early stages of the disorder, sufferers are typically overactive, constantly busy, and exercise much of the time. As weight loss continues, they become tired and weak, the skin becomes dry, lanugo hair (fine, downy hair) grows on the body, and normal hair becomes thinner. Starvation causes certain biochemical disorders and disrupts the balance of sex hormones, leading to amenorrhea in many cases.

Most people with anorexia eat very little and are very choosy about their food. Sometimes they have food binges and then make themselves

FEATURES OF ANOREXIA NERVOSA

- Weight loss
- Overactivity and obsessive exercising
- Tiredness and weakness
- Lanugo (babylike) hair on body, thinning of hair on head
- Extreme choosiness over food
- Binge eating
- Induced vomiting
- Use of laxatives to promote weight loss

vomit or take *laxative drugs* or *diuretic drugs* to promote weight loss (see *Bulimia*). Such behavior occurs because they often feel intensely hungry, even though they may deny this. Food and weight dominate thinking to an extreme degree. Sufferers have a distorted body image and "see" themselves as much fatter than they really are. Drug abuse and alcohol abuse occasionally occur.

TREATMENT

Hospital treatment is often necessary to help the sufferer return to a normal weight. Treatment is usually based on a closely controlled refeeding program, combined with individual *psychotherapy* or *family therapy*. Unless a strict watch is kept on feeding, patients tend to hide or throw away food. Occasionally, a system of rewards is used: the more weight gained, the more privileges given to the patient. Drugs may be needed if there is a depressive or other illness. *Chlorpromazine* is often helpful in the early stages to calm patients and to promote weight gain.

OUTLOOK

Sufferers may need to continue psychotherapy for months or years after they have achieved a more normal weight. Relapses are common whenever there is the slightest stress. About 50 percent of all patients treated for anorexia nervosa in a hospital continue to have symptoms for many years; 5 to 10 percent later die from starvation or suicide.

Anorgasmia

Inability to achieve orgasm (see *Orgasm, lack of*).

Anosmia

Loss of *smell*.

A

Anoxia

A medical term that means literally a complete absence of oxygen within a body tissue—for example, the brain or a muscle. Anoxia causes a disruption of cell *metabolism* (chemical activity) and cell death unless corrected within a few minutes.

Anoxia is very rare, occurring during cardiopulmonary arrest or asphyxiation, whereas *hypoxia* (the reduction of oxygen supply to a tissue) is a more common problem.

Antacid drugs

COMMON DRUGS

Aluminum hydroxide Magnesium hydroxide Magnesium trisilicate Sodium bicarbonate

> **WARNING**
> Antacid drugs should not be taken regularly except under medical supervision as they may suppress the symptoms of a more serious disorder or provoke serious complications.

Drugs taken to relieve *indigestion, heartburn, esophagitis* (inflammation of the esophagus), *acid reflux* (regurgitation of stomach acids into the esophagus), and *peptic ulcer.*

TYPES
Antacid drugs usually contain compounds of *magnesium* or *aluminum,* which have a long-lasting effect, or *sodium bicarbonate,* which produces a rapid, short-lived effect. Some antacid drugs also contain alginates, dimethicone, or a local anesthetic.

HOW THEY WORK
Antacid drugs neutralize stomach acids, an action that helps prevent or relieve inflammation and pain in the upper digestive system.

Antacid drugs also give the stomach lining time to heal when it has been damaged by a peptic ulcer and is therefore sensitive to normal amounts of stomach acid.

Alginates included in antacid preparations help to protect the esophagus against acid reflux. Dimethicone may possibly relieve *flatulence,* and local anesthetics may numb the pain of esophagitis.

POSSIBLE ADVERSE EFFECTS
Aluminum may cause constipation and magnesium may cause diarrhea—these effects may be avoided if a preparation contains both ingredients. Sodium bicarbonate may cause fluid retention and flatulence. Antacid drugs interfere with the absorption of

many drugs and a physician's advice should be sought before taking them with other medication.

Antepartum hemorrhage

Vaginal bleeding after the 28th week of pregnancy.

CAUSES AND INCIDENCE
Antepartum hemorrhage is most commonly due to a problem with the placenta, the organ in the uterus that sustains the developing fetus. The problem may be *placenta previa,* in which the placenta is positioned abnormally close to the birth canal; placental abruption (detachment of part of the placenta from the wall of the uterus); or bleeding from the edge of a normally sited placenta. Bleeding can also be caused by *cervical erosion* or other disorders of the cervix or vagina.

Antepartum hemorrhage occurs in about 3 percent of all pregnancies.

SYMPTOMS
The bleeding is often painless but there may be abdominal pain if the placenta becomes partly separated from the uterus.

INVESTIGATION AND TREATMENT
Admission to hospital is necessary for investigation and treatment. The fetus' heartbeat is monitored to assess the baby's condition. The position of the placenta is located by *ultrasound scanning* (a vaginal examination is not performed as this could damage a low-lying placenta).

In some cases, it is necessary only to keep a careful watch on the conditions of the woman and her baby. If bleeding is severe, the woman is given an *intravenous infusion* and possibly *blood transfusions.* Immediate delivery (possibly by *cesarean section*) may be necessary at times to prevent the baby from becoming starved of oxygen.

When delivery is not necessary, the woman usually stays in hospital for at least 48 hours. If the woman is considered to be at risk of further bleeding, which could endanger her or the baby, she may have to stay in hospital until delivery. Otherwise, if the bleeding has stopped and the conditions of woman and baby are considered satisfactory, the woman is allowed to go home—though her condition is carefully monitored for the remaining weeks of the pregnancy.

COMPLICATIONS
Because of good obstetric care, mortality of women and babies today is low. Death of the baby is more likely than maternal death; infant death may be caused by lack of oxygen or by prematurity if bleeding triggers labor.

Anterior

Relating to the front of the body. In human *anatomy,* the term is synonymous with *ventral.*

Anthelmintic drugs

COMMON DRUGS

Niclosamide Niridazole Piperazine Pyrantel Thiabendazole

A group of drugs used to treat *worm infestations.* Different types of anthelmintic drugs are used to treat infestation by different types of worms.

One or two doses of anthelmintic drugs usually kill or paralyze worms in the intestines, preventing them from gripping the intestinal walls and causing them to pass out of the body in the feces. To hasten this process, laxative drugs are occasionally prescribed with anthelmintics.

Anthelmintic drugs help kill worms in other tissues by making them more vulnerable to attack by the *immune system.* Once these worms have been killed, they may require surgical removal along with any cysts that the worms have produced.

Possible adverse effects of anthelmintic drugs include nausea, vomiting, abdominal pain, rash, headache, and dizziness.

Anthracosis

An old term for coal worker's *pneumoconiosis,* a lung disease caused by inhalation of large amounts of coal dust over a period of many years.

Anthralin

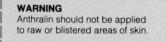

> **WARNING**
> Anthralin should not be applied to raw or blistered areas of skin.

An ointment or cream used to treat *psoriasis* (a skin disorder caused by excessive skin cell production). Anthralin slows the rate at which skin cells multiply; its action can be increased by ultraviolet light therapy (see *Phototherapy*).

POSSIBLE ADVERSE EFFECTS
Anthralin can cause redness and irritation of the skin, which may be relieved by topical corticosteroids. Normal skin near areas of psoriasis may be protected by petroleum jelly.

Since anthralin may stain clothes and, temporarily, the skin and hair, one should wear old clothes and gloves when applying this drug.

Anthrax

A serious bacterial infection of livestock that occasionally spreads to humans. The most common form of anthrax in humans is cutaneous anthrax, which affects the skin. Another form, pulmonary anthrax, affects the lungs.

CAUSES AND INCIDENCE

Anthrax is caused by a bacterium, *BACILLUS ANTHRACIS*, which produces spores that can survive dormant for many years in soil and animal products but are capable of reactivation.

Animals become infected by grazing on contaminated land. People may become infected via a scratch or sore if they handle materials from infected animals. Pulmonary anthrax occurs as a result of inhaling large numbers of spores contained in infected animal fibers.

Anthrax has not occurred in Canada since 1961, but serious epidemics have occurred in some developing countries, usually as a result of lapses in control programs.

SYMPTOMS AND TREATMENT

In cutaneous anthrax, a raised, itchy area develops at the site of entry of the spores, progressing to a large blister and finally to a black scab, with swelling of the surrounding tissues. Cutaneous anthrax is readily treatable with *penicillin* in its early stages. Without treatment, the infection may spread to lymph nodes and the bloodstream, and may be fatal.

Pulmonary anthrax causes severe breathing difficulty and is fatal in nearly all instances.

Antianxiety drugs

A group of drugs used to relieve symptoms of *anxiety*. *Benzodiazepine drugs* and *beta-blocker drugs* are the two main types of antianxiety drugs. Other drugs that may occasionally be used to treat anxiety include *antidepressant drugs*.

WHY THEY ARE USED

Antianxiety drugs are used to provide temporary relief from anxiety when it limits a person's ability to cope with everyday life. In most cases, the underlying disorder is best treated by *counseling*, *psychotherapy*, or other forms of therapy.

Antianxiety drugs are sometimes used to calm a person before surgical treatment (see *Premedication*) or before a public performance.

HOW THEY WORK

Benzodiazepines promote mental and physical relaxation by reducing nerve activity in the brain; for this reason, they may also be prescribed to treat insomnia. Beta-blockers work by reducing the physical symptoms of anxiety, such as shaking and palpitations.

Antiarrhythmic drugs

A group of drugs used to treat different types of *arrhythmia* (irregular heartbeat). Antiarrhythmic drugs include *beta-blocker drugs, calcium channel blockers, digitalis drugs, disopyramide, lidocaine, procainamide,* and *quinidine*. The specific drug prescribed by the physician depends on the type of arrhythmia being treated.

WHY THEY ARE USED

An arrhythmia can reduce the pumping efficiency of the heart, causing breathlessness, dizziness, and chest pain. Antiarrhythmic drugs relieve these symptoms and, in some cases, restore normal heartbeat.

HOW THEY WORK

The heart's pumping action is governed by electrical impulses. Some antiarrhythmic drugs work by altering these impulses within or on their way to the heart. Others affect the response of the heart muscle to the impulses received.

Antibacterial drugs

A group of drugs used to treat infections caused by *bacteria*. Antibacterial drugs share the actions of *antibiotic drugs* but, unlike antibiotics, these drugs have always been produced synthetically. The largest group of antibacterial drugs are the *sulfonamide drugs*, used mainly for the treatment of *urinary tract infection*.

Antibiotic drugs

COMMON DRUGS

Aminoglycosides
Gentamicin Streptomycin

Cephalosporins
Cefaclor Cephalexin Cephradine

Penicillins
Amoxicillin Ampicillin Flucloxacillin Phenoxymethylpenicillin

Tetracyclines
Doxycycline Minocycline Oxytetracycline Tetracycline

Others
Erythromycin Neomycin

WARNING
You must inform your physician of any previous allergic reaction to an antibiotic drug.

A group of drugs used to treat infections caused by *bacteria*. Originally obtained from molds and fungi (the first group was derived from *PENICILLIUM*), antibiotic drugs are now produced synthetically.

TYPES

Many antibiotic drugs belong to one of four main types: *aminoglycoside drugs, cephalosporin drugs, penicillin drugs,* and *tetracycline drugs*.

Some antibiotic drugs are effective against only certain types of bacteria. Others, known as broad-spectrum antibiotics, are effective against a wide range of bacteria. The choice of antibiotic drug depends on the type of bacteria and on the site of the infection. This choice is most effectively made by growing a culture of the bacteria and checking its sensitivity to various types of antibiotic.

More than one antibiotic drug may be prescribed to increase the efficiency of treatment and to reduce the risk of antibiotic resistance.

WHY THEY ARE USED

Antibiotic drugs are used to treat bacterial infections. They are also used to prevent infection if a person's *immune system* is impaired or if there is a risk of *endocarditis* (inflammation of the lining of the heart).

ANTIBIOTIC RESISTANCE

Some bacteria develop resistance to a previously effective antibiotic drug. Resistance may occur if a type of bacteria develops a method of growth that is not disrupted by the effects of the drug or if it begins to produce an *enzyme* that breaks down or inactivates the drug.

Resistance is most likely to develop during long-term treatment or if a person fails to take an antibiotic drug as directed by the doctor. Alternative antibiotic drugs are available to treat some bacteria that are resistant to the more commonly prescribed types of antibiotic drugs.

POSSIBLE ADVERSE EFFECTS

Most antibiotic drugs can cause nausea, diarrhea, or a rash, as well as adverse effects typical of particular types. Antibiotic drugs may disturb the normal balance in the body between certain types of bacteria and fungi, leading to proliferation of the fungi that cause oral, intestinal, or vaginal *candidiasis* (thrush). Some people occasionally experience a severe allergic reaction to antibiotic drugs, resulting in facial swelling, itching, or breathing difficulty. If this happens, stop taking the drug and see your physician immediately.

HOW ANTIBIOTICS WORK

Antibiotic drugs are either bactericidal (killing bacteria) or bacteriostatic (halting bacterial growth, allowing the immune system to cope with the infection). Penicillin drugs and cephalosporin drugs are bactericidal; these drugs work by disrupting bacterial cell walls.

Bactericidal antibiotics
These cause the bacterial cell wall to disintegrate; water is taken into the cell, which expands and then bursts, killing the bacteria.

Antibody

A protein that is manufactured by certain lymphocytes (types of white blood cell) to neutralize an *antigen* (foreign protein) in the body. Bacteria, viruses, and other microorganisms commonly contain many antigens; antibodies formed against these antigens help the body neutralize or destroy the invading microorganisms. Antibodies may also be formed in response to *vaccines*, thereby giving immunity against some infections. Antibodies are also known as *immunoglobulins*.

In some cases, inappropriate or excessive formation of antibodies leads to illness. The body's response to certain substances may lead to *allergy*, as in *asthma* or some types of *eczema*. Antibodies against antigens in skin grafts or organ transplants may result in rejection. In some disorders, antibodies are formed against the body's own tissues, resulting in an *autoimmune disorder*; examples of this type of disorder include some forms of *arthritis* and the *collagen diseases*. (See also *Immune response*.)

Antibody, monoclonal

An artificially produced *antibody* that neutralizes only one specific *antigen* (foreign protein).

Monoclonal antibodies are produced in the laboratory by stimulating the growth of a large clone of antibody-producing cells. (A clone is a group of cells that are genetically identical, or an individual member of such a group.) In effect, this cloning process enables antibodies to be tailor-made so that they will react with a particular antigen.

Monoclonal antibodies are used in the study of human cells, hormones, microorganisms, and in the development of new vaccines. They are also being used experimentally in the diagnosis of some forms of cancer, such as *lymphoma*. In addition, research is being carried out on the use of monoclonal antibodies to treat certain cancers: the antibodies can be directed against specific cancer cells and can, in theory, be used to carry lethal substances, such as radioactive molecules or toxins, to these target cells.

Anticancer drugs

COMMON DRUGS

Cytotoxic
Azathioprine Chlorambucil
Cyclophosphamide Doxorubicin Etoposide
Fluorouracil Lomustine Melphalan
Mercaptopurine Methotrexate Procarbazine

Sex hormone-related
Aminoglutethimide Ethinyl estradiol
Medroxyprogesterone Megestrol
Nandrolone Tamoxifen

Drugs used to treat *cancer*. Anticancer drugs are particularly useful in the treatment of *lymphomas, leukemias,* and cancer affecting the ovary or testis. These drugs are sometimes used after surgery or *radiation therapy*.

TYPES

Most anticancer drugs are cytotoxic drugs (drugs that kill or damage cells).

Others are synthetic forms of sex hormones and substances related to these hormones (e.g., *androgen drugs, estrogen drugs,* and *progesterone drugs*).

Anticancer drugs are often prescribed in combination to maximize their effects. The choice of drugs depends on the type of cancer, its stage of development, and the general health of the patient.

HOW THEY WORK

All anticancer drugs kill cancer cells by preventing them from growing and dividing. Some cytotoxic drugs work by damaging the cells' *DNA* (genetic material). Others block the chemical processes in the cell that are necessary for growth.

Sex hormones stimulate the growth of certain cancers (e.g., estrogen stimulates some types of breast cancer). Substances related to these hormones may inhibit growth by blocking their stimulatory effect. The growth of other cancers is sometimes disrupted by a synthetic sex hormone given in high doses. Cancer of the prostate gland, for example, may be treated with the estrogen drug *diethylstilbestrol* or *DES*.

POSSIBLE ADVERSE EFFECTS

In the early stages of treatment, nausea, vomiting, and diarrhea may occur; in some cases, these effects may be sufficiently serious to make hospitalization necessary.

Anticancer drugs may alter the rate at which noncancerous cells grow and divide. This effect may cause alopecia (hair loss) and reduce the number of blood cells produced by the bone marrow, causing *anemia*, increased susceptibility to infection, and/or abnormal bleeding. Regular blood tests are usually carried out to monitor blood-cell production.

To minimize adverse effects, anticancer drugs are usually given in short courses with time between each course to enable noncancerous cells to recover from the drugs' effects.

Anticholinergic drugs

COMMON DRUGS

Atropine Belladonna Benztropine
Dicyclomine Hyoscyamine Ipratropium
Orphenadrine Procyclidine Propantheline
Scopolamine

A group of drugs that block the effects of *acetylcholine*, a chemical released from nerve endings in the parasympathetic division of the *autonomic nervous system*. Acetylcholine triggers activity in a number of cells by relax-

HOW ANTICHOLINERGICS WORK

Acetylcholine combines with a receptor on the cell's surface. This interaction stimulates activity in that cell (e.g., contraction of a muscle fiber or secretion of a fluid). Anticholinergic drugs block the stimulatory action of acetylcholine by combining with the acetylcholine receptors. This action produces, for example, muscle relaxation (e.g., in the bladder, intestine, and bronchi) and dries up secretions in the mouth and lungs. Anticholinergic drugs are used to treat asthma.

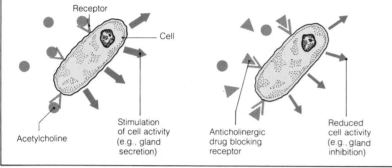

Receptor · Cell · Acetylcholine · Stimulation of cell activity (e.g., gland secretion)

Anticholinergic drug blocking receptor · Reduced cell activity (e.g., gland inhibition)

ing some muscles, tightening others and affecting the release of saliva. Thus it increases secretions in the mouth and lungs, and slows the heartbeat.

WHY THEY ARE USED

Anticholinergic drugs are used in the treatment of *irritable bowel syndrome*, urinary *incontinence*, *Parkinson's disease*, *asthma*, and *bradycardia* (abnormally slow heartbeat). They are also used to dilate the pupil before an examination of, or surgical procedure on, the eye. Anticholinergic drugs are also helpful as a *premedication* before general *anesthesia* and in the treatment of *motion sickness*.

Anticholinergic drugs may cause dry mouth, blurred vision, urinary retention, and confusion.

Anticoagulant drugs

COMMON DRUGS

Heparin Warfarin

> **WARNING**
> Many drugs, such as ASA and alcohol, may increase the risk of an anticoagulant drug causing abnormal bleeding. Always consult your physician before taking any other drug during anticoagulant treatment.

A group of drugs used to treat and prevent abnormal *blood clotting*. They are used to treat *thrombosis*, and *stroke* or *transient ischemic attack* (stroke symptoms lasting less than 24 hours). Anticoagulant drugs are also pre-scribed to prevent abnormal blood clotting after major surgery (especially heart valve replacement) or during hemodialysis (see *Dialysis*).

HOW THEY WORK

Heparin increases the activity in the blood of antithrombin III, an enzyme that blocks the activity of other enzymes—known as clotting factors—that are needed for blood to clot. This drug is given by injection and begins to work within a few hours. Most other anticoagulant drugs are taken by mouth and take longer before they become effective. They work by reducing the production of some of the clotting factors.

By disrupting the blood clotting mechanism, anticoagulant drugs prevent an abnormal blood clot from forming. When a blood clot already exists, anticoagulant drugs stop it from enlarging and reduce the risk of an *embolus* breaking off and blocking another blood vessel. Anticoagulant drugs, however, do not dissolve blood clots that have already formed. *Thrombolytic drugs* are needed for that.

POSSIBLE ADVERSE EFFECTS

Anticoagulant drugs in high doses may cause abnormal bleeding in different parts of the body. As a result, regular *blood clotting tests* are carried out to monitor treatment.

Anticonvulsant drugs

COMMON DRUGS

Carbamazepine Clonazepam Diazepam Ethosuximide Phenobarbital Phenytoin Primidone Valproic acid

> **WARNING**
> Never suddenly stop taking an anticonvulsant drug after long-term treatment; the dose should be reduced gradually or symptoms may return.

A group of drugs used in the treatment of *epilepsy* and other types of *seizure*. Anticonvulsant drugs are taken on a regular basis to reduce the frequency and severity of seizures and as an emergency treatment to stop a prolonged seizure.

Anticonvulsant drugs are also administered to prevent seizures following a serious head injury or some types of brain surgery; they may be given to a child with a high fever who has a history of febrile seizures (see *Convulsion, febrile*). The choice of drug is largely determined by the type of seizure. Long-term treatment may require use of more than one type of anticonvulsant drug.

HOW THEY WORK

Seizures are caused by an abnormally high level of electrical activity in the brain. Anticonvulsant drugs have an inhibitory effect that neutralizes this excessive electrical activity and thereby prevents its spread throughout areas of the brain.

POSSIBLE ADVERSE EFFECTS

Anticonvulsant drugs may produce various adverse effects, including reduced concentration, impaired memory, poor coordination, and fatigue. The doctor will try to establish a dose that prevents seizures but minimizes adverse effects. Regular monitoring of blood levels of the drug may be needed to achieve this.

Antidepressant drugs

COMMON DRUGS

Tricyclics
Amitriptyline Amoxapine Clomipramine Doxepin Imipramine Trazodone

Monoamine oxidase inhibitors (MAOIs)
Isocarboxazid Phenelzine Tranylcypromine

Others
Lithium Fluvoxamine Tryptophan

> **WARNING**
> Food and drink containing tyramine (e.g., cheese and red wine) and certain drugs may produce a dangerous rise in blood pressure if taken during treatment with an MAOI. Always tell your physician if you are taking an MAOI.

Drugs used in the treatment of *depression*. The two main types are tricyclic antidepressant drugs and monoamine oxidase inhibitors.

HOW THEY WORK

Some antidepressant drugs trigger the release of chemicals in the brain that stimulate nerve activity. Others, notably tricyclic antidepressants and monoamine oxidase inhibitors, prolong the active life of these chemicals after their release. Antidepressant drugs usually take at least 10 days to have any beneficial effect and up to eight weeks to become fully effective.

POSSIBLE ADVERSE EFFECTS

Most antidepressant drugs can cause dry mouth, blurred vision, dizziness, drowsiness, constipation, and difficulty in passing urine; these symptoms often improve as treatment continues. An overdose of an antidepressant drug may cause abnormal heart rhythm, seizures, coma, and, occasionally, death.

Antidiarrheal drugs

COMMON DRUGS
Adsorbent agents
Kaolin Methylcellulose
Others
Codeine Diphenoxylate
Loperamide Psyllium

> **WARNING**
> Do not take antidiarrheal drugs regularly except under medical supervision because they may mask a serious underlying disorder.

A group of drugs used to treat *diarrhea*. Some antidiarrheal drugs, including bulking agents, are adsorbent substances; others, including narcotic antidiarrheals, reduce the activity of the intestines.

WHY THEY ARE USED

Antidiarrheal drugs may be recommended if diarrhea persists for more than 24 to 48 hours. They are often prescribed while the cause of persistent diarrhea is being investigated, especially if the diarrhea is severe and debilitating. Antidiarrheal drugs are also given to help regulate bowel action in people who have had a *colostomy* or *ileostomy*.

HOW THEY WORK

Many adsorbent antidiarrheal drugs are believed to work by taking in the toxic substances that cause diarrhea, making the feces more solid. Bulking agents, such as methylcellulose, adsorb water from the feces.

Drugs that reduce the activity of muscles in the intestinal wall slow the passage of feces and allow more time for water to be absorbed into the bloodstream. As a result, both the fluidity and frequency of bowel movements are reduced.

POSSIBLE ADVERSE EFFECTS

Antidiarrheal drugs may cause constipation. In cases of diarrhea caused by an infection, antidiarrheal drugs may delay recovery by slowing the elimination of microorganisms.

Bulking agents may cause intestinal obstruction if they are used without drinking sufficient water or if the bowel is narrowed.

Prolonged use of a narcotic antidiarrheal drug may cause physical dependence (see *Drug dependence*), producing nausea, abdominal pain, and diarrhea if the drug is suddenly stopped. *Loperamide* is chemically similar to narcotic antidiarrheals, but does not have a narcotic effect.

Antidiuretic hormone

See *ADH*.

Antidote

A substance that neutralizes or counteracts the effects of a poison. The antidote for acid is alkali, and vice versa. A chemical antidote works by combining with a poison to form an innocuous substance, or in some way blocking or diverting the action of the poison. A mechanical antidote prevents the absorption of poison into the blood from the stomach and intestine.

Anti-D(Rh$_o$) immune globulin

An *antiserum* that contains antibodies against Rhesus (Rh) D factor (a substance present on the red blood cells of people who have Rh-positive blood). It is given to a woman who has Rh-negative blood after she has given birth to a baby whose blood is Rh positive, which may occur if the baby's father is Rh positive.

Anti-D(Rh$_o$) immune globulin is also given to a pregnant woman with Rh-negative blood after she has had an *amniocentesis*, bleeding episode, *miscarriage*, or *abortion*, or in other instances in which she might have been exposed to fetal blood cells. The injected antibodies destroy any red blood cells from the fetus that have entered the woman's bloodstream. This precaution is important in preventing or reducing the risk that the woman will form her own antibodies against Rh-positive blood, which might adversely affect a subsequent

pregnancy. (See also *Hemolytic disease of the newborn* and *Rh incompatibility*.)

Antiemetic drugs

COMMON DRUGS
Anticholinergics
Hyoscine
Antihistamines
Dimenhydrinate Meclizine Promethazine
Phenothiazines
Chlorpromazine Perphenazine
Prochlorperazine Promethazine
Thiethylperazine
Others
Metoclopramide

> **WARNING**
> An antiemetic drug should not be taken regularly except under medical supervision as it may mask a serious underlying disorder.

A group of drugs used to treat *nausea* and *vomiting* caused by *motion sickness*, *vertigo*, *Meniere's disease*, *radiation therapy*, or certain drugs (especially *anticancer drugs*). Some antiemetic drugs are also used to treat severe vomiting during pregnancy.

Antiemetic drugs are seldom prescribed to treat food poisoning because it is believed that vomiting enables the body to rid itself of harmful substances.

HOW THEY WORK

Some antiemetic drugs reduce nerve activity at the base of the brain and thereby suppress the vomiting reflex. *Antihistamine drugs* and also *anticholinergic drugs* reduce the vomiting associated with vertigo by suppressing nerve activity in the balance center in the inner ear. Other antiemetic drugs prevent vomiting by relaxing the muscles in the lower part of the stomach and so enabling the stomach contents to pass from the stomach into the small intestine.

POSSIBLE ADVERSE EFFECTS

Many antiemetic drugs cause drowsiness. Some must not be taken during pregnancy because they may damage the developing fetus.

Antifreeze poisoning

Most antifreeze contains ethylene glycol or methanol (methyl alcohol), both of which are poisonous. Antifreeze poisoning is rare. Most cases occur as a result of accidental swallowing.

SYMPTOMS AND TREATMENT

Drinking antifreeze initially produces the same effects as alcohol intoxication, but vomiting, stupor, seizures, and coma may follow within a few hours; acute *kidney failure* may occur within 24 to 36 hours. Blindness is a possibility if the antifreeze contains methanol.

Any person believed to have drunk antifreeze needs immediate medical attention. Until such help arrives, small amounts of alcohol (approximately two shots of liquor) should be given if the person is conscious; alcohol reduces the rate at which antifreeze is metabolized and becomes toxic in the body.

Hospital treatment may include pumping out the stomach (see *Lavage, gastric*) and giving *diuretic drugs*, alcohol, and bicarbonate (by drip into a vein) to correct excess acidity in the body fluids. Hemodialysis (see *Dialysis*) may be required to remove ethylene glycol from the blood and to treat kidney failure.

Antifungal drugs

COMMON DRUGS

Amphotericin B Clotrimazole Econazole Flucytosine Griseofulvin Ketoconazole Miconazole Nystatin Tolnaftate

A group of drugs prescribed to treat infections caused by *fungi*. Antifungal drugs are commonly used to treat different types of *tinea*, including tinea pedis (athlete's foot) and tinea capitis (scalp ringworm). They are also used to treat *candidiasis* (thrush) and rare fungal infections (such as *cryptococcosis*) which affect internal organs.

Antifungal preparations are available in various forms: tablets, lozenges, liquids, creams, injections, and vaginal suppositories.

HOW THEY WORK

Antifungal drugs damage the cell walls of fungi, causing chemicals essential for normal cell function and growth to escape. The fungal cells are unable to survive without these chemicals and die.

POSSIBLE ADVERSE EFFECTS

Preparations applied to the skin, scalp, mouth, or vagina may occasionally increase irritation. Antifungal drugs given by mouth or injection may cause more serious side effects, including liver or kidney damage.

Antigen

A substance that can trigger an *immune response*, resulting in production of an *antibody* as part of the body's defense against infection and disease. Many antigens are foreign proteins (those not found naturally in the body); they include parts of microorganisms, toxins, and tissues from another person used in organ transplantation. Sometimes, harmless substances (e.g., pollen) are misidentified as potentially harmful antigens by the immune system, resulting in an allergic response (see *Allergy*).

Antihistamine drugs

COMMON DRUGS

Astemizole Azatadine Chlorpheniramine Mebhydrolin Promethazine Terfenadine Trimeprazine Triprolidine

> **WARNING**
> Do not drive or operate potentially dangerous machinery while taking an antihistamine drug until you are certain that the treatment is not causing dizziness or drowsiness or impairing your coordination.

A group of drugs that block the effects of *histamine*, a chemical released during allergic reactions (see *Allergy*).

WHY THEY ARE USED

Antihistamine drugs are used in the treatment of *urticaria* (hives) and other rashes to relieve itching, swelling, and redness. Drugs of this type are also used in the treatment of allergic *rhinitis* (hay fever) to relieve sneezing and a runny nose.

Antihistamine drugs are sometimes included in *cough remedies* and *cold remedies* because they dry up nasal secretions and suppress the nerve centers in the brain that trigger the cough reflex. Antihistamines are also used as *antiemetic drugs* because they suppress the vomiting reflex.

Because many antihistamine drugs have a sedative effect, they are sometimes used to induce sleep, especially when itching keeps the sufferer awake at night. The most recently introduced antihistamines have very little sedative effect.

Antihistamine drugs are usually given by mouth but they may be given by injection in an emergency to aid in treating *anaphylactic shock* (a severe allergic reaction).

HOW THEY WORK

Antihistamine drugs block the effect of histamine on tissues such as the skin, eyes, and nose. Without drug treatment, histamine would dilate (widen) small blood vessels, resulting in redness and swelling of the surrounding tissue due to leakage of fluid from the circulation. Antihistamines also prevent histamine from irritating nerve fibers, which would otherwise cause itching.

POSSIBLE ADVERSE EFFECTS

Many antihistamines cause drowsiness and dizziness. However, the latest generation of antihistamines have virtually no soporific effect. Other possible side effects of antihistamines include loss of appetite, nausea, dry mouth, blurred vision, and difficulty passing urine.

Antihypertensive drugs

COMMON DRUGS

ACE inhibitors
Captopril Enalapril

Beta-blockers
Atenolol Loratidine Metoprolol Oxprenolol Propranolol

Calcium channel blockers
Diltiazem Nifedipine Verapamil

Diuretic drugs
Chlorthalidone Hydrochlorothiazide

Vasodilator drugs
Hydralazine Minoxidil Prazosin

Others
Clonidine Methyldopa

> **WARNING**
> Never stop taking antihypertensive drugs suddenly as this may cause a dangerous rise in blood pressure.

A group of drugs that are used in the treatment of *hypertension* (high blood pressure) to prevent the development of complications such as *stroke, myocardial infarction* (heart attack), *heart failure* (reduced pumping efficiency), and kidney damage.

HOW THEY WORK

Beta-blocker drugs reduce the force of the heartbeat, thereby lowering the pressure of blood flow into the circulation. *Diuretic drugs* increase the amount of salts and water excreted in the urine, although the way in which they lower the blood pressure is not entirely clear.

Other types of antihypertensive drugs cause the blood vessels to dilate (widen), which decreases the resistance to blood flow and thereby lowers the blood pressure.

POSSIBLE ADVERSE EFFECTS

Apart from the side effects typical of specific groups, all antihypertensive drugs may cause dizziness and fainting initially through lowering the blood pressure too much. Determining proper dosage may take time.

Anti-inflammatory drugs

Drugs that reduce the symptoms and signs of *inflammation*. (See *Analgesic drugs; Corticosteroid drugs; Nonsteroidal anti-inflammatory drugs.*)

Antimalarial drugs

See *Malaria.*

Antiperspirant

COMMON DRUGS
Aluminum chloride Aluminum chlorhydrate

A substance applied to the skin in the form of a lotion, cream, or spray to reduce excessive sweating.

WHY IT IS USED

An antiperspirant is used to prevent the accumulation of sweat, especially in the armpits. When sweat remains on the skin, it creates a moist environment in which bacteria can thrive. The bacteria break down chemicals in the sweat, causing body odor (sweat itself is almost odorless).

High concentrations of antiperspirants are sometimes prescribed to treat *hyperhidrosis* (abnormally profuse sweating). Results of this treatment are variable.

HOW IT WORKS

An antiperspirant reduces the production of sweat by the sweat glands and blocks the ducts that drain sweat onto the surface of the skin.

POSSIBLE ADVERSE EFFECTS

Antiperspirants may cause skin irritation and a burning or stinging sensation. Such effects are more common when high concentrations are used. If the irritation persists when a lower dose is used, treatment should be stopped to prevent *dermatitis*. (See also *Deodorants.*)

Antipsychotic drugs

COMMON DRUGS
Phenothiazines *Chlorpromazine Fluphenazine Perphenazine Thioridazine Trifluoperazine*
Others *Haloperidol Lithium Thiothixene*

A group of drugs used to treat *psychoses* (mental disorders involving loss of contact with reality), particularly *schizophrenia* and *manic-depressive illness*. Antipsychotic drugs enable many people suffering from mental illness to live relatively normal lives outside mental institutions.

Antipsychotic drugs are also used to calm or sedate people with other mental disorders (such as *dementia*) who have become highly agitated or aggressive.

Antipsychotic drugs include *phenothiazine drugs* and *lithium*, which is used specifically to treat the symptoms of *mania* (abnormal elation and overactivity).

HOW THEY WORK

Most antipsychotic drugs block the action of *dopamine*, a chemical that stimulates nerve activity in the brain. Lithium is thought to reduce the release of *norepinephrine* in the brain.

POSSIBLE ADVERSE EFFECTS

Most antipsychotic drugs can cause drowsiness, lethargy, *dyskinesia* (jerky movements of the mouth, face, and tongue), and *parkinsonism* (symptoms similar to those of Parkinson's disease). Other possible side effects include dry mouth, blurred vision, and difficulty passing urine. Lithium may cause nausea, diarrhea, tremor, rash, weight gain, and weakness of the muscles.

Antipyretic drugs

Drugs that reduce fever, such as ASA and acetaminophen.

Antirheumatic drugs

COMMON DRUGS
Corticosteroid drugs *Dexamethasone Prednisolone*
Immunosuppressant drugs *Azathioprine Chlorambucil*
Others *Auranofin Chloroquine Gold Penicillamine*

A group of drugs used in the treatment of *rheumatoid arthritis* and types of arthritis caused by other *autoimmune disorders* (disorders in which the body's immune system attacks its own tissues)—for example, systemic *lupus erythematosus*. Antirheumatic drugs are prescribed for active disease when *nonsteroidal anti-inflammatory drugs* (NSAIDs) fail to relieve pain and stiffness in the joints, or when the disease is causing progressive deformity and disability.

HOW THEY WORK

Antirheumatic drugs limit the damage caused by the immune system by suppressing either the production or activity of white blood cells. Each type of drug works in a different way, but all antirheumatics damp down the inflammation caused by the autoimmune reaction and also slow degeneration of the cartilage that lines joints.

The effectiveness of each type of antirheumatic drug varies according to the individual. Beneficial effects do not usually appear for several weeks after starting drug treatment, so patience is essential.

POSSIBLE ADVERSE EFFECTS

All antirheumatic drugs may cause serious adverse effects. For example, *gold*, which many consider the most effective, and *penicillamine* may cause rashes, blood disorders and kidney damage; the prolonged use of *chloroquine* may damage the eyes; and *immunosuppressant drugs* may cause blood disorders. In view of the seriousness of these risks, regular medical examinations, including blood and urine tests, are carried out during treatment to monitor toxic effects.

Antiseptics

Chemicals applied to the skin to destroy bacteria and other microorganisms and thus prevent *sepsis* (infection). Antisepsis (the use of antiseptics to prevent infection) is not the same as asepsis, which is the creation of a germ-free environment (see *Aseptic technique*). Antiseptics are milder than *disinfectants*, which decontaminate inanimate objects but are too strong to be used on the body.

Antiseptic fluids are generally used for bathing wounds, whereas creams are applied to wounds before they are dressed. Among the more commonly used antiseptics are *iodine*, *hydrogen peroxide*, and *chlorhexidine*.

Antiserum

A preparation containing antibodies that combine with specific *antigens* (foreign proteins), usually components of microorganisms (such as viruses or bacteria). Such antibody-antigen interaction leads to the inactivation or destruction of the microorganisms. Antiserum samples are usually prepared from the blood of animals who have been injected with killed, or live but harmless, strains of particular viruses or bacteria.

Antiserum is usually used, along with *immunization*, as an emergency treatment when someone has been exposed to a dangerous infection such as *rabies* and has not previously been immunized against the infection. The antiserum helps to provide some immediate protection against the infective microorganisms while full immunity is developing. However, such measures are not as effective in preventing disease as earlier (pre-exposure) immunization.

Antisocial personality disorder

Failure to conform to social norms of behavior. The category of antisocial personality is relatively new and was devised to provide clear guidelines for diagnosing psychiatric disorder. In the past, people displaying antisocial behavior were classified in a number of ways, for example as "sociopaths" or "psychopaths," but it was argued that these labels described character traits rather than specific illnesses that brought about changes in personality or behavior.

DIAGNOSIS

For a person to be diagnosed as suffering from this type of disorder, the antisocial behavior must have started before the age of 15 and must not be a result of *mental handicap* or obvious illness. Since there must be evidence of persistent disturbance over a period of time, the term cannot be used to describe anyone under 18 years of age. For a positive diagnosis, there must be evidence of disturbances in all the following areas of the individual's life: performance at work or school; childhood behavior; personal life; and personal relationships.

In the first area, signs of disturbance include constant job changes; persistent unemployment for no good reason; regular absences from work; and poor school performance. For a positive rate in the second area, at least three of the following must have occurred: truancy; rule breaking; expulsion from school; lying; stealing; running away from home; excessive drinking; juvenile court appearances; or precocious sexual activity. A positive rating in the third area is given if two or more of the following have occurred: crimes; separation or divorce; fighting; regular drunkenness; money troubles; or periods of homelessness. In the fourth area, a positive rating is given if there is an inability to form or maintain close relationships with family, friends or sexual partners that seems to be due to a basic lack of concern for others.

TREATMENT

The aim of treatment is to alter behavior; this may include living in *therapeutic communities*, *behavior therapy*, various forms of *psychotherapy*, and participation in community help programs. There is a clear overlap with legal punishment, since criminal activity is common, but the debate as to whether people with antisocial personality disorder are "bad" or "mad" remains unresolved.

Antispasmodic drugs

COMMON DRUGS

Belladonna Dicyclomine Peppermint oil

A group of drugs that relax spasm in smooth (involuntary) muscle in the wall of the intestine or bladder. Antispasmodic drugs are used in the treatment of *irritable bowel syndrome* and *irritable bladder*.

Antispasmodic drugs may have an anticholinergic action (that is, they work by blocking the action of *acetylcholine*, a neurotransmitter chemical released from nerve endings that stimulates muscle contraction).

Possible adverse effects of antispasmodic drugs include dry mouth, blurred vision, and difficulty passing urine. (See also *Anticholinergic drugs*.)

Antitoxin

Any of a variety of commercially prepared substances, each of which contains *antibodies* that can combine and neutralize the effect of a specific toxin released into the bloodstream by bacteria (such as those that cause *tetanus* and *diphtheria*).

Antitoxins are prepared from the blood of animals or humans that have been exposed to particular toxins (either by inoculation or as a result of suffering from the disease) and have therefore produced antibodies against the toxins.

Antitoxins are usually administered by injection into a muscle, under the supervision of a physician. Occasionally, an antitoxin may cause an allergic reaction; rarely, it causes an *anaphylactic shock* (a severe allergic reaction) requiring emergency treatment.

Antitussive drugs

A group of drugs that prevent or relieve a *cough,* either by suppressing the coughing reflex or helping to loosen and get rid of excess sputum. (See *Cough remedies*.)

Antivenin

 A specific treatment for snake, scorpion, spider, or other venomous animal bites or stings. Antivenin is prepared by inoculating animals, usually horses, with small but increasing amounts of venom from a particular poisonous animal. This provokes the production of *antibodies* that will neutralize the poisons in the venom. A preparation of these antibodies can then be produced from samples of the horse's blood.

Antiviral drugs

COMMON DRUGS

Acyclovir Amantadine Idoxuridine Trifluridine Zidovudine

A group of drugs used in the treatment of infection by *viruses*. Drugs that kill viruses have proved difficult to develop because viruses live only within body cells and there is a danger that antiviral drugs will damage the host cells as well as the virus. To date, no drugs have been developed that can effectively eradicate viruses and cure the illnesses that they cause.

Immunization is at present more important than drug treatment in fighting serious viral infections. However, some drugs have already proved useful in tackling a few viral infections, particularly those caused by *herpes* viruses. Antiviral drugs reduce the severity of these infections but may not eliminate them completely, so attacks may recur. Other antiviral drugs are currently being developed and used (e.g., to treat *AIDS*).

HOW THEY WORK

Most antiviral drugs destroy viruses by disrupting chemical processes necessary for viruses to grow and multiply within cells. Some antiviral drugs prevent viruses from actually penetrating cells.

POSSIBLE ADVERSE EFFECTS

Antiviral drugs used in treating AIDS carry a high risk of causing anemia due to bone marrow damage. Most other antiviral drugs rarely cause side effects. Antiviral creams may irritate the skin. Antiviral drugs given by mouth or injection can cause nausea and dizziness, and, rarely, in long-term treatment, kidney damage.

Antral irrigation

Irrigation of the maxillary antrum (also called the maxillary sinus), one of the nasal sinuses, to diagnose and treat persistent *sinusitis*.

WHY IT IS USED

Antral irrigation is used when sinusitis persists after drug treatment (usually with *antibiotic drugs* and *decongestant drugs*) has failed to provide a cure. The procedure enables the physician to get a positive diagnosis of infection, and it sometimes also cures the infection.

The normal drainage channel from the antrum into the nose is usually at least partly blocked in chronic sinusitis, causing infected material to build up within the cavity. Antral irrigation creates a temporary opening that allows the contents to be flushed out through the natural opening.

HOW IT IS DONE

In antral irrigation, a cannula (hollow, flexible tube) is inserted into the antrum, guided by a trocar (sharp, pointed rod). The trocar is inserted into the nostril and pushed through the bony side wall of the nose into the antrum. The trocar is then withdrawn, leaving the cannula in place. At this point, a syringe is attached to the cannula and the contents of the sinus are sucked out and sent to the laboratory for bacteriological culture to identify the organism responsible for the infection and to test its sensitivity to various antibiotics.

A large syringe filled with warm saline (salt solution) is attached to the cannula and the antrum is thoroughly washed out by injecting the solution into the cavity and causing it to flow out through the natural sinus opening. Washing out is repeated until the fluid is clear.

RESULTS

Unless sinusitis has been present for so long that permanent damage to the mucosa (lining of the sinus) has occurred, antral irrigation may be curative. However, if the infection fails to disappear after a period of several weeks, and an irrigation confirms that the antrum is still infected, surgery to enlarge the drainage channel may be required.

Anuria

Complete cessation of urine output. Such total failure to pass urine is an indication of a serious problem in the urinary tract because some urine is produced even when a person is severely dehydrated.

Anuria may be caused by a severe malfunction of the kidneys, but a much more common cause is a complete blockage to the flow of urine—due, for example, to enlargement of the prostate gland (see *Prostate, enlarged*), a *bladder tumor*, or a stone (see *Calculus, urinary tract*). Failure of urine production by the kidneys may be due to oxygen depletion as a result of reduced blood flow through the kidneys, as occurs in *shock*, or to severe kidney damage caused by a disease such as *glomerulonephritis*.

Anuria requires urgent investigation to establish the cause and to allow treatment, such as rehydration, or removal of the blockage, to begin. Without treatment, anuria leads to *uremia* (excess urea and other waste products in the blood) and death.

Anus

The canal at the end of the alimentary tract through which feces are expelled from the body. About 4 cm long, the anus is an extension of the rectum as it passes backward and downward through the pelvic floor. The orifice at the end of the anal canal is open only during defecation—at other times it is kept closed by the muscles of the anal sphincter. These muscles are arranged in two layers, the internal sphincter, which cannot be controlled voluntarily, and the external sphincter, which can be relaxed at will for defecation. (See also *Digestive system*.)

Anus, cancer of

A rare cancer of the skin of the anus. Possible early signs of anal cancer are swelling at the outside of the anus accompanied by bleeding and discomfort. Surgical removal of the cancer is the usual treatment.

Anus, imperforate

A rare *congenital* abnormality, detected and treated at birth, in which the anal opening appears to be covered over.

TYPES

Classification of the two main types of imperforate anus, high and low, depends on whether or not the bowel ends above or below the pelvic floor. In the high type, the anal canal fails to develop and there is no connection between the rectum and the anus. Many of the normal anal structures, such as the muscles, are missing. This type of imperforate anus is often associated with other abnormalities, especially of the urinary organs. In the low type, there may be only a layer of skin covering the anal opening.

TREATMENT

Treatment for high imperforate anus involves surgery to open up the end of the rectum and join it to the anus. This operation is usually successful and the long-term outlook is good. In some cases of this disorder, a *colostomy* may be needed.

Treatment for low imperforate anus usually involves surgical removal of the skin over the anus. In addition, *anal dilatation* (a procedure to enlarge the anus) may be needed for several months afterward.

DISORDERS OF THE ANUS

Most anal disorders are minor but they may cause considerable discomfort and concern. Many are aggravated by constipation, and may be helped by regular toilet habits, an increased intake of fluids, whole-grain products, fruits, and vegetables to soften the feces, and the use of glycerin suppositories.

CONGENITAL DEFECTS

Imperforate anus is an uncommon birth defect in which the anus is sealed (see *Anus, imperforate*).

In *anal stenosis*, the anus is too narrow to allow the normal passage of feces. This is sometimes a congenital abnormality, but it can also result from scarring after surgery for another disorder.

INJURY

Anal fissures originate from small tears in the lining of the anus, usually as a result of straining to pass hard, dry feces.

TUMORS

Cancer of the skin around the anus is rare (see *Anus, cancer of*).

OTHER DISORDERS

Hemorrhoids are enlarged blood vessels under the lining of the anus and may cause bleeding during defecation, itching, and pain.

An *anal fistula* is an abnormal tunnel connecting the inside of the anal canal with the skin surrounding the anus. These fistulas usually result from an abscess in the wall of the anus.

Itching of the anus (pruritus ani) may be a direct result of another disorder, such as an anal fistula, hemorrhoids or *pinworm* infestation.

INVESTIGATION

Investigation of anal disorders is usually by visual inspection, sometimes including *proctoscopy* (use of an internal viewing tube), and digital examination (feeling with a finger). Sometimes a biopsy (specimen of tissue for analysis) or swab may be taken for bacteriological culture.

STRUCTURE OF THE ANUS

The anus is a canal at the end of the alimentary tract, with internal and external sphincters to open and close the orifice.

Rectum

Internal sphincter muscle

External sphincter muscle

Anxiety

An unpleasant emotional state ranging from mild unease to intense fear. An anxious person usually feels a sense of impending doom, although there is no obvious threat, and has certain physical and psychological symptoms. A certain amount of anxiety is normal and serves to improve performance. Anxiety becomes a symptom when it starts to inhibit thought and to disrupt normal everyday activities.

SYMPTOMS AND SIGNS

The most common physical symptoms relate to the chest. They include palpitations (awareness of a more forceful or faster heartbeat), throbbing or stabbing pains, a feeling of tightness and inability to take in enough air, and a tendency to sigh or over breathe (see *Hyperventilation*).

Muscle tension leads to headaches, spasms in the neck, back pains, grasping too tightly, and an inability to relax. Restlessness, tremor of the hands, and a sense of tiredness are

also common. A pins and needles sensation or spasm of the arms sometimes follows hyperventilation.

Gastrointestinal symptoms include dryness of the mouth, a feeling of distention, diarrhea, nausea, changes in appetite, constant belching, and difficulty swallowing. Some sufferers may actually vomit or have severe pain mimicking serious illness.

Other symptoms include sweating, blushing, pallor, dizziness, lightheadedness, yawning, and a frequent need to urinate or defecate.

People with anxiety usually have a constant feeling that something bad is going to happen. They may fear that they have a chronic or dangerous illness (a fear reinforced by their physical symptoms) or worry about the health or safety of family and friends. Fear of losing control is also common. Anxiety often leads to increasing dependence on others, irritability, a sense of fatigue, and a state of being easily frustrated. Inability to relax may lead to difficulty getting to sleep and constant waking during the night. Frightening dreams often occur.

Strange but common symptoms are *depersonalization* (the sense of being cut off from oneself) or *derealization* (the sense of being cut off from the world). These symptoms can begin suddenly and last for a long time, leading some people to fear they are becoming insane.

Symptoms of anxiety usually result from an *anxiety disorder*, or are part of another psychological disorder, such as *hypochondriasis*, *depression*, or a type of *psychosexual disorder*.

CAUSES

Three different areas of research have contributed theories for causes of anxiety. Physiological measurements show that anxious individuals have a raised level of *arousal* in the central nervous system, which makes them react more excitedly and adapt more slowly to events. This leads to physical symptoms, such as palpitations, which themselves are unpleasant and reinforce the anxiety.

Psychoanalytical ideas derive from Freud, who coined the term "anxiety neurosis" and believed that anxiety originates from repressed, unresolved childhood experiences. Originally, anxiety was thought to be due to unsatisfied sexual needs, but a better understanding of the importance of *bonding* and of child-parent separations has now led to theories that are based on the fear of losing loved objects. Unconscious conflict can also lead to anxiety.

Behavioral psychologists describe anxiety as a learned response to, for example, pain or mental discomfort. Initially, anxiety drives people to improved performance, but eventually the anxious response becomes a deeply conditioned habit that cannot be controlled and is brought on by the slightest difficulty. Anxiety thus comes to impair performance and thought processes.

TREATMENT

People suffering from anxiety may be helped by reassurance or *counseling*, and, in more severe cases, *psychotherapy* or drug treatment.

Anxiety disorders

A group of mental illnesses in which symptoms of *anxiety* are the main feature. Anxiety disorders include a number of specific syndromes, although there is considerable overlap among them and boundaries are not always clear.

Anxiety disorders are common, affecting roughly 4 percent of the population, mainly young adults; the disorders occur equally in men and women and heredity is a contributing factor. Symptoms tend to vary during the course of the illness.

TYPES

Generalized anxiety disorder (the traditional "anxiety neurosis") is diagnosed if the patient has had at least one definite period of anxiety, accompanied by at least one physical or psychological symptom that impairs normal activity. *Panic disorders* are characterized by sudden, intense attacks of panic (extreme, unreasonable fear and anxiety). *Phobias* are dominated by irrational fears that lead to avoidance of certain situations or objects, such as open spaces or spiders. *Post-traumatic stress disorder* is associated with a serious specific event, such as *rape* or a major accident, and symptoms include reliving the event in dreams and a general feeling of numbness and lack of involvement. The principal features of *obsessive-compulsive disorder* are recurrent and persistent thoughts, and ritualized, repetitive behavior.

TREATMENT

Treatment of anxiety disorders is most effective when there is an identifiable and justified reason for stress. Treatment is more successful in people who have stable underlying personalities. Reassurance, *counseling*, and *psychotherapy* are used, as are *antianxiety drugs* (especially *benzodiazepine drugs*), which help reduce agitation.

A

Aorta

The main *artery* of the body. The aorta arises directly from the left ventricle (the main pumping chamber of the *heart*) and supplies oxygenated blood to all other arteries except the pulmonary artery (which carries deoxygenated blood from the right side of the heart to the lungs).

DISORDERS

Like other arteries, the aorta can become narrowed as a result of *atherosclerosis* (fat deposits on the walls), which often causes *hypertension* (high blood pressure). There are also specific aortic disorders, notably *coarctation of the aorta* (a condition in which the aorta is abnormally narrow at birth) and *aortitis* (inflammation of the wall of the aorta).

Both aortitis and atherosclerosis can cause an aortic *aneurysm* (ballooning of the vessel wall), which may require surgery to correct impaired blood flow and to remove the risk of rupture and fatal blood loss. (See also *Arteries, disorders of; Circulatory system.*)

Aortic insufficiency

Leakage of blood through the aortic valve (one of the *heart valves*), resulting in a backflow of blood into the left ventricle (the main pumping chamber of the heart).

CAUSES

Failure of the aortic valve to close correctly may be due to a *congenital* abnormality. Another cause of aortic insufficiency is *aortitis* (inflammation of the aorta). Sometimes, the aortic valve leaflets are destroyed by bacterial *endocarditis*, a condition that occurs in intravenous drug users. Aortic insufficiency is also found in untreated *syphilis* and is associated with *ankylosing spondylitis* (a disorder affecting the spine), and *Marfan's syndrome* (a congenital disorder of connective tissues). *Rheumatic fever* was once a common cause of aortic insufficiency but is now rare. *Atherosclerosis* (fat deposits on the walls of arteries) is associated with aortic insufficiency and also with *aortic stenosis* (narrowing of the aortic valve).

SYMPTOMS AND SIGNS

Aortic insufficiency may not cause any symptoms. It is sometimes found during a routine medical examination; the doctor hears a murmur (abnormal heart sound) over the front of the chest wall to the left of the sternum (breastbone).

The heart compensates for the backflow of blood into the left ventricle by working harder, until the combina-

LOCATION AND STRUCTURE OF THE AORTA

From its origin at the left ventricle, the aorta passes upward, curves behind the heart, and runs downward, passing through the thorax (chest) and into the abdomen, where it terminates by dividing into two common iliac arteries. The aorta is thick-walled and large in diameter (about 2.5 cm at its origin) to cope with the high pressure and large volume of blood that passes through it. The thick walls of the aorta have an elastic quality that helps even out the peaks and troughs of pressure that occur with each heartbeat.

Aortic valve

Thorax

Abdomen

Common iliac artery

Arteries to head and neck

Artery to arm

Aorta

tion of hypertrophy (muscle thickening) and dilatation (ballooning) of the left ventricle wall eventually leads to *heart failure* (reduced pumping efficiency); this, in turn, results in breathing difficulty and *edema* (accumulation of fluid).

DIAGNOSIS

A *chest X ray* may show white patches of calcium in the area of the aortic valve, an enlarged heart, and widening of the aorta. An *ECG* (measurement of the electrical activity of the heart) may show evidence of thickening of, and strain on, the left ventricle.

Echocardiography (imaging of the heart structures by measuring the pattern of reflection of sound waves from them) will show the diameter of the valve opening and the diameter of the aortic ring, a thickening of the wall of the left ventricle, and reduced movement of the aortic valve. Doppler echocardiography shows the blood flow through the valve.

A cardiac catheter (flexible tube inserted into the heart via blood vessels) is sometimes used to demonstrate the degree of incompetence; a radiopaque substance is injected into the heart through the catheter and X-ray pictures are then taken (see *Catheterization, cardiac*).

TREATMENT

Heart failure resulting from aortic insufficiency can be treated with *di-*

uretic drugs to remove retained fluid from the lungs. *Heart valve surgery* to replace the damaged valve may eventually be necessary, but often not until many years after the condition was first diagnosed.

Aortic stenosis

Narrowing of the opening of the aortic valve (one of the *heart valves*), causing obstruction of blood flow into the circulation. This makes the heart work harder and causes the muscle in the wall of the left ventricle (the main pumping chamber) to thicken.

CAUSES

The most common cause is deposition of calcium on the aortic valve, usually associated with *atherosclerosis* (fat deposits). Aortic stenosis may also be due to a *congenital* abnormality. Another cause is *cardiomyopathy* (heart muscle disease) in which thickening of the heart muscle may lead to subaortic stenosis (narrowing within the pumping chamber just below the valve). In the past, *rheumatic fever* was a common cause of heart valve damage; today it is rare.

SYMPTOMS AND SIGNS

Aortic stenosis may not cause any symptoms. It is sometimes found during a routine medical examination; the doctor hears a murmur (abnormal heart sound) over the front of the chest wall to the right of the sternum (breastbone) and sometimes up into the neck. Symptoms, when they do occur, include fainting attacks, lack of energy, chest pain on exertion due to *angina pectoris*, and breathing difficulty. Other features include a weak pulse and *cardiomegaly* (enlargement of the heart) at a late stage.

DIAGNOSIS

A *chest X ray* may show white patches of calcium in the area of the aortic valve. The heart may also appear enlarged on an X ray.

An *ECG* (measurement of the electrical activity of the heart) may show evidence of thickening of, and strain on, the left ventricle.

Echocardiography (imaging of the heart structures by measuring the pattern of reflection of sound waves from them) usually reveals the diameter of the valve opening and thickness of the valve leaflets, abnormal movement within the aortic valve, and thickening of the walls of the left ventricle. Doppler echocardiography can confirm and measure the reduced flow through the valve.

A cardiac catheter (a flexible tube inserted into the heart through blood vessels) can be fitted with a pressure-measuring device to measure the degree of aortic stenosis; the difference in pressure on either side of the valve reflects the severity of the stenosis (see *Catheterization, cardiac*).

TREATMENT

Before developments in *heart valve surgery*, the outlook for people with aortic stenosis was gloomy; once symptoms developed, the predicted life span was only a year or so. Now, provided that valve replacement is performed before irremediable damage to the left ventricle occurs, the outlook is good.

Aortitis

Inflammation of the aorta, the large artery that carries blood from the heart to supply all parts of the body except the lungs. Aortitis is a rare condition that occurs in people with *arteritis*

(inflammation of the arteries) or untreated *syphilis* and in some people with *ankylosing spondylitis* (an inflammatory disorder affecting both the joints between the vertebrae of the spine and between the spine and the pelvis).

Aortitis may cause part of the aorta to widen and its walls to become thinner. This may then lead to the formation of an *aneurysm* (ballooning of the artery), which may burst and cause severe, sometimes fatal, blood loss. Aortitis may also damage the ring surrounding the aortic valve in the heart, leading to *aortic insufficiency*, which allows regurgitation of blood back to the heart and may eventually result in *heart failure*.

Aortography

An imaging procedure by which the *aorta* (the main artery leaving the heart) and its branches can be seen on X-ray film after injection of a contrast medium (a substance that is opaque to X rays) into a artery.

WHY IT IS DONE

Aortography is used to detect aortic *aneurysm* (ballooning of the aorta) and assess the severity of *peripheral vascular disease* before surgery.

HOW IT IS DONE

Contrast medium is usually injected into the aorta through a fine catheter (flexible plastic tube) inserted either into the femoral artery at the groin or into the brachial artery on the inside of the elbow. In people with severe arterial disease, the major arteries may be blocked and the contrast medium may have to be injected through a hollow needle directly into the aorta within the lower abdomen.

COMPLICATIONS

There is a small risk of a reaction to the contrast medium. Damage to a vessel during puncture or catheterization can also occur.

Aperient

A mild *laxative drug*.

Apgar score

A system devised by Virginia Apgar, an American anesthetist, to assess the condition of a newborn baby. Five features are scored at 1 minute and at 5 minutes after birth. The features scored are respiratory effort, heart rate, color, muscle tone, and reaction to nasal stimulation. Most important are the infant's attempts to breathe and the infant's heart rate. In general, if these two features are satisfactory, the others will be as well.

Each feature is scored from 0 to 2, making a total of 10 possible points. A low total score of 0 to 3, which will occur if the baby does not breathe or if the heart rate is too slow, means the baby needs urgent resuscitation. A middle score (4 to 6) indicates that the baby may need medical help. A high score (7 to 10) indicates a well baby.

Parents should not attach undue importance to the Apgar score. It was originally intended to try to quantify the vast changes a newborn goes through in the first minutes of life and to help direct appropriate care.

Aphakia

The absence of the crystalline *lens* from the eye. Aphakia occurs if the lens has been surgically removed, as after *cataract surgery*, or if it has been destroyed by a penetrating injury and subsequently absorbed into the aqueous humor (the fluid within the front part of the eyeball).

Aphakia causes severe loss of focusing in the affected eye or eyes and calls for correction by lens implants, contact lenses, or glasses.

Aphasia

Strictly, a complete absence of previously acquired language skills, caused by a brain disorder that affects the ability to speak and write, and/or the ability to comprehend and read. The term aphasia is also sometimes used interchangeably with the term dysphasia (which more specifically

APGAR CHART

Sign	0	1	2
Color	Blue, pale	Body pink; extremities blue	Completely pink
Respiratory effort	Absent	Weak cry; irregular breathing	Good strong cry; regular breathing
Muscle tone	Limp	Bending of some limbs	Active motion; limbs well flexed
Reflex irritability	No response	Grimace (on nasal stimulation)	Cry
Heart rate	Absent	Slow (below 100 beats per minute)	Over 100 beats per minute

describes disturbance rather than absence of these language skills).

The term aphasia should not be used to describe language difficulties caused by disorders of parts of the body involved in the mechanics of speech (see *Dysarthria; Dysphonia*), or by defective hearing or sight.

Related disabilities that may occur, either as a feature of aphasia or, more rarely, by themselves, are *alexia* (inability to recognize words) and *agraphia* (writing difficulty).

CAUSES

A *stroke* or a *head injury* is the most common cause of brain damage leading to aphasia.

Language function within the brain lies in the dominant cerebral hemisphere (see *Cerebrum*). Two particular areas in the dominant hemisphere, called Broca's and Wernicke's areas (named after their discoverers), and the pathways connecting the two are known to be important in language skills. Damage to these areas is the most common cause of aphasia.

TYPES AND SYMPTOMS

BROCA'S (EXPRESSIVE) APHASIA Damage to Broca's area causes difficulty in the expression of language. Speech is nonfluent, slow, labored, with loss of normal rhythm. The few words uttered do tend to be meaningful. Writing may also be impaired.

WERNICKE'S (RECEPTIVE) APHASIA Damage to Wernicke's area causes difficulty in comprehension. Speech is fluent but, because of the impaired comprehension, its content is disturbed, with many errors in word selection and grammar, indicating that "internal speech" is impaired. Writing is also impaired and spoken or written commands are not understood.

GLOBAL APHASIA In global aphasia there is a total or near total inability to speak, write, or understand spoken or written words. This is usually caused by widespread damage to the dominant cerebral hemisphere.

NOMINAL APHASIA This is restricted to a difficulty in naming objects or in finding words, although the person may be able to choose the correct name from several offered. Nominal aphasia may be caused by generalized cerebral dysfunction or damage to specific language areas.

TREATMENT AND OUTLOOK

Some recovery from aphasia is usual after a stroke or head injury, although the more severe the aphasia, the less the chances of recovery. *Speech therapy* is the main treatment. (See also *Speech; Speech disorders.*)

Language function and the brain
Damage to two particular areas (and the pathways between them) in the dominant cerebral hemisphere results in aphasia.

Apheresis

Also called pheresis, a procedure in which blood is withdrawn from a donor and then reinfused after selected components, such as platelets, white blood cells, or plasma, have been separated and removed. (See also *Blood donation.*)

Aphonia

Total loss of the voice, usually sudden in onset and caused by emotional stress. A physician examining the larynx (voice box) would see that the vocal cords fail to meet as normal when the patient tries to speak, although they come together when the person coughs. Otherwise, there is no detectable abnormality in the larynx.

There is no treatment other than reassurance and *psychotherapy*. The sufferer's voice usually returns as suddenly as it disappeared.

Disease of, or damage to, the larynx usually causes only partial loss of voice production (see *Dysphonia*).

Aphrodisiacs

Substances which are claimed to stimulate erotic desire and enhance sexual performance. Aphrodisiacs are named after Aphrodite, the ancient Greek goddess of love, beauty, and fertility.

Various substances have been used as "love potions" over the centuries—honey, ginseng, ginger, strychnine, rhinoceros horn, and oysters, among many others. In fact, no substance has a proven aphrodisiac effect, although virtually anything may produce the desired results if the person taking it believes strongly enough that it will

work. *Alcohol* can encourage sexual desire by removing inhibitions, but a high blood alcohol level can impair sexual performance.

Probably the best known "aphrodisiac" is Spanish fly, which consists of powdered, dried beetles of the species *LYTTA VESICATORIA*. The active ingredient, cantharidin, irritates the lining of the bladder and urethra (the tube between the bladder and outside) and may, in some cases, cause a man to develop *priapism* (a painful, persistent erection). Spanish fly is potentially dangerous; some men have died as a result of using it.

Other substances used for their purported aphrodisiac effects include *marijuana*, yohimbine (a chemical obtained from the bark of the West African yohimbe tree), and *amyl nitrite*. There is no scientific evidence that any of these is effective, and amyl nitrite may reduce blood pressure to dangerously low levels.

The male sex hormone *testosterone* is sometimes regarded as a sexual stimulant. In normal men, it has no effect on sexual desire or potency but does reduce sperm production. In men who have a testosterone deficiency, however, the hormone may restore both libido and potency.

Apicectomy

Surgical removal of the tip of a tooth root. Apicectomy may be required as part of *root canal treatment*.

Aplasia

Incomplete or severely reduced growth and development of any organ or tissue. For example, in bone marrow aplasia, the rate of cell division in the bone marrow is considerably reduced, leading to diminished formation of blood cells of one or all types (see *Anemia, aplastic*). A number of birth defects—for example, the presence of one or more stunted limbs (see *Phocomelia*)—are a result of incomplete organ formation during prenatal development.

Aplastic anemia

See *Anemia, aplastic*.

Apnea

Cessation of breathing, either temporarily (for a few seconds to a minute or two) or for a prolonged period.

CAUSES

Breathing is an automatic process controlled by the respiratory center in the brain stem. The respiratory center sends nerve impulses that regulate contractions of the diaphragm and muscles in the chest wall, thereby controlling the rate and depth of breathing.

Prolonged apnea can occur if the brain stem is damaged by a *stroke*, by a *transient ischemic attack* (symptoms of stroke lasting less than 24 hours), or by a *head injury*. Prolonged apnea can also occur as an effect of certain drugs or as the result of *airway obstruction*, usually by food, drink, vomit, or a small inhaled object.

Deliberate temporary apnea occurs during *breath-holding attacks* and when swimming underwater. Nondeliberate temporary apnea can also occur, usually during sleep (see *Sleep apnea*).

Another type of apnea occurs in *Cheyne-Stokes respiration*; this is characterized by cycles of deep, rapid breathing alternating with episodes of breathing stoppage.

INVESTIGATION AND TREATMENT
Apnea requires investigation and treatment of the underlying cause. Treatment may be aimed at relieving any airway obstruction. It may also include the use of respiratory stimulants if the respiratory center in the brain stem is affected.

Apocrine gland
A gland that discharges cellular material in addition to the fluid it secretes. The term is usually applied to the type of *sweat glands* that appear in hairy areas of the body after puberty.

Aponeurosis
A wide sheet of tough, fibrous tissue that acts as a tendon (i.e., attaches a muscle to a bone or a joint).

Apoplexy
An outdated term for a *stroke*, resulting in sudden loss of consciousness, paralysis, or loss of sensation.

Apothecary
An obsolete term for a *pharmacist*.

Appendectomy
Surgical removal of the appendix to treat acute *appendicitis* (inflammation of the appendix).

WHY IT IS DONE
Appendectomy is carried out to prevent an inflamed appendix from bursting and causing *peritonitis* (inflammation of the peritoneum, the lining of the abdominal cavity) or an abdominal abscess.

Acute appendicitis is often difficult to diagnose and sometimes, because of the dangerous complications that can develop from the condition, a *laparotomy* (an exploratory operation on the abdomen) is performed even when appendicitis is only suspected. If a laparotomy is performed, the appendix, which has no apparent useful function in humans, is removed even if it is normal, to prevent the possibility of appendicitis developing in future.

About 24,000 appendectomies are done in Canada each year. More than half these operations are done on people aged 15 to 24.

HOW IT IS DONE
If there is time before the operation, the patient is started on a course of antibiotic drugs to prevent the operative wound from becoming infected, a serious risk in appendectomy. Next, the surgeon makes a small incision in the abdomen and removes the appendix (see box).

If the appendix has burst, the infected area of the abdominal cavity is washed out with saline (salt solution) and a plastic drainage tube is inserted through another small incision to drain off pus. Antibiotics may also be given to prevent peritonitis.

COMPLICATIONS
Possible complications are infection of the incision wound in the abdominal wall, an abscess at the site from which the appendix was removed, or localized peritonitis.

RECOVERY PERIOD
Following an uncomplicated appendectomy, the patient is usually able to drink and to eat light food within 24 hours. If a drainage tube has been inserted, it is removed after about 48 hours; the wound seals itself. Normally, the patient can go home after two or three days. Stitches are removed seven to 10 days after the operation (an outpatient procedure). Normal physical activities can usually be resumed after two or three weeks. Recovery may take much longer if there are complications.

Appendicitis
Acute inflammation of the appendix, which is a common cause of abdominal pain and *peritonitis* (inflammation of the lining of the abdominal cavity) in children and young adults.

CAUSES
The cause is usually not known, but appendicitis is sometimes due to obstruction of the appendix by a lump of feces or, occasionally, by worms in *pinworm infestation*. The closed end of the appendix beyond the obstruction becomes inflamed, swollen, and infected. This may lead to *gangrene* (tissue death) in the appendix wall, which may perforate (burst).

INCIDENCE
Appendicitis is the most common abdominal surgical emergency in de-

---

PERFORMING AN APPENDECTOMY
The patient is given a general anesthetic. A small incision is made in the lower right abdomen, above the groin, revealing the cecum (the chamber that links the small and large intestine), to which the appendix is attached.

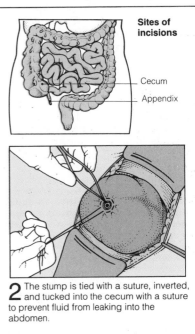

Sites of incisions

Cecum

Appendix

1 The appendix is then carefully and gently brought to the surface of the abdomen, clamped, tied off at the base (where it joins the cecum), and cut off.

2 The stump is tied with a suture, inverted, and tucked into the cecum with a suture to prevent fluid from leaking into the abdomen.

veloped countries, a sharp contrast to developing countries where the operation is comparatively rare.

SYMPTOMS

The first symptom is usually vague discomfort just above and around the navel. Within a few hours this gradually develops into a sharper, more localized pain. This pain is usually most intense in the lower right-hand side of the abdomen.

Symptoms may differ if the appendix is not in the most common position. For example, if the appendix descends behind the cecum, appendicitis may cause little abdominal pain but produce severe pain if the physician performs a *rectal examination*. If the appendix impinges on the ureter, the urine may become bloodstained.

Other possible symptoms of appendicitis are slight fever, loss of appetite, nausea, vomiting, a coated tongue, and foul breath, sometimes preceded by constipation. Anyone who has sudden abdominal pain and other symptoms of appendicitis should consult a physician without delay.

DIAGNOSIS

Diagnosis can sometimes be difficult because the symptoms of appendicitis are similar to those of many other abdominal disorders. Mesenteric adenitis, which is common in childhood and often follows a viral respiratory tract infection, has symptoms and signs that resemble those of appendicitis. Disorders of the right *fallopian tube* and *ovary*, *Crohn's disease*, and right-sided *pyelonephritis* (inflammation of the kidney) can also mimic appendicitis. Sometimes a *laparotomy* (surgical investigation of the abdomen) is necessary to confirm or exclude a diagnosis of appendicitis.

COMPLICATIONS

If treatment is delayed, an inflamed appendix may perforate, releasing its contents into the abdomen. At this point, the pain abruptly ceases, but the perforation leads inevitably to peritonitis. In some cases, the omentum (fold of peritoneum covering the intestines) envelops the inflamed appendix; this prevents the spread of infection and results in a localized abscess around the appendix. Peritonitis or an abscess causes a fever (sometimes with chills) as well as increasing pain and tenderness in the abdomen. This pain first appears a few hours to a day or so after the appendix ruptures.

TREATMENT

The usual treatment is *appendectomy* (surgical removal of the appendix). If an abscess of the appendix is suspected, drainage of the abscess and an appendectomy may be delayed until the infection has been treated by large doses of antibiotic drugs.

Appendix

A narrow, small, finger-shaped tube that branches off the large intestine. The appendix has no known function. In adults it is usually about 9 cm long, with a thick wall, narrow cavity, and a lining similar to that of the intestine. It contains a large amount of lymphoid tissue, which provides a defense against local infection.

The appendix projects out of the cecum (the first part of the colon) at the lower right-hand side of the abdomen. It may lie behind or below the cecum, or in front of or behind the ileum (part of the small intestine). The position of a person's appendix partly determines the set of symptoms produced by acute *appendicitis* (inflammation of the appendix).

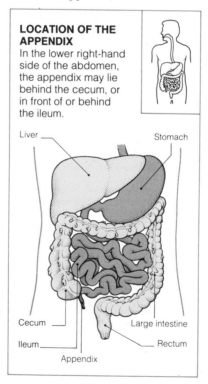

LOCATION OF THE APPENDIX

In the lower right-hand side of the abdomen, the appendix may lie behind the cecum, or in front of or behind the ileum.

Liver

Stomach

Cecum

Large intestine

Ileum

Rectum

Appendix

Appetite

A desire for food; a pleasant sensation felt in anticipation of eating, as opposed to *hunger*, a disagreeable feeling caused by the need for food.

Appetite, which is regulated by two parts of the *brain* (the *hypothalamus* and the cerebral cortex), is learned by enjoying a variety of foods that smell, taste, and look good. Ideally, it combines with hunger to ensure that the correct amount of a wide range of foods is eaten to stay healthy, to provide proper nutrition for growth in children, and to maintain a proper weight in adults.

Appetite may be lost as a result of various disorders, both physical and psychological (see *Appetite, loss of*).

Appetite, loss of

Known medically as anorexia, loss of appetite is usually temporary and due to an emotional upset or minor feverish illness. However, persistent loss of appetite may be a symptom of a more serious underlying physical or psychological disorder and requires investigation by a physician.

CAUSES

In adolescents and young adults, loss of appetite may be due to *anorexia nervosa* (a disorder characterized by a refusal to eat), or to the abuse of drugs, particularly *amphetamine drugs*. *Depression* or *anxiety* can cause loss of appetite at any age. Loneliness may be the chief culprit, where elderly people are concerned.

Among possible physical causes are a *stroke*, *brain tumor*, or a *head injury* that has damaged the *hypothalamus* or cerebral cortex, the parts of the brain that control appetite. Other physical causes include intestinal disorders, such as *gastritis* (inflammation of the stomach lining, which is common in alcoholics), *stomach cancer*, and *gastric ulcer*, and liver disorders, such as *hepatitis*. Many infectious diseases (*influenza*, for example) can also cause loss of appetite.

Between the ages of about 2 and 4, some children go through a phase of refusing food. If there are no other symptoms, this period of food refusal should be regarded as a normal part of child development.

For a person who is otherwise healthy, a period of two or three days without food is not harmful, provided that plenty of nonalcoholic fluids are drunk. However, if there are other health problems, particularly *diabetes mellitus*, or if regular medication is being taken, a physician should always be consulted.

All cases of loss of appetite that last for more than a few days should be investigated by a physician. Appetite generally returns to normal once any underlying illness has been treated. (See also *Appetite stimulants*.)

Appetite stimulants

There are no known drugs that safely and effectively stimulate the appetite. Lost appetite usually returns when an underlying illness subsides. A variety of drugs (including alcohol and elixirs containing small quantities of iron, quinine, and strychnine) have been prescribed, but these are rarely effective when there is an underlying physical illness.

Appetite suppressants

COMMON DRUGS

Diethylpropion Fenfluramine Phentermine

These drugs are generally not recommended.

A group of drugs that reduce the desire to eat. Appetite suppressants may be used in the treatment of *obesity*, along with advice on diet and exercise. Some appetite suppressants are nervous system stimulants that are thought to suppress appetite by affecting the *hypothalamus* (part of the brain). Others are bulking agents that, when taken with water before a meal, swell in the stomach to give a feeling of fullness.

POSSIBLE ADVERSE EFFECTS

Adverse effects include dry mouth, dizziness, palpitations, nervousness, restlessness, and difficulty getting to sleep. These symptoms usually disappear after a few days of treatment. Bulking agents may cause flatulence, abdominal pain, and a bloated feeling.

Taking a stimulant appetite suppressant regularly for longer than about six weeks may lead to dependence (see *Drug dependence*). Newer appetite suppressants are less addictive than the *amphetamine drugs* that used to be prescribed.

Apraxia

An inability to carry out purposeful movements despite normal muscle power and coordination. Apraxia is caused by damage to nerve tracts within the cerebrum (the main mass of the brain) that translate the idea for a movement into an actual movement. People with apraxia usually know what they want to do but appear to have lost the ability to recall from memory the sequence of actions necessary to achieve the movement. The damage to the cerebrum may be caused by a direct *head injury*, infection, *stroke*, or *brain tumor*.

TYPES AND SYMPTOMS

Various forms of apraxia are known, each related to damage within dif-

ferent parts of the brain. A person with ideomotor apraxia is unable to carry out a spoken command to make a particular movement—for example, to lick his or her lips—but at other times can be seen making precisely the same movement unconsciously.

Agraphia (difficulty in writing) and expressive *aphasia* (severe difficulty in expressing language) are special forms of apraxia.

TREATMENT AND OUTLOOK

Recovery from events such as a stroke or head injury, and from accompanying syndromes such as apraxia, is highly variable. In most cases, some deficit remains, and it may require considerable effort and patience to relearn lost skills.

APUD cell tumor

A growth, sometimes called an apudoma, composed of cells that produce various hormones. These cells—amine precursor uptake and decarboxylation (APUD) cells—occur in different parts of the body. The cells are similar wherever they are found.

Some tumors of the thyroid gland, pancreas, and lungs are APUD cell tumors, as are a *carcinoid* tumor and *pheochromocytoma* (a type of nonmalignant adrenal tumor).

Arachnodactyly

Long, thin, spiderlike fingers and toes that sometimes occur spontaneously but are characteristic of *Marfan's syndrome*, an inherited connective tissue disease.

Arachnoiditis

An uncommon condition characterized by chronic inflammation and thickening of the arachnoid mater, the middle of the three *meninges* (membranes that cover and protect the brain and spinal cord).

Arachnoiditis may develop up to several years after an episode of *meningitis* (infection of the meninges) or a *subarachnoid hemorrhage* (bleeding beneath the arachnoid). It may be a feature of *syphilis* or of *ankylosing spondylitis* (a disorder affecting the spine). Arachnoiditis may also result from injury or follow procedures, such as *myelography*, in which radiopaque dye is injected into the spinal canal. Usually, however, no cause is found.

The signs and symptoms vary with the extent of the disorder. Arachnoiditis may cause headaches, epileptic seizures, blindness, or slowly progressive spastic paralysis (difficulties with movements due to increased

muscle tension) that may affect both legs or all four limbs. There is no effective treatment.

ARC

Abbreviation for *AIDS-related complex*. (See also *AIDS*.)

Arcus senilis

A gray-white ring near the edge of the *cornea* (the transparent front part of the eyeball) that occurs in most elderly people. The ring overlies the outer rim of the iris and is encircled by a narrow zone of unaffected cornea. Arcus senilis is caused by degeneration of fatty material within the cornea.

Arcus senilis
The arcus senilis is the lighter ring that overlies the edge of the iris (the colored part of the eye).

Arcus senilis develops gradually during adult life, usually starting in the lower part of the cornea, then appearing in the upper part, and eventually affecting the sides to form a complete ring. The ring never spreads to the center, does not affect eyesight, and is not believed to be related to health in any way.

A similar phenomenon in the young is called arcus juvenilis; this condition may be associated with *hyperlipidemias* (a group of disorders in which fat levels in the blood are abnormally high).

Aroma therapy

A range of treatments using aromatic oils extracted from plants. Many ancient civilizations, particularly the Chinese, documented the use of essential oils in treating different disorders. Recently, interest in aroma therapy has been rekindled along with other forms of *alternative medicine*. Practitioners claim that aroma therapy can be used to treat a range of disorders, but that it is particularly effective in *psychosomatic* and stress-related conditions.

The patient describes his or her symptoms to the therapist, who chooses the most appropriate oil or oils from a prepared range. The oil is applied in small quantities through massage or is inhaled or incorporated into creams or lotions. Very occasionally the oil is taken internally.

There is no conclusive scientific evidence that the benefits are greater than those that can be achieved by the power of suggestion.

Arousal

The awakening of a person from unconsciousness or semiconsciousness. The term arousal is also used to describe any state of heightened awareness, such as that caused by sexual stimulation or fear. Arousal is regulated by the reticular formation in the *brain stem*.

Arrhenoblastoma

A rare tumor of the ovary, also called andreoblastoma, that occurs in young women. Although the tumor is benign, it secretes *androgen hormones* (male sex hormones) that cause *virilization* (the development of male sex characteristics). Treatment is by surgical removal of the affected ovary.

Arrhythmia, cardiac

An abnormality of the rhythm or rate of the *heartbeat*. Arrhythmia is caused by a disturbance in the electrical impulses within the *heart* (see box above). Any isolated irregular beat is called an *ectopic beat* (which does not necessarily indicate the presence of an abnormality).

TYPES

Arrhythmias can be divided into two main groups: the tachycardias, in which the rate is faster than normal (more than 100 beats per minute), and the bradycardias, in which the rate is slower than normal (fewer than 60 beats per minute). The rhythm may be regular, as in the normal heartbeat, with each beat of the atria (upper chambers) being followed by one beat of the ventricles (lower chambers), or it may be irregular. The beat may originate at the sinoatrial node or in some other area of the heart.

TACHYCARDIAS In *sinus tachycardia*, the rate is raised (100 to 160 beats per minute), the rhythm is regular, and the beat originates in the sinoatrial node. *Supraventricular tachycardia* is faster (with a rate of 120 to 200 beats

CARDIAC ARRHYTHMIA

Any disorder that interferes with the generation or transmission of impulses through the heart's electrical conducting system (below) can lead to a disturbance of cardiac rate or rhythm. These ECG recordings show two kinds of arrhythmia: sinus bradycardia and atrial fibrillation.

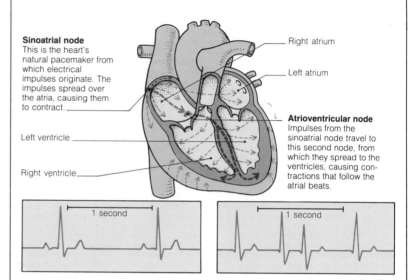

Sinoatrial node
This is the heart's natural pacemaker from which electrical impulses originate. The impulses spread over the atria, causing them to contract.

Left ventricle

Right ventricle

Right atrium

Left atrium

Atrioventricular node
Impulses from the sinoatrial node travel to this second node, from which they spread to the ventricles, causing contractions that follow the atrial beats.

1 second

1 second

Sinus bradycardia
The heart rate is slow but the rhythm normal, with each atrial beat (small rise) followed by a ventricular beat (spike). Sinus bradycardia is common in athletes, but can also be caused by hypothyroidism.

Atrial fibrillation
The atria beat rapidly and irregularly. Ventricular beats (spikes) do not follow each atrial beat and are irregularly spaced. This arrhythmia is common in the elderly and in people with hyperthyroidism.

per minute), the rhythm is regular, and the beat may arise anywhere in the conducting tissue above the ventricles. When rapid, irregular heartbeats (120 to 200 beats per minute) originate in the ventricles, it is called *ventricular tachycardia*.

In *atrial flutter*, the atria beat regularly and very rapidly (200 to 400 beats per minute), but not every impulse reaches the ventricles, which beat at a rate of about 100 to 200 beats per minute. Totally uncoordinated beating of the atria at about 300 to 500 beats per minute is called *atrial fibrillation* and produces completely irregular ventricular beats.

Ventricular fibrillation is a form of cardiac arrest in which the ventricles twitch very rapidly in a completely disorganized manner.

BRADYCARDIAS A slow, regular beat is called *sinus bradycardia*. In *heart block*, the conduction of electrical impulses through the heart muscle is partly or completely blocked, leading to slow, irregular beating. Periods of bradycardia may alternate with periods of tachycardia (see *Sick sinus syndrome*).

CAUSES

A common cause of arrhythmia is *coronary artery disease*. In this condition, vessels supplying blood to the heart are narrowed by *atheroma* (fatty deposits) and are unable to supply sufficient blood to the conducting tissue, which becomes damaged as a result. Arrhythmias due to coronary artery disease come on more frequently after a *myocardial infarction* (heart attack).

Sinus tachycardia may be a normal response to exercise or stress; likewise, sinus bradycardia often occurs in healthy athletes.

Caffeine and other drugs can cause tachycardia in some individuals. *Amitriptyline* and some other *antidepressant drugs* can cause serious cardiac arrhythmias if taken in high doses.

SYMPTOMS

Sudden onset of tachycardia can cause palpitations, in which the individual becomes aware of an abnormally fast heartbeat. Any sudden arrhythmia can cause faintness or dizziness due to reduction of blood flow to the brain. If a bradycardia reduces the flow of blood to the lungs, breathing difficulty may occur. If there is underlying heart disease, arrhythmia may lead to *angina pectoris* (chest pain due to reduced blood supply) or *heart failure*.

DIAGNOSIS

The physician makes a preliminary assessment by feeling the patient's pulse and listening to the heart. The type of arrhythmia is confirmed by an *ECG*, which shows the pattern of electrical activity within heart muscle. In some cases, if the arrhythmia is intermittent, it may be necessary to make continuous ECG recordings for 24 hours using a portable monitor.

TREATMENT

Many different drugs can be used to treat arrhythmias (see *Antiarrhythmic drugs*). When an arrhythmia occurs suddenly after a myocardial infarction, *defibrillation* (application of a short electric shock to the heart) may be necessary to restore the heartbeat to normal.

Artificial *pacemakers* can be used to stimulate heartbeats in cases of heart block. Pacemakers usually consist of a small generating unit implanted under the skin of the chest wall that passes electrical impulses to the heart by means of electrodes.

Arrowroot

A starchy substance obtained from the roots of the West Indian plant *MARANTA ARUNDINACEA*. Traditionally, arrowroot was mixed to a paste with milk or water for use as an easily digestible invalid or baby food.

Arsenic

A metallic element that occurs naturally in its pure form and in various chemical compounds. The term arsenic is also popularly used to refer to the poisonous compound arsenic trioxide.

Arsenic is present in trace amounts in water and many foods and, as a result, most people have minute quantities in their bodies, particularly in their hair and skin.

POISONING

Arsenic has been used intentionally to murder, particularly in fiction, but most poisoning occurs through accidental ingestion, particularly in rural areas, where arsenic is an important constituent of some pesticides. Industrial poisoning from arsenic is nowadays quite rare.

Arsenic poisoning may be acute or chronic. Acute poisoning primarily affects the lining of the intestine and causes the sudden onset of painful symptoms. The victim experiences nausea, vomiting (sometimes with blood in the vomit), diarrhea, excessive sweating, and burning of the throat, followed by collapse and death if the poisoning is not treated.

Chronic poisoning is usually first noticeable as weakness, tiredness, scaly skin, *keratosis* (thickening of the skin), "raindrop" pigmentation of the skin, and swelling of the lining of the mouth. *Neuropathy* (degeneration of nerves) then sets in, producing tingling and then numbness in the hands and feet. Prolonged absorption of arsenic may cause cancer of the skin and lungs.

INVESTIGATION AND TREATMENT

Arsenic poisoning, once suspected, may be confirmed by analysis of the urine. Treatment of acute poisoning includes washing out the stomach (see *Lavage, gastric*), replacement of lost fluids, treatment for *shock* and pain, and administration of dimercaprol, a drug that helps remove the poison from the body. Chronic poisoning is also treated with dimercaprol.

Arterial reconstructive surgery

An operation to repair arteries that are narrowed, blocked, or weakened.

WHY IT IS DONE

Arterial reconstructive surgery is most often performed to repair arteries narrowed or blocked by *atherosclerosis* (fatty deposits on artery walls). The procedure is also used to repair *aneurysms* (ballooning of blood vessels), which may be *congenital* or due to atherosclerosis. Arterial reconstructive surgery can also be used to repair arteries that have been damaged as a result of injury.

HOW IT IS DONE

A narrowed or blocked section of artery can be bypassed by sewing in a length of vein—usually taken from the patient's leg—above and below the constricted area. This technique is commonly used for coronary arteries (see *Coronary artery bypass*).

For damaged arteries elsewhere in the body, it is more common to cut out the affected section and replace it with an artificial tube or a section of vein taken from another part of the body.

OUTLOOK

Arterial reconstructive surgery is generally successful, depending on the age and health of the patient. Reconstruction of the *aorta* (the main artery carrying blood from the heart) has an operative death rate of up to 5 percent, but the risks associated with rupture of an untreated aneurysm are greater. (See also *Angioplasty, balloon; Endarterectomy*.)

Arteries, disorders of

Disorders of the arteries may take the form of abnormal narrowing (which reduces blood flow and may cause tissue damage), complete obstruction (which may cause tissue death), or abnormal widening and thinning of an artery wall (which may cause rupture of the blood vessel).

TYPES

ATHEROSCLEROSIS This disorder, in which fat deposits build up on the lining of the artery wall, affects most adults to some extent and is the most common arterial disease. Atherosclerosis can involve arteries throughout the body, including the brain (see *Cerebrovascular disease*), the heart (see *Coronary artery disease*), and the legs (see *Peripheral vascular disease*). Atherosclerosis is the main type of *arteriosclerosis*, a group of disorders that cause thickening and loss of elasticity of artery walls.

HYPERTENSION High blood pressure is another common cause of thickening and narrowing of arteries. Hypertension predisposes people to coronary artery disease and increases the risk of a *stroke* or *kidney failure*.

ARTERITIS This term refers to a group of disorders in which inflammation of artery walls causes narrowing and sometimes blockage.

ANEURYSM This thinning and ballooning of an artery wall may be due to a congenital defect or to atherosclerosis. An aortic aneurysm may result from *aortitis* (inflammation of the aorta wall), which may be part of a generalized arteritis or, rarely today, due to untreated syphilis.

THROMBOSIS A thrombus (blood clot) may form within an artery, causing partial or complete obstruction of the blood flow. Thrombosis occurs most commonly in areas that have already been damaged by atherosclerosis or aneurysm.

EMBOLISM This is the term for obstruction of an artery by an embolus (usually a fragment of thrombus that has broken off from a larger vessel or from the wall of the heart, although it may consist of fat particles from a bone fracture or an air bubble that has formed as a result of a decompression accident in a diver).

RAYNAUD'S DISEASE This is a disorder involving intermittent spasm of small arteries in the hands and feet, usually due to cold. The obstruction to blood

A

flow causes a change in skin color, numbness, and pins and needles. Occasionally, if the obstruction lasts, skin damage and an ischemic ulcer (see *Ischemia*) may result.

DIAGNOSIS AND TREATMENT

For the diagnosis and treatment of disorders affecting the arteries, see individual entries on specific disorders.

Arteriography

Another name for *angiography*, a technique for imaging blood vessels.

Arteriole

A blood vessel that branches off an *artery*. Arterioles themselves branch to form *capillaries*. Arterioles are intermediate in size and structure between arteries and capillaries. Arterioles have a high proportion of smooth muscle in their walls, and their nerve supply enables them to be narrowed or widened to meet decreases or increases in the blood-flow needs of the tissues they supply.

Arteriopathy

Any abnormal condition or disorder of an artery. (See *Arteries, disorders of.*)

Arterioplasty

Surgical repair of an artery (see *Arterial reconstructive surgery*).

Arteriosclerosis

A group of disorders that cause thickening and loss of elasticity of artery walls. *Atherosclerosis* is the most common type of arteriosclerosis. Other types include medial arteriosclerosis (in which muscle and elastic fibers from the lining of large- and medium-sized arteries are replaced by fibrous tissue) and Monckeberg's arteriosclerosis (in which there are deposits of calcium in the lining of arteries).

Arteriovenous fistula

An abnormal communication or malformation between an artery and a vein. An arteriovenous fistula may be present at birth or may result from injury or infection. A fistula can also be created surgically to provide an easy route of access into the bloodstream. This procedure is useful for people receiving *dialysis*.

If the fistula is close to the skin surface, it may cause a small, pulsating swelling. If several fistulas are present in the lungs, they can impair the uptake of oxygen into the blood, causing *cyanosis* (blue skin color), breathing difficulty during exertion, and sometimes *coughing up blood*.

If an isolated fistula is causing symptoms, it is usually cut away and the ends of the blood vessels stitched. If there are large numbers of fistulas, surgery is not practicable. Some arteriovenous malformations in inaccessible areas of the brain are treated by *radiation therapy*.

Arteritis

Inflammation of an artery wall, causing narrowing or complete obstruction of the affected artery, reduced blood flow, and, in some cases, *thrombosis* and damage to tissues.

Buerger's disease is an arteritis that affects the limbs, causing pain, numbness, and, in severe cases, *gangrene*.

Periarteritis nodosa, a serious *autoimmune disorder* (a disorder in which the body's defense mechanisms attack its own tissues), can affect arteries in any part of the body, especially the heart and kidneys. It may also cause symptoms such as abdominal and testicular pain, chest pain, breathing difficulty, and tender lumps under the skin.

Temporal arteritis affects arteries in the scalp over the temples, causing headache and scalp tenderness; if the retinal artery is affected, there is a risk of permanent blindness.

A very rare type of arteritis is Takayasu's arteritis, which is thought to be an autoimmune disorder. This disorder usually affects young women and involves the arteries that branch from the first part of the *aorta* into the neck and arms.

Artery

A blood vessel that carries blood away from the *heart*. Systemic arteries carry blood pumped from the left ventricle (lower chamber) of the heart to all parts of the body except the lungs. The largest sytemic artery (in fact, the largest artery in the body) is the *aorta*, which emerges directly from the left ventricle; other major systemic arteries branch off from the aorta.

The pulmonary arteries carry blood from the right ventricle of the heart to the lungs. Pulmonary arteries are shorter, thinner-walled, and contain blood under a lower pressure than systemic arteries.

STRUCTURE AND FUNCTION

Arteries are pliable tubes with thick walls that enable them to withstand the high blood pressure to which they are subjected on each heartbeat.

The structure of arteries helps even out the peaks and troughs of blood pressure caused by the heartbeat, so that the blood is flowing at a relatively

STRUCTURE OF AN ARTERY

An artery's walls consist of three layers: a smooth, inner lining, a thick, muscular, elastic, middle layer, and a tough, fibrous outer covering. Veins have thinner walls and most contain valves.

Artery

Thin, elastic layers

Tough, outer layer

Muscular, middle layer

Inner coat

Vein

Inner coat

constant pressure by the time it reaches the smaller blood vessels. These smaller vessels include the *arterioles*, which branch directly off the artery. The arterioles connect to the even smaller *capillaries*, which carry blood to each cell of the body. (See also *Arteries, disorders of.*)

Arthralgia

A term meaning pain in the joints or in a single joint. (See also *Arthritis; Joint.*)

Arthritis

Inflammation of a joint, characterized by pain, swelling, and stiffness. Arthritis is not a single disorder but the name for joint disease from a number of causes. The arthritis may involve one joint or many, and can vary in severity from a mild ache and stiffness to severe pain and, later, joint deformity.

TYPES AND CAUSES

OSTEOARTHRITIS Also known as degenerative arthritis or osteoarthrosis, this is the most common type of arthritis. It results from wear and tear on the joints, although metabolic, genetic and other factors may also contribute.

It evolves in middle age, and most commonly troubles people who are 60 years or older.

RHEUMATOID ARTHRITIS The most severe type of inflammatory joint disease, rheumatoid arthritis is an *autoimmune disorder* in which the body's *immune system* acts against and damages joints and surrounding soft tissues. Many joints—most commonly those in the hands, wrists, feet, and arms—become extremely painful, stiff, and deformed. Typically, the symptoms occur in people younger than those with osteoarthritis and it is more common in women.

STILL'S DISEASE Also called juvenile rheumatoid arthritis, this disorder is most common in children under the age of 4. It usually clears up after a few years, but even then may stunt growth and leave the child with permanent deformities.

SERONEGATIVE ARTHRITIS This is a group of disorders that cause symptoms and signs of arthritis in a number of joints, although blood test results for rheumatoid arthritis are negative. Seronegative arthritis can be associated with skin disorders (such as *psoriasis*), inflammatory intestinal disorders (such as *Crohn's disease*), or autoimmune disorders.

INFECTIVE ARTHRITIS Also known as septic or pyogenic arthritis, this joint disease is caused by the invasion of bacteria into the joint from a nearby infected wound or from *bacteremia* (infection in the bloodstream). The infected joint usually becomes warm and red as well as painful and swollen. In countries where *tuberculosis* is widespread, infective arthritis may result from invasion of the joint by tubercle bacilli.

Arthritis may also occur as a complication of an infection elsewhere in the body, such as *chickenpox*, *rubella* (German measles), *mumps*, *rheumatic fever*, or *gonorrhea*; it may also be a complication of *nonspecific urethritis*, in which case the joint inflammation forms part of *Reiter's syndrome*.

ANKYLOSING SPONDYLITIS In this arthritis of the pelvic joints and the spine, the joints linking the vertebrae (spinal bones) become inflamed and the vertebrae fuse. This type of arthritis may also involve other joints, usually the hips and knees.

GOUT This disorder is associated with a form of arthritis in which uric acid (one of the body's waste products) accumulates in joints in the form of crystals, causing inflammation. Gout usually affects one joint at a time.

DIAGNOSIS
The diagnosis is made from the patient's symptoms and signs. To discover the cause, fluid may be withdrawn through a needle from an affected joint. This fluid may then be examined microscopically for the presence of microorganisms, or uric acid or other crystals. Sometimes a *culture* is made from the fluid so that it can be analyzed for any infection.

X rays may be carried out to reveal the type and extent of joint damage. *Blood tests* can reveal the presence of proteins typical of rheumatoid arthritis; a high level of uric acid indicative of gout; or sometimes a high *ESR* (erythrocyte sedimentation rate), indicating inflammation.

TREATMENT
There are specific treatments for the different types of arthritis—for example, *antibiotic drugs* for septic arthritis, *anti-inflammatory drugs* for treating rheumatoid arthritis and osteoarthritis, and *allopurinol* for gout. Many other drugs are used to treat different forms of arthritis, but none seems able to effect a cure.

In a severe attack of arthritis affecting several joints, a few days' bed rest will help settle the inflammation; individual joints can be splinted to reduce the pain, and heat and supervised exercises help keep joint deformity to a minimum. Obese people with arthritis in weight-bearing joints should lose weight.

Diseased joints that have become extremely painful, unstable, or deformed may require *arthroplasty* (replacement of a joint with an artificial substitute) or *arthrodesis* (fusion of the bones in a joint).

OUTLOOK
Arthritis has many forms and varies widely in its effects. Only a few sufferers become severely disabled. Most are able to lead productive lives, although activities may need to be modified to preserve joint function.

Arthritis in the hands
Severely deformed joints in the hands of an elderly woman who is suffering from rheumatoid arthritis.

Arthrodesis
A surgical procedure in which the two bones in a diseased joint are fused to prevent the joint from moving.

WHY IT IS DONE
If pain and deformity in a diseased joint—caused, for example, by *rheumatoid arthritis*—cannot be relieved by drugs, splinting, and *physiotherapy*, or if a joint has become unstable (usually as the result of an injury), some form of surgery is required. In most cases, the operation of first choice is *arthroplasty* (reconstruction of a diseased joint using artificial replacements), because this procedure retains movement in the joint. However, when arthroplasty is not feasible or fails, arthrodesis may be used.

HOW IT IS DONE
A local anesthetic may be all that is required for a small joint, such as a finger joint. Otherwise, a general anesthetic is used. The technique of the operation varies according to the joint being treated, but in most cases cartilage (smooth, shock-absorbing tissue) is removed from the ends of the two bones, along with a surface layer of bone from each. The two ends are then joined so that, when fresh bone cells grow, the ends will fuse. The bones may need to be kept in position with plates, rods, or screws; a *bone graft* may also be carried out in some cases.

In arthrodesis of the knee or ankle, additional immobilization of the joint—by transfixing it with pins inserted through the skin—may be necessary to keep the area stable until healing is complete.

RECOVERY PERIOD
Complete union of the bones can take up to six months but is usually much quicker. In some cases the bones fail to fuse, but often this is irrelevant because fibrous tissue fills the gap between them and provides the same effect and strength as bone fusion.

OUTLOOK
One advantage of arthrodesis over arthroplasty is that, once performed, it needs no regular surveillance or further care; the patient can be reasonably certain that the problem with the joint has been solved permanently.

Arthrography
A diagnostic technique in which the interior of a damaged joint is X-rayed after injection of a radiopaque solution (a solution visible on X ray) into the joint. The procedure is gradually being replaced by *MRI*, *ultrasound scanning*, and *arthroscopy*.

A

Arthrogryposis
See *Contracture*.

Arthropathy
A medical term for *joint* disease.

Arthroplasty
Replacement of a joint or part of a joint by metal or plastic components. *Hip replacements* were the first operations of this type to be introduced and are still the most successful and most frequently performed. Replacement of other joints, including the knee (see *Knee joint replacement*), finger (see *Finger joint replacement*), shoulder, and elbow, is also routine.

Surgery to replace crippled natural joints with artificial ones is increasingly used for arthritic conditions.

The first attempts to replace part of a damaged hip joint with an artificial substitute were made in the 1930s. In the 1960s, hip replacement operations were revolutionized by developments on three fronts. First, metal and plastic materials were developed that were strong enough to allow a good level of activity while being to some extent self-lubricating; second, cement was used to help fix the artificial joint to the bones; and third, the risk of infection in the joint—a very serious complication—was greatly reduced by the use of *antibiotic drugs*. In many hospitals the surgery is performed in an operating room in which the air is filtered and all members of the surgical team wear sterile, all-enveloping clothing.

These principles have now been applied to the full range of replacement joints. Engineers and orthopedic surgeons are still developing and improving replacements for the knee and shoulder, which are more complex than the hip.

Arthroscopy
Inspection through an *endoscope* (a viewing tube) of the interior of a joint, usually for the purpose of diagnosing a condition affecting that joint. Arthroscopy has rapidly become one of the most frequently performed procedures in orthopedic surgery, thanks to the development of modern lens systems and brighter lighting by means of fiberoptics.

WHY IT IS DONE
Arthroscopy is most frequently used to inspect the inside of the knee joint. Many conditions affecting the knee do not show up on X rays and are difficult to diagnose on the basis of symptoms alone. Arthroscopy allows the sur-

HOW ARTHROSCOPY IS DONE
The procedure is usually performed under general anesthesia, but sometimes a *nerve block* is used. The joint is distended by injecting air or a saline solution; the instrument is inserted into the joint through a small skin incision. While watching through the endoscope, the surgeon can probe or lift structures to check for damage.

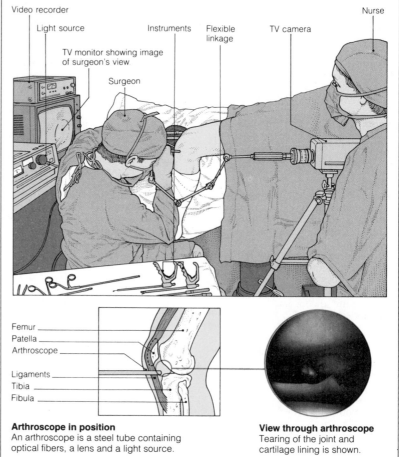

Video recorder

Light source

TV monitor showing image of surgeon's view

Surgeon

Instruments

Flexible linkage

TV camera

Nurse

Femur
Patella
Arthroscope
Ligaments
Tibia
Fibula

Arthroscope in position
An arthroscope is a steel tube containing optical fibers, a lens and a light source.

View through arthroscope
Tearing of the joint and cartilage lining is shown.

geon to see the surfaces of the bones that come into contact in the joint, the ligaments and cartilages within the joint, and the synovial membrane that lines the internal surface of the joint capsule. Specimens of these structures can be removed for examination and analysis.

A new and exciting development is the application of arthroscopic surgery techniques. Instruments that fold down as they are passed through a channel in the arthroscope enable surgeons to carry out some procedures that formerly necessitated opening up the knee. Procedures include removal of damaged cartilage, repair of torn cartilage and ligaments, and shaving or drilling the surface of the patella (kneecap). Arthroscopic surgery substantially reduces the time a patient needs to stay in hospital, and the time an athlete is unable to participate in his or her sport.

Artificial insemination
The introduction of semen into the cervix (opening of the uterus) by means of an instrument instead of by sexual intercourse, with the aim of inducing conception and pregnancy.

TYPES
There are two principal types of artificial insemination.

AIH (artificial insemination using the husband's semen) is the use of semen from the woman's permanent sexual partner. It is usually employed for couples who are unable to have intercourse, either because of psychosexual difficulties, such as impotence, or because of physical injury or deformity. Occasionally, AIH may be used when the husband has a low sperm count or a low volume of ejaculate, or if factors such as antibodies in the woman's genital tract create a hostile environment for the sperm. It is also used when semen has been stored from a man who is to undergo treatment (such as chemotherapy) that may make him sterile.

Donor insemination, sometimes called AID (artificial insemination of a donor's semen), is the use of semen from an anonymous donor. It is available to couples if the man is infertile, has a genetic disease, or may be a carrier of such a disease. It may also be used by a woman who wants children but has no male partner.

HOW IT IS DONE

Both AIH and AID are carried out at centers that are specially staffed and equipped to obtain and store semen and to carry out the insemination. Fresh semen may be used for AIH, but all semen from anonymous donors is frozen in liquid nitrogen and stored pending test results. Only donors who are in good health are chosen, and they are also usually screened for as many physical and mental disorders as possible. The semen is tested for any infection-causing microorganisms. Most centers screen for the *hepatitis B* virus and all centers screen for *AIDS*.

To prevent the transmission of AIDS through insemination, all stored semen is placed in quarantine until the donor is shown to be HIV antibody negative after two tests six months apart.

Despite all these precautions, there is no fail-proof safeguard against the use of sperm from unwitting carriers of genetic diseases.

Insemination is carried out by injecting semen into the woman's cervix with a small syringe. Two or three inseminations are carried out during the two to four optimum days for conception in the woman's menstrual cycle and, unless pregnancy occurs, this procedure is repeated for up to five more cycles.

RESULTS

When fresh semen is used, the success rate of artificial insemination in bringing about pregnancy over a six-month period is 60 to 70 percent. With semen that has been frozen, the success rate is 55 percent.

Artificial kidney

The common name for the machine used in *dialysis*.

Artificial respiration

Forced introduction of air into the lungs of someone who has stopped breathing (see *Respiratory arrest*). Artificial respiration may be administered by the mouth-to-mouth or mouth-to-nose method. It may also be given by the use of ventilating equipment administered by anesthetists (see *Ventilation*).

WHY IT IS DONE

Artificial respiration should be started as soon as possible after someone has stopped breathing; delay in breathing for four to six minutes can cause brain damage or death. When someone has stopped breathing, there is no rise and fall movement of the chest or abdo-

A

FIRST AID: ARTIFICIAL RESPIRATION

1 If someone stops breathing, send for medical help, but start resuscitation immediately. Lay the victim on his or her back on a rigid surface. If there are no signs of neck injury, gently tilt the victim's head backward to open the airway. Do this by pressing down on the forehead with one hand while lifting the chin with the fingers of the other hand.

2 Sometimes a victim's breathing is restored when the airway is opened by this head tilt, chin lift maneuver. Look, listen and feel to see if this has happened. See if the chest rises and falls. Place your ear and cheek close to the victim's nose and mouth to hear and feel exhaled air. If none of these signs are present, the victim is not breathing and needs artificial respiration right away.

3 Using the hand you have on the victim's forehead, pinch the nose shut by sealing the nostrils with your thumb and index finger. Take a deep breath, seal your mouth around the victim's mouth, and deliver two full breaths of air, allowing for full deflation of the victim's chest before giving the second breath. Maintain the head tilt, chin lift throughout, or air may not enter the lungs.

4 Remove your mouth. Check the carotid pulse for seven seconds by placing your index and middle fingers in the hollow between the Adam's apple and the side muscles of the neck. If there is a pulse, but the victim is not breathing, continue giving one breath every five seconds until breathing is restored or medical help arrives.

men, the face changes color, becoming grayish or blue-gray, and no exhaled breath can be felt. If no pulse can be felt in the neck, external cardiac compressions should be carried out in conjunction with artificial respiration (see *Cardiopulmonary resuscitation*).

When breathing is weak or shallow, movements of the chest are minimal and hardly any breath can be felt. If breathing is not restored, the brain is deprived of oxygen; permanent brain damage or death can result.

HOW IT IS DONE

MOUTH-TO-MOUTH RESUSCITATION This is the simplest and most effective method of introducing air into a victim's lungs (see illustrated box).

MOUTH-TO-NOSE RESUSCITATION If the victim has a facial injury, it may be difficult for you to breathe into his or her mouth. In such cases, follow steps 1 and 2 shown in the box. Use your thumb and index finger to close the victim's mouth. Take a deep breath and seal your mouth around the victim's nose. Blow strongly into the nose. Remove your mouth and hold the victim's mouth open with your hand, so that air can escape. Repeat as for mouth-to-mouth resuscitation every five seconds.

RESUSCITATION OF YOUNG CHILDREN For children age 1 year and older, artificial respiration is performed as for adults. For a child between 1 and 8 years of age, deliver a smaller breath than you would for an adult and give a breath every four seconds.

RESUSCITATION OF BABIES

The method of resuscitating an infant 12 months of age or younger is basically the same method used for adults, except that you will find it easier to seal your mouth over both the mouth and nose of the infant. When tilting the head, do not tip the infant's neck back very far because an infant's neck and airway are more fragile than an adult's. Blow two gentle puffs of air into the lungs followed by one breath every three seconds (20 breaths per minute) until the child's chest starts to rise.

Artificial sweeteners

Synthetic substitutes for sugar used by people on slimming diets, by diabetics, and by the food industry. Although saccharin and aspartame are often recommended for use in slimming diets, they are of questionable value because they do not reduce the craving for sweet foods. In Canada, saccharin and cyclamate are available as table-top sweeteners only;

neither of these substances may be used as additives in products manufactured by the food industry.

TYPES

SACCHARIN is 500 to 600 times sweeter than sugar (sucrose), although it has a sour after-taste and provides no calories. It is not suitable for use in baking. Saccharin has been associated with bladder cancer in animal experiments but the risk of associated cancer in humans is negligible.

CYCLAMATE is about 30 times as sweet as sugar, and provides no calories. Unlike saccharin, it can be used in baking without going bitter. Cyclamate was banned as a commercial food additive because it was suspected of causing cancer in animals.

ASPARTAME is about 200 times sweeter than sugar—although its sweetness is destroyed by prolonged heating—and it is virtually calorie free and without adverse effects in normal quantities. Excessive amounts, however, may cause neurological disorders.

SORBITOL is a sugar substitute that occurs naturally in certain fruits. It is a sugar alcohol which has no effect on the teeth and is used in "sugar-free" sweets and chewing gums. It is used by diabetics but its high calorie value—about 490 per 100 g—makes it unsuitable for use in slimming diets. One problem with using sorbitol is that its slow absorption from the intestine into the bloodstream may cause diarrhea by drawing fluid into the intestine.

ASA

See *Acetylsalicylic acid*.

Asbestos-induced diseases

A variety of diseases caused by the inhalation of asbestos fibers. Asbestos is a fibrous mineral formerly used a great deal as a heat- and fire-resistant insulating material. It is also used in brake linings and gaskets. Its use for insulation has declined dramatically over the past 20 years.

TYPES

ASBESTOSIS In this condition, widespread fine scarring occurs in the lungs; this tends to progress even when exposure to asbestos is discontinued. The disease causes breathlessness and a dry cough, eventually leading to severe disability and death.

Asbestosis develops only in people who have been heavily exposed to asbestos, such as asbestos miners, workers in asbestos factories, and workers who handle insulation materials. The period from first exposure

to development of the disease is seldom less than 10 years and is usually much longer. Diagnosis is by chest X ray, which shows widespread shadowing of the lung if asbestosis is present. Asbestosis increases the risk of developing *lung cancer* about fivefold in smokers and nonsmokers alike; the combination of cigarette smoking and asbestosis leads to death from lung cancer in about one third of sufferers.

In Canada, about 10 deaths a year are attributed to asbestosis.

MESOTHELIOMA This is a malignant tumor of the *pleura* (the membrane that surrounds the lungs) or the *peritoneum* (the membrane that lines the abdominal cavity and covers the abdominal organs). In the pleura, mesotheliomas cause pain and breathlessness; tumors in the peritoneum cause enlargement of the abdomen and intestinal obstruction.

There is no treatment for the condition, which usually leads to death within one or two years. The average interval between the first exposure to asbestos and death is between 20 and 30 years. The condition almost exclusively affects those who have worked with blue or brown asbestos; the risk with white asbestos is almost nil.

BILATERAL DIFFUSE PLEURAL THICKENING In this condition, the outer and inner layers of the pleura become thickened, and excess fluid may accumulate in the cavity between them. This combination restricts the ability of the lungs to expand, resulting in shortness of breath. The condition may develop after even short exposure to asbestos.

PLEURAL PLAQUES These are areas of thickening, called plaques, confined to the outer layer of the pleura. Pleural plaques do not cause symptoms or

Asbestos fiber in lung
Asbestos is a fibrous mineral that can cause lung disease if inhaled.

A

disability but are detectable on X rays. The plaques occur commonly in people who have had substantial exposure to asbestos; detection does not usually take place until 20 or more years after first exposure. Sometimes, plaques appear after only a short duration of exposure. Although pleural plaques indicate past exposure to asbestos, they do not indicate a higher than normal risk of developing other asbestos-related diseases.

Asbestosis

See *Asbestos-induced diseases*.

Ascariasis

Infestation with the worm *ASCARIS LUMBRICOIDES*. Ascariasis is common worldwide, especially in the tropics. The causative parasite is a pale, cylindrical, tapered roundworm, between 15 and 35 cm in length in adult form, which lives in the small intestine of its human host. One or several worms may be present, but symptoms usually occur only in people with heavy worm infestations.

INCIDENCE AND CAUSES

Ascariasis affects up to 80 to 90 percent of the population in poorer countries, where children living in rural areas are prone to heavy infestations. The disease is spread by ingestion of worm eggs from soil contaminated by human feces or from uncooked food contaminated with soil containing eggs. In some dry, windy climates, airborne eggs may be swallowed after being blown into the mouth. The eggs hatch in the intestine, eventually developing into adults, which produce more eggs that are excreted in the feces. The full cycle of the infestation is shown in the diagram.

There are a few small endemic centers of ascariasis in Canada, but this disease is primarily an imported infection. It may be present in up to 10 percent of some immigrant groups, but this prevalence usually decreases in a year or so due to treatment and natural loss of infection.

SYMPTOMS

Light infestations may cause either no symptoms or occasional nausea, abdominal pain, and irregular bowel movements. A worm may be passed via the rectum or vomited.

A heavy load of worms may compete with the host for food, leading to malnutrition and anemia, which in children can retard growth.

DIAGNOSIS AND TREATMENT

Ascariasis is diagnosed by finding the worm's eggs during microscopic

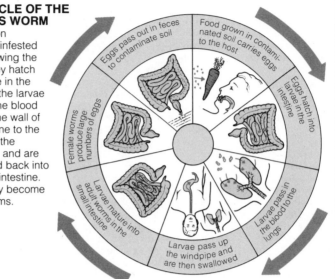

LIFE CYCLE OF THE ASCARIS WORM

The person becomes infested by swallowing the eggs. They hatch into larvae in the intestine; the larvae travel in the blood through the wall of the intestine to the lungs, up the windpipe, and are swallowed back into the small intestine. There they become adult worms.

Eggs pass out in feces to contaminate soil

Food grown in contaminated soil carries eggs to the host

Eggs hatch into larvae in the intestine

Female worms produce large numbers of eggs

Larvae mature into adult worms in the small intestine

Larvae pass in the blood to the lungs

Larvae pass up the windpipe and are then swallowed

examination of a person's feces or, occasionally, finding that an adult worm has been passed in the feces.

The worm infestation is treated with *anthelmintic drugs*, such as *piperazine* (which is highly effective in a single dose). The worms are passed via the rectum some days after the drug is taken. The patient usually makes a complete recovery.

Ascites

An excess of fluid in the peritoneal cavity—the space between the two layers of membrane, or peritoneum, that line the inside of the abdominal wall and the outside of the abdominal organs. As much as several litres of fluid may be present, causing abdominal swelling.

CAUSES

Ascites may occur in any condition that causes generalized *edema* (excessive accumulation of fluid in the body tissues). The most important of these conditions are congestive *heart failure, nephrotic syndrome*, and *cirrhosis* of the liver. Ascites may occur in *cancer* if metastases (secondary growths) from lung, breast, or intestinal tumors are deposited on the surface of the peritoneum. Ascites also occurs when *tuberculosis* affects the abdomen.

In addition to abdominal swelling and discomfort, ascites may cause breathing difficulty due to pressure on, and immobilization of, the diaphragm, the sheet of muscle that separates the thorax (chest) from the abdomen.

DIAGNOSIS

Ascites is detected during physical examination by a physician. Diagnosis of the cause involves removing and analyzing a sample of ascitic fluid via a sterile needle inserted through the abdominal wall. The fluid is examined under the microscope for malignant cells. Its color, turbidity (cloudiness), and chemical composition also help identify whether the cause of the ascites is inflammation or a condition such as cirrhosis.

TREATMENT

Treatment depends on the precise cause of the ascites, but in many cases includes bed rest, and fluid and salt (sodium) restriction. Alcohol must not be taken by the patient if liver disease is implicated. *Diuretic drugs*, particularly *spironolactone*, may be prescribed.

If the ascites causes discomfort or breathing difficulty, fluid can be drained from the peritoneal cavity.

Ascorbic acid

The chemical name for *vitamin C*.

Aseptic technique

The creation of a germ-free environment, mainly by the use of *sterilization*, to protect a patient from infection. Aseptic sterilization is distinct from antisepsis, which is the destruction of germs by chemicals (known as *antiseptics*).

WHY IT IS DONE

Aseptic technique is needed for any procedure in which there is a danger of introducing infection into the body.

The patient can be contaminated by microorganisms from four main sources: other people, his or her own body, instruments, and the air.

Aseptic technique is used for all surgery in an operating room and for other minor surgical procedures, such as inserting a urinary catheter or stitching a wound. Aseptic technique is also needed when caring for patients suffering from diseases, such as *leukemia*, in which the *immune system* is suppressed and the body's natural defenses against infection are reduced as a result.

HOW IT IS DONE

All people who come in contact with the patient must scrub their hands and wear presterilized gowns and disposable gloves and masks. Instruments are sterilized beforehand in an *autoclave* (a chamber containing pressurized steam) and placed ready for use on a cart that is covered with sterile material.

The area of the patient that is to be operated on is cleaned with antiseptic solutions of *iodine* or *hexachlorophene*, and the surrounding skin is covered with sterile drapes. In addition, before operations on the intestine, the bowel is cleared by giving *laxative drugs* and also sometimes an *enema* to prevent any contamination of the abdominal area by feces.

When using aseptic technique, care is taken to place used, possibly contaminated, instruments well away from sterile instruments and dressings. In an operating room it is important to keep the air and the room scrupulously clean. The windows remain closed and the only air that enters the room is through a special ventilation system that purifies the air and maintains it at a preset humidity. (See also *Isolation*.)

Aspergillosis

An infection caused by aspergillus, a fungus which grows in decaying vegetation; spores of this fungus are usually present in the air all the year round. Aspergillus is harmless to healthy people but causes trouble in certain circumstances. It may grow as a fungus ball in people whose lungs have been damaged by *tuberculosis* and cause coughing up of blood. In some people with *asthma*, aspergillus grows in the mucus in the bronchi and causes worsening of symptoms and areas of lung collapse. Aspergillus may also cause serious and often fatal infection in people with reduced resistance to infection, particularly those being treated by *anticancer drugs* for leukemia or other forms of cancer, or by *immunosuppressant drugs* to prevent the rejection of transplanted organs.

Aspermia

See *Azoospermia*.

Asphyxia

The medical term for suffocation. Asphyxia may be caused by obstruction of a large airway, usually by a foreign body (see *Choking*), by insufficient oxygen in the surrounding air (as occurs when a closed plastic bag is put over the head), or by poisoning with a gas such as carbon monoxide that interferes with the uptake of oxygen into the blood.

The person initially breathes more rapidly and strongly to try to overcome the lack of oxygen in the blood. There is also an increase in heart rate and blood pressure.

TREATMENT

First-aid treatment consists of *artificial respiration* after first moving the person into the open air and clearing the airway of any obstruction. Untreated asphyxia causes death.

Aspiration

The withdrawal of fluid or tissue from the body by suction. The term also refers to the act of breathing in a foreign body, usually food or drink.

Aspiration *biopsy* is the removal of tissue or fluid for examination by suction through a needle attached to a syringe. The procedure is commonly used to obtain cells from a fluid-filled cavity (such as a breast cyst). It is also used to obtain cells from the bone marrow (see *Bone marrow biopsy*), or from internal organs, when a narrow needle is guided to the site of the biopsy by *CT scanning* or *ultrasound scanning*. The cells obtained are examined under a microscope.

Aspiration pneumonia is inflammation of the lungs due to inhalation of foreign material (e.g., vomit or infected respiratory secretions).

Aspirin

See *Acetylsalicyclic acid*.

Assay

Analysis or measurement of a substance to determine its presence or effects. A qualitative assay determines only whether a substance is present, whereas a quantitative assay determines the actual amount present.

Biological assays (called bioassays) are concerned mainly with measuring the responses of an animal or specific organ to particular substances. They are used, for example, to assess the effects of a drug or to measure hormone levels. (See also *Immunoassay*; *Radioimmunoassay*.)

Astereognosis

An inability to recognize objects by touch when they are placed in one hand—even though there is no defect of sensation in the fingers or any difficulty holding the object. Testing for astereognosis is part of any detailed examination of the central nervous system. Astereognosis is either left-sided or right-sided; tactile recognition is normal on the other side. If both sides are affected, the condition is called tactile *agnosia*.

Astereognosis and tactile agnosia are caused by damage to parts of the cerebrum (main mass of the brain) concerned with recognition by touch.

Asthenia

An old term meaning loss of strength and energy (see *Weakness*).

Asthenia, neurocirculatory

See *Cardiac neurosis*.

Asthma

Recurrent attacks of breathlessness, characteristically accompanied by wheezing, especially when exhaling, and varying in severity from hour to hour and day to day. The illness often starts in childhood and tends to improve or clear up in early adulthood. The familiar form of asthma is more correctly called bronchial asthma; this use of the full name distinguishes it from a condition associated with wheezing caused by heart failure (see *Asthma, cardiac*).

Although asthma frequently begins early in life (most sufferers have their first attack before the age of 5), it can develop at any age.

CAUSES

Bronchial asthma can be classified into two main types: extrinsic, in which an allergy (usually to something inhaled) triggers an attack, and intrinsic, in which there is no apparent external cause for the asthma.

The most common *allergens* responsible for extrinsic asthma are pollens, which often also cause allergic *rhinitis* (hay fever), house dust, house-dust mites, animal fur, feathers, and dander (tiny particles shed from animal skin, fur, or feathers). Extrinsic asthma may also be triggered by a viral or bacterial respiratory infection, by exercise (especially in cold air), by tobacco smoke or other air pollutants, or by allergy to a particular food or drug.

Intrinsic asthma tends to develop later in life than extrinsic asthma, with the first attack often following a respiratory tract infection. Stress or anxiety may precipitate attacks.

PREVALENCE

About one in 20 of the overall population is asthmatic but the prevalence among children is much greater—about one in 10.

Heredity is a major factor in the development of extrinsic asthma. Asthma seems to be becoming more common in developed countries.

SYMPTOMS

Asthmatic attacks vary greatly in their severity, ranging from mild breathlessness to *respiratory failure*. The main symptoms of asthma are breathlessness, wheezing, a dry cough sometimes brought on by exercise, and a feeling of tightness in the chest.

During a severe attack, breathing becomes increasingly difficult, caus-

ing sweating, rapid heartbeat, and great distress and anxiety. The sufferer cannot lie down or sleep, may be unable to speak, breathes rapidly, and wheezes loudly.

In a very severe attack, the low amount of oxygen in the blood may cause *cyanosis* (bluish discoloration) of the face, particularly the lips, and the skin may become pale and clammy. Such attacks may be fatal.

PREVENTION

Although there is no cure for asthma, attacks can be prevented to a large extent. For sufferers from extrinsic asthma, tests are available to discover whether any of the common allergens is responsible for triggering attacks; if a specific cause is discovered, steps can be taken to avoid it. For example, if the house-dust mite is responsible, mattresses, pillows and quilts (in which the mites flourish) should be enclosed in airtight plastic covers and the home should be kept as free from dust as possible.

Hyposensitization (a course of injections of the allergen) has limited results. Much more successful in pre-

venting attacks are prophylactic (preventive) drugs, such as *sodium cromoglycate* and inhaled *corticosteroid drugs*. To be effective, they must be taken several times daily, usually through an inhaler.

TREATMENT

Once an attack has started, a prophylactic drug has limited effects and a *bronchodilator drug*, such as *salbutamol*, is needed to relax and widen the airways. Bronchodilator drugs are usually inhaled from small pressurized aerosol cans (see illustration). The technique of inhalation is very important. For young children and those who have difficulty with aerosols, inhalers that deliver the drug in the form of a mist or powder make the procedure easier. Oral *theophylline* preparations may also be used to prevent or treat attacks. Long-term treatment with oral corticosteroids may be necessary for people with chronic continuing asthma if all other treatments have failed.

EMERGENCY PROCEDURE

Most attacks of asthma either pass naturally or can be controlled by use

---

THE CAUSE OF ASTHMA

Breathlessness and wheezing in asthma is caused by narrowing of the bronchioles (small airways in the lungs). Asthma can be triggered by a wide variety of stimuli, including exercise, infection, pollen, and dust, which would have no effect on non-asthmatic people.

Inflammation of the linings of these bronchioles causes an increased production of sputum (phlegm), which makes the obstruction worse. A dry cough often develops as the sufferer attempts to clear the airways.

Effect of asthma on the lungs

Trachea

Bronchus

TREATMENT OF AN ASTHMA ATTACK

Attacks are treated by inhalation of a bronchodilator drug from an inhaler or from a nebulizer.

INHALER

Pressurized canister

Mouthpiece

Using an inhaler
To use the inhaler correctly, exhale first; then take in a slow, deep breath while you release the drug by depressing the canister. Two puffs should increase air flow within 15 minutes.

Obstructed bronchiole
Before treatment, airflow is obstructed by a narrowing of the bronchiole.

Healthy bronchiole
Inhalation of the bronchodilator widens the bronchiole and improves airflow.

Grass

Tree

Molds

J F M A M J J A S O N D

Seasonal asthma
When symptoms occur only during a few months, the cause is likely to be allergy to pollen or spores.

of a bronchodilator. In some cases, however, an attack may be so severe that it fails to respond to the recommended dose of the drug. In this case, the dose should be repeated. If it has no effect, a doctor should be consulted or the person taken to hospital.

Emergency treatment at home or in hospital may include the administration of oxygen, a corticosteroid, and a bronchodilator through a nebulizer or an intravenous injection of *aminophylline*. If these measures are ineffective (which is rare), the patient has to be put on a *ventilator*, which forces air or oxygen under pressure into the lungs.

OUTLOOK

More than half of the children who suffer from asthma grow out of it completely by the age of 21; in a proportion of the remainder, attacks become less severe as they grow older. With modern drug treatment, even people who suffer repeated attacks as adults can expect to live a normal life. In most cases, quality of life need not be impaired (demonstrated by the success of world-class athletes who have had asthma). However, a small minority continue to suffer from disabling asthma despite being on optimum treatment. Severe cases may be hospitalized frequently.

Asthma, cardiac

Breathing difficulty caused by accumulation of fluid in the lungs that causes bronchospasm and wheezing. This response is usually due to reduced pumping efficiency of the left side of the heart (see *Heart failure*), causing congestion and increased pressure within the blood circulation through the lungs, and the accumulation of fluid in the lungs.

Although cardiac asthma has a different cause from the more familiar bronchial asthma, the two conditions have similar symptoms, including wheezing and breathing difficulty. A chest X ray may show fluid in the lungs. Treatment is primarily for heart failure but may include use of bronchodilator drugs.

Astigmatism

A condition in which the front surface of the cornea does not conform to the normal "spherical" curve. Although the eye is perfectly healthy, the corneal surface has discrepancies in its curvature, with the result that magnifying power in one direction is greater than in the other.

A minor degree of astigmatism is normal and glasses are not necessary

to correct it. More severe astigmatism causes blurring of lines set at a particular angle. A person with astigmatism might see horizontal lines clearly but vertical lines blurred, or the blurring may occur in an oblique meridian.

TREATMENT

Ordinary spherically curved spectacle lenses cannot correct astigmatism. Correction requires lenses with little optical power in the "normal" meridian but greater curvature in other meridians. These "cylindrical" lenses must be framed at a precise angle.

Hard contact lenses can bridge over the anomalous corneal curve and present an even spherical surface for focusing; they give excellent vision in astigmatism. Ordinary soft lenses tend to mold to the astigmatic curve.

Astringent

COMMON DRUGS

Aluminum acetate Potassium permanganate Silver nitrate Zinc sulfate

A substance that causes tissue to dry and shrink by reducing its ability to absorb water. Astringents are widely used in *antiperspirants* and skin tonics. They are also used to promote healing of broken or inflamed skin. Astringent drugs are used to treat *otitis externa* (inflammation of the ear canal) and watering of the eye due to minor irritation. Astringents may cause burning or stinging when applied.

Astrocytoma

A type of malignant *brain tumor*. Astrocytomas are the most common type of *glioma*, a tumor arising from the glial (supporting) cells within the nervous system, and are composed of cells called astrocytes.

Astrocytomas most commonly develop within the cerebrum (the main mass of the brain). Although all types are very serious, they are classified in four grades (I to IV) according to their rate of growth and malignancy. A grade I astrocytoma is a slow-growing tumor that may spread widely throughout the brain but may be present for many years before causing symptoms. A grade IV astrocytoma is a very fast-growing tumor that causes rapid development of disabling symptoms.

Symptoms are similar to those caused by other types of brain tumor. Diagnostic tests include *CT scanning* or *MRI* and, often, *angiography*. Few astrocytomas can be completely surgically removed.

Asylum

An outdated term for an institution that provides care for those who are mentally ill.

Asymptomatic

A medical term that means without *symptoms*—those indications of illness noticed by the patient (as distinct from *signs*, which are observed by the physician). Examples of conditions that may be asymptomatic include *hypertension* (high blood pressure), which is usually discovered during a routine blood pressure test, and *diabetes mellitus*, which is often diagnosed from a blood or urine test. Most disorders are asymptomatic in their early stages. In the case of *cancer*, much effort has been made to devise screening tests to detect tumors at their early, asymptomatic stage.

Asystole

A term meaning absence of the heartbeat (see *Cardiac arrest*).

Ataxia

Incoordination and clumsiness, affecting balance and gait, limb or eye movements, and/or speech.

CAUSES

Ataxia may be caused by damage to the *cerebellum* (part of the brain concerned with coordination) or to the nerve pathways that carry information to and from the cerebellum. Possible causes include injury to the brain or to the spinal cord. In adults, ataxia may be caused by drug or *alcohol intoxication* (the most common cause), by a *stroke* or *brain tumor* affecting the cerebellum or brain stem, by a disease of the balance organ in the ear, or by *multiple sclerosis* or other types of nervous system degeneration. In rare cases, ataxia is a result of untreated *syphilis*. In children, causes include acute infection, brain tumors, and the inherited condition *Friedreich's ataxia*.

SYMPTOMS

Symptoms depend on the site of damage within the nervous system, although an awkward gait is common to most forms. The typical ataxic gait is lurching and unsteady, like that of a drunk person, with the feet widely placed. If the damage is to nerves that carry sensory information from joints and muscles to the cerebellum, sensory ataxia results. In such cases, the person's unsteadiness is worse when the eyes are closed. Damage to parts of the brain stem concerned with controlling eye movements often causes *nystagmus* (jerky eye movements).

Damage to the cerebellum itself usually causes slurred speech as well as an unsteady gait. Sometimes, if damage is confined to one side of the cerebellum, incoordination is confined to the limbs on the same side and is often accompanied by a tremor in the limbs during purposeful movements. When walking, the person often has a tendency to veer or fall toward the affected side. Other features may include decomposition of complex actions into their component parts, producing jerky movements, and "overshoot" when attempts are made to touch or pick up objects.

DIAGNOSIS AND TREATMENT
Discovery of the cause of ataxia may be helped by *CT scanning* or *MRI*. Treatment depends on the cause.

Atelectasis
Collapse of part or all of a lung caused by obstruction of the bronchus (the main air passage through the lung) or the bronchioles (smaller air passages). When this happens, air already in the lung cannot be breathed out and, instead, is absorbed into the blood, leading to the collapse of all or part of the lung. After collapsing, the lung loses its elasticity and cannot take in air; consequently, the blood passing through it can no longer absorb oxygen or dispose of carbon dioxide.

In an adult, atelectasis is usually not life-threatening, because unaffected parts of the lung (or, if the whole lung has collapsed, the other lung) expand to compensate for the loss of function in the collapsed area. However, when a lung collapses in a newborn baby—because mucus has blocked a bronchus—the baby's life is at risk. (For lung collapse caused by a perforation of the outer covering of the lung, see *Pneumothorax*.)

CAUSES AND INCIDENCE
Obstruction of a bronchus is usually due to one of four mechanisms. First, secretions of mucus in the bronchus or bronchioles may accumulate and cause blockage. This can happen after an abdominal or chest operation that has made coughing difficult due to pain; in a baby at birth; in *asthma*; or in certain infections, such as *pertussis* (whooping cough) in children or chronic *bronchitis* in adults.

Second, an accidentally inhaled *foreign body*, such as a peanut, may stick in the bronchus; this is more common in children than in adults. Third, a benign or malignant *tumor* in the lung may block the bronchus. Fourth, enlarged lymph nodes (which

occur in *tuberculosis*, other lung infections, or some forms of *cancer*) may exert pressure on the airway.

SYMPTOMS, DIAGNOSIS, AND TREATMENT
The main symptom is breathing difficulty. There may also be a cough and chest pain, depending on the underlying cause.

The condition is diagnosed by physical examination of the chest and *chest X rays*. Treatment is aimed at the cause of the blockage. If the cause is an accumulation of mucus, the patient will be given chest *physiotherapy*, including encouragement to clear the chest by coughing or deep breathing and use of *postural drainage*.

Once the obstruction has been removed, the collapsed lung usually reinflates gradually, although some areas of it may be permanently damaged or scarred.

Atenolol
A *beta-blocker drug* commonly used in the treatment of *hypertension* (high blood pressure), *angina pectoris* (chest pain due to impaired blood supply to heart muscle), and certain types of *arrhythmia* (irregular heartbeat).

Atheroma
Fatty deposits on the inner lining of an artery that can cause *atherosclerosis*.

Atherosclerosis
A disease of the arterial wall in which the inner layer thickens, causing narrowing of the channel and thus impairing blood flow.

The narrowing is due to the development of raised patches called plaques in the inner lining of the arteries. These plaques consist of a substance called atheroma, a mixture of low-density lipoproteins (see *Fats and oils*), decaying muscle cells, fibrous tissue, clumps of blood platelets, *cholesterol*, and sometimes calcium; they tend to form in regions of turbulent blood flow and are found most often in people with high concentrations of cholesterol in the bloodstream. The number and thickness of plaques increase with age, causing loss of the smooth lining of the blood vessels and encouraging *thrombus* (abnormal blood clot) formation. Sometimes, a fragment of thrombus breaks off and forms an *embolus*, which travels through the bloodstream and blocks smaller vessels.

INCIDENCE
Atherosclerosis is responsible for more deaths in Canada than any other condition. Atherosclerotic heart dis-

ease involving the coronary arteries is the most common single cause of death, accounting for one third of all deaths (see *Coronary artery disease*); atherosclerotic interference with blood supply to the brain (causing *stroke*) is the third most common cause of death after cancer. Atherosclerosis also causes a great deal of serious illness by reducing the blood flow in other major arteries, such as those to the kidneys, legs, and intestines.

CAUSES
Certain risk factors increase the probability that atherosclerosis will develop. These risk factors are cigarette smoking, *hypertension* (high blood pressure), male gender, obesity, physical inactivity, a high level of cholesterol in the blood, poorly controlled *diabetes mellitus*, family history of arterial disease, and, possibly, an anxious or aggressive personality.

The risk of atherosclerosis increases with age, probably in part because of the length of time it takes for the plaques to develop. The influence of gender is illustrated by comparing men with premenopausal women: in the group aged 35 to 44, coronary artery disease kills six times as many men as women.

PREVENTION
Modifications of the risk factors, especially early in adult life, can markedly reduce the probability that atherosclerosis will develop or can at least delay its manifestations. Smoking should be stopped, blood pressure checked regularly, and hypertension treated. Diet should be low in saturated fats and obesity should be avoided. If cholesterol levels remain high despite a low-fat diet, drug therapy to reduce the cholesterol levels may be warranted. Meticulous control of diabetes mellitus is important. Regular exercise is of great value in maintaining the health and efficiency of the heart and circulation.

SYMPTOMS
Unfortunately, atherosclerosis produces no symptoms until the damage to the arteries is severe enough to restrict blood flow. Restriction of blood flow to heart muscle due to atherosclerosis can cause *angina pectoris*. Restriction of blood flow to the muscles of the legs causes intermittent *claudication* (pains in the legs brought on by walking and relieved by rest). Narrowing of the arteries supplying blood to the brain may cause *transient ischemic attacks* (symptoms and signs of a *stroke* lasting less than 24 hours) and episodes of dizziness.

A

A medical history and examination will reveal much about the health of the circulation, but special investigation may be necessary. Blood flow in an artery can be investigated by *angiography* (X rays after injection of a radiopaque substance), *Doppler* ultrasound scanning, or *plethysmography* (a technique that produces a tracing of the pulse pattern).

TREATMENT
Medication is unsatisfactory in treating atherosclerosis because the damage has already been done. *Anticoagulant drugs* have been used to try to minimize secondary clotting and embolus formation, but have little or no effect on the progress of the disease. *Vasodilator drugs* are helpful in providing symptom relief but are of no curative value.

Surgical treatment may be recommended for people who are unresponsive to medical treatment or who have a high risk of suffering serious complications. Balloon *angioplasty* may be used to open up narrowed vessels and improve blood supply. The blood supply to the heart muscle can be restored by *coronary artery bypass* surgery. Large atheromatous and calcified arterial obstructions can be removed by *endarterectomy*, and entire segments of diseased peripheral vessels can be replaced by woven plastic tube grafts (see *Arterial reconstructive surgery*).

Athetosis
A nervous system disorder, characterized by slow, writhing, involuntary (uncontrollable) movements, most often seen in the head, face, neck, and limbs. The movements commonly include facial grimacing, with contortions of the mouth and lips. Often, the affected person also has difficulty balancing and walking. In some cases the muscles are flaccid (floppy), and in others they are spastic (tense).

Very commonly, athetosis is combined with *chorea* (involuntary fidgety movements)—a combination called choreoathetosis. Both conditions arise from damage to the *basal ganglia*, clusters of nerve cells deep within the brain that are concerned with the control of movements. Causes include damage to the brain prior to or around the time of birth (see *Cerebral palsy*), *encephalitis* (brain infection), degenerative disorders such as *Huntington's chorea*, or the use of certain drugs such as *phenothiazine drugs* or *levodopa* derivatives. If drug treatment is the cause, the abnormal movements may stop when the drug is withdrawn.

Athlete's foot
A common skin condition in which the skin between the toes becomes itchy and sore, may crack and peel away, and occasionally blisters. The webs between the fourth and fifth toes are most often involved. Athlete's foot is rare in young children and is asso-

Athlete's foot
The typical appearance shows fissuring in the cleft between the fourth and fifth toes. There is usually an annoying itch.

ciated with wearing shoes and sweating; the condition is rare where most people go barefoot.

CAUSES
Athlete's foot is usually caused by a dermatophyte (a type of fungal) infection, known medically as tinea pedis, but may be caused by bacteria. Secondary infection occurring through skin cracks is bacterial.

TREATMENT
Athlete's foot sometimes clears up without medication. Careful drying of the affected area is necessary; wearing dry cotton socks or sandals may help. Disinfecting the floors of showers and locker rooms helps control the spread of infection.

Most fungal infections respond to treatment with *antifungal drugs*, such as tolnaftate, miconazole, or an undecenoate compound.

ARTERIAL DEGENERATION IN ATHEROSCLEROSIS
Atherosclerosis is narrowing of the arteries caused by plaques on their inner linings. These plaques are composed mainly of fats deposited from the bloodstream. They disrupt the normal flow of blood through the affected artery. Men are affected earlier than women because premenopausal women are protected by natural estrogen hormones.

RISK FACTORS

| Cigarette smoking |
| Hypertension |
| Male gender |
| Obesity |
| Physical inactivity |
| Diabetes mellitus |
| Heredity |
| Aggressive personality |

X ray showing atherosclerosis
The leg arteries shown here appear as bright channels. One is narrowed at a point corresponding to the dark gap.

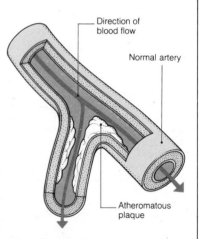

Direction of blood flow

Normal artery

Atheromatous plaque

Atherosclerotic artery
A deposit of atheromatous plaque disrupts normal blood flow through the artery at the point where it branches. This occurs because of the greater level of turbulence in this area.

Atony

Complete loss of tension in a muscle, so that the muscle is completely flaccid (floppy). Atony can occur in some nervous system disorders or after injury to nerves. The arm muscles may become atonic after injury to the *brachial plexus* (nerve roots in the neck passing into the arm).

Atopy

A predisposition to allergic reactions (see *Allergy*). Atopic individuals tend to suffer from allergic-based disorders, such as *asthma*, *eczema*, *urticaria* (hives), and allergic *rhinitis* (hay fever). The mechanism that causes the predisposition is not fully understood, although various theories have been proposed.

There is a distinct genetic, or inherited (familial), basis to atopy—the relatives of atopic individuals are much more likely than the average person to be atopic (even after allowance is made for bias caused by similarities of environment).

ATP

The abbreviation for adenosine triphosphate, the chief energy-carrying chemical in the body. (See also *ADP*; *Metabolism*.)

Atresia

The *congenital* absence or closure of a body opening or canal, caused by a failure of development while in the uterus. Examples are *biliary atresia*, in which the bile ducts between the liver and duodenum are absent; *esophageal atresia*, in which the esophagus comes to a blind end; pulmonary atresia, in which the pulmonary artery between the right side of the heart and the lungs is closed off; and anal atresia (see *Anus, imperforate*), in which the anal canal is narrowed and shut off. Most forms of atresia require surgical correction early in life.

Atrial fibrillation

A type of irregular heartbeat (see *Arrhythmia, cardiac*) in which the atria (upper chambers of the heart) beat irregularly and very rapidly (300 to 500 beats per minute). Not all these beats pass through the atrioventricular node (the impulse carrier between the atria and the ventricles, the lower chambers of the heart). As a result, the ventricles beat irregularly at a rate of 80 to 160 beats per minute.

CAUSES

Atrial fibrillation can occur in almost any long-standing heart disease in which there is enlargement of the atria. It is common in rheumatic heart disease (see *Rheumatic fever*), *thyrotoxicosis* (overactivity of the thyroid gland), and atherosclerotic heart disease.

SYMPTOMS AND SIGNS

Sudden onset of atrial fibrillation can cause *palpitations* (awareness of fast heartbeat) or *angina pectoris* (chest pain due to reduced blood supply). The inefficient pumping action of the heart in *heart failure* can reduce the output of blood into the circulation by as much as 30 percent. Blood clots in the atria may enter the bloodstream and become lodged in an artery (see *Embolism*). This is most serious when it affects the main artery to the lungs, causing *pulmonary embolism*, or an artery in the brain, causing *stroke*.

DIAGNOSIS

The pulse is irregular in rate and strength and does not correspond with the heart rate; many heartbeats audible at the heart fail to reach the wrist because the heart has contracted prematurely when only partly filled with blood. The diagnosis of atrial fibrillation is confirmed by an *ECG*.

TREATMENT

The first step usually is to control the heart rate by giving *digoxin* or, in certain instances, intravenous *verapamil*. If the fibrillation is of recent onset, treatment is directed at remedying the cause—for example, treatment for thyrotoxicosis, or replacement of heart valves damaged by rheumatic heart disease. Atrial fibrillation of recent onset can often be reversed by *defibrillation* (application of a short electric shock to the heart).

If atrial fibrillation is long-standing, or is combined with severe heart disease, the likelihood of reversing it is small. In this case, control of the heart rate with digoxin is continued and *beta-blocker drugs* are sometimes also used. *Anticoagulant drugs* may also be given to reduce the risk of embolism.

Atrial flutter

A type of irregular heartbeat (see *Arrhythmia, cardiac*) in which the atria (upper chambers of the heart) beat very rapidly at 200 to 400 beats per minute. At these rates the atrioventricular node, the conducting mechanism between the atria and the ventricles (lower chambers of the heart), is unable to respond to every beat. As a result, the ventricles beat only once to every two, three, or four beats of the atria. The condition generally occurs in people over 40 who have severe heart disease.

Some people with atrial flutter have no symptoms; others may complain of palpitations (an awareness of a fast heartbeat). The condition can lead to *heart failure* (reduced pumping action of the heart) or *angina pectoris* (chest pain due to reduced blood supply).

When treatment is urgent, *defibrillation* (application of a short electric shock to the heart) may be effective. For nonurgent treatment, *digoxin* may be prescribed.

Atrial natriuretic peptide

A substance produced in the muscular wall of the atria (upper chambers of the heart). It is released into the bloodstream in response to an increase in atrial muscle tension caused, for example, by *heart failure* or by some types of *hypertension*.

Atrial natriuretic peptide increases the amount of sodium excreted in the urine; sodium draws water out with it, decreasing the volume of water in the circulation and helping to lower the blood pressure. Atrial natriuretic peptide also lowers the blood pressure by causing blood vessels to dilate (widen) so that blood can flow more easily.

Children with congenital heart disorders causing heart failure (see *Heart disease, congenital*) have high levels of atrial natriuretic peptide. These levels fall after successful surgery to correct the abnormality.

Atrium

Either of the two (right and left) upper chambers of the *heart*.

ANATOMY OF THE ATRIUM

The left atrium receives oxygenated blood from the pulmonary veins; the right atrium receives deoxygenated blood from the venae cavae.

Superior vena cava

Pulmonary veins

Right atrium

Left atrium

Atrophy

Shrinkage or wasting away of a tissue or organ due to a reduction in the size or number of its cells. Atrophy is commonly caused by disuse (such as when a limb has been immobilized in a plaster cast) or by inadequate cell nutrition due to poor blood circulation. Atrophy may also occur during prolonged serious illness, when the body needs to use up the protein reserves in the muscles. Other, less common, causes include nerve damage that partly or completely immobilizes part of the body, and lack of a specific *enzyme* or *hormone* needed to stimulate growth of a cell or an organ.

Atropine

ANTICHOLINERGIC

Tablet Injection Eye-drops

Prescription needed

A drug derived from *belladonna*. Atropine is used to treat *iritis* (inflammation of the iris) and *corneal ulcer*. It is also used in young children to dilate (widen) the pupil of the eye for the purpose of examination.

Atropine is commonly given as a *premedication* before general *anesthesia* to reduce secretions from the lungs and is also used as an emergency treatment for *bradycardia* (abnormally slow heartbeat).

Atropine is occasionally prescribed for its antispasmodic effects. It is sometimes combined with an *antidiarrheal drug* to relieve abdominal cramps accompanying diarrhea.

POSSIBLE ADVERSE EFFECTS
Adverse effects include dry mouth, blurred vision, abnormal retention of urine, and, in the elderly, confusion. Atropine eye drops are rarely given to adults because they cause disturbance of vision lasting two to three weeks and may precipitate acute *glaucoma* in a susceptible person.

Attachment

An affectionate bond between individuals, especially between parent and child (see *Bonding*), or between a person and an object, as in the case of a young child and a security object such as a blanket or a doll. The attachment gives emotional satisfaction. The term attachment is also used to note the joining of a muscle or tendon to a bone. In dentistry, it describes anything that attaches or stabilizes a partial denture.

Attending physician

A physician who has the primary responsibility for care of a patient in hospital (see *Intern; Resident physician*).

Audiogram

A graph produced as a result of certain *hearing tests* that shows the hearing threshold—that is, the minimum audible decibel level (loudness)—for each of a range of sound frequencies.

Audiology

The study of hearing, especially of impaired hearing that cannot be corrected by drugs or surgery. Audiologists can train people to overcome problems related to hearing loss, but cannot treat infection or disease.

Audiometry

Measurement of the sense of hearing. The term often refers to specific *hearing tests* in which a machine is used to produce sounds of a defined intensity (loudness) and frequency (pitch) and in which the hearing in each ear is measured over the full range of normally audible sounds.

Auditory nerve

Also called the acoustic nerve, the part of the *vestibulocochlear nerve* (the eighth *cranial nerve*) concerned with the sense of hearing.

Aura

A peculiar "warning" sensation that precedes or marks the onset of a *migraine* attack or of a seizure in a person suffering from *epilepsy*.

A migraine attack may be preceded by a feeling of elation, unusual well-being, excessive energy, or drowsiness. The sufferer comes to recognize these as warning signs of an attack. Thirst or a craving for sweet foods may develop. An attack of migraine may also be heralded by flashing lights seen before the eyes, blurred or tunnel vision, or difficulty in speaking. Weakness, numbness, or tingling of one half of the body may occur. As these symptoms subside, the migraine headache pain begins.

An epileptic aura may be a distorted perception, such as a hallucinatory sound or smell, or a sensation of movement in part of the body. One type of attack (in people with *temporal lobe epilepsy*) is often preceded by a vague feeling of discomfort in the upper abdomen, sometimes accompanied by borborygmi (rumbling, gurgling bowel sounds) and followed by a sensation of fullness in the head.

Auranofin

A *gold* preparation used as an *antirheumatic drug* in the treatment of *rheumatoid arthritis*. Auranofin, unlike other gold preparations, is effective when taken by mouth.

Auricle

Another name for the pinna, the external flap of the *ear*. The term was also once used as a synonym for *atrium* (one of the two upper chambers of the heart). Earlike appendages of the atria are still called auricles.

Auriscope

An instrument for examining the ear, also called an *otoscope*.

Auscultation

The procedure of listening to sounds within the body to assess the functioning of an organ or to detect the presence of disease. The sounds are heard through a stethoscope.

To listen to the heart, the physician places the stethoscope at four points on the chest, corresponding to the location of the heart valves. With the patient sitting up, in a semireclining position, or lying on his or her left side, the physician listens for any abnormality in the rate and rhythm of the heartbeat and for heart *murmurs* or other abnormal *heart sounds* that might indicate a heart defect.

When listening to the lungs, the physician places the stethoscope on many different areas of the front and back of the chest. The patient breathes normally and then takes deep breaths while the doctor compares the sounds of the air movement on the left and right sides. Abnormal breath sounds may indicate *pneumonia, bronchitis,* or *pneumothorax*. Additional sounds (called crepitations) that resemble crackling or bubbling are caused by fluid in the lungs. Wheezing sounds result from spasm of the airways, usually as a result of *asthma*. In *pleurisy*, a scratching sound can be heard, produced by inflamed areas of the lung rubbing together.

The physician may also test for vocal resonance by asking the patient to whisper something. The sound produced is louder if there is pus in the lung (e.g., as a result of pneumonia) because sound is transmitted better through an affected, pus-containing lung than through normal air-containing lung tissue.

Blood vessels near the skin surface (usually the carotid artery in the neck, the abdominal aorta, and the renal

PROCEDURE FOR AUSCULTATION

A physician's examination often includes auscultation—listening to sounds within the body using a stethoscope. Some organs make sounds during normal functioning.

Examples are the movement of fluid through the stomach and intestine, the opening and closing of heart valves, and the flow of air through the lungs and airways. However, the presence of abnormal sounds usually indicates disease of that tissue. The obstetrician listens to the baby's heartbeat as part of routine examination during pregnancy.

STETHOSCOPE

The heart
The stethoscope is usually placed at four places on the chest overlying the sites of the heart valves. The physician listens for the presence of murmurs, clicks, and extra heart sounds that may indicate disease of a heart valve.

Using a stethoscope
The end is held against the skin. The diaphragm picks up most noises, while the bell detects quiet, deep noises.

Carotid artery and abdominal aorta
The physician may listen to the flow of blood through a blood vessel that passes just beneath the skin. The presence of bruits (sounds of turbulence) usually indicates abnormal narrowing or widening of an artery.

The abdomen
The physician may listen to the abdomen for the sounds made by movement of fluid through the intestine. A disorder of the intestine may cause these sounds to be absent, abnormal, or very loud.

The lungs
The physician places the stethoscope over several different areas of the chest and back to listen to sounds made during breathing. The presence of crackles and dry or moist wheezes indicates various types of lung disease.

artery) may be listened to for bruits (sounds made by turbulent or abnormally fast blood circulation). Such sounds occur when blood vessels are narrowed (e.g., by fatty deposits in *atherosclerosis*) or widened (e.g., by an *aneurysm*), or when heart valves are narrowed or damaged (e.g., by *endocarditis*).

The abdomen is auscultated for borborygmi (loud rumbling, gurgling sounds made by the movement of air and fluid in the intestine) and for abnormal bowel sounds. The former may have no significance; the latter may indicate *intestinal obstruction*.

Autism

A condition in which a child is unable to relate to people and situations and may show an obsessive resistance to any change.

INCIDENCE

Nearly three times more boys than girls are affected by this rare disease, which seems more common among the higher social classes. Autism is by definition evident before the age of 30 months and is usually apparent within the first year of life.

CAUSES

The precise causes of autism are unknown, but evidence points to a physical basis. Because about one quarter of autistic children have signs of a neurological disorder and because epileptic seizures develop at adolescence in nearly one third of sufferers, it is likely that there is a subtle form of brain damage.

The earlier theory that lack of warmth from parents was a cause of autism is now rejected.

SYMPTOMS AND SIGNS

Often, autistic children are normal for the first few months of life before becoming increasingly unresponsive to parents or other stimuli. The first sign may be an inability to fix on the mother's face. Resistance to being cuddled may cause the child to scream to be put down when picked up.

The child remains aloof from parents and other people and fails to form relationships. He or she avoids eye-to-eye contact, has a preference for playing alone, and is often indifferent to the feelings of others and to social conventions.

Extreme resistance to change of any kind is an important feature. The child reacts with severe tantrums to alteration in routine or interference with activities. Rituals develop in play and often the child becomes attached to unusual objects or collections, or obsessed with one particular topic or idea. This wish for sterile "sameness" makes it very difficult to teach the autistic child new skills.

Delay in speaking is very common. The autistic child lacks the ability to understand or copy speech or gestures and responds to sounds inappropriately. Even when speech is acquired, it is immature, unimaginative, and has a robotlike sound. The child often makes up words.

There may be other behavioral abnormalities, such as walking on tiptoe, flicking or twiddling fingers for hours on end, rocking, self-injury, sudden screaming fits, and *hyperactivity*. Unusual fears and difficulty in learning manual tasks are also common in autistic children.

Despite all these bizarre symptoms, appearance and muscular coordination are normal. Some autistic children have an isolated special skill, such as an outstanding rote memory or musical ability.

TREATMENT

There is no known effective treatment. Special schooling, support and *counseling* for parents and families, and sometimes *behavior therapy* (e.g., to reduce violent self-injury) can be helpful. Medication is useful only for specific problems, such as *epilepsy*.

OUTLOOK

Outlook depends on intelligence and language ability. Only about one sixth of autistic children can lead any form of independent life; the majority need special, sometimes institutional, care.

Autoclave

An apparatus that produces steam at high pressure within a sealed chamber; the resulting high temperature of the water vapor destroys microorganisms. Autoclaving is used in hospitals as a means of sterilizing surgical equipment (see *Sterilization*).

Autoimmune disorders

Any of numerous disorders, including *rheumatoid arthritis*, insulin-dependent *diabetes mellitus*, and systemic *lupus erythematosus*, caused by a reaction of the individual's *immune system* against the organs or tissues of his or her own body.

The function of the immune system is to respond to invading microorganisms (for example, bacteria or viruses) by producing antibodies or sensitized lymphocytes (types of white blood cell) that will recognize and destroy the invaders. Autoimmune disorders occur when these reactions inexplicably take place against the body's own cells and tissues, producing a variety of disorders.

The disease-producing processes in autoimmunity are termed *hypersensitivity* reactions, of which there are several types. These reactions are similar to the reactions that occur in *allergy* except that in autoimmune disorders the hypersensitivity response is to the body itself rather than to an outside substance.

CAUSES

The immune system normally distinguishes "self" from "nonself." Some lymphocytes are capable of reacting against self, but these lymphocytes are generally suppressed. Autoimmune disorders occur when there is some interruption of the normal control process, allowing lymphocytes to escape from suppression, or when there is an alteration in some body tissue so that it is no longer recognized as "self" and is consequently attacked as if it were an invader.

The exact mechanisms causing these changes are not fully understood, but bacteria, viruses, and drugs may play a role in triggering an autoimmune process in someone who already has a genetic (inherited) predisposition. It is speculated that the usual inflammatory response of tissues to these agents somehow provokes an abnormal "sensitization" response to the tissues involved.

AUTOIMMUNE DISORDERS

Autoimmune disorders are a group of conditions in which the immune system attacks the body's own tissues as if they were foreign substances. The reasons why these disorders develop are unclear but genetic factors may play a role. Women are more often affected than men. An individual who has one autoimmune disorder may develop others.

An autoimmune disorder may primarily affect a specific organ or cell type, or may affect various organs. The following are examples of conditions that are, or are thought to be, autoimmune.

Specific (organs or cells affected)
Addison's disease (adrenal glands)
Autoimmune hemolytic anemia (red blood cells)
Autoimmune chronic active hepatitis (liver)
Autoimmune infertility (sperm or ovary)
Diabetes mellitus type 1 (pancreas)
Goodpasture's syndrome (lung and kidney)
Graves' disease (thyroid gland)
Hashimoto's thyroiditis (thyroid gland)
Idiopathic thrombocytopenic purpura (platelets)
Myasthenia gravis (muscle receptors)
Pernicious anemia (stomach lining)
Vitiligo (melanocytes)

Nonspecific
Behçet's syndrome
Rheumatoid arthritis
Sjögren's syndrome
Systemic lupus erythematosus

TYPES

Autoimmune processes can have various results—for example, slow destruction of a particular type of cell or tissue, stimulation of an organ into excessive growth, or interference in its function. Organs and tissues frequently affected by autoimmune processes include the endocrine glands (such as the thyroid, pancreas, and adrenal glands), components of the blood (such as the red blood cells), and the connective tissues, skin, muscles, and joints.

Specific autoimmune disorders are frequently classified into organ-specific and non-organ-specific types. In organ-specific disorders, the autoimmune process is directed mainly against one organ. Examples (with the organ affected) include *Hashimoto's thyroiditis* (thyroid gland), pernicious *anemia* (stomach), *Addison's disease* (adrenal glands), and insulin-dependent *diabetes mellitus* (pancreas).

In non-organ-specific disorders, autoimmune activity is widely spread throughout the body. Examples are systemic *lupus erythematosus* (SLE), *rheumatoid arthritis*, and *dermatomyositis*. Some autoimmune diseases fall between the two types. Sometimes, patients may experience several organ-specific or non-organ-specific diseases simultaneously. However, there is little overlap between the two ends of the spectrum.

TREATMENT

The first principle in treating any autoimmune disorder is to correct any major deficiencies. This may involve replacing hormones, such as thyroxin or insulin, that are not being produced by a gland. Alternatively, it may involve replacing components of the blood by transfusion.

The second principle is to diminish the activity of the immune system; this necessitates a delicate balance, controlling the disorder while maintaining the body's ability to fight disease in general. The drugs most commonly used are *corticosteroid drugs*. More severe cases can be treated with other more powerful *immunosuppressant drugs* such as cyclophosphamide, methotrexate, and azathioprine, but all of these drugs can damage rapidly dividing tissues, such as the bone marrow, and so are used with caution.

Drugs that act more specifically on the body's immune system (for example, by blocking a particular hypersensitivity reaction) are being researched and developed.

Automatism
A state in which behavior is not controlled by the conscious mind. The individual carries out movements and activities without being aware of doing so, and later has no clear memory of what happened. Episodes of automatism, which is uncommon, start abruptly and usually last a few seconds or minutes at the most.

Automatism may be the main symptom of *temporal lobe epilepsy*; this diagnosis can be confirmed by *EEG*. Other causes include *dissociative disorders, hysteria, alcohol intoxication, drug abuse,* and *hypoglycemia* (low blood sugar level).

Autonomic nervous system
The part of the *nervous system* that controls the involuntary, seemingly automatic, activities of organs, blood vessels, glands, and a variety of other tissues in the body. The autonomic nervous system consists of a network of nerves divided into two parts: the sympathetic nervous system and the parasympathetic nervous system.

In general, the sympathetic nervous system heightens activity in the body—quickening the heartbeat and breathing rate as if it were preparing the body for a *fight or flight response*. The parasympathetic system has the opposite effect.

The two systems act in conjunction and normally balance each other. However, during exercise or at times of stress or fear, the activity of the sympathetic system predominates, while during sleep the parasympathetic system exerts more control.

SYMPATHETIC NERVOUS SYSTEM
The sympathetic nervous system consists of two chains of nerves that pass from the spinal cord throughout the body to the organs and other structures they control. Into these tissues the nerve endings release the *neurotransmitter* chemicals *epinephrine* and *norepinephrine*. The sympathetic nervous system also stimulates the release of epinephrine from the adrenal glands into the bloodstream.

Among the most important effects produced by the neurotransmitters of the sympathetic nervous system are acceleration and strengthening of the heartbeat, widening of the airways, widening of the blood vessels in muscles, and narrowing of the blood vessels in the skin and abdominal organs (to increase blood flow through the muscles). In addition, the neurotransmitters decrease the activity of the digestive system, dilate the pupils of the eyes, and produce the contractions in the male urethra by which semen is ejaculated at orgasm.

PARASYMPATHETIC NERVOUS SYSTEM
The parasympathetic nervous system is composed of one chain of nerves that passes from the brain and another that leaves the lower spinal cord. The nerves are distributed to the same organs and structures that are supplied by the nerves of the sympathetic system. The parasympathetic nerves release the neurotransmitter *acetylcholine*, which has effects opposite to those produced by epinephrine and norepinephrine. The parasympathetic system also helps to produce and maintain erection of the penis.

EFFECT OF DRUGS
Certain disorders can be treated by giving drugs that affect the autonomic nervous system. *Anticholinergic drugs*, for example, block the effect of acetylcholine, which can reduce muscle spasms in the intestine. *Beta-blocker drugs* block the action of epinephrine and norepinephrine on the heart and thus slow the rate and force of its beat. (See box, p. 146.)

Autopsy
Postmortem examination of a body by a pathologist, usually soon after death. It always includes microscopic examination; sometimes biochemical and toxicologic analyses are done as well. Most autopsies are done in hospitals (with permission of the next of kin) to advance medical knowledge. If death was due to violence, was unexpected, was possibly due to malpractice, or was from an apparent cause for which the person was not under medical care, a coroner or medical examiner may order an autopsy. In some provinces death in an institution or jail must be investigated by autopsy.

Autosuggestion
Putting oneself into a receptive hypnotic-type state as a means of stimulating the body's ability to help itself. The idea that symptoms could be relieved merely through attitude was put forth by the Frenchman Emile Coué at the end of the 19th century. He observed that, if people accepted a physician's suggestion that a treatment would be effective, it was often enough to make it so. He thought that it might be possible for people to make suggestions to themselves with equally effective results.

As an aid to achieving the necessary relaxed state for successful autosuggestion, Coué advocated repetition of the catchphrase "Every day in every way, I am getting better and better." Although autosuggestion enjoyed only brief popularity, some techniques used today are based on its premise. For example, in one method used to control anxiety symptoms, people are taught muscular relaxation (*biofeedback*) techniques and then learn to summon up calming imagery or pleasant thoughts.

Aversion therapy
An outdated form of *behavior therapy* in which unpleasant stimuli, such as electric shocks, are applied to suppress unwanted behavior. It has been used to help treat self-injurious behavior in people who are mentally handicapped. Other forms of therapy are, in general, now considered to be more appropriate.

Aviation medicine
The medical speciality concerned with the physiological effects of flight and the causes and treatment of medical problems during air travel. Aviation medicine includes assessment of the fitness of aircrew and sometimes of passengers to fly, the management of medical emergencies in the air, the consequences of special types of flight (e.g., in helicopters, high-altitude aircraft and spacecraft), and the investigation of aircraft accidents.

EFFECTS OF REDUCED OXYGEN
Increasing altitude causes a fall in air pressure and with it a fall in the pressure of oxygen. *Hypoxia* (a seriously reduced oxygen concentration in the blood and tissues) is a serious threat to anyone who flies at altitude.

If aircraft cabins were not pressurized, the oxygen saturation of the blood would fall from nearly 100 percent on the ground to about 80 percent at 3,000 m. To avoid the development of hypoxia, airliners are kept at a pressure equivalent to an altitude of about 1,800 m during flight, although the cruising altitude may be as high as 12,000 m (even higher in Concorde). This means that the cabin pressure is about 30 percent less than at ground level but much higher than the outside pressure during flight. Any sudden failure of the aircraft's pressure hull leads to a rapid fall in cabin pressure, with a risk of hypoxia and *decompression sickness*. Rapid decompression in civil aircraft is extremely rare, but passengers and crew are provided with oxygen masks for use in emergencies while the aircraft descends to a safe altitude.

A

FUNCTIONS OF THE AUTONOMIC NERVOUS SYSTEM

The autonomic nervous system is responsible for controlling the involuntary body functions, such as sweating, digestion, and heart rate. The system affects smooth muscles, such as those of the airways and the intestine, rather than the striated muscles, which are under the body's voluntary control.

SYMPATHETIC SYSTEM

Dilates pupils

Inhibits salivation

Dilates bronchi

Accelerates heart rate

Inhibits gastric juice production

Inhibits digestive process

Relaxes bladder muscles

Contracts rectum

PARASYMPATHETIC SYSTEM

Contracts pupils

Stimulates salivation

Constricts bronchi

Slows heart rate

Stimulates gastric juice production

Speeds up digestive process

Contracts bladder muscles

Relaxes rectum

Medulla oblongata

Cranial nerves

Cervical nerves

Ganglia chain

Thoracic nerves

Lumbar nerves

Stimulates secretion of epinephrine and norepinephrine

Sacral nerves

Spinal cord

The autonomic nervous system

The autonomic nervous system is divided into two systems: the sympathetic nervous system and the parasympathetic nervous system. The sympathetic system is primarily concerned with preparing the body for action; it predominates at times of stress or excitement. The sympathetic system stimulates functions such as heart rate and sweating, and dilates the blood vessels to the muscles so that more blood is diverted to them. Simultaneously, it subdues the activity of the digestive system. In contrast, the parasympathetic nervous system is concerned mainly with the body's everyday functions such as digestion and the excretion of waste products; this system dominates during sleep. The parasympathetic system slows the heart rate and stimulates the organs of the digestive tract. Most of the time, activity is balanced between the two systems, with neither dominating. Both systems play an important part in sexual arousal and orgasm in both men and women.

ANXIETY AND HYPERVENTILATION

Hypoxia or, more commonly, anxiety during flight can lead to *hyperventilation* ("overbreathing"), in which increased breathing efforts result in excess loss of carbon dioxide. This alters the acidity of the body and gives rise to symptoms such as tingling around the mouth, muscle spasms, and light-headedness.

Quite often the symptoms of hyperventilation are themselves likely to increase anxiety.

Although flying can be an exhilarating experience, many people are anxious at some stage of a flight; others suffer an acute fear of flying and may need mild preflight sedation. If symptoms of hyperventilation develop, the treatment is to rebreathe air from a paper bag held over the nose and mouth, which reduces the loss of carbon dioxide.

DECOMPRESSION SICKNESS

Aviator's decompression sickness has the same causes as the condition that affects scuba divers and deep tunnel workers. It is not a risk for passengers on normal flights, except when there is a marked, rapid depressurization in the cabin or when a passenger has recently been exposed to pressure changes (usually through scuba diving, which is best avoided in the 24 hours before a flight).

PRESSURE EFFECTS ON BODY CAVITIES

The changes in altitude or cabin pressure during a flight affect the body's gas-containing cavities, principally the middle ears, facial sinuses, lungs, and intestines. When pressure drops during ascent, the volume of gas in these cavities increases; on descent, the gas volume decreases as pressure outside the body rises.

On ascent, unless there is a catastrophic fall in pressure, air from the lungs is harmlessly released via the trachea (windpipe), air in the large intestine and stomach can also escape freely (although trapped gas in the small intestine can give rise to a feeling of fullness), and air in the middle ears and sinuses can leave via ducts linking them to the back of the nose.

It is during descent that pressure changes in the ears and sinuses may fail to keep up with cabin repressurization. Unless preventive measures are taken, this may lead to pain and, rarely, damage (see *Barotrauma*).

ACCELERATION AND DECELERATION

The accelerative forces experienced by civil aircraft passengers are mild, even during takeoff and descent, and no precautions are necessary other than the wearing of a seat belt. Military aircraft pilots, on the other hand, may experience severe accelerations and must wear special suits and use a reclined seat to prevent pooling of blood in the feet, which would cause immediate loss of consciousness.

OTHER EFFECTS

Motion sickness is usually less of a problem for air than for road or sea travelers. Passengers prone to motion sickness may benefit from taking an antimotion sickness preparation.

Air travel allows the rapid crossing of several time zones within a short period, which can affect sleep-waking cycles, causing *jet lag*.

FITNESS TO FLY

Most aircraft passengers are well able to tolerate travel in the comfort of a pressurized cabin. Those with preexisting disorders, however, are advised to seek medical advice before undertaking a journey by air, especially if the condition is likely to be made worse by even the mild hypoxia induced at normal cabin pressures.

AVIATION MEDICINE SPECIALISTS

Most large airlines have a medical department staffed by physicians specially trained in aviation medicine, who are responsible for the health care of the airline staff. The physicians also give advice on the transportation of sick passengers, the provision of training and equipment to deal with illness during a flight, and the maintenance of airline hygiene.

Avitaminosis

Any condition that results from an insufficiency of one or more *vitamins*. Avitaminosis (also called hypovitaminosis) may be due to an inadequate dietary intake of vitamins, or a digestive disorder that causes *malabsorption* (impaired absorption of nutrients from the intestine).

Avulsed tooth

A tooth that has become completely dislodged from its socket as the result of an accident. The tooth should be carried to the dentist immediately in a glass of milk or cool water, or in a loosely wrapped, damp cloth. The dentist will reimplant the tooth into the socket as rapidly as possible, and immobilize it with a splint (see *Reimplantation, dental*). If the tooth is reimplanted within 30 minutes of the accident, and the patient is young, it will reattach itself to the socket in 90 percent of cases.

Avulsion

The tearing away of a body structure from its point of attachment.

Avulsion may be due to an injury—for example, when a severe ankle

CONDITIONS AFFECTING PASSENGER SUITABILITY FOR AIR TRAVEL

Conditions	Comments
Lung disease (such as chronic bronchitis or emphysema) Severe anemia Heart condition (such as angina pectoris, heart failure, or recent heart attack)	The lowered cabin pressure (and thus the oxygen level) at higher altitudes aggravates an already impaired ability to oxygenate the blood and/or tissues and may cause severe respiratory distress or collapse. Seek your physician's advice. Flying may be possible if you are able to walk 50 metres without breathlessness or chest pain.
Recent stroke	Seek your physician's advice. You may need to wait some weeks before flying.
Recent surgery to inner or middle ear, abdomen, chest, or brain; a recently collapsed lung or a fractured skull	Seek your physician's advice. You may need to wait before flying to avoid damage to your hearing mechanism from the expansion of gas trapped in the chest, abdomen, or skull.
Pregnancy	No flying after 34 to 36 weeks on most airlines.
Newborn baby	An infant should not fly until at least 48 hours old.
Psychiatric disorder	May need trained escort.
Infectious disease, terminal illness, or vomiting	May be refused entry to aircraft. Check with airline.

sprain stretches ligaments on the outside of the ankle, causing a small fragment of bone to be torn away from the fibula (outer lower leg bone).

Avulsion may also be performed deliberately as part of a surgical procedure. In the surgical treatment of *varicose veins*, for example, the stripping of veins from the leg is described as an avulsion.

Axilla
The medical name for the armpit.

Axon
The thin, elongated part of a *neuron* (nerve cell) that conducts nerve impulses. Many axons in the body are covered with a fatty *myelin* sheath.

Ayurvedism
See *Indian medicine*.

Azatadine
An *antihistamine drug* used in the treatment of *urticaria* (hives) and insect bites to relieve itching, swelling, and redness of the skin. Azatadine is also given to relieve nasal congestion and runny eyes which often occur with allergic *rhinitis* (hay fever).

Possible adverse effects include dry mouth and blurred vision. Azatadine has a strong sedative effect, so it may cause drowsiness.

Azathioprine

IMMUNOSUPPRESSANT

Tablet Injection

Prescription needed

An *immunosuppressant drug* used in the treatment of severe *rheumatoid arthritis* and other *autoimmune disorders* (disorders in which the *immune system* attacks the body's own tissues). Azathioprine is prescribed when other treatments (e.g., *corticosteroid drugs* and other *antirheumatic drugs*) fail to slow the progress of the disease or to improve symptoms. Azathioprine is also used to prevent organ rejection after *transplant surgery*.

HOW IT WORKS

Azathioprine reduces the efficiency of the body's immune system by preventing lymphocytes (types of white blood cells) from multiplying. Lymphocytes destroy foreign proteins (those not normally found in the body) and, in autoimmune disorders, attack body proteins that the immune system considers to be foreign.

POSSIBLE ADVERSE EFFECTS

Abnormal bleeding and increased susceptibility to infection may occur as a result of reduced blood cell production by the bone marrow; regular blood tests are carried out to monitor these effects.

Azoospermia
The absence of sperm from semen; an important cause of *infertility* in males. Azoospermia may be caused by a disorder present at birth or may develop later in life. The condition is thought to affect about one male in 100.

CAUSES

Congenital azoospermia may be the result of a chromosomal abnormality, such as *Klinefelter's syndrome* (the presence of an extra sex chromosome); failure of the testes to descend into the scrotum; absence of the vasa deferentia (the ducts that carry sperm from the testes to the seminal vesicles, the sacs where sperm is stored before ejaculation); or *cystic fibrosis*, a genetic disease affecting the lungs and pancreas that may also cause defects of the vasa deferentia. *Orchitis* caused by mumps may result in azoospermia or oligospermia (fewer than normal numbers of sperm).

In some males, azoospermia is due to puberty failing to take place, usually because the pituitary gland produces insufficient follicle-stimulating hormone (*FSH*), which is necessary for sperm production. In other males, puberty occurs but the testes fail to function properly. This disorder may also cause azoospermia.

The most common cause of azoospermia in later life is *vasectomy*, the sterilization operation in which the vasa deferentia are cut and tied off. Another cause is blockage of the ducts, which may follow a *sexually transmitted disease*, *tuberculosis*, or surgery on the groin (usually performed to repair a *hernia* or to lower undescended testes in a boy).

Azoospermia can also develop because of a temporary or permanent failure of the testes to produce sperm. This can follow *radiation therapy*, accidental radiation exposure, treatment with certain drugs (particularly *anticancer drugs* and the antidiarrheal drug *sulfasalazine*), and prolonged exposure to heat, insecticides, or industrial chemicals. In some cases, production of sperm ceases permanently for no known reason.

DIAGNOSIS

The diagnosis is made by analyzing at least two samples of semen, given a month apart, for the presence of sperm. Other tests are carried out to discover or confirm the cause. Blood samples are analyzed for evidence of chromosomal abnormalities or measured for levels of FSH. *Biopsy* analysis of cells from the testes will show whether or not sperm are being produced; absence of sperm from the semen when biopsy results are normal indicates blockage of the ducts.

TREATMENT AND OUTLOOK

Injections of FSH may cause puberty to develop, and surgery can sometimes unblock ducts closed by infection. Most other causes of azoospermia are untreatable and a sufferer who wishes to become a parent must do so by *artificial insemination* of his partner with donor sperm or must adopt a child.

AZT
The abbreviation for azidothymidine, the former name for *zidovudine*.

B

Babinski's sign

A reflex movement in which the big toe bends upward when the outer edge of the sole of the foot is scratched. In adults, Babinski's sign indicates damage or disease of the brain or the spinal cord. In babies, Babinski's sign is a normal reflex.

Baby blues

A common name for a mild form of depression that may occur after childbirth. Such depression almost always disappears without treatment, but can occasionally develop into a more serious depressive illness. (See *Postpartum depression*.)

Bacilli

Rod-shaped *bacteria*. Bacilli are responsible for many diseases, including tuberculosis, pertussis (whooping cough), tetanus, typhoid fever, and diphtheria (see *Infectious disease*).

Bacitracin

ANTIBIOTIC		
Powder Injection Ointment		

Ointment available over-the-counter

An *antibacterial drug* active against many of the bacteria that cause skin and eye infections. Bacitracin is often used in combination with other antibiotics, such as neomycin and polymyxin B. It is usually applied to the skin as a powder or ointment and to the eye in the form of an ointment. Because it is not absorbed into the bloodstream when taken by mouth, it is given by injection when used to treat a severe infection. Bacitracin may cause kidney damage, so it is generally used only for severe infections that have not responded to other antibiotics.

Back

The area between the shoulders and the buttocks. The back is supported by the spinal column (see *Spine*), which is bound together by ligaments and supported by muscles that also control posture and movement.

DISORDERS

Problems involving the back are numerous. They arise from a number of causes affecting the spine, and can involve disorders of bones, muscles, ligaments, tendons, nerves, and joints in the spine. These disorders can cause *back pain*. (See also *Spine* disorders box.)

Backbone

See *Spine*.

Back pain

Most people suffer from back pain at some time in their lives. In many cases, no exact diagnosis is made because the pain gets better with rest and because *analgesic drugs* (painkillers) are used before any tests, such as *X rays*, are performed. In such cases, physicians use the term "nonspecific back pain."

CAUSES

Nonspecific back pain is one of the largest single causes of working days lost through illness in Canada. People most likely to suffer from back pain are those whose jobs involve much heavy lifting and carrying, or those who spend long periods sitting in one position or bending awkwardly. Overweight people are also more prone to back pain—their backs carry a heavier load and they tend to have weaker abdominal muscles, which help provide back support.

Nonspecific back pain is thought to be due to a mechanical disorder affecting one or more structures in the back. The disorder may be the result of a ligament strain, a muscle tear, damage to a spinal facet joint, or prolapse of an intervertebral disk.

In addition to pain from a damaged structure, spasm of surrounding muscles will cause additional pain and tenderness over a wider area and can cause temporary *scoliosis* (abnormal sideways curvature of the spine).

Abnormalities of a facet joint and *disk prolapse* (slipped disk) can both cause *sciatica* (pain in the buttock and down the back of the leg into the foot), resulting from pressure on a sciatic nerve root as it leaves the spinal cord. Coughing, sneezing, or straining will increase the pain. Pressure on the sciatic nerve can also cause pins and needles in that leg, and weakness in muscles activated by the nerve. Rarely, pain may radiate down the femoral nerve at the front of the thigh.

Osteoarthritis in the joints of the spine can cause persistent back pain. *Ankylosing spondylitis* (an inflammatory disorder in which arthritis affects the spine) causes back pain and stiffness with loss of back mobility. *Coccygodynia* (pain and tenderness at the base of the spine) may occur after a fall in which the coccyx has struck the ground, during pregnancy, or spontaneously for unknown reasons.

Fibrositis is an imprecise term sometimes used to describe pain and tenderness in muscles. It may affect the back. Fibrositis is often worse in cold and damp weather and is occasionally associated with feeling unwell. Unlike other causes of back pain, fibrositis is not accompanied by muscle spasm or restriction of back movement. It often improves when treated with *nonsteroidal anti-inflammatory drugs*.

Pyelonephritis can cause back pain with pain and tenderness in the loin, fever, chills, and pain when passing urine. Cancer in the spine can cause persistent back pain that disturbs sleep and is not relieved by rest.

SELF-HELP

Back pain and sciatica may improve by resting on a firm mattress or board. Analgesic drugs and the application of heat to the back can help relieve pain. However, if pain persists, is very severe, or is associated with weakness in a leg or problems with bladder control, a physician should be consulted without delay.

INVESTIGATION

Examination of the back may show tenderness in specific areas and loss of mobility of the back. Weakness or loss of sensation in the legs implies pressure on a nerve root, which requires prompt investigation.

X rays of the spine may show narrowing between the intervertebral disks, osteoarthritis, *osteoporosis*, ankylosing spondylitis, compression fracture, stress fracture, *bone cancer*, or *spondylolisthesis* (displacement of vertebrae). X rays will not reveal ligament, muscle, facet joint, or disk damage. To reveal pressure on a nerve root (due to disk prolapse, for example), *myelography*, *CT scanning*, or *MRI* is performed.

TREATMENT

If a specific cause is found for back pain, treatment will be for that cause. Acute nonspecific back pain is treated with periods of rest and use of analgesic drugs. Chronic nonspecific back pain is more difficult to treat. Treatment may include *ASA* and related drugs, *nonsteroidal anti-inflammatory*

B

BACKACHE Pain and/or stiffness in the back that may be continuous or intermittent.

Of recent origin

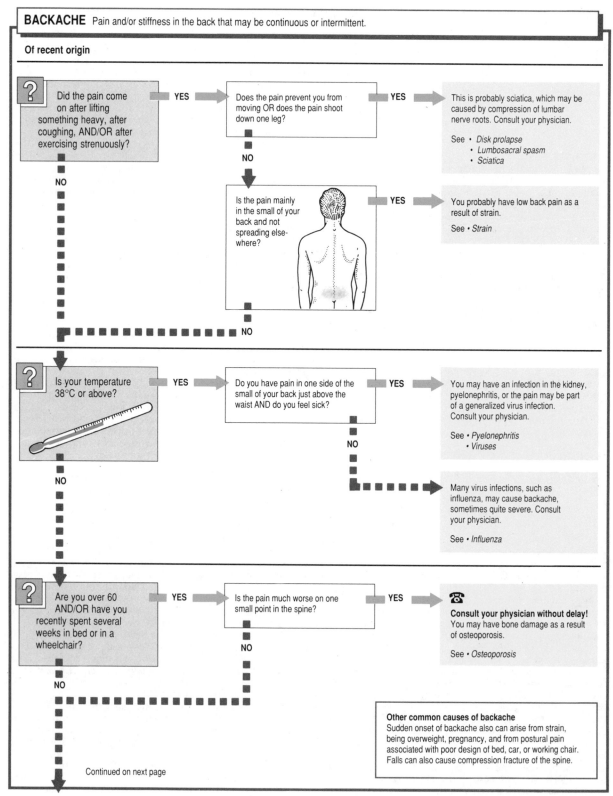

Did the pain come on after lifting something heavy, after coughing, AND/OR after exercising strenuously?

YES → Does the pain prevent you from moving OR does the pain shoot down one leg?

YES → This is probably sciatica, which may be caused by compression of lumbar nerve roots. Consult your physician.

See • Disk prolapse
• Lumbosacral spasm
• Sciatica

NO

Is the pain mainly in the small of your back and not spreading else-where?

YES → You probably have low back pain as a result of strain.

See • Strain

NO

NO

Is your temperature 38°C or above?

YES → Do you have pain in one side of the small of your back just above the waist AND do you feel sick?

YES → You may have an infection in the kidney, pyelonephritis, or the pain may be part of a generalized virus infection. Consult your physician.

See • Pyelonephritis
• Viruses

NO

Many virus infections, such as influenza, may cause backache, sometimes quite severe. Consult your physician.

See • Influenza

NO

Are you over 60 AND/OR have you recently spent several weeks in bed or in a wheelchair?

YES → Is the pain much worse on one small point in the spine?

YES → ☎

Consult your physician without delay!
You may have bone damage as a result of osteoporosis.

See • Osteoporosis

NO

NO

Other common causes of backache
Sudden onset of backache also can arise from strain, being overweight, pregnancy, and from postural pain associated with poor design of bed, car, or working chair. Falls can also cause compression fracture of the spine.

Continued on next page

B

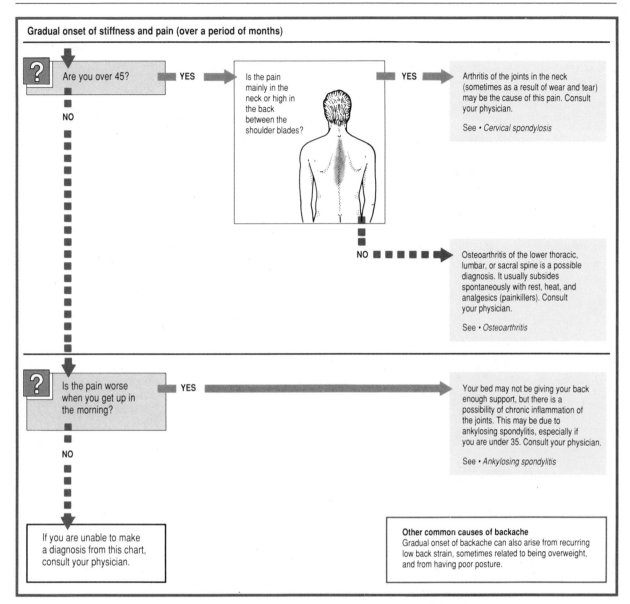

Gradual onset of stiffness and pain (over a period of months)

? Are you over 45? → **YES** →

Is the pain mainly in the neck or high in the back between the shoulder blades? → **YES** →

Arthritis of the joints in the neck (sometimes as a result of wear and tear) may be the cause of this pain. Consult your physician.

See • *Cervical spondylosis*

NO

NO →

Osteoarthritis of the lower thoracic, lumbar, or sacral spine is a possible diagnosis. It usually subsides spontaneously with rest, heat, and analgesics (painkillers). Consult your physician.

See • *Osteoarthritis*

? Is the pain worse when you get up in the morning? → **YES** →

Your bed may not be giving your back enough support, but there is a possibility of chronic inflammation of the joints. This may be due to ankylosing spondylitis, especially if you are under 35. Consult your physician.

See • *Ankylosing spondylitis*

NO

If you are unable to make a diagnosis from this chart, consult your physician.

Other common causes of backache
Gradual onset of backache can also arise from recurring low back strain, sometimes related to being overweight, and from having poor posture.

---

drugs, or *muscle-relaxant drugs*; *acupuncture* or spinal injection; or exercise, spinal *manipulation*, wearing a surgical *corset*, or spinal surgery.

Baclofen

MUSCLE RELAXANT

Tablet   Liquid

Prescription needed

A *muscle relaxant drug* that blocks nerve activity in the spinal cord. Baclofen relieves muscle spasm and stiffness that have been caused by injury to the brain or spinal cord, by a *stroke*, or by neurological disorders such as *multiple sclerosis*. Baclofen does not cure the underlying disorder but often allows *physiotherapy* to be more effective, and makes walking and performing tasks with the hands easier.

To reduce the risk of adverse effects, such as drowsiness and muscle weakness, the dose of the drug is usually increased slowly under medical supervision until the desired effect is achieved. People age 60 and over have an increased likelihood of adverse effects, such as confusion.

Bacteremia

The presence of bacteria in the bloodstream. Bacteremia occurs for a few hours after many minor surgical operations and may also occur with infections such as tonsillitis.

In people with abnormal heart valves, due to a congenital defect or to scarring from previous rheumatic fever, the bacteria may cause *endocarditis* (inflammation of the heart lining and valves). If bacteremia affects a person whose *immune system* has been weakened by illness or a major surgical operation, *septicemia* and *septic shock* may follow.

BACK PAIN

Most people experience back pain some time in their lives, but in most cases it is not serious and the problem corrects itself before investigation takes place. However, some kinds of back pain can be related to a specific disorder. In the diagram below, you will find the most common sites affected by back pain.

Osteoarthritis
Pain and stiffness in the back due to degeneration of the joints between the vertebrae in one (or more) of the cervical, thoracic, or lumbosacral regions.

Fibrositis
Pain and tenderness in the larger back muscles.

Nonspecific back pain
Pain that commonly affects the lower back but may occur in other parts due to ligament, muscle, joint, or disk damage.

Pyelonephritis
Pain in the loin due to infection of the kidney.

Sciatica
Pain in the buttock and down the back of the leg into the foot due to pressure on a nerve.

Coccygodynia
Pain and tenderness at the base of the spine, sometimes after a fall.

REDUCING STRAIN ON THE BACK

Don't push a heavy object in front with straight arms; this puts strain on the back.

Do push backward; the strain is taken by the legs instead.

Don't slouch; the lower back is pushed out at an angle, resulting in strain.

Do sit up straight, with the spine resting against the chair back.

Don't lift with straight legs and curved back; this puts strain on the lower back.

Do lift with the back straight and knees bent, which transfers strain to the legs.

Bacteria

A group of single-celled *microorganisms*, some of which cause disease. Commonly known as "germs," bacteria have been recognized as a cause of disease for over a century, but it is still not fully understood why some people become ill while others remain well when exposed to the same sources of infection. Abundant in the air, soil, and water, most bacteria are harmless to humans. Some, indeed, are beneficial, such as those that live in the intestine and help break down food for digestion. Bacteria that cause disease are known as pathogens.

Bacteria were discovered by Antonj van Leewenhoek in the 17th century following development of the microscope, but it was not until the mid-19th century that the French scientist Louis Pasteur established beyond doubt that they were the cause of many diseases.

TYPES
Pathogenic (disease-producing) bacteria are classified, on the basis of shape, into three main groups: cocci (spherical); bacilli (rod-shaped); and spirochetes or spirilla (spiral-shaped).

Among the wide range of diseases caused by cocci are pneumonia, tonsillitis, bacterial endocarditis, meningitis, toxic shock syndrome, and various skin disorders.

Diseases caused by bacilli include tuberculosis, pertussis (whooping cough), tetanus, typhoid fever, diphtheria, salmonellosis, shigellosis (bacillary dysentery), Legionnaires' disease, and botulism.

Bacteria from the third, and smallest group, the spirochetes, are responsible for syphilis, yaws, leptospirosis, and Lyme disease.

GROWTH, MOVEMENT, REPRODUCTION
The bacteria that colonize the human body thrive in warm, moist condi-

tions. Some are aerobic—that is, they require oxygen to grow and multiply—and so they are most commonly found on the skin or in the respiratory system. Anaerobic bacteria thrive where there is no oxygen—deep within tissue or wounds.

Many bacteria are naturally static and, if they move around the body, do so only in currents of air or fluid. Some, however, such as salmonella (responsible for food poisoning and typhoid) are highly motile, moving through fluid by lashing with their flagella (whiplike, filamentous tails).

Bacteria reproduce by dividing into two cells, which in turn divide, and so on. Under ideal conditions (exactly the right temperature and sufficient nourishment for all cells), this division can take place every 20 minutes, an extremely rapid rate of reproduction. After only six hours, a single bacterium can have multiplied to form a colony of more than 250,000 bacteria. This seldom happens, however, because ideal conditions rarely occur and in a healthy individual the *immune system* destroys invading bacteria.

As well as dividing, some types of bacteria—such as clostridia (responsible for botulism, tetanus, pseudomembranous colitis, and anthrax)—multiply in a more restricted way, by each producing a spore. A spore is a single new bacterium, protected by a tough membrane, that can survive high temperatures, dry conditions, and lack of nourishment.

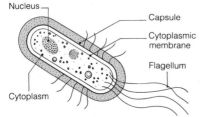

Magnified bacterium
A typical bacterial cell enlarged to approximately 20,000 times its normal size.

Staphylococcus
(causes boils)

Streptococcus
(causes sore throat)

Salmonella typhosa
(causes typhoid fever)

Spirochaeta
(causes syphilis)

Common types of bacteria

HOW BACTERIA ENTER THE BODY
Bacteria can enter through the lungs if droplets breathed, coughed, or sneezed out by an infected person are inhaled. Diseases caught thus include diphtheria, and pertussis.

The digestive tract can become infected if contaminated food is eaten. Bacteria may be present in food at its primary source, or brought to it by flies or by people preparing it with contaminated hands.

Microorganisms that enter the genitourinary system include those causing sexually transmitted diseases (e.g., syphilis, pelvic inflammatory disease, and gonorrhea).

Bacteria can penetrate the skin in various ways: through hair follicles (which may cause boils); through superficial wounds, such as cuts or abrasions (which may lead to erysipelas); or through deep wounds (as in the case of tetanus).

HOW BACTERIA CAUSE DISEASE
Bacteria produce poisons that are harmful to human cells. If they are present in sufficient quantity and the affected person is not immune to them, disease results. Some bacteria release poisons known as endotoxins, which can cause fever, hemorrhage, and shock. Others produce exotoxins, which account for the major damage in diseases such as diphtheria, tetanus, and toxic shock syndrome.

RESISTANCE BY THE BODY
The body's first means of preventing invasion by harmful bacteria are the substances hostile to bacteria in the skin, lining of the respiratory tract, digestive tract, and genitourinary system. The eyes are protected by an enzyme in the tears, and the stomach secretes hydrochloric acid, which kills many of the bacteria found in food and water.

If the bacteria break through these defenses, two types of white blood cell attack them: neutrophils engulf and destroy many of the bacteria, and lymphocytes produce antibodies against them. The antibodies attack the bacteria directly. After an infection, antibodies remain in the blood for a considerable time—many years in the case of typhoid and scarlet fever—so that any further attacks of the disease are usually prevented or are mild.

TREATMENT OF BACTERIAL DISEASE
The response of the immune system to bacterial illness is sometimes enough by itself to bring about recovery, but in many cases medical treatment is necessary. The main form of

treatment is *antibiotic drugs*, given either by mouth or by injection. Some, such as penicillin, are bactericidal (destroy the invading bacteria); others, such as tetracycline, are bacteriostatic (prevent them from multiplying further), permitting the immune system to overcome the invaders.

Some diseases—among them diphtheria, tetanus, botulism, and gas gangrene—are treated by the injection of an antiserum. This is a fluid taken from the blood of a person or a horse who has been given a series of immunizing injections and whose blood therefore contains antibodies against the disease organisms.

Superficial inflammation and infected wounds may be treated with antiseptic solutions.

PREVENTION
Immunity to certain bacterial diseases (for example, diphtheria, typhoid, pertussis and tetanus) can be acquired by active *immunization* (injection with weakened or killed forms of the bacteria or their poisons).

People with infections should take steps to prevent their spread; those with respiratory infections should keep away from crowded places to prevent the possibility of droplet infection, and should always use a handkerchief when coughing or sneezing. Food handlers should be meticulous about their health and personal hygiene.

Any wound should be washed with an antiseptic solution to destroy bacteria, and then covered with a clean, dry dressing. (See also *Infectious disease*.)

Bactericidal
A term used to describe any substance that kills bacteria. (See *Antibacterial drugs*; *Antibiotic drugs*.)

Bacteriology
The study of *bacteria*, particularly of the types that cause disease. The pioneer of this science was the French scientist Louis Pasteur (1822-1895), who was the first to prove that bacteria are the cause and not the result of illness. He was followed by the German physician Robert Koch (1843-1910), who not only discovered a large number of the bacteria responsible for particular diseases but also laid down the principles for isolating and identifying disease-producing bacteria on which modern bacteriology is based.

METHODS OF IDENTIFYING BACTERIA
To discover which bacterium is causing a disease, it must be isolated. A throat swab or a specimen of urine,

CULTURING AND TESTING BACTERIA

1 The bacteria are introduced onto a nutrient plate (i.e., agar or blood agar) and incubated at body temperature.

2 Any bacteria present multiply rapidly to form visible colonies that can be studied under the microscope and identified by different patterns of growth.

3 To test sensitivity to specific antibiotics, disks of different antibiotics are placed within the colonies of bacteria.

4 Any clear areas around each disk indicate that the bacteria are being killed by a particular antibiotic.

feces, blood, spinal fluid, sputum, or pus is first taken from an infected person. This material is then examined by one of three main methods.

STAINING The application of special stains makes it possible to look at and differentiate bacteria under the microscope. In a sample treated with Gram's stain, for example, staphylococci or streptococci bacteria turn purple, whereas many other types, such as salmonella, turn red.

CULTURE For this method of examination, the sample material is introduced into a nutrient, where the bacteria multiply and can be identified by their appearance and growth requirements. Different antibiotics are introduced and their effects studied to see which will be effective in treating the infection (see box).

ANTIBODY TESTING This is done by extracting serum from the blood of an infected person and adding it to a sample of the type of bacteria suspected of causing the infection. If the suspicion is correct, antibodies against the bacteria already present in the serum will visibly clump together with the bacteria in the sample.

Bacteriostatic

A term used to describe a substance that stops the growth or multiplication of bacteria. (See *Antibacterial drugs; Antibiotic drugs*.)

Bacteriuria

The presence of *bacteria* in the urine. A small, harmless number of bacteria may be found in the urine of many healthy people, so bacteriuria is of significance only if more than 100,000 bacteria are present in each millilitre of urine, or if 100 white blood cells (pus cells) per millilitre are present.

Bad breath

See *Halitosis*.

Bagassosis

An occupational disease affecting the lungs of workers who handle moldy bagasse (the fibrous residue of sugarcane after the juice has been extracted). Bagassosis is one cause of allergic *alveolitis*, a reaction of the lungs to inhaled dust that contains fungal spores.

Acute attacks usually develop four to five hours after inhalation of dust. The symptoms may include shortness of breath associated with wheezing, fever, headache, and cough; typically they last no more than 24 hours. Repeated exposure to dust may lead

to permanent lung damage, chronic sickness, and weight loss. Protective measures taken by industry have now made the disease rare.

Baker's cyst

A firm, walnut-sized, fluid-filled lump behind the knee. A Baker's cyst is caused by increased pressure within the knee joint due to a buildup of fluid in a disorder such as *rheumatoid arthritis*. The cyst is created by a backward "ballooning out" of the synovial membrane covering the knee joint.

Most Baker's cysts are painless. Some disappear spontaneously, perhaps after many months. Occasionally, a cyst may rupture, causing fluid to seep down between the layers of the calf muscles. A ruptured cyst may produce pain and swelling.

Diagnosis may be assisted by *arthrography* (imaging of the joint with X rays after injection of a radiopaque substance). Treatment may consist simply of a supportive bandage. In some cases, surgical removal of the cyst is required.

Balance

The ability to remain upright and move without falling over. Keeping one's balance is a complex process that relies on a constant flow of information about body position to the brain. Integration of this information and a continual flow of instructions from the brain enable various parts of the body to perform the changes needed to maintain balance.

Information about body position comes from three sources: the eyes, which give visual information about the body's position relative to its surroundings; sensory receptors (called proprioceptors) in the skin, muscles, and joints, which provide information about the position and movement of the different parts of the body; and the three semicircular canals of the labyrinth in the inner ear, which detect the direction and speed of head movements. The part of the brain called the cerebellum collates this information and instructs muscles to contract or relax to maintain balance.

DISORDERS

Various disorders can affect balance, particularly disorders of the inner ear, such as *labyrinthitis* (inflammation of the labyrinth of the ear) and *Meniere's disease* (abnormally high pressure of fluid in the labyrinth). In some cases, *otitis media* (inflammation of the middle ear) may also affect the inner ear and disturb the patient's balance.

In addition to loss of balance, these disorders often cause *dizziness* or *vertigo*, and impaired hearing.

Damage to nerve tracts in the spinal cord, which carry information from proprioceptors, may occur as a result of spinal tumors, disorders of the circulation, nerve degeneration due to deficiency of vitamin B_{12}, or, rarely, tabes dorsalis (a complication of *syphilis*). These disorders produce a distinctive, wide-based, clumsy gait.

A tumor or stroke that affects the cerebellum may cause not only clumsiness of the arms and legs, but also speech disorders and other features of impaired muscular coordination.

Balanitis

Inflammation of the glans (head) of the penis and foreskin. The main symptom is a painful or itchy penis, and the entire area may be red and moist. Causes include infection with bacteria or fungi, *phimosis* (tight foreskin), or irritation by chemicals in clothing or contraceptive cream. Infection may be the result of poor hygiene, but fungal infections such as *candidiasis* (thrush) are usually contracted from a sexual partner.

Washing the penis (including under the foreskin), applying a soothing cream (your physician will recommend one), and taking a course of *antibiotic drugs* will relieve the symptoms. If balanitis recurs frequently, or if the cause is phimosis, *circumcision* (removal of the foreskin) may be recommended.

Baldness

See *Alopecia*.

Balloon catheter

A flexible tube with a balloon at its tip, which, when inflated, keeps the tube in place or applies pressure to an organ or vessel.

USES

The oldest and simplest type, the Foley catheter, is used to drain urine from the bladder. This catheter is passed into the bladder and sterile water is then pumped into one channel to inflate the balloon, which prevents the catheter from dropping out. Urine flows out of the bladder through a second channel.

Balloon catheters are sometimes used when a blood vessel has been blocked by a blood clot. The end of the catheter is passed through the clot, the balloon is inflated, and, when the catheter is withdrawn, the balloon pulls the clot out with it. This procedure is called balloon *embolectomy*.

TYPES OF BALLOON CATHETER

- Irrigation tube for fluid to wash out bladder
- Sterile water tube
- Tube to drain urine from bladder

Embolectomy catheter

Inflatable balloon

Urinary catheter

A type of balloon catheter with a sausage-shaped balloon is used to expand narrowed arteries. Maneuvered to the narrowest section, it is inflated and deflated a few times. In many cases this technique, known as balloon *angioplasty*, avoids the need for surgery, although narrowing of the vessel may recur.

Another use of the balloon catheter is to treat bleeding *esophageal varices* (widened veins in the lower part of the esophagus), a life-threatening complication of some kinds of liver disease. The tube is passed down the esophagus and into the stomach, where a balloon at the tip keeps the tube in position. Another balloon higher up the tube is inflated to compress the vein walls; this usually stops or controls the bleeding until the patient can be prepared for surgery.

Another type of balloon can be placed by a narrow catheter into a blood vessel, inflated with a quick-setting durable material, detached, and left in permanent position, thereby completely shutting off blood flow in that vessel. These catheters are used to control bleeding or to starve a tumor of its blood supply.

Balm

A soothing or healing medicine applied to the skin.

Bandage

A strip or tube of fabric used to keep *dressings* in position, to apply pressure, to control bleeding, or to support a sprain or strain.

Roller bandages are the traditional type and are still the most widely used. Tubular gauze bandages are a newer type that are in many ways quicker and easier to apply than roller bandages. They are, however, more expensive than roller bandages and require a special applicator. Tubular gauze bandages are mainly used for small cuts, grazes, and burns on parts of the body that are awkward to bandage, such as a finger. Triangular bandages are used to make *slings* to support limbs. (See also *Wounds*.)

Barbiturate drugs

COMMON DRUGS

Amobarbital Pentobarbital
Phenobarbital Secobarbital
Thiopental

WARNING

Barbiturates may be habit forming; if taken with large amounts of alcohol, they may cause death.

A group of *sedative drugs* that work by depressing activity within the brain. Barbiturates were formerly in wide use as *antianxiety drugs*, *sleeping drugs*, and *anticonvulsant drugs*. Today, their use is strictly controlled because they are habit-forming and widely abused. An overdose can be fatal.

WHY THEY ARE USED

Phenobarbital is still often used as an anticonvulsant drug in the treatment of *epilepsy*, and thiopental remains a drug of choice for inducing anesthesia (see *Anesthesia, general*). However, *benzodiazepine drugs* and other non-barbiturate drugs have now largely replaced barbiturates in the treatment of sleeplessness and anxiety. Barbiturates which are occasionally used today to induce sleep include amobarbital, pentobarbital, and secobarbital.

HOW THEY WORK

The sedative action of barbiturate drugs is produced by the drug molecules blocking the conduction of stimulatory chemical signals between nerve cells in the brain and reducing the ability of the cells to respond.

Barbiturates, especially phenobarbital, also reduce the sensitivity of brain cells to abnormal electrical activity. This action is beneficial in the treatment of epilepsy because it reduces the likelihood of seizures.

B

FIRST AID: APPLYING BANDAGES

TUBULAR BANDAGE

1 Cut a length of tube gauze about two and a half times the length of the finger and put it all onto the applicator. Push the applicator over the finger and hold on to the end of the gauze.

2 Still holding the gauze end on the finger, gently pull back the applicator, leaving the tube of gauze in position. Then twist it once or twice, but not more, or you may impair circulation.

3 Push the applicator back onto the finger; again, hold onto the two gauze ends, then pull it off again leaving two layers in position. Secure the ends of the gauze with tape.

ROLLER BANDAGE

1 Place the end of the bandage on the arm and hold it firmly while you make a straight turn with the rolled end to secure it.

2 Work up the limb, making a series of spiral turns so that each successive turn covers two thirds of the previous one.

3 Complete the bandaging with a straight turn, cut off the spare bandage roll, and secure the end with a safety pin, adhesive tape, or bandage clip.

Bandaging equipment
Shown (from left) are crepe roller bandages, a bandage clip, gauze roller bandages, safety pins, a tubular bandage applicator, a roll of tubular bandage, and a triangular bandage.

POSSIBLE ADVERSE EFFECTS

Adverse effects include excessive drowsiness, staggering gait, and, in some cases among the very young and old, excitability. The depressant effect of barbiturates on the brain (including suppression of the respiratory center) is dangerously increased by alcohol.

Barbiturates are likely to produce *drug dependence* if used for longer than a few weeks; withdrawal effects (which may include sleeplessness, twitching, nightmares, and convulsions) may occur when regular treatment is suddenly stopped. Tolerance, in which increasingly large doses are needed to produce the same effect, often develops.

Barium X-ray examinations

A group of procedures used to detect and follow the progress of some diseases of the gastrointestinal tract. Powdered barium sulfate mixed with water is passed into the part of the tract that needs to be examined and X-ray pictures of the area are taken. Because barium, a metallic element, is opaque to X rays, it provides an image of the tract on the X-ray film.

WHY THEY ARE DONE
Barium X rays are among the studies used to diagnose the cause of swallowing difficulty, abdominal pain, bloodstained vomit, bleeding from the rectum, a change in bowel habits, persistent diarrhea or constipation, and unexplained weight loss.

Disorders that can be detected by barium X rays include narrowing or inflammation of the esophagus, disorders of the swallowing mechanism, hiatal hernia, stomach and duodenal ulcers and tumors, inflammatory bowel disease, diverticular disease, Crohn's disease, celiac disease, and tumors or polyps in the colon. In many instances, barium X rays have been replaced or supplemented by *endoscopy.*

HOW THEY ARE DONE
Barium X-ray examinations are generally carried out on an outpatient basis. No anesthetic is required. A fluorescent screen connected to the X-ray machine enables the radiologist to follow the progress of the barium through the gastrointestinal tract, and to see any abnormalities outlined by the barium. Permanent records of the examination are provided by X-ray photographs or video recordings.

Because barium sulfate liquid dries out as its water content is absorbed in the colon, it often causes constipation. Patients may therefore need a fiber-rich diet, should drink plenty of fluids and, in some cases, may need laxatives to get rid of the chemical.

TYPES OF EXAMINATION

Different types of barium X-ray examination are used to investigate the gastrointestinal tract.

BARIUM SWALLOW, BARIUM MEAL, BARIUM FOLLOW-THROUGH These are used to investigate disorders of the upper gastrointestinal tract: barium swallow for the esophagus, barium meal for the lower esophagus, stomach, and duodenum, and barium follow-through for the small intestine.

In a barium swallow examination, the patient usually takes in enough air with the barium to facilitate double-contrast imaging. If a double-contrast barium meal examination is required, it is necessary to give carbonated barium, usually with gas-producing tablets or granules. Double-contrast imaging is usually not possible for a follow-through examination because it is too difficult to introduce air into the small intestine.

BARIUM X-RAY PROCEDURES

BARIUM SWALLOW, MEAL, AND INTESTINAL FOLLOW-THROUGH

1 No food or drink is permitted for six to nine hours beforehand

2 At the examination, the patient swallows a glass of barium mixed with a flavored liquid, or is given a piece of bread or a biscuit soaked in barium if a disorder of the swallowing mechanism is being investigated.

3 The X-ray technician then takes X-ray pictures. For a barium swallow, the patient stands; for a barium meal, the patient lies on the table in different positions; for a barium follow-through, the patient lies on the right side and X rays are taken at intervals until the barium has progressed through the small intestine.

BARIUM SMALL-BOWEL ENEMA

1 No food or drink is permitted for nine hours beforehand.

2 At the examination, the patient lies down and the radiologist passes a fine tube through the mouth or nose, down through the stomach and duodenum, and into the small intestine.

3 Barium is then passed down the tube directly into the small intestine.

BARIUM ENEMA

1 For successful examination, the large intestine needs to be as empty and clean as possible, since feces can obscure or simulate a polyp or tumor. For this reason the patient's intake of food and fluids is sometimes restricted for a few days before the examination, and laxatives are given.

2 The patient lies facedown on the X-ray table.

3 The radiologist introduces barium into the intestine through a tube inserted into the rectum.

X-RAY TECHNIQUES
There are two different techniques.

Double-contrast technique
Air, as well as barium liquid, is introduced into the tract. As a result, the barium does not fill the tract but forms only a film on its inner surface. This provides an image of small, surface abnormalities that would not be visible using the single-contrast technique.

Single-contrast technique
The section of intestine is filled with barium liquid, which provides an outline image that shows up prominent abnormalities.

Barium swallow and meal take about 10 minutes to perform; follow-through may last up to five hours.

BARIUM SMALL-BOWEL ENEMA Also called enteroclysis, this single-contrast X-ray technique provides a more detailed examination of the small intestine than the barium follow-through because more barium reaches the area. Sedation may be necessary because the procedure, which takes 20 to 25 minutes, can cause discomfort.

BARIUM ENEMA This technique is used to investigate disorders of the lower gastrointestinal tract: the large intestine and rectum. For a single-contrast image, the large intestine is filled with diluted barium liquid. For a double-contrast examination, a smaller quantity of more concentrated barium liquid is introduced, followed by air. The whole procedure lasts about 20 minutes, and in most cases causes only mild discomfort.

After the examination, a small amount of barium is expelled from the body immediately, and the rest is excreted later in the feces.

Barotrauma

Damage or pain, mainly affecting the middle *ear* and facial *sinuses*, caused by the effects of a change in surrounding air pressure. Air travelers are by far the largest group at risk, but scuba divers also face similar problems (see *Scuba-diving medicine*).

CAUSE

When an aircraft ascends to cruising height, cabin pressure is usually reduced by about one third (to a pressure equivalent to an altitude of about 1,800 m). A "popping" sensation may be felt as air, trapped at ground-level pressure in the middle ears and facial sinuses, escapes via the eustachian tubes and sinus ducts (which, respectively, link the middle ears and sinuses to air passages at the back of the throat).

When the aircraft descends, cabin pressure is increased again and becomes greater than the pressure within the ears and sinuses. Some pain may be felt as the eardrum is pushed inward. To ease this, air needs to be reintroduced into the middle ears and sinuses to equalize the internal and external pressures. This "ear clearing" can be achieved by vigorous swallowing or by forcibly breathing out with the mouth closed and the nose pinched (the Valsalva maneuver).

If the sinus ducts or eustachian tubes are blocked with mucus, as com-

Increased air pressure

Eardrum bulging inward

Reduced air pressure

Blocked eustachian tube

Mechanism of barotrauma
The diagram above shows the location of the middle ear, and pressure changes when the eustachian tube is blocked and there is an increase in surrounding air pressure.

monly occurs during a head cold, equalizing pressure by using the ear-clearing methods described above may be difficult or impossible. Minor damage can occur if pressure equalization is prevented or delayed, or if the Valsalva maneuver is carried out over-enthusiastically. The damage usually involves rupture of tiny blood vessels in the walls of the middle ears, or in the membranes lining the inside of the sinuses.

Changes in pressure sufficient to rupture the eardrum are unlikely to occur during ordinary commercial flights but rupture may be suffered by scuba divers or high altitude pilots (see *Eardrum, perforated*).

PREVENTION

Anyone with a severe head cold should avoid flying if possible. If flying is unavoidable, a nasal spray containing a *decongestant drug* should be used shortly before aircraft descent. Air travelers should also know how to perform the Valsalva maneuver. Infants should be breast- or bottle-fed during descent; the baby's sucking and swallowing has the same effect as the Valsalva maneuver.

SYMPTOMS

Pain in the ears, or over the cheekbones and forehead, during aircraft descent is a warning of pressure differences. Minor pressure damage in the middle ear, called barotraumatic otitis, may cause continued pain, some hearing loss, and *tinnitus* (ring-

ing in the ears) for a few days; pressure damage within the facial sinuses, called barotraumatic sinusitis, may also cause pain, and possibly a discharge of mucus or blood.

TREATMENT

In most cases, no treatment is necessary and symptoms wear off within hours or a couple of days. However, if an infection is present, these symptoms may become worse and persist for several days. If sinus pain persists or a discharge from the nose is noticed, symptoms that suggest infection, medical advice should be sought. Treatment may be required. (See also *Aviation medicine*.)

Barrier cream

A cream used to protect the skin against the effects of irritant substances and of excessive exposure to water. (See also *Sunscreens*.)

Barrier method

A method of preventing pregnancy by blocking the passage of sperm to the uterus, for example, by using a condom or a diaphragm. (See *Contraception, barrier methods of*.)

Barrier nursing

The nursing technique by which a patient with an infectious disease is prevented from infecting others (see *Isolation*).

Bartholin's glands

A pair of oval, pea-sized glands whose ducts open into the vulva (the folds of flesh that surround the opening of the vagina). During sexual arousal these glands secrete a fluid that helps to lubricate the vulval region.

DISORDERS

Infection of Bartholin's glands causes bartholinitis, in which an intensely

BARTHOLIN'S GLANDS
These glands are located on each side of the entrance to the vagina.

Vagina

Vulva

Bartholin's glands

Anus

painful red swelling forms at the opening of the ducts. Treatment is with *antibiotic drugs, analgesic drugs* (painkillers), and warm baths.

If infection produces an *abscess*, the affected gland is cut open and drained, usually under general anesthesia. Should abscesses recur, an operation may be performed, either to convert the duct into an open pouch (see *Marsupialization*), or to remove the gland completely.

If an infection narrows the duct by scarring, the gland may not be capable of emptying, and a Bartholin's cyst, a painless swelling of the duct, may form. The cyst may become repeatedly infected, in which case marsupialization or removal of the gland is needed. Even if both the Bartholin's glands are removed or destroyed by infection, other glands in the vagina are capable of secreting adequate amounts of lubricants.

Basal cell carcinoma

A type of skin cancer that occurs most commonly on the face or neck, also known as a rodent ulcer. The cells of the tumor closely resemble, and are possibly derived from, cells in the basal (innermost) skin layer.

INCIDENCE
Basal cell carcinoma is the most common skin cancer. Without treatment, the growth gradually invades and bites deeper into surrounding tissues. Fortunately, basal cell carcinomas virtually never spread to other parts of the body.

Fair-skinned people over 50 are the most commonly affected (dark and black-skinned people are affected only rarely). The incidence is much higher among people living in sunny climates, especially those with outdoor occupations; in parts of Arizona and Texas, for example, and in Queensland, Australia, more than half the white population has had a basal cell carcinoma by the age of 75.

CAUSE
Direct skin damage from the ultraviolet radiation in sunlight is thought to be the cause in most cases. Dark-skinned people are protected by the larger amount of *melanin* (a pigment that absorbs ultraviolet radiation) in their skin.

SYMPTOMS
More than 90 percent of basal cell carcinomas occur on the face, often at the side of an eye or on the nose, but the tumor can appear virtually anywhere on the body. It starts as a small, flat nodule and grows slowly, even-

tually breaking down at the center to form a shallow ulcer with raised edges. Diagnosis is confirmed by microscopic examination of a sample of cells from the tumor.

PREVENTION
Individuals at risk, particularly fair-skinned people, should avoid overexposure to strong sunlight by wearing protective clothing and sun hats, and using *sunscreen* preparations containing para-aminobenzoic acid (*PABA*).

TREATMENT AND OUTLOOK
The tumor can be destroyed by *cryosurgery* or *radiation therapy* or it may be removed surgically. Treatment usually results in a complete cure, although new tumors may develop in people who do not take adequate preventive measures. (See also *Melanoma, malignant; Squamous cell carcinoma; Sunlight, adverse effects of*.)

Basal ganglia

Paired nerve cell clusters in the *brain*, deep within the cerebrum (main mass of the brain) and upper part of the brain stem. The basal ganglia play a vital part in producing smooth, continuous muscular actions and in stopping and starting movement.

Disease or degeneration of the basal ganglia and their connections may lead to the appearance of involuntary movements, trembling, and weakness, as occur in *Parkinson's disease*.

Baseball finger

Injury to the fingertip from a heavy blow that forces the tip into a bent position. Baseball finger, also called mallet finger, can occur in any sport where a ball (e.g., a baseball, softball, football, or basketball) strikes the finger in this way.

The sudden bending of the extended finger may tear the tendon on the back of the finger, or, if the tendon doesn't "give," pull off a fragment of bone. In either case, the fingertip is bent.

The condition is treated with an external splint or the insertion of a temporary wire through the bones to hold the finger straight. The injury heals over two to three months.

Battered baby syndrome

Injuries to a child that suggest repeated physical assault. Such injuries often include bruises, burns, and fractures. Usually the full extent of past injuries is apparent only when the child is examined medically and the complete skeleton is X-rayed. (See *Child abuse*.)

B-cell
See *Lymphocyte*.

BCG vaccination

B

A vaccine that provides immunity against *tuberculosis*. BCG is prepared from an artificially weakened strain of bovine (cattle) tubercle bacilli, the microorganisms responsible for the disease. The initials BCG stand for "bacille Calmette-Guérin," after the two Frenchmen who developed the vaccine in 1906.

WHY IT IS DONE
In Canada, BCG vaccine is administered to selected groups such as infants, native peoples, certain immigrants, and persons such as health care workers repeatedly exposed to tuberculosis. It is used only when other measures to prevent the disease prove ineffective.

HOW IT IS DONE
Except in newborn babies, a *tuberculin test* is performed first and only those with negative reactions (no immunity) are vaccinated. The vaccine is usually injected into the upper arm. About six weeks later a small pustule appears. This normally heals completely, leaving a small scar. An occasional complication is development of a chronic ulcer because the pustule fails to heal.

Beclomethasone

A *corticosteroid drug* prescribed as a nasal spray to relieve the symptoms of allergic *rhinitis* (hay fever) and as an inhaler to treat *asthma*. Beclomethasone controls nasal symptoms by reducing inflammation and mucus production in the nose. In asthma, it helps to reduce wheezing and coughing by reducing inflammation in the bronchi. It also reduces the severity and frequency of asthma attacks. However, once an attack has started, beclomethasone will not help relieve symptoms because it takes up to a few days to have any effect.

Beclomethasone is given primarily to people whose asthma does not respond to *bronchodilator drugs* alone. Adverse effects may include hoarseness, throat irritation, and, rarely, fungal infections in the mouth. Irritation may be prevented by thoroughly rinsing the mouth and gargling with water after each inhalation.

Beclomethasone is also prescribed as a cream or ointment to treat skin inflammation caused by *eczema*.

Becquerel

A unit of radioactivity (see *Radiation units box*).

Bed bath

A method of washing a person who is confined to bed. To give a bed bath, wash and dry a small area at a time, keeping the rest of the person covered to prevent chilling.

Bedbug

 A flat, wingless, brown insect 5 mm long and 3 mm wide. Bedbugs live in furniture, especially beds, and floors during the day and emerge at night to feed on humans by sucking blood. They are not known to transmit any diseases but their bites cause itching sores that may become infected.

Bedpan

A metal, plastic, or fiber container into which a patient confined to bed can defecate and, if female, urinate. Male patients use a *urinal* for urination. In the past, bedpans and urinals were used routinely, but today, unless the patient is immobile, the use of the toilet or a bedside *commode* is considered to be less stressful.

Bed rest

A term used to describe periods spent in bed. It may be an essential part of treatment in certain illnesses, such as rheumatic fever, and for some types of injuries, such as a fractured vertebra or a slipped disk. Prolonged bed rest may involve various risks for the patient, among them muscle wasting, *bedsores*, weakness, depression, and loss of calcium leading to bone demineralization and urinary tract *calculi* (stones). People recovering from an operation are at special risk of developing deep vein thrombosis (see *Thrombosis, deep vein*) and, especially if elderly, of contracting *pneumonia*. To prevent these problems, patients today are encouraged to be physically active while in bed and to get out of bed sooner than in the past.

Bedridden

A term used to describe a person who is unable to leave bed due to illness or injury. People most likely to be bedridden are the very elderly, the terminally ill, and those paralyzed as the result of an accident.

Beds, hospital

Special beds for nursing sick or injured patients may be used in hospitals and sometimes at home.

TYPES

STANDARD HOSPITAL BED This bed is made of metal to allow it to be disinfected, mounted on wheels for ease of movement, jointed to allow tilting in any direction, and adjustable in height. The higher position is used for nursing procedures; the lower position allows the patient to get in and out of bed easily. A firm mattress provides support for the patient while various procedures are being performed.

TURNING FRAMES These beds, including the Stryker frame and the Foster frame, enable patients with extensive burns, multiple injuries, pelvic and spinal fractures, or spinal cord injuries to be turned with a minimum of handling and without disturbing body alignment. The patient lies prone or supine on a canvas-covered frame. When turning is required, a second canvas is placed on top of the patient, both canvases (with the patient sandwiched between) are rotated through 180 degrees, and the top canvas is then removed.

REVOLVING CIRCULAR BED This bed is used for the same purposes as manual turning frames, but allows the patient to be placed in a variety of sitting or standing positions at any angle between vertical and horizontal. It is particularly useful for patients with spinal cord injury who may develop hypotension (lowered blood pressure) when sitting or placed upright after being immobilized in a horizontal position for a prolonged period. Gradual rehabilitation of patients is also facilitated because they can adjust gradually from lying flat to standing upright, while remaining supported.

AIRBEDS AND WATERBEDS Beds with air- or water-filled mattresses can help prevent bedsores by providing uniform support for the patient's whole body.

PREVENTING BEDSORES

Once a bedsore has developed it will heal only if pressure on it is minimized, so good nursing care of a bedridden, immobile patient is crucial. The patient's position should be changed at least every two hours and it is important to wash and dry pressure areas carefully, especially if there is incontinence. Barrier creams can be used for additional protection.

Air flow

Ripple bed mattress
A rippling effect is created by pumping air in and out of the mattress, so stimulating the circulation.

Cushions and pillows
These can be used to relieve pressure by placing them between the knees and under the shoulder.

Sheepskins
A sheepskin under the buttocks and bootees under the heels relieve pressure.

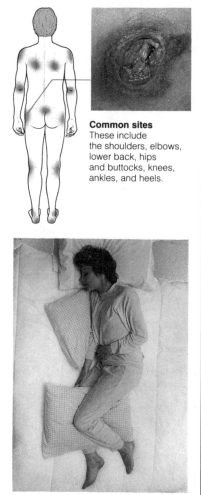

Common sites
These include the shoulders, elbows, lower back, hips and buttocks, knees, ankles, and heels.

Airbeds are more commonly used than waterbeds because they are lighter and more comfortable for patients. A modern type of airbed, the ripple bed, has a small motor that alternately fills and empties coils inside the mattress with air, creating a rippling effect. The continuous motion stimulates the patient's circulation, which, it is claimed, helps to keep the skin healthy and less susceptible to bedsores.

BALKAN FRAME This is used for the attachment of traction apparatus. It incorporates a hanging bar so that the patient can pull himself or herself up.

Bedsores

Also known as decubitus ulcers or pressure sores, these are ulcers that develop on the skin of patients who are bedridden, unconscious, or immobile. They commonly affect victims of *stroke* or *spinal injuries* that result in a loss of sensation. Constantly wet skin, caused by *incontinence*, may also be a contributory factor.

Bedsores start as red, painful areas that become purple before the skin breaks down, developing into open sores. Once the skin is broken, the sores often become infected, enlarged and deeper, and are very slow to heal.

TREATMENT
Deep, chronic ulcers may require treatment with *antibiotic drugs*, packing with plastic foam, and possibly *plastic surgery*. New medications for preventing and treating bedsores are constantly being evaluated.

Bed-wetting

The common name for poor bladder control at night. (See *Enuresis*.)

Bee stings

See *Insect stings*.

Behavioral problems in children

Behavioral problems occasionally occur in all children; specialist management is called for when they become frequent and disrupt school and/or family life. *Enuresis* (bed-wetting), sleep difficulties, *tantrums*, feeding difficulties, truancy, disobedience, stealing, jealousy, aggressive attitudes toward siblings, *alcohol intoxication*, and *drug abuse* are all common problems. When a particular form of disturbed behavior continues for a long time or forms part of a larger pattern, it becomes a cause for concern. Almost inevitably, however, stressful external events, such as moving home, changing schools, peer pressure, birth of a sibling, divorce, remarriage, hospitalization, chronic disease in the family or child, unemployment, or death in the family may produce periods of problem behavior.

MANAGEMENT
BABIES Most problems resolve themselves over a matter of months; your physician will discuss any concerns you may have. (See also *Colic, infantile; Crying in infants; Feeding, infant*.)

TODDLERS Parents need to be realistic and consistent in their expectations, and should encourage a degree of decision sharing. Consistent and appropriate discipline should be exercised. Toilet-training should be delayed until a child is physically and emotionally ready. Separations from parents and changes in activity should be carefully planned. Parents who exercise adequate self-control provide the best model for a toddler who is having difficulty controlling explosive feelings. (See also *Breath-holding attacks; Head-banging; Toilet-training*.)

EARLY CHILDHOOD Parents should take a positive approach and concentrate on rewarding good behavior rather than punishing bad behavior, which tends to exaggerate difficulties or create new ones. Close cooperation is needed between home and playgroup/school because children often behave badly in only one place. (See also *Nightmares; Thumb-sucking*.)

TYPES OF PROBLEM, BY AGE

Babies up to 18 months	Sleeping and feeding difficulties, colic, crying
Toddlers and small children 1-4 years	Head-banging, tantrums, biting, breath-holding attacks, separation anxiety, poor social interaction, difficulty changing from one activity to another, toilet-training problems
Early childhood 4-8 years	Nail-biting, thumb-sucking, aggression, clinginess, anxiety about illness and death, nightmares, enuresis
Middle childhood/ adolescence 9-18 years	Lying, stealing, smoking, truancy, disobedience, aggression, low achievement in school, drug or alcohol use, running away, sexual promiscuity

MIDDLE CHILDHOOD/ADOLESCENCE Firm, but not punitive, parental treatment can help the child at this stage. If the child's difficulties persist and there are stressful family events, it may be useful to seek professional advice. Drug or alcohol abuse (or suspicion that they are taking place) requires immediate medical attention.

OUTLOOK
Parents who find a baby difficult to care for may find they can cope better when the child is older. When an older child's behavior is linked to a deterioration in the family situation, improvements can be expected when the circumstances improve. Whether family problems persist or are resolved, professional advice should be sought if the child's behavior continues to be difficult. Even when the family situation is satisfactory, worried parents can often benefit from professional advice.

Behaviorism

An American school of *psychology* founded by John Broadus Watson early in this century. He argued that, because behavior, rather than experience, was all that could be observed in others, it should constitute the sole basis of psychology.

Behavior therapy

A collection of techniques, based on psychological theory, for changing abnormal behavior or treating anxiety. Behavior therapy can be effective in the treatment of phobic and obsessional disorders and certain kinds of sexual and marital problems.

The concept of behavior modification originated with animal psychologists, but the techniques have been expanded and refined by clinical psychologists in the last decade. Treatment relies on two basic ideas: that exposure to a feared experience under safe conditions will render it less threatening, and that desirable behavior can be encouraged by using a system of rewards. Aversion therapy—using punishment to discourage undesirable behavior—was used in the past, particularly in the treatment of alcoholics and drug addicts, but was found to be ineffective in the long term.

TYPES
EXPOSURE THERAPY Also called desensitization, this consists of exposing the patient in stages to the cause of his or her anxiety. At the same time, the patient is taught to cope with anxiety symptoms by using relaxation tech-

niques. The intensity of the anxiety-provoking stimulus is gradually increased until eventually the patient is able to deal with the full situation.

FLOODING Instead of being introduced to the cause of the phobia in stages, the patient is confronted with the anxiety-provoking stimulus at once, but with the support of the therapist. The patient remains in this situation until his or her feelings of anxiety eventually disappear.

RESPONSE PREVENTION The patient is prevented from carrying out an obsessional task. This technique is used in combination with other methods.

MODELING The therapist acts as a model for the patient, performing the anxiety-provoking activity first, so that the patient may copy.

HOW IT IS USED

TREATMENT OF PHOBIC DISORDERS This treatment is dependent on exposure therapy, through which the patient is helped to face the feared situation. In agoraphobia (fear of open spaces), for example, the therapist accompanies the sufferer on a short journey, providing emotional support. The sufferer may use relaxation techniques to help cope with anxiety. Gradually, the distance traveled from home is increased, and the therapist withdraws from the treatment as the sufferer gains confidence.

Similar techniques of gradual exposure may also help people with animal phobias, flying phobias, or other phobias in which there is a specific fear.

TREATMENT OF OBSESSIONAL RITUALS This consists of three different aspects: prevention, exposure, and modeling. For example, a patient with a hand-washing compulsion would be prevented from carrying out the washing rituals. At the same time, exposure to materials that the patient might consider contaminated is encouraged, the therapist acting as a model by touching the "contaminated" objects first.

TREATMENT OF MARITAL AND SEXUAL PROBLEMS This is based on *marital counseling*; partners rewarding each other for pleasing or helpful behavior. (See also *Sex therapy*.)

Behçet's syndrome

A rare disorder in which the main symptoms are recurrent mouth ulcers, genital ulceration, and inflammation of the eye. There may also be rashes, arthritis, and venous thrombosis (abnormal clot formation in veins). Less common features are intestinal ulcers, arterial disease, inflammation of the testis and epi-

didymis, and neuropsychiatric symptoms. The condition was first described by the Turkish dermatologist Hulusi Behçet (1889-1948).

The cause of the disorder is unknown. The diagnosis relies on one or more of the three main symptoms being present.

Often treatment is difficult and may require *corticosteroid drugs* or *anticancer drugs*. The condition frequently becomes chronic.

Belching

The noisy return of air from the stomach through the mouth. Swallowing air is usually a nervous habit of which the person is unaware. It also may be a result of eating or drinking too much too quickly.

Each time a person belches, he or she swallows air, which makes further belching more likely. Sometimes, belching helps alleviate discomfort caused by indigestion. During pregnancy, belching briefly helps relieve nausea and heartburn, which disappear after delivery of the baby.

Belladonna

An extract of the deadly nightshade plant, containing *alkaloids* including *atropine*, which has been used medicinally since ancient times. Women used to apply belladonna to their eyes to dilate the pupils (the name in Italian means beautiful lady). In modern medicine, belladonna alkaloids are used as *antispasmodic drugs* to treat gastrointestinal disturbances. (See also *Anticholinergic drugs*.)

Bell's palsy

The most common form of *facial palsy*.

Bends

A popular term for *decompression sickness*, especially for the severe bone and joint pains that are a common symptom in divers who rise to the surface too rapidly.

The origin of the term "bends" is uncertain, but it may have referred to the diver being literally bent double in pain, or to the slight easing of pain, which may be achieved by flexing an affected joint.

Benign

The term used to describe a relatively mild form of a disease. For example, a benign tumor will not spread throughout the body, whereas a *malignant* or cancerous tumor may do so if not removed at an early stage.

Benzodiazepine drugs

COMMON DRUGS

Chlordiazepoxide
Diazepam Oxazepam

Among the best-known and most widely prescribed drugs in the world, benzodiazepines are used mainly as *tranquilizer drugs* for the control of symptoms due to *anxiety* or *stress* and as *sleeping drugs* for *insomnia*.

WHY THEY ARE USED

For the treatment of anxiety, benzodiazepines are given for short periods to promote mental and physical relaxation. They reduce feelings of agitation and restlessness, slow mental activity, and relax the muscles.

Most benzodiazepine drugs have a strong sedative effect and help to relieve insomnia. They cause drowsiness and sleep when given in a higher dose than that used to treat anxiety.

Benzodiazepines are also used in the management of alcohol withdrawal and in the control of *epilepsy*.

HOW THEY WORK

Benzodiazepines promote sleep and relieve anxiety by depressing brain function. By interfering with chemical activity in the brain and nervous system, they reduce the communication between nerve cells. This leads to a reduction in brain activity, in proportion to the amount of drug taken.

POSSIBLE ADVERSE EFFECTS

Minor adverse effects include daytime drowsiness, dizziness, and forgetfulness. Benzodiazepines may also cause unsteadiness and slow reactions, thus impairing the ability to drive or operate machinery.

The main risk of benzodiazepines is that regular users may become psychologically and physically dependent on them. For this reason, they are usually given for courses of two to three weeks or less. When benzodiazepines are stopped suddenly, withdrawal symptoms, such as excessive anxiety, nightmares, and restlessness, may occur. When they are taken for longer than two weeks, they should be withdrawn gradually under medical supervision.

Benzodiazepine drugs have been abused for their sedative effect.

Benzoyl peroxide

An *antiseptic* agent used in the treatment of *acne*.

Bereavement

The emotional reaction following the death of a loved relative or friend. A

B

bereaved person's feelings will vary in intensity according to his or her level of maturity and the nature of emotional problems or conflict in the bereaved person prior to the loss. Also involved is the nature and quality of the bereaved person's relationship with the deceased and the kind of relationship they shared before the death. The expression of grief is individual to each person, but there are recognized stages of bereavement, each characterized by a particular attitude.

STAGES OF BEREAVEMENT

Numbness, hallucinations, and an unwillingness to recognize the death are defense mechanisms against admitting, and therefore accepting, the loss and associated pain. Numbness is the pervading feeling that enables the bereaved person to get through the funeral arrangements and family gatherings. This stage may last from three days to three months. Often, the reality of the death does not penetrate completely at this time, and many people continue to behave as if the dead person were still alive. Hallucinations, too, are a common experience among the recently bereaved. They may consist of a sense of having seen or heard the dead person, or of having been aware of his or her presence. This can be comforting for some people, disturbing for others.

Depression is a reaction to loss. Once the numbness wears off and the bereaved person can know and feel that a loss has occurred, he or she may be overwhelmed by feelings of anxiety, anger, and despair that can develop into a depressive illness (see *Depression*). Gastrointestinal disturbances and *mental disorders* may occur and there is a risk of attempted suicide. An increase in the intake of alcohol, tranquilizers, and other drugs is common, as are insomnia, malaise, agitation, and tearfulness.

Gradually, but usually within two years, the bereaved person adjusts to the loss and begins to make positive plans for the future. This process can involve periods of pain and despair, alternating with periods of enthusiasm and interest; eventually, positiveness usually triumphs over despair. Research suggests, however, that the death of a spouse may increase the mortality for people in every age group, although there is little consistent information on the length of survival after widowhood. Survival may depend on whether a bereaved person can develop other relationships.

SUPPORT AND COUNSELING

Family and friends can often provide the support a bereaved person needs, but sometimes other factors impede the recovery process. Outside help may be required and may be given by a social worker, member of the clergy, or self-help group. For some people, however, the care of a psychiatrist is necessary when depression, apathy, and lethargy obstruct recovery. In these cases, specialized *counseling* and *psychotherapy* should be encouraged by family and friends. (See also *Stillbirth*.)

Beriberi

A metabolic disorder caused by a lack of thiamine (vitamin B_1) in the diet. In developed countries, the illness is seen only in people who are starving or on an extremely restricted diet (such as alcoholics). Breast-fed babies can develop beriberi if their mother's milk is seriously deficient in thiamine due to severe dietary restriction.

CAUSES

Thiamine, found in whole-grain cereals, meat, green vegetables, potatoes, and nuts, is essential for the metabolism of carbohydrates. Without it, the brain, nerves, and muscles (including the heart muscle) are unable to function properly.

INCIDENCE

Beriberi occurs among underfed populations. It was once a major problem in the Far East among people subsisting on rice from which the thiamine-rich outer layer had been removed, but improved milling and a better overall diet has led to a dramatic decline in the disorder.

SYMPTOMS AND SIGNS

Two forms of the illness—"dry" and "wet" beriberi—are recognized. In dry beriberi, the thiamine deficiency mainly affects the nerves and skeletal muscles. Symptoms include numbness, a burning sensation in the legs, and wasting of the muscles. In severe cases, the patient becomes emaciated, virtually paralyzed, and bedridden.

In wet beriberi, the main problem is *heart failure* (inability of the heart to keep up with its task of pumping blood). This in turn leads to congestion of blood in the veins, and *edema* (swelling caused by fluid accumulation) in the legs, and sometimes also in the trunk and face. Other symptoms include poor appetite, rapid pulse, and breathlessness. As the heart failure worsens, breathing becomes difficult and, without medical treatment, the patient will die.

DIAGNOSIS AND TREATMENT

The diagnosis is usually obvious from the symptoms and environmental factors; it can be confirmed by a test of the levels in the blood of lactic and pyruvic acids, which accumulate because carbohydrates cannot be completely metabolized.

Treatment consists of thiamine, given orally or by injection, which brings a rapid and complete cure. Since other vitamin deficiencies are also likely, a permanent improvement in diet is also needed.

Berylliosis

An occupational disease caused by the inhalation of dust or fumes containing beryllium, a metallic element which, with its compounds, is used in high-technology industries, such as nuclear energy, electronics, and aerospace.

Short exposure to high concentrations of beryllium may lead to severe *pneumonitis* (lung inflammation), which is characterized by coughing and breathlessness. Lengthy exposure to smaller concentrations may lead to more permanent lung and liver damage. The lung changes may lead eventually to severe breathlessness after the slightest exertion.

Treatment with *corticosteroid drugs* can help alleviate the symptoms but does not alter the course of the illness. Prevention requires adequate protection against the inhalation of beryllium fumes.

Beta-blocker drugs

COMMON DRUGS

Cardioselective
Acebutolol Atenolol Metoprolol

Noncardioselective
Nadolol Oxprenolol Pindolol Propranolol

> **WARNING**
> Do not suddenly stop taking a beta-blocker; a severe recurrence of your previous symptoms and a significant rise in blood pressure may result.

A group of drugs, also known as beta-adrenergic blocking agents, prescribed principally to treat heart disorders. They have been used since the 1960s and although other, newer drugs have been found to treat many of the conditions for which they are effective, beta-blockers are still prescribed widely today.

WHY THEY ARE USED

Beta-blocker drugs are used in the treatment of *angina pectoris* (chest pain

HOW BETA-BLOCKERS WORK

Beta-blockers block beta-receptors—specific sites on body tissues where *neurotransmitters* (chemicals released from nerve endings) bind. There are two types of beta-receptor: beta$_1$-receptors found in heart tissue and beta$_2$-receptors found in the lungs, blood vessels, and other tissues. At these receptors, two chemicals, epinephrine and norepinephrine, are released from nerve endings in the *sympathetic nervous system*, the part of the involuntary nervous system that enables the body to deal with stress, anxiety, and exercise. These neurotransmitters bind to beta-receptors to increase the force and speed of the heartbeat, to dilate the airways to increase air flow to the lungs, and to dilate blood vessels.

Cardioselective beta-blockers combine predominantly with beta$_1$-receptors; noncardioselective beta-blockers combine with both types.

Beta-blockers slow heart rate and reduce the force of contraction of heart muscle. These effects can be used to slow a fast heart rate and regulate abnormal rhythms.

Beta-blockers prevent angina pectoris attacks by reducing the work performed by the heart muscle and so the heart's oxygen requirement. High blood pressure is reduced because the rate and force at which the heart pumps blood into the circulation is lowered.

The effect of blocking beta-receptors on muscles elsewhere in the body is to reduce the muscle tremor of anxiety and an overactive thyroid gland. Beta-blockers can help to reduce the frequency of migraine attacks by preventing the dilation of blood vessels surrounding the brain, which is responsible for the headache. In glaucoma they lower pressure in the eye by reducing fluid production in the eyeball.

Cardioselective beta-blockers
These beta-blockers occupy beta$_1$-receptors on heart tissue and have only a mild effect on beta$_2$-receptors in the bronchi of the lungs. These drugs are used in the treatment of heart disorders to reduce the work load of the heart,

thus slowing the rate and reducing the force of contractions. They are less likely than other beta-blockers to cause breathing difficulty.

Types of beta-receptors
Beta$_1$-receptors occur mainly in the heart muscle; beta$_2$-receptors are found in the lungs, blood vessels, and certain tissues. Beta-blocker drugs bind to beta-receptors, thereby blocking neurotransmitters.

Key
- Beta$_1$-receptor
- Beta$_2$-receptor
- Neurotransmitter
- Beta-blocker
- Blocked beta-receptor

due to insufficient oxygen reaching the heart muscle), *hypertension* (high blood pressure), and cardiac *arrhythmia* (irregular heartbeat). Beta-blockers are sometimes given after a *myocardial infarction* (heart attack) to reduce the likelihood of further damage to the heart muscle.

Beta-blockers may also be given to prevent *migraine* attacks and to reduce the physical symptoms of *anxiety* (such as palpitations, tremor, and excessive sweating). They may be given to control symptoms of *thyrotoxicosis* (overactive thyroid gland). A beta-blocker is sometimes given in the form of eye drops to treat *glaucoma* (raised fluid pressure in the eyeball) by lowering the fluid pressure.

HOW THEY WORK
See explanatory box.

POSSIBLE ADVERSE EFFECTS
By reducing heart rate and air flow to the lungs, beta-blockers may reduce an individual's capacity for strenuous exercise, although this may not be noticed if physical activity is already limited by heart problems.

Beta-blockers may worsen the symptoms of *asthma*, *bronchitis*, or other forms of lung disease. They may also reduce the flow of blood to the limbs and thus aggravate *peripheral vascular disease*.

If long-term treatment with beta-blockers is abruptly withdrawn, there may be a sudden severe recurrence of the patient's symptoms and a significant rise in blood pressure. These problems can be avoided by gradually decreasing the dose.

Betahistine
A drug used to treat *Meniere's disease* (a disorder of the inner ear). Taken regularly, betahistine reduces the frequency and severity of the attacks of nausea and vertigo that characterize this condition. Betahistine is thought to work by reducing pressure in the inner ear, possibly by improving blood flow in the small blood vessels. Adverse effects are rare but may include headache and nausea.

Betamethasone

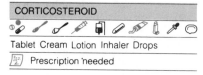

CORTICOSTEROID

Tablet Cream Lotion Inhaler Drops

Prescription needed

A *corticosteroid drug* used to treat inflammation. Betamethasone is applied to the skin to treat *eczema* and *psoriasis*. Regular inhalation of this drug can reduce the severity and frequency of *asthma*. Betamethasone is also prescribed to treat allergic *rhinitis* (hay fever).

Betamethasone is taken by mouth to treat severe cases of asthma and *arthritis*. It is also occasionally used to reduce cerebral edema (swelling of the brain) and in mothers about to deliver prematurely, to lessen the baby's risk of developing *respiratory distress syndrome*.

POSSIBLE ADVERSE EFFECTS
Adverse effects are unlikely to occur when betamethasone is inhaled or used as ear drops. This is because the dose that reaches the bloodstream is low. A higher dose may be absorbed when the drug is applied to the skin and for this reason betamethasone should be applied only sparingly and for short periods. Even when used with caution, betamethasone can cause thinning of the skin. It may also aggravate a skin infection and is therefore sometimes prescribed with an *antibiotic drug*. Taking betamethasone tablets for a prolonged period or in high doses can cause adverse effects typical of other corticosteroid drugs.

Bezoar
A ball of food and mucus, vegetable fiber, hair, or other indigestible material, in the stomach. Bezoars are rare in adults except after partial *gastrectomy* (removal of part of the stomach). Trichobezoars (composed of hair) may form in children or emotionally disturbed adults who nibble at, or pull out and swallow, their hair.

Bezoars can cause loss of appetite, constipation, nausea and vomiting, and abdominal pain. If they pass into the intestines, they may cause an obstruction (see *Intestine, obstruction of*). Bezoars are diagnosed by means of a *barium X-ray examination* or *endoscopy* (passing a viewing tube down the digestive tract), and are removed by washing out the stomach (see *Lavage, gastric*), by use of a pincer attachment on the endoscope, by surgery, or by use of drugs that break down the protein portion of the bezoar.

A low-fiber diet may help prevent recurrent bezoars in affected adults. (See also *Foreign body*.)

Bi-
The prefix meaning two or twice, as in bilateral (two-sided).

Bicarbonate of soda
See *Sodium bicarbonate*.

Biceps muscle
The name, meaning "two heads," given to a muscle originating at one end as two separate parts, which then fuse. The biceps in the upper arm bends the arm at the elbow and rotates the forearm; the biceps at the back of the thigh bends the leg at the knee and extends the thigh.

LOCATION OF BICEPS
There are four biceps muscles in the body—one in each upper arm and one on the back of each thigh.

Two heads of biceps

Biceps muscle

Humerus

Ulna   Radius

Bicuspid
A term meaning to have two cusps (curved, pointed structures). It is used, for example, to describe certain *heart valves* and as an alternative name for a premolar tooth (see *Teeth*).

Bifocal
This term is used to describe a spectacle lens with two different focal lengths. Glasses with bifocal lenses make corrections for both close and distant vision.

Bilateral
A term that means affecting both sides of the body, or affecting both organs if they are paired (for instance, both ears in bilateral deafness).

Bile
A greenish-brown liquid secreted by the *liver*. It carries away waste products formed in the liver and also helps to break down fats in the small intestine so that they can be digested.

The waste products in bile include the pigments *bilirubin* and biliverdin, which give the liquid its greenish-brown color. The other main constituents of bile are bile salts and *cholesterol*. Bile salts aid in the breakdown and absorption of fats.

Bile passes out of the liver via the bile ducts and is then concentrated and stored in the gallbladder until, after a meal, it is expelled and enters the duodenum by way of the common bile duct. At the end of the small intestine, most of the bile salts are reabsorbed into the bloodstream to be recycled into bile again by the liver. Bile pigments are normally excreted from the body in the feces, which they color dark brown. (See also *Biliary system*; *Cholestyramine*.)

Bile duct
Any of the ducts by which *bile* is carried from the liver, first to the gallbladder and then to the duodenum (the first section of the small intestine).

STRUCTURE
The bile duct system starts as tiny tubular canals called canaliculi that surround the liver cells and collect the bile. The canaliculi join together to form a network of bile ducts of increasing size, which emerge from the liver, on the underside, as the two hepatic ducts.

These ducts join within or just outside the liver to form the common hepatic duct. Shortly after the junction, another duct, known as the cystic duct, branches off to the gallbladder, which lies in a hollow on the undersurface of the liver. The continuation of the common hepatic duct past the junction with the cystic duct is known as the common bile duct. This leads directly into the duodenum. (See also *Biliary system*.)

Bile duct cancer
See *Cholangiocarcinoma*.

Bile duct obstruction
A blockage or constriction of any of the ducts that carry bile from the liver to the gallbladder and then to the duodenum (see *Biliary system*).

The obstruction results in *cholestasis* (accumulation of bile in the liver), and the development of *jaundice* due to accumulation of *bilirubin* in the blood. Prolonged bile duct obstruction over many years can lead to secondary *biliary cirrhosis*, a serious type of advanced liver disease.

CAUSES

The bile ducts can become blocked or narrowed for a variety of reasons. Perhaps the most common cause is *gall-stones*, which have usually formed in the gallbladder and escaped into the common bile duct.

A tumor of the pancreas (see *Pancreas, cancer of*) may compress the lower end of the common bile duct. Occasionally, cancers of other organs may spread to the biliary system and cause obstruction. *Cholangiocarcinoma* (cancer of the bile ducts) is a very rare cause of blockage.

Bile duct obstruction is a rare side effect of certain drugs, such as tranquilizers, antibacterials, and sex hormones. It may also be caused by trauma, such as injury during gallbladder operations, by *cholangitis* (inflammation of the bile ducts), and, very rarely, by the entry of various flukes or worms into the ducts.

SYMPTOMS

All patients develop "obstructive" jaundice, which is characterized by pale-colored feces (due to lack of the normal bilirubin content) and dark urine (due to excess bilirubin content) as well as a yellow skin color. Some patients also complain of itching, caused by the presence of bile salts in the skin.

Other symptoms depend on the cause of the biliary obstruction—for example, abdominal pain with gallstones, or weight loss with many types of cancer.

DIAGNOSIS AND TREATMENT

Liver function tests may suggest an obstruction, the site of which can be confirmed by *ultrasound scanning* and *cholangiography* or *ERCP*.

If bile duct obstruction is due to a drug, the drug should be discontinued. In other cases, an obstruction can sometimes be removed by surgery or by means of an attachment to an *endoscope* (viewing instrument) passed down the digestive tract and up the common bile duct.

When the obstruction is due to a cancer that is too advanced for surgical removal, the obstruction is usually bypassed to relieve the jaundice. This may be done by joining a loop of intestine either to the gallbladder or to the biliary system above the blockage. Alternatively, a tube may be pushed through the blockage, either from the intestinal side using an endoscope, or with catheters from the liver side of the duct (using X rays to track the catheters). The tube is left in place for bile to flow through.

Bilharziasis

An alternative name for the tropical parasitic disease *schistosomiasis*.

Biliary atresia

A rare disorder, present from birth, in which the bile ducts, either outside or inside the liver, fail to develop or have developed abnormally. As a result, bile cannot flow through the ducts to the duodenum (the first part of the small intestine) and becomes trapped in the liver (see *Cholestasis*). Unless the atresia is treated, secondary *biliary cirrhosis* will develop and may prove fatal.

The main signs of biliary atresia are deepening *jaundice*, usually beginning a week after birth, and the passing of dark urine and pale feces.

DIAGNOSIS AND TREATMENT

If biliary atresia is suspected, blood tests and a *liver biopsy* (removal and microscopic examination of a small sample of liver tissue) are performed. If these tests show that the baby's jaundice is not due to a different cause, such as *hepatitis*, an operation may be performed to examine the liver and bile ducts directly. If this confirms the diagnosis of biliary atresia, surgery is carried out to bypass the ducts by joining a loop of small intestine directly to the liver. If this fails, or if the jaundice recurs, a *liver transplant* is the only possible treatment.

Biliary cirrhosis

An uncommon form of liver *cirrhosis* that results from disease or defects of the bile ducts. There are two types: primary and secondary biliary cirrhosis. Both types are characterized by *cholestasis* (accumulation of bile in the liver), which impairs liver function.

PRIMARY BILIARY CIRRHOSIS

In this type of biliary cirrhosis, the bile ducts within the liver become inflamed and are destroyed. The cause is unknown, but the disease seems to be associated with a malfunction of the *immune system*. Middle-aged women are the group most commonly affected.

The first symptom is itching, followed later by *jaundice*, an enlarged liver, and sometimes abdominal pain, fatty diarrhea, and *xanthomatosis* (the appearance of fatty deposits under the skin). *Osteoporosis* may develop. Over a number of years the patient may develop other symptoms of liver cirrhosis and *liver failure*.

The disease is diagnosed by *liver function tests*, by *liver biopsy*, and by *cholangiography* or *ERCP*. Drug treatment has been aimed mainly at relieving symptoms, such as itching, and minimizing complications. A *liver transplant*, if available, provides the only long-term cure.

SECONDARY BILIARY CIRRHOSIS

This results from prolonged *bile duct obstruction* or *biliary atresia* (absence or abnormality of the bile ducts from birth). The symptoms and signs include abdominal pain and tenderness, liver enlargement, fevers and chills, and sometimes blood abnormalities. Treatment is as for bile duct obstruction or biliary atresia.

Biliary colic

A severe pain in the upper right quadrant of the abdomen usually caused by the gallbladder's attempts to expel *gallstones* or the movement of a stone in the bile ducts. The pain is extremely severe and often lasts for up to an hour. It may mimic the pain of a heart attack and may radiate to the right shoulder or penetrate through to the centre of the back.

Injections of an *analgesic drug* (painkiller) and an *antispasmodic drug* may be given to relieve the colic. Tests such as *cholecystography* or *ultrasound scanning* are usually carried out to determine whether gallstones are definitely present; if they are, *cholecystectomy* (surgical removal of the gallbladder) may be considered.

Biliary system

The organs and ducts by which *bile* is formed, concentrated, and carried from the *liver* to the duodenum (the first part of the small intestine). Bile removes waste products from the liver and carries bile salts, necessary for the breakdown and absorption of fat, to the intestine.

Bile is secreted by the liver cells and collected by a system of tubes that mirrors the blood supply to the organ. This network of bile-drainage channels carries the bile out of the liver by way of the hepatic ducts, which join together to form a common duct that opens into the duodenum at a controlled orifice called the ampulla of Vater. Bile does not pass directly into the duodenum but is first concentrated and then stored until needed in the gallbladder, a pear-shaped reservoir lying in a hollow under the liver, to which it gains access by way of the cystic duct.

When food is eaten, the presence of fat in the duodenum causes the secretion of a hormone, which opens the ampulla of Vater and causes the gallbladder to contract, squeezing stored bile via the cystic and common bile ducts into the duodenum. In the duodenum, bile salts emulsify the fat, breaking it down to a kind of milk of microscopic globules.

DISORDERS

The main disorder of the gallbladder is the formation of *gallstones*, which can have multiple complications affecting the entire biliary system (see *Gallbladder* disorders box). The main disorders

of the bile ducts are congenital *biliary atresia* (absence or abnormality of the bile ducts from birth) and *bile duct obstruction*, which may itself be caused by gallstones or by other causes. Bile duct obstruction can have important complications affecting the liver.

Biliousness

A term commonly and erroneously used to describe nausea or vomiting.

More accurately, however, biliousness describes a condition in which bitter bile is brought up to the mouth from the stomach.

Bilirubin

The main pigment found in *bile*. Bilirubin is produced by the breakdown of *hemoglobin*, the pigment in red blood cells. Bilirubin is the yellow pigment associated with *jaundice*. Products

---

FUNCTION OF THE BILIARY SYSTEM

The system consists of the bile ducts leading from the liver and gallbladder, the gallbladder itself, and associated structures. The system drains waste products from the liver into the duodenum and aids the process of fat digestion through controlled release of fat-emulsifying agents (contained within bile).

FAT DIGESTION

1 Dietary fat passes from the stomach to the duodenum in the form of large droplets.

2 Bile released into the duodenum contains salts that disperse the fat into smaller droplets.

3 The fats are now more easily broken down by an enzyme, lipase, made by the pancreas, and absorbed through the intestinal lining.

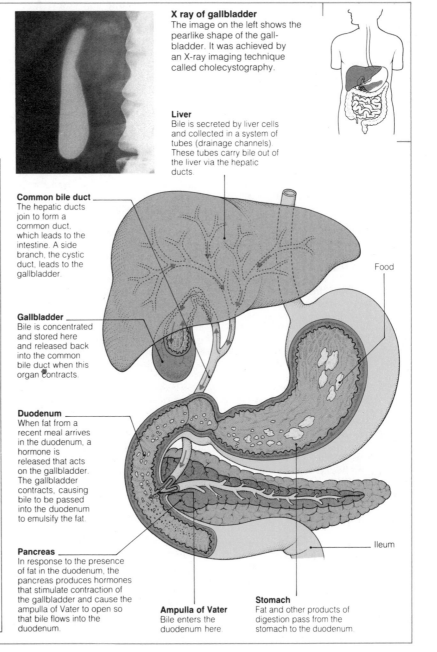

X ray of gallbladder
The image on the left shows the pearlike shape of the gallbladder. It was achieved by an X-ray imaging technique called cholecystography.

Liver
Bile is secreted by liver cells and collected in a system of tubes (drainage channels). These tubes carry bile out of the liver via the hepatic ducts.

Common bile duct
The hepatic ducts join to form a common duct, which leads to the intestine. A side branch, the cystic duct, leads to the gallbladder.

Gallbladder
Bile is concentrated and stored here and released back into the common bile duct when this organ contracts.

Duodenum
When fat from a recent meal arrives in the duodenum, a hormone is released that acts on the gallbladder. The gallbladder contracts, causing bile to be passed into the duodenum to emulsify the fat.

Pancreas
In response to the presence of fat in the duodenum, the pancreas produces hormones that stimulate contraction of the gallbladder and cause the ampulla of Vater to open so that bile flows into the duodenum.

Ampulla of Vater
Bile enters the duodenum here.

Stomach
Fat and other products of digestion pass from the stomach to the duodenum.

Food

Ileum

B

formed from the breakdown of bilirubin are responsible for the brown color of feces.

Billings' method

A technique (also called the mucus inspection method) in which a woman notes changes in her normal vaginal discharge to predict the time of ovulation for purposes of *contraception* or *family planning*.

Billroth's operation

A type of partial *gastrectomy* in which the lower part of the stomach is removed. Devised by the Viennese surgeon Theodor Billroth, it was the first successful stomach operation and is still one of the standard operations for treating *peptic ulcer* and certain types of stomach tumor.

Binet test

The first *intelligence test* that attempted to measure higher mental functions rather than more primitive abilities, such as reaction times. It was devised by Alfred Binet and Theodor Simon for French schoolchildren in 1905.

Bio-

A prefix that describes a relationship to life, as in biology, the science of life.

Bioavailability

The amount of a drug that enters the bloodstream and thus reaches the tissues and organs throughout the body, usually expressed as a percentage of the dose given. In this way, the effectiveness of various means of administration or types of preparation can be compared. For instance, intravenous administration produces 100 percent bioavailability since the drug is injected directly into the bloodstream. Drugs given by mouth have a much lower bioavailability, because only a proportion of the drug can be absorbed through the digestive system; some drugs may be broken down in the liver before reaching the general circulation.

Preparations with equal bioavailabilities are described as bioequivalent. (See also *Drug*.)

Biochemistry

A science that studies the chemistry of living organisms, including human beings. The human body is made up of millions of cells that require nutrients and energy, and which grow, multiply, and die. The chemical processes involved in providing cells with energy, eliminating their wastes, repairing damage, cell growth, and normal and abnormal cell division are all studied by biochemists.

Life is maintained by a huge number of chemical reactions that are carried out inside cells and that link together in a complex way. These reactions together make up the *metabolism* of the body. The reactions which produce energy and break down food and body structures are termed catabolism, and those which build up body structures and store away food are termed anabolism. Overall, large-scale regulation of all these processes is a function of *hormones* (chemicals secreted into the bloodstream by the *endocrine glands*), whereas regulation of individual metabolic reactions is carried out by *enzymes* (biological catalysts).

Some vital chemical processes occur in every cell in the body. Other chemical processes are confined to specialized cells that make up the tissues of particular organs; for example, liver cells store and chemically modify the digestion products of food, and kidney cells help to control the amounts of various substances in the blood (such as certain minerals), as well as regulating the amount of fluid in the body.

There is a constant interchange between fluids, which move in and out of cells, and blood and urine. As a consequence, biochemists can learn about the chemical changes going on inside cells from measurements of the various minerals, gases, enzymes, hormones, and proteins in blood and urine. Such tests are used to make diagnoses, to screen people for disease, and to monitor the progress of a disease and its treatment. The most important biochemical tests are *blood tests* (such as *liver function tests*), *kidney function tests*, and *urinalysis*.

Biofeedback training

A technique in which a person uses information about a normally unconscious body function, such as blood pressure, to gain conscious control over that function.

WHY IT IS USED

Biofeedback training may help in the treatment of various stress-related conditions, including certain types of *hypertension* (high blood pressure), *anxiety*, and *migraine*.

HOW IT IS DONE

The physician connects the patient to a recording instrument that can measure one of the unconscious body activities: blood pressure, pulse rate, body temperature, muscle tension, the amount of sweat on the skin, brain waves, or stomach acidity. The patient receives information (feedback) on the changing levels of these activities from alterations in the instrument's signals—a flashing light, a fluctuating needle, or a sound changing its tone.

After some experience with the technique, the person starts to become aware of how he or she is feeling whenever there is a change in the recording instrument's signal. *Relaxation techniques* may also be used to bring about a change in the signal; the response of the biofeedback machine may indicate which methods of relaxation are most effective.

With time, the patient learns to change the signals at will, by consciously controlling the body function being tested. Once acquired, this control can be exercised without the instrument.

Biomechanical engineering

A discipline that applies engineering principles and methods to the human body to explain how it functions and to treat disorders. Joint movements, the reaction of bone to stress, and the flow of blood are among the body activities that can be looked at in terms of these principles. Practical applications include the design of artificial joints, plaster casts, kidney dialysis machines, and artificial heart valves.

Biopsy

A diagnostic test in which tissue or cells are removed from the body for examination under the microscope. Most biopsies are minor procedures that require no sedation, but some require local or general anesthesia. Biopsy is an accurate method of diagnosing many illnesses, including cancer. The term biopsy is also commonly used for the cell or tissue sample itself (although the term biopsy specimen is more correct).

WHY IT IS DONE

Microscopic examination of tissue (*histology*) or of cells (*cytology*) usually gives a correct diagnosis. Biopsy is valuable for discovering whether a tumor is benign or malignant, since a malignant tumor usually has many features that clearly distinguish it from a benign tumor.

In the case of a malignant tumor, biopsies of the surrounding tissue and the lymph nodes can be done to determine whether the cancer has spread. Another important use of biopsies is to determine the cause of unexplained infections and inflammations.

HOW IT IS DONE

INCISIONAL BIOPSY This consists of cutting away a small piece of skin or muscle for analysis. Usually only a local anesthetic is required.

NEEDLE BIOPSY A needle is inserted through the skin and into the organ or tumor to be investigated. The needle may be fitted with a cutting tip to help remove a piece of tissue for examination. Aspiration biopsy is another type of needle biopsy in which the cells that are sucked from a tumor are examined cytologically. Usually, only a local anesthetic is required.

Until recently, if the target area could not be felt through the skin, or the organ was not accessible by endoscopic biopsy (see below), the physician would have to work blindly, relying only on experience and a knowledge of anatomy, so that deep-needle biopsy was almost never done. Today, guided biopsy, using *ultrasound scanning* or *CT scanning* to precisely locate the tissue to be biopsied and follow the progress of the needle, makes the procedure far more accurate, safe, and productive. In addition, the recent use of very fine needles for biopsies allows for safe sampling of tumors in organs such as the salivary glands and pancreas, in which sampling with larger needles was considered dangerous.

ENDOSCOPIC BIOPSY An *endoscope* (viewing tube) is passed into the organ to be investigated and an attachment (such as forceps to remove tissue or brushes to remove cells) is used to take a sample.

The procedure, which usually requires sedation, is used to take samples from the lining of accessible hollow organs and structures, such as the lungs, bladder, esophagus, stomach, and colon.

OPEN BIOPSY This is part of an operation, usually requiring a general anesthetic, in which the surgeon opens a body cavity, such as the chest or abdomen, to reveal a diseased organ or tumor, and removes a sample of tissue. Open biopsy is carried out when neither guided nor endoscopic biopsy is possible, or when it is likely that the organ or tumor will require removal. Prompt analysis of a tissue sample can enable the surgeon to decide whether to remove the entire diseased area immediately, so making a second operation unnecessary.

EXCISIONAL BIOPSY If a lump is found in the skin or an organ, such as the

BIOPSY PROCEDURES

NEEDLE (ASPIRATION) BIOPSY

1 The area is usually first numbed with local anesthetic, although occasionally a general anesthetic is required. A needle attached to a syringe is then inserted into the cyst or tumor to be investigated and cells are sucked out to be examined cytologically.

2 Before examination, the fluid is sometimes spun at high speed in a centrifuge and a small amount is placed on a slide.

3 The cells are then fixed (preserved) and finally stained for viewing. The cytologist examines individual cells for abnormalities, paying particular attention to the size, shape, and structure of the nucleus.

Cells as seen through microscope

INCISIONAL BIOPSY

1 The area is first numbed with a local anesthetic and a section of tissue is cut away. The wound is then stitched.

2 The tissue is then embedded in wax so that it is given a firm consistency suitable for slicing. This process usually takes 24 hours.

3 The tissue is then cut into ultra-thin slices and transferred to a slide. The pathologist conducts an examination, looking for distortion or alteration of tissue structure.

Tissue sample as seen through microscope

ENDOSCOPIC BIOPSY

If an area of abnormal tissue is to be removed for further examination, the forceps attachment, shown here, is passed through an endoscope to remove the piece of tissue.

Endoscope

Forceps attachment

The forceps attachment is removing a tissue sample from a stomach.

B

breast, the surgeon may remove the lump completely and send the whole specimen for laboratory examination. If an abnormality is detectable only by an imaging technique, such as *mammography*, injected dye or fine wire probes may be used to identify the abnormal area for the surgeon.

OBTAINING A RESULT

When immediate diagnosis is essential (e.g., to enable breast cancer to be operated on without delay), the biopsy sample is prepared for preliminary microscopic examination in a few minutes by freezing or by smearing cells onto slides.

The sample may also be prepared for later, more detailed examination. For a tissue sample, this usually involves embedding the sample in wax and then *staining* it with dyes to show up structures more clearly or to identify particular constituents, such as *antibodies* or *enzymes*. In special cases, a biopsy sample may be examined under an electron *microscope*—for example, to determine the origin of certain tumors.

In the investigation of infections and inflammations, a tissue sample may be tested with specific antibodies. In some cases, a tissue *culture* may be required.

Many of the more specialized techniques for preparing biopsy specimens prolong the time required to make an exact diagnosis but allow for greater accuracy and more precise information about the outlook for patients with certain diseases.

Biorhythms

A term used to describe physiological functions that vary in a rhythmic way (e.g., the menstrual cycle, which repeats itself approximately every 28 days in fertile women).

Most biorhythms are based on a daily or circadian (24-hour) cycle. Our bodies are governed by an internal clock, itself regulated by *hormones* (chemicals secreted into the bloodstream by the *endocrine glands*). Periods of sleepiness and wakefulness may be affected by the level of melatonin, secreted by the pineal gland in the brain. Release of melatonin is stimulated by darkness and suppressed by light. When the normal regular division between night and day is distorted by air travel to a distant time zone, the body's internal clock is disrupted and the result is *jet lag* (the symptoms of which could theoretically be relieved by the administration of melatonin).

Cortisol, secreted by the adrenal glands, also reflects the sleeping and waking states, being low in the evening and high in the morning.

The applications of biorhythms are still being explored. For example, many asthmatics feel worse in the morning due to the cyclic release of hormones. This finding has implications for the management of their condition, and research groups are studying the optimum time of day for the administration of *bronchodilator drugs* and other drugs that interact with body functions that undergo rhythmic variations.

Bipolar disorder

An illness characterized by swings in mood between opposite extremes (see *Manic-depressive illness*).

Birth

See *Childbirth*.

Birth canal

The passage, extending from the cervix (neck of the uterus) to the introitus (vaginal opening), through which the baby passes during *childbirth*.

Birth control

Limitation of the number of children born, either to an individual or within a population. Most people in developed nations now practice birth control; as a result, their population growth rates have decreased. Furthermore, in some countries, political and social pressures are applied to couples in an attempt to reduce population growth. Nevertheless, the total world population is still increasing rapidly (see box).

WORLD POPULATION

The rapid rate of population growth is a major problem. Reduction in infant and child mortality, due to better sanitation and disease control, has increased the number of people reaching their reproductive years. Because the world's population is doubling every 35 years, the task of adequately feeding, educating, and employing people is becoming increasingly difficult.

World population growth
The chart on the right shows growth from 1750 to 1990.

Distribution by continent
The diagram below shows the 1990 population of each continent, given also as percentages of total world population.

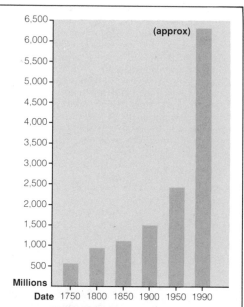

Date 1750 1800 1850 1900 1950 1990

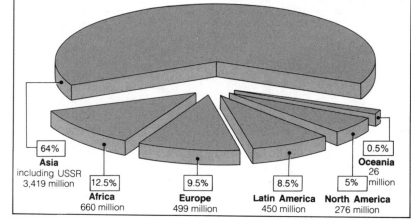

64%
Asia
including USSR
3,419 million

12.5%
Africa
660 million

9.5%
Europe
499 million

8.5%
Latin America
450 million

5%
North America
276 million

0.5%
Oceania
26 million

Family planning allows men and women to choose if and when to have children; *contraception* and abortion (see *Abortion, induced*) can prevent unwanted pregnancies.

Birth defects

Abnormalities obvious at birth or detectable early in infancy. Also called congenital defects, they encompass both minor abnormalities, such as *birthmarks,* and serious disorders such as *spina bifida* (a failure of the spinal column to close completely). Heart defects, about 3,700 a year, top Canada's list of serious birth abnormalities. The next most common disorders, with the annual incidence in parentheses), are genital defects, mostly in males (2,700); clubfoot (2,250); and defective fingers, bones, and muscles (1,650).

CAUSES
Birth defects may have a variety of different causes, but unknown factors also play a part. Among the recognized causes of birth defects are the following.

CHROMOSOME DEFECTS Some children are born with more or fewer than the normal 23 pairs of *chromosomes* (threadlike structures in cell nuclei that carry the information necessary for normal development)—or there are extra or missing parts of chromosomes (see *Chromosomal abnormalities*). In *Down's syndrome,* for example, where there is an extra chromosome, there is a higher incidence of congenital heart disease and intestinal defects.

GENETIC OR HEREDITARY DEFECTS These may be inherited from one or both parents (see *Genes; Genetic disorders*). Examples of genetic defects obvious at birth are *achondroplasia* and *albinism.*

DRUGS AND OTHER HARMFUL AGENTS Certain drugs can damage the fetus if taken by the mother during early pregnancy, the most notorious examples being *thalidomide,* a sedative widely prescribed in the late 1950s and early 1960s, and *isotretinoin,* used to treat acne. Thalidomide is no longer licensed in Canada, and isotretinoin should be given to women only if they are prepared to avoid becoming pregnant during the period of treatment.

Smoking by the mother can harm the fetus; some constituents of tobacco smoke diminish the baby's growth. Alcohol can have a similar effect and may also affect the development of the brain and face (see *Fetal alcohol syndrome*).

Drugs and chemicals that can harm the fetus in this way are collectively called *teratogens.*

IRRADIATION Irradiation of the embryo in early pregnancy—for example, if a woman is X-rayed before the pregnancy is recognized or if she receives *radiation therapy* for cancer—can cause abnormalities. However, great care is taken to prevent radiation from reaching the embryo if a woman is known to be (or might be) pregnant.

Radiation damage to the unborn child may also occur from atomic radiation or radioactive fallout (following a nuclear explosion or leak from a nuclear reactor). Heavy doses of radiation, as occurred at Hiroshima in 1945 for example, can cause serious mental and physical handicaps at birth. Even very small doses of radiation increase the child's risk of developing *leukemia* later in life (see *Radiation, hazards of*).

MATERNAL INFECTIONS Certain illnesses during pregnancy can cause birth defects. If a woman who has not been immunized against *rubella* (German measles) contracts the disease during the first three months of pregnancy, there is a 50 percent chance that her child will suffer brain, eye, ear, or heart abnormalities. Other types of infection, such as *toxoplasmosis,* may cause inflammation of the eyes, liver, spleen, and various other organs in the fetus.

PHYSICAL FACTORS IN THE UTERUS If the developing baby has too little fluid around it, its limbs may become distorted. *Talipes* (clubfoot) is thought to occur in this way.

Apart from defects of known cause, many others occur, the causes of which are unknown. Among the more common are abnormalities of the brain and spinal cord. In the embryo these structures develop from a simple, fluid-filled tube of nerve tissue. Interference in its development can lead to *spina bifida* with or without *hydrocephalus.*

The heart and blood vessels in a fetus develop from what in the embryo is a central muscular tube. If development of the cardiovascular system is impaired, a congenital heart disorder may result—for example, patent ductus arteriosus, septal defect, coarctation of the aorta, or transposition of the great vessels (see *Heart disease, congenital*).

Other common defects include *cleft lip and palate,* both of which result from a failure of the two halves of the fetal face and palate to join completely.

PREVENTION
Steps can be taken to minimize the risk of an abnormal child being born. For example, before starting a family,

genetic counseling should be obtained if either parent has relatives who have genetic or hereditary abnormalities. All women should make sure they are immune to rubella.

A woman should not smoke during pregnancy and should drink alcohol in moderation only. Unless prescribed by a doctor, drugs of any kind should be avoided during the first three months of pregnancy.

Various tests may be carried out when there is a possibility that a fetus may have some defect. Tests include *amniocentesis* (taking a sample of amniotic fluid from the uterus), blood tests to detect the level of *alpha-fetoprotein* (AFP) in the mother, *chorionic villus sampling* (removing a sample of tissue from the placenta), and *ultrasound scanning.*

Birth injury

Damage sustained during birth. All babies suffer at least minor trauma, such as abrasions or minor bruising. Bruising and swelling of the scalp during a vaginal delivery is sometimes marked (see *Cephalhematoma*).

More serious injury can occur, particularly if the baby is born prematurely or if the baby has difficulty passing through the mother's birth canal—for example, in a difficult *breech delivery.* Birth injuries are less common today, however, partly because more babies are delivered by *cesarean section.*

In breech deliveries, nerves in the shoulder region are sometimes injured, causing temporary paralysis in the arm. The face, likewise, may be paralyzed temporarily if the facial nerve is traumatized by forceps. Fractures of bones, such as the clavicle (collarbone), humerus (upper arm bone), and femur (thighbone), are another hazard of difficult deliveries. The bones usually heal easily.

Many cases of *cerebral palsy, mental retardation,* and *epilepsy* were once attributed to birth injury, but it is now considered that most of these problems are due to prenatal factors. Poor nutrition, smoking, maternal alcohol intake, bleeding during pregnancy, and prematurity are among the factors that can lead to brain damage or abnormal brain development. (See *Birth defects; Brain damage*.)

Birthmark

An area of discolored skin present from birth. The most common birthmarks are *moles* and freckles; these and other types of melanocytic *nevus*

B

(various flat, brown to blue-gray skin patches) are malformations of pigment cells.

Strawberry marks (bright red, usually protuberant areas) and port-wine stains (purple-red, flat, often large areas) are *hemangiomas* (malformations of blood vessels). Strawberry marks often increase in size in the first year but 90 percent disappear after the age of 9 years. Port-wine stains seldom fade.

Unsightly moles can be removed from late childhood onward by *plastic surgery*. Some port-wine stains can now be caused to fade by *laser treatment*; such treatment is best undertaken after the age of about 17 years. The most successful results have been in young adults.

Very rarely, a mole may develop into a type of skin cancer called a malignant *melanoma*. A mole that is large or irregular or suddenly starts to change shape, to darken or bleed, or to be tender, painful or itchy is cause for suspicion.

Birthmark
Strawberry marks—a common type of birthmark caused by malformation of blood vessels—are usually bright red, protuberant, and spongy.

Birth weight

The average full-term infant weighs 3.4 kg at birth. Few babies weigh less than 2.5 kg or more than 4.5 kg.

A baby's birth weight depends on a number of factors, including the size and ethnic origin of the parents. Small parents tend to have small babies. Asian infants tend to be smaller than white or black infants. Baby boys weigh, on average, slightly more than baby girls.

Babies who weigh less than 2.5 kg at birth are classified as being of low birth weight. About one half of these babies are small due to *prematurity*— that is, they were born before the 37th week of pregnancy. Others are small because they have been undernourished in the uterus, where the placenta was insufficient, for example,

because the mother had *preeclampsia* or smoked heavily during pregnancy.

Oversized babies are often born to mothers who have *diabetes mellitus*.

During the first few weeks of life, babies may lose up to 10 percent of their birth weight, but thereafter should steadily gain weight.

Bisexuality

Sexual interest in members of both sexes that may or may not involve sexual activity. Between what are regarded as being the two ends of the human sexuality spectrum—exclusive heterosexuality and exclusive homosexuality—there exists a continuous spectrum of bisexuality. Sexuality is determined by a person's sexual desires as well as his or her actual sexual behavior. Thus, the term bisexual includes those who suppress homosexual desires and behave exclusively as heterosexuals.

Sexual preference may vary during a person's lifetime. Alfred Kinsey, who conducted a broad study of human sexual habits in the United States during the 1940s, developed a scale that allowed him to rate the relative amounts of heterosexual and homosexual activity and/or responses during different periods in an individual's life. He concluded that, at some stage in their adult life, half the population engaged in both heterosexual and homosexual activity, or reacted sexually to persons of both sexes.

Bismuth

A metal, salts of which are used in tablets to treat *peptic ulcer* and in suppositories to treat *hemorrhoids* (piles). Bismuth salts adhere to ulcers of the stomach and duodenum and form a protective coating over them, thus promoting healing.

Bismuth preparations taken by mouth may color the feces black, simulating the presence of blood. The tongue may darken and occasional nausea and vomiting may also occur. Long-term treatment is avoided because of the risk of brain damage.

Bite

See *Occlusion*.

Bites, animal

Any injury inflicted by the mouthparts of an animal—from the tiny puncture wounds of bloodsucking insects to the massive injuries caused by shark or crocodile attacks. For discussion of special problems caused by bites of venomous snakes, spiders,

insects, and other venomous animals, see *Insect bites*; *Snakebites*; *Spider bites*; *Venomous bites and stings*.

INCIDENCE
The greatest number of animal attacks worldwide come from dogs, mainly strays. In Canada about 100,000 people annually are bitten badly enough by animals to seek hospital treatment. A few deaths each year result from dog bites, and occasionally from the bites of other domestic animals, such as horses, cattle, and pigs.

Wild animals that have killed or caused serious injuries to humans include lions, tigers, elephants, rhinoceroses, hippopotamuses, buffaloes, bears, wolves, hyenas, and wild pigs. Small mammals, such as rodents, cause less extensive injury but many such creatures have razor-sharp teeth and there is a high risk of infection from any bites they inflict.

About 100 shark attacks occur worldwide each year, of which half are fatal. In Africa, more than 1,000 people die annually from crocodile attacks. Other aquatic creatures capable of inflicting a serious bite include barracudas, piranhas, and moray and conger eels.

THE MAIN HAZARDS
TISSUE DAMAGE The biological function of the mouth is to obtain food and prepare it for digestion. Teeth, especially those of carnivores, are well adapted to tearing, crushing, and macerating tissues and bones, and can inflict severe and extensive mechanical injury.

BLOOD LOSS Severe injuries and lacerations to major blood vessels can lead to loss of a large amount of blood and physiological *shock*.

INFECTION An animal's mouth is heavily populated with bacteria and other microorganisms that thrive on food residue and debris. These organisms can produce serious secondary infection, especially in wounds where there is already extensive tissue damage. *Tetanus* is a particular hazard of animal bites.

RABIES In Canada any animal may potentially harbor the *rabies* virus and transmit it through infected saliva. A bat was the source of Canada's last rabies fatality—in Alberta in 1985. Only 21 persons have died of rabies in Canada since reporting began in 1925. But some 4,000 to 5,000 persons receive post-exposure treatment each year, half because of rabies-suspected pets—34 percent dogs, 16 percent cats. Approximately 13 percent are treated following exposure to suspect foxes. About 4,000 cases of rabies in animals are confirmed each year. Of these approximately 84 percent are in Ontario and about 12 percent in Saskatchewan. Some 80 percent of Agriculture Canada's laboratory-confirmed cases of animal rabies are found in wild creatures, close to 13 percent in farm animals, and less than 8 percent in pets. The fact that several people may have contact with one pet accounts for the numbers treated because of contact with pets, which form such a small percentage of the rabid population.

TREATMENT

Medical advice should be sought for all but minor injuries—or if there is any possibility of rabies. Treatment usually includes wound cleaning and examination (under anesthesia, if necessary). The wound will usually be left open and dressed, rather than stitched, because closing the wound tends to encourage the multiplication of bacteria that have been transmitted by the bite. Preventive antibiotic treatment, and an antitetanus injection, may also be given.

If possible, the animal that inflicted the bite should be held and checked for rabies. Sometimes, an antirabies vaccine or serum may need to be given. (See also *Bites, human*.)

Bites, human

Wounds caused by one person biting another. In general, these wounds are more serious than animal bites due to a higher complication and infection rate. People bite each other more often than might be supposed—commonly in the course of fights, as part of a general pattern of *child abuse*, or during sexual play.

HAZARDS

Human bites rarely cause serious tissue damage or blood loss. However, infection from any microorganisms in the mouth is as likely, or even more likely, than with animal bites, particularly if the bite is deep. There is a risk of *tetanus* infection.

The viruses responsible for *hepatitis B*, *herpes simplex*, *AIDS*, and *rabies* are present in the saliva of those affected by these illnesses. Transmission of hepatitis B and AIDS by a bite is a theoretical hazard. Human cases of rabies are extremely rare, and the risk of being bitten by a human victim would be generally confined to physicians and nurses caring for the patient.

Treatment for any bite that penetrates the skin is as for *Bites, animal*.

Black death

The medieval name for *bubonic plague*. One feature of the disease is bleeding that occurs beneath the skin, causing dark blue or black bruises. This, along with the fact that in medieval times the disease was fatal in more than 50 percent of cases, accounts for the name.

Black eye

The bruised appearance of the skin around the eye, usually following an injury. Any direct blow damages the many small blood vessels beneath the skin, causing blood to leak and collect there.

Because the skin around the eyes is loose and transparent, bruising is darker in this area than on other parts of the body. A cold compress held over the eye will help to relieve the discomfort.

Blackhead

A semisolid, black-capped plug of greasy material blocking the outlet of a sebaceous (oil-forming) gland in the skin. Blackheads occur most commonly on the face, chest, shoulders, and back, alone or in groups, and are associated with increased sebaceous gland activity, which is normal in adolescents. Blackheads are a characteristic feature of certain types of *acne*.

Blackout

A common term for loss of consciousness (see *Fainting*).

Black teeth

See *Discolored teeth*.

Blackwater fever

An occasional and life-threatening complication of falciparum *malaria* (the most dangerous form of malaria). The condition is brought on by a sudden increased rate of destruction of red blood cells. The breakdown products of the cells find their way via the kidneys into the urine and cause it to darken, hence "blackwater." Other symptoms include loss of consciousness, fever, chills, and vomiting.

Bladder

The hollow, muscular organ in the lower abdomen that acts as a reservoir for *urine*. The adult bladder can hold half a litre or more of urine. It lies behind the pubic bone, hidden within and protected by the bony pelvis.

The bladder walls consist of muscle and an inner lining called urinary epithelium. At the back are the two

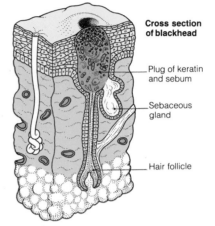

Cross section of blackhead

Plug of keratin and sebum

Sebaceous gland

Hair follicle

ureters, which carry urine to the bladder from the kidneys. At the lowest point of the bladder—the neck—is the opening into the urethra; this is normally kept tightly closed by a ring of muscle (the urethral sphincter).

FUNCTION

The bladder's function is to collect and store urine until it can be expelled from the body at a suitable time.

Full control over bladder function takes several years to develop. In infants, emptying of the bladder is an entirely automatic or *reflex* reaction. When the bladder fills and stretches beyond a certain point, signals are sent to the spinal cord. Nerve signals from the spinal cord then cause the urethral sphincter to relax and the main bladder muscle to contract, thus expelling urine via the urethra.

As the child grows, he or she gradually develops the ability to delay emptying. Stretching of the bladder is registered consciously (as discomfort) in brain centers, which, if desired, can then send nerve signals suppressing the emptying reflex. Eventually, however, the bladder becomes so full and stretched that the urge to pass urine is overwhelming.

Children vary in the age at which they achieve perfect bladder control and, in particular, night-time control. Most children are dry at night by the age of five years, but some take longer (see *Enuresis*).

Defective bladder function, leading to problems such as involuntary emptying of the bladder and complete or partial *urinary retention*, can have a variety of causes. (See *Bladder disorders box*.)

Bladder cancer

See *Bladder tumors*.

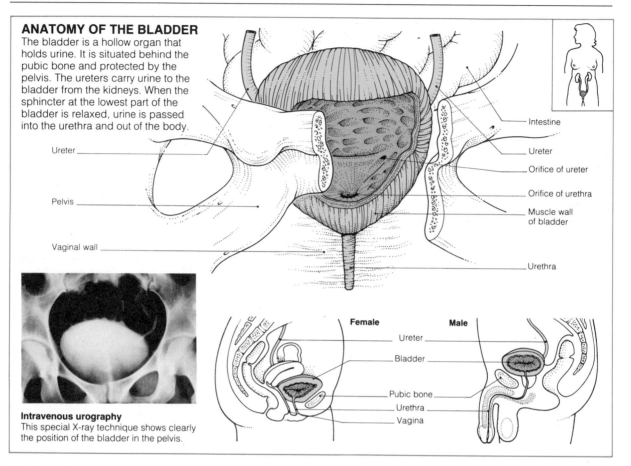

ANATOMY OF THE BLADDER

The bladder is a hollow organ that holds urine. It is situated behind the pubic bone and protected by the pelvis. The ureters carry urine to the bladder from the kidneys. When the sphincter at the lowest part of the bladder is relaxed, urine is passed into the urethra and out of the body.

Ureter

Pelvis

Vaginal wall

Intestine

Ureter

Orifice of ureter

Orifice of urethra

Muscle wall of bladder

Urethra

Intravenous urography
This special X-ray technique shows clearly the position of the bladder in the pelvis.

Female   Male

Ureter

Bladder

Pubic bone

Urethra

Vagina

Bladder tumors

Growths originating in the inner lining of the bladder. Many bladder tumors are *papillomas* (small wart-like growths), which tend to recur, and eventually may become cancerous. Other, more malignant growths tend to spread inward, into the bladder cavity, but may also spread through the bladder wall to nearby organs, such as the rectum, colon, prostate gland, or uterus, and to the lymph glands and pelvic bones.

Bladder cancers account for about 7 percent of all cancers in men (3,500 new cases a year) and 2.5 percent of all cancers in women (1,200 new cases a year). The average age at diagnosis is 65 years.

Certain groups are at increased risk, notably smokers and workers in the dye and rubber industries. Exposure to carcinogenic substances used in these industries or in tobacco smoke is the presumed cause in these groups. Bladder cancer is also common in areas of the tropics where the parasitic infection *schistosomiasis* is prevalent.

PREVENTION

Avoiding smoking is the principal means of reducing the personal risk. The incidence of occupational bladder cancer has been reduced by protective measures in the industries concerned and by screening of those who have been exposed in the past.

SYMPTOMS

Hematuria (blood in the urine) is the main symptom. Passing urine is usually painless, but a bladder infection may develop, and the passage of urine then becomes painful and frequent. Sometimes, a tumor may obstruct the entry of a ureter into the bladder, causing back pressure and pain in the kidney region, or may obstruct the urethral exit, causing difficulty in passing urine.

DIAGNOSIS AND TREATMENT

Bladder tumors are investigated by *cystoscopy* (passage of a slim viewing tube up the urethra into the bladder) and by *biopsy* (removal of a sample of tissue for microscopic analysis). Early tumors are usually cut out or treated by *diathermy* (heat destruction) via the cystoscope. Tumors recur in at least 60 percent of cases, so regular follow-up cystoscopy is necessary. Recurrences may be treated surgically or with a solution of *anticancer drugs* introduced into the bladder.

In the case of a more widely spread cancer, treatment is usually by *radiation therapy*, though if this fails, more drastic surgery to remove the bladder (see *Cystectomy*) may be necessary.

OUTLOOK

This varies according to what stage the growth has reached when first diagnosed. If a tumor is diagnosed and treated early, the long-term prospects are excellent. However, if cancer has spread beyond the bladder wall, the chances of survival for more than five years are poor.

Bleaching, dental

A cosmetic procedure for lightening some types of *discolored teeth*, including nonvital "dead" teeth. The surface of the affected tooth is painted with chemical oxidizing agents and then exposed to ultraviolet light.

DISORDERS OF THE BLADDER

The most important causes of bladder problems are infection, tumors, *calculi* (stones), or impairment of the bladder's nerve supply.

INFECTION

Infection of the bladder, better known as *cystitis*, is particularly common in women, mainly because of the much shorter female urethra, which provides less of a barrier to bacteria. In men, infection is usually associated with obstruction to the flow of urine from the bladder by, for example, tumors of the bladder or an enlarged prostate gland. In some parts of the tropics, the parasitic worm infection *schistosomiasis* (bilharziasis) is a common cause of bladder problems.

TUMORS

Bladder tumors may be benign or malignant and are more common in men than in women. They are usually painless in the early stages and may cause *hematuria* (blood in the urine) or obstruction to the outflow of urine from the bladder. The latter may also be caused by a tumor or enlargement of the prostate and result in partial or complete *urine retention* and stagnation in the bladder.

Tumors of the spinal cord may affect the nerves controlling the bladder, leading either to retention or *incontinence*.

CALCULI

Calculi (stones) in the bladder, caused by the precipitation from solution of substances present in the urine, are an uncommon problem. They mainly affect men and usually result from urinary retention and/or a long-standing urinary tract infection. In some other parts of the world, such as Southeast Asia, they are more common and are often associated with a low-protein diet.

Cancer
● a growth that can arise from any part of the bladder wall

Urethral stricture
● narrowing that can be due to infection or trauma

Infection
● causing inflammation of bladder wall

Stone
● can block urethral opening

Enlarged prostate
● causing slow urination

INJURY

Injury to the bladder is uncommon. It may occur, however, if the pelvis is fractured when the bladder is full. Such injury typically occurs in traffic accidents. The bladder ruptures and urine leaks into the abdominal and pelvic cavities.

Damage to the nerves involved in bladder control may severely disrupt bladder filling and emptying, causing either incontinence or urinary retention, depending on the site of the injury. The most common cause of such damage is spinal cord injury due to road traffic accidents. Nerves that control the bladder may also be damaged by a prolapsed intervertebral disk.

OTHER DISORDERS

Disturbance of bladder control can also result from nerve degeneration found in conditions such as *diabetes mellitus*, *multiple sclerosis*, or *dementia*.

An unstable or *irritable bladder* is a common condition in which the urge to empty the bladder occurs frequently. It is not fully understood but is sometimes associated with a *urinary tract infection* or prolapse of the uterus. Many other underlying conditions, most com-

monly tension or anxiety, can cause frequent urination.

Failure to achieve bladder control by the age of 3 or 4 is termed *enuresis* (bed-wetting); this may be due to a treatable physical cause, such as urinary tract infection, or to emotional problems but more often results from delayed maturation of the nervous system.

INVESTIGATION

Various methods are used to investigate bladder disorders. Urinary tract infection is diagnosed by culturing a urine sample. The bladder can be viewed directly by *cystoscopy*. X-ray studies include micturating *cystourethrography*, which normally shows only the bladder and urethra, and intravenous *urography*, which shows the whole urinary tract except the urethra. *Cystometry* measures bladder capacity in relation to pressure.

Bleeding

Loss of blood from the *circulatory system* caused by damage to the blood vessels or by a *bleeding disorder*. Bleeding may be visible (external) or concealed (internal). Rapid loss of more than 10 percent of the blood volume can cause symptoms of shock.

CAUSES

The most common cause of bleeding is an injury. The speed with which blood flows from a cut depends on the type of blood vessel damaged: blood usually oozes from a capillary, flows from a vein, and spurts from an artery. If an injury does not break open the skin, blood collects around the damaged blood vessels close under the skin to form a *bruise*.

Damage to internal blood vessels may be the result of inflammation, infection, an ulcer, or a tumor. Any lost blood that mixes with other bodily fluids such as sputum (phlegm) or urine will be noticed quite readily; bleeding in the digestive tract may make vomit or feces appear darker than usual because the blood is partially digested. Sometimes, internal bleeding is not discovered until severe *anemia* develops.

Bleeding that is not caused by injury usually requires medical investiga-

B

tion. The obvious exceptions are an occasional minor *nosebleed* and bleeding during *menstruation*. The amount of blood lost during menstruation varies from woman to woman and from month to month. Menstrual blood loss is only a problem if it is very heavy or frequent, when it might lead to iron-deficiency anemia.

Bleeding disorders

A group of conditions characterized by bleeding in the absence of injury or by abnormally prolonged and excessive bleeding after injury.

Bleeding disorders result from defects in the mechanisms by which bleeding is normally stopped (see *Blood clotting*). These mechanisms are blood coagulation, plugging of damaged blood vessels by platelets, and constriction of blood vessels.

Defects in the coagulation system tend to cause deep bleeding into the gastrointestinal tract, the muscles, and the joint cavities. Defects of the platelets or blood vessels usually produce superficial bleeding into the skin, gums, or lining of the intestine or urinary tract. However, bleeding may occur anywhere in the body with any type of bleeding defect.

COAGULATION DEFECTS
These disorders usually result from deficiencies of the enzymes (called coagulation factors) that take part in blood clotting, or from the enzymes being abnormal. Blood-clot formation is very slow and the clots are weak and do not seal blood vessels securely. Coagulation defects may be congenital (present from birth) or acquired later in life.

CONGENITAL The principal congenital coagulation defects are *hemophilia, Christmas disease,* and *von Willebrand's disease*. In each of these, one of the coagulation factors is either absent from the blood or is present in only small amounts.

Hemophilia and Christmas disease are similar disorders, resulting from deficiencies of two different coagulation factors, called factor VIII and factor IX, respectively. The inheritance of these disorders is sex-linked (see *Genetic disorders*), which means that only males are affected. About 10 persons per 100,000 have hemophilia and about two persons per 100,000 have Christmas disease.

Von Willebrand's disease is also an inherited disorder in which there is a factor VIII defect, but one that affects both sexes roughly equally. About five persons per 100,000 are affected.

Individuals with bleeding disorders may suffer from bruising, internal bleeding, abnormally heavy menstrual periods, and excessive bleeding from wounds. In severe cases, sufferers may bleed recurrently into joints such as the knee.

ACQUIRED Deficiencies of coagulation factors may develop at any age as a result of severe liver disease, digestive system disorders that prevent the absorption from the diet of *vitamin K* (required to make some coagulation factors), or the use of *anticoagulant drugs*, such as warfarin, that prevent normal production of coagulation factors. As with congenital bleeding disorders, a severe bleeding tendency may result.

One particularly complex coagulation disorder is disseminated intravascular coagulation (DIC), which may be triggered by any of a variety of circumstances. In DIC, there is aggregation of platelets and clotting within small blood vessels. Subsequently, coagulation factors are used and broken up in the blood faster than they can be replaced by the liver, and severe bleeding may result. Paradoxically, anticoagulant drugs are sometimes used to interfere with clotting activity in this condition, but in most cases this very serious condition does not improve until the underlying problem (for example, infection or cancer) is brought under control.

Coagulation defects are investigated by *blood-clotting tests* such as the prothrombin time. Treatment is based on giving the patient transfusions of the missing coagulation factor or factors in fresh blood or fresh frozen plasma. Research is being carried out to prepare these factors synthetically, but for the time being, the factors are obtained from human blood. Transmission of some viral infections (e.g., *hepatitis B* and *HIV* infection) has occurred in the past, but blood is now checked for harmful viruses and discarded if necessary. Blood products are also heat-treated in an attempt to destroy viruses.

PLATELET DEFECTS
Bleeding may occur if there are too few platelets in the blood—a condition called *thrombocytopenia*. The main feature of this disorder is surface bleeding into the skin and gums, causing multiple small bruises.

Occasionally, the platelets are present in normal numbers but function abnormally, with resultant bleeding. Defects of platelet function may be inherited, may be associated with the use of certain drugs (including *ASA*), or may be a complication of certain bone marrow disorders such as myeloid *leukemia*.

Platelet defects are investigated by tests, such as measuring bleeding time and clotting time, and various other tests of platelet aggregation (clumping). Whatever the cause, the main treatment consists of transfusions of platelets from single donors or from "pools" (obtained from several normal blood transfusions). The transfusions need to be given every one to three days until the underlying defect has been corrected and the body is again producing its own healthy platelets.

BLOOD VESSEL DEFECTS
In rare cases, abnormal bleeding is caused by a blood vessel defect. In the past, *scurvy* (a disorder caused by vitamin C deficiency) was a common and often fatal disorder of this type, affecting sailors, polar explorers, and anyone with a diet lacking fresh fruit and vegetables. Today, mild scurvy is occasionally seen in elderly people on a poor diet.

Elderly people and patients on long-term courses of *corticosteroid drugs* may suffer mild abnormal bruising due to loss of skin support to the smallest blood vessels. Treatment is rarely required.

Bleeding gums
See *Gingivitis*.

Bleeding, treatment of
Part of the body's response to internal or external loss of blood is to constrict the damaged blood vessels and to cause blood to clot at the site of injury. At the same time, blood flow may be reduced in the skin and muscles to make sure that the brain, kidneys, and other vital organs are adequately supplied. Loss of a large volume of blood quickly causes a dramatic fall in blood pressure, accompanied by weakness, confusion, pallor, and sweating as the body tries to compensate; this state is known as *shock*.

First aid measures have two objectives: to minimize blood loss and to help the body cope with the loss. In most cases, bleeding can be stopped, or at least slowed, by direct pressure (see box).

PROFESSIONAL TREATMENT
When bleeding is severe, intravenous infusions of saline solution and plasma preparations may be given to help replace fluids lost from the circulation. If a large amount of blood is

lost, *blood transfusion* may also be required. Large wounds may need closing with sutures (stitches), which are effective in stopping bleeding from scalp injuries and also reduce the extent of scarring. If bleeding within the abdomen is suspected following an accident, *CT scanning* and/or exploratory surgery may be needed. If bleeding within the skull is compressing the brain, a hole will be drilled in the skull to relieve the pressure.

Severe bleeding may require treatment in the operating room. During operations, bleeding from small blood vessels is controlled by clamping them with forceps and then either tying them or sealing them by *diathermy* (the application of a high-frequency electric current).

Blepharitis

Inflammation of the eyelids, with redness, irritation, and scaly skin at the lid margins. The patient may complain of burning and discomfort in the eyes and flakes or crusts may be found on the lashes. Occasionally, the surface of the eye may also be inflamed and red. In some cases, the roots of the eyelashes become infected, and small ulcers form. Blepharitis is common, tends to recur, and is sometimes associated with dandruff of the scalp or eczema.

The problem can often be cleared up by removing the scales with cotton wool moistened with warm water. Blepharitis of the lid margins frequently recurs, especially after periods of stress or illness, or when aggravated by dust or tobacco smoke, and requires further treatment. Ulcerated eyelids need medical attention. Severe cases of blepharitis may lead to *corneal ulcers*. Various eye drops reduce discomfort even though they cannot prevent recurrences.

Blepharoplasty

A cosmetic operation to remove wrinkled, drooping skin from the upper and/or lower eyelids. The operation is usually done under local anesthesia and takes about one and a half hours. The patient can usually go home the same day.

WHY IT IS DONE

As a person grows older, the skin loses some of its fat, and much of its elasticity, becoming droopy and creased. This process may be accelerated by worry or sudden weight loss. As a result, the eyelids become baggy. Removing the excess skin can greatly improve appearance.

FIRST AID: TREATING BLEEDING

SIMPLE CUT

1 Wash your hands before dealing with the cut. Then, if the cut has dirt in it, rinse it lightly under lukewarm running water until it is clean, being careful not to touch the spout.

2 Dab the cut gently with sterile gauze to dry it. Then dress the cut with an adhesive dressing.

DEEP CUT

1 Raise the injured part and support it. Put a sterile dressing on the wound and apply firm pressure to control bleeding.

2 If blood seeps through, do not remove the dressing as this may disturb clots and restart bleeding. Put other dressings on top of the first one and bandage all dressings snugly.

HOW IT IS DONE

On the upper lids a horizontal fold of skin is removed from the center of each lid so that the resultant scar runs in a natural crease line. On the lower lids the incision is made just below the eyelashes, so that the scar will be in the shadow of the lashes and extend into a smile wrinkle. The baggy skin is pulled upward and outward, the excess is removed, and the wound is then stitched.

RECOVERY PERIOD

After the operation, ice packs and pads soaked with witch hazel solution are applied to both eyes, to reduce swelling and bruising. The patient is advised to repeat these applications at home. Swelling usually subsides within three days but bruising may last for as long as two weeks.

Some of the stitches are removed three to five days after the operation, the rest seven to 10 days after. The scars usually fade to fine, unnoticeable marks after six to 12 months.

Blepharospasm

Involuntary, prolonged contraction of one of the muscles that control the eyelids, causing the eyes to close. It may be

Appearance before (inset) and after
Blepharoplasty involves removal of a crescent-shaped section of skin and underlying fat from each eyelid.

B

due to *photophobia* (abnormal sensitivity of the eyes to light), *blepharitis* (inflammation of the eyelids), *anxiety*, or *hysteria*. Treatment is aimed at remedying the cause.

Blind loop syndrome

A condition in which abnormal feces occur due to a redundant area or dead end (blind loop) in the small intestine. Blind loop syndrome is characterized by *steatorrhea* (pale yellow, foul-smelling, fatty, bulky feces that are difficult to flush away), together with general sickness, tiredness, and weight loss. The syndrome is usually the result of surgery but may be *congenital* (present at birth).

The blind loop interferes with the normal flow of bowel contents, resulting in stagnation. Bacteria other than the usual dominant inhabitants of the bowel proliferate in the loop and spread into other areas of the intestine, where they interfere with the absorption of nutrients, including fat and vitamin B_{12}.

Antibiotic treatment, usually with a *tetracycline drug*, may be successful. If not, surgery to remove the blind loop usually cures the condition.

Blindness

Inability to see. Generally, the term blindness refers to a severe loss of *vision* that cannot be corrected with ordinary *glasses*. Precise definitions of blindness and of partial sight vary. In Canada, blindness is usually defined as a *visual acuity* of 6/60 or less in the better eye, or

a *visual field* of no more than 20 degrees in the better eye. Partial sight is a lesser degree of visual disability, which affects employment or normal living.

INCIDENCE
It is estimated that more than 40 million people in the world are partially or totally blind. *Vitamin A* deficiency alone accounts for blindness in millions of children living in developing countries of Africa, Asia, and South America.

In Canada, about 500,000 persons have significantly impaired vision.

CAUSES
Blindness may result from injury, disease, or degeneration of the eyeball, of the optic nerve or nerve pathways connecting the eye to the brain, or of the brain itself.

EYEBALL Normal vision depends on the uninterrupted passage of light from the front of the eye to the light-sensitive retina at the back. Anything that prevents light from reaching the retina can cause blindness.

Various disorders may impair the transparency of the cornea at the front of the eye. In *Sjögren's syndrome*, an inability to produce tears leads to *keratoconjunctivitis sicca*, which, if severe, causes the cornea to cloud over. Other causes of a cloudy cornea include vitamin A deficiency, accidental chemical damage, infections, and injury. *Corneal ulcers* can also cause blindness because they leave scars after healing. The most common causes of such ulcers are severe attacks of certain infections,

among them *ophthalmia* neonatorum (inflammation of the conjunctiva in newborn babies), *trachoma* (most common in hot, overcrowded regions), *herpes simplex*, and bacterial ulcers.

Inflammation of the iris, ciliary body, or choroid—a condition known as *uveitis*—can cause loss of vision. The inflammation may occur in association with *tuberculosis*, *sarcoidosis*, *syphilis*, *toxocariasis*, or *toxoplasmosis*, but often occurs for no known reason.

Cataract (cloudiness of the lens) is a common cause of blindness. It is usually the result of the lens becoming less transparent in old age, but is occasionally present from birth or develops in childhood.

Diabetes mellitus, *hypertension*, or injury can cause bleeding into the cavity of the eyeball. In *hyphema*, blood enters the aqueous humor (watery substance in front of the lens). *Vitreous hemorrhage* is bleeding into the jellylike vitreous humor behind the lens.

Disorders of the retina are a common cause of blindness. They include age-related *macular degeneration* (degeneration of the central area of the retina, which occurs in old age), *retinopathy* due to diabetes or hypertension, *retinal artery occlusion* or *retinal vein occlusion* (blockage of the blood flow to or from the retina), *retinal detachment*, tumors such as *retinoblastoma* and malignant *melanoma* of the eye, and *retinal hemorrhage* (bleeding into the retina), caused by diabetes, hypertension, vascular disease, or injury.

AIDS FOR THE BLIND

There are many ways in which life can be made easier for the blind person, and there are now a number of specially designed and adapted devices available. These include braille writers, mathematical apparatus, and home appliances, as well as aids for helping the blind person get around outside the home.

Liquid level indicator
This device measures liquid being poured into a cup or glass. Two sets of prongs are connected to a bleeper. A short set of prongs measures almost to the top, while the long set measures small amounts in the bottom. A bleep sounds when the liquid makes contact with the prongs.

Pocket watch
Strengthened hands and raised dots make it easier for a blind person to "read" numerals: three dots are at 12, two are at 3, 6, and 9, and one is at each of the other hour positions.

Pocket braille maker
This frame produces braille on one side of the paper. A special pointed stylus is used to make the braille indentations; a stencil keeps the stylus in the right place. The braille can be read without removing the paper from the frame.

In *glaucoma*, another common cause of blindness, excessive pressure in the eyeball causes degeneration of nerve fibers at the front end of the optic nerve. The most common type of glaucoma can cause loss of side vision, which may not be noticed until the disease is well advanced.

OPTIC NERVE AND NERVE PATHWAYS The light energy received by the retina is transformed into nerve impulses that travel along the optic nerve and nerve pathways into the brain. Conduction of these impulses may be impaired by pressure from a tumor in the orbit (the bony cavity that contains the eyeball) or in the brain; by interference with the blood supply to the optic nerve, caused by diabetes mellitus, hypertension, a tumor, injury, or *temporal arteritis*; by *optic neuritis* (inflammation of the optic nerve that may occur in *multiple sclerosis*); by toxic amblyopia, which is caused by the poisonous effects of certain chemicals; or by nutritional deficiency amblyopia, which is caused by a lack of certain essential nutrients in the diet.

BRAIN Nerve impulses from the retina eventually arrive in a region of the *cerebrum* (main mass of the brain) called the visual cortex. Here, the nerve impulses are analyzed and interpreted to provide conscious images. Blindness can be caused if there is pressure on the visual cortex from a *brain tumor* or *brain hemorrhage*, or if a *stroke* reduces the blood supply to the cortex.

Finally, apparent blindness may be related to *hysteria*, a reaction to severe stress in which physical symptoms develop without any physical cause, or to *malingering*.

DIAGNOSIS AND TREATMENT
Anyone who suffers a loss of vision, whether partial or complete, should consult a doctor immediately. Various types of *vision tests* can be done.

Often, the cause can be ascertained by direct examination of the eye, including ophthalmoscopy, slit-lamp examination, tonometry, and perimetry. Electrical activity produced in the brain following visual stimulation can be measured by visual potentiometry (see *Evoked responses*). The age and medical history of the patient, the patient's account of the development of the sight loss, and other signs and symptoms, may provide important clues to the diagnosis. In a few cases, *ultrasound scanning*, *CT scanning*, or *MRI* may be performed to look for any abnormalities in the eyes, orbits, structures around the optic nerves, or brain. *Fluorescein angiography* (a technique for photo-graphing the vessels of the eye) may be used to study the retina and choroid. Treatment depends on the underlying cause. If the loss of vision cannot be corrected, the patient may then be registered as legally blind or partially sighted. Certain services and benefits may then be available. (See also *Eye*; *Vision, loss of*.)

Blind spot

The small, oval-shaped area on the retina of the eye where the optic nerve joins the eyeball. The area is not sensitive to light because it has no light receptors (nerve endings responsive to light). To demonstrate the presence of the blind spot, mark an X on a piece of paper and a dot 15 cm to the right. While holding the paper at arm's length, shut your left eye and look at the X with your right eye. Slowly move the paper toward you until the dot disappears. This is the point at which the image of the dot has fallen on your right eye's blind spot.

Blister

A collection of fluid beneath the outer layer of the skin that forms a raised area, which is usually oval or circular in shape. Large blisters (any that are more than 1 cm in diameter) are sometimes called bullae; small blisters are sometimes called vesicles.

The fluid in a blister is serum that has leaked from blood vessels in underlying skin layers after minor damage. The fluid is usually sterile and the blister provides valuable protection to the damaged tissue.

CAUSES
Common causes of blisters are *burns* (including *sunburn*) and friction—for example, from an ill-fitting shoe.

A number of skin diseases can also cause blisters. These include *eczema*, *impetigo*, *erythema multiforme*, and *epidermolysis bullosa*, the bullous disorders *pemphigoid*, *pemphigus*, and *dermatitis herpetiformis*, and some types of *porphyria*.

Small blisters develop at an early stage in the rashes of the viral infections *chickenpox*, *herpes zoster* (shingles), and *herpes simplex*; these blisters contain infectious virus particles that may spread the infection.

TREATMENT
A blister is best left to heal on its own. It should not be burst, because the underlying damaged tissue could become infected. In the case of large, troublesome, or unexplained blisters, consult your physician. Bullous disorders are potentially serious.

Blocked nose

See *Nasal congestion*; *Nasal obstruction*.

Blocking

Inability to express true feelings or thoughts, usually as a result of emotional or mental conflict. In Freudian-based psychotherapies, blocking is regarded as originating from repression of painful emotions in early life. Successful treatment is thought to depend on putting patients in touch with these unconscious feelings.

A very specific form of thought blocking occurs in *schizophrenia*. In this disorder, trains of thought are persistently interrupted involuntarily, to be replaced by new ones that are totally unconnected with the first. (See also *Psychotherapy*.)

Blood

The sticky red fluid that circulates in our veins, arteries and capillaries. Its main function is to act as the body's transport system, but blood also plays an important role in the defense against infection.

The body of the average-sized adult has about 5 litres of blood. At rest, roughly this same volume of blood is pumped each minute by the heart via the arteries to the lungs and all other tissues, then returned to the heart in veins, in a continuous circuit (see *Circulatory system*). During exercise, the heart may pump blood at a rate of 30 litres or more a minute.

Almost half the volume of blood consists of *blood cells*; these include red

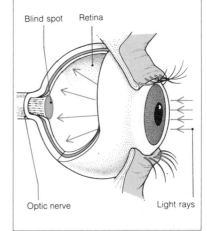

LOCATION OF BLIND SPOT
The blind spot is a minute area on the retina that lacks light receptors and so is not light sensitive.

Blind spot   Retina

Optic nerve   Light rays

B

B

blood cells (or erythrocytes), white blood cells (or leukocytes), and platelets (or thrombocytes). The remainder of the blood volume is a watery, straw-colored fluid called plasma, which contains dissolved proteins, sugars, fats, salts, and minerals.

BLOOD CELLS

The main function of red blood cells is to act as containers for *hemoglobin* (a pigmented protein that contains iron). Hemoglobin carries oxygen from the lungs to the tissues, where the oxygen is exchanged for the waste product carbon dioxide (see *Respiration*). White blood cells play an important part in the defense against infections and cancers, and also contribute to inflammation (see *Immune system*). Platelets are essential to the arrest of bleeding and to the repair of damaged blood vessels. The platelets clump together to block small holes in blood vessels, and the clumps release chemicals that begin the process of *blood clotting*.

PLASMA

Blood plasma is a straw-colored fluid, consisting mainly of water (95 percent), with a salt content very similar to that of seawater. Levels of the many other dissolved constituents in plasma vary from time to time. Measurements of these constituents are useful to physicians in the diagnosis of disease (see *Blood tests*; *Liver function tests*). Important constituents of plasma include the following.

NUTRIENTS These are transported to the tissues after absorption from the intestinal tract or after release from storage depots such as the liver. Nutrients include sugars (principally glucose), fats, amino acids (required by cells to make proteins), and various vitamins and minerals. Immediately after a meal rich in fats, the blood plasma has a milky appearance as a consequence of its high fat content.

WASTE PRODUCTS The main waste product of tissue metabolism is *urea* (produced by the breakdown of proteins), which is transported in the plasma to the kidneys; abnormally high blood urea levels occur in *kidney failure*. The waste product from the destruction of hemoglobin is a yellow pigment called *bilirubin*. This is normally removed from the plasma by the liver and excreted in the *bile*. Bilirubin levels become abnormally high in liver disease, or in hemolytic *anemia*, in which there is excessive destruction of red blood cells.

PROTEINS These include substances, such as fibrinogen, that are involved in the processes of blood coagulation, and others that act to inhibit coagulation (see *Blood clotting*). Plasma proteins, such as *immunoglobulins* (also called *antibodies*), and *complement*, are part of the immune system. Another important plasma protein is *albumin*. The large size of the protein molecules prevents them from escaping from the blood into the tissues; this helps to keep water in the blood (by a mechanism called osmotic pressure) and thus maintain blood volume.

HORMONES These are chemical messengers produced by various glands of the *endocrine system* and transported in the blood to their target organs.

Blood cells

Cells present in blood for most or part of their life span. These include red blood cells, which make up about 40 percent by volume of normal blood, and white blood cells and platelets, which make up less than 5 percent of the total volume.

All types of blood cells are formed in the bone marrow by a series of divisions from one type of cell called a stem cell.

RED BLOOD CELLS

These are also called RBCs, red blood corpuscles, or erythrocytes. They carry oxygen from the lungs to the tissues, where they exchange the oxygen for the waste product carbon dioxide (see *Respiration*).

FORMATION Red blood cells are formed from stem cells in the bone marrow by a process (called erythropoiesis) that takes about five days. Their formation requires an adequate supply of nutrients, including iron, amino acids, and the vitamins B_{12} and folic acid. The rate at which RBCs are formed is influenced by a hormone called erythropoietin, which is produced by the kidneys.

Immature red blood cells just released into the bloodstream from the marrow are called reticulocytes; over a period of two to four days, these develop into mature red blood cells. Reticulocytes are easily recognized in blood by means of special staining techniques, and a count of their numbers provides physicians with a helpful estimate of the rate at which RBCs are being formed.

STRUCTURE AND FUNCTION One cubic millimetre of blood contains about 5 million red blood cells, each of which is disk-shaped, about 0.0075 mm in diameter, and much thicker around the edge than at the center. This shape gives each cell a relatively large surface area, which helps it absorb and release oxygen molecules, and allows the cell to distort as it squeezes through narrow blood vessels.

Each red blood cell is packed with large quantities of *hemoglobin*, a pigmented protein that contains iron. Hemoglobin is highly efficient at "binding" (combining chemically) with oxygen when the oxygen concentration is high (in the lungs), and at releasing the oxygen when the oxygen concentration is low (in the tissues). Oxyhemoglobin, formed when oxygen combines with hemoglobin, is responsible for the bright red coloration of oxygenated blood (which flows mainly through arteries). Most venous blood is darker in color, because it contains the unbound (deoxygenated) form of hemoglobin.

Each red blood cell also contains *enzymes*, minerals, and sugars, which provide energy for the cell's *metabolism* and maintain its shape, structure, and elasticity. The surface structure of red blood cells varies slightly among individuals, and this provides the basis for classifying blood into groups (see *Blood groups*).

AGING AND DESTRUCTION The normal life span of red blood cells in the circulation is about 120 days. (Blood in blood banks must be discarded after three to four weeks, by which time the proportion of dead cells has reached significant levels.) As red blood cells age, their internal chemical machinery wears out, they lose elasticity, and they become trapped in small blood vessels in the spleen and other organs; they are then destroyed by a type of white blood cell called a macrophage. Most components of the hemoglobin molecules are reused, but some are broken down to form the waste product *bilirubin*.

DISORDERS Abnormalities can occur in the rate at which RBCs are formed or destroyed, in their numbers in the blood, and in their shape, size, and hemoglobin content, causing various forms of *anemia* and *polycythemia* (see *Blood* disorders box, p.184).

WHITE BLOOD CELLS

These are also called WBCs, white blood corpuscles, or leukocytes; their principal role is to protect the body against infection and to fight infection when it occurs. White blood cells are bigger than red blood cells (up to 0.015 mm in diameter) but much less numerous (about 7,500 per cubic millimetre of blood). They generally spend a much shorter part of their life span than red blood cells in the blood itself.

There are three main types of white blood cells, called granulocytes, monocytes, and *lymphocytes*.

GRANULOCYTES White blood cells of this type are also called polymorphonuclear leucocytes. Under the microscope, they are seen to contain granules and have an oddly shaped nucleus. Granulocytes are themselves of three types, called neutrophils, basophils, and eosinophils. Of these, the most important are neutrophils, which are responsible for isolating and destroying invading bacteria (pus consists largely of neutrophils). The action of neutrophils in "swallowing" bacteria has led to their being called phagocytes (literally "engulfing cells"). Neutrophils remain in the blood for only about six to nine hours before moving through blood vessel walls into the tissues, where they survive for a few more days. Eosinophils play a part in allergic reactions and increase in numbers in response to certain parasitic infections. Basophils are involved in inflammatory and allergic reactions.

MONOCYTES These cells are also a type of phagocyte; they circulate in the bloodstream for about six to nine days and play an important part in the *immune system*.

LYMPHOCYTES Many of these are formed in the lymph nodes rather than the bone marrow. They play a central role in the immune system, roving around the body between the bloodstream, the lymph nodes, and the channels between the lymph nodes.

T-type lymphocytes are responsible for the delayed hypersensitivity phenomena (see *Allergy*) and produce substances known as lymphokines, which affect the function of many cells. T-type lymphocytes also moderate the activity of other lymphocytes called B-type cells. These B-type lymphocytes form the *antibodies* that protect us against second attacks of certain diseases (such as measles). Individual lymphocyte cells may survive for anywhere between three months and 10 years.

DISORDERS The *leukemias* are disorders in which there is a disorganized proliferation of WBCs in the bone marrow. WBCs may also be too few in number (see *Blood* disorders box, p.184). In *AIDS*, certain T-lymphocytes are infected by *HIV* (the AIDS virus), which results in dysfunction of the immune system, and increased risk of certain types of infection and cancers.

PLATELETS

These are the smallest type of blood cell (0.002 mm to 0.003 mm in diameter), more numerous than white cells but less numerous than red cells (about 250,000 per cubic millimetre of blood). Like other blood cells, they originate from stem cells in the bone marrow. Platelets survive in blood for about nine days.

FUNCTION Platelets circulate in the blood in an inactive state, but under certain circumstances they begin to stick to blood vessel walls and adhere to each other. These activities play a very important part in the arrest of bleeding and in *blood clotting*. The same processes can also lead to the unwanted formation of thrombi (clots) in intact blood vessels (see *Thrombosis*), and to fatty deposits on blood-vessel walls (see *Atherosclerosis*).

Because of their role in clot formation, platelets are sometimes also called thrombocytes.

CONSTITUENTS OF BLOOD

Blood is pumped around the body in veins and arteries, transporting oxygen from the lungs to the tissues, and carbon dioxide from the tissues to the lungs. Blood also carries nutrients such as sugars, fats, and proteins that have been absorbed from the intestine, and hormones produced by a variety of glands. Waste products that are released from cells are carried in the blood to be broken down in the liver or excreted from the kidneys.

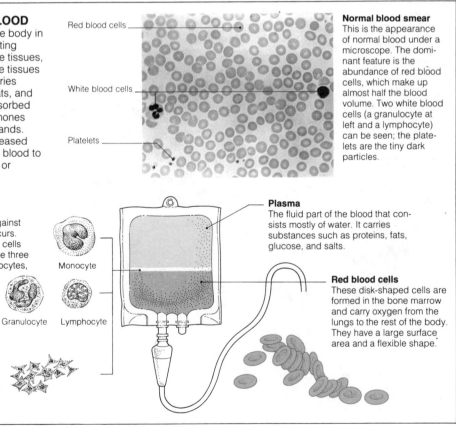

Red blood cells

White blood cells

Platelets

Normal blood smear
This is the appearance of normal blood under a microscope. The dominant feature is the abundance of red blood cells, which make up almost half the blood volume. Two white blood cells (a granulocyte at left and a lymphocyte) can be seen; the platelets are the tiny dark particles.

White blood cells
These cells protect the body against infection and fight it when it occurs. They are bigger than red blood cells but fewer in number. Each of the three main types (granulocytes, monocytes, and lymphocytes) plays a different role in dealing with infection.

Monocyte

Granulocyte   Lymphocyte

Platelets
The smallest type of blood cell produced in the bone marrow; they play an important part in blood clotting.

Plasma
The fluid part of the blood that consists mostly of water. It carries substances such as proteins, fats, glucose, and salts.

Red blood cells
These disk-shaped cells are formed in the bone marrow and carry oxygen from the lungs to the rest of the body. They have a large surface area and a flexible shape.

B

DISORDERS Abnormal platelets, or a lack of platelets in the blood, can lead to some types of *bleeding disorder*.

BLOOD CELLS IN DIAGNOSIS
Microscopic examination of blood preparations may reveal not only blood cell abnormalities characteristic of various diseases, but also healthy variations in the numbers of white blood cells produced in response to infections. For example, the number of neutrophils is raised in response to bacterial infections. The same is also true of lymphocytes in some viral infections.

The numbers, shapes, and appearance of the various types of blood cell are of great value to physicians in the diagnosis of disease (see *Blood count*; *Blood film*).

Blood clotting

Solidification of blood. Blood begins to clot within seconds of the skin being cut. The clot helps seal the damaged blood vessels, which also constrict to keep blood loss to a minimum. Blood clotting is not always helpful, however. Thrombi (clots) formed inside major blood vessels are the cause of many heart attacks, strokes, and other disorders (see *Thrombosis*).

The blood clotting process has two parts: the activation and clumping of platelets in the blood; and the formation of fibrin filaments, which enmesh the platelets as well as red and white cells. (See box below.)

To prevent the formation of clots inside healthy blood vessels, the blood also contains mechanisms that act to discourage clotting and to dissolve clots. These balance the proclotting mechanisms; normally, the balance is tipped in favor of clot formation only when a blood vessel is damaged.

PLATELET AGGREGATION
Platelets have to be "activated" before they will clump together. This occurs when they come into contact with damaged blood vessel walls or with artificial surfaces (such as glass), when blood flow is turbulent, or when platelets are acted on by certain chemicals secreted into the blood.

Once activated, platelets first become sticky, adhering to surfaces. They then change shape from disks into spiny spheres, enmeshing with each other. Finally, they release chemicals that activate other platelets, start process of fibrin formation, and cause blood vessels to contract.

FIBRIN FORMATION
This process, also called coagulation, is triggered by chemicals released either by activated platelets or by tissues following injury. It results from a complex series of reactions in the blood plasma called the coagulation cascade. With each step in the cascade, a coagulation factor in the plasma is converted from an inactive to an active form. The active form of the factor then activates several molecules of the next factor in the series—and so on until, in the final step, a factor called fibrinogen is converted into fibrin.

Provided all the participating factors are present, the activation of just one molecule of the first factor in the series can lead to the explosive production of up to 30,000 molecules of fibrin at the site of injury.

The factors involved in the coagulation cascade are numbered I, II, and V to XIII. Factor I is fibrinogen and factor II, its immediate precursor in the cascade, is called prothrombin. Most coagulation factors are made in the liver. An adequate supply in the diet of *vitamin K*, found in green vegetables, is required for the manufacture of certain factors.

HOW BLOOD CLOTS

Clotting describes the solidification of blood anywhere in the body. Clotting occurs almost immediately at the site of a cut and helps limit blood loss by sealing damaged blood vessels. However, if abnormal clotting occurs in major blood vessels, heart attacks, strokes, and other disorders may occur. The clotting process has two main parts— platelet activation and the formation of fibrin filaments.

Red blood cells enmeshed in fibrin filaments
Fibrin is formed by a chemical change from a soluble protein, fibrinogen, which is present in the blood. The fibrin molecules aggregate to form long filaments, which enmesh blood cells (see left) to form a solid clot. The conversion of fibrinogen to fibrin is the last step of the "coagulation cascade," a series of reactions in the blood triggered by tissue injury and platelet activation.

Platelet   Fibrin

Clot
Epidermis
Dermis
White blood cell
Red blood cell

1 Platelets are activated by coming into contact with damaged blood vessel walls, where they become sticky and then clump at the site of injury and adhere to the damaged blood vessel wall.

2 Chemicals released by platelets and damaged tissues stimulate coagulation factors within the blood to form filaments of fibrin at the site of injury.

3 The fibrin filaments enmesh the platelets along with red and white blood cells.

4 Once the cut blood vessel is plugged by the mass of fibrin, platelets, and red and white blood cells, the fibrin filaments contract to form a solid clot.

ANTICLOTTING MECHANISMS

Separate mechanisms act to prevent unwanted platelet activation and fibrin formation.

Platelet activation is inhibited mainly by a substance called prostacyclin (a type of *prostaglandin*), which is secreted by the walls of healthy blood vessels.

Fibrin formation is discouraged by various mechanisms. First, a number of inhibitory enzymes (types of protein) circulating in the blood neutralize activated coagulation factors. The most important of these is called antithrombin III. Second, a further series of enzymes is activated at the same time as the coagulation cascade. These enzymes form a substance called plasmin that breaks down fibrin (see *Fibrinolysis*). In addition, blood flow tends to discourage coagulation by washing away active coagulation factors from areas where they are being formed, and the liver deactivates any excess coagulation factors.

DEFECTS AND DISORDERS

Defects can occur for a wide variety of reasons in the clotting (or anticlotting) mechanisms, tipping the balance either in favor of a tendency to bleed or to form clots.

Some people carry a genetic defect that prevents them from making sufficient amounts of one of the coagulation factors. In other cases, abnormally few platelets are produced, insufficient vitamin K (which is required to make certain coagulation factors) is absorbed from the diet, or excessive amounts of the enzymes that inhibit coagulation are produced. Any of these conditions may result in a tendency to bleed excessively (see *Bleeding disorders*).

On the other hand, sometimes the balance is tipped abnormally in favor of coagulation and clotting. Possible causes include an increase in the levels of coagulation factors (as can occur in late pregnancy or when using some oral contraceptives), a decrease in the level of enzymes that inhibit coagulation (as can occur in some forms of liver disease), or a sluggish blood flow through a particular area. The result may be thrombosis (abnormal clot formation).

Conditions in which there is a tendency for clot formation are often treated with *anticoagulant drugs* such as heparin or warfarin. Heparin exerts its anticoagulant effect by increasing the activity of antithrombin III, which neutralizes activated coagulation factors; warfarin works by disrupting the production of coagulation factors by inhibiting the action of vitamin K. Because of the delicate balance between the clotting and anticlotting mechanisms in blood, the use of anticoagulant drugs must be monitored frequently to prevent the development of severe bleeding.

Blood-clotting tests

Tests performed to screen for and diagnose *bleeding disorders*. These disorders usually result from deficiencies or abnormalities of platelets or of blood coagulation factors (see also *Blood clotting*).

Bleeding disorders caused by low numbers of platelets are detected by a *blood count* in conjunction with a test of the bleeding time.

Bleeding time may be measured by nicking the skin of the ear or the forearm and timing the interval before bleeding stops. The normal range is three to eight minutes.

Reduced platelet activity results in a prolonged bleeding time.

Various tests are used to assess the activity of blood coagulation factors, the most frequently performed being prothrombin time and activated partial thromboplastin time (named after two coagulation factors). The time taken for the patient's blood to clot is measured after addition of calcium and other substances that promote the coagulation process; the results are compared with the time taken for normal blood to clot under the same conditions. Abnormal results may indicate deficiency of a specific coagulation factor, as occurs in *hemophilia*, or of many coagulation factors, as occurs in liver disease.

Anticoagulant drug therapy is designed to prolong the prothrombin time or the clotting time and to reduce the risk of *thrombosis* (abnormal clotting) in susceptible people. Anyone taking anticoagulation drugs should have regular clotting tests to ensure that the dosage is not excessive, which could cause bleeding.

Blood count

Also called full blood count, this test measures hemoglobin concentration, and the numbers of red blood cells, white blood cells, and platelets in 1 cu. mm of blood. The proportion of various white blood cells is measured and the size and shape of red and white cells is noted.

A blood count is the most commonly performed blood test. It is important for diagnosing *anemia* or conditions in which the number of blood cells is abnormally high (such as white blood cells in *leukemia*) or abnormally low (such as platelets in *thrombocytopenia*).

About 1 to 2 ml of blood is required for a blood count, which is usually performed by an automatic analyzer.

Blood culture

See *Culture*.

Blood donation

The process of giving blood so that it can be used in *blood transfusion*. In most cases, whole blood is taken from the donor and broken down later into components for storage. Recently, a new method called apheresis has been introduced, which involves extracting only a specific blood component from the donor. Donation time, with medical check and recovery periods included, is about 45 minutes for whole blood, while apheresis takes about one hour for plasma and two hours for platelets and white cells.

Any healthy adult can potentially be a blood donor. Volunteer donors are first interviewed about their medical history. Anyone who has had *anemia, cancer*, types of heart disease, *malaria*, or *hepatitis*, or who has been exposed to *HIV* (the *AIDS* virus) may be disqualified. Pregnant women are also disqualified. A blood sample usually taken from a finger or earlobe is then tested for anemia; body temperature, pulse, and blood pressure are also checked.

Most regular donors of whole blood give blood twice a year. Donors may safely give plasma by apheresis 26 times in a six-month period. Platelet donors may make 24 donations a year; white cell donors, however, are limited to 12 donations a year.

HOW IT IS DONE

WHOLE BLOOD DONATION While the donor lies down and relaxes, a needle attached to a tube is inserted into the forearm. Up to 500 ml of blood (about one tenth of the total volume in the circulation) is slowly withdrawn into a plastic bag containing anticoagulant to prevent the blood from clotting. Most people feel no effects from giving blood. A few may feel faint or sick and should rest or lie down for a few minutes. All donors should avoid strenuous exercise for about five hours afterward and should drink plenty of water and fruit juices.

The Canadian Red Cross Society tests all donated blood for hepatitis B virus, syphilis, and antibodies to HIV.

B

DISORDERS OF THE BLOOD

Abnormalities can occur in any of the components of blood—the red blood cells (RBCs), white blood cells (WBCs), platelets, and numerous constituents of plasma.

Anemia (a deficiency of the red cell pigment *hemoglobin* and a consequent reduction in the blood's oxygen-carrying capacity) is by far the most common blood disorder. It has many different possible causes. In *polycythemia* there are too many red blood cells. In *leukemia* excessive numbers of abnormal white blood cells crowd out the normal cells from the bone marrow.

Defects in the platelets and in the clotting mechanisms may lead to any of various *bleeding disorders*. Unwanted clot formation (*thrombosis*) may result from circumstances that overactivate the blood-clotting mechanisms.

Deficiencies of the proteins in blood plasma include hypo-albuminemia (*albumin* deficiency) and agammaglobulinemia (gamma-globulin deficiency). Known causes of blood disorders include the following.

GENETIC DISORDERS

In these disorders there is an inherited abnormality in the production of some component of blood. People with *sickle cell anemia* and *thalassemia* produce an abnormal type of hemoglobin that makes their red blood cells more fragile; those with *hemophilia* fail to produce enough of one of the factors involved in blood clotting. Disorders of this kind are present from birth and continue throughout life.

Sickle cell anemia
In this genetic (inherited) disorder, the red blood cells are abnormally fragile and have a characteristic sickle shape.

NUTRITIONAL DISORDERS

Loss of regular amounts of blood over an extended period may mean that iron (required to make hemoglobin) is lost faster than it can be replaced in the diet (see *Anemia, iron-deficiency*).

If insufficient amounts of the vitamins B_{12} or folic acid reach the bone marrow, it produces fewer red blood cells, which are abnormally large (see *Anemia, megaloblastic*). The vitamin deficiency may be due to a poor diet or, more often in developed countries, to a failure to absorb vitamin B_{12} correctly from the intestinal tract.

INFECTION

Multiplication of bacteria in the blood is termed *septicemia*.

Many other microorganisms (i.e., viruses, fungi, protozoa, and other parasites) may infect the blood at some stage in their life cycle. Some organisms (notably those responsible for *malaria*) may actually attack and destroy red blood cells and so cause anemia (see *Anemia, hemolytic*).

TUMORS

All types of leukemia are the result of a type of cancer of the bone marrow, causing overgrowth of abnormal white blood cells and destruction of the healthy marrow. In polycythemia vera, a similar process occurs, except that mainly red cells are produced to excess. Another type of bone marrow cancer called *multiple myeloma* can cause an excess of certain proteins in the blood plasma.

POISONS

Carbon monoxide directly impairs the functioning of red blood cells by displacing oxygen bound to hemoglobin within the cells. Lead poisoning causes defective red blood cell production. Some snake and spider venoms destroy red cells and/or provoke clotting. Septicemia describes the multiplication of bacteria in the blood; *toxemia* describes the presence of metabolic poisons in the blood.

DRUGS

Certain drugs can cause blood abnormalities as a side effect. For example, co-trimoxazole, thiazide diuretics, and carbimazole may depress the production of white blood cells and/or platelets; chloramphenicol and sulfonamides may depress all blood

Cold agglutinin disorder
This is a rare blood disorder in which the body develops antibodies to its own red blood cells, causing them to clump together. This effect is especially marked in cold conditions when the clumps of cells reduce blood flow to the limbs.

cell production; methotrexate and phenytoin may interfere with red cell production.

Too high a dose of *anticoagulant drugs* can cause a bleeding tendency through excessive disruption of clotting mechanisms.

RADIATION

High doses of radiation (received at the time of therapy or from nuclear explosions or radioactive leaks from nuclear reactors) can severely damage the bone marrow, causing depression of all blood cell production (see *Anemia, aplastic*).

OTHER DISORDERS

Albumin—an important protein in the blood plasma—may become deficient due to liver disease (reduced production) or kidney disease (loss of albumin in the urine).

Liver disease may also cause *hyperbilirubinemia* (excess bilirubin in the blood), anemia, and deficiencies of some clotting factors. Kidney disease causes *uremia* (excess urea in the blood), sometimes anemia (possibly due to decreased production of the hormone erythropoietin), and changes in blood chemistry.

INVESTIGATION

Blood disorders are investigated principally by various *blood tests*, such as the *blood count, blood smear*, and *blood-clotting tests*, and by *bone marrow biopsy*.

The blood will not be used for transfusion if any of these is present. After being classified into blood groups, the blood is stored in a blood bank, either whole or separated into its different components (see *Blood products*).

APHERESIS This technique allows only a blood component, such as plasma, platelets, or white cells, to be withdrawn from the circulation. For example, with one type of machine about 500 ml of the donor's blood is taken from one arm, circulated through a closed, sterile separator system, and then returned to the other arm minus the particular component being collected. This withdrawal and return is repeated six to eight times, and collects an amount of component that would normally require six to eight donors.

Because only a single donor may be required to provide a patient with a sufficient quantity of a particular component, the risk of reaction or hepatitis transmission is reduced.

Blood donor

See *Blood donation*.

Blood film

A test that involves smearing a drop of blood onto a glass slide so that it can be examined under a microscope. For this procedure, the blood film is stained with special dyes to make the blood cells show up more clearly.

The shape and appearance of blood cells are inspected for any abnormality, such as sickle-shaped red blood cells in *sickle cell anemia* or abnormal lymphocytes in infectious *mononucleosis*. The relative proportions of the different types of white blood cells can also be counted. This examination, called a differential white cell count, may be helpful in diagnosing infection or *leukemia*.

Blood films are also used in diagnosing infections, such as *malaria*, in which the parasites can be seen inside the red blood cells.

Blood films are usually done together with a full *blood count*.

Blood gases

A test for determining the acidity-alkalinity (pH) and the concentrations of oxygen, carbon dioxide, and bicarbonate in the blood.

Blood oxygen and carbon dioxide values are useful in diagnosing and monitoring *respiratory failure*. Bicarbonate and acidity reflect the *acid-base balance* of the body. This may be disturbed in conditions such as diabetic ketoacidosis, ASA poisoning, hyperventilation (overbreathing), or repeated vomiting.

Modern apparatus can quickly measure blood gases using a few drops of blood. Blood for analysis is usually taken from an artery rather than from a vein and possibly from the interior of the heart.

Blood groups

Systems of classifying blood according to the different marker proteins on the surface of red blood cells. These marker proteins—called *antigens*—affect the ability of the red blood cells to provoke an *immune response*. Blood group typing is essential for safe *blood transfusion*.

TYPES

ABO GROUPS Attempts in the 19th century and earlier at transfusing blood from one living person to another were sometimes successful but sometimes caused serious illness and even death. In 1900 the German pathologist Karl Landsteiner began mixing blood taken from different people and found that some mixtures were compatible while others were not. He discovered two types of antigens on the surface of the red blood cells—these he called A and B. According to whether a person's blood contains one or other antigen, both, or neither, it is classified as type A, B, AB, or O. Landsteiner found that the fluid part of some people's blood contained *antibodies*—anti-A and/or anti-B—that reacted with the antigens. People with the A antigen (blood group A) have anti-B antibodies; people with the B antigen (blood group B) have anti-A antibodies; those with both the A and B antigens (blood group AB) have no anti-A or anti-B antibodies; people with no A or B antigens (blood group O) have both anti-A and anti-B antibodies. A person cannot safely be transfused with blood of a group containing antigens to which he or she has antibodies (see *Bloof group* table, p.186).

In Canada, the most common of the ABO blood groups is O, followed by A, then B, and finally AB. The precise frequency of each group differs between races.

RHESUS FACTORS Another blood-group system, the Rhesus system (Rh factors), was discovered in 1940 by Landsteiner during experiments on Rhesus monkeys. This system involves several antigens, the most important of which is factor D. This factor is found in the blood of 85 percent of people, who are called Rh positive, while 15 percent lack the factor and are Rh negative. Individuals are therefore classed as, for example, "O positive" or "AB negative" on the basis of their ABO and Rh blood groups.

The importance of this group relates mainly to pregnancy in Rh-negative women since, if the baby is Rh positive, the mother may form antibodies against the baby's blood (see *Rhesus incompatibility*). An Rh-negative mother is therefore given antibodies directed against factor D after delivery to prevent her developing anti-D antibodies, which might cause *hemolytic disease of the newborn* in subsequent Rh-positive infants.

Transfusion of Rh-positive blood into an Rh-negative patient can cause a serious reaction if the patient has had earlier blood transfusions containing the Rh antigen.

OTHER GROUPS

Since the discovery of the ABO and Rh factors, about 400 other antigens have been identified, but these rarely cause transfusion problems.

USES

TRANSFUSION AND CROSS MATCHING The ABO and Rh groups are used to categorize blood stored in blood banks. If, for example, a patient who is A positive needs a transfusion, he or she can be given A-positive blood from the bank. In practice, however, each unit (about 500 ml) of blood to be given is first tested against a small sample of the patient's blood to exclude the small possibility that the two might be incompatible because of a reaction due to one of the other blood groups. This test is known as cross matching and takes a short time to perform. In an emergency, however, unmatched blood of the appropriate group may need to be given.

INHERITED DISORDERS Some blood groups are associated with particular disorders. For example, blood group A is more common in people suffering from cancer of the stomach, while blood group O is more common in those with peptic ulcer.

PATERNITY CASES The blood group of an individual is determined by the genes inherited from his or her parents. Identification of blood group can be used in a paternity case to establish that a man could not have been the father of a particular child. It cannot be shown positively that a man is the father by blood grouping, but, with genetic analysis, paternity can now be proved with virtual certainty (see *Paternity testing*).

BLOOD GROUP COMPATIBILITY

Recipient blood group	Donor blood group			
	A	B	AB	O
A	▲	●	●	▲
B	●	▲	●	▲
AB	▲	▲	▲	▲
O	●	●	●	▲

Key ▲ Compatible ● Incompatible

CRIMINAL INVESTIGATION Blood found at the scene of a crime can be grouped according to the various red blood cell antigens present. New techniques of genetic analysis allow identification of the blood of a suspect with virtual certainty (see *Genetic fingerprinting*).

ANTHROPOLOGY The ABO blood groups are found in all people, but the frequency of each group varies with race and geographical distribution. Study of blood groups can therefore aid anthropologists in investigating, for example, the origins and migrations of various populations.

Blood level

The concentration of a given substance in the blood plasma or serum. Sodium, potassium, and glucose levels are commonly measured in routine *blood tests*. The police may order the measuring of blood alcohol levels, or blood alcohol concentration (BAC), in connection with traffic offenses. For this purpose, the legal limit in Canada is 80 mg of alcohol per 100 ml of blood, a reading of 0.08 on a breathalyzer.

Blood loss

See *Bleeding, treatment of.*

Blood poisoning

A common name for *septicemia* with *toxemia*, a serious, often life-threatening illness caused by multiplication of bacteria and their formation of toxins (poisons) in the bloodstream. Septicemia may be a complication of an infection (e.g., an infected wound or burn). It was formerly a feared and fatal complication of childbirth (see *Puerperal fever*). In some infective conditions, *septic shock* may be caused by toxins released by bacteria. The mortality rate of septicemia used to be high but has been substantially reduced by treatment with *antibiotic drugs* and by intensive therapy for shock. (See also *Bacteremia*.)

Blood pressure

The pressure exerted by the flow of blood through the main arteries. Blood pressure rises and falls as the heart responds to the varying demands made by the body during different activities, such as exercise, stress, and sleep. Two types of pressure are measured. Systolic, the highest, is the pressure created by the contraction of the heart muscle and the elastic recoil of the aorta (the main artery leaving the heart) as blood surges through it. Diastolic pressure (the lowest) is recorded during relaxation of the ventricles between beats; it reflects the resistance of all the small arteries in the body and the load against which the heart must work. The pressure wave transmitted along the arteries with each heartbeat is easily felt as the *pulse*.

MEASURING BLOOD PRESSURE
Blood pressure is measured using a *sphygmomanometer*. This instrument consists of a cuff with an air bladder connected to a tube and bulb (for pumping air into the bladder), and a gauge for indicating the air pressure being exerted. The soft rubber cuff of the sphygmomanometer is inflated around the upper arm until it is tight enough to stop the flow of blood in the main artery in the arm. The cuff is then gradually deflated until, by listening to the artery through a *stethoscope*, the blood can first be heard as a beat forcing its way along the artery. This is recorded as the systolic pressure. The cuff is then deflated further until the beat disappears and the blood flows steadily through the now open artery—giving the diastolic pressure.

In special circumstances, blood pressure may also be measured by miniature devices attached to an artery or by a continuous recording for 24 hours or more while a person leads his or her daily life.

Blood pressure is recorded by giving the systolic pressure and diastolic pressure, expressed as millimetres of mercury (mm Hg). This unit was adopted because the earliest equipment used a glass column filled with mercury to measure the pressure directly. Today, some sphygmomanometers use a spring gauge with a round dial. A healthy young adult has

CHANGES IN BLOOD PRESSURE

Raised or lowered blood pressure can be caused by various factors. During pregnancy it tends to rise but then returns gradually to its previous level after birth. Certain drugs also affect blood pressure as a side effect. During the day (below) a normal person's blood pressure fluctuates according to activity. Hypertension (abnormally high blood pressure) is treated with weight loss, sodium restriction, drugs, and modification of life-style.

Waking and getting up cause blood pressure to rise.

Vigorous exercise raises blood pressure.

Getting tense or smoking makes blood pressure rise.

Systolic

Diastolic

S

D

Time 7 am 8 9 10 11 12 1 pm 2

a blood pressure reading of about 110/75 (i.e., 110 mm Hg systolic and 75 mm Hg diastolic). This often rises normally with age, to about 130/90 at age 60. Abnormally high blood pressure is known medically as *hypertension*; abnormally low pressure is termed *hypotension*.

Blood products

After *blood donation*, blood is stored either whole or separated into its various components. Each product has a particular use in *blood transfusion*.

WHOLE BLOOD
This is used to restore blood volume after sudden severe bleeding—as may occur, for instance, after a traffic accident or during major surgery. Whole blood keeps for only three to four weeks after donation.

PACKED RED CELLS
These are prepared by removing part of the liquid plasma. Concentrated red cells are used to treat patients with some forms of chronic *anemia* that have not responded to drug treatment. The red cells provide the necessary hemoglobin without overloading the recipient with fluid, which can result in, or aggravate, *heart failure*. Concentrated red cells can also be used to treat babies with *hemolytic disease of the newborn*.

WASHED RED CELLS
This is blood that has had the white blood cells and/or plasma proteins removed, thus reducing the chances of an allergic reaction occurring in patients, such as those with chronic anemia, who require transfusions over a long period.

FROZEN RED CELLS
Red cells can be preserved for long periods if stored at very low temperatures. This technique is valuable in preserving red cells belonging to rare blood groups.

PLATELETS
Platelets play an important part in normal blood clotting. Their low level in some blood disorders causes patients to bruise easily and to suffer from internal bleeding. Patients with such disorders may benefit from transfusions of platelets that have been extracted from whole blood and then concentrated. If necessary, platelets from several donors can be given during one transfusion.

WHITE BLOOD CELLS
Granulocytes, a type of white blood cell, can be separated from normal blood, or from the blood of patients with chronic myeloid (granulocytic) *leukemia*, who have an excess of these cells. Patients with life-threatening infections accompanied by low levels of granulocytes may be treated with granulocytes if they are not responding to antibiotic drugs.

FROZEN FRESH PLASMA
This is prepared by separating and freezing plasma as soon as possible after blood has been collected. Because fresh plasma is rich in clotting factors, it is used to correct many types of bleeding disorder.

PLASMA PROTEIN SOLUTIONS
The liquid part of any whole blood not used within three weeks of collection can be converted into a concentrated solution of albumin (the main protein in plasma). The solution can be stored for long periods. Its chief use is in treating *shock*, resulting from severe blood loss, until whole blood compatible with the patient's blood group becomes available. Purified albumin preparations are used to treat *nephrotic syndrome* (a kidney disorder causing albumin loss in the urine) and chronic liver disease (in which production of albumin is deficient).

CLOTTING FACTORS
Concentrates of clotting factors VIII and IX can be prepared for the treatment of *hemophilia* and *Christmas disease*. Because blood from many donors is required to produce one small batch of clotting factor, it must be heat-treated to reduce the risk of *hepatitis* or *AIDS* virus transmission.

IMMUNOGLOBULINS
Immunoglobulins (also called antibodies) occur in the blood of healthy individuals who have recovered from the common viral diseases. These nonspecific immunoglobulins can be taken from the blood plasma, concentrated, and given by injection (see *Immunoglobin injection*) to protect, by passive *immunization*, people who are unable to produce their own antibodies or who are likely to be exposed to *hepatitis A*. Nonspecific immunoglobulins can also be given intravenously in large doses to treat certain *autoimmune disorders*, such as thrombocytopenic *purpura*.

Specific antibodies (taken from patients who have recovered from a particular infection or who have been specifically immunized against one) are given as passive immunization to protect especially susceptible patients from specific infections. For example, varicella-zoster virus antibodies are given to children with leukemia who are exposed to chickenpox, and pseudomonas antibodies are given to patients suffering from burns.

Anti-D immunoglobulin, a type of specific antibody, is obtained from the blood of patients sensitized to the Rh blood group factor. If anti-D immunoglobulin is given to an Rh-negative mother within 60 hours of her giving birth to an Rh-positive baby, it will prevent *hemolytic disease of the newborn* occurring in any other babies she might have.

Blood smear
See *Blood film*.

Blood tests
Analysis of a sample of blood to give information on its cells and proteins and any of the chemicals, antigens, antibodies, and gases that it carries. Since blood is the main transport system of the body, such tests can be used to check on the health of major organs, as well as on respiratory function, hormonal balance, the immune system, and metabolism.

TYPES
HEMATOLOGICAL TESTS These involve looking at the components of the blood itself, including examination of the numbers, shape, size, and appearance of blood cells, and testing the function of clotting factors. The most important hematological tests are *blood count*, *blood film*, *blood clotting tests*, and *blood group* tests.

BIOCHEMICAL TESTS These measure chemicals in the blood, such as glucose, sodium, potassium, uric acid, urea, enzymes, gases, digested foods, and drugs. (See *Acid-base balance*; *Kidney function tests*; *Liver function tests*.)

MICROBIOLOGICAL TESTS These look for microorganisms in the blood, such as bacteria, viruses, fungi, and parasites, and the antibodies formed against them. (See *Culture*; *Immunoassay*.)

HOW THEY ARE DONE
The most convenient site for taking a blood sample is a vein at the bend in the elbow. A tourniquet is applied to the upper arm, and the blood is withdrawn through a needle into a syringe. The procedure causes only mild discomfort. Up to 20 ml of blood may be required, but, as the circulation contains 4 to 5 litres, loss of this small proportion has no harmful effect. If only a few drops are needed, they may be obtained by pricking a finger. Rarely, tests may require a sample of arterial blood, which is taken from the elbow, wrist, or groin; this is a more difficult procedure and causes some discomfort.

The sample may be allowed to clot, leaving its clear serum for examina-

B

tion, or an anticoagulant may be added to allow study of the cells and clotting factors. The sample is then sent to the laboratory, where one or more of the hundreds of available tests are carried out. In some laboratories, modern computerized analyzers are used to perform many different tests simultaneously on one small sample of blood. The printed results compare each value with the accepted normal range for that test. Each laboratory produces its own normal ranges that depend on the method and the ingredients of the test, and sometimes on the age and sex of the patient. Some tests may be performed at the bedside or in a physician's consulting room. Some, such as blood glucose, may be performed by patients on themselves.

Blood transfusion

The infusion of large volumes of blood or blood components directly into the bloodstream, performed mainly to remedy severe blood loss or to correct chronic anemia.

Before the discovery of the major *blood groups* earlier this century, blood transfusion was a hazardous undertaking, often causing severe reactions and even death. Growing knowledge of the complex properties of blood and its components has now made transfusion a safe procedure, although still not without possible complications.

WHY IT IS DONE
Blood transfusion may be needed by a patient who has bled severely after an accident or who has lost a lot of blood during an operation. It may also be required after internal bleeding—for example, from a bleeding *peptic ulcer*. Chronic *anemia* that does not respond to medication may require treatment by blood transfusion (for example, in conditions such as *thalassemia* and *leukemia*).

In an exchange transfusion, nearly all of the recipient's blood is replaced by donor blood. It is most often needed in *hemolytic disease of the newborn*, when abnormally high levels of bilirubin in the blood might cause brain damage.

CROSS MATCHING Before a transfusion, blood must be cross matched to ensure compatibility. This procedure involves taking a sample of the recipient's blood, identifying the blood groups, and matching it with suitable donor blood. This is done by mixing some of each blood sample and examining it to make sure there are no *antibodies* in the recipient's plasma that

would damage the donor blood cells. Blood can usually be cross matched in one hour or less. If the patient is losing blood very rapidly, it may not be possible to wait. In this case, O Rh-negative (universal donor) blood that has not been cross matched, plasma protein solution, or a plasma substitute may be given until tested blood becomes available.

HOW IT IS DONE
Blood is transfused into an arm vein. Usually, each unit (about 500 ml) of blood is given over one to four hours; in an emergency 500 ml may be given in a couple of minutes. The amount of blood the patient requires depends on how much has been lost or on the severity of anemia. During transfusion, the patient's pulse, blood pressure, and temperature are measured regularly, and, if there is any sign of an adverse reaction, the transfusion is stopped.

COMPLICATIONS
If blood has not been cross matched reliably, antibodies in the recipient's blood may cause incompatible donor cells to hemolyze (burst). The most severe reactions can result in *shock* or *kidney failure*. Less severe reactions can produce fever, chills, a rash, or delayed anemia. Transfusion reactions can also occur as a result of allergy to transfused white cells, plasma proteins, or platelets.

Infections, such as with *HIV* (the AIDS virus), *hepatitis B*, *syphilis*, and *malaria*, can occur if donor blood has not been adequately screened. All blood for transfusion is now carefully tested and the risk of infection is extremely small.

In elderly or severely anemic patients, transfusion can overload the circulation, leading to heart failure. *Diuretic drugs*, which cause fluid loss, may need to be given simultaneously to avoid this. In patients with chronic anemia who require regular transfusion over many years, excess iron may accumulate (a condition called hemosiderosis) and cause damage to various organs, such as the heart, liver, and pancreas. Dangerous buildup of iron can be relieved by giving the drug deferoxamine.

Blood transfusion, autologous

The use of a person's own blood, donated on an earlier occasion, for *blood transfusion* during or after surgery. Autologous transfusion is used to avoid the risk that blood from another donor might be infected.

WHY IT IS DONE
Autologous transfusion eliminates the slight but serious risk of infecting a recipient with HIV (the AIDS virus) or the *hepatitis* virus from contaminated blood. It also eliminates the less significant risk of transmitting *cytomegalovirus*, *malaria*, and *syphilis*.

Another advantage of autologous transfusion is that there is no risk of a transfusion reaction occurring as a result of incompatibility between donor and recipient blood.

Autologous transfusion has been used illegally by people associated with professional sports. Carried out just before a sporting event, "blood doping" increases the oxygen-carrying capacity of the circulation and thus improves stamina.

HOW IT IS DONE
Blood can be withdrawn (in the same way as for *blood donation*) in several sessions at least four days apart and up to three days before surgery is planned. A total of up to about 3.5 litres of blood can be removed and stored. Iron tablets are prescribed to ensure that the bone marrow produces replacement blood cells.

Blood vessels

A general term for arteries, veins, and capillaries. (See *Circulatory system*.)

Blue baby

An infant with a cyanotic (bluish) complexion, especially of the lips and tongue, caused by a relative lack of oxygen in the blood. This is usually due to a structural defect of the heart or of the major arteries leaving the heart. The defect allows some of the deoxygenated blood returning to the right side of the heart to be pumped straight back into the general circulation instead of first going to the lungs to receive oxygen, or results in too little blood passing into the lungs because of a blocked or narrowed pulmonary artery. Such defects may need to be corrected surgically. (See *Heart disease, congenital*.)

Blue bloater

A term used by physicians to describe the appearance of some patients with lung disease (see *Lung disease, chronic obstructive*).

Blue Cross

A private, non-profit corporation that offers a range of health insurance plans for hospitalization, prescription drugs, medical and dental care. Blue Cross insurance can be obtained voluntarily, or is offered through employment plans. It provides coverage in addition to *Medicare*.

Blurred vision

A common term used to indicate indistinct, fuzzy, or misty visual images. Blurred vision should not be confused with *double vision* (diplopia). Blurred vision can occur in one or both eyes, for episodes of varying lengths of time, and can develop gradually or suddenly. Sometimes only part of the field of vision is affected. Any change in vision should be brought to the attention of your physician.

CAUSES

Blurred vision is most commonly due to refractive errors—*myopia* (nearsightedness), *hypermetropia* (farsightedness), and *astigmatism* (unequal curvature of the front of the eye). These defects can easily be rectified by glasses or contact lenses.

Many people notice gradual changes in near vision from the age of 40 onward—their vision for close work becomes progressively less sharp, causing problems with small print and the need for reading glasses or bifocals for close-up reading to correct the blur. This is due to *presbyopia* (decreased ability to focus near objects). If a person has been nearsighted, he or she may simply need to take off the glasses to see close objects after the age of 40.

Vision may be impaired, or blindness caused, by damage, disease, or abnormalities affecting the tear film, cornea, iris, lens, aqueous humor, vitreous humor, retina, or the nerve pathways behind the eye. These nerve pathways may be damaged by a tumor, *head injury*, or *stroke*.

Blushing

Brief reddening of the face and sometimes the neck caused by widening of the blood vessels that are close to the surface of the skin. Blushing is usually an involuntary reaction to embarrassment. In some women, blushing is a feature of the *hot flashes* that occur during the *menopause*. Flushing of the face occurs in association with *carcinoid syndrome*.

Body contour surgery

Operations performed to remove excess fat, skin, or both, from various parts of the body, especially the abdomen, thighs, and buttocks. Diet and exercise are the proper means of reducing the fat content of the body, and surgery is not a substitute. Operations may improve appearance where accumulations of fat or excess skin persist in certain areas after successful weight control.

TYPES

ABDOMINAL WALL REDUCTION In this reshaping operation, often called abdominoplasty, excess skin and fat are removed from the abdomen. The operation may benefit people who retain an excess of skin following weight loss or pregnancy.

Abdominal wall reduction is carried out under general anesthesia and requires a hospital stay of two to three days. The surgeon makes a horizontal "bikini" incision in the skin as low down on the abdomen as possible, then cuts upward between the fat and muscle layers. The flap of skin and fat is pulled down and the excess is removed. Sometimes, when the amount to be removed is particularly large, a vertical incision is required in addition to the horizontal one. In many cases, the umbilicus (navel) must be moved to a higher position because it has been pulled down with the flap. At the end of the operation, the skin is stitched together. Drains are inserted into the wound and left in place for several days to prevent the risk of blood or serum collecting, which can lead to infection.

To minimize the size of the scar or scars, the patient should avoid tension on the wound and walk with the trunk slightly flexed for several weeks. Despite taking care, the final scar is often not as narrow as the patient and surgeon would like.

REDUCTION OF THIGHS AND BUTTOCKS For thigh reduction, excess fat and skin are removed through an incision along the "stocking-seam line." For buttock reduction, the scar is planned to lie in the crease line separating the thighs and buttocks. In both cases, the scars are often wide and unattractive, and the reduction seldom satisfies the patient. There is also a risk of complications. The skin surrounding the wound often dies, leading to infection and delayed healing, which may necessitate skin grafting.

SUCTION LIPECTOMY To overcome the problem of noticeable scars, instruments have been developed to remove fat through "key-hole" incisions. A suction instrument is inserted through a small skin incision and moved back and forth under the skin to break up large areas of fat, which can then be sucked out through the instrument. However, because of the plentiful blood supply within the fat, there may be significant blood and fluid loss, which must be treated by the surgeon to prevent shock or anemia. In addition, the total amount of fat that can be removed at one time is limited. Suction lipectomy is useful in improving the appearance of people who have localized areas of excess fat, but cannot be used as a substitute for weight control. Minor irregularities and dimpling of the skin commonly occur after surgery.

Body odor

The smell caused by sweat on the skin surface. Sweat itself has no odor, but, if it remains on the skin for a few hours, bacterial decomposition may lead to body odor. The sweat may also smell strongly after garlic, curry, or other spicy foods have been eaten. Bacterial decomposition of sweat occurs most noticeably in the armpits and around the genital area, because the *apocrine glands* in these areas contain proteins and fatty materials favorable to the growth of bacteria. Sweat from other areas of the body is mainly salt water, which does not encourage bacteria to grow. Feet are an exception because they are under warm, airless conditions for many hours—the perfect environment for bacteria and fungi to flourish.

PREVENTING BODY ODOR

If body odor is a problem, the most effective treatment is to wash all over at least once daily. After washing, the use of a deodorant containing an antiperspirant will prevent sweat from reaching the surface of the skin.

Boil

An inflamed, pus-filled area of skin, usually an infected hair follicle (the tiny pit from which a hair grows). Common sites include the back of the neck and moist areas such as the armpits and groin. A more severe and extensive form occurs when several boils form a *carbuncle*.

The usual cause of boils is infection with the bacterium STAPHYLOCOCCUS AUREUS. Some people carry this organism in their noses or other sites, but often the source of an infection cannot be traced.

SYMPTOMS

A boil starts as a red, painful lump. As it swells it fills with pus and becomes rounded, with a yellowish tip (head). Recurrent boils may occur in people with known or unrecognized *diabetes mellitus* or other conditions in which general body resistance to bacterial infection is impaired.

B

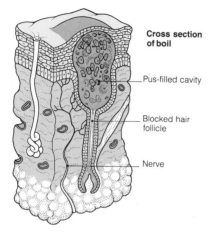

Cross section
of boil

— Pus-filled cavity

— Blocked hair
follicle

— Nerve

TREATMENT

Do not burst a boil, as this may spread the infection. A hot compress applied every two hours will relieve discomfort and hasten possible drainage and healing. Showering, instead of bathing, reduces the chance of spreading the infection.

If the boil is large and painful, consult your physician. He or she may prescribe an antibiotic, or may open the boil with a sterile needle to allow the pus to drain. Large boils occasionally need to be lanced with a surgical knife, usually using local anesthesia.

Bolus

A soft mass of chewed food that is produced by the action of the tongue, teeth, and saliva. In this form, food is easily swallowed and passed through the esophagus.

The term bolus is also used to describe a drug dose that is rapidly injected into a vein.

Bonding

The process by which a strong psychological and emotional tie is established between a parent and newborn child. Bonding is essential for a baby's healthy emotional development.

Ideas about bonding were developed from studies of geese, monkeys, and other animals. Goslings were observed attaching themselves to and following the first moving object they saw after birth. Monkeys deprived of their mothers failed to develop normal parental instincts. However, most monkeys in the experiment developed normally when they were given an inanimate mother substitute, especially if this was a furry one that could be held and cuddled.

Bonding is a reciprocal process in which baby and parent respond to

each other's gestures and expressions. A failure to bond may occur if a baby is ill or premature and has to be separated from his or her parents (by being placed in an incubator directly after birth), but such babies usually bond normally if given special attention at a later stage. Bonding problems may occur if a new parent's own early family experiences failed to provide a good model of parent-infant interaction. However, such people can be taught successful ways to interact with their newborns.

Lack of bonding may increase the risk of neglect or *child abuse* in adult life and may also lead to delayed emotional development, depression, and inability to develop satisfactory relationships in adulthood.

Most studies of the process indicate that working mothers may bond as successfully as nonworking mothers and that children can fare well with more than one primary caregiver (of either sex) as long as all caregivers are loving and consistent.

The bonding process
By maintaining eye-to-eye and frequent physical contact, bonding gradually becomes established.

Bonding, dental

Dental techniques that use plastic resins and veneers made of acrylic or porcelain to repair, restore, or improve the appearance of damaged or defective (*teeth*). Dental bonding is sometimes used as an alternative to crowning (see *Crown, dental*), and may also be used as a preventive technique to protect the teeth.

WHY IT IS DONE

Bonding techniques are sometimes suitable for treating teeth that are badly stained, chipped, broken, or malformed. Bonding may also be used to fill the gaps between teeth that are too widely spaced, or to rebuild decayed back teeth. In some cases, bonding is performed before the attachment of *orthodontic ap-*

pliances. Bonding can be used as a protective measure when the roots of the teeth are exposed or when teeth are particularly sensitive to changes in temperature. Plastic sealants are sometimes applied as a preventive measure, to prevent the buildup of bacteria in the deep grooves of the back teeth.

HOW IT IS DONE

There is usually no need for anesthesia during bonding procedures.

The dentist begins by applying a weak acid solution to the tooth—a technique sometimes known as acid-etching. This roughens the surface of the tooth so that it will hold the resin, which is applied to the tooth in liquid form.

If a portion of a tooth needs rebuilding, or is missing completely, the resin can be shaped on the tooth. The resin is then hardened either chemically or by the application of a special light. The bonded surface is then smoothed and polished. If bonding is carried out on badly stained or highly visible teeth, a porcelain or acrylic veneer may be applied over the resin.

RESULTS

Bonding can improve both the structure and the appearance of teeth. Typically, however, the procedure must be repeated after about five years. Bonding materials are weaker than natural tooth enamel and thus chip more easily. Bonded teeth may also become stained by certain types of food and drink. Because bonding materials are less hard-wearing than the materials used for dental crowns, crowning may sometimes be a more suitable technique for the repair of badly damaged back teeth.

Bone

The structural material of the *skeleton*. Bone contains calcium and phosphorus, which make it hard and rigid; the arrangement of fibers in bone makes it resilient and strong.

STRUCTURE

The surface of bone is covered with periosteum, a thin membrane that contains a network of blood vessels and nerves. Beneath the periosteum is a hard, dense shell that is known as compact, ivory, or cortical bone. Inside this shell the bone has a mesh-like structure and is known as spongy, cancellous, or trabecular bone. The central cavity found in some bones and the spaces in spongy bone contain a fatty tissue, *bone marrow*, in which the red cells, platelets, and most white blood cells are formed.

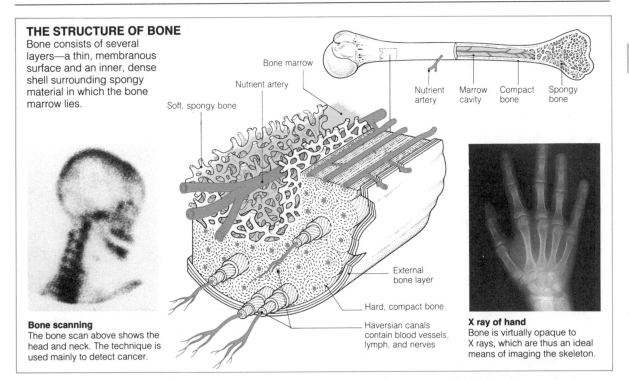

THE STRUCTURE OF BONE
Bone consists of several layers—a thin, membranous surface and an inner, dense shell surrounding spongy material in which the bone marrow lies.

Bone marrow

Nutrient artery

Soft, spongy bone

Nutrient artery

Marrow cavity

Compact bone

Spongy bone

External bone layer

Hard, compact bone

Haversian canals contain blood vessels, lymph, and nerves

Bone scanning
The bone scan above shows the head and neck. The technique is used mainly to detect cancer.

X ray of hand
Bone is virtually opaque to X rays, which are thus an ideal means of imaging the skeleton.

The hard structural bone underneath the periosteum is formed of columns of bone cells; each column has a central hollow called a haversian canal. These canals are important for the nutrition, growth, and repair of the bone. The direction of the canals corresponds with the mechanical forces acting on the bone. Bone is insensitive; any sensation comes from the nerves in the periosteum.

FUNCTIONS
The bones of the skeleton provide a rigid framework for the muscles; parts of the skeleton protect the body's organs (the heart and lungs in the bony thoracic cavity, the brain in the skull, and the uterus and bladder in the bony pelvis). Bones, together with the joints and muscles, form the locomotor system.

GROWTH
The growth of bone is a balance between the activity of its two constituent cells, osteoblasts and osteoclasts. Osteoblasts encourage deposition of the mineral calcium phosphate on the protein framework of the bone. Osteoclasts remove mineral from the bone. The actions of these cells are controlled by hormones: growth hormone secreted by the pituitary gland, the sex hormones estrogen and testosterone, the adrenal hormones, parathyroid hormone, and the thyroid

hormone thyrocalcitonin. These hormones also maintain the calcium level in the blood within close limits; any fall below the normal range affects the nerves and muscles.

Most bones begin to develop in the embryo during the fifth or sixth week of pregnancy, when they take the form of cartilage. This cartilage begins to be replaced by hard bone, in a process known as *ossification*, at around the seventh or eighth week of pregnancy; the process is not complete until early adult life. At birth many bones consist mainly of cartilage, which will ossify later. The *epiphyses* (the growing ends of the long bones) are separated from the bone shaft by the epiphyseal plate. Some bones, such as some skull bones, do not develop from cartilage and are known as membranous bones.

Bone abscess
A localized collection of pus in a bone (see *Osteomyelitis*).

Bone cancer
Malignant growth in bone. Bone cancer may originate in the bone itself (primary bone cancer); more commonly, it occurs as a result of cancer spreading from elsewhere in the body (secondary bone cancer). The cancerous growth replaces bone, causing

pain and sometimes swelling. It also makes the bone more likely to fracture without preceding injury. Bone cancer that affects the spine may cause collapse or crushing of vertebrae (spinal bones), damaging the spinal cord, and thus causing weakness or paralysis of one or more limbs.

PRIMARY BONE CANCER
All forms of primary bone cancer are rare. The type that occurs most often is *osteosarcoma*, which most frequently affects the leg bones of children and young adults. Symptoms of osteosarcoma are pain, tenderness, and swelling, typically just above or just below the knee. X rays, bone scans (see *Bone imaging*), and *biopsy* may be used to confirm the diagnosis.

Other types of primary bone cancer include *chondrosarcoma* (originating from cartilage) and *fibrosarcoma* (from fibrous tissue). Bone cancer can also start in the bone marrow (see *Ewing's sarcoma*; *Multiple myeloma*).

The treatment of osteosarcoma, chondrosarcoma, and fibrosarcoma depends on the extent to which the disease has spread. If it remains confined to bone, amputation may be recommended. Alternatively, radiation therapy or chemotherapy, or both, may be used to control the tumor. With modern *anticancer drugs*, the outlook has improved.

B

SECONDARY BONE CANCER

Secondary, or metastatic, bone cancer is more common than primary bone cancer; it usually occurs later in life. The cancers that spread readily to bone are those of the breast, lung, prostate, thyroid, and kidney. Bone metastases occur commonly in the spine, pelvis, ribs, and skull.

In secondary bone cancer, pain is usually the main symptom and is often worse at night. Affected bones are abnormally fragile and may fracture, even without preceding injury. Such a fracture (a pathological fracture) may be the first indication that a person has cancer.

Imaging studies will confirm the presence of secondary bone cancer. If the original site of the cancer is not obvious, further tests may be needed to identify it.

Secondary bone cancers from the breast and prostate often respond to hormone therapy. Growth of prostate tumors may be inhibited with estrogen or hypothalamic hormones and in some breast tumors by *hormone antagonists*. Sometimes the most effective treatment is removal of the ovaries, testes, or adrenal glands. Fractures may require orthopedic surgery, including the use of pins and plates inserted in the bone.

Bone cyst

An abnormal cavity in a bone, usually filled with fluid. Bone cysts typically develop at one end of a long bone. The presence of a cyst is often discovered by chance after there has been a bone fracture at the site of the cyst. A minor operation that involves scraping the cyst and filling the cavity with bone chips usually cures the condition.

Bone graft

An operation in which a small piece of bone is taken from one part of the body to repair bone damage in another part. The bone graft is attached to the defective bone, and provides a protein that stimulates bone growth. Although the bone graft itself eventually dies, when first transplanted it acts as a scaffold upon which new bone can grow.

WHY IT IS DONE

A bone graft has four main uses: to encourage a fracture to heal, to restore bone lost through injury, to replace bone removed surgically because of disease, and to provide a peg to join the bones of a diseased or unstable joint. A bone graft may also be used in cosmetic surgery to improve the shape of the face and skull.

HOW IT IS DONE

The bone from which the graft is to be taken is exposed and a portion removed. The most common sources are the iliac crests (upper part of the hip bones). These bones contain a large amount of the inner, spongy bone, which is especially useful for getting grafts to "take." Other sources are the ribs, which provide curved bone, and the ulna (in the forearm), which provides excellent bone pegs.

The bone that needs treatment is exposed and the graft fixed to it with screws or wires. After the area has been stitched, a plaster cast is applied to keep the graft in place.

RECOVERY PERIOD

Bruising and pain at the site from which the graft was taken clear up within a week or two, and the only large scars left are those where bone has been taken from the iliac crests. X rays are taken to check the progress of healing, which usually is well under way after about six weeks.

Most bone graft operations succeed in permitting formation of new bone as strong and efficient as the old.

Bone imaging

Techniques for providing pictures that show the structure or function of bones, used for the detection of disease or injury.

TYPES

Because X rays are more fully absorbed by bone than by other tissues, X-ray images show bone structure clearly. This makes them ideal for diagnosing fractures and injuries and also for revealing tumors and infections that cause changes in bone structure. A more detailed examination of small changes or abnormalities hidden by surrounding structures is provided by *tomography* (taking X-ray pictures at different depths of the structure being examined) or by *CT scanning*. *MRI* shows tumors and infections and the effect of diseased bone on surrounding muscles, ligaments, and fat. Either CT scanning or

---

DISORDERS OF THE BONE

Bone is affected by the same types of disorders as other body tissues, but its hard, rigid structure makes for extra complications. If a bone receives a direct blow or suffers from repeated stress it may *fracture*. If it becomes infected (for instance, due to *osteomyelitis* or a *bone abscess*), the resulting inflammation may interfere with the blood supply, leading to death of part of the bone.

GENETIC DISORDERS

Several genetic (inherited) conditions may affect bone growth; these include *achondroplasia* and *osteogenesis imperfecta*. Such disorders often result in *short stature*.

NUTRITIONAL DISORDERS

Lack of calcium and vitamin D in the diet may result in *rickets* in children and *osteomalacia* in adults; in both conditions the bones become soft and lose their shape.

HORMONAL DISORDERS

If the pituitary gland produces excess growth hormone before puberty, there is an overgrowth of bones and other organs leading to *gigantism*. Excess parathyroid hormone causes *bone cysts*. *Osteoporosis* is also frequently due to other hormonal disturbances.

TUMORS

Several different types of benign and malignant growth can affect bones (see *Bone cancer; Bone tumor*).

DEGENERATION

Degenerative disorders of bone become more common in old age. In *osteoarthritis* there is wearing of the bone surface in a number of joints.

AUTOIMMUNE DISORDERS

Here the body's *immune system* attacks its own tissues. The main autoimmune disorder that may affect bones is *rheumatoid arthritis*.

OTHER DISORDERS

Paget's disease involves thickening of the outer layer of the bones while the inside becomes spongy.

INVESTIGATION

Bone disorders are investigated by techniques such as *X rays*, *CT scanning*, and *radionuclide scanning*, by *biopsy*, and by biochemical *blood tests* to look for any abnormalities in the levels of hormones or nutrients such as calcium and vitamin D.

MRI is useful in looking for *disk prolapse* (slipped disk) in people with low back pain.

Radionuclide scanning is used to reveal bone function by showing the rate of blood flow to the bone and of cell activity within it. The technique is used mainly to determine whether cancer has spread to bone. It can also give useful information on bone injuries, infections, tumors, arthritis, and metabolic disorders, such as *rickets*, that affect bone.

Bone marrow

The soft fatty tissue found in bone cavities; it may be red or yellow. Red bone marrow is a blood-producing tissue present in all bones at birth. During the teens, it is gradually replaced in some bones by less active yellow marrow. In adults, red marrow is confined chiefly to the spine, sternum (breastbone), ribs, clavicles (collarbones), scapulae (shoulder blades), pelvis (hipbones), and skull bones.

Red bone marrow is the factory for most of the *blood cells*—all of the red cells and platelets and most of the white cells. Stem cells (cells whose descendants specialize into different cell types) within the red marrow are stimulated to form blood cells by erythropoietin, a hormone originating in the kidney. The blood cells go through various stages of maturation in the red marrow before they are ready to be released into the circulation. Yellow marrow is composed mainly of connective tissue and fat. If the body needs to increase its rate of blood formation, some of the yellow marrow will be replaced by red.

Sometimes marrow fails to produce sufficient numbers of normal blood cells, as occurs in aplastic anemia (see *Anemia, aplastic*) or when marrow has been displaced by tumor cells. In other cases, marrow may overproduce certain blood cells, as occurs in *polycythemia* and *leukemia*.

Bone marrow biopsy

A procedure to obtain a sample of cells from the bone marrow (aspiration biopsy) or a small core of bone with marrow inside (trephine biopsy). The sample is usually taken from the sternum (breastbone) or the iliac crests (upper part of the hipbones).

Microscopic examination of the bone marrow gives information on the development of the various components of blood and on the presence of cells foreign to the marrow. It is useful in the diagnosis of many blood disorders, including *anemia, leukemia,* bone marrow failure, and certain infections. It can also show whether bone marrow has been invaded by *lymphoma* (a cancer of lymphatic tissue) or cells from other tumors.

Trephine biopsy requires a long, thick needle for removal of the bone core, usually from the iliac crest. Trephine biopsy is used when tumor growth makes aspiration impossible, or when the bone marrow structure needs to be examined.

Bone marrow biopsy may be performed repeatedly to monitor the response of a disease to treatment.

Bone marrow transplantation

The technique of using normal bone marrow to replace malignant or defective marrow in a patient. In allogeneic bone marrow transplantation (BMT), healthy bone marrow is taken from a donor who has a very similar tissue type to the recipient's—usually a brother or sister. In autologous BMT the patient's own bone marrow is used. Either type of transplantation is performed only in centers that specialize in this procedure.

WHY IT IS DONE
Because the procedure itself carries certain risks, BMT is used only in the treatment of potentially fatal blood and immune system disorders, including severe aplastic anemia (see *Anemia, aplastic*), *leukemia*, severe combined immunodeficiency (see *Immunodeficiency disorders*) and some inborn errors of metabolism (see *Metabolism, inborn errors of*).

HOW IT IS DONE
ALLOGENEIC BMT Blood samples are taken from the patient and the prospective donor to assess compatibility of tissue types.

Before transplantation is carried out, all of the recipient's marrow (healthy and diseased) must first be destroyed. This is achieved by treatment in the form of *cytotoxic drugs* or radiation. Destroying the marrow prevents rejection of the donated cells and also kills any cancer cells present. After this has been done, the patient is nursed in a single room with reverse *isolation* facilities to minimize the risk of infection. The procedure for removing bone marrow from a donor and transplanting it into the patient is shown in the illustrated box, page 194.

AUTOLOGOUS BMT Bone marrow is taken from the patient (usually a person who has a malignant disease) while his or her disease is in remission (not active) and stored by *cryopreservation* (a tissue-freezing technique). Before freezing, the marrow is sometimes treated in an attempt to eliminate any remaining malignant cells. However, this method remains experimental for most conditions. If the disease recurs, the stored bone marrow can then be thawed and reinfused into the patient, after first destroying all his or her bone marrow as in allogeneic BMT.

COMPLICATIONS
Infection can be a major problem during the recovery period, and isolation nursing procedures must continue for about four to six weeks until the new marrow is producing adequate numbers of white blood cells.

In allogeneic BMT, the other dangerous complication is the rejection process known as *graft-versus-host disease* (GVHD). GVHD occurs when lymphocytes in the donor bone marrow recognize their new host (recipient) environment as foreign. Symptoms include rash, jaundice, and diarrhea. *Immunosuppressant drugs*, such as *cyclosporine* and *corticosteroid drugs*, prevent and treat rejection. The risk of GVHD may be reduced by removing the T-cells from the bone marrow with monoclonal antibodies (see *Antibody, monoclonal*) before it is reinfused.

Complications may continue to arise for long periods after a bone marrow transplant.

Bone tumor

A swelling occurring in a bone. Bone tumors may be malignant (see *Bone cancer*) or benign (noncancerous).

Benign bone tumors are classified into different types. The most common is an *osteochondroma*, a mixed swelling of bone and cartilage that often begins in childhood. Other types are *osteoma*, a smooth, rounded bone swelling, and chondroma, which is made up of cartilage cells and occurs mainly in the hands or feet (see *Chondromatosis*). Osteoma and chondroma are painless and may affect any bone in the body.

No treatment is necessary unless the tumor becomes very large or unsightly, or causes symptoms by pressing on other structures (such as arteries or nerves). In such cases, the tumor can be removed surgically.

Another type of benign bone tumor is an osteoclastoma (also called a giant cell tumor). This tumor, which usually occurs in the arm or leg of a young adult, is tender and painful. For these reasons, and for appearance, such tumors should be removed.

B

PERFORMING A BONE MARROW TRANSPLANT

Normal bone marrow is used to replace malignant or defective marrow. In the allogeneic procedure, healthy marrow is taken from a donor. In the autologous procedure, the patient's own healthy marrow is used.

With one sibling there is a 25% chance of finding a compatible donor.

With three siblings there are three opportunities for a 25% chance of finding a donor.

Finding a donor
The more siblings one has, the greater the chance of finding a donor. With three or more siblings, the chances are good.

HOW IT IS DONE

1 Before transplantation, all the recipient's marrow is destroyed by treatment with drugs or radiation. Destroying the marrow kills any cancer cells.

3 After aspiration, the bone marrow is transfused intravenously into the patient. The bone marrow cells find their way through the circulation into the patient's marrow cavities, where they start to grow.

SITES OF BONE MARROW

Red or yellow in color, bone marrow is a soft, fatty tissue found in the cavities of bones. In newborn babies, red bone marrow is present in all bones; during the teen years, most is replaced by yellow marrow. The marrow used for transplants is red.

Bone marrow

Soft, spongy bone

Hard, compact bone

Bone marrow seen under the microscope

Surgeon

Assistant

2 Using general anesthesia, bone marrow is aspirated from the donor's iliac crests and/or sternum. Only 20 to 50 ml is removed, since the transplanted marrow grows quickly to occupy the bone spaces.

Anesthetist

ASPIRATION BIOPSY

A hollow aspiration needle is introduced into the bone (iliac crests or sternum). A stylet (a thin, sharp lance) is passed through the needle and advanced (using small, twisting movements) through the bone cortex. The stylet is removed. Bone marrow is sucked out from the cortex into a syringe connected to the needle.

Stylet

Aspiration needle

Syringe

Sternum

Iliac crest

Booster
A follow-up dose of *vaccine* given to reinforce the effect of a first course.

Borborygmi
A name for the audible bowel sounds that are a normal part of the digestive process. They are caused by movement of air and fluid through the intestine. In some people they may be accentuated during times of anxiety.

Borborygmi may be affected by some disorders of the *intestine*, and physicians listen to the bowel sounds as an aid to diagnosis.

Borderline personality disorder
A form of personality disorder falling between neurotic and psychotic levels. The person with a borderline personality disorder is usually incapable of maintaining stable relationships. Mood changes are often rapid and inappropriate. Frequent, angry outbursts are common, as are impulsive, self-damaging acts such as gambling, shoplifting, or suicide attempts.

Bornholm disease
One of many names for epidemic *pleurodynia*, an infectious viral disease that is characterized by severe chest pains and fever.

Bottle-feeding
A method of infant feeding using a formula based on modified cow's milk. Although *breast-feeding* is preferable and recommended where possible, parents sometimes choose bottle-feeding. With bottle-feeding, there is no fluctuation in the quality or quantity of the milk, and the baby's intake can be measured and regulated as required.

PREPARING THE FEEDING
The formula must be measured accurately and mixed with water to the correct strength as indicated on the container. The proportions of protein, fat, lactose (milk sugar), and minerals are similar to those in human milk and vitamins are added. No extra milk powder, sugar, or cereal should be added to the feeding.

It is essential that strict rules of hygiene be observed when preparing infant feedings because bacteria thrive in warm milk. All equipment must be cleaned thoroughly and sterilized using one of two methods.

ASEPTIC STERILIZATION
This technique involves sterilizing all bottles, nipples, and caps before use by immersing them in boiling water and storing them in an antiseptic solution such as sodium hypochlorite. The feeding is then prepared using boiled water and can be used immediately after it cools to a lukewarm temperature.

TERMINAL STERILIZATION
This method involves sterilizing the prepared milk along with the bottles in a special steam sterilizing unit or saucepan. Up to six feedings—enough for one day—may be prepared at once and stored in the refrigerator. The feeding may be warmed for use by standing the bottle in a pan of hot water, or by placing it in an electric warmer. Do not use a microwave oven; this method of warming may alter the nutritional value of the feeding. Any unused milk must be discarded immediately.

PROBLEMS
If feedings are carefully prepared, equipment sterilized, and bottles given with warmth and cuddling, problems should be rare. However, parents should guard against overfeeding; the correct amount for an infant is based on his or her weight and expected weight for age. There is some variation in infant requirements, however.

A more serious long-term problem for some bottle-fed infants concerns proteins and peptides found in cow's milk, but not in breast milk. Early exposure to these may sensitize the infant to cow's milk protein and result in allergic reactions in later life. If there is a history of allergy in the family, feeding an infant with a non-milk protein formula may be recommended to prevent an allergic reaction in the child; consult your physician. (See also *Feeding, infant*.)

Botulism
A rare but serious form of poisoning caused by eating improperly canned or preserved food contaminated with a toxin produced by the bacterium *CLOSTRIDIUM BOTULINUM*. The toxin causes progressive muscular paralysis and other disturbances of the central and peripheral nervous system.

CAUSES AND INCIDENCE
CLOSTRIDIUM BOTULINUM is found in soil and untreated water in most parts of the world and is harmlessly present in the intestinal tracts of many animals, including fish. It produces spores that resist boiling, salting, smoking, and some forms of pickling. These spores, which multiply only in the absence of air, cannot normally infect humans, but thrive in improperly preserved or canned food where they produce the toxin. If such food is eaten, absorption of even minute amounts of toxin can lead to severe poisoning. Botulism is rare in Canada, but a few cases a year do occur.

SYMPTOMS AND TREATMENT
Symptoms appear between eight and 36 hours after eating contaminated food. There may be difficulty swallowing and speaking, nausea, vomiting, and double vision. Prompt treatment with an antitoxin reduces the risk of death. (See *Food poisoning*.)

BOTTLE-FEEDING
The parent's back should be supported firmly with feet flat on the floor. The baby should be cradled snugly with the head supported well above the level of the stomach. Eye contact should be maintained.

Types of bottle
Bottles, and their nipples, come in various shapes and sizes. Some come ready-filled with formula.

Technique
The bottle must be kept tilted and the flow of milk maintained at a good rate but not so fast as to cause choking.

Bowel

A common name for the large and/or small *intestines*.

Bowel movements, abnormal

See *Feces, abnormal*.

Bowel sounds

See *Borborygmi*.

Bowen's disease

A rare skin disorder that sometimes becomes cancerous. The disorder consists of a flat, regular-shaped patch of red, scaly skin, usually on the face or hands. Treatment consists of removing the diseased patch of skin surgically or destroying it by freezing or *cauterization*. The disorder is unlikely to recur.

Some physicians believe that a person who has had Bowen's disease is at increased risk of developing cancer of the lung, kidney, or large intestine later in life.

Bowleg

An outward curving of bones in the legs. Bowlegs are common in very young children and are a normal part of development. The curve usually straightens as the child grows, but, if the bowing is severe, is on one side only, or persists beyond the age of 6, a physician should be consulted. An operation may be needed to correct the condition.

Rarely, leg deformity is a result of bone disease, particularly *rickets* (a vitamin D deficiency) in children.

Brace, dental

See *Orthodontic appliances*.

Brace, orthopedic

An appliance worn to support part of the body or to hold it in a fixed position. An orthopedic brace may be used to correct or halt the development of a deformity, to aid mobility, or to relieve pain. (See *Caliper splint; Corset; Splint*.)

Brachialgia

Pain or stiffness in the arm. Brachialgia is often accompanied by pain, tingling, or numbness of the hands or fingers, and weakness of hand grip. It may indicate an underlying disorder such as *frozen shoulder* or nerve compression from *cervical osteoarthritis* (arthritis in the bones of the neck).

Brachial plexus

A collection of large nerve trunks that pass from the lower part of the cervical spine (in the neck) and the upper part of the thoracic spine (in the chest) down the arm. These nerve trunks divide into the musculocutaneous and axillary, median, ulnar, and radial nerves which both control muscles in and receive sensations from the arm and hand.

INJURIES

Injuries to the brachial plexus are an important and fairly common cause of partial or complete loss of movement and sensation in the arm. Damage to the brachial plexus sometimes occurs during birth, with an increased risk in *breech delivery*. In adults, a common cause of brachial plexus injury is a fall from a motorcycle.

Injury is usually a forcible separation of the neck and shoulder, due to a fall pushing the shoulder downward or to a blow to the side of the neck that stretches or tears upper nerve roots in the plexus. Damage to these roots causes paralysis in muscles of the shoulder and elbow.

Injury to lower nerve roots in the plexus, causing paralysis of muscles in the forearm and hand, can result from a forcible blow that lifts the arm and shoulder upward.

In severe injuries, both the upper and the lower nerve roots of the brachial plexus are damaged, producing complete paralysis of the arm.

Paralysis may be temporary if the stretching was not severe enough to tear nerve fibers.

TREATMENT Treatment of a brachial plexus injury depends on the extent and severity of nerve damage. Possible investigational procedures include *EMG* (electromyography) to demonstrate which nerves are still intact, and *myelography* (X-ray examination of the spinal cord after injection of a contrast medium).

Nerve roots that have been torn can be repaired by nerve grafting, a *microsurgery* procedure often performed with good results. However, if a nerve root has become separated from the spinal cord, surgical repair will not be successful.

In the event of permanent paralysis of a particular group of muscles in the arm, function can be improved by a muscle or *tendon transfer* operation to provide an alternative structure to perform a particular movement. *Physiotherapy*, with exercises continued at home, helps restore function after a successful nerve graft operation and can also help to reduce *contractures* in paralyzed muscles.

OTHER DISORDERS

Apart from injuries, the brachial plexus may be affected by the presence of a *cervical rib* (extra rib), infections, tumors, or *aneurysms*.

Bradycardia

An adult heart rate of below 60 beats per minute. Most people have a heart rate of between 60 and 100 beats per minute, the average being 72 to 78. Many athletes and healthy people who exercise regularly and vigorously have perfectly normal bradycardia. In others, however, bradycardia may indicate an underlying disorder such as *hypothyroidism* (underactivity of the thyroid gland) or *heart block*. Bradycardia may also occur as a result of taking *beta-blocker drugs*.

Profound or sudden bradycardia may cause a drop in blood pressure and symptoms such as loss of energy, weakness, and fainting attacks. Bradycardia occurs in a *vasovagal attack*, a condition in which the vagus nerve slows the heart rate, dilates blood vessels, and causes fainting.

Braille

A system of embossed dots that enables blind people to read and write. It was developed by the Frenchman Louis Braille and is now accepted for all written languages, music, mathematics, and science.

The braille system is based on six raised dots, which can be arranged in different combinations. There are two types. In Grade I, each symbol represents an individual letter or punctuation mark. In Grade II, symbols represent common letter combinations or words. This second form is more widely used.

Example of Grade 1 braille
In this system, each letter is represented by its own pattern of dots.

Brain

The major organ of the *nervous system*, located in the *cranium* (skull). The brain is the organ of thought, speech, and emotion, but its primary role in humans—just as in animals—is as the body's control center.

The brain and spinal cord constitute the *central nervous system* (CNS). The CNS controls basic functions such as heart rate, breathing, and body temperature. The brain receives, sorts, and interprets sensations from the

STRUCTURE OF THE BRAIN

The brain has three main parts—the brain stem (an extension of the spinal cord), the cerebellum, and the forebrain, much of which consists of the two large cerebral hemispheres. Each hemisphere consists of an outer layer, or cortex, which is rich in nerve cells and called gray matter, and inner areas rich in nerve fibers, called white matter. The surface of each hemisphere is thrown into folds called gyri separated by fissures called sulci. The two hemispheres are linked by a thick band of nerve fibers, the corpus callosum. Deep within the forebrain are various central structures, which include the thalamus, hypothalamus, basal ganglia, and pituitary gland.

The brain has a consistency like jelly and, in adults, weighs about 1.4 kg. It is protected by membranous coverings, the meninges, within the skull.

Lobes

These are broad surface regions of each hemisphere that are named after the overlying bones of the skull. The four main regions are the frontal, parietal, temporal, and occipital lobes.

Special areas

Some brain areas are associated with specific functions—for example, the occipital lobe with vision, and the cerebellum with balance and coordination. Touch and pressure sensation is perceived within the postcentral gyrus. Muscle movements are controlled from the precentral gyrus; speech is controlled from an area in the frontal lobe of the dominant hemisphere.

Angiography

This technique makes blood vessels clearly visible. The angiogram above shows the carotid artery and its branches.

Magnetic resonance imaging

This technique is used mainly to reveal abnormalities that are otherwise undetectable. In the MRI scan above, the white mass to the upper right is a tumor.

CT scanning

The CT scan above shows a "slice" through the head. The nose and eyeballs are visible at the right; the small circular area in the center is the brain stem.

B

nerves that extend from the CNS to every other part of the body; it initiates and coordinates the motor output involved in activities such as movement and speech.

Three main structures are easily recognized: the *brain stem, cerebellum,* and, above the brain stem, the large forebrain, much of which consists of the *cerebrum* (see *Brain* structure box, p. 197). Extending from the brain are 12 pairs of *cranial nerves*; some of these have a sensory function, some a motor function, and some are both sensory and motor.

BRAIN STEM AND CEREBELLUM

These parts of the brain are the oldest in evolutionary terms, and their structure and function differ little between humans and other mammals. The brain stem is concerned mainly with control of vital functions, such as breathing and blood pressure, and the cerebellum with muscular coordination, balance, and posture.

Both these brain regions operate below the level of consciousness by *reflex* action, a system by which particular stimuli or patterns of stimuli evoke preprogrammed or automatic responses. The brain stem and cerebellum receive sensory information (about temperature, pressure, position, or pain) from sensory receptors scattered throughout the body. They then transmit the appropriate response—for example, to muscles in the blood vessels or limbs to change blood pressure and flow or alter posture.

FOREBRAIN

The forebrain consists of a central group of structures and nerve nuclei (nerve cell groups) above the brain stem and, enclosing these, the relatively huge cerebrum.

CENTRAL STRUCTURES These act mainly as links between parts of the cerebrum above and brain stem below. They include the two egg-shaped *thalami,* which serve as relay stations for sensory information passing toward the cerebrum. Beneath them, the *hypothalamus* is a tiny region involved in the regulation of body temperature, thirst, and appetite; it also influences sexual behavior, aggression, and sleep. The hypothalamus has close connections with the *pituitary gland,* which produces hormones that affect other glands and in this way controls growth, sexual development, metabolism, fluid balance, and numerous other physiological variables. Encircling the thalami, a further complex of nerve centers, called the *limbic system,* is thought to be involved in the handling of emotions, some memory functions, and the processing of olfactory (smell) sensations.

CEREBRUM The two hemispheres that make up the cerebrum project upward and outward from the center of the forebrain to form an almost continuous egg-shaped mass. The cerebrum constitutes nearly 70 percent of the weight of the entire nervous system.

The surfaces of the hemispheres are folded into deep clefts so that only one third of the total surface is visible. Certain of the sulci (fissures) separating gyri (folds) are particularly noticeable and divide the surface into distinct lobes—occipital, parietal, temporal, and frontal—named after the main bones of the skull that overlie them. The two halves of the cerebrum are connected by the corpus callosum.

The cerebral cortex (the outer surface of the cerebrum) consists of gray matter, with nerve cells arranged in six layers. This is the region concerned with conscious thought, sensation, and movement. It operates in a similar way to the more primitive parts of the brain, except that incoming sensory information undergoes a far more detailed analysis. Various conscious processes, such as perception, memory, thought, and decision-making, take place between the reception of sensory information and the output of a motor response. Actions initiated by output from the cortex—speech, movement, writing—can be extremely complex in form.

Beneath the cortex, much of the cerebrum consists of tracts of nerve fibers forming white matter; these tracts connect various areas of the cortex to each other and to nerve centers in the center of the forebrain and brain stem. Deeper within the hemispheres are groups of cells named the *basal ganglia*; they are connected to the brain stem and cerebellum and are involved in relaying and modifying motor output from the cerebral cortex, signaling and coordinating movements to skeletal muscles.

Though the cerebrum is symmetrical in appearance, some higher activities such as speech and writing are controlled from one cerebral hemisphere, the dominant one. In right-handed people this is the left hemisphere; even in left-handed people the left side is usually dominant. The nondominant side plays an important role in visual/spatial orientation and may also be involved in artistic/creative thought.

PROTECTION AND NOURISHMENT

The whole of the brain and spinal cord is encased in three layers of membranes, called the *meninges.* The *cerebrospinal fluid* circulates between two of these layers and also within the four main brain cavities called *ventricles* (one in each cerebral hemisphere, a third in the center of the forebrain, and a fourth in the brain stem). This cerebrospinal fluid helps nourish the brain and also helps cushion it from injury when the head is moved quickly or receives a blow.

The brain as a whole also has an extensive blood supply. Blood comes from a circle of arteries fed by the internal *carotid arteries* (which run up each side of the front of the neck to enter the base of the skull) and from two vertebral arteries that run parallel to the spinal cord. The brain receives about 20 percent of the heart's output of blood. (See also *Brain* disorders box on facing page.)

Brain abscess

A collection of pus, surrounded by inflamed tissues, within the brain or on its surface. Along with *brain tumors* and other space-occupying brain abnormalities, abscesses cause symptoms due to raised pressure within the skull and local damage to nerve tracts. The most common sites of brain abscesses are the frontal and temporal lobes of the *cerebrum* in the forebrain.

CAUSES AND INCIDENCE

Brain abscesses may follow head injury but most cases result from the spread of infection from elsewhere in the body. Approximately 40 percent of abscesses result from middle ear or sinus infections. Other causes include infection following a penetrating brain injury, and blood-borne infection, most commonly in patients with acute bacterial *endocarditis* or some types of *immunodeficiency disorders.* Abscesses due to blood-borne infection are often multiple.

SYMPTOMS

The commonest symptoms are headache, drowsiness, and vomiting. There may also be visual disturbances, fever, epileptic seizures, and symptoms due to local brain damage—for example, partial paralysis or speech disturbances.

DIAGNOSIS AND TREATMENT

The diagnosis is suggested by *CT scanning* or *MRI* (magnetic resonance imaging) of the brain. Treatment consists of a high dosage of antibiotics and usually surgery. A hole may need

DISORDERS OF THE BRAIN

Defects and disorders of the brain have much the same causes as disease in other body organs. One special feature of the brain, however, is that it is packed inside a rigid casing, the skull, so any space-occupying *brain abscess, brain tumor*, or *hematoma* (large blood clot) following a *head injury* or *brain hemorrhage* creates raised pressure that impairs the function of the whole brain. Another special feature is that brain cells destroyed through injury or disease cannot be replaced, so the loss in function can be more difficult to reverse.

Some diseases and defects in the brain are localized in a small region and may thus have a specific effect—for example, *aphasia* (speech loss). More often, damage is more diffuse and, because the brain has so many related functions, the symptoms can be varied and numerous.

CONGENITAL DEFECTS

Babies may be born with brain defects due to genetic or chromosomal disorders, as in *Down's syndrome, Tay-Sachs disease*, or *cri du chat syndrome* (all of which are associated with mental deficiency). Structural defects that arise during fetal development may be fundamental and untreatable, as in *microcephaly* (small head), or fatal, as in *anencephaly* (congenital absence of the brain). Others are potentially correctable, even while the fetus is still in the uterus, as in *hydrocephalus* (water on the brain).

IMPAIRED BLOOD AND OXYGEN SUPPLY

These are two of the most important causes of brain dysfunction because brain cells can survive only a few minutes without oxygen. *Hypoxia* (lack of oxygen) affecting the brain as a result of asphyxiation during the process of birth is one of the causes of *cerebral palsy*. Later in life, cerebral hypoxia can result from an accident such as choking or from arrest of breathing and heartbeat following electrocution or drowning.

From middle age onward, the most important affliction of the brain is *cerebrovascular disease* impairing blood supply to one or several brain regions. If an artery within the brain becomes blocked or ruptures leading to hemorrhage, the result is a *stroke*.

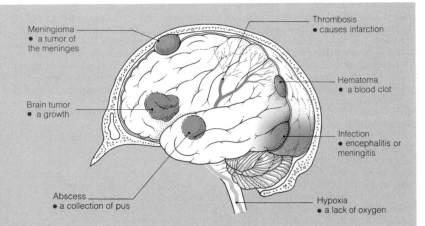

INJURY

Although protected by the skull, the brain may be damaged by heavy blows to the head or following skull fracture as a result of falls, high-speed impacts, bullet wounds, or other physical violence (see *Head injury*).

INFECTION

Infection within the brain, called *encephalitis*, or of the membranes surrounding the brain, called *meningitis*, is uncommon today. Meningitis is usually caused by a bacterial infection. Encephalitis can be caused by any one of numerous viruses, of which the best known and most dangerous are the *rabies* and *herpes simplex* viruses.

An abscess (localized pocket of infection) in the brain may result from spread of infection from the ear, sinuses, or elsewhere in the body (see *Brain abscess*).

TUMORS

Tumors that affect the brain may be primary (arising from tissues inside the skull) as in *gliomas, meningiomas, acoustic neuromas*, and *pituitary tumors*, or secondary (arising from cancer cells that have spread through the bloodstream from tumors in the lungs, breasts, or elsewhere). See *Brain tumors*.

DEGENERATION

Multiple sclerosis, a progressive disease of unknown cause in which the nerve sheaths (composed of myelin) are destroyed, starts most commonly in early adulthood.

Degenerative brain diseases, such as *Alzheimer's disease* (a type of dementia) and *Parkinson's disease*, are particularly important causes of disability among the elderly.

OTHER DISORDERS

Disorders characterized by their symptoms rather than any obvious cause include *migraine, narcolepsy* (excessive episodic sleepiness), and idiopathic *epilepsy* (epilepsy of unknown cause), though epileptic seizures can also have specific causes, such as a tumor.

Disorders of thought, emotion, or behavior are generally described as psychiatric or *mental illnesses*. Often, there is no obvious physical brain defect or disorder, although, with many important mental illnesses, such as *depression* and *schizophrenia*, there seems to be an underlying disturbance of brain chemistry. Some psychiatric illnesses, collectively called organic *brain syndromes*, by definition have a physical cause.

INVESTIGATION

Many different procedures may be used to investigate disorders of the brain. A full *physical examination* will include assessment of brain function by means of tests of mental abilities and state, sensation, movement, muscle tone, and reflexes. Electrical activity within the brain may be measured by means of an *EEG*. Physical abnormalities may be looked for using *brain imaging* techniques, such as *angiography, CT scanning*, or *MRI*. A *lumbar puncture* may be performed to look for evidence of bleeding or infection.

to be made in the skull (see *Craniotomy*), and the abscess is then cut open and drained of pus.

OUTLOOK

Brain abscesses prove fatal in about 10 percent of cases, and the remaining patients often suffer some residual impairment of brain function. *Epilepsy* is common, so *anticonvulsant drugs* are often prescribed after removal or drainage of the abscess.

Brain damage

Degeneration or death of nerve cells and tracts within the brain. Damage may be localized to particular areas of the brain—causing specific defects of brain function, such as loss of coordination or difficulty with speech—or may be more diffuse, causing mental or severe physical handicap.

DIFFUSE DAMAGE

The most important cause of diffuse brain damage is prolonged cerebral *hypoxia* (insufficient oxygen reaching the brain). This may occur during birth; a baby's brain cannot tolerate a lack of oxygen for more than about five minutes. At any age, hypoxia may result from *cardiac arrest* (heart stoppage) or *respiratory arrest* (cessation of breathing), or from causes such as poisoning, drowning, or *status epilepticus* (prolonged convulsions).

Diffuse damage may also occur through the accumulation in the brain of substances poisonous to nerve cells—as in untreated *phenylketonuria* or *galactosemia*, or as a result of inhaling or ingesting environmental pollutants such as compounds of lead or mercury (see *Minamata disease*).

Other possible causes include infections of the brain, such as *encephalitis* or, very rarely, brain damage following *immunization*.

LOCALIZED DAMAGE

Localized brain damage may occur as a result of *head injury*, especially penetrating injury, at any age. It may occur later in life as a result of a *stroke, brain tumor*, or *brain abscess*.

At birth, local damage to the *basal ganglia* (nerve cell centers deep within the brain) caused by a raised blood level of *bilirubin* (formed from the destruction of blood cells in *hemolytic disease of the newborn*) leads to a condition called *kernicterus*. This condition is characterized by disorders of movement and sometimes by mental deficiency. The basal ganglia may also be damaged by carbon monoxide.

SYMPTOMS AND TREATMENT

Brain damage that occurs before, during, or after birth may result in *cerebral palsy*, a condition characterized by paralysis and abnormal movements, and often associated with *mental retardation* and sometimes *deafness*.

Victims of head injury, stroke, or other causes of localized or diffuse brain damage may also be left with any of a range of handicaps, including disturbances of movement, speech, or sensation, mental handicap, or epileptic seizures.

Nerve cells and tracts in the brain and spinal cord do not recover their function if they have been destroyed (nerves in the limbs or trunk regenerate slowly after being cut or crushed). Nevertheless, some degree of improvement may be expected after brain damage as the victim learns to use other parts of the brain and other muscle groups in the body.

Treatment toward this goal often involves teamwork on the part of physicians and specialists in other health-related disciplines, such as *physiotherapy, speech therapy*, and *occupational therapy*.

Brain death

The irreversible cessation of all functions of the entire brain, including the *brain stem*. The recognition of brain death, as defined above, has allowed physicians to certify death in situations where the lungs and heart continue to function (with machine assistance) but where death has occurred based on the absence of brain function. (See also *Death*.)

Brain hemorrhage

Bleeding within or around the brain, caused either by injury or by spontaneous rupture of a blood vessel. There are four possible types: *subdural hemorrhage, extradural hemorrhage, subarachnoid hemorrhage*, and *intracerebral hemorrhage*.

CAUSES AND SYMPTOMS

Extradural and subdural hemorrhages usually result from a blow to the head (see *Head injury*); symptoms may include headache, drowsiness, confusion, and the development of paralysis on one side of the body. These symptoms may develop within hours in extradural hemorrhage but much more slowly (over weeks or months) in subdural hemorrhage. Hospital investigation and treatment is urgently required.

Subarachnoid and intracerebral hemorrhages usually occur spontaneously (i.e., without any head injury) and are the result of rupture of *aneurysms* or small blood vessels in the brain. Middle-aged and elderly persons with untreated *hypertension* (high blood pressure) are at highest risk. Subarachnoid hemorrhage is characterized by a sudden violent headache and/or sudden loss of consciousness. Intracerebral hemorrhage is one of the three main types of *stroke*; symptoms may include collapse, speech loss, and paralysis of the muscles of the face or of an arm or leg. Subarachnoid and intracerebral hemorrhages are medical emergencies.

SITES OF BRAIN HEMORRHAGE

Hemorrhages within the skull fall into four main categories—extradural, subdural, subarachnoid, and intracerebral hemorrhages—according to the site of the bleeding in relation to the brain and its protective coverings, the meninges. The causes and effects of the bleeding and the outlook for the patient vary among the categories.

Skin
Subcutaneous layer
Skull
Dura mater
Arachnoid
Pia mater
Brain
Subarachnoid

Extradural   Subdural   Intracerebral

Intracerebral hemorrhage
This brain section shows a mass of blood in the left hemisphere.

Brain imaging

Techniques that provide pictures of the brain; they are used to detect injury or disease. Computerized scanning has brought tremendous growth in this field during the past decade.

TYPES

CONVENTIONAL X RAYS The simplest and longest established method of obtaining images of the brain is to take *X-ray* films. Such films reveal distortion or erosion of the bony skull caused by a fracture, *brain tumor, aneurysm,* or *brain abscess.* Unless the brain substance itself is calcified in a localized area due to disease, plain X-ray techniques cannot detect disease of the brain matter.

Angiography involves injecting a contrast medium that shows up on X rays into one of the arteries supplying the brain, and then taking X-ray pictures. This technique shows up the blood vessels in the brain, and is used to investigate *subarachnoid hemorrhage,* aneurysms, abnormalities of the blood vessels, and other disorders of the circulation.

SCANNING TECHNIQUES *CT scanning* was first conceived in 1971 specifically to study the brain. Unlike conventional X rays, this method gives images of the brain substance. It gives especially clear pictures of the ventricles (the fluid-filled cavities of the brain) and can reveal tumors, blood clots, strokes, aneurysms, and abscesses. Contrast medium is often administered to help differentiate normal from abnormal brain tissue.

MRI produces better images of the brain than CT scanning. It is especially helpful in showing tumors of the posterior fossa (back of the skull). MRI does not involve radiation.

Radionuclide scanning uses radioactive isotopes to detect tumors, abnormalities of blood vessels, and other lesions. For most purposes, radionuclide scanning has been replaced by CT scanning and MRI.

Ultrasound scanning is used only in premature or very young babies because ultrasound waves cannot penetrate the bones of a mature skull. Ultrasound scanning is particularly useful in detecting *hydrocephalus* and ventricular hemorrhage in premature babies and, because no radiation is involved, repeated scans can be performed safely.

PET scanning combines the administration of radionuclides with CT scanning and provides information about the levels of activity in different parts of the brain.

Brain stem

A stalk of nerve tissue that forms the lowest part of the brain and links with the spinal cord. The brain stem acts partly as a highway for messages traveling between other parts of the brain and spinal cord, but also connects with 10 of the 12 pairs of *cranial nerves* and controls basic functions, such as breathing, vomiting, and eye reflexes. The activities of the brain stem are below the level of consciousness and operate largely on an automatic basis.

STRUCTURE

From the spinal cord upward, the brain stem consists of three main parts, called the medulla, pons, and midbrain. Attached to the back of the brain stem is a separate part of the brain, the *cerebellum,* which is concerned principally with balance and coordinated movement. Running longitudinally through the middle of the brain stem is a canal, which widens in the pons and medulla to form the fourth *ventricle* (cavity) of the brain, which contains the circulating *cerebrospinal fluid.*

MEDULLA The medulla resembles a thick extension of the spinal cord. It contains the nuclei (nerve cell centers) of the ninth to 12th cranial nerves, by which it receives and relays taste sensations from the tongue and relays signals to muscles involved in speech and in tongue and neck movements. It also contains the vital centers—groups of nerve cells involved in the automatic regulation of heartbeat, breathing, blood pressure, and digestion—and sends and receives information regarding these functions via the 10th cranial or *vagus nerve.*

Many of the nerve tracts running through the medulla cross over in its lower portion so that the right side of the body links up with the left side of the brain and vice versa.

PONS The pons is considerably wider than the medulla and contains thick bundles of nerve fibers that connect with the cerebellum, which lies directly behind. The pons also contains the nuclei for the fifth to eighth cranial nerves and thus relays sensory information from the ear, face, and teeth, as well as the signals that move the jaw, adjust facial expressions, and produce some eye movements.

MIDBRAIN The midbrain is the smallest section of the brain stem, above the pons. It contains the nuclei of the third and fourth cranial nerves, which control eye movements and the size and reactions of the pupil. It also contains

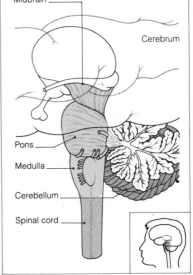

LOCATION OF THE BRAIN STEM
The brain stem is a 7.5-cm-long stalk of nerve cells and fibers that joins the upper spinal cord to the rest of the brain.

Midbrain

Cerebrum

Pons

Medulla

Cerebellum

Spinal cord

cell groups such as the substantia nigra and red nuclei, which are involved in the smooth coordination of limb movements.

RETICULAR FORMATION Scattered throughout the brain stem are numerous nerve cell groups collectively known as the reticular formation. The reticular formation is believed to act as a watchdog on sensory information entering the brain, alerting the higher brain centers to new or important sensory stimuli that may require a conscious response. Our sleep/wake cycle is controlled by the reticular formation, and many *sleeping drugs* and *stimulant drugs* are believed to exert their actions through their effects on this part of the brain.

DISORDERS

The brain stem is susceptible to the same disorders that afflict the rest of the central nervous system (see *Brain disorders box,* p. 199). Damage to the medulla's vital centers is rapidly fatal, while damage to the reticular formation may cause *coma.* Damage to specific cranial nerve nuclei can have specific effects—*facial palsy* in the case of the seventh cranial (facial) nerve and tongue-wasting with the 12th cranial (hypoglossal) nerve. Degeneration of the substantia nigra in the midbrain is thought to be a cause of *Parkinson's disease.*

Brain syndrome, organic

Any disturbance of a person's consciousness, intellect, or mental functioning that is of organic (physical) as opposed to psychiatric origin. Possible causes of the syndrome include degenerative diseases such as *Alzheimer's disease*, metabolic imbalances, infections, certain drugs, toxins, vitamin deficiencies, or the effects of injury, *stroke*, or tumor.

SYMPTOMS

In acute organic brain syndrome, symptoms range from slight confusion to stupor or *coma*, and may also include restlessness, disorientation, memory impairment, hallucinations, and delusions (see *Delirium*). The chronic form results in a progressive decline in intellect, memory, and behavior (see *Dementia*).

TREATMENT

Treatment relies on discovering and, if possible, dealing with the underlying cause. Treatment is more likely to be successful with the acute form. In chronic cases, irreversible *brain damage* may already have occurred. (See also *Psychosis*.)

Brain tumor

An abnormal growth in or on the brain. Although not always malignant, all brain tumors are serious because of the buildup of pressure in the brain and compression of adjoining brain areas that occur as the tumor expands.

TYPES

Brain tumors may be primary growths arising directly from tissues within the skull, or metastases (secondary growths) spread via the bloodstream from tumors elsewhere in the body, most commonly from tumors in the lung or breast.

The cause of primary brain tumors is not known. About 60 percent are *gliomas* (frequently malignant), which arise from the brain substance. Other primary tumors include *meningiomas*, arising from the meningeal membranes that cover the brain; *acoustic neuromas*, arising from the acoustic nerve; and *pituitary tumors*, arising from the pituitary gland. All of these tumors are benign.

Certain types of primary brain tumors mainly affect children and are often situated in the back of the brain. These include two types of glioma called *medulloblastoma* and cerebellar *astrocytoma*.

Secondary growths, or metastases, are always malignant and may be found in more than one organ.

INCIDENCE

In Canada, about 2,000 cases of primary brain tumor are reported yearly and there are about 1,300 deaths from brain tumor each year. They occur most commonly around the age of 50 years, although a significant number of children are also affected; each year about 50 Canadian children die from a primary brain tumor.

SYMPTOMS

Brain tumors cause symptoms by several mechanisms. Compression of brain tissue or nerve tracts within the vicinity of the tumor may cause muscle weakness, loss of vision, or other sensory disturbances, speech difficulties, and, in about 20 percent of cases, epileptic seizures. The presence of an expanding tumor can increase pressure within the skull, causing headache, vomiting, visual disturbances, and impairment of mental functioning. If the circulation of cerebrospinal fluid is obstructed by the tumor, *hydrocephalus* may result.

DIAGNOSIS

Many different techniques are used to locate the site of a brain tumor and to establish the extent of its spread. The most important are *CT scanning*, *MRI*, special X-ray studies, and *angiography*.

TREATMENT

When possible, tumors are removed by surgery after opening the skull (see *Craniotomy*), but many malignant growths are inaccessible or too extensive for removal. The outlook in these cases is poor; fewer than 20 percent of patients survive for a year after the initial diagnosis. In cases where a tumor cannot be completely removed, as much of it as possible will be cut away to relieve pressure in the brain. *Radiation therapy* or *anticancer drugs* may also be given.

Corticosteroid drugs are often prescribed to reduce the swelling of tissue around a tumor, thus temporarily relieving symptoms.

Bran

The fibrous outer covering of grain. Eating bran regularly, either in breakfast cereals or added to food, raises the *fiber* content of the diet. This helps prevent *constipation* and thus reduces the risk of intestinal disease.

Branchial disorders

A group of disorders resulting from abnormal development of the branchial arches in the *embryo*. Branchial disorders include branchial cyst and branchial fistula.

A branchial cyst is a soft swelling, about 2 to 5 cm across, that appears on the side of the neck in early adult life. The swelling contains a puslike or clear fluid that is rich in cholesterol. Diagnosis is made by identifying cholesterol crystals in a few drops of the fluid drawn from the cyst by means of a needle and syringe. Treatment is by surgical removal.

A branchial fistula is an abnormal passage between the back of the throat and the external surface of the neck, where it appears as a small hole usually noted at birth. If the hole in the neck does not extend to the back of the throat, it is termed a branchial cleft sinus; it may be present at birth or may form if a branchial cyst becomes infected and ruptures. A branchial fistula or cleft sinus may discharge mucus or pus, in which case the fistula or sinus may be removed surgically.

Braxton Hicks' contractions

Short, relatively painless contractions of the uterus during pregnancy. In early pregnancy, Braxton Hicks' contractions may be felt by a physician performing an internal examination. In late pregnancy, they may be felt by the woman and seen by looking at the abdomen. Sometimes they are mistaken for labor pains, although they occur as isolated contractions, have no effect on the cervix, and are not as uncomfortable as the contractions of true labor.

Breakbone fever

A tropical, mosquito-spread, viral illness also called *dengue*. One symptom of the illness is severe joint and muscle pain, hence the name "breakbone."

Breakthrough bleeding

Vaginal bleeding or staining ("spotting") between menstrual periods when taking an *oral contraceptive*, especially a low-dose preparation. Breakthrough bleeding is most common during the first few months of taking the pill, when the body is adjusting to alterations in hormone levels. Loss of blood during pregnancy, or when an oral contraceptive is not being taken, may be a symptom of a serious underlying disorder (see *Vaginal bleeding*).

Breast

In addition to its primary function of nourishing a baby with milk, the female breast is a secondary *sexual characteristic*, and is regarded by society as a symbol of femininity, beauty, and eroticism. Size, shape, and appearance vary from one woman to another. The male breast is an immature version of the female breast.

STRUCTURE

The female breast consists mainly of 15 to 20 lobes of milk-secreting glands embedded in fatty tissue. The ducts of these glands have their outlet in the nipple, which is surrounded by the areola, the circular area of pigmented skin. The breast contains no muscle, but bands of fine ligaments that weave between the fat and lobules are attached to the skin and determine the breast's height and shape.

The skin over the breast is somewhat smoother, thinner, and more translucent than over much of the rest of the body. The areola skin is particularly thin, and contains sweat glands, sebaceous glands, and hair follicles. The nipple is very sensitive to touch; contraction of its muscle fibers results in erection, which is a sign of sexual arousal or cold.

The size and shape of the breasts of mature women not only vary between individuals, but also at different times—during the menstrual cycle, during pregnancy and lactation, and after the menopause.

FUNCTION

During pregnancy, estrogen and progesterone, secreted by the ovary and placenta, cause the milk-producing glands to develop and become active and the nipple to enlarge in preparation for *breast-feeding*. Just before or after childbirth the glands in the breast produce a watery fluid called colostrum, which contains proteins and antibodies to protect the newborn baby against infection. Within about three days the colostrum is replaced with milk, whose production is stimulated by the hormone prolactin, released from the anterior pituitary gland.

BREAST DEVELOPMENT

The breasts start to grow from mammary buds when the fetus is about five months old. At birth there is a nipple with rudimentary milk ducts. At *puberty*, a girl's breasts begin to develop—the areola swells and the nipple enlarges. This is followed by an increase in glandular tissue and fat, which enlarge the breast. Eventually, the breast becomes rounded and the areola flattens.

Breast abscess

A collection of pus in the mammary gland, usually in a woman who is lactating (producing milk). Breast abscesses develop if acute *mastitis* (inflammation of the breast, usually due to infection) is not treated promptly with *antibiotic drugs*. They occur most commonly during the first month after a woman's first delivery.

SYMPTOMS

The initial symptoms are of acute mastitis: the breasts become increasingly tense and tender, and the woman may also develop fever and chills. The abscess develops in one area, which becomes very firm, red, and extremely painful.

TREATMENT AND PREVENTION

Simple *analgesic drugs*, such as acetaminophen, provide some pain relief. The abscess is treated by surgical incision and drainage of the pus under general anesthesia. A drainage tube may be left in the wound for a couple of days after surgery. The operation rapidly relieves the pain, and healing takes place quickly. Infrared heat treatment may help speed up the healing process.

Breast infections can be prevented by cleaning and drying the breasts carefully after each feed. Breast abscesses are less likely to occur if the breasts are emptied regularly, making engorgement (overfilling) and the development of mastitis less likely.

Breastbone

A common name for the *sternum*.

Breast cancer

The most common cancer in women. About one woman in 20 will develop a form of breast cancer at some time in her life. The disease causes about 5,000 deaths a year. Fewer than one in every 100 cases of breast cancer occur in men.

Mortality from breast cancer (taking account of age) has hardly changed this century, but, in the early 1980s, research studies in Sweden and the Netherlands suggested that deaths could be cut by about one third by mammographic screening of whole populations of women. Other studies

THE FEMALE BREAST

The breast is made up of lobes of glands set in fatty tissue, the ducts of which have their outlet at the nipple. The areola contains sweat glands, sebaceous glands, and hair follicles.

Fat
Skin
Areola
Nipple
Milk duct
Lobules
Pectoral muscle

A mammogram
An X ray of a healthy breast. The white, thready areas are fibrous tissues that support the fat nodules.

DISORDERS OF THE BREAST

Problems involving the breasts are usually minor and respond readily to treatment. The most important causes of problems are infection, tumors, and hormonal disturbance.

INFECTION

This is uncommon except during breast-feeding. Nursing mothers may suffer from *mastitis* (inflammation of the breast), usually due to a blocked milk duct. An *abscess* may follow if mastitis is not treated.

TUMORS

A *breast lump* may be a *cyst* (a fluid-filled sac), a *fibroadenoma* (a thickening of the milk-producing tissue) or other benign tumor, or more rarely, *breast cancer*.

HORMONAL DISORDERS

It is common for women to notice that before *menstruation* their breasts become bigger and lumpy. Such lumps shrink when menstruation is over. More common are breast pain and tenderness, which often occur just before menstruation or as a result of taking hormones. Hormonal disorders may, rarely, cause *galactorrhea* (abnormal milk production).

In men, *gynecomastia* (abnormal breast development) may result from hormonal disturbance or treatment with certain drugs.

INVESTIGATION

Disorders of the breast may be discovered during *breast self-examination* or by your physician during a physical examination. Special investigations for the breast are *biopsy* and *mammography*.

Fibroadenoma
● a common benign tumor

Cancer
● a malignant growth

Cyst
● a collection of fluid

Abscess
● a collection of pus

Nipple discharge

Galactorrhea
● abnormal production of milk

Mastitis
● inflammation of tissue

indicate the great importance of breast examination by women and their physicians in diagnosing breast cancer in its early stages. Most deaths from breast cancer occur because the disease has already spread beyond the breast when first detected.

CAUSES

Current theories of the cause of breast cancer are focused on hormonal influences. The incidence of breast cancer is known to be raised in women whose menstrual periods began when they were young and those whose menopause was late; in those who had no children or had their first child in their late 20s or 30s; and in those with mothers or sisters who had breast cancer. Diet also plays a part. The disease is rare in Japan, which has a low-fat diet, but Japanese women living in North America and eating a North American diet have the same rate of breast cancer as North Americans. Tall, heavy women have more breast cancer than short, thin ones. Breast cancer may also be more common in women who have had certain types of nonmalignant tumors removed from their breasts.

Several research studies in the late 1980s suggested that prolonged use of oral contraceptives might increase the risk of a woman developing breast cancer before the age of 35. However, such tumors are rare, so if there is any increase in breast cancer due to the pill, the overall effect is small. Furthermore the risk is balanced by the pill's effect in lowering the incidence of cancer of the ovary and uterus. Breast cancer has not become any more common in Europe or North America in the 20 years since the introduction of the pill.

SYMPTOMS

The most common site of a malignant breast tumor is the upper, outer part of the breast. The lump is usually felt rather than seen and in most cases is not painful. Other symptoms include a dark discharge from the nipple, retraction (indentation) of the nipple, and an area of dimpled, creased skin over the lump. In 90 percent of the cases only one breast is affected.

DIAGNOSIS

Monthly examination of the breasts (see *Breast self-examination*) should enable a woman to detect at an early stage any new or changed *breast lump* or any change in her nipples. Routine breast examination is carried out when women attend hospital for other complaints. In addition, *mammography* (X ray of the breasts) is recommended for high-risk women (i.e., women with a family history of breast cancer) at age 40 and should be repeated every three to five years thereafter, or sooner if advised. Mammography is also of value for all women over 50 years old.

A woman who discovers a lump in her breast should report it to her physician immediately. A mammogram may be appropriate at this time. If the physician suspects that the lump is merely a *cyst* (a fluid-filled tissue sac), it can be aspirated (i.e., the fluid can be withdrawn) and may disappear. Where there is a possibility that the lump may be a malignant tumor, a *biopsy* will be carried out. This may be an outpatient procedure in which breast tissue is withdrawn with a hollow needle, causing little discomfort, or an operation to remove all or part of the lump; in either case the suspect tissue will be examined under the microscope. If cancer is discovered, blood tests, X rays, and scanning will determine whether the disease has spread to other parts of the body, such as the bones or liver.

TREATMENT

Surgical removal of the tumor achieves a cure (as defined by survival for 20 years) in one third of women with early breast cancer. Studies have shown survival is not improved by extensive operations (such as radical *mastectomy*); many surgeons recommend lumpectomy (simple removal of the tumor), combined with *radiation therapy* and/or *anticancer drugs*. The treatment given depends on the woman's age, the size of the tumor, whether or not there are signs of spread to the lymph nodes under the arm, and the sensitivity of the tumor cells to hormones as determined in the laboratory by a technique called estrogen receptor testing.

Secondary tumors in other parts of the body, which may be present at the time of the initial diagnosis or may develop years after apparently successful treatment, are treated with anticancer drugs and hormones. Such treatment usually relieves symptoms and prolongs life.

OUTLOOK

If cancer is treated early, the outlook is optimistic; either a complete cure or years of good health can be expected. Regular checkups are needed to detect any recurrence or cancer in the other breast. Breast self-examination should be carried out monthly and mammograms should be performed periodically. If the cancer recurs, it can be controlled for years by drugs, *radiation therapy*, and, in some cases, further surgery.

Breast enlargement
See *Mammoplasty*.

Breast-feeding
The natural method of infant feeding from birth to weaning. Human milk contains the ideal balance of nutrients for the human baby and provides valuable antibodies to protect the child against infections, such as *gastroenteritis*. Breast-feeding also provides the mother and child with a physical closeness that establishes and strengthens the psychological bond between them.

HOW TO BREAST-FEED

Ideally, the baby should be put to the breast as soon after delivery as possible. Once sucking has begun, the mother should ensure that the whole of the areola (the dark area around the nipple) is in the baby's mouth. This helps to stimulate the milk flow and can prevent soreness caused by the baby chewing on the nipple. In the first few days after birth, the baby should be encouraged to suck frequently, but for only a few minutes at a time. This provides him or her with valuable colostrum, and also stimulates the breasts so that a consistent and plentiful milk supply is established. During the first few weeks a baby should be fed on demand to make sure that the milk supply is maintained. Babies may want to feed from once every hour or two, to once every three or four hours.

PROBLEMS

Engorged breasts are common in early lactation; they are uncomfortable and can prevent the baby from sucking properly. Expression of milk, either manually or with a *breast pump*, usually solves the problem.

Sore or cracked nipples, often a problem in the early weeks, may be relieved by using a nipple shield. Alternatively, the milk may be expressed and given by bottle.

A possible complication of breast-feeding is infection leading to an abscess, indicated by soreness and inflammation on the surface of the breast. Early treatment with *antibiotic drugs* may mean that breast-feeding can continue.

Sometimes breast-feeding problems have an emotional basis. A few women regard their breasts as having a primarily sexual function and find the whole feeding process distasteful. Others fear feeding may spoil the shape of their breasts and may resent the intensive commitment to the child that breast-feeding requires.

A woman whose baby always seems unsatisfied after feeding may doubt the quality or quantity of her milk. If she is in good health, eating a nutritious diet, and getting enough rest, then her milk supply should be adequate, and she may simply need reassurance and encouragement. Sometimes, despite continuing efforts by the mother, the baby remains hungry or the process of feeding is painful. A change to *bottle-feeding* or supplementing the breast with the bottle is the likely answer, and should not be seen as failure or a reason for guilt. (See also *Feeding, infant*.)

Breast lump
Any mass, cyst, or swelling that can be felt in the breast tissue. At least 80 percent of lumps are benign; the remainder are malignant (see *Breast cancer*). All breast lumps need to be checked by a physician.

CAUSES AND TYPES

The most common cause of a breast lump is *fibroadenosis* (also known as chronic mastitis or fibrocystic disease), in which one or more cysts (fluid-filled tissue sacs) develop. Occurring mainly between the ages of 30 and 50, fibrocystic disease usually causes one or both breasts to become lumpy and tender in the week or so before a menstrual period starts.

Another common cause of a breast lump is found most often in young women and usually results in a single lump called a *fibroadenoma*. This benign growth is usually round, firm, and rubbery, causes no pain, and can be moved about beneath the skin using the fingertips.

There are also several less common forms of breast lump: breast cancer, lipoma, intraductal papilloma, and cystosarcoma phylloides. A lipoma is a benign, painless tumor, made up of fatty tissue, that sometimes changes the size of the breast.

An intraductal papilloma is a wart-like growth within a duct of the milk-

---

MANAGING BREAST-FEEDING

The mother should wear comfortable, loose, front-opening clothes and a nursing bra that provides good support. She should rest her back, firmly cradling the baby in the crook of her arm, with the baby's head well above stomach level.

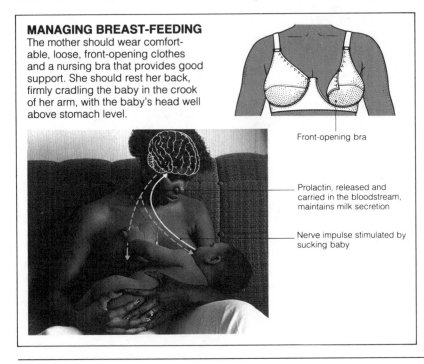

Front-opening bra

Prolactin, released and carried in the bloodstream, maintains milk secretion

Nerve impulse stimulated by sucking baby

producing glands. The most common symptom is a discharge from the nipple; the discharge may be clear, dark or bloody. There may also be a pea-sized lump beneath the nipple. Intraductal papillomas are harmless but may become malignant.

A cystosarcoma phylloides is a rare tumor of connective tissue that can grow to an enormous size very quickly. It is usually benign and only rarely becomes malignant.

SEEKING MEDICAL ADVICE

All women should examine their breasts regularly each month (see *Breast self-examination*) to detect any significant changes. If a new lump or any change in a long-standing lump is detected, or if there is any discharge from a nipple, it should be reported to a physician.

DIAGNOSIS AND TREATMENT

Since a physical examination cannot reveal whether or not a growth is benign, *mammography* and/or *biopsy* (analysis of a sample of tissue removed either by needle aspiration or by surgery) will be arranged.

Cysts can be drained in a simple outpatient procedure. Other lumps can be removed surgically. (For the treatment of malignant tumors, see *Breast cancer*.)

Breast pump

A simple device, consisting of a rubber bulb and a glass or plastic tube and reservoir, that is used to draw milk from the breasts. The pump is used to relieve overfull breasts during early lactation and to express milk for future use. Most pumps are hand-operated, although an electrically operated version is also available.

Breast reconstruction

See *Mammoplasty*.

Breast reduction

See *Mammoplasty*.

Breast self-examination

A visual and manual examination of the breasts carried out by a woman to detect lumps and other changes that might indicate the presence of early breast cancer. Although *mammography* (breast X ray) has been shown to be more effective, self-examination still has an important part to play and should be carried out at about the same time every month.

WHY IT IS DONE

Breast cancer is the leading cause of death among women aged 35 to 54 years. It is curable, however, if diag-nosed at an early stage. Self-examination allows early changes and small lumps (less than 1 cm in diameter) to be detected, and enables treatment to be undertaken when the chances of cure are greatest.

Breast tenderness

Soreness or tenderness of the breasts, often accompanied by a feeling of fullness in one or both breasts. Breast tenderness is relatively common just before menstruation (see *Premenstrual syndrome*), in early pregnancy, or during lactation.

Most cases of breast tenderness are thought to be due to hormonal changes (particularly increased levels of estrogen or progesterone) affecting the cells of the breast, causing them to retain excess fluid. This explains why *oral contraceptives* cause, or worsen breast tenderness in some women. Conversely, very low dose oral contraceptives may reduce tenderness in others. Tenderness during lactation may be due to engorgement with milk or to *mastitis* (inflammation of breast tissue as a result of infection).

At other times, and in the absence of other symptoms (such as a *breast lump, nipple discharge*, or hot, inflamed skin over the breast), breast tenderness is unlikely to be due to a serious underlying disorder. *Breast cancer* is usually painless.

EXAMINING YOUR BREASTS

1 Once a month after your period, examine your breasts. With arms by your side, look in a mirror and get to know their general appearance, shape, and size. Be alert to changes.

2 Raise each arm in turn above your head, looking for changes in appearance. Turn from side to side, looking at the outline of the breasts for any changes.

3 Gently squeeze the nipples to see whether there is any discharge.

4 Examine the skin surface for peculiarities. Orange-peel texture could indicate the presence of a lump.

5 Lie on your back with a pillow under your shoulders and head, one arm by your side. Using the flat of your hand, work around the outer parts of the breast in a clockwise direction.

6 Raise your arm above your head and examine the inner parts of the breast. Stretching the tissue makes detection of lumps easier. Feel also along the top of the collarbone and into the armpit.

Breath-holding attacks

Periods during which an infant or toddler holds his or her breath, usually as an expression of pain, frustration, or anger. It is thought that children may unconsciously bring on these attacks to exert control over their parents.

The child usually begins to cry, expels air from the lungs, and then holds his or her breath, becoming red or even blue in the face after a few seconds. The child may faint temporarily, but breathing quickly resumes as a natural reflex, ending the attack. Breath-holding sometimes results in twitching that resembles a seizure. Although breath-holding attacks may be alarming to parents, they are usually harmless.

CAUSES AND INCIDENCE

Breath-holding attacks occur in 1 to 2 percent of toddlers. They are most common between the ages of 1 and 2 years, particularly in children with determined personalities. Children at this age are just beginning to see themselves as individuals and are trying to determine the full extent of their power over the environment. They may quickly learn that breath-holding attacks annoy or frighten parents, and may then use them as a means of manipulation.

MANAGEMENT

Breath-holding attacks should be ignored as far as possible. If the child is rewarded by gaining increased attention from parents, then he or she will continue to have the attacks. As soon as the child realizes there is nothing to be gained, the attacks will stop. Firm, patient, and consistent handling will help prevent attacks. Parents who are anxious about their child's breath-holding should consult a physician for advice, but attacks will usually stop in any case by the time the child is 4.

Breathing

The process by which air passes into and out of the lungs to allow the blood to take up oxygen and dispose of carbon dioxide. Since breathing is controlled by the respiratory center in the brain stem, it is done instinctively; no conscious effort is needed to inhale and exhale air. However, the depth and rate at which we breathe can be altered voluntarily.

During exercise, when the heart and muscles need more oxygen, reflexes lead to a rapid increase in the breathing rate. This can vary in an adult from 13 to 17 breaths per minute at rest up to 80 breaths per minute during vigorous exercise. A newborn breathes at a rate of approximately 40 breaths per minute.

HOW AIR ENTERS THE LUNGS

When air is inhaled (inspiration), the diaphragm, which is dome shaped when relaxed, contracts and flattens. The muscles between the ribs contract and pull the rib cage upward and outward. This movement increases chest volume, causing the lungs to expand and suck in air. When air is exhaled (expiration), the chest muscles and diaphragm relax, causing the rib cage to sink and the lungs to contract, squeezing out air.

The lungs do not fill completely during inhalation or empty completely during exhalation. In normal, quiet breathing, only about one tenth of the air in the lungs passes out to be replaced by the same amount of fresh air. This new air (tidal volume) mixes with the stale air (residual volume) already held in the lungs.

A man's lungs hold up to about 6 litres of air, and a woman's lungs about 4.25 litres. At rest, about 400 ml of air is taken into the lungs during normal inspiration; a deep breath can take in as much as 3 to 4 litres of air. (See also *Respiration*.)

Breathing difficulty

Distressed breathing that includes a change in the rate and depth of breathing. Breathing difficulty may occur when the effort required to breathe is increased, or when breathing movements are causing pain. Symptoms that may accompany breathing difficulty include a feeling of tightness in the chest, coughing, wheezing, or chest pain.

CAUSES

Breathing difficulty may be caused by any condition that affects the flow of air into and out of the lungs, the transfer of oxygen from lungs to the blood, the circulation of blood through the lungs, or control of breathing by the brain stem. Breathing difficulty can occur either at rest, or when more oxygen is needed by the body during exercise or illness.

LACK OF FITNESS The heart and lungs of an unfit person cannot respond adequately when there is an increased

B

BREATHING

Inhalation and exhalation occur between 13 and 17 times a minute at rest, and up to 80 times a minute during vigorous exertion. A normal, resting inhalation takes in about 400 ml of air; a deep breath, up to 4 litres.

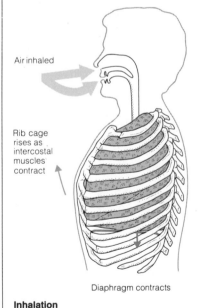

Air inhaled

Rib cage rises as intercostal muscles contract

Diaphragm contracts

Inhalation
Air is drawn into the lungs as the intercostal muscles (between the ribs) contract, causing the rib cage to rise, and the diaphragm contracts and flattens.

Air exhaled

Rib cage falls as intercostal muscles relax

Diaphragm relaxes

Exhalation
Air is expelled from the lungs as the intercostal muscles relax, causing the rib cage to fall, and the diaphragm relaxes and resumes its domed shape.

B

BREATHING DIFFICULTY Rapid breathing, or pain or tightness in the chest that makes you aware of your breathing.

? Has the breathlessness come on suddenly? **YES →**

Do you have pain in the chest AND/OR is breathing painful? **YES →** See • *Chest pain*

NO ↓

NO ↓

WARNING
If someone is having severe difficulty breathing AND/OR if there is a bluish coloring around the lips, this is an EMERGENCY requiring immediate medical attention.

Is your temperature 38°C or above AND/OR do you have a cough? **YES →**

☎
Call your physician without delay!
A chest infection, such as pneumonia or acute bronchitis, is the likely cause of your symptoms. This can be dangerous, especially for the elderly, the very young, and those in poor health.

See • *Bronchitis*
      • *Pneumonia*

NO ↓

Have you been awakened at night by an attack of breathlessness AND/OR have you been coughing up frothy white or pink sputum (phlegm)? **YES →**

☎
Call your physician without delay!
A dangerous build-up of fluid in the lungs, perhaps as a result of heart disease, is a possibility. Sit upright in a chair and try to stay calm; this will make breathing easier for you until help arrives.

See • *Edema*

NO ↓

Have you recently been confined to bed through illness or injury? **YES →**

☎ **EMERGENCY!**
GET MEDICAL HELP NOW!
A blood clot in the lung is a possibility, especially if you have also coughed up bloody sputum (phlegm).

See • *Pulmonary embolism*

NO ↓

Has the attack of breathlessness come on at a time when you are feeling tense or under great stress? **YES →**

☎
Call your physician without delay!
Panic attacks caused by severe anxiety often result in hyperventilation. If this is the first time you have experienced such symptoms, or if you are in any doubt as to the cause, call your physician now.

See • *Hyperventilation*
      • *Panic attack*

NO ↓

Continued on next page

Do you cough up thick, gray or greenish-yellow sputum (phlegm) most days?

YES → **Do you smoke?**

YES → Chronic bronchitis, emphysema, or pneumonia may be the cause, especially if you have had periods of wheezing in the past. Consult your physician.

See • *Bronchitis*
    • *Lung disease, chronic obstructive*
    • *Pneumonia*

NO → **Do you work, or have you worked, in a dusty atmosphere – for example, in a mine or quarry?**

YES → A reaction to coal dust in the lungs or another dust disease is a possibility. Consult your physician.

See • *Pneumoconiosis*

NO

Has your breathing become increasingly difficult over the past weeks or months?

YES → **Do your ankles look unusually puffy AND/OR do they pit when you press them with your finger?**

YES → You may have congestive heart failure. Consult your physician.

See • *Heart failure*

NO

NO

Does your work involve regular contact with grain or other crops AND/OR caged birds or animals?

YES → A fungal infection of the lungs, alveolitis or farmer's lung (caused by allergy to inhaled particles in moldy houseplants, grain, or hay) or bird-breeder's lung (allergic reaction to inhaled dust containing bird proteins) can cause breathlessness often accompanied by coughing. Consult your physician.

See • *Alveolitis*
    • *Histoplasmosis*

NO

WARNING
Sudden breathlessness associated with wheezing is usually due to asthma. Other possibilities include blockage of an airway from some inhaled object or the sudden worsening of congestive heart failure. If you have not had any previous attacks of wheezing, you should get medical help immediately. If you know you have asthma but your standard treatment does not relieve the attacks within one hour, get medical help immediately.

If you are unable to make a diagnosis from this chart, consult your physician.

---

need for oxygen, so the extra effort causes discomfort. This can be overcome by fitness training.

EXCESS WEIGHT Overweight people often experience difficulty in breathing during exertion; this occurs partly because they are unfit and partly because of the increased effort needed to carry their excess weight. In Pickwickian syndrome, the breathing center in the brain stem of very obese people does not function efficiently, which results in irregular patterns of breathing.

ANXIETY Severe anxiety during times of stress or tension can bring on attacks of *hyperventilation*. These attacks are associated with a feeling that it is impossible to get a good breath, which in turn leads to further overbreathing.
BRAIN STEM DAMAGE Damage to the breathing center in the brain stem due to a *stroke* or a *head injury* can reduce or increase breathing activity. This may also happen as a side effect of certain drugs. In certain instances, breathing may need *ventilator* assistance.
ALTITUDE Being at high altitude can

cause a person to become breathless because there is less oxygen present in the surrounding air, making it necessary for the lungs to work harder to provide the body with sufficient oxygen. Swelling of the brain and fluid in the lungs are serious features of altitude sickness (see *Mountain sickness*).
ANEMIA In all types of anemia, there is insufficient *hemoglobin* to carry oxygen around the body. If anemia is severe, the lungs need to work harder to supply the body with oxygen, resulting in breathlessness.

B

CIRCULATION DISORDERS Breathing difficulty intensified upon exertion may be caused by a reduced circulation of blood through the lungs. This may be due to *heart failure* (reduced pumping efficiency of the heart), to *pulmonary embolism* (blockage of blood vessels in the lungs by blood clots), or to *pulmonary hypertension* (increased pressure in the arteries in the lungs).

AIRWAYS BLOCKAGE Breathing difficulty due to airflow obstruction may be caused by chronic *bronchitis* (in which mucus and thickened walls block the airways), by *asthma* or an allergic reaction (in which there is narrowing of the air passages), or by *lung cancer* (if the tumor blocks a large airway).

LUNG DAMAGE Breathing difficulty may also be due to inefficient transfer of oxygen from the lungs into the bloodstream. Temporary damage to lung tissue may be due to *pneumonia, pneumothorax* (collapsed lung), *pulmonary edema* (fluid in the lung), or *pleural effusion* (fluid around the lung). Permanent lung damage may be due to *emphysema*, a condition in which the walls of the *alveoli* (small air sacs in the lungs) are destroyed.

PAIN Any pain in the chest that is made worse by chest or lung movement can make normal breathing difficult and painful. A fractured rib, for example, results in pain at the fracture site during breathing or movement of the torso. *Pleurisy* is associated with pain in the lower chest and often in the shoulder tip of the affected side.

SKELETAL DISORDERS Abnormalities of the skeletal structure of the thorax (chest), such as severe *scoliosis* or *kyphosis* (conditions in which there are abnormal curvatures of the spine), may cause breathing difficulty by impairing normal movements of the rib cage.

Breathing exercises

Techniques for learning to control the rate and depth of breathing. Breathing exercises are used for therapeutic purposes and to aid in *relaxation*.

WHY THEY ARE DONE

PHYSIOTHERAPY Breathing exercises are sometimes recommended for people with chronic chest diseases, such as chronic *bronchitis*. They can also help people with *anxiety disorders* who breathe too deeply and rapidly and as a result disturb the chemical makeup of their blood.

Breathing exercises are important after surgery, because postoperative patients often breathe shallowly and avoid coughing because of pain. In

Hand lying on chest should hardly move

Hand lying on stomach should rise first

Practicing breathing
This exercise can be done unsupervised. A second person may apply gentle pressure to the chest or abdomen to help you become aware of the muscle groups used.

these circumstances, poor air exchange and the buildup of secretions can lead to collapse of segments of the lung or to collapse of a lobe of the lung, particularly in patients who are overweight or who smoke. Deep breathing promotes coughing and keeps the lungs clear.

RELAXATION In *yoga*, deep rhythmic breathing is used to achieve a state of relaxation. During *childbirth*, breathing exercises relax the mother and also help to control contractions and reduce pain.

HOW THEY ARE DONE

Breathing exercises aim to teach people to inhale through the nose, while expanding the chest, and then to exhale fully through the mouth, while contracting the abdominal muscles. (See also *Physiotherapy*.)

Breathlessness

Rapid, shallow breathing to provide the body with sufficient oxygen. Breathlessness occurs as a normal response to exercise or exertion. It may also occur as a result of some underlying disorder (see *Breathing difficulty*).

Breech delivery

A birth in which the baby's bottom emerges before the head.

By around the 32nd week of pregnancy, most babies have assumed a head-down position in the uterus, but about 3 to 4 percent take up a breech presentation, with the head at the top of the uterus. Often, one of two twins may present as a breech. At 34 weeks, some obstetricians try to turn a baby with a breech presentation into the head-down position.

If this attempt fails, the baby is left in the breech presentation until delivery. A breech delivery adds to the problems of both mother and baby because the baby's bottom does not push its way through the birth canal as efficiently as the head. Usually, an *episiotomy* is performed in such situations to ease the baby's passage, and obstetric *forceps* are commonly used to ensure smooth emergence of the infant's head.

If a baby with a breech presentation has a large head or if the mother's pelvic girdle is small, delivery by *cesarean section* may be decided upon before she goes into labor.

Some obstetricians recommend cesarean section for most breech babies, particularly if the baby is a footling presentation (feet-first) or if a woman has not had a previous vaginal delivery, as there is an increased risk of *birth injury*. In other instances, the decision regarding cesarean section is based on the results of a series of investigations including X *rays* and *fetal heart monitoring*.

Assistant's hand presses on top of uterus to help ease the baby out

Delivering a breech baby
The buttocks are delivered first and then the legs. An episiotomy may be performed before the head is delivered.

Bridge, dental

False teeth (usually no more than four) attached to natural teeth on either side of a gap left by a missing tooth or teeth. A bridge is fitted to enable the person to bite properly and to speak clearly, and to avoid problems resulting from shifting or drifting of the remaining natural teeth.

Bridges for the front of the mouth are usually made of gold alloy faced with porcelain. Bridges for the back of the mouth are commonly made of gold or gold alloy without a facing. Unlike a *denture*, a bridge has no baseplate (artificial gum) and cannot be removed by the wearer.

B

FITTING THE BRIDGE

The most common type of bridge consists of one or more false teeth attached to a crown on each side of a gap. The natural teeth are shaped to receive the crowns, which are then cemented into place.

1 Two complete teeth are missing. A bridge of two false teeth and three crowns can be attached.

2 The three healthy teeth are shaped so that they can receive the crowns on either side of the gap.

3 A cast-metal subframe made from an impression is tried out in the mouth and any necessary alterations are made.

4 The finished bridge is in position, showing the new porcelain teeth cemented to the metal base.

Bright's disease

Another name for *glomerulonephritis*, a kidney disease that was first described by Dr. Richard Bright (1789-1858), a physician at Guy's Hospital, London.

Brittle bones

Bones with an increased tendency to fracture. Brittle bones are a feature of the disorder *osteoporosis* (thinning of the bones), which is common in women after the menopause, and may occur in people who are confined to bed, who are taking *corticosteroid drugs*, or who are suffering from certain hormonal disorders. In *osteomalacia* (a disorder caused by deficiency of *vitamin D*), the bones become soft and have an increased tendency both to become deformed and to fracture.

A rare cause of brittle bones and frequent fractures is the inherited connective tissue abnormality *osteogenesis imperfecta* (sometimes called brittle-bone disease).

Broken tooth

See *Fracture, dental*.

Broken veins

See *Telangiectasia*.

Bromides

Substances formerly prescribed as *sedative drugs* in the treatment of *anxiety* or as *anticonvulsant drugs* in the treatment of *epilepsy*. Bromides are no longer prescribed because of their unpleasant side effects, which include loss of sex drive, acne, tremor, lack of coordination, and confusion.

Bromocriptine

A drug that inhibits the secretion of the hormone *prolactin* by the anterior pituitary gland.

WHY IT IS USED

Bromocriptine is helpful in treating disorders associated with excessive prolactin production. Such conditions include *galactorrhea* (abnormal milk production by the breast), some types of female and male infertility, severe premenstrual breast discomfort, and benign pituitary tumors, including *prolactinomas* and tumors that cause *acromegaly* (abnormal tissue and bone growth). Bromocriptine can also be used to suppress lactation in women who do not wish to breast-feed.

A few years after its development in the 1960s, bromocriptine was also found to be effective in relieving the symptoms of *Parkinson's disease*. Its characteristics are almost identical to *dopamine*, the chemical that is lacking in the brains of Parkinson's victims. Bromocriptine is now widely used to treat patients in advanced stages of the disease when other drugs have failed or are unsuitable.

ADVERSE EFFECTS

Nausea and vomiting are the most common adverse effects. Low doses are unlikely to cause serious adverse effects but ulceration of the stomach occurs in rare cases. High doses may cause drowsiness and confusion.

Bronchiectasis

A lung disorder in which one or more bronchi (the air passages leading from the trachea) are distorted and stretched, and have damaged linings. Bronchiectasis is most common in childhood and results in chronic infections that may persist into later life.

CAUSES AND INCIDENCE

Bronchiectasis was formerly common and was usually caused by childhood chest infections such as measles, pertussis (whooping cough), tuberculosis, or severe bacterial pneumonias. As these infections are now prevented by *immunization* and controlled by *antibiotic drugs*, the incidence of bronchiectasis has dropped markedly.

SYMPTOMS

The main symptom of chronic lung infection in bronchiectasis is a cough that produces green or yellow sputum (phlegm) containing pus and occasionally flecks of blood. The sputum sometimes causes bad breath. If the disease is extensive, it causes shortness of breath.

DIAGNOSIS AND TREATMENT

The diagnosis is usually made from the symptoms. The extent of damage to the bronchi can be determined by *chest X rays* or by *bronchography* (an imaging technique).

Symptoms can usually be controlled by antibiotic drugs and by *postural drainage*; the patient is taught to lie in a position that allows pus and fluid to drain from the affected areas of lung so that they can be coughed up more easily.

If severe symptoms persist despite these measures, surgery may be recommended to remove the damaged lung areas.

Bronchiolitis

An acute viral infection of the lungs, mainly affecting babies and young children. This infection causes the bronchioles (the smaller airways in the lungs that branch off from the bronchi) to become inflamed.

CAUSES AND INCIDENCE

The most common cause is the respiratory syncytial virus (RSV), but other viruses may also be responsible. Adult bronchiolitis may follow bronchitis, brought on by an influenza virus. The viruses responsible can be transmitted in airborne droplets, and a virus that may cause only a moderate infection in an adult can cause severe bronchiolitis in an infant. People with head or chest infections should therefore minimize contact with babies.

SYMPTOMS

The symptoms are a cough, rapid breathing, fever, and, in severe cases, a cyanotic (bluish) complexion due to shortage of oxygen. The physician will often hear rales (bubbling noises) in the lungs through a stethoscope.

TREATMENT

If a child's cold and cough suddenly worsen, with rapid and labored breathing, a physician should be consulted. In the more severe cases, the child may be admitted to hospital, where (after X rays and sputum tests have ruled out bacterial pneumonia) *oxygen therapy* and *physiotherapy* (to clear mucus from the bronchioles) can be given. The child may be put on an artificial ventilator. Treated promptly, a child usually recovers within a few days. Antibiotic drugs are ineffective against the viral infection, but may prevent any secondary bacterial infection. Adults with bronchiolitis are commonly treated with corticosteroid drugs.

Bronchitis

Inflammation of the bronchi, the airways that connect the trachea (windpipe) to the lungs, resulting in a cough that may produce considerable quantities of sputum (phlegm). Two forms of the disease are recognized—acute and chronic. Both are common in smokers.

Bronchitis, acute

A form of *bronchitis* that develops suddenly and usually clears up within a few days except in people with a low resistance to infection.

CAUSES AND INCIDENCE

Acute bronchitis is usually a complication of a viral infection such as a cold or influenza, but may also be caused by the effect of air pollutants. Bacterial infection may cause acute bronchitis or may occur as a further complication of acute bronchitis when this has other causes. Attacks occur most often in winter. Smokers, babies, the elderly, and people with lung disease are particularly susceptible.

SYMPTOMS

The inflammation of the mucosal lining of the bronchi causes swelling and congestion, and pus is formed. The principal symptoms are wheezing, shortness of breath, and a persistent cough that produces yellow or green sputum. There may also be discomfort behind the sternum (breastbone) and a raised temperature.

TREATMENT

Symptoms may be relieved by humidifying the lungs, either using a humidifier in the home, or by inhaling steam directly (taking care to avoid burns). Drinking plenty of fluids helps loosen the sputum so that it can be coughed up more easily.

Most acute bronchitis clears up without further treatment, causing no further trouble. Complications, such as *pneumonia* and *pleurisy*, develop only in exceptional cases. However, a physician should be consulted in any

of the following circumstances: if there is severe breathlessness, if there is no improvement after three days, if blood is coughed up, if the temperature is above 38.3°C, or if the patient has underlying lung disease.

If the physician suspects there is a bacterial infection, *antibiotic drugs* will be prescribed, but these are of no use if the infection is caused by a virus.

Bronchitis, chronic

A form of *bronchitis* in which sputum is coughed up on most days during at least three consecutive months in at least two consecutive years. The disease commonly results in widespread narrowing and obstruction of the airways in the lungs. It often coexists with (and may contribute to the development of) another lung disease, *emphysema*, in which the alveoli (air sacs) in the lungs become distended (widened). Chronic bronchitis and emphysema together are sometimes called chronic obstructive lung disease (COLD) or chronic obstructive airways disease (COAD).

CAUSES

Smoking, the main cause, stimulates the production of mucus in the lining of the bronchi and thickens the bronchi's muscular walls and those of the bronchioles (smaller airways in the lungs), resulting in narrowing of these air passages. The passages then become more susceptible to infections, causing further damage.

SYMPTOMS AND COMPLICATIONS

The symptoms are the same as in acute bronchitis—cough, breathless-

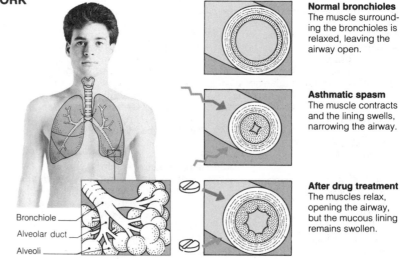

HOW BRONCHODILATORS WORK

When bronchioles become narrow following contraction of the muscle layer and swelling of the mucous lining, the passage of air is impeded. Bronchodilator drugs relax the muscles surrounding bronchioles by acting on the nerve signals that govern muscle activity. Sympathomimetic and anticholinergic drugs interfere with nerve signals passed to the muscles through the autonomic nervous system. Sympathomimetics enhance the action of neurotransmitters that encourage muscle relaxation. Anticholinergics block the neurotransmitters that trigger muscle contraction. Xanthine drugs relax muscle in the bronchioles by a direct effect on the muscle fibers, but their precise action is not known.

Bronchiole
Alveolar duct
Alveoli

Normal bronchioles
The muscle surrounding the bronchioles is relaxed, leaving the airway open.

Asthmatic spasm
The muscle contracts and the lining swells, narrowing the airway.

After drug treatment
The muscles relax, opening the airway, but the mucous lining remains swollen.

ness, and, rarely, chest pain—except that they are persistent instead of clearing up, and there is usually no fever. This persistence of symptoms also distinguishes the disease from chronic *asthma*, in which wheezing and breathlessness vary in severity from hour to hour and day to day.

As the disease progresses, often with the development of emphysema, the lungs become more resistant to the flow of blood, resulting in *pulmonary hypertension* (increased pressure in the arteries supplying blood to the lungs) and strain on the right side of the heart, as it must increase its work to pump blood through the lungs. The patient may suffer severe breathlessness. Sometimes, *heart failure* develops, further reducing the oxygen in the blood and causing a cyanotic (bluish) complexion. *Edema* (swelling caused by fluid collection) then develops in the legs and ankles due to the back pressure in blood vessels as a result of the heart failure.

People with chronic bronchitis usually have two or more episodes of acute viral or bacterial infection of the lungs every winter. Occasionally, blood may be coughed up, requiring medical investigation to exclude the possibility of *lung cancer*.

PREVENTION
A reduction in atmospheric pollution in towns and cities over the last few decades has reduced the incidence of chronic bronchitis, but the most important preventive measure is for people to stop (or never to start) smoking, as this is by far the most important cause of the disease. Waiting until symptoms develop may be too late to halt its course.

DIAGNOSIS AND TREATMENT
Before starting treatment, the physician may decide to investigate the severity of the patient's condition by *chest X rays, blood tests, sputum* analysis, and *lung function tests*.

To relieve breathlessness, the physician may prescribe an inhaler containing a *bronchodilator drug* (a drug that relaxes and widens the bronchi). Certain patients may benefit from inhaling oxygen from oxygen cylinders or an oxygen concentrator kept at home. Efforts may be made to help the patient cough up sputum. *Antibiotic drugs* may be given to treat or prevent bacterial lung infection.

The disease often shows an inexorable progression, with increasing shortness of breath leading to early retirement; eventually the sufferer may become housebound.

Bronchoconstrictor

A substance that causes constriction (narrowing) of the airways in the lungs. Bronchoconstrictors, such as *histamine* or methyl choline, are sometimes given by inhalation to provoke an attack of *asthma* (in order to confirm the diagnosis), or to test the effectiveness of a *bronchodilator drug*.

Bronchodilator drugs

COMMON DRUGS

Sympathomimetics
Ephedrine Epinephrine Fenoterol Isoproterenol Orciprenaline Salbutamol Terbutaline

Anticholinergics
Ipratropium

Xanthines
Aminophylline Oxtriphylline Theophylline

WARNING
If your inhaler is not helping your symptoms, call your physician.

A group of drugs that widen the bronchioles (small airways in the lungs) to increase the flow of air and improve breathing. Narrowing of the airways may be caused by contraction of the bronchiole walls and/ or by congestion with mucus.

Three main groups of drugs are used as bronchodilators: sympathomimetic drugs, *anticholinergic drugs*, and xanthine drugs. Sympathomimetic drugs are primarily used for the rapid relief of breathing difficulty. Anticholinergic and xanthine drugs are more often used for the long-term prevention of attacks of breathing difficulty.

Drugs can be given by *inhaler*, in tablet form, or, in severe cases, by *nebulizer* (a type of inhaler that uses air and/or oxygen under pressure to propel a watery suspension of the drug into the lungs) or by injection.

WHY THEY ARE USED
Bronchodilator drugs are used to improve airflow into the lungs, especially in the treatment of *asthma* and chronic *bronchitis*.

HOW THEY WORK
The action of bronchodilators is described in the box opposite.

POSSIBLE ADVERSE EFFECTS
Sympathomimetic drugs may cause palpitations and trembling. Anticholinergic drugs may cause dry mouth, blurred vision, and difficulty passing urine. Xanthine drugs may cause headaches and palpitations.

Inhaled bronchodilator drugs are not absorbed by the body in large amounts and serious side effects are therefore uncommon. However, because of the possible effect of sympathomimetic and xanthine drugs on heart rate, these drugs are prescribed cautiously for people who have heart problems, high blood pressure, or an overactive thyroid gland. Anticholinergic drugs may not be suitable for men who have enlarged prostate glands or for people who have a tendency to glaucoma.

Bronchography

An X ray procedure for examining the bronchi, the main air passages of the lungs. Bronchography was formerly used to diagnose the *bronchiectasis*, but has now been largely replaced by other imaging techniques, such as *CT scanning* or lung *tomography*, and by the use of *bronchoscopy*.

HOW IT IS DONE
After the patient has been given mild sedation and/or a local anesthetic, contrast medium (a substance opaque to X rays) is introduced into the lung through a hollow flexible tube (either a cannula or a bronchoscope). X-ray pictures are then taken of the bronchi to detect any abnormalities. When the procedure is finished, the contrast medium is partly coughed up by the patient and partly absorbed into the bloodstream.

Bronchopneumonia

The most common form of *pneumonia*. Bronchopneumonia differs from the other main type of pneumonia (lobar pneumonia) in that the inflammation is spread throughout the lungs in small patches rather than being confined to one lobe. Bronchopneumonia is often the actual cause of death in patients who are chronically ill from other conditions.

Bronchoscopy

Examination or treatment of the bronchi, the main airways of the lungs, by means of a hollow tube or a fiberoptic *endoscope* (viewing tube with a light and lens attached).

WHY IT IS DONE
The two main uses of bronchoscopy are to aid in diagnosing and treating certain lung disorders. Apart from inspecting the bronchi for abnormalities, diagnostic procedures include collecting samples of mucus, obtaining cells from the outermost distant airways of the lungs, and taking biopsy specimens (small samples of tissue), all for analysis or microscopic examination. The bronchoscope is

also sometimes used in a type of X-ray investigation called *bronchography*.

Among the various forms of treatment possible are removing thick secretions of mucus or inhaled foreign bodies, destroying growths, and sealing off damaged blood vessels. The last two are carried out by *laser therapy*, *diathermy*, or *cryosurgery* (a tissue freezing technique) by means of attachments to the bronchoscope.

Bronchospasm

Temporary narrowing of the bronchi (airways into the lungs) caused by contraction of the muscles in the walls of the bronchi, by inflammation of the lining of the bronchi, or by a combination of both.

Contraction and relaxation of the airways is controlled by the autonomic nervous system. Contraction may also be caused by the release of substances during an allergic reaction.

When the airways are narrowed, flow of air out of the lungs causes wheezing or coughing. The most common cause of bronchospasm is *asthma*, though other causes include respiratory infection, chronic lung disease (including *emphysema* and chronic *bronchitis*), *anaphylactic shock*, or an allergic reaction to chemicals.

Bronchus

A large air passage in a lung. Each lung has one main bronchus, originating at the end of the trachea (windpipe). This main bronchus divides into smaller branches known as segmental bronchi, which further divide into bronchioles.

Bronchus, cancer of

See *Lung cancer*.

Brown fat

A special type of fat, found in infants and some animals, but not in healthy adults. It is located between and around the scapulae (shoulder blades) on the back. Brown fat is a source of energy and helps infants to maintain a constant body temperature.

Brucellosis

A rare bacterial infection, caught from farm animals and dairy products, that may cause a feverish illness.

CAUSES AND INCIDENCE

The disease is caused by various species of *BRUCELLA*, which may be transmitted to humans from affected cattle, goats, and pigs. Farm workers, veterinary surgeons, and people who work in slaughterhouses have the

---

PERFORMING BRONCHOSCOPY

There are two kinds of bronchoscope. The rigid type is passed into the bronchi via the mouth and requires anesthesia. The flexible, fiberoptic bronchoscope (a narrower tube formed from light-transmitting fibers) can be inserted through either the mouth or nose. It is used after giving only a mild sedative and/or local anesthetic and it reaches farther into the lungs. Both types of bronchoscope can be fitted with forceps, and the instrument also has attachments for performing laser therapy and cryosurgery. (See also *Endoscopy*.)

Bronchoscope

Trachea

Lung

View through bronchoscope

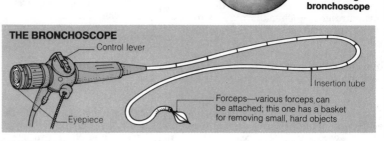

THE BRONCHOSCOPE

Control lever

Insertion tube

Forceps—various forceps can be attached; this one has a basket for removing small, hard objects

Eyepiece

---

highest risk of infection. The bacteria enter the bloodstream through a cut or are breathed in.

In countries where milk pasteurization is not the rule, the disease can be caught by drinking milk or by eating unpasteurized dairy products, including cheese. There have been no outbreaks of brucellosis in Canada in recent years; sporadic cases, usually in dairy workers, are occasionally reported.

SYMPTOMS

Acute brucellosis consists of a single bout of high fever, shivering, aching, and drenching sweats, which last for a few days. Other symptoms include headache, poor appetite, backache, weakness, and depression. Untreated severe cases may lead rarely to potentially fatal complications, such as *pneumonia* or *meningitis*.

In chronic brucellosis, bouts of the illness recur over months or years.

DIAGNOSIS AND TREATMENT

A definite diagnosis of brucellosis is made from blood tests. The disease is treated by bed rest and *antibiotic drugs*.

Bruise

A discolored area under the skin, caused by leakage of blood from damaged capillaries (tiny blood vessels). At first, the blood appears blue or black; then the breakdown of *hemoglo-*

---

bin turns the bruise yellow. To reduce the pain and swelling of a large bruise, place a cloth soaked in ice-cold water over it for 10 minutes.

If a bruise does not fade after about one week, or if bruises appear for no apparent reason or are severe after only minor injury, a physician should be consulted as these may be indications of a *bleeding disorder*. (See also *Black eye*; *Purpura*.)

Bruits

The sounds made in the heart, arteries, or veins when blood circulation becomes turbulent or flows at an abnormal speed. This happens when blood vessels become narrowed by disease (as in *arteriosclerosis*), when heart valves are narrowed or damaged (as in *endocarditis*), or if blood vessels dilate (as in an *aneurysm*). Bruits are usually heard through a *stethoscope*.

Bruxism

Rhythmic grinding or clenching of the teeth that usually occurs during sleep but may be done unconsciously when a person is awake. Bruxism may develop at any age. The chief underlying causes are emotional stress and minor discomfort or unevenness when the teeth are brought together.

Continued bruxism may cause wearing away and loosening of the teeth, and stiffness in the jaw. If the underlying problems cannot be resolved, a biteplate worn at night will minimize the damage.

Bubonic plague
The most common form of *plague*, characterized by the development of a bubo (swollen lymph node) in the groin or armpit early in the illness.

Buccal
An anatomical term, from the Latin word for cheek, that means relating to the cheek or mouth.

Buck teeth
Prominent upper incisors (front teeth), which protrude from the mouth and are often splayed out at an angle to each other. Apart from the usually undesirable appearance, buck teeth are easily damaged and may be susceptible to decay because they are not moistened by saliva.

CAUSES
The malpositioning of the teeth is probably an inherited trait rather than acquired (for example, by faulty eating habits). Often, the person's upper jaw is relatively large compared with the lower jaw, and the lips do not close over and exert a controlling influence on the position of the teeth. Rarely, the malpositioning may be the result of an abnormally large tongue gradually displacing the teeth forward. Often, there is an overall crowding of teeth within the upper jaw in persons with this condition.

Buck teeth formerly occurred in conjunction with mouth breathing due to enlarged *adenoids*, but this has become less common.

TREATMENT
Orthodontic treatment involves gradually coaxing the teeth back into position with a removable brace (see *Brace, dental*), or, in more extreme cases, with a fixed *orthodontic appliance*. To create room for the incisors, other crowded teeth may sometimes need to be extracted.

Budd-Chiari syndrome
A rare disorder in which the veins draining blood from the liver become blocked or narrowed. Blood then accumulates in the liver, which swells. The blockage leads to serious *liver failure*, and to *portal hypertension* (back pressure in the blood vessels due to abnormally slow blood flow through the liver).

Treatment is aimed at removing the cause of the vein obstruction—which

may be a blood clot, pressure on the veins from a liver tumor, or a congenital abnormality of the veins. In most cases, however, treatment has only a limited effect, and unless a *liver transplant* can be performed, most patients die within two years.

Buerger's disease
A rare disorder, also called thromboangiitis obliterans, in which the arteries, nerves, and veins in the legs, and sometimes those in the arms, become severely inflamed. Narrowing of the arteries blocks off blood supply to the patient's toes and fingers, thus eventually causing *gangrene* (tissue death).

The disease occurs mainly in men under the age of 45 who smoke heavily. Most have a history of *phlebitis* (vein inflammation). The main symptom is pain in the hands and feet. In cold conditions, sufferers' hands turn white, then blue, and then red (see *Raynaud's phenomenon*).

Sufferers must stop smoking to halt progress of the disease. *Vasodilator drugs* (drugs that widen blood vessels) may be prescribed, but are rarely, if ever, effective. If gangrene develops, the affected limb, toes, or fingers usually have to be amputated.

Bulimia
An illness characterized by bouts of gross overeating usually followed by self-induced vomiting. These activities are often performed secretly so the exact prevalence of the disorder is not easy to assess. Most sufferers are girls or women between the ages of 15 and 30.

CAUSES
Bulimia is often, although not always, a variant of *anorexia nervosa*, a disorder in which dieting is carried out to excess. In both disorders, the sufferer has a morbid fear of fatness. After months or years of eating sparsely, a person with anorexia nervosa may develop a constant craving for food and begin to binge—but the fear of becoming overweight remains and prompts the self-induced vomiting. Sometimes, large doses of *laxative drugs* are used as well as, or instead of, vomiting in an effort to expel food as quickly as possible.

Occasionally, a woman may develop bulimia without a previous history of anorexia.

SYMPTOMS
People with bulimia may be of normal weight or be only slightly underweight, although some are extremely

thin. Bingeing and vomiting may occur once or several times a day. In severe cases, repeated vomiting can lead to dehydration and loss of potassium from the body, causing symptoms such as weakness and cramps. The gastric acid in vomit may damage the teeth. The sufferer is often highly distressed about her compulsive behavior and as a result may be depressed and sometimes suicidal.

TREATMENT AND OUTLOOK
The sufferer must first be persuaded to accept treatment. This is similar to the treatment for anorexia nervosa and includes supervision and regulation of eating habits, and, sometimes *psychotherapy* and/or *antidepressant drugs*. In many patients there is a risk of relapse weeks or even months after treatment has ended.

Bulla
A large air- or fluid-filled bubble, usually in the lungs or skin.

Lung bullae in young adults are usually congenital defects (abnormalities present from birth). In later life, lung bullae develop in patients with the lung disease *emphysema* as the alveoli (tiny air sacs in the lungs) become distended and join together. Skin bullae are simply large, fluid-filled *blisters*.

Bunion
A thickened, fluid-filled *bursa* (pad), overlying the joint at the base of the big toe. A bunion can become inflamed and very painful. The underlying cause of the bunion is *hallux valgus*, in which the joint at the base of big toe projects outward while the tip of the toe turns inward.

TREATMENT
Without treatment, any bunion will get worse. To remedy a small bunion, wear properly fitting shoes and a special toe pad that straightens the big toe and keeps it in position. Large bunions may require surgery.

Buphthalmos
A large, prominent eyeball in an infant, resulting from increased pressure inside the eyeball due to congenital *glaucoma*. Treatment usually involves surgery to reduce pressure, otherwise the child's sight is progressively damaged.

Burkitt's lymphoma
A cancer of lymph tissues, common in the tropics, that is characterized by an enlarging tumor or tumors within the jaw or abdomen, or both.

B

HOW BUNIONS FORM

A bunion results from rubbing of a shoe against an abnormal outward projection of the joint at the base of the big toe (a hallux valgus), leading to irritation and inflammation. The joint abnormality is often itself due to the wearing of narrow, pointed shoes with high heels, although it can also result from an inherited weakness in the joint.

Valgus deformity of the joint between the first metatarsal bone and the adjoining phalanx.

INCIDENCE
Burkitt's lymphoma is confined almost exclusively to children living in low-lying, moist, tropical regions of Africa and New Guinea. However, a few cases of the disease have occurred among a wider age group in North America and Europe.

CAUSE
The growths are believed to be an abnormal response to a common virus, the Epstein-Barr virus. The distribution of the disease in Africa closely follows that of *malaria*; it is now believed by most researchers that malaria in childhood may alter the body's immune response to the Epstein-Barr virus, which triggers growth of the lymphoma.

TREATMENT
Anticancer drugs or *radiation therapy* give complete or partial cure of the disease in about 80 percent of cases. (See also *Lymphoma*.)

Burns
Each year some 7,000 Canadians are burned badly enough to require admission to hospital, and on any one day they occupy about 260 hospital beds. Burns are most common in children and older people; many are due to accidents in the home, most of them preventable by commonsense precautions and devices such as fire alarms.

TYPES
Skin is a living tissue, and even brief heating above 49°C damages its cells. FIRST-DEGREE BURNS cause reddening of the skin and affect only the epidermis, the top layer of the skin. Such burns heal quickly, but the damaged skin may peel away after a day or two. *Sunburn* is a common example of a first-degree burn.

SECOND-DEGREE BURNS damage the skin more deeply, causing the formation of blisters. However, some of the dermis (deep layer of the skin) is left to recover, and as a result these burns usually heal without scarring, unless they are very extensive.

THIRD-DEGREE BURNS destroy the full skin thickness. The affected area will look white or charred, and, if the burn is very deep, muscles and bones may be exposed. Even if very localized, third-degree burns will need specialist treatment and possibly skin grafts to prevent scarring.

ELECTRICAL BURNS can cause extensive damage with minimal external skin damage. Because the electric current may also cause heart damage, electrical burns always require evaluation by a physician.

EFFECTS AND COMPLICATIONS
Extensive first-degree burns (such as sunburn) cause pain, restlessness, headache, and fever, but are not life-threatening.

In second- or third-degree burns affecting more than 10 percent of the body surface, the victim will be in a state of *shock*, with lowered blood pressure and a rapid pulse. This is caused by the loss of large quantities of fluid (and its constituent proteins) from the burned area. Shock may be fatal if not treated by intravenous fluid replacement.

When the skin is burned, it can no longer protect the body from contamination by airborne bacteria. The infection of extensive burns may cause fatal complications if effective treatment with antibiotic drugs is not available.

Victims who have inhaled smoke may develop swelling and inflammation of the lungs and may need specialist care for burns of the eyes and respiratory passages. Autopsies consistently show that people who die in burning buildings usually suffocate long before their bodies are burned.

PROFESSIONAL TREATMENT
The burn is either lightly dressed with an antibacterial dressing or left exposed to promote healing, with every effort made to keep the skin area scrupulously clean by reverse *isolation* nursing. If necessary, analgesic drugs (painkillers) are given, and antibiotic drugs are prescribed if there is any sign of the wound being infected. Shock is treated by intravenous fluids through a drip inserted into a vein, usually in the arm.

For extensive second-degree burns, *skin grafts* are used early in the treatment to minimize scarring. Patients suffering from third-degree burns always require skin grafting if scarring is to be avoided. Extensive burns may require repeated operations by a plastic surgeon.

Length of hospital stay can vary from a few days in some cases to many weeks in the case of severe and extensive burns. Patients with extensive burns are usually treated at a specialist burn center. (See illustrated box on facing page.)

Burping
Another term for *belching*.

Burr hole
A hole made in the skull by a special drill with a rounded tip (burr). The hole is made to relieve pressure on the brain, often resulting from the accumulation of blood between the inside of the skull and the brain after a *head injury*. The burr hole relieves the potentially fatal pressure by allowing the blood to drain.

Several burr holes may be made as part of a *craniotomy*, in which a section of the skull is removed to allow access to the brain and surrounding tissues.

Bursa
A fluid-filled pad that acts as a cushion at a pressure point in the body—often near a joint, where a tendon or muscle crosses bone or other muscles. The

CARE OF BURN PATIENTS

Burn patients need specialized nursing care. Sterile linen should be used with sterile starch powder sprinkled on it. Drafts should be avoided and room humidity should be controlled. The revolving circular bed is useful in the treatment of burn patients since it can be moved into many different positions and stopped at any angle.

The revolving circular bed

Skin surface area
This is a rough guide to what percentage each area represents of the total skin area (percentages do not total 100 due to rounding).

7%
2.5%
4% 4%
26%
3% 3%
3% 3%
9.5% 9.5%
5% Buttocks
7% 7%
3.5% 3.5%

Epidermis
Dermis
Sweat gland
Hair follicle
Subcutaneous fat
Nerve
1st
2nd
3rd

Degrees of burns
Burns are divided into three categories. First-degree burns affect the epidermis and skin may peel; second-degree burns cause blisters; third-degree burns destroy the whole of the skin's thickness and require special treatment.

FIRE-RELATED DEATHS IN CANADA IN 1987

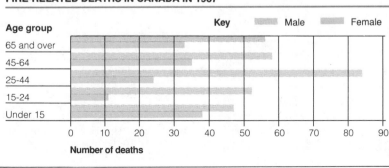

Age group	Key: ▨ Male ▨ Female
65 and over	
45-64	
25-44	
15-24	
Under 15	

0 10 20 30 40 50 60 70 80 90
Number of deaths

---

important bursae are around the knee, elbow, and shoulder.

A *bunion* is a thickened bursa at the base of the big toe.

Bursitis

Inflammation of a *bursa*, causing pain and swelling due to accumulation of fluid. Bursitis is usually the result of pressure, friction, or slight injury to the membrane surrounding the joint. Less commonly, it may be caused by bacterial infection.

TYPES

Prepatellar bursitis ("housemaid's knee") is caused by prolonged kneeling on a hard surface, tibial tubercle bursitis ("clergyman's knee") from kneeling on a more upright surface, and olecranon bursitis ("student's elbow") from prolonged pressure of the elbow point against a desk or table. Another common form is subdeltoid bursitis (affecting the shoulder), which, if left untreated, may result in *frozen shoulder*.

TREATMENT

Rest is the usual treatment. Bursitis usually subsides after a few days as the fluid is reabsorbed into the bloodstream. Application of an ice pack may help relieve pain. Bacterial bursitis usually requires treatment with *antibiotic drugs*.

If swelling persists, a physician may drain the bursa using a needle and syringe and apply a pressure bandage for a few days to stop the fluid from reforming. An injection of a *corticosteroid drug* may also be given.

In rare, recurrent cases, bursectomy (a minor operation to remove the bursa) may be performed. Under general anesthesia, a small incision is made in the skin over the bursa, and the lining of the bursal sac is completely removed to prevent it from regrowing.

Bypass surgery

Procedures to bypass the blockage or narrowing of an artery or vein or any part of the digestive system.

TYPES

Arteries can become blocked or narrowed in *atherosclerosis*. Most often affected are the carotid arteries (in the neck), the coronary arteries (in the heart), and the iliofemoral arteries (leading to the legs). Obstructions can be bypassed using sections of artery or vein (taken from the patient) or using synthetic tubing.

Surgeons have attempted to bypass blocked arteries in the brain by joining points above the blockage to an artery

FIRST AID: TREATING BURNS

MINOR BURNS

1 Immerse the burned area immediately in cold, running water.

2 Or apply a cold-water compress (a clean towel or handkerchief) until the pain diminishes.

3 Remove any watches, bracelets, rings, belts, or constricting clothing from the area before it begins to swell.

4 Dress the area with a clean (if possible, sterile), nonfluffy material.

MAJOR BURNS

1 If a person's clothing is on fire, douse the victim with water or wrap him or her in a blanket and place on the ground.

2 Do not remove clothing that is stuck to the wound, but cover any exposed burned areas with a dry, clean, nonfluffy cloth to stop infection; secure with a bandage.

DO NOT
- use adhesive dressings on burns
- apply butter, oil, or grease
- apply lotions or creams
- prick blisters with a pin or otherwise interfere with the injured area
- use fluffy materials on wounds

in the neck. Known as extracranial-intracranial bypass, this procedure has had little success, and is now rarely used.

Veins are bypassed most often in patients with diseases of the liver that cause portal hypertension (increased pressure in the veins draining the intestinal tract) and bleeding esophageal varices (enlarged veins in the lower esophagus). These bypasses are called *shunts*.

Intestinal bypasses are most commonly employed in patients with cancer. If tumor growth is too extensive for surgical removal, symptoms may be relieved by joining the sections of intestine at either side of the blockage. An obstructed bile duct may be diverted into the intestine lower down the digestive tract.

Intestinal bypass operations for the treatment of *obesity* have largely been replaced in recent years by operations to reduce the capacity of the stomach. (See also *Arterial bypass*; *Coronary artery bypass*.)

Byssinosis

An industrial disease of the lungs caused by an unknown agent in the dust produced during the processing of flax, cotton, hemp, or sisal.

Byssinosis, once a common problem among cotton mill workers in Britain and the United States, has become less prevalent due to preventive measures such as better dust control. The decline of the textile industry has also helped lower the incidence in Britain and North America, but the disease remains common in India and other developing countries.

SYMPTOMS

Byssinosis produces a feeling of tightness in the chest and shortness of breath that may become chronic. At first, symptoms are most pronounced at the start of the working week, but gradually they become troublesome on every working day.

In chronic byssinosis (the risk of which is considerably increased by smoking), the sufferer is short of breath even when away from work. *Respiratory failure* may develop when lung damage has become extensive, but this is quite uncommon.

TREATMENT AND PREVENTION

Bronchodilator drugs and other drugs used to treat *asthma* may relieve symptoms, but the answer to the problem is prevention. This is achieved by treatment of raw textiles before processing, reduction of dust levels, and the wearing of face masks.

Cachexia

An appearance of profound illness and severe weight loss. Cachexia is usually caused by extreme starvation or by a serious underlying disease such as cancer or tuberculosis.

Cadaver

A dead human body used as a source of transplant organs or preserved for anatomical study and dissection.

Cadmium poisoning

The toxic effects of cadmium, a tinlike metal. Poisoning due to the inhalation of cadmium dust or fumes is an industrial hazard, the effects of which vary according to the duration and severity of exposure. Acute exposure may lead to *pneumonitis* (inflammation of the lungs). Exposure over a long period can lead to urinary tract *calculi* (stones), *kidney failure*, or *emphysema* (a form of permanent lung damage).

Cadmium poisoning may also be caused by eating vegetables grown in cadmium-rich soil or by consuming food or drink that has been stored in cadmium-lined containers. Cadmium is known to accumulate in the body (especially in the kidneys) throughout life. Although cadmium has been implicated in the development of high blood pressure in animals, a causative link has not been proved in humans.

Minute amounts of cadmium may be of some value in animal diets.

Café au lait spots

Coffee-colored patches on the skin. Café au lait spots are usually oval in shape, may measure several centimetres across, and may develop anywhere on the skin. The presence of a only a few such spots is usually of no significance. Larger numbers of café au lait spots may be a sign of *neurofibromatosis*, a hereditary disorder of the sheaths that surround nerve fibers. In neurofibromatosis, café au lait spots are commonly accompanied by multiple small nodules in and on the skin.

Caffeine

A *stimulant drug* that occurs naturally in coffee beans, tea leaves, cocoa beans, and cola nuts commonly used in drinks. Caffeine is used in some drug preparations.

Caffeine in drinks generally produces unpleasant side effects, such as agitation and tremors, only when consumed in large quantities or by particularly sensitive individuals. People who regularly consume large amounts of caffeine (e.g., more than five cups of coffee per day) often find that their *tolerance* to the substance has increased, making it necessary for them to increase their intake to obtain the equivalent stimulant effect. They may also suffer withdrawal symptoms, such as tiredness, headaches, and irritability, if they go without caffeine for even as little as a few hours.

Because of its stimulant effect, caffeine can improve short-term athletic performance, but its use is forbidden in pill or injectable form prior to amateur athletic competition. Caffeine levels in the body can be monitored by a urine concentration test.

CAFFEINE LEVELS (mg per cup)	
Tea, weak	50
Tea, strong	80
Coffee, weak	80
Coffee, strong	200
Cocoa	10-17
Cola	43-75

The strength and method of preparation determine exact amounts of caffeine present (in milligrams per cup).

EFFECTS OF CAFFEINE ON THE BODY

Caffeine has a stimulant effect on all organs and tissues. It acts directly on individual cells by affecting their chemical reactions, and indirectly by increasing the release from the adrenal glands of epinephrine and norepinephrine, hormones that stimulate cell activity.

Brain
Small amounts of caffeine stimulate the brain cells, helping to reduce drowsiness and fatigue. Concentration is improved and reactions are speeded up. Large amounts cause overstimulation, anxiety, irritability, and restlessness. This is why consuming caffeine before going to bed can cause insomnia and a hangover in the morning, with excessive fatigue and drowsiness on waking.

Skeletal muscles
Stimulation by caffeine may improve their performance during exercise, but excessive stimulation of the skeletal muscles can cause twitching.

Heart
With small amounts of caffeine, the heart muscle is stimulated, augmenting its pumping action. This causes the blood to circulate faster and blood pressure to increase for a short time. Too much caffeine results in overstimulation of the heart muscle and can result in palpitations.

Stomach
While small amounts of caffeine can actually help digestion by increasing production of stomach acid, too much can cause abdominal pain and nausea.

Kidneys
Caffeine action on the kidneys increases the production of urine.

C

Caffeine is often included in various drug preparations, particularly in combination with certain *analgesic drugs* (painkillers). However, its value is questionable, because it does not enhance the painkilling effect. Caffeine is combined with *ergotamine* in several drugs for the early preventive treatment of migraine attacks. (See also *Drug dependence* and *Sports, drugs and*.)

Calamine

A pink substance consisting of zinc oxide and iron oxide that is applied to the skin in the form of ointments, lotions, or dusting powders. Calamine has a protective, cooling, and drying effect, and is used to relieve skin irritation and itching. It is sometimes combined with a local anesthetic (see *Anesthesia, local*), a *corticosteroid drug*, or an *antihistamine drug*. Bandages impregnated with calamine are sometimes used to protect leg ulcers.

Calcaneus

The heel bone. The calcaneus is one of the tarsal bones and is the largest bone in the *foot*.

DISORDERS

The calcaneus may be fractured as a result of falling from a height onto the heels. Minor fractures usually do not cause problems and are treated by putting the foot and leg in a cast. A more serious fracture, with compression of the bone, may cause permanent damage to the joints involved in turning the foot in and out, leading to pain and stiffness that are aggravated by walking.

The *Achilles tendon* is fixed to the back of the heel bone and controls the up and down movement of the foot. The point at which the tendon joins the bone may be strained by excessive or prolonged stress from the pull of the tendon—for example, in some *running injuries*. In children this area of bone is still growing and occasionally becomes inflamed and painful (see *Osteochondrosis*).

Tendons of the sole of the foot are fixed under the heel bone; the associated muscles are important in supporting the arches of the foot. Inflammation around these tendons (as in plantar *fasciitis*) causes pain and tenderness under the heel when standing or walking.

A calcaneal spur (a bony protrusion from this part of the calcaneus) occurs in some people with plantar fasciitis and also sometimes in people with healthy feet.

LOCATION OF THE CALCANEUS
This is the largest tarsal bone, projecting backward beyond the leg bones.

Talus

Metatarsals

Calcaneus

Calcification

The deposition of calcium salts in body tissues. Calcification is part of the normal process of bone and teeth formation and is necessary for the healing of fractures. Calcification can occur in an injured muscle and is common in arteries affected by *atherosclerosis*. It may also occur if the blood calcium level is raised as a result of a disorder of the *parathyroid glands*.

Calcification, dental

The deposition of calcium crystals in developing teeth. Calcium and phosphorus salts are carried in the blood supply to the teeth, where the crystals make up 96 percent of tooth enamel and 70 percent of dentin. Calcification of primary teeth begins in the fetus between three and six months' gestation; calcification of permanent teeth (other than the wisdom teeth) begins before age 4.

Abnormal calcification occurs in amelogenesis imperfecta, an inherited disorder of the enamel involving incomplete calcification (see *Hypoplasia, enamel*). Another cause of abnormal calcification is the absorption of high levels of fluoride (see *Fluorosis*).

Calcinosis

A condition in which there is abnormal deposition of *calcium* salts in various tissues, such as the skin, muscles, or *connective tissues*. The abnormal calcium deposits form nodules within the affected tissues. Calcinosis tends to be associated with an underlying connective tissue disorder, such as *scleroderma* or *dermatomyositis*.

The term "calcinosis" is usually combined with another word to signify which part of the body is affected—for example, calcinosis cutis affects the skin. (See also *Calcification*.)

Calcitonin

A hormone produced by the *thyroid gland*. Calcitonin helps to control the level of *calcium* in the blood by slowing the rate at which calcium is lost from the bones.

WHY IT IS USED

A synthetic form of calcitonin is used to treat *Paget's disease*, in which the bones grow abnormally and become deformed, causing pain and an increased risk of fracture. Given by injection, calcitonin halts abnormal bone formation in about a week and can relieve pain within a few months.

Calcitonin is also used to treat *hypercalcemia* (abnormally high levels of calcium in the blood) caused by overactivity of the *parathyroid glands* or by cancer of the bone. Calcitonin helps relieve the nausea and vomiting that result from hypercalcemia by quickly reducing the level of calcium in the blood. Calcitonin may be prescribed in conjunction with a *corticosteroid drug* that also decreases the calcium level in the blood.

POSSIBLE ADVERSE EFFECTS

Calcitonin does not usually cause any troublesome adverse effects. Gastrointestinal reactions, such as nausea, vomiting, and diarrhea, usually diminish with continued use.

Calcium

The most abundant mineral in the body, with several important functions. Calcium is essential for the functioning of cells, for muscle contraction, for the transmission of nerve impulses from nerve endings to muscle fibers, and for blood clotting. In the form of calcium phosphate it makes up the hard basic constituent of teeth and bones. An average-sized person carries about 0.9 to 1.1 kg of calcium, mostly in the bones.

The main dietary sources of calcium are dairy products, eggs, fish (when the bones are eaten), and some vegetables (e.g., green, leafy vegetables). Calcium may be added to flour.

CONTROL OF CALCIUM LEVELS

Vitamin D and certain hormones help control the overall amount of calcium in the body by regulating the amount of calcium absorbed from food, and the amount removed from the body by the kidneys (which filter excess calcium from the blood and excrete it in the urine).

Control of calcium levels is achieved by the actions of two hormones: parathyroid hormone (produced by the *parathyroid glands*) and calcitonin (produced by the *thyroid gland*). Normally the blood plasma carries less than 0.1 percent of the body's total amount of calcium—the optimum amount for the efficient functioning of cells throughout the body. When the level of calcium in the blood falls to a low level, the parathyroid glands release more parathyroid hormone, which raises the blood calcium level by helping to release calcium from the enormous reservoir in the bones. When the blood calcium level rises to a high level, the thyroid gland releases more calcitonin, which counteracts the effects of parathyroid hormone and lowers the calcium level.

DISORDERS OF CALCIUM METABOLISM

Abnormally high or low levels of calcium in the blood may seriously disrupt cell function, particularly in muscles and nerves. Having too much calcium in the blood is called *hypercalcemia* and having too little is called *hypocalcemia*. (See also *Calcium channel blockers; Mineral supplements*.)

Calcium channel blockers

COMMON DRUGS

Diltiazem Nifedipine Verapamil

A relatively new class of drugs used in the treatment of *angina pectoris* (chest pain arising from an inadequate blood supply to heart muscle), *hypertension* (high blood pressure), and certain types of cardiac *arrhythmia* (irregular heartbeat).

HOW THEY WORK

In the treatment of angina pectoris and high blood pressure, calcium channel blockers work by interfering with muscle contraction. They prevent the movement of calcium across the membrane that lines muscle cells, which is an essential part of the mechanism of muscle contraction. This action decreases the work of the heart in pumping blood, reduces the pressure of blood flow through the body, and improves the circulation of blood through heart muscle.

Calcium channel blockers also slow the passage of nerve impulses through heart muscle, which helps correct certain types of arrhythmia.

POSSIBLE ADVERSE EFFECTS

Adverse effects of calcium channel blockers are mainly related to their action of increasing blood flow through tissues. These effects include headaches, facial flushing, and dizziness (usually on standing). Such effects, however, generally disappear with continued treatment.

Calculus

A deposit on the teeth (see *Calculus, dental*) or a small, hard, crystalline mass formed from substances occurring in fluid, such as bile, urine, or saliva. The usual sites for such calculi are the salivary ducts, the gallbladder and bile ducts (see *Gallstones*), and the kidneys, ureters, or urinary bladder (see *Calculus, urinary tract*). Far more men than women suffer from kidney stones. Whatever the site, stones may be symptomless or may cause severe pain and may then need to be treated (by being dissolved, shattered, or surgically removed). (See *Urinary tract calculi* box, p. 222.)

Calculus, dental

A hard, crustlike deposit found on the crowns and roots of teeth. Also known as tartar, calculus is formed when mineral salts from saliva are deposited in existing *plaque*. These minerals, mainly calcium and phosphorus, make up about 70 percent of the calculus; the rest is organic material and bacteria.

TYPES

Supragingival calculus, which forms above the gum margin on the crowns of teeth, is usually white or yellowish. It commonly occurs on the inside surfaces of the lower incisors and on the outer surfaces of the upper molars—areas close to the duct openings of the salivary glands.

Subgingival calculus, which forms below the gum margin, is more evenly distributed around all the teeth. Possibly because of breakdown products of blood from the gums, subgingival calculus is brown or black, and is visible if the gum is gently parted from the tooth. It may show through the gum as a dark area.

Both types of calculus are hard and are therefore difficult to remove; the subgingival variety may be more difficult to remove because of its location and degree of calcification.

EFFECTS AND TREATMENT

Being porous, calculus is impossible to keep clean and continually becomes covered by plaque. The irritant effect of toxins in plaque and calculus causes progressive inflammation and destruction of the gums and supporting structures of the teeth (see *Periodontitis*). Calculus should be completely removed on a regular basis by professional *scaling*. Careful *oral hygiene*, professional cleaning, and elimination of stagnation areas, such as poorly finished fillings, should diminish or slow its recurrence.

Calculus, urinary tract

A stone in the kidneys, ureters, or bladder, caused by precipitation from solution of the substances in urine.

INCIDENCE

The incidence of stones varies in different parts of the world. Kidney and ureteral stones are more common than bladder stones in developed countries, whereas bladder stones are relatively more common in developing countries.

Kidney or ureteral stones are three times more common in men than in women and the incidence is highest in the summer months, perhaps because the urine is more concentrated because of loss of fluid in sweat. Stones tend to be a recurrent problem; about 60 percent of patients treated for a stone develop another one within seven years.

COMPOSITION AND CAUSES

KIDNEY AND URETERAL STONES There are various types of kidney and ureteral stones. In the majority of cases, there is no identifiable underlying cause, although mild chronic dehydration (for example, due to inadequate water consumption in a hot climate) may play a part, as may a prolonged period of confinement to bed.

About 70 percent of kidney and ureteral stones consist mainly of calcium oxalate and/or phosphate. Oxalate is an end product of body *metabolism* and is present naturally in the urine. The salt it forms with calcium dissolves poorly. An abnormally high level of oxalate in the urine predisposes to stone formation and may be related to a diet containing food or drinks with a high oxalic acid content (for example, rhubarb, spinach, leafy vegetables, and coffee). Stones containing calcium are in some cases the first evidence of a disturbance of metabolism associated with *hyperparathyroidism* (overactivity of the parathyroid glands).

About 20 percent of calculi are termed infective stones and are linked with chronic *urinary tract infection*. These calculi consist of a combination of calcium, magnesium, and ammonium phosphate and are associated with a high ammonium content and alkalinity of the urine produced by the action of bacteria on urea (a substance in urine). In the kidney, an infective stone may fill the entire network of urine-collecting ducts and the top part of the ureter, forming a large, oddly shaped "staghorn" calculus.

Stones consisting mainly of uric acid comprise about 5 percent of the

C

C

total and may occur in people with *gout*, people with some cancers, and people with chronic *dehydration*. Other types of stone occasionally occur. Those formed from the amino acid cystine affect people with cystinuria (an inherited *metabolic disorder*).

BLADDER STONES In poorer countries, bladder stones usually develop as a result of a diet that is low in phosphate and protein. In developed countries, they usually result from obstruction to the flow of urine from the bladder and/or a long-standing urinary tract infection. The composition of bladder stones varies according to the acidity or alkalinity of the urine, but in Canada the most common type consists of calcium oxalate.

SYMPTOMS

The most common symptom of a stone in the kidney or ureter is *renal colic* (a severe pain in the loin). The most common symptom of a bladder stone is difficulty in passing urine.

DIAGNOSIS

Investigation of a suspected calculus usually starts with examination of the urine, which may reveal red blood cells and the presence of crystals. The degree of acidity or alkalinity of the urine may reflect the type of stone involved. About 90 percent of urinary tract calculi are visible on X rays, which show the site of the stone; this can be confirmed by intravenous or retrograde *urography*. These special X-ray techniques also indicate any obstruction of the urinary tract above the stone, which can be monitored by *ultrasound scanning*. If a metabolic disorder is a suspected cause of the stone, chemical analysis of the blood and urine may be performed to look for high levels of calcium, phosphate, urate, or cystine.

TREATMENT

Renal colic is treated with bed rest, a narcotic analgesic drug (painkiller), and adequate fluid intake to encourage passing of the stone through the ureter, bladder, and urethra. The majority of stones less than 5 mm in diameter are passed in the urine at home with relatively few problems.

In the case of larger stones, or if an infection or obstruction to urinary flow is present, surgical treatment may be needed to prevent damage to the kidney. The traditional method of removing stones from the ureter or the junction between the ureter and kidney is by surgery under general anesthesia. Stones in the bladder and lower ureter can be crushed and removed by *cystoscopy* (passage of a slim viewing tube and crushing device up the urethra into the bladder) or by ureterorenoscopy (passage of a similar tube into the ureter).

In recent years, new methods for removing kidney and ureteral stones have been developed and have dramatically changed the way in which stones are treated. Ultrasonic *lithotripsy* involves the use of an ultrasonic probe, which is inserted into the body through a telescopic tube to help break up stones that are too large to be removed whole. A more advanced treatment is the extracorporeal shockwave lithotriptor, which disintegrates kidney stones by focusing shock waves on them from outside the body.

If a stone is thought to have developed because of a metabolic disorder, the patient may be prescribed a diet, and possibly drugs, to lower the content in the urine of the substance from which the stone is formed; it may also be necessary to maintain a high fluid intake. These methods may act to dissolve an existing stone and may help prevent recurrences.

Stones associated with hyperparathyroidism are treated by methods appropriate to their location; in most cases a parathyroid gland tumor is responsible for the condition and this is removed.

Calendar method

A method of *contraception*, also called the rhythm method, that entails abstaining from sexual intercourse around the time of ovulation, which is predicted on the basis of the length of previous menstrual cycles.

The calendar method is unreliable because a woman's cycle may vary, and thus the time of ovulation can be estimated only approximately. There are now more scientific and effective contraceptive methods of this type. (See *Contraception, natural methods of*.)

Calf muscles

The muscles extending from the back of the knee to the heel. The *gastrocnemius muscle* starts behind the knee and forms the bulky part of the calf. Under it is the soleus muscle, which

---

URINARY TRACT CALCULI

Symptoms vary according to the site of the stone. Small stones in the kidney often cause no symptoms until they start to pass down the ureter, resulting in *renal colic*, a sudden pain in the flank that moves toward the groin. The pain is acute, sharp, and intermittent and may cause nausea and vomiting. There may also be hematuria (blood in the urine). Bladder stones, which affect men far more often than women, can cause difficulty in passing urine, a poor flow rate, and dribbling. Some stones may be associated with recurrent episodes of *urinary tract infection*. Any obstruction to urine flow may result in rapid kidney damage and acute severe infection termed *pyelonephritis*.

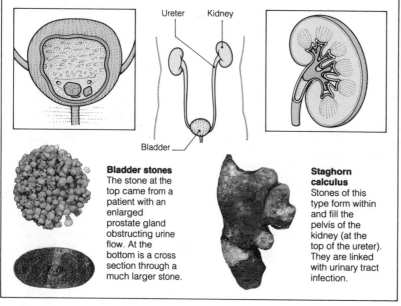

Ureter Kidney

Bladder

Bladder stones
The stone at the top came from a patient with an enlarged prostate gland obstructing urine flow. At the bottom is a cross section through a much larger stone.

Staghorn calculus
Stones of this type form within and fill the pelvis of the kidney (at the top of the ureter). They are linked with urinary tract infection.

starts lower down from the back of the *tibia* (shin). These muscles join to form the *Achilles tendon*, which connects them to the calcaneus (heel). See illustration below.

Contraction of the calf muscles pulls the heel up to produce a springing movement through the toes. This movement is important in walking, running, jumping, and hopping.

Pain can occur because of *cramp*, *sciatica* (inflammation of the sciatic nerve), or, more rarely, deep vein *thrombosis*. The calf muscles may be affected by *claudication* (a cramplike pain brought on by walking and quickly relieved by rest).

Caliper splint

An orthopedic device used to exert control on a deformed leg or to support a leg weakened by a muscular disorder, making it possible for the person to stand and walk. For example, a person who has lost the ability to flex the foot upward, and, as a result, drags the toes on the ground with each step, can be fitted with a splint that keeps the foot permanently at right angles to the leg and thus allows walking.

A caliper splint consists of one or two vertical metal rods attached to leather or metal rings worn around the limb. A caliper splint extending only below the knee is sufficient to control the position of the ankle. Longer splints may be jointed to allow knee movement.

LOCATION OF CALF MUSCLES
The gastrocnemius and soleus join to form the Achilles tendon.

Gastrocnemius muscle

Soleus muscle

Achilles tendon

Calcaneus

Callosity
See *Callus, skin*.

Callus, bony

A diffuse growth of new soft *bone* that forms around a healing *fracture*. The callus is eventually replaced by stronger bone with a more organized structure. A callus can sometimes be felt as a lumpy deformity around a fracture site and is visible on an X ray. Presence of a callus provides evidence that healing has started. As healing continues, the original shape of the bone is restored.

Callus, skin

An area of thickened skin, caused by regular or prolonged pressure or friction. Manual laborers develop calluses on the palms of their hands, joggers on the soles of their feet, and guitarists on the tips of their fingers.

Calluses may also develop if body weight is borne unevenly—for example, if there is a persistent deformity affecting one foot. A *corn* is a callus on a toe.

TREATMENT
If a callus on the foot becomes troublesome or painful, a podiatrist should be consulted. He or she can pare away layers of thickened skin with a scalpel. Calluses caused by foot deformities almost always recur unless the underlying problem is corrected—either surgically or by using a molded insole in the shoe.

Caloric test

A method of discovering whether a person with *vertigo* (dizziness) and hearing loss has a diseased labyrinth (part of the inner ear).

The outer ear canal of one ear is briefly flooded with water at different temperatures above and below normal body temperature. This flooding sets up convection currents in the semicircular canals situated within the inner ear.

If the labyrinth is normal, *nystagmus* (rapid reflex flickering of the eyes) occurs for a predictable period. If the labyrinth is diseased, nystagmus will either not occur or will stop sooner than normal. The presence and duration of the nystagmus may be observed directly or be recorded electrically using the technique of *electronystagmography*.

Calorie

A measure of energy. Strictly, one calorie is the amount of energy needed to raise the temperature of 1 g

Performing a caloric test
The physician floods the outer ear with water at different temperatures and watches for reflex flickering of the eyes.

of water by 1°C. In medicine and dietetics, the energy content of foods and the energy used to perform various activities is sometimes measured in units called kilocalories, which are equal to 1,000 calories. These two units are often confused because both are referred to as calories. However, the medical unit is abbreviated as Cal or kcal, whereas the ordinary, "small" calorie is abbreviated as cal.

When the daily calorie intake is the same as the amount of energy expended, a person's weight usually remains constant. If intake exceeds expenditure, weight is usually gained; if expenditure exceeds intake, weight is usually lost. In general, fats contain the most calories per unit weight. (See also *Calorimetry; Diet and disease*.)

Calorie requirements
See *Energy requirements*.

Calorimetry

The measurement of the *calorie* (energy) value of foodstuffs or the energy expenditure of a person.

Direct calorimetry is the usual method of calculating the calorie value of small amounts of a particular foodstuff. This calorie value may then be converted to the number of calories in a typical serving. After being weighed and placed in a special sealed container, called a bomb calorimeter, the food is ignited; the calorimeter is then immersed in a known volume of water. The rise in the temperature of the water when the foodstuff is completely burned up is used to calculate the calorie value.

Energy production in humans is more easily measured indirectly. It has been found that every litre of oxygen taken into the body produces 4,800 calories of energy. Therefore, to calculate energy production, it is only necessary to measure oxygen uptake. This can be done by comparing the percentage of oxygen in inspired and expired air.

Canada Health Act

A federal law that establishes the criteria and conditions provinces and territories must meet before they can receive the federal transfer payments that partially support hospital, physician, and other health care services.

Canadian Dental Association

Canadian dentists' national organization. It represents the provincial dental associations in dealings with the federal government, and helps develop national positions on dental practice, education, and research.

Canadian Medical Association

The national association of Canada's physicians, 41,000 (85 percent) of whom are members. Its mission: to protect and improve the general health of Canadians, to maintain high standards of medical education and professional ethics; to promote high quality, effective health care available to all Canadians; and to present the profession's views as effectively as possible to the public and to government. The CMA also represents and coordinates the work of 10 *provincial medical associations/societies*, which deal directly with the various provincial governments.

The CMA offers its members scientific publications, economic information, and guidelines on a number of topics. It does not licence or discipline members. The CMA is financed primarily by membership dues, and receives no financial support from any government.

Canadian Nurses Association

The national organization of professional nurses, with more than 130,000 members. It represents Canadian nurses in dealings with the federal government, represents provincial nurses' associations, and acts to influence public policy in the interests of nurses, and patients.

Cancer

Any of a group of diseases in which symptoms are due to the unrestrained growth of cells in one of the body organs or tissues. Malignant tumors most commonly develop in major organs, such as the lungs, breasts, intestines, skin, stomach, or pan-

CANCER-CAUSING AGENTS

The table gives a rough estimate of the proportion of cancer deaths that can be attributed to various specific agents or behaviors. Smoking is particularly implicated in lung and bladder cancers, and alcohol in cancers of the tongue, pharynx, and esophagus. Sexual and reproductive behavior affects the risk of cervical cancer (the more sexual partners a woman has, the higher the risk) and of breast cancer (having children while relatively young protects against this cancer). Note the importance of dietary factors.

CANCER-CAUSING AGENTS

Agent	% of cancer deaths
Natural constituents of food	35
Tobacco	30
Sexual and reproductive history	7
Occupational hazards	4
Alcohol	3
Food additives	1
Other	20

creas, but they may also develop in the nasal sinuses, the testes or ovaries, or the lips or tongue. Cancers may also develop in the blood cell-forming tissues of the bone marrow (the *leukemias*) and in the lymphatic system, muscles, or bones.

Cancers are not the only type of abnormal growth, or *neoplasm*. However, a cancer differs from a *benign tumor* in two important ways. As it grows, it infiltrates the tissues around it and may block passageways, destroy nerves, and erode bone. Cells from the cancer may spread via the blood vessels and lymphatic channels to other parts of the body, where these *metastases* form new, satellite tumors.

INCIDENCE

Cancer is a process that has affected humans since prehistoric times and is just as common in domestic and farm animals, birds, and fish. Just over 100,000 new cases are reported annually in Canada. At 52,000 deaths a year, it is the second most common cause of death after coronary artery disease. Put another way, 24 percent of males and 21 percent of females alive today will eventually die of cancer. It is also Canada's leading cause of *potential years of life lost*. Apart from childhood cancers, which may be associated with events during pregnancy, such as exposure to radiation, most adult cancers are a feature of the aging process.

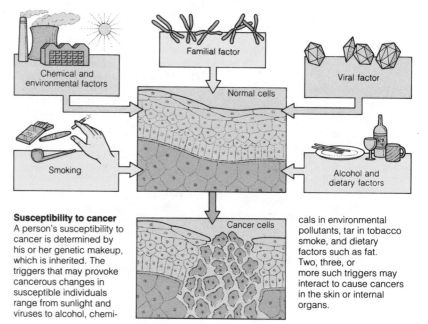

Susceptibility to cancer
A person's susceptibility to cancer is determined by his or her genetic makeup, which is inherited. The triggers that may provoke cancerous changes in susceptible individuals range from sunlight and viruses to alcohol, chemi-

cals in environmental pollutants, tar in tobacco smoke, and dietary factors such as fat. Two, three, or more such triggers may interact to cause cancers in the skin or internal organs.

C

INCIDENCE OF CANCER

The likelihood of cancer developing varies with age. A 20-year-old has a very low likelihood of it developing by the age of 30, but the risk roughly doubles between 30 and 40, and doubles again for each decade thereafter. Whatever the cause of death in someone aged 90, careful examination of the internal organs will often reveal a small cancer that may not have caused any symptoms. Localized cancer of the prostate is an almost universal finding in elderly men. Thus, while cancer seems to be much more common than in the past, this is mostly due to the increasing numbers of old people in the population.

CANCER WARNING SIGNS

Cancer may cause a variety of minor symptoms. Any that persist for several days should be checked by a physician. The earlier a cancer is diagnosed, the better the chance of there being a cure.

Rapid weight loss without apparent cause
A scab, sore, or ulcer that fails to heal within three weeks
A blemish or mole that enlarges, bleeds, or itches
Severe recurrent headaches
Difficulty swallowing
Persistent hoarseness
Coughing up bloody sputum (phlegm)

Persistent abdominal pain
Change in shape or size of testes
Blood in urine, with no pain on urination
Change in bowel habits
Lump or change in breast shape
Bleeding or discharge from nipple
Vaginal bleeding or spotting between periods or after menopause

5-YEAR SURVIVAL FROM ALL FORMS OF CANCER

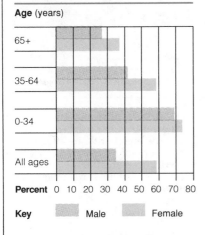

Age (years)

Percent 0 10 20 30 40 50 60 70 80

Key Male   Female

The percentages refer to people of both sexes and all ages diagnosed as having cancer at the start of a five-year period. The better survival among women is due mainly to the better prognosis of breast cancer compared to lung cancer, which affects twice as many men as women. Improved treatment of childhood cancers, such as leukemias, accounts for the better survival of young people.

HOW CANCER AFFECTED CANADIAN MEN IN 1989

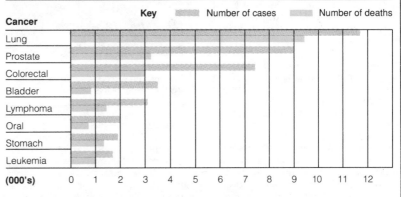

Key Number of cases   Number of deaths

Cancer: Lung, Prostate, Colorectal, Bladder, Lymphoma, Oral, Stomach, Leukemia

(000's) 0 1 2 3 4 5 6 7 8 9 10 11 12

HOW CANCER AFFECTED CANADIAN WOMEN IN 1989

Key Number of cases   Number of deaths

Cancer: Breast, Colorectal, Lung, Uterus (body), Lymphoma, Ovary, Uterus (cervix), Leukemia

(000's) 0 1 2 3 4 5 6 7 8 9 10 11 12

The bars indicate the number of new cancer cases in 1989. The shaded sections indicate deaths from a particular cancer that year. Note that lung cancer is by far the most likely cancer to be fatal. It is also the most preventable. (Not included are *Squamous cell cancers* of the skin, which are almost never fatal.)

C

CAUSES

The growth of a cancer begins when the *oncogenes* (genes controlling cell growth and multiplication) in a cell or cells are transformed by agents known as *carcinogens*.

Once a healthy cell is transformed into a tumor-forming type (malignant transformation), the change in its oncogenes is passed on to all offspring cells. A small group of abnormal cells is thus established, and these abnormal cells divide more rapidly than the normal surrounding cells. Usually the abnormal cells show a lack of *differentiation*—that is, they no longer perform the specialized task of the cells of their host tissue—and may escape the normal control of hormones and nerves. Thus, they are in effect parasites, contributing nothing to their host tissue but continuing to consume nutrients from it.

Years may pass before the growth of cells becomes large enough to cause symptoms, although the rate of growth varies according to the tissue of origin. Current estimates suggest that some cancers of the lung and breast may be present for well over five years before they cause symptoms. During this "occult" phase, metastases may be seeded in the liver, lungs, bones, or brain, and, in these circumstances, a purely surgical cure is impossible because the cancer has already spread far beyond the primary site of origin.

SYMPTOMS

The range of symptoms produced by cancers is vast. The symptoms depend on the site of the growth, the tissue of origin, and the extent of the growth. Symptoms may be a direct feature of the growth (e.g., lumps or skin changes) or they may be derived from obstruction or bleeding into passageways, such as the lung airways, gastrointestinal tract, or urinary tract, or from disruption of the function of a vital organ. Tumors pressing on or disturbing nerve tracts can cause nervous system disorders and pain. Some tumors lead to the overproduction of hormones, with complications and effects far distant from the site of the growth. Unexplained weight loss is a common feature.

Some important warning signals that always warrant investigation by a physician are shown in the *Incidence of cancer* box on page 225.

DIAGNOSIS

Both the means of diagnosing cancer at an early stage (when the chances of cure are highest) and the range of

TREATMENT OF CANCER

The treatment of many cancers is still primarily surgical; excision of an early tumor will often give a complete cure. Because there may be small, undetectable metastases at the time of operation, surgery is commonly combined with *radiation therapy* and *anticancer drugs*. The aim of these treatments is to suppress, or arrest, the rate of cell division in any tumor cells left after surgery. Anticancer drugs often have unpleasant side effects because it is sometimes difficult to target specific drugs effectively, and normal cells and tissues may be disrupted along with the tumor cells.

Before radiation therapy
The photograph shows a skin cancer in front of the ear before treatment.

After radiation therapy
This was the appearance a few weeks later, after a course of radiation therapy.

treatments available have improved dramatically in the past decade.

Screening tests (for early breast cancer, cancer of the cervix, and intestinal cancer) have reduced mortality from these tumors. For most tumors, however, diagnosis generally occurs after the appearance of symptoms, is based on the physician's examination of the patient, and is confirmed by microscopic examination of tissue cells obtained by *biopsy* (cancer cells look different from normal cells). New scanning and imaging techniques give more information while causing less discomfort to the patient.

There are four main types of tests: cytology tests, imaging techniques, chemical tests, and direct inspection (see chart facing page).

OUTLOOK

Almost half of all cancers are today cured completely, and cure and survival rates for various years after diagnosis continue to improve. For disease of certain organ systems, the diagnosis of a cancer may actually provide a better outlook than some of the alternative diagnoses. Cure and survival

rates and the chances of recurrence do, however, differ markedly according to the organ or tissue affected.

For more information on cancers of individual organs—their incidence, causes, symptoms, treatment, and outlook—refer to the organ in question (e.g., *Breast cancer; Lung cancer; Stomach cancer*).

Cancerphobia

An intense fear of developing cancer, out of proportion to the actual risk, so that the sufferer's behavior and lifestyle are significantly altered. A cancerphobic person becomes convinced that any symptoms (e.g., skin problems, constipation, or difficulty in swallowing) are signs of cancer and seeks medical advice. Instead of paying sensible attention to diet and prevention (such as giving up smoking), he or she adopts extreme behavior (for example, prolonged washing rituals, avoidance of social contact, bizarre eating habits) typical of *obsessive-compulsive disorder*. *Psychotherapy* or *behavior therapy* may be of benefit. (See also *Phobia*.)

TYPES OF CANCER TEST

Cytology tests	These tests reveal the shedding of abnormal cells. One example is the *cervical smear test*, an investigation in which cells are scraped from the cervix and examined microscopically to	detect potential or early cancer of the cervix. Another example is the urine cytology test, periodically carried out on those working in manufacturing industries where bladder cancer is a known risk.
Imaging techniques	These can sometimes reveal early cancerous changes in tissue. A notable example is the special low-dose X-ray technique used in *mammography* to detect early cancer of the breast. Research	with *ultrasound scanning*, which produces images of internal organs, suggests that it may provide a means of screening for cancer of the ovary.
Chemical tests	These tests can reveal the presence of substances that are indicative of cancer—for example, microscopic amounts of blood in	the feces, and high levels of the enzyme acid phosphatase in the blood.
Direct inspection	Inspection of the interior of organs subject to cancer is usually carried out with an *endoscope* (a tube with a viewing lens), which is passed into the organ to be examined. Examples of this technique are	*colonoscopy*, *gastroscopy*, *cystoscopy*, and *laparoscopy*. These procedures are usually carried out only when clinical suspicion has been aroused.

Cancer screening

Tests carried out on groups of people to detect cancer at an early stage. To warrant their use, screening tests must have a high rate of accuracy, must be safe, and must cause minimal discomfort. There must also be an effective treatment available. Screening tests are most effectively carried out among people who are particularly susceptible to cancer.

In theory, screening might be expected to detect cancers in an early, treatable stage, and tests have been developed for cancers of the cervix, breast, ovary, gastrointestinal tract, bladder, and prostate gland. Screening for cancer of the cervix is important because this treatable cancer is relatively slow-growing in its early stages. *Mammography* and *breast self-examination* are valuable for detecting breast cancer.

Unfortunately, some cancers, such as those of the lung and stomach, which have a tendency to spread rapidly and are rarely cured by surgery or radiation, cannot be detected before they cause symptoms.

Cancrum oris

A condition, also called *noma*, in which ulcers and tissue destruction occur within and around the mouth. It commonly affects malnourished children in poor tropical countries.

Candidiasis

Infection by the fungus CANDIDA ALBICANS, also known as thrush or moniliasis. It most commonly affects the vagina but also affects other areas of mucous membrane, such as the mouth.

CAUSES AND INCIDENCE
The fungus that causes candidiasis is normally present in the vagina and mouth. Its growth is kept under control by the bacteria usually present in these organs. If a course of *antibiotic drugs* destroys too many of the bacteria, or if the body's resistance to infection is lowered, the fungus may multiply excessively.

Certain disorders, notably *diabetes mellitus*, and the hormonal changes that occur in pregnancy or when a woman is taking *oral contraceptives*, may also encourage growth of the CANDIDA ALBICANS fungus.

Candidiasis can be contracted by sexual intercourse with an infected partner. It is much more common in women than in men. Candidal infection of the penis is uncommon but is more likely to occur in men who have not been circumcised.

Candidiasis may spread from the genitals or mouth to other moist areas of the body. It may also affect the gastrointestinal tract, especially in people who have impaired immune systems. In infants, candidiasis sometimes occurs in conjunction with *diaper rash*.

SYMPTOMS
Vaginal candidiasis may cause a thick, white, "cottage cheese" discharge from the vagina and/or vaginal itching and irritation. There may also be discomfort when passing urine. However, some women have no symptoms. In men, infection of the penis usually causes *balanitis* (inflammation of the head of the penis).

Oral candidiasis produces sore, creamy-yellow, raised patches in the mouth. Candidiasis that affects the skin folds or the diaper area takes the form of an itchy red rash with flaky white patches.

DIAGNOSIS AND TREATMENT
Candidiasis is diagnosed by examination of a sample of the white discharge or patches. Treatment is with an *antifungal drug*, such as nystatin, clotrimazole, miconazole, or econazole nitrate. Drugs are usually prescribed in the form of vaginal suppositories or creams to be applied to the affected area. Simultaneous treatment of sexual partners is recommended to prevent reinfection.

Treatment is usually successful but the condition tends to recur. People with a tendency to skin candidiasis should keep the skin as dry as possible, and women who take *oral contraceptives* may be advised to consider changing to another, nonhormonal, method of contraception.

Canine tooth

See *Teeth*.

Cannabis

Psychoactive preparations derived from the hemp plant CANNABIS SATIVA. (See *Marijuana*.)

Cannula

A plastic or metal tube with a smooth, unsharpened tip for inserting into a blood vessel, lymphatic vessel, or body cavity in order to introduce or withdraw fluids.

To insert a cannula, the physician first punctures the site with a long, thin needle, slides the cannula over it, and then withdraws the needle. Alternatively, he or she may insert a trocar (sharp-pointed rod) inside the cannula and remove it once the vessel has been entered.

Cannulas are frequently used for *blood transfusions* and *intravenous infusions* and for draining *pleural effusions*. In certain circumstances, such as when blood is required for testing over a period of time, the cannula may be left in place for several days.

C

Cap, contraceptive

A barrier method of contraception in the form of a latex rubber device placed directly over the cervix to prevent sperm from entering. (See *Contraception, barrier methods of*.)

Capgras' syndrome

The *delusion* (false belief) that a relative or close friend has been replaced by an impostor. Also known as the "illusion of doubles," Capgras' syndrome is seen most frequently in paranoid *schizophrenia*, but also occurs in organic disorders (see *Brain syndrome, organic*) and *affective disorders*.

Capillary

Any of the vessels that carry blood between the smallest arteries, or arterioles, and the smallest veins, or venules (see *Circulatory system*). Capillaries form a fine network throughout the body's organs and tissues. It is through the thin capillary walls that blood and cells exchange their constituents (see *Respiration*).

Capillaries have a diameter of approximately 0.008 mm—not much wider than the red blood cells that flow through them. The capillary walls are permeable to substances such as oxygen, glucose, carbon dioxide, and water, which can thus move freely between the blood and the tissue fluid that surrounds all cells.

STRUCTURE OF CAPILLARIES

These minute blood vessels have permeable walls to allow transfer of oxygen, glucose, and water from blood to tissues.

Pseudopodia of a white blood cell

Oxygen, glucose, and water

Carbon dioxide, waste products, and excess water

Red blood cell

The capillaries are not open to blood flow all the time; they open and close according to different organs' requirements for oxygen and nutrients. Thus, when a person is running, most of the capillaries in the leg muscles are open, but at rest many are closed. The opening and closing of skin capillaries plays an important role in *temperature* regulation. Blood flow through each capillary is controlled by a tiny circle of muscle at its entrance.

DISORDERS

A direct blow to the body may rupture the thin capillary walls, resulting in bleeding under the surface of the skin and causing swelling and bruising.

Capillaries become more fragile in the elderly, in people taking high doses of *corticosteroid drugs*, and in sufferers from *scurvy* (vitamin C deficiency). All such people have a tendency to *purpura* (small blue-purple areas of bleeding under the skin).

Capillary *hemangiomas* are benign tumors of the capillary wall that may cause a red patch of variable size and shape on the skin or mucous membranes. Such hemangiomas may be congenital (present at birth) or they may develop later in life.

Capping, dental

See *Crown, dental*.

Capsule

An anatomical structure enclosing an organ or body part; examples include the capsules of the liver, kidneys, joints, and eye lenses.

The term capsule is also used to describe a hard or soft shell, usually made of gelatin, containing a drug. Capsules are taken by mouth and have two main advantages over solid tablets. Firstly, their elongated shape makes them easier to swallow. Secondly, they make it easier for patients to take solid or liquid medications that would otherwise have an unpleasant taste or smell.

Some capsules have a special coating to prevent the release into the stomach of drugs that may have an irritant effect. Others are designed to release their contents into the small intestine at a slow, steady rate so that a drug need be taken less frequently than if it was in the form of a conventional capsule or tablet.

Capsulitis

Inflammation of a capsule around an organ or other body part. Inflammation of the capsule of the shoulder joint is a feature of *frozen shoulder*.

Captopril

The first member of a new class of drugs, the *ACE inhibitors*, used in the treatment of *hypertension* (high blood pressure) and *heart failure*.

Caput

The Latin word for head. The term caput is also used to refer to the face, skull, and all associated organs, to the origin of a muscle, or to any enlarged extremity, such as the caput femoris, the head of the femur (thighbone). However, the term most commonly refers to the caput succedaneum, a soft swelling in the scalp of newborn babies. The swelling occurs as a result of pressure on the baby's head during labor and usually disappears after a few days.

Carbachol

A pupil-constricting drug, which acts like *acetylcholine*. It is primarily used in treating glaucoma.

Carbamazepine

ANTICONVULSANT
Tablet Liquid
📋 Prescription needed

An *anticonvulsant drug*, introduced in 1960, chemically related to the tricyclic *antidepressant drugs*.

WHY IT IS USED

Carbamazepine reduces the likelihood of seizures caused by abnormal nerve signals in the brain and is mainly used in the long-term treatment of *epilepsy*. It has less of a sedative effect than many other anticonvulsant drugs.

Carbamazepine is also prescribed to relieve *neuralgia* (the intermittent severe pain caused by damage to, or irritation of, a nerve). Carbamazepine is occasionally prescribed to treat certain psychological or behavioral disorders, such as *mania*.

POSSIBLE ADVERSE EFFECTS

There may be some sedative effect, especially if alcohol is consumed.

Carbenoxolone

An *ulcer-healing drug* that is used to treat stomach ulcers. Carbenoxolone is thought to work by stimulating the production of mucus that forms a protective coating over the lining of the stomach. Carbenoxolone is also given in the form of a special capsule for the treatment of duodenal ulcers; the capsule releases the active drug in the duodenum after it has passed through the stomach. A gel containing carbenoxolone is also available for the relief of mouth ulcers.

Adverse effects of carbenoxolone are usually caused by a loss of potassium or an increase in sodium levels in the body and include headache and muscle weakness.

Carbohydrates

A group of compounds composed of carbon, hydrogen, and oxygen which supply the body with its main source of energy.

TYPES AND SOURCES

There are two groups: available carbohydrates, which are metabolized (chemically changed) in the body, and unavailable carbohydrates, which can not be broken down by human digestive *enzymes*.

Monosaccharides	glucose, galactose, fructose
Disaccharides	sucrose, lactose, maltose
Polysaccharides	starch cellulose

Types of carbohydrates
Monosaccharides are the simplest, consisting of a single saccharide molecule. Disaccharides consist of two saccharide molecules linked together. Polysaccharides consist of a long chain of many saccharide molecules. The most important carbohydrate is starch.

The available carbohydrates include starches (complex carbohydrates) and sugars (simple carbohydrates) and are found in cereals, root crops, and fruits. The unavailable carbohydrates include cellulose and hemicellulose, which pass through the body virtually unchanged and make up the bulk of what is known as dietary fiber (see *Fiber, dietary*).

The term refined carbohydrate usually refers to sucrose refined from cane or beet, with no other nutrients. Corn starch (cornflour) is another refined carbohydrate, consisting of pure starch with no other nutrients.

CARBOHYDRATE METABOLISM

The monosaccharides or simple sugars—glucose (grape sugar), galactose (a milk sugar), and fructose (fruit sugar)—are absorbed into the bloodstream unchanged; the disaccharides (double sugars) such as sucrose and lactose (a milk sugar) have to be broken down to the simple sugars first, and so do the starches.

The monosaccharides (principally glucose) are then absorbed through the intestinal wall and into the bloodstream for distribution throughout the body. Certain cells, such as brain cells and red blood cells, must have a constant supply of glucose to survive. Some of the glucose is used immediately by these cells, which "burn" it in a series of biochemical reactions to generate energy (see *Metabolism*). The rest of the glucose is conveyed to the liver, muscles, and fat cells where it is converted into *glycogen* (animal starch) and fat for storage. When more energy is needed, this glycogen is converted back to glucose, which re-enters the bloodstream for distribution around the body.

Fat cannot be converted to glucose but can be burned as fuel to conserve glucose. Unlike glucose, galactose and fructose cannot be used directly by the body's cells and so must first be converted by the liver to glucose; thereafter, the fate of this glucose is the same as that of glucose absorbed directly into the bloodstream from the intestine.

When the blood glucose level is high, such as after a meal, carbohydrate metabolism is primarily controlled by *insulin*, a hormone secreted by the *pancreas*. Insulin restores the glucose level to normal by stimulating its uptake by the liver, muscles, and adipose cells for storage as glycogen and fat. In the disorder *diabetes mellitus*, carbohydrate metabolism is disturbed by a deficiency of insulin, and carbohydrates cannot enter most cells for storage.

The action of insulin is balanced by that of *glucagon*, another hormone produced by the pancreas. When the blood sugar level is low—for example, after fasting overnight or after exercise—insulin secretion diminishes and glucagon stimulates the conversion of glycogen to glucose for release into the bloodstream. Epinephrine and corticosteroid hormones produced by the *adrenal glands* at times of stress also act to raise the blood sugar level.

Carbon

A nonmetallic element that is present in all organic molecules (the fundamental molecules of all living organisms), such as *proteins*, *fats*, and *carbohydrates*, and also in some inorganic molecules, such as *carbon dioxide*, *carbon monoxide*, and *sodium bicarbonate*. Pure carbon is the major constituent of diamonds, coal, *charcoal*, and graphite (pencil lead).

C

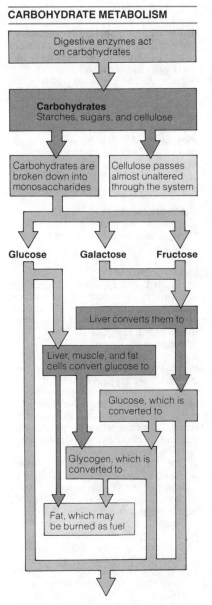

CARBOHYDRATE METABOLISM

Digestive enzymes act on carbohydrates

Carbohydrates
Starches, sugars, and cellulose

Carbohydrates are broken down into monosaccharides

Cellulose passes almost unaltered through the system

Glucose   Galactose   Fructose

Liver converts them to

Liver, muscle, and fat cells convert glucose to

Glucose, which is converted to

Glycogen, which is converted to

Fat, which may be burned as fuel

Glucose is absorbed into the bloodstream for distribution throughout the body or is used directly by body cells.

Carbon dioxide

A colorless, odorless gas. Carbon dioxide is present in small amounts in the air and is an important by-product of normal *metabolism* in the body. Carbon dioxide consists of one carbon atom (symbol C) linked to two oxygen atoms (symbol O) and has the chemical formula CO_2. When it is cooled and compressed, carbon dioxide forms a white solid, *dry ice*, which is important in *cryosurgery*.

Carbon dioxide is a waste product of metabolic reactions that break down various substances, especially carbohydrates and fats, to generate energy. Waste carbon dioxide is carried by the blood to the lungs, where it is released and breathed out. One of the factors controlling the rate of breathing is the level of carbon dioxide in the bloodstream. When a person exercises, the amount of carbon dioxide produced increases, and the resultant high level in the bloodstream causes the person to breathe more rapidly to eliminate the carbon dioxide and to take in more oxygen.

Carbon monoxide

A colorless, odorless, poisonous gas. Carbon monoxide is present in the exhaust fumes of oil- or gasoline-powered engines and is also produced by inefficient burning of coal, gas, oil, or bottled gas in domestic heating appliances. It consists of one carbon atom (chemical symbol C) linked to one oxygen atom (symbol O) and has the chemical formula CO.

POISONING

Carbon monoxide is poisonous because it binds with *hemoglobin* (the oxygen-carrying molecule in red blood cells) and prevents it from carrying oxygen. As a result, the tissues are deprived of oxygen and asphyxiation occurs. Continued inhalation of the gas may lead to permanent brain damage or even death.

The initial symptoms of carbon monoxide poisoning—which may sometimes be mistaken for those of food poisoning—are dizziness, headache, nausea, and faintness. The most important step in first-aid treatment is to take the victim into the fresh air; continued exposure to the gas will lead to loss of consciousness. If the victim has stopped breathing, give *artificial respiration* and get emergency medical aid. Even if the victim seems to recover completely when taken into the fresh air, it is advisable for him or her to consult a physician to make certain that there are no long-term effects.

Carbon tetrachloride

A colorless, poisonous, volatile liquid with a characteristic odor. Carbon tetrachloride is not available for retail sale, but is present in some home dry-cleaning fluids and is sometimes used as an industrial solvent. It consists of one carbon atom (symbol C) linked to four chlorine atoms (symbol Cl) and has the chemical formula CCl_4.

Carbon tetrachloride is a dangerous chemical; it can produce dizziness, mental confusion, and liver and kidney damage if it is inhaled or drunk. Symptoms of poisoning include abdominal pain, nausea, headache, and convulsions.

Carbuncle

A cluster of interconnected *boils* (painful, pus-filled, inflamed hair roots). Carbuncles are usually caused by the bacterium *STAPHYLOCOCCUS AUREUS*; they generally begin as single boils, then spread. Common sites are the back of the neck and the buttocks.

Carbuncles are less common than single boils. They mainly affect people who have a lowered resistance to infection, in particular, people with *diabetes mellitus*.

TREATMENT

Anyone with a carbuncle should see a physician, who will usually prescribe an *antibiotic drug*. The application of hot *compresses* may encourage the pus-filled heads of the boils to burst and thus relieve pain. After the boils have burst, the carbuncle should be covered with a dressing until it has healed completely. Occasionally, incision and drainage (with removal of the core of the carbuncle) are necessary if drainage and healing do not occur on their own.

Carcinogen

Any agent capable of causing *cancer*, such as tobacco smoke, high-energy radiation, or asbestos fibers.

CHEMICAL CARCINOGENS

Chemicals are the largest group of carcinogens. Among the most important are polycyclic aromatic hydrocarbons (PAHs), which occur in tobacco smoke, pitch, tar fumes, and soot. Exposure to PAHs may lead to cancer of the respiratory system or skin. Other major chemical carcinogens are certain aromatic amines. These are used principally in the chemical and rubber industries and may cause bladder cancer after prolonged exposure.

PHYSICAL CARCINOGENS

The best-known physical carcinogen is high-energy *radiation*, including nuclear radiation and X rays. High doses of high-energy radiation destroy individual cells (an effect utilized in *radiation therapy* to destroy tumors), and very high doses may kill people within a few hours. Lower doses may not kill cells but may sometimes cause malignant changes.

Radiation affects most easily those cells which divide quickly—for example, the precursors of white blood cells in the bone marrow, so causing leukemia.

Exposure over many years to ultraviolet radiation in sunlight can cause skin cancer, particularly in people who are fair-skinned.

Asbestos fibers are another known physical cause of cancer. White asbestos may cause lung cancer, particularly in workers who are exposed to the fibers for long periods, who already have *asbestos-induced diseases* of the lungs, and who smoke. Blue asbestos and, to a lesser extent, brown asbestos can cause *mesothelioma* (a tumor of the membranes that surround certain body cavities and organs).

BIOLOGICAL CARCINOGENS

Very few biological agents cause cancer in humans. *SCHISTOSOMA HAEMATOBIUM*, one of the blood flukes responsible for the tropical disease *schistosomiasis*, can cause cancer of the bladder, where it lays its eggs. *ASPERGILLUS FLAVUS*, a fungus that contaminates stored grain and peanuts, produces the poison *aflatoxin*, which is believed to be a cause of liver cancer.

Certain viruses have been associated with cancer. The papilloma virus is believed to play a part in the causation of cancer of the cervix, the hepatitis B virus has been implicated in liver cancer, and the Epstein-Barr virus is considered to be a factor in the causation of *Burkitt's lymphoma*, a malignant tumor of the jaw and abdomen which occurs mainly among children in Africa. *Kaposi's sarcoma* is probably associated with a virus (possibly cytomegalovirus). Although not caused directly by *HIV* (the *AIDS* virus), Kaposi's sarcoma is seen more frequently in individuals who have HIV infection.

SCREENING

Canada follows international guidelines for screening substances thought to be carcinogenic that might be marketed to the public. Such substances could be found in chemicals, cosmetics, drugs and food. One major preliminary test is to expose a certain strain of bacteria to the substance, and, if *mutation* (genetic change) occurs in the bacteria, the substance is regarded as a suspect carcinogen. It is then tested on laboratory animals, such as rats. If an increased incidence of tumors occurs in the test animals, no license is usually granted to manufacture the substance for public sale.

AVOIDING CARCINOGENS

In industry, known carcinogens are

either banned or allowed only if their use is considered essential, if exposure to them is strictly limited, and if regular medical screening is provided for workers using them, as, for example, in the nuclear fuel industry and hospital X-ray departments.

Outside industry, the individual is exposed to very few known, unavoidable, high-risk carcinogens. However, given the long latent period from exposure to the development of cancer for most carcinogens, it would be prudent to regard handling of any chemical repeatedly as something to be done with the maximum of care. (See also *Carcinogenesis*.)

Carcinogenesis

The development of a *cancer* (a malignant tumor) caused by the action of certain chemicals, viruses, constituents of the diet, radiation, or unknown factors on cells that are primarily normal.

Cancer-causing factors are called *carcinogens*. Carcinogens are believed to alter the *DNA* (genetic material) within cells, particularly the structure of certain genes called *oncogenes* which normally control the growth and division of cells. An altered cell divides abnormally rapidly and passes on the changes in its genetic material to all its offspring cells. Thus, a group of cells becomes established that is not affected by the body's normal restraints on growth.

Carcinoid syndrome

A rare condition characterized by bouts of facial flushing, diarrhea, and wheezing. Carcinoid syndrome is caused by an intestinal or lung tumor, called a carcinoid, that secretes excess quantities of the hormone serotonin.

Symptoms usually occur only if the tumor has spread to the liver, or arises from the lung.

DIAGNOSIS AND TREATMENT
Carcinoid syndrome is diagnosed by measuring the level of a breakdown product of serotonin in the urine.

The condition is sometimes treated by surgical removal of the tumor from the intestine or lung, and from the liver as well, if possible. In most cases, surgical treatment is unlikely to be helpful, and in these circumstances symptoms may be relieved by drugs that block the action of serotonin.

Carcinoma

Any malignant tumor (*cancer*) arising from cells in the covering surface layer or lining membrane of a body organ.

A carcinoma is thus distinguished from a *sarcoma*, which is a cancer arising in bone, muscle, or connective tissue. Carcinomas include all the most common cancers of the lungs, breast, stomach, skin, cervix, colon and rectum (parts of the large intestine). The terms cancer and carcinoma tend to be used interchangeably but are not strictly synonymous.

Carcinomatosis

The presence of malignant tissue in many different sites of the body due to the spread of cancer cells from an original malignant tumor.

SYMPTOMS
The sufferer experiences weight loss, lack of energy, and other symptoms depending on the site of the *metastases* (secondary or offspring tumors). Metastases in the lungs may cause coughing or breathlessness; in the liver they may cause jaundice.

DIAGNOSIS AND TREATMENT
A diagnosis of carcinomatosis may be confirmed by *X rays* or by *radionuclide scanning* of the bones and lungs, by biochemical tests, or during an operation or postmortem examination. An operation to remove the primary (original) tumor will not help someone with carcinomatosis unless the primary tumor is producing a hormone that is directly stimulating growth of the metastases. *Anticancer drugs* or *radiation therapy* may be given to deal with the metastases, sometimes following surgery for removal of a primary carcinoma.

Metastases associated with some cancers (of the testis, prostate, and thyroid glands) may be treated with drugs or hormones, and a prolonged abatement of symptoms, and even cure, is now common. Metastases from lung and intestinal cancers are less responsive to treatment and, in such cases, the outlook is not good.

Cardiac arrest

A halt in the pumping action of the heart due to cessation of its rhythmic, muscular activity.

CAUSES
The most common cause is a *myocardial infarction* (heart attack), but other causes include *respiratory arrest*, *electrical injury*, *hypothermia*, loss of blood, drug overdose, and *anaphylactic shock*.

DIAGNOSIS AND TREATMENT
A person with cardiac arrest collapses suddenly, with loss of consciousness, and absence of pulse and breathing. A person who is breathing cannot have suffered from a cardiac arrest.

An absolutely certain diagnosis can be made only by measuring the electrical activity of the heart by *ECG*, but *cardiopulmonary resuscitation* should be started immediately to minimize the risk of brain damage.

As soon as adequate help arrives— most hospitals have a cardiac arrest team on standby—the diagnosis can be confirmed by ECG. This test distinguishes between *ventricular fibrillation* and *asystole*, which are the two types of heart muscle disturbance that can lead to cardiac arrest.

Ventricular fibrillation is the random, uncoordinated contraction of individual heart muscle fibers. This may be corrected by *defibrillation* (an electric shock to the heart).

Asystole is the complete absence of heart muscle activity and is more difficult to reverse. It may respond to intravenous injection of *epinephrine* and calcium or in extreme cases to direct injection of epinephrine into the heart. An electrical *pacemaker* may also stimulate the heart in asystole.

In all cases of cardiac arrest the balance of the chemical constituents of the blood is disturbed, making the blood more acidic; an intravenous infusion of sodium bicarbonate is usually given to correct this. Other drugs, such as lidocaine, can also be administered intravenously to stabilize the heart muscle.

OUTLOOK
Between one fifth and one third of patients whose heartbeat is restored after cardiac arrest recover sufficiently to leave hospital (however, a substantial number of these die within the following year). In the remainder, the damage to the heart or brain is too extensive for recovery to be possible.

Cardiac massage

See *Cardiopulmonary resuscitation*.

Cardiac neurosis

Excessive anxiety or fear about the condition of the heart. It usually occurs after a *myocardial infarction* (heart attack) or heart surgery but may also occur in people who have had no previous heart trouble.

The sufferer experiences symptoms that mimic those typical of heart disease—chest pain, tightness in the chest, lethargy, palpitations, and breathlessness—and may be reluctant to exercise or to return to work for fear of bringing on these symptoms. Examination and investigation of the heart by a physician will reveal no physical cause for the symptoms.

C

C

Psychotherapy may help the patient overcome fears and anxieties. If it does not, the patient may not be able to return to a normal, active life.

Cardiac output

The volume of blood pumped by the heart in a given time (usually per minute). Cardiac output can be used as a measure of how efficiently the heart is working. At rest, a healthy adult heart pumps between 2.5 and 4.5 litres of blood per minute; during exercise this figure may rise to as much as 30 litres per minute. A low figure during exercise is a sign that the heart muscle is damaged or that major blood loss has occurred.

Cardiac stress test

A type of *fitness test* carried out on people who experience chest pain, breathlessness, or palpitations during exercise. The test is used to determine whether the patient has *angina pectoris* and signs of *coronary artery disease*. A cardiac stress test may also be performed in conjunction with *radionuclide scanning* to identify any damaged areas of heart muscle.

HOW IT IS DONE

The patient is attached to an *ECG* machine, which records the pattern of the heart's electrical activity. He or she then performs an exercise, such as walking on a treadmill. A diagnosis of angina is confirmed if there are specific changes in the wave pattern shown on the *ECG* recording as the intensity of exercise is increased.

The test is performed under close medical supervision, with resuscitation facilities immediately available. If at any time the patient suffers chest pain, becomes breathless, or feels sick, the test is stopped immediately.

Cardiology

The study of the function of the *heart*; the investigation, diagnosis, and medical treatment of disorders of the heart and blood vessels, especially *atherosclerosis* and *hypertension*.

Anatomically and physiologically, the heart occupies a central position in the body. It has a single function—to pump blood first to the lungs and then to the rest of the body—but the sequence of events in each heart contraction is complex.

Reduced pumping efficiency of the heart can have various underlying causes, including *arrhythmias*, *coronary artery disease* (in which the blood supply to the heart muscle is impaired), *cardiomyopathy* (in which the

muscle itself is abnormal), and *heart valve disorders*.

Disease of the lungs and blood vessels can also have adverse effects on heart function. Some babies are born with structural defects of the heart and/or major blood vessels that emerge from that organ (see *Heart disease, congenital*).

Heart disorders are the leading cause of death in Canada. The study of the heart in health and disease is thus a large part of the training of every physician; general practitioners are familiar with the treatment of patients with common disorders, such as coronary artery disease and hypertension.

For more expert investigation and treatment, a person with a heart problem may be referred to a cardiologist (heart specialist), who may perform tests such as *echocardiography*, and detailed interpretation of ECGs (electrocardiograms) and *chest X rays*. A cardiologist may, in turn, refer a patient to a cardiovascular surgeon if surgical treatment is necessary.

The past 10 years have seen rapid advances in the understanding of heart disease, its causes, its investigation, and its treatment.

Cardiomegaly

Enlargement of the heart. In some cases, cardiomegaly takes the form of hypertrophy (thickening) of the heart muscle; in others, it takes the form of dilatation (increase in volume) of one or more of the heart chambers.

CAUSES

Hypertrophy of the heart muscle occurs in any condition where the heart has to work harder than normal to pump blood around the body. Such conditions include *hypertension* (increased blood pressure), which causes the wall of the left ventricle (main pumping chamber) to thicken; *pulmonary hypertension* (increased blood pressure in the lungs), in which the wall of the right ventricle thickens; and one type of *cardiomyopathy* (disease of the heart muscle), in which either or both ventricles may thicken.

Dilatation of a heart chamber may be due to heart valve incompetence (failure of a valve to close properly after a contraction). For example, in *aortic insufficiency*, failure of the aortic valve to close completely allows blood to flood back from the aorta into the left ventricle after each contraction, eventually enlarging the chamber. Certain types of cardiomyopathy can also lead to swelling of a chamber.

SYMPTOMS

There are no symptoms until enlargement reaches a point where the heart is no longer capable of coping with additional stress (for example, as a result of exercise or infection). This reduces the efficiency of the heart as a pump and leads to *heart failure*, causing breathlessness and swelling of the legs and hands.

DIAGNOSIS AND TREATMENT

Cardiomegaly is diagnosed by physical examination, *chest X ray*, and *ECG* (measurement of electrical impulses in the heart). Treatment is directed at the underlying disorder.

Cardiomyopathy

Any disease of the heart muscle that causes a reduction in the force of heart contractions and a resultant decrease in the efficiency of circulation of blood through the lungs and to the rest of the body. The disease may have an infectious, metabolic, nutritional, toxic, autoimmune, or degenerative cause, but in many cases the cause is unknown.

TYPES

Cardiomyopathies fall into the following three main groups: hypertrophic, dilated, and restrictive.

Hypertrophic cardiomyopathy is usually a familial (inherited) disorder of unknown cause in which there is abnormality of the heart muscle fibers.

In dilated cardiomyopathy, muscle cell metabolism (chemical activity) is abnormal, and the walls of the heart tend to dilate (balloon out) under pressure. The cause of the abnormal cell metabolism is unknown.

Restrictive cardiomyopathy is triggered by scarring of the endocardium (the inner lining of the heart) or by *amyloidosis* (infiltration of the muscle with a starchlike substance).

Heart muscle disorders may also be due to poisoning (e.g., by excessive consumption of alcohol) or to a vitamin or mineral deficiency (e.g., lack of vitamin B_1).

INCIDENCE

Cardiomyopathies are less common than other types of heart disease. The specific incidence of the different types is unknown because in many cases of cardiomyopathy there are few or no symptoms. Sometimes the damage to the heart muscle is discovered only at an autopsy after the individual has died from an unrelated cause.

SYMPTOMS AND SIGNS

Symptoms usually include fatigue, chest pain, and palpitations due to an increased awareness of the heartbeat

C

Chest X ray showing cardiomyopathy
The heart has become much enlarged, due to the heart muscle abnormality.

or to an abnormal heart rhythm such as *atrial fibrillation* (rapid, uncoordinated contractions of the upper chambers of the heart). *Heart failure* (reduced pumping efficiency) can cause breathing difficulty and edema (swelling) of the legs and hands.

DIAGNOSIS

A *chest X ray* usually shows enlargement of the heart outline. An *ECG* (measurement of electrical activity in the heart) often shows enlarged electrical impulses on the tracing due to heart muscle hypertrophy.

The diagnosis can be confirmed by examining a *biopsy* sample of heart muscle under the microscope to show muscle cell abnormalities.

TREATMENT

If, as is often the case, the cause remains unknown, there is no specific treatment. Treatment of symptoms may include the use of *diuretic drugs* to control heart failure and *antiarrhythmic drugs* to correct abnormal heart rhythm. For those with alcoholic cardiomyopathy, stopping all intake of alcohol is essential. *Immunosuppressant drugs* are occasionally helpful.

In many cases, heart muscle function steadily deteriorates, and the only option left is a *heart transplant*.

Cardiopulmonary resuscitation

The administration of the lifesaving measures of external cardiac compression massage and mouth-to-mouth resuscitation (see *Artificial respiration*) to someone collapsing with *cardiac arrest* (cessation of heartbeat).

It is vital to restore the circulation of oxygen-carrying blood to the brain as quickly as possible because permanent brain damage is likely if the brain is starved of oxygen for more than three to four minutes.

WHEN TO GIVE CARDIOPULMONARY RESUSCITATION

Before starting cardiopulmonary resuscitation it is important to establish that the victim has suffered a cardiac arrest and has not simply fainted. A person who has had a cardiac arrest will be unresponsive and have no (or very slight) breathing motions. Skin color will be extremely pale, or bluegray, especially around the lips. The person's heart will not seem to be beating. No pulse will be felt in the wrist or neck, and no heartbeat will be heard when listening to the chest. (If the collapsed person is breathing, no matter how slowly, then the heart will probably still be beating, even if no pulse can be felt.)

HOW TO GIVE CARDIOPULMONARY RESUSCITATION

See illustrated box, page 234.

Cardiotocography

See *Fetal heart monitoring*.

Cardiovascular

A term that means pertaining to the heart and blood vessels.

Cardiovascular disorders

Disorders of the heart, blood vessels, and blood circulation. (See *Heart disorders box; Arteries, disorders of; Veins, disorders of*.)

Cardiovascular surgery

The branch of surgery concerned with the heart and blood vessels. Cardiovascular surgery includes operations to prevent or repair damage caused, for example, by congenital heart disease (see *Heart disease, congenital*), *atherosclerosis* (fat deposits on arterial walls), or a *myocardial infarction* (heart attack). Procedures performed include *heart valve surgery, coronary artery bypass*, and *heart transplant*.

Cardioversion

Another name for *defibrillation*.

Carditis

A general term for inflammation of any part of the heart or its linings. Carditis may be one of three kinds: a *myocarditis* (inflammation of the heart muscle), usually caused by a viral infection; an *endocarditis* (inflammation of the internal lining of the heart

chambers and heart valves) usually due to a bacterial infection; or a *pericarditis* (inflammation of the outer lining of the heart), possibly with *effusion* (collection of fluid). The latter is usually due to a viral or bacterial infection, but may be associated with a *myocardial infarction* (heart attack) or, occasionally, may be caused by an *autoimmune disorder*, such as systemic *lupus erythematosus* (SLE).

Caries, dental

Tooth decay; the gradual erosion of enamel (the protective covering of the tooth) and dentin (the substance beneath the enamel).

CAUSES

Plaque is the main cause of tooth decay (see *Causes of tooth decay* box, p. 235). The most common sites of initial decay are areas where plaque easily becomes trapped, such as the grinding surfaces of the back teeth (which contain numerous minute grooves), the lateral (side) edges of adjacent teeth, and near the gum line.

INCIDENCE

An encouraging sign in most Western countries over the past 10 to 15 years has been the significant decline (of 35 to 50 percent) in dental caries among children. The evidence suggests that, of the various factors probably responsible, the most important is water *fluoridation*, which strengthens enamel. The addition of *fluoride* to toothpaste has also played a part.

SYMPTOMS

Early decay does not usually cause any symptoms. The chief symptom of advanced decay is toothache, which may be aggravated by eating very sweet, hot, or cold food. Decay may also cause bad breath.

TREATMENT

Treatment consists of drilling away the area of decay and filling the cavity (see *Filling, dental*) with either dental amalgam (a mercury alloy) or cement (a composite resin that matches the color of the tooth).

In cases of advanced decay, it may be necessary to remove the infected pulp (the central, living part of a tooth) and replace it with a filling (see *Root canal treatment*) or to extract the tooth (see *Extraction, dental*).

PREVENTION

Our modern diet makes it unlikely that we can completely avoid dental caries even by taking the most scrupulous preventive measures. However, it is possible to reduce the risk of caries considerably by consuming less sugar and other refined carbohydrates

C

FIRST AID: CARDIOPULMONARY RESUSCITATION

1 First make sure the airway is clear. Then look and listen for signs of breathing. Listen for air escaping and feel for air flow. Feel for the pulse.

2 If the victim is breathing, place in the *recovery position*. If the victim is not breathing, place on a hard surface and start mouth-to-mouth resuscitation.

3 Pinch the victim's nose shut, take a breath, seal your lips around the mouth, and blow. Your breath contains enough oxygen for the victim's needs.

4 If breathing does not restart and you cannot detect a pulse or heartbeat, start cardiac compression. Press with the heel of one hand placed on top of the other.

5 It is vital to apply pressure at the correct point—the lower part of the breastbone. Keep the pressure well clear of the victim's ribs.

6 If you are on your own, the rate of compression should be 80 per minute, with two breaths given after every 15 compressions.

WARNING

Cardiopulmonary resuscitation (CPR) is a life-support technique that is used in a medical emergency when the victim is not breathing and when it is possible that his or her heart has stopped beating.

A victim's breathing can be restored effectively at the time of the crisis by following instructions in the *Artificial respiration* entry, but such is not the case with CPR, which requires training, skill, and practice. Serious damage could be done by the untrained. For this reason, cardiac compression, and all phases of cardiopulmonary resuscitation, should be learned through formal instruction. Refresher courses are also recommended.

WITH TWO RESCUERS
If two rescuers are available, one should perform cardiac compression and the other mouth-to-mouth resuscitation (one breath to five compressions). Sixty compressions should be given per minute, with 1 to 1.5 seconds pause after every five compressions.

and by practicing good oral hygiene, such as regular toothbrushing.

Sweet food should be eaten only at mealtimes; snacks between meals should be limited. From the beginning of a child's life, careful attention to diet is essential to minimize the harmful effects of refined carbohydrates. Babies should not be given a bottle of milk, fruit juice, or other sugar-containing liquid to comfort them or get them to sleep; this habit can cause extensive early tooth decay.

Teeth need brushing thoroughly each day with fluoride toothpaste, and dental floss should be used to clean between the teeth. A dentist should be visited regularly for checkups. (See also *Oral hygiene*.)

Carisoprodol
A *muscle relaxant* useful for minor muscle spasm, pain and rigidity. It can cause dizziness and drowsiness.

Carotene

An orange pigment which is found in carrots, tomatoes, and various other colored plants, including leafy green vegetables.

Most of the carotene absorbed from food is converted in the walls of the intestine to *vitamin A*, which is essential for normal vision and the health of the skin and other organs.

Excessive intake of carotene-containing foods, especially carrots, results in carotenemia (abnormally high blood levels of carotene). This condition is harmless, but does cause yellowing of the skin, especially of the palms and soles. It can be differentiated from jaundice because the eyes remain white. The abnormal pigment rapidly disappears if carrots or other such carotene-containing plants are omitted from the diet.

Some recent research indicates that carotene may have some protective effect against certain types of cancer but this is far from proven.

Carotid artery
Any of the four principal arteries of the neck and head. There are two common carotid arteries (left and right), each of which divides into two main branches (internal and external).

The left common carotid artery arises from the *aorta* (main blood vessel leading from the heart) just above the heart, and runs up the neck on the left side of the *trachea* (windpipe). Just above the level of the *larynx* (voice box) it divides into two, forming the

CAUSES OF TOOTH DECAY
The primary cause of tooth decay is dental *plaque*, a sticky substance that forms on the teeth. Plaque consists of food remains, mucus-saliva by-products, and the bacteria that live in the mouth. The bacteria feed mainly on the fermentable carbohydrates (simple sugars and starches) in food, and, in breaking them down, create an acid that gradually destroys enamel, forming a cavity. If the process is not checked, the dentin is eroded next, enlarging the cavity and enabling the bacteria to invade the pulp at the center of the tooth.

Severe dental caries
Example of caries affecting the necks of several upper and lower teeth.

1 Acid produced in the breakdown of food gradually destroys enamel, forming a cavity.

2 Unchecked, decay spreads to the dentin.

3 The cavity continues to enlarge, enabling the bacteria to invade exposed pulp at the tooth's center.

4 If untreated, the infected pulp will die and the tooth will be destroyed.

left internal carotid and the left external carotid arteries. The right common carotid artery arises from the subclavian artery, which branches off the aorta, and then follows a similar path to the left common carotid, but on the other side of the neck.

The external carotid arteries have multiple branches, which supply most of the tissues in the face, scalp, mouth, and jaws. The internal carotid arteries enter the skull to supply the brain (via cerebral branches) and eyes (via ophthalmic branches). At the base of the brain, branches of the two internal carotids and the basilar artery join to form a ring of blood vessels called the circle of Willis. Narrowing of these vessels may be associated with *transient ischemic attack* (TIA), while obstruction causes a *stroke*.

The carotid arteries have two specialized sensory regions in the neck, called the carotid sinus and the carotid body. The former monitors blood pressure; the latter monitors the oxygen content of the blood.

Carpal tunnel syndrome
Numbness, tingling, and pain in the thumb, index, and middle fingers that often worsens at night. The condition may affect one or both hands and is sometimes accompanied by weakness in the thumb.

CAUSES AND INCIDENCE
The condition results from pressure on the median nerve where it passes into the hand via a gap (the "carpal tunnel") under a ligament at the front of the wrist. The median nerve carries sensory messages from the thumb and some fingers and also motor stimuli to the muscles in the hand; damage to the nerve causes sensory disturbances, particularly numbness or tingling, and weakness.

Carpal tunnel syndrome occurs most commonly among middle-aged women, usually for no obvious reason. It also occurs more commonly than average during pregnancy, in women who have just started using *oral contraceptives* or who suffer from *premenstrual syndrome*, and in men or

C

LOCATION OF CAROTID ARTERY
The common carotid on each side divides to form internal and external branches.

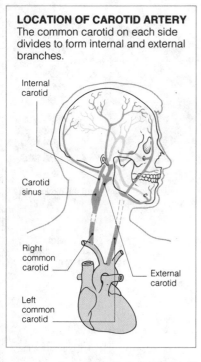

women who suffer from *rheumatoid arthritis*, *myxedema*, or *acromegaly*.

DIAGNOSIS AND TREATMENT
The diagnosis may be confirmed by measuring the passage of nerve impulses through the median nerve to the muscles of the hand. The condition often disappears without treatment. Resting the affected hand at night in a splint may alleviate symptoms. If symptoms persist, a small quantity of a *corticosteroid drug* may be injected under the ligament in the wrist. If this fails to help, surgical cutting of the ligament may be performed to relieve the pressure on the nerve.

Carrier
A person who is able to pass on a disease to others without actually suffering from it. Carriers may transmit infectious diseases to others, or may pass on inherited diseases to their offspring.

A carrier who harbors potentially harmful bacteria or viruses may unknowingly transmit an infectious disease such as typhoid fever or hepatitis B. The carrier may never have had symptoms of the disease, or may have had an infection in the past with apparently complete recovery.

Inherited disease may be transmitted if a parent who shows no signs of having a particular disease carries a gene for it. For example, a woman who carries the gene for the bleeding disorder hemophilia does not have the disease herself but may pass the gene on to some of her children; if one of her sons receives the gene, he will develop hemophilia.

Car sickness
See *Motion sickness*.

Cartilage
A type of connective tissue (a material that holds body structures together). Cartilage is not as hard as *bone* but nevertheless forms an important structural component of many parts of the skeletal system, such as the *joints*. Much of the fetal skeleton is formed entirely of cartilage, which is then gradually converted to bone by a process known as *ossification*.

Cartilage consists of specialized cells called chondrocytes embedded in a matrix, or ground substance, that comprises varying amounts of *collagen*, a gellike substance. There are three main types of cartilage: hyaline, fibrocartilage, and elastic, each with a different proportion of collagen and each with different functions.

TYPES
Hyaline cartilage is a tough, smooth tissue that lines the surfaces of joints, such as the knee, providing an almost frictionless layer over the bony parts of the joint. If the lining becomes worn (as occurs in *osteoarthritis*) or damaged, joint movement may be painful or severely restricted.

Fibrocartilage contains a large amount of collagen and is solid and very strong. It makes up the intervertebral disks between the bones of the spine and the shock-absorbing pads of tissue that are found in joints.

Elastic cartilage is soft and rubbery. It is found in various structures, notably the outer ear and the *epiglottis*.

Cast
A rigid casing applied to a limb or other part of the body to hold a broken bone or dislocated joint so that it will heal in the correct position. Most casts are made using bandages impregnated with plaster of Paris. The bandages are applied wet to the injured part and harden as they dry. Modern fiberglass casts are stronger and lighter than plaster but are more expensive and difficult to apply. Casts are removed using an electric saw that cuts through the cast but does not damage the skin.

A back slab is a type of cast that covers only half the affected limb and

TYPES OF CARTILAGE
The three main types contain different proportions of collagen and differ in their toughness and elasticity.

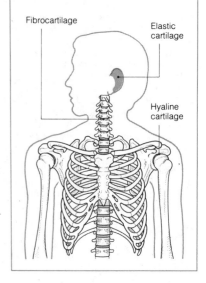

is held in place with straps. A back slab is used if swelling at the site of injury is likely, or as a temporary measure pending the insertion of a pin to secure a broken bone.

Castor oil
A colorless or yellow-tinged oil obtained from the leaves of the castor oil plant. When given orally, castor oil irritates the lining of the small intestine and within two to six hours causes a powerful *laxative* action that completely empties the bowel. This effect helps in preparing patients for X rays of the intestine. Castor oil should not be used as a regular treatment for *constipation* because of its extremely strong and rapid effects.

Zinc and castor oil ointment is a soothing, moistening cream used to treat conditions such as diaper rash.

Castration
The removal of the testes (see *Orchiectomy*) or ovaries (see *Oophorectomy*).

Castration is performed to remove a diseased organ or to reduce the amount of *testosterone* (male hormone produced in the testes) or *estrogen* (female hormone produced in the ovaries) in the body. The procedure may be used in the treatment of breast and prostate cancers because estrogen stimulates the growth of some breast cancers and testosterone stimulates the growth of cancer of the prostate. Castration in adulthood has no immediate effect on libido (sexual desire), although libido may be reduced in the long term.

In former times, castration was performed to preserve the high-pitched voices of boy singers and to emasculate male slaves who guarded harems.

Catalepsy
A physical state in which the muscles of the face, body, and limbs are maintained in a semirigid position. Catalepsy may last for many hours, during which time neither the expression nor the bodily position will alter, no matter how uncomfortable. Attempts to change the person's position will meet with resistance or the unyielding adoption of a new position. Catalepsy occurs mainly in people with *schizophrenia*, *epilepsy*, or a *conversion disorder*, but may also be caused by brain disease and some drugs.

Cataplexy
A sudden loss of muscle tone, causing the victim to collapse, without any loss of consciousness. Cataplexy usually lasts for a few seconds and is triggered by emotions, particularly laughter. A rare cause of sudden involuntary falls, cataplexy occurs almost exclusively in those suffering from *narcolepsy* and other *sleep disorders*.

Cataract
Loss of transparency of the crystalline *lens* of the *eye*. Cataract is due to changes in the delicate protein fibers within the lens, similar to the changes that occur in cooked egg whites.

Cataract never causes complete blindness, because even a densely opalescent lens will still transmit light. However, with increasing loss of transparency, the clarity and detail of the image is progressively lost. Even at a fairly advanced stage, a cataract may not be apparent to an external observer, and it is only when the front part of the crystalline lens becomes densely opaque that whiteness is visible in the pupil.

Cataract usually occurs in both eyes, but in most cases one eye is more severely affected than the other.

INCIDENCE
Most cataracts occur in elderly people. In fact, almost everyone over the age of 65 has some degree of cataract, but usually the opacification is minor and often confined to the edge of the lens, where it does not interfere with vision. Opacification tends to progress with age, so that the majority of people over 75 have minor visual deterioration from cataract.

CAUSE
Most cataracts in the elderly have no known cause but they are so common that they might be considered a part of the normal aging process. With age, the center of the lens becomes progressively harder and the permeability of the lens capsule increases.

Congenital cataract (a cataract that is present from birth) may be due to infection of the mother early in pregnancy, especially with the *rubella* (German measles) virus, or to the toxic effects of drugs taken during pregnancy. Congenital cataract may also occur in infants who have *Down's syndrome* or a variety of rare genetic conditions, such as *galactosemia*.

Cataract may be caused by direct injury to the eye, and is almost inevitable if a foreign particle enters the crystalline lens. Cataract is common in people with *diabetes mellitus* and may develop at an early age if blood sugar levels are very high. Other possible causes of cataract include prolonged intake of *corticosteroid drugs*, poisoning by substances such as naphthalene (found in mothballs) or ergot (formed in stored grain contaminated by a certain type of fungus). Many types of radiation, including infrared, microwave, and X rays, can cause a cataract to develop.

SYMPTOMS
Cataract is entirely painless and causes only visual symptoms. The onset of these symptoms is almost imperceptible, and progress is nearly always very slow.

The main symptom is progressive loss of visual acuity (increased blurring of vision). Increased density in the lens often produces an increase in its light-refracting power so that the person concerned becomes nearsighted. This may temporarily permit a person who was previously farsighted to read without using his or her reading glasses.

Color values are often disturbed, with dulling of blues and accentuation of reds, yellows, and oranges; the full perception of color is strikingly restored after surgery. Often the opacities in the lenses cause scattering of light rays and, even at a fairly early stage, this may seriously affect night driving. Many people with cataracts, however, are barely aware of these effects and notice only that they cannot see as well as before.

TREATMENT
If normal clear images are to be perceived, the opacified lens must be removed surgically and the refracting power of the eye restored by a spectacle lens, a contact lens, or by a replacement lens implanted during the operation. Provided the eye is otherwise healthy, *cataract surgery* gives excellent results in most cases.

Cataract surgery
Removal of an opacified lens, or *cataract*, from the eye to restore sight. Cataract extraction is most often performed as soon as the opacification of the lens has developed to a point where the person feels it seriously impairs his or her vision.

WHY IT IS DONE
Once a cataract has developed, changes to the lens are irreversible and vision can be restored only by removing the opacified lens and replacing it with an artificial lens. In the past, patients were forced to wear very strong, highly magnifying ("pebble") glasses, which were often uncomfortable and caused distortion at the edges of the narrowed field of vision. By replacing the removed lens with a tiny plastic implant, fixed permanently in the eye during the operation, the need to use such thick glasses can now usually be avoided.

HOW IT IS DONE
Each surgeon uses a slightly different technique, but a typical cataract operation is described in the illustrated box on page 238.

Sometimes the whole lens is removed, in its capsule, by means of a probe that can be made to freeze to the lens (the lens may first be loosened by means of a digestive enzyme injected into the front chamber of the eye). In this case, the lens is replaced by an implant that either clips into the pupil or is fitted in front of the iris. Another technique involves placing the implant within the capsule of the lens, after removing all its contents; the implant is supported by loops or flanges which keep it in a central position. Alternatively, the implant may be placed in front of the pupil.

By taking preoperative measurements of the curvature of the cornea and (using an ultrasonic method) of the length of the eye, it is often possible to calculate the power of the implant lens needed to restore normal vision to the patient. Some patients, however, continue to need to wear glasses after the operation, at least for reading.

C

PROCEDURE FOR CATARACT SURGERY

In a normal, healthy lens there is no interference with the passage of light rays. Even with peripheral opacities, vision is not limited until the central zone is affected. Dense nuclear opacities, such as that shown right, result in deteriorating vision and cannot be restored to transparency; hence the need for surgical replacement.

Dense, nuclear cataract

Normal lens

Peripheral cataract

1 In preparation for surgery, measurements are taken of the cornea and of the length of the eye, in order to calculate the power of the lens implant needed to restore vision fully. The operation may be performed using general or local anesthesia; there is no pain in either case. Instruments of remarkable delicacy and precision are used to carry out the procedure, usually with the help of microscope magnification.

2 Before the operation, drops are used to widen the pupil so that most of the front surface of the lens is exposed. An incision is made around the upper edge of the cornea using an instrument with a diamond tip.

3 A small quantity of a clear gel (sodium hyaluronate) is injected to maintain a space between the back of the cornea and the lens.

4 A large part of the center of the front capsule of the lens is then removed and the hard nucleus of the lens carefully removed. The soft remaining parts of the lens are then cleared away, leaving the back of the capsule.

Artificial lens

Plastic loop

5 The artificial implant is slipped into the natural lens capsule; plastic loops hold it in place. The corneal incision is sewn up with fine nylon thread about half the diameter of a human hair.

There are, however, some cataract patients for whom intraocular lens implants are unsuitable. This group consists mainly of people with a history of other eye disease. Some surgeons also advise against intraocular lenses in young people because the life span of the implant has not been established. Contact lenses can offer these people excellent vision post-operatively, and many people now wear such lenses.

RECOVERY PERIOD

Most patients can leave hospital within a couple of days of the operation. In some cases, the patient may be discharged on the same day, provided that facilities for specialist supervision during the next few days are available.

The corneal incision takes about a month to heal, but it is usually about two months before the corneal curvature has ceased to alter. Glasses may not be fitted until then.

The results of treatment are usually excellent provided no other cause of visual deterioration is present.

Catarrh

Inflammation of a *mucous membrane* causing an increase in the amount of mucus secreted. Catarrh is usually due to infection or to allergy, and may affect the nose (see *Rhinitis*), the middle ear (see *Glue ear*), or the sinuses (see *Sinusitus*).

Catatonia

A state characterized by abnormalities of movement and posture. An affected person appears to be awake but makes no voluntary movements. He or she may adopt rigid, often bizarre, postures, which may be maintained against resistance. Catatonia is a feature of a rare form of *schizophrenia* and also occurs in some types of brain disease.

Catharsis

A term meaning purification. Catharsis is used to refer to the process of evacuation of the bowels. In *psychoanalytic theory*, it refers to the process of expressing or acting out feelings and memories that were previously repressed. The term was originally used in psychiatry by Sigmund Freud, who believed that the revival of "forgotten" memories and the expression of the emotions associated with them could bring relief from anxiety, tension, and other symptoms.

The patient may be hypnotized or given drugs to bring on a suggestive state that allows the traumatic memory to be recalled and the emotions associated with the memory to be openly expressed. *Psychodrama*, which involves dramatic re-creation of events, is another method used to help patients achieve emotional release. This method is claimed to be particularly successful in the treatment of *posttraumatic stress disorder*.

Cathartic

A term that means having the power to purify or cleanse. A cathartic is a drug that stimulates movement of the bowels (see *Laxative drugs*).

Catheter

A tube used to drain or inject fluid, or to apply pressure to a vessel. Catheters are commonly used to drain urine from the bladder (see *Catheterization, urinary*). Other types are used to sample blood from the heart or to inject dye into the blood vessels during X-ray screening (see *Catheterization, cardiac*). Catheters are also used to unblock or widen obstructed blood vessels, or to control bleeding. (See also *Balloon catheter*.)

Catheterization, cardiac

A diagnostic test in which a fine, sterile *catheter* (tube) is introduced into the heart, via a blood vessel, to investigate its condition.

The technique is used to diagnose and assess the extent of congenital heart disease (see *Heart disease, congenital*) and *coronary artery disease*. It is also used to diagnose as well as to treat some disorders of the *heart valves* (see *Valvuloplasty*). Cardiac catheterization enables the pressure within the heart chambers to be measured, blood samples to be taken, and samples of tissue from the heart lining to be removed for analysis.

Cardiac catheterization may cause temporary disturbance of the heart rhythm and is therefore used only to investigate disorders that might become life-threatening.

HOW IT IS DONE

The procedure, which causes little discomfort, is performed under local anesthesia. A small incision is made in an artery or vein through which the catheter is introduced. The tube is passed along the blood vessel and into the heart. Catheterization of the left side of the heart is carried out via an artery in the thigh or elbow. Investigation of the right side of the heart is performed via a vein in the patient's groin or elbow.

Once the catheter is in position, it can be used to measure blood pressure within the heart, to withdraw blood to measure its oxygen content, or to inject a *radiopaque* substance into the heart so that X rays of the heart cavities can be taken.

After the catheter has been removed, the blood vessel through which it was passed may be repaired with stitches or simply tied off.

Catheterization, urinary

Insertion of a sterile *catheter* (tube) into the bladder to drain urine.

WHY IT IS DONE

Urinary catheterization is most often performed when a person is unable to empty the bladder normally or is suffering from incontinence (see *Incontinence, urinary*). Patients with urinary incontinence associated with neurological disorders may be given permanent catheters or are taught to carry out self-catheterization.

Urinary catheterization may be necessary during certain operations in which a full bladder might obstruct the surgeon's view of surrounding

organs. The procedure is also carried out to allow careful monitoring of urine production by patients who are critically ill. Urinary catheterization is performed too for tests of bladder function, such as *cystometry* and micturating *cystourethrography*.

HOW IT IS DONE

There are two principal techniques: urethral catheterization (described in the illustrated box below) and suprapubic catheterization.

Suprapubic catheterization is used if it is not possible to pass a catheter up the urethra (e.g., if the urethra is abnormally narrow). The skin of the lower part of the abdomen is cleaned with an antiseptic solution and a local anesthetic is injected under an area of skin overlying the bladder. A small incision is then made with a scalpel blade and a suprapubic catheter is inserted into the bladder through the abdominal wall.

RISKS

There is a risk that urinary catheterization may lead to *urinary tract infection* even though the procedure is performed under sterile conditions.

CATHETERIZATION OF THE BLADDER

The catheter is usually passed into the bladder through the urethra. Before this is done, the physician or nurse cleans the surrounding area with antiseptic solution to avoid introducing infection into the urinary tract. The procedure usually takes about 10 minutes.

Fitting a catheter
The catheter is passed up the urethra until urine flows down it, indicating that the tip is in the bladder.

Self-retaining type
If the catheter is to remain in the bladder, a self-retaining type is used. This catheter has a balloon at its tip that can be inflated and filled with sterile water.

CAT scanning

An abbreviation for computerized axial tomographic scanning, more commonly known as *CT scanning*.

Cat-scratch fever

An uncommon disease that usually develops after a scratch or bite by a cat and is thought to be due to infection with a type of small bacterium (which has not yet been identified) transmitted by the cat. The cat itself is not ill. Three quarters of cases occur in children, and the disorder is most common in autumn and winter.

SYMPTOMS

Symptoms usually appear three to 10 days after a bite or scratch. In some cases there is no apparent break in the skin, although contact with a cat is sometimes reported. The main sign of illness is a swollen lymph node near the scratch. The node may become painful and tender and, in rare cases, may produce a discharge. A small, infected blister sometimes develops at the original site of skin injury. A fever, rash, and headache may also occur.

DIAGNOSIS AND TREATMENT

The diagnosis is confirmed by *biopsy* (removal of a small tissue sample for microscopic analysis) of the swollen lymph node and by the results of a skin test. Analgesic drugs (painkillers) may be needed to relieve fever and headache. A severely infected lymph node or blister may have to be surgically drained. In most cases, the illness clears up completely within two months. There is no need to destroy the cat.

Cats, diseases from

Cats carry various parasites and infectious organisms that can be spread to humans. Some are specific to cats, others affect dogs as well. A well-cared for cat poses no serious threat to human health, but cat owners should be aware of possible problems.

SPECIFIC DISEASES

Rabies is the most serious disorder that can be contracted from an infected cat. Sudden unexplained aggression in a cat should be cause for suspicion. Have the animal examined by your vet. Anyone who is bitten by a cat (or any other mammal) should see a physician immediately.

Cat-scratch fever is an uncommon illness that usually follows the scratch or bite of a cat. The suspected cause of the illness is a small bacterium that has not yet been identified.

Cats commonly carry the protozoan (single-celled parasite) TOXOPLASMA GONDII, which is the cause of *toxoplasmosis*. A form of the parasite is present in the cat's feces. In most cases, the infection causes few or no symptoms, but, if a woman is infected during pregnancy, the parasites may gain access, via the placenta, to the fetus. Infections in early pregnancy can lead to spontaneous abortion or severe malformation; infections that occur later in pregnancy can cause nervous system disorders and sometimes blindness in early childhood. Pregnant women should not change cat litter boxes.

Cat feces may also carry eggs of the cat roundworm, a possible cause of *toxocariasis*. In rare cases, a larva from an ingested roundworm egg may migrate to and lodge in an eye, causing deterioration of vision or even blindness. This most commonly occurs in children who have been playing in soil or sand that is contaminated by dog or cat feces infected with roundworm eggs.

Of the more common problems, a substantial number of *tinea* (ringworm) fungal infections of the skin—particularly scalp ringworm—probably come from cats. Unlike dogs, cats are little affected by the fungus, but its presence can be demonstrated by examining the fur under ultraviolet light, which causes fluorescence of infected skin and hairs.

Bites from cat *fleas* are common; many bites blamed on midges and mosquitoes are actually caused by fleas. The fleas may jump onto humans to feed, particularly in warm weather and if the cat is absent. Flea bites are most common around the ankles and lower leg.

Some people develop allergic reactions to dander (tiny scales derived from animal skin and fur and present in the air) and consequently may suffer from *asthma* or *urticaria* when a cat is in the house.

PREVENTION

Serious diseases from cats are easily avoided by good hygiene—in particular, thorough washing of the hands if there is any chance they have been contaminated by cat feces. Young children should be discouraged from playing with cats and other animals, except under supervision, until they have become aware of the risks of poor hygiene. Animals that are obviously ill should be seen by a veterinary surgeon, and routine health care should include regular worming and flea treatment.

Cauda equina

A collection of nerve roots that descends from the lower part of the *spinal cord* and occupies the lower third of the spinal canal (the central space within the spine). This "spray" of nerves resembles a horse's tail.

Caudal

Denoting a position toward the lower end of the spine. Caudal literally means "of the tail."

HOW CATS TRANSMIT INFECTION

There are three main routes by which an infection or parasitic disease may be spread.

Direct contact
Mites or fungi from the animal's fur may be transferred.

In feces
Worm eggs or parasites contained in feces may contaminate fingers or food.

Bites or scratches
Microorganisms contained in the cat's mouth or on its claws may be transmitted by a bite or scratch.

C

Caudal block

A type of *nerve block* in which a local anesthetic is injected into the lower part of the spinal canal (the central space within the spine). Caudal block is sometimes used for obstetric and gynecological procedures.

Cauliflower ear

A painful, swollen, distortion of the pinna (ear flap) resulting from blows or friction that have caused bleeding within the soft cartilage framework. The condition occurs most commonly in boxers.

TREATMENT

If the ear swells after injury, an ice pack should be used to reduce the swelling. In severe cases, a physician should be consulted. Blood can be drained from the ear using a needle and syringe, and a pressure bandage applied. Despite these measures, repeated injury may lead to a severely distorted ear, and plastic surgery is sometimes needed to improve the appearance.

Example of cauliflower ear
Deformity of the shape of the ear, with loss of normal folds of skin.

Causalgia

A persistent, burning pain, usually in an arm or leg. The skin overlying the painful area may be red and tender or may be blue, cold, and clammy.

Causalgia usually occurs as the result of injury to a nerve by a deep cut, limb fracture, or gunshot wound. In some cases, the pain may be aggravated by emotional factors or even by normal sensations, such as touch or a cold breeze.

Treatment is usually unsatisfactory but a few patients benefit from *sympathectomy*, an operation in which nerves are severed.

Caustic

A term applied to any substance that has a burning or corrosive action on body tissues or has a burning taste. An example is caustic soda, the common name for sodium hydroxide.

Caustic substances can destroy body tissues and therefore should not be used without adequate protection, such as rubber gloves. If a caustic chemical is spilled onto the skin or splashed into the eye, wash it off immediately with a gentle stream of running water, taking care not to wash the chemical onto other areas of skin or into the other eye.

Cauterization

The application of a heated instrument or a *caustic* chemical to tissues in order to destroy them, to stop them from bleeding, or to promote healing within them.

In the past, heat was widely used to destroy *hemorrhoids* (piles), to treat *cervical erosion*, and to stop bleeding during operations. Cauterization has now been largely replaced by *electrocoagulation* (the use of high-frequency electric current), which is more efficient and easier to use. Chemicals such as silver nitrate are still used to destroy *warts*.

Cavernous sinus thrombosis

Blockage by a *thrombus* (abnormal blood clot) of a venous sinus (widened channel for venous blood) deep within the skull behind an eye socket. Cavernous sinus thrombosis usually occurs as a complication of a bacterial infection in an area drained by the veins entering the sinus. At first, only the veins behind one eye are affected but, within two or three days, the thrombosis may spread to the sinus behind the other eye. This serious condition has become rare since the advent of *antibiotic drugs* to treat bacterial infections.

CAUSES

Among the infections that can lead to cavernous sinus thrombosis are *cellulitis* (a severe skin infection) of the face; infections of the mouth, eye, or middle ear; *sinusitis* (infection of the air spaces of the facial skull); and *septicemia* (infection in the bloodstream). Picking at a small, infected pimple at the angle of the nose may also spread infection to the sinus.

Rarely, the thrombosis is caused by a tumor pressing on the veins or by *polycythemia* (an excessive concentration of red cells in the blood).

SYMPTOMS

The patient is usually critically ill. The symptoms are severe headache, high fever, pain in and above the affected

Cavernous sinus thrombosis behind eye socket

Cavernous sinus

Thrombus

Thrombus in cavernous sinus
The cavernous sinus is found behind the eye socket, deep within the skull.

eye, and loss of sensation in the cornea and on the forehead due to pressure on the fifth cranial nerve. There may also be evidence of *proptosis* (protrusion of the eyeball) due to swelling around and behind the eye. The patient's vision may become blurred and eye movements paralyzed due to pressure on the optic nerve and on other cranial nerves controlling the muscles that move the eyes.

TREATMENT

Treatment is with antibiotic drugs to treat the infection and *anticoagulant drugs* to prevent the blood clot enlarging. Treatment can save vision in the affected eye or eyes; if untreated, blindness will result, and the infection may prove fatal.

Cavity, dental

A hole in a tooth, commonly caused by dental caries (see *Caries, dental*).

Cecum

The first and widest part of the large intestine. The cecum is joined to the *ileum* (the last part of the small intestine) and to the ascending *colon*. Projecting from the cecum is the short tube known as the *appendix*. (See also *Digestive system*.)

Cefaclor

A common cephalosporin-type antibiotic drug. (See *Cephalosporin drugs*.)

Celiac disease

An uncommon condition, known also as gluten enteropathy, in which the

C

lining of the small intestine is damaged by gluten, a protein found in wheat, rye, and certain other cereals. The damage causes *malabsorption* (failure to absorb nutrients from the intestine), and the affected person loses weight and also suffers from deficiencies of some vitamins and minerals. This can lead to *anemia* and skin problems. The feces are bulky and foul-smelling and contain large amounts of fat and other nutrients.

CAUSE

Damage to the intestinal lining seems to be due to *hypersensitivity* (an abnormal immunological response). The *immune system* becomes sensitized to gluten and reacts in the same way as it would to an infection or foreign body. The abnormal reaction is limited to the intestinal lining, and the practical result is that the villi (frondlike projections) from the lining become flattened, seriously impairing the absorption of nutrients.

INCIDENCE

The proportion of people affected by celiac disease differs greatly among different populations. In the west of Ireland the incidence is 300 per 100,000; in North America, it is 60 per 100,000, while the disease is almost unknown in Africa and Asia.

Celiac disease tends to run in families—relatives of patients are much more likely than other people to have the disease themselves—which suggests that genetic factors may be involved (see *Genetic disorders*).

SYMPTOMS AND SIGNS

The severity of the disease varies, and many people who suffer some damage to the intestinal lining never develop symptoms.

In babies, symptoms usually develop within six months of the introduction of gluten into the diet. The feces become bulky, greasy, pale, and offensive smelling, and the baby loses weight, becomes listless and irritable, and produces a lot of intestinal gas, which makes the abdomen swell. Defective absorption of iron may lead to anemia (see *Anemia, iron-deficiency*). Defective absorption of folic acid (a vitamin) may lead to megaloblastic anemia (see *Anemia, megaloblastic*). Vomiting may occur, and sometimes the baby develops acute diarrhea and may thus become dehydrated and seriously ill.

In adults, symptoms usually develop gradually over months or years. Symptoms may include vague tiredness, breathlessness, weight loss, diarrhea, vomiting, abdominal pain,

and swelling of the legs. Some patients develop a chronic, distinctive rash called *dermatitis herpetiformis*.

DIAGNOSIS

A firm diagnosis is made by means of jejunal *biopsy*, in which a small sample of tissue is taken from the lining of the upper small intestine via a tube passed through the stomach under X-ray guidance. Three biopsies may be performed over a period of time—one when the patient is eating a diet that contains gluten, another when he or she is on a gluten-free diet, and a third when gluten is again introduced into the diet. A change in the intestinal lining during the second and third stages indicates that gluten is causing the illness. Tests on the blood, urine, and feces may be performed to show the level of malabsorption.

TREATMENT AND OUTLOOK

The only treatment required is a lifelong gluten-free diet; all foods containing wheat, rye, or barley must be avoided (many sufferers are also advised to avoid oats).

Specially manufactured substitute foods, including gluten-free bread, flour, and pasta, are available. There is no restriction on meat, fish, eggs, dairy products, vegetables, fruit, rice, and corn.

Within a few weeks of the start of a gluten-free diet, symptoms clear up and the sufferer starts to regain lost weight and to enjoy normal health.

Cell

The basic structural unit of the body. Each person consists of billions of cells, structurally and functionally integrated to perform the nearly infinite number of complex tasks necessary for life.

There is enormous variation among cells in the body. For example, mature red blood cells are only about 0.0075 mm in diameter and are so highly specialized for their function of transporting oxygen that they lack some of the internal structures normally found within other cells, such as a nucleus. In contrast, individual nerve cells may be 1 m or more in length and are specialized to perform their function of transmitting electrochemical messages (nerve impulses).

Despite detailed differences, most human cells are basically similar in structure. Each cell is an invisibly small bag containing a fluid material called cytoplasm, surrounded by an outer "skin" called the cell membrane. Within the cytoplasm are the nucleus (except in red blood cells) and various

other specialized structures, which are known collectively as organelles.

CELL MEMBRANE

Formed from a double layer of fatty material and proteins, the cell membrane envelops and holds the cell together. Its other main function is to regulate the passage of materials into and out of the cell, thereby enabling useful substances (such as nutrients and oxygen) to enter the cell, and waste materials (such as carbon dioxide) and substances for use elsewhere in the body (hormones, for example) to leave it. Small molecules can pass freely through the cell membrane, but larger molecules require special molecular transport systems to cross the membrane.

NUCLEUS

The control center of the cell, the nucleus governs all major activities and functions. The nucleus exerts its influence by regulating the amount and types of *proteins* made in the cell. Proteins have two main functions. Large, structural proteins make up the tough building materials of the body (such as muscle fibers). Smaller proteins called *enzymes* regulate all functions and activities of the cell.

The *chromosomes* (genetic material of the cell), in the form of the *nucleic acid* known as *DNA*, are situated in the nucleus. This DNA contains the instructions for *protein synthesis*. These instructions are conveyed into the cytoplasm by a type of *RNA*, another nucleic acid. Particles called ribosomes in the cytoplasm play a major part in decoding these instructions for the purpose of protein synthesis.

OTHER ORGANELLES

In addition to the nucleus, the cell contains various other organelles, each with a specific role.

The endoplasmic reticulum is a single sheet of membrane twisted into complex folds. The sheet has rough and smooth areas. Rough endoplasmic reticulum is covered with tiny round "beads"—the ribosomes that help produce proteins.

Once completed, the proteins are transferred to another membrane system, the Golgi apparatus, which resembles a series of stacked plates. Here protein structures are modified and packaged into vesicles budded from its surface.

Energy is generated from the breakdown of sugars and fatty acids by organelles called mitochondria. These are shaped like coffee beans and have a complex, folded inner surface. Cells which have high energy require-

C

CELL TYPES

Despite their fundamental similarities, the cells of the body are differentiated to perform specific tasks, such as carrying oxygen (red blood cells), destroying invading microorganisms (white blood cells), manufacturing hormones (secretory cells in glands), and so on. Some cells (nerve cells, for instance) cannot be replaced once destroyed, while other cells (those that form fingernails, for instance) continue to function even after death. Cells can be grouped into four main types according to their underlying similarities.

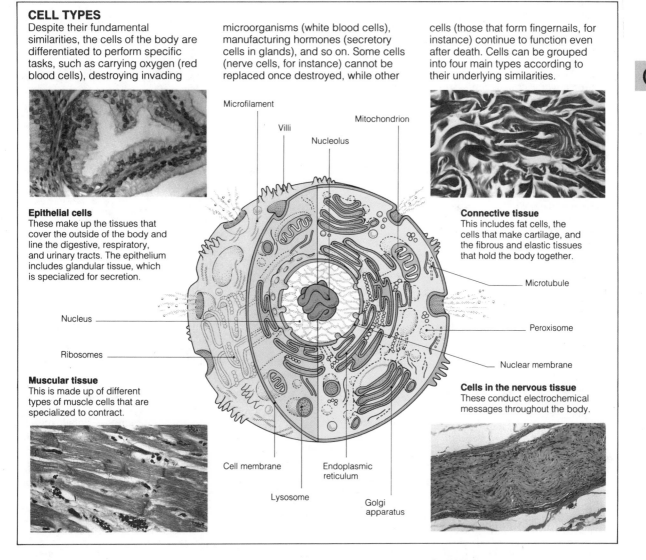

Epithelial cells
These make up the tissues that cover the outside of the body and line the digestive, respiratory, and urinary tracts. The epithelium includes glandular tissue, which is specialized for secretion.

Muscular tissue
This is made up of different types of muscle cells that are specialized to contract.

Connective tissue
This includes fat cells, the cells that make cartilage, and the fibrous and elastic tissues that hold the body together.

Cells in the nervous tissue
These conduct electrochemical messages throughout the body.

Labels on diagram: Microfilament, Villi, Nucleolus, Mitochondrion, Nucleus, Ribosomes, Cell membrane, Lysosome, Endoplasmic reticulum, Golgi apparatus, Microtubule, Peroxisome, Nuclear membrane

---

ments, such as muscle or liver cells, have a large number of mitochondria.

Many cell processes involve substances that would damage the cell if they came into contact with the cytoplasm, so they are contained within special vesicles called lysosomes and peroxisomes. Lysosomes are the cell's major digestive structures in which enzymes break down large particles, such as bacteria. Peroxisomes neutralize toxic substances.

CYTOPLASM
Modern techniques for studying the structure of cells have shown that the cytoplasm contains a network of fine tubes (microtubules) and filaments (microfilaments) known as the cytoskeleton. This network gives the cell a definite shape and allows it to move. In addition, microfilaments support microvilli (small projections from the surface of the cell), which help to increase the surface area of the cell. Microfilaments also form micromuscles, which can produce contractions and movements of the cell.

Cell division

The processes by which cells multiply. There are two main types of cell division, *mitosis* and *meiosis*. The former gives rise to daughter cells that are identical to the parent cell. The latter gives rise to egg and sperm cells, which differ from their parent cells in that they have only half the normal number of *chromosomes*.

Cellulitis

A bacterial infection of the skin and underlying tissues, most commonly caused by streptococci bacteria entering via a wound.

SYMPTOMS
The face, neck, or legs are the usual sites. The affected area is hot, tender, and red, and the patient may be feverish and have chills.

Untreated cellulitis complicating a wound may progress to *bacteremia* and *septicemia* or, occasionally, to *gangrene*. Before the advent of *antibiotic drugs*, cellulitis was an occasional cause of death. Facial infections may spread to the eye socket. Very rarely, cellulitis occurs after childbirth and may spread to the pelvic organs.

C

Any form of cellulitis is likely to be more severe in people with reduced resistance to infections, such as people with *diabetes mellitus* or any type of *immunodeficiency disorder*.

TREATMENT

The usual treatment is a *penicillin* antibiotic (or *erythromycin* in the case of patients who are allergic to penicillin). Drugs may have to be taken for up to two weeks to clear an infection. (See also *Erysipelas*.)

Celsius scale

A temperature scale in which the melting point of ice is zero degrees (0°C) and the boiling point of water is 100 degrees (100°C). On this scale, normal body temperature is 37°C (equivalent to 98.6°F). The scale is named after the Swedish astronomer Anders Celsius (1701-1744).

Centigrade is an obsolete name for the same scale.

To convert a Celsius temperature to Fahrenheit, multiply by 1.8 (or nine fifths), then add 32. To convert Fahrenheit to Celsius, subtract 32 then multiply by 0.56 (or five ninths). (See also *Fahrenheit scale*.)

0°C	37°C	100°C
32°F	98.6°F	212°F

Cementum

The bonelike tissue that surrounds the root of a tooth (see *Teeth*).

Centigrade scale

The obsolete name for the *Celsius scale*.

Central nervous system

The anatomical term for the brain and spinal cord, often abbreviated as CNS. The central nervous system works in tandem with the *peripheral nervous system* (PNS), which consists of all the nerves that carry signals between the CNS and the rest of the body.

The overall role of the CNS is to receive sensory information from organs, such as the eyes, ears, and receptors within the body, analyze this information, and then initiate an appropriate motor response (for example, contracting a muscle).

The analytical stage may be very short and simple for information that goes no further than the spinal cord or lower areas of the brain (see *Reflex*), but may be complex and prolonged for information that reaches higher, conscious brain centers.

In anatomical terms, the CNS consists of nerve cells or neurons and supporting tissue; the PNS is made up of nerve fibers extending from cells in the CNS. In functional terms, injury or disease affecting the CNS usually causes permanent disability, whereas recovery is sometimes possible after repairing damage to the PNS. (See also *Nervous system*.)

Centrifuge

A machine that separates the different components of a body fluid, such as blood or urine, so that they can be analyzed as an aid to diagnosis. The liquid is placed in a container that is spun at high speed around a central axis, and the centrifugal force (force moving away from the center) separates groups of particles of varying density. Blood, for example, can be separated into red cells, white cells, and its remaining constituents.

Cephalexin

A common cephalosporin-type antibiotic drug. (See *Cephalosporin drugs*.)

Cephalhematoma

An extensive, soft swelling on the scalp of a newborn infant, caused by bleeding into the space between the cranium (skull) and its overlying fibrous covering (the periosteum or pericranium). The swelling is due to pressure on the baby's head during delivery, causing rupture of small blood vessels.

Although possibly alarming, a cephalhematoma is not serious and no treatment is necessary. However, the cephalhematoma should not be handled unnecessarily. The swelling gradually subsides as the blood clot is reabsorbed, although this may take many weeks.

Cephalic

Relating to the head, as in cephalic presentation, the head-first appearance of a baby in the birth canal.

Cephalosporin drugs

COMMON DRUGS

Cefaclor Cefadroxil Cefamandole Cefazolin Cefotoxamine Cefuroxime Cephalexin Cephradine

A group of *antibiotic drugs* derived from the fungus CEPHALOSPORIUM ACREMONIUM. Cephalosporin drugs were discovered in Sardinia in 1948. A large number of synthetic cephalosporin drugs have since been

Bilateral cephalhematoma
This baby was born with a cephalhematoma on both sides of the scalp at the back of the head. The red line superimposed on the photograph indicates the normal outline of the head.

produced, the most recent of which are effective against a wide range of infections. Some cephalosporins are effective only if injected.

WHY THEY ARE USED

Cephalosporins are widely used to treat infections of the ear, throat, and respiratory tract. They are also particularly useful in the treatment of *urinary tract infections* (which are often caused by bacteria that are resistant to penicillin-type antibiotics) and are used to treat *gonorrhea* that is resistant to other antibiotics. Cephalosporins are also sometimes used after surgery to reduce the incidence of wound infections.

The drugs in this group may be used in patients allergic to penicillin-type antibiotics. However, approximately 10 percent of those people allergic to penicillins are also found to be allergic to cephalosporins.

HOW THEY WORK

Cephalosporins interfere with the development of bacterial cell walls and inhibit the production of protein within the bacterial cells. As a result, the bacterial cells disintegrate and the bacteria die. However, some types of bacteria produce an enzyme (a protein that stimulates chemical reactions) called beta-lactamase that can inactivate some of the older varieties of cephalosporin drugs. The newer drugs in the group are not affected by this enzyme.

POSSIBLE ADVERSE EFFECTS

Some people who take cephalosporins develop an allergic reaction causing rash, itching, and fever. In very rare cases, *anaphylactic shock* (a severe allergic reaction that causes collapse) may occur.

C

Cerebellar ataxia

Jerky, staggering gait and other uncoordinated movements caused by disease or damage to the *cerebellum*. Other features include *dysarthria* (slurred speech); hand tremor and "overshoot" when an attempt is made to touch something; and *nystagmus* (abnormal jerky eye movements).

Possible causes include *stroke, multiple sclerosis, brain tumor,* damage caused by *alcohol dependence,* and degeneration of the cerebellum due to a hereditary disorder.

Cerebellum

A region of the brain concerned primarily with the maintenance of posture and balance and with the coordination of movement.

STRUCTURE

The cerebellum is a rounded structure located behind the *brain stem,* to which it is linked by thick nerve tracts. The cerebellum accounts for about 11 percent of the whole brain weight and, with its convoluted surface, appears similar to the *cerebrum* (the main mass of the brain).

Outwardly, the cerebellum consists of two hemispheres flanking the vermis, which is a small protrusion from the brain stem. The cortex (outer part) of the hemispheres consists of numerous parallel ridges separated by deep fissures, so that only one sixth of the surface is visible. From the inner side of each hemisphere, three nerve fiber stalks, or peduncles, arise; these link up with different parts of the brain stem. All the signals between the cerebellum and the rest of the brain travel along these nerve tracts.

Microscopically, a cross section of the cerebellum shows the nerve fibers from these tracts fanning out toward the convoluted cortical surface. The cortex itself consists of gray matter (interconnected nerve cells) arranged in three main layers. Prominent in the middle layer are large cells called Purkinje's cells, each of which may interconnect with up to 100,000 other cells.

FUNCTION

Via its connections to the brain stem, the cerebellum receives information from organs such as muscle tendons and the balance organ in the inner ear. Much of this information concerns the body's posture and the state of contraction or relaxation of its muscles. Using this information, the cerebellum, working in concert with the *basal ganglia* (nerve cell clusters deep within the brain), fine-tunes the orders sent to muscles from the motor cortex in the cerebrum, resulting in smoothly coordinated movements and balance.

DISORDERS

Disease or damage to the cerebellum may result in *cerebellar ataxia,* characterized by jerky, staggering gait, slurred speech, and other uncoordinated movements. *Alcohol intoxication* impairs cerebellar function and thus may produce symptoms similar to those of cerebellar disease.

Cerebral hemorrhage

Bleeding within the brain caused by rupture of a blood vessel. (See *Intracerebral hemorrhage.*)

Cerebral palsy

A general term for disorders of movement and posture resulting from damage to a child's developing brain in the later months of pregnancy, during birth, in the newborn period, or in early childhood. These disorders are nonprogressive (i.e., the disability does not increase with time).

A child with cerebral palsy may suffer from *spastic paralysis* (abnormal stiffness and contraction of groups of muscles), *athetosis* (involuntary writhing movements), or *ataxia* (loss of coordination and balance). The degree of disability is highly variable, ranging from slight clumsiness of hand movement and gait to complete immobility. Other nervous system disorders, such as hearing defects or epileptic seizures, may be present. Many affected children are also mentally retarded, although some are of normal or high intelligence.

One to six children per 1,000 have some form of cerebral palsy, although the incidence varies between countries. There has been only a slight reduction in cases in the past 20 years.

CAUSES

In more than 90 percent of cases the damage occurs before or at birth. Probably the most common cause is cerebral *hypoxia* (poor oxygen supply to the brain).

A maternal infection spreading to the baby within the uterus is an occasional cause. A rare cause is *kernicterus,* which results from an excess of bilirubin (bile pigment) in babies with *hemolytic disease of the newborn.* The baby is severely jaundiced, and the bile pigment damages the *basal ganglia* (nerve cell clusters in the brain concerned with control of movement).

Following birth, possible causes of disorders include *encephalitis* (inflammation of the brain) or *meningitis* (inflammation of the brain's protective coverings), *head injury,* or *intracerebral hemorrhage* (bleeding within the brain).

SYMPTOMS

Cerebral palsy may not be recognized until well into the baby's first year. Sometimes, some of the infant's muscles are initially hypotonic (floppy), and the parents may notice that the baby in some way does not "feel right" when held. There may also be feeding difficulties. Delay in sitting up without support is another early sign.

Most affected children fall into one of two groups—a spastic group, in which the muscles of one or more limbs are permanently contracted and stiff, thus making normal movements very difficult, and a smaller, athetoid group, characterized by involuntary writhing movements.

Children in the spastic group may be affected by diplegia (in which all four limbs are affected, but the legs more severely than the arms), hemiplegia (in which the limbs on just one side of the body are affected, usually the arm worse than the leg), or by quadriplegia (in which all four limbs are severely affected, not necessarily symmetrically). In each case, muscle stiffness begins to appear from the age of about 6 months onward. Normal balance is disrupted and the limbs

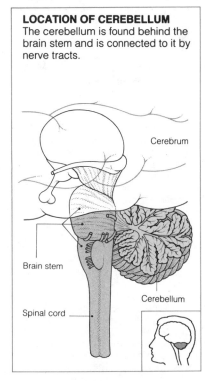

LOCATION OF CEREBELLUM
The cerebellum is found behind the brain stem and is connected to it by nerve tracts.

Cerebrum

Brain stem

Cerebellum

Spinal cord

C

settle in abnormal positions—for example, in children with diplegia the affected legs cross in scissorlike fashion, and in those with hemiplegia the affected arm is tucked up at the side of the body, with both the elbow and wrist bent.

The diplegic child has delayed development in many movement skills and has difficulty learning to walk. In hemiplegia the limbs on the affected side grow slowly; there may be some sensory deficiency from the affected side of the body.

In quadriplegia, it may be difficult to know whether the child's arms or legs are the worst affected; mental retardation is usually severe. Often, the child never learns to walk.

Mental retardation, with an IQ below 70, occurs in about three quarters of all children with cerebral palsy, but the exceptions are important and occur particularly among athetoids; many athetoids and some diplegics are highly intelligent.

The features of most types of cerebral palsy change as the child gets older, often for the better with patience and skilled treatment.

DIAGNOSIS

Parents of babies who are "at risk" from cerebral palsy—for example, babies born prematurely or those who have had particularly difficult births—are generally encouraged to take the child more frequently for routine checkups by a physician, who will test with particular care for any abnormalities in the baby's muscle tone and reflexes, and for any delay in reaching various developmental milestones (see *Child development*). The diagnosis may rely on a combination of abnormalities being present.

TREATMENT

Although cerebral palsy is incurable, much can be done to help children affected by it. Abilities need to be recognized and developed to the full, as much stimulation as possible should be offered, and loving patience must be shown.

Physiotherapy is required to teach an affected child how to develop muscular control and maintain balance. This therapy is often given initially at a special school or clinic and then continued at home, possibly with the use of special equipment.

Inadequate speech can be helped greatly by *speech therapy*. For children who cannot speak at all, sophisticated techniques and devices have been developed to teach them how to communicate nonverbally.

Every attempt is made to place children with mild cerebral palsy in normal schools, but those who are severely affected need the special help and facilities that are available at schools for the physically and/or mentally handicapped.

OUTLOOK

Children with only moderate disability have a near-normal life expectancy and, with the help of social services, most of those who can move around and communicate effectively grow up to lead a relatively independent life.

Cerebral thrombosis

The formation of a *thrombus* (blood clot) in an artery in the brain. The clot may completely block the artery, cutting off the supply of blood, nutrients and oxygen to a region of the brain, causing a *stroke*.

Cerebrospinal fluid

A clear, watery fluid that circulates between the ventricles (cavities) within the brain, the central canal in the spinal cord, and the space between the brain and spinal cord and their protective coverings, the meninges. Cerebrospinal fluid contains dissolved glucose (sugar), proteins, and salts, and some lymphocytes (white blood cells).

The fluid functions as a shock-absorber, helping to prevent or minimize damage to the brain and spinal cord after a blow to the head or back.

Examination of cerebrospinal fluid, usually obtained by *lumbar puncture*, is important in the diagnosis of many conditions affecting the brain and spinal cord, including *meningitis* and *subarachnoid hemorrhage*.

Accumulation of cerebrospinal fluid within the skull during fetal development or in infancy may cause the skull to become enlarged—a condition known as *hydrocephalus*.

Cerebrovascular accident

Sudden rupture or blockage of a blood vessel within the brain, causing serious bleeding and/or local obstruction to blood circulation, and leading to features of nervous system disturbance commonly called a *stroke*.

Blockage may be due to *thrombosis* (clot formation) or to *embolism* (a fragment or air bubble carried in the blood). Rupture of different blood vessels may cause different patterns of bleeding—such as *intracerebral hemorrhage* (bleeding within the brain) or *subarachnoid hemorrhage* (bleeding around the brain).

Cerebrovascular disease

Any disease affecting an artery within, and supplying blood to, the brain—for example, *atherosclerosis* (narrowing of the arteries) or constitutional defects or weaknesses in arterial walls causing *aneurysm* (a balloonlike swelling in an artery). The disease may eventually lead to a *cerebrovascular accident* (sudden blockage or rupture of a blood vessel), which most commonly leads to the features of *stroke*. Extensive narrowing of blood vessels throughout the brain can be a cause of *dementia*.

Cerebrum

The largest and most developed part of the brain, and the site of most conscious and intelligent activities. The cerebrum consists of two large outgrowths from the upper part of the brain stem (an extension of the spinal cord) called the cerebral hemispheres. Together these outgrowths form an almost continuous mass that envelops much of the rest of the brain.

For size relative to body weight, and also for sophistication, the human cerebrum is unmatched in the animal kingdom, except arguably by that of some marine mammals, such as dolphins. Its complexity dwarfs that of the most advanced man-made machines and, although its structure and function are understood in broad terms, much of its workings remain a complete mystery.

STRUCTURE

Like the rest of the brain, the cerebrum consists of billions of interconnected nerve cells, arranged in layers or in clusters called nuclei, together with nerve fibers, the long filamentous outgrowths from nerve cells along which electrical messages (nerve impulses) pass to other cells. These fibers are organized into bundles, or nerve tracts, like electrical cables. Both the nerve cells and their fibers lie in a matrix of supporting cells, called glial cells, which provide both physical support and some metabolic requirements (e.g., energy, nutrients, or structural components) for the nerve cells.

Each cerebral hemisphere contains a central cavity, called a ventricle, which is filled with *cerebrospinal fluid*. Much of the rest of each hemisphere falls into three main layers: an inner layer surrounding the ventricle and consisting of clusters of nerve cells called the basal ganglia; a middle layer of "white matter" consisting mainly of tracts of nerve fibers; and an outer surface layer, known as the cerebral cortex or "gray matter," which is about 1 cm deep and consists of several layers of interconnected nerve cells.

The surface of each hemisphere is thrown into a series of folds, called gyri, separated by fissures called sulci; much of the cortex is hidden within the folds. Broad surface regions, or lobes, of each hemisphere are named after overlying bones; the four main regions are the frontal, parietal, temporal, and occipital lobes.

The pattern of cortical folding is not precisely the same for everyone, but some of the gyri and sulci are constant and easily recognized on the surface of any brain. They have been given names by anatomists. The parietal and frontal lobes, for example, are separated by the central sulcus, and the temporal lobe from the frontal by the sylvian fissure. The longitudinal fissure is a deep cleft running front to back over the entire surface of the cerebrum, thus separating the two hemispheres. By reference to such landmarks, the location of any point on the surface of the cortex can be specified with some precision.

The nerve fibers forming much of the white matter in each hemisphere are of three main types: association fibers that link areas of cortex within a single hemisphere; projection fibers that link areas of the cortex to central brain structures and to the brain stem below; and commissural fibers, collected into a thick band called the corpus callosum, that link the two hemispheres. A continuous stream of information, in the form of electrical impulses, flows along these fibers between groups of nerve cells.

FUNCTION

Much of the sensory information from organs such as the eyes and ears and from sensory receptors in the skin has its final destination in the cerebral cortex, where it is sorted, analyzed, and generally integrated until finally it is perceived as images, sound, touch sensations, and the like. Different levels of analysis are thought to correspond to the distinct layers of neurons in the cortex, with full conscious sensation probably occurring only in the top few layers.

Certain sensory modalities are specifically located within particular cortical regions—for example, visual perception is located within a part of the occipital lobe called the visual cortex. If this part of the brain is seriously damaged, vision is lost completely.

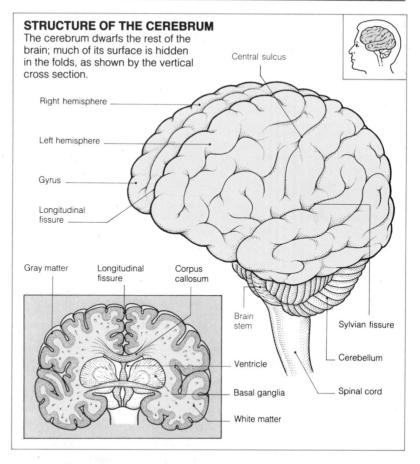

STRUCTURE OF THE CEREBRUM

The cerebrum dwarfs the rest of the brain; much of its surface is hidden in the folds, as shown by the vertical cross section.

Central sulcus

Right hemisphere

Left hemisphere

Gyrus

Longitudinal fissure

Gray matter

Longitudinal fissure

Corpus callosum

Brain stem

Sylvian fissure

Ventricle

Cerebellum

Basal ganglia

Spinal cord

White matter

Touch and pressure sensations are consciously perceived along the postcentral gyrus, immediately behind the central sulcus that divides the frontal and parietal lobes.

Other cortical regions, mainly in the temporal lobe, are associated with auditory (hearing), olfactory (smell), and gustatory (taste) sensations, although less specifically so. If these areas are destroyed, sensation is dulled considerably, but not lost altogether. This would seem to indicate that some primitive sensations (e.g., smell and pain) may be perceived below the level of the cortex.

In addition to sensory areas, there are also specific "motor" areas concerned with the initiation of signals for movement by the skeletal muscles. The main motor area of the cortex is in the frontal lobe, along the precentral gyrus, immediately in front of the central sulcus. Again, it seems that not all movements are initiated from the cortex. Some learned, semiautomatic program of movement, such as those for walking, are delegated to lower brain regions, leaving the cortex free to deal with newly formulated, skilled movements.

Linked to the more clearly defined sensory and motor areas are association areas of the cortex, which integrate information from various senses. The association areas also perform functions such as comprehension and recognition, memory storage and recall, arithmetical calculation, thought and decision-making, or are involved in the conscious experience of emotions. Whereas many of the sensory and motor areas are on both sides of the cerebrum (serving the opposite side of the body), some of these other cortical functions are localized to one hemisphere. The "dominant" hemisphere (the left in almost all right-handed and many left-handed people) tends to control logical functions such as word comprehension, language, speech, and numeration, whereas the nondominant hemisphere is concerned with spatial relationships and emotional responses such as color appreciation.

C

In general, the more complex the function, the less well localized it is. However, the areas responsible for the comprehension of words (heard and read) and for language expression are located within clearly defined areas of the dominant hemisphere. The comprehension region (Wernicke's area) is close to the part of the cortex concerned with sound perception; the region concerned with language expression (Broca's area) is close to the motor region controlling the muscles used in speech.

Of all the regions of the cerebrum, the functions of the frontal lobe are the least understood, and for this reason it is sometimes termed a "silent area." Information on the activity of this and some other areas derives mainly from study of the symptoms of local damage or disease.

DISORDERS

Damage to the cerebrum may be the result of direct physical trauma (see *Head injury*), *intracerebral hemorrhage* or other forms of *stroke*, *brain tumors*, *encephalitis* (inflammation of the brain), or to some types of poisoning, nutritional deficiency, and degenerative processes.

Damage to particular regions may cause specific syndromes. Examples are mental apathy and self-neglect (or other personality change) resulting from frontal lobe damage, or the loss of sensory discrimination, tactile *agnosia* (loss of the ability to recognize objects by touch), and geographic disorientation (losing one's way even in a familiar area), which may occur with parietal lobe injury. Disease of the temporal lobe may cause *amnesia* (loss of memory), strange hallucinations of smell, sight, and sound, and *aphasia* (loss of the ability to comprehend or express language) if the dominant hemisphere is affected. Specific visual defects result from damage to the occipital lobe.

Often, however, cerebral disease causes nonspecific symptoms such as epileptic convulsions or headaches making diagnosis difficult.

Cerumen

The waxlike yellowish substance commonly found in the external ear canal (see *Earwax*).

Cervical

Relating to the neck or to the cervix (neck of the uterus).

Cervical cancer

See *Cervix, cancer of*.

Cervical erosion

A condition affecting the cervix (neck of the uterus) in which a layer of cells more characteristic of those found in the inner lining of the cervix appears on its outside surface—as though the cervix had been turned inside out. The layer of cells contains many that are column-shaped and of a glandular (mucus-forming) type. The term "erosion" is something of a misnomer as there is no loss of tissue or ulceration of the cervix. The cervix may, however, be more fragile and have a tendency to bleed and secrete more mucus than normal.

CAUSES

Some women are born with cervical erosion and have no symptoms. Other possible causes of the condition include injury to the cervix during labor (which may cause glandular tissue to appear on the outer surface of the cervix during healing) and long-term use of *oral contraceptives*.

SYMPTOMS

Most women with cervical erosion have no or few symptoms. Those that do have symptoms usually complain of a vaginal discharge, especially in the week prior to a period, or bleeding between periods or after intercourse. Inspection of the cervix shows a reddened area on the surface that may bleed easily when touched. This appearance needs to be distinguished from cervical cancer by means of a *cervical smear test* and perhaps *colposcopy* (examination of the cervix with a viewing instrument).

TREATMENT

Only women with symptoms need to be treated. Treatment by local destruction of glandular tissue includes *cauterization*, *cryosurgery* (freezing), *diathermy* (heat destruction), or *laser treatment*. The areas of destroyed glandular tissue are replaced in time by a layer of normal squamous (flat) cells.

Cervical incompetence

Abnormal weakness of the cervix (the neck of the uterus) that can result in recurrent *miscarriages*. Normally, the cervix remains closed until labor begins. However, if the cervix is incompetent, it may gradually widen from about the 12th week of pregnancy onward because of the weight of the fetus within the uterus, or may suddenly open during the middle third of pregnancy.

CAUSES AND SYMPTOMS

Cervical incompetence may be suspected if a woman has had two or more miscarriages after the 14th week of pregnancy. About one fifth of women who have recurrent miscarriages have cervical incompetence.

The obstetrician may be able to detect the cervical widening by performing an internal pelvic examination. The condition may also be diagnosed by *ultrasound scanning*.

TREATMENT

When a woman with cervical incompetence becomes pregnant, a suture (stitch) is tied, like a purse string, around the cervix. This is performed during the fourth month of pregnancy under an epidural or general anesthetic. After the operation, the patient stays in the hospital for a few days, and may be advised to rest frequently in bed throughout the remainder of the pregnancy. The suture is left in position until the pregnancy is at or near full term. It is then cut so that the mother can deliver the baby normally.

Cervical mucus method

A form of contraception based on periodic abstinence from intercourse according to the changes in the mucus secreted by a woman's cervix. (See *Contraception, natural methods of*.)

Cervical osteoarthritis

A degenerative disorder, also known as cervical spondylitis, that affects the joints between the cervical vertebrae (bones in the neck).

Because the degenerative changes are associated with aging, the condition mainly affects middle-aged and elderly people. An X ray of almost everyone over the age of 50 would

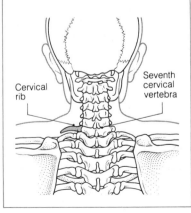

LOCATION OF CERVICAL RIB
The overdeveloped seventh cervical vertebra forms a rib parallel to a normal one.

Cervical rib

Seventh cervical vertebra

show some evidence of cervical osteoarthritis, but most people have no symptoms, or only minor ones.

Occasionally, the degeneration may be started by an injury—for example, a whiplash neck injury sustained in a road traffic accident.

SYMPTOMS

The main symptoms are pain and stiffness in the neck. Pressure on nerves passing between the affected vertebrae may cause pain in the arms and shoulders, numbness and tingling in the hands, and a weak grip. Symptoms tend to flare up from time to time, with intervening periods of only mild discomfort.

Other symptoms include dizziness, unsteadiness, double vision and headache brought on by turning the head. These symptoms are caused by pressure on blood vessels running through the vertebrae up to the brain. Rarely, pressure on the spinal cord itself can cause weakness or even paralysis in the legs, and loss of bladder control.

DIAGNOSIS AND TREATMENT

People who have persistent minor symptoms or symptoms that are becoming worse should consult their physician. X rays and possibly other tests will be performed.

Treatment of severe neck pain and stiffness may include rest, *heat treatment*, supporting the neck in a collar, *traction* of the neck, and the use of *analgesic drugs* (painkillers). *Physiotherapy*, including *diathermy*, ultrasound, massage, and exercises to improve neck posture and movement, is useful when the pain has eased. People with pressure on the spinal cord may benefit from a surgical procedure to relieve pressure on the cord (see *Decompression, spinal canal*).

Cervical rib

A *congenital* abnormality in which the lowest of the seven cervical vertebrae (neck bones) has overdeveloped to form a *rib*. The cervical rib lies parallel to and above the first normal rib. The abnormality varies from a small bony swelling to a fully developed rib and may occur on one or both sides. The cause is unknown.

SYMPTOMS

Often, the cervical rib is discovered only when an X ray of the chest or neck is taken for some unrelated reason. Symptoms may develop in early adult life, when the rib begins to press on the lower part of the *brachial plexus* (the group of nerves passing from the spinal cord into the arm), causing pain, numbness, and pins and nee-

dles in the forearm and hand. These symptoms can often be relieved by changing the position of the arm.

DIAGNOSIS AND TREATMENT

An X ray will show the presence of a cervical rib, but other possible causes of pain and tingling in the hand or arm (such as *carpal tunnel syndrome* or a *disk prolapse*) still need to be excluded.

Symptoms due to a cervical rib can sometimes be reduced by exercises. Severe or persistent symptoms may require surgical removal of the rib.

Cervical smear test

A test to detect abnormal changes in the cells of the cervix (the neck of the uterus) and thus to prevent the devel-

---

PROCEDURE FOR A CERVICAL SMEAR

The procedure is risk-free and the smear test itself takes only a few seconds. It should be done as a matter of routine within six months of first having sexual intercourse, and then six to 12 months after. Thereafter, it should be performed at approximately three-yearly intervals.

EQUIPMENT USED

Speculum · Plastic gloves · Spatula · Glass slides · Fixative

1 The woman lies, preferably on her back, with her arms relaxed. Her legs should be bent up and relaxed so that the knees fall open.

2 The vagina is held open with a speculum; a spatula is used to scrape away some cells, which are examined under the microscope.

Normal cells as seen under the microscope

Abnormal cells as seen under the microscope

opment of cervical cancer (see *Cervix, cancer of*). This is also known as a Pap test for George Papanicolaou, the pathologist who devised it.

WHY IT IS DONE

The test offers a 95 percent chance of detecting dysplasia (abnormal cell changes) which, if not discovered and treated, could become cancerous.

Cervical smears can also detect viral infections of the cervix, such as *herpes simplex* and wart virus infection (see *Warts, genital*).

WHEN IT IS DONE

A woman should have a cervical smear within six months of first having sexual intercourse. A second smear should be performed six to 12 months later (because of the small chance of missing an abnormality on one smear) and, if no abnormality is found, subsequently at approximately three-yearly intervals for the remainder of her life.

More frequent tests may be needed in women who change sex partners often or whose partner changes sex partners frequently.

Most family planning clinics and well woman clinics perform cervical smears; women may also be tested by their general practitioners.

RESULTS

If the cells in the cervix appear normal, no further treatment is required. If the cells appear abnormal, the smear is graded according to the cervical intra-epithelial neoplasia (CIN) classification system: CIN1 (mild dysplasia), CIN2 (moderate dysplasia), or CIN3

(severe dysplasia/early cancer). All abnormal smears are followed either by repeat smears or by *colposcopy* (examination of the cervix with a viewing instrument) and *biopsy* (removal of small samples of tissue for microscopic analysis) of any suspicious areas. There are two types of cervical biopsy: punch and cone (see illustration below).

Areas confirmed as abnormal by biopsy are treated by *electrocoagulation* or *laser* (both of which use heat to destroy tissue) or by *cryosurgery* (which uses cold to destroy tissue). Treatment is sometimes carried out at the same time as colposcopy if the abnormal area is small and well-defined. If a woman is pregnant, treatment is usually delayed until after delivery.

If colposcopy is not available, or if the extent of the severe dysplasia cannot be identified, treatment is by *cone biopsy*, an operation to remove a core of cervical tissue.

Cervical spondylosis

An alternative name for *cervical osteoarthritis*.

Cervicitis

Inflammation of the cervix (the neck and outlet of the uterus). Cervicitis is usually due to a vaginal infection or a sexually transmitted disease, such as *gonorrhea, chlamydial infection*, or genital *herpes*. Cervical infection may also follow injury to the cervix during childbirth or surgery on the uterus. There are acute and chronic forms of cervicitis.

SYMPTOMS

Acute cervicitis is often symptomless and may not be discovered until the cervix is examined for some other reason. The cervix is inflamed and there may be a discharge from it.

Chronic cervicitis may produce a vaginal discharge, bleeding from the vagina after sexual intercourse or between periods, and pain low in the abdomen, sometimes felt only during sexual intercourse.

COMPLICATIONS

Untreated cervicitis can spread to cause *endometritis* (inflammation of the lining of the uterus), *salpingitis* (inflammation of the fallopian tubes), or *pelvic inflammatory disease*.

If a pregnant woman has cervicitis, her baby may be infected during delivery, resulting in neonatal *ophthalmia* (an eye infection leading to blindness) or, less commonly, in *pneumonia* caused by chlamydial infection.

DIAGNOSIS AND TREATMENT

A woman with the symptoms described should see her physician, who will probably examine her cervix and take swabs of any discharge so that the microorganism responsible for the discharge can be identified.

Treatment is with *antibiotic drugs*, especially a *tetracycline* or *penicillin drug*, or with an *antiviral drug*, such as *acyclovir*, depending on the cause of infection. If symptoms persist, the inflamed area of the cervix may be cauterized by *electrocoagulation, cryotherapy*, or *laser treatment* to destroy the infected tissue.

BIOPSY OF THE CERVIX

If a woman has recurrent abnormal smears, colposcopy and biopsy of suspicious areas will be performed. If the abnormal area cannot be seen completely by colposcopy, a larger sample of tissue is removed by cone biopsy. This procedure is used for treatment as well as diagnosis.

View of cervix
The photograph shows the end-on appearance of the cervix after a biopsy specimen has been taken from its tip.

Punch biopsy
If regions of the cervix look abnormal, but not serious enough for full biopsy, minute fragments of the cervix are removed for examination.

Cone biopsy
Using general anesthesia, a cone-shaped piece of the cervix (containing an area with abnormal cells) is removed with a scalpel. The resulting crater is repaired by stitching flaps of tissue over the wound. Alternatively, the wound may be left open and diathermy or freezing used to stop any bleeding. Lasers (left) may be used to destroy abnormal tissue.

Cervix

A small, cylindrical organ, several centimetres in length and less than 2.5 cm in diameter, comprising the lower part and neck of the uterus. The cervix separates the body and cavity of the uterus from the vagina. Running through the cervix is a canal, through which sperm can pass from the vagina into the uterus and through which blood passes during *menstruation*. The cervical canal forms part of the birth canal during *childbirth*.

The bulk of the cervix consists of fibrous tissue with some smooth muscle. This tissue makes the cervix into a form of sphincter (circular muscle) and allows for the great adaptability in its size and shape required during *pregnancy* and childbirth.

FUNCTION

After puberty, mucus is secreted from glandular cells in the canal. The function of this mucus is to assist the entry of sperm into the upper cervix, which acts as a sperm reservoir. In the middle of the menstrual cycle, this mucus becomes less viscous and more favorable for the passage of sperm. Within the cervix, the sperm are protected and provided with energy by the mucus.

During pregnancy, the internal muscular fibers increase in size, thus lengthening the cervix, which acts as a barrier for retention of the fetus. Toward the end of pregnancy there is a general shortening of the cervix in readiness for labor and delivery. During labor the central canal widens to up to 10 cm in diameter to allow the baby to pass from the uterus. Soon after childbirth the muscles in the cervix contract and the canal returns to its original size.

Cervix, cancer of

Cancer of the cervix (neck of the uterus) is one of the most common cancers affecting women worldwide, and in many areas is becoming more common. Untreated, it may spread to most of the organs in the pelvis. The chances of cure depend very much on what stage the cancer has reached when first detected.

TYPES

Cervical cancer has well-defined precancerous stages. Before any cancer appears, abnormal changes in cells on the surface of the cervix, referred to as dysplasia, can be detected by a *cervical smear test*. Mild dysplasia may later revert to normal, but any woman who has an abnormal cervical smear should undergo further investigation

and possible follow-up smears. If more severe dysplasia or early cancer is detected, it can be treated and cured completely.

CAUSES

There are two main types of cervical cancer. Both can occur before or after the *menopause*.

SQUAMOUS TYPE This is by far the most common type of cervical cancer and is almost certainly the result of some process that occurs during sexual intercourse, possibly involving an infectious organism acquired from the male partner. Recent evidence suggests that the organism responsible for squamous cancer is a strain of the human papillomavirus (wart virus). A woman in a sexual relationship with a man who has genital warts (see *Warts, genital*) has about a one in three risk of developing a precancerous condition of the cervix.

There are more than 40 different strains of human papillomavirus, but traces of "high risk" strains, especially HPV16 and HPV18, have been found in 90 percent of squamous-type cervical cancers and in 50 to 70 percent of precancerous conditions.

Other factors are also known to predispose a woman to cancer of the cervix. Smokers are at higher risk than nonsmokers, possibly because smoking impairs the *immune system* (natural defenses against infection) and thus allows entry and proliferation of a causative virus.

An alternative explanation is that the chemical *carcinogen* in cigarettes is absorbed into the bloodstream and excreted into the cervical secretions. Additional evidence in favor of this theory is the observation of various researchers that the incidence of cervical cancer is affected by the smoking habits of women's male partners.

The sexual behavior of a woman and her male partner or partners strongly influences her chances of developing the disease. The earlier a woman and/or her partner first started having sex, and the greater the number of sexual partners they have had, the higher the risk that she will develop a precancerous condition.

ADENOCARCINOMA The causes of this much rarer type of cervical cancer are unclear. Both sexually active women and those who have never had intercourse are susceptible.

INCIDENCE

About 1,500 new cases of cervical cancer are diagnosed in Canada each year, and about 400 deaths are reported from this cause. In the past

20 years both the incidence and the death rate from this form of cancer have been declining steadily. This trend should continue as cervical smear screening becomes more efficient and widespread.

SYMPTOMS

The precancerous stages cause no symptoms whatsoever. Symptoms of the malignant stage are also initially few. Eventually, a woman will notice vaginal bleeding or a bloodstained discharge at unexpected times—between periods, after intercourse, or after the menopause.

If left untreated, the cancer spreads from the cervical surface into the deeper parts of the cervix and then out into the pelvic tissues, causing pain. Eventually the cancer spreads to the bladder, rectum, and surrounding pelvic tissue.

DIAGNOSIS

The precancerous stages can be detected only by a cervical smear test

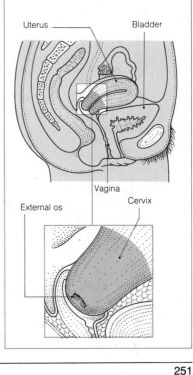

ANATOMY OF THE CERVIX
The cervix contains a central canal for passage of sperm and menstrual blood, and for childbirth. Both the canal and outer surface of the cervix are lined with two types of cells: mucus-secreting glandular cells and protective squamous cells.

Uterus — Bladder

Vagina

External os — Cervix

C

DISORDERS OF THE CERVIX

The cervix (neck of the uterus), with its central position in the female reproductive tract, is susceptible to injury, infections, and tumors.

INJURY

Minor injury to the cervix is common during childbirth, especially if labor has been prolonged or if forceps have been used to deliver the baby's head. These injuries usually take the form of a laceration (tear) in the side wall. Usually they can be repaired immediately after delivery, but rarely they may extend into the tissues surrounding the uterus and lead to internal bleeding, requiring major surgery.

Injury may also occur if the cervical canal is excessively dilated (widened) in the process of an abortion, especially if the woman has not had children. However, the risk of such injury is extremely small if the abortion is carried out in a well-equipped hospital or clinic by a qualified gynecologist.

When an injury does occur, there is a danger that the muscle fibers within the cervix will be damaged or weakened, leading to a condition called *cervical incompetence*. The ability of the cervix to retain a fetus in the uterus is impaired, with a risk of miscarriage unless the weakness is repaired.

INFECTION

Cervical infections are common and usually sexually transmitted, but may cause no or few symptoms. *Gonorrhea* and *chlamydial infections* are the two most frequent and are sexually transmitted. These infections may spread to the lining of the uterus or to the fallopian tubes with a risk of causing infertility (see *Cervicitis; Endometritis; Salpingitis*).

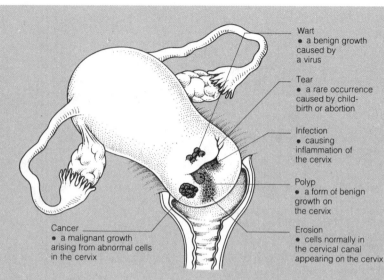

Wart
• a benign growth caused by a virus

Tear
• a rare occurrence caused by childbirth or abortion

Infection
• causing inflammation of the cervix

Polyp
• a form of benign growth on the cervix

Erosion
• cells normally in the cervical canal appearing on the cervix

Cancer
• a malignant growth arising from abnormal cells in the cervix

Trichomoniasis is another common infection affecting the vagina and cervix; it is also sexually transmitted and caused by a protozoan parasite.

Viral infections of the cervix are becoming more common, especially those due to the human papilloma or wart virus and the herpes simplex virus. These infections are sexually transmitted and are associated with warts or herpetic ulcers in other parts of the reproductive tract (see *Warts, genital; Herpes, genital*). Both have been linked to cancerous and precancerous conditions of the cervix.

TUMORS

Growths may be benign or malignant (cancerous). The former are usually present in the form of a polyp.

Malignant growths are always preceded by changes in the surface layer of cells, called cervical dysplasias. These changes can be detected by a cervical smear test and alert the gynecologist to the need for

possible further investigation and treatment to prevent a cancer from developing (see *Cervix, cancer of*).

OTHER DISORDERS

Mucus-forming cells typical of those usually found in the cervical canal may appear as a layer on the outer surface of the cervix, causing a tendency to bleed. This condition is readily treated (see *Cervical erosion*).

INVESTIGATION

Investigation is by means of an internal examination (see *Pelvic examination*), a *cervical smear test*, and, in cases of suspected cancer or a precancerous condition, a *colposcopy*.

or by *colposcopy* (inspection of the cervix with a viewing instrument). All sexually active women are advised to have a cervical smear test soon after their first experience of sexual intercourse, again six to 12 months later, and at intervals of approximately three years thereafter.

Diagnosis of more advanced stages may be made from a cervical smear, colposcopy, *cone biopsy*, or from a physician seeing areas of ulceration or cauliflowerlike growths on the cervix after symptoms are experienced.

TREATMENT

If a persistent area of abnormality or localized early cancer is diagnosed and can be seen in its entirety, destruction is by *electrocoagulation, diathermy,* or *laser treatment* (all of which use heat), or by *cryosurgery* (which uses cold). All methods except diathermy can usually be carried out painlessly under local anesthesia. Success rates for complete removal after one application of laser or diathermy are about 95 percent. If a woman is pregnant, treatment of pre-

cancerous conditions or early cancer is usually delayed until after delivery.

If an area of abnormality or cancer has spread into the cervical canal, close inspection of a cone biopsy may show that this procedure has removed all the diseased tissue. In all other cases of spreading cancer, treatment will depend on the extent of the spread, the age of the patient, and the physician's recommendation for surgery or *radiation therapy*.

In more advanced cases, when the tumor has spread to the organs of the pelvis, radiation therapy is given. In certain specialized centers, radical surgical techniques may be employed for selected patients, in which the bladder, vagina, cervix, uterus, and rectum may all be removed.

Survival rates (five or more years after treatment) are about 50 to 80 percent for early spreading cancer, whether treated by surgery or radiation therapy. For later-stage disease, survival rates drop to 10 to 30 percent, but improve to about 30 to 50 percent among those selected patients who undergo radical surgery.

Cesarean section

An operation to deliver a baby from the uterus through a vertical or horizontal incision in the abdomen. Cesarean section is performed when it is impossible or dangerous to deliver the baby vaginally. In the past 25 years the number of cesarean sections performed in Canada has risen from 6 percent to 18 percent of all births.

HOW IT IS DONE

The procedure for performing a cesarean section is shown in the illustrated box (see overleaf).

RECOVERY PERIOD

After the operation, the mother is given *analgesic drugs* (painkillers) as required. She is usually allowed to take fluids after 12 hours and to eat after 24 hours. The recovery period tends to be quicker if *epidural anesthesia* rather than general anesthesia (see *Anesthesia, general*) is used. Provided there are no problems, the usual hospital stay is around a week after the operation.

Cestodes

The scientific name for tapeworms—a group of long, flat, multisegmented parasites. (See *Tapeworm infestation*.)

Chagas' disease

An infectious parasitic disease found only in parts of South and Central America and spread by certain insects commonly called "cone-nosed" or "assassin" bugs. The disease is named after the Brazilian physician Carlos Chagas (1879-1934).

The parasites responsible for Chagas' disease are single-celled organisms called trypanosomes, very similar to those that cause *sleeping sickness* in Africa. They live in the bloodstream and can also affect the heart, intestines, and nervous system.

Symptoms include swelling of the lymph nodes and fever. Long-term complications include damage to the heart. Treatment is unsatisfactory. A drug called nifurtimox kills trypanosomes in the blood but has unpleasant side effects.

Chalazion

A round, painless swelling in the upper or lower eyelid, sometimes known as a meibomian cyst. The swelling is caused by obstruction of one of the meibomian glands that lubricate the edge of the eyelids. If the swelling is large, pressure on the cornea at the front of the eye can cause blurring of vision.

Chalazions can occur at any age and are particularly common in people suffering from the skin conditions *acne, rosacea,* or seborrheic *dermatitis*. If the cyst becomes infected, the eyelid becomes more swollen, red, and painful. About one third of chalazions disappear without any treatment, but large cysts usually need to be removed surgically (from behind the eyelid) under local anesthetic.

Chancre, hard

An ulcer, usually on the genitals, that develops during the first, or primary, stage of the sexually transmitted disease *syphilis*.

Chancroid

A sexually transmitted disease found mainly in the tropics; it is characterized by painful ulcers on the genitals and enlarged lymph nodes in the groin. Also known as soft chancre or soft sore, the disorder is caused by the bacterium HAEMOPHILUS DUCREYI.

The infection is very rare in Canada; most cases occur in sailors or travelers who have had contact with prostitutes in tropical countries.

Prompt treatment with *antibiotic drugs* is usually effective. If the disease is not treated, abscesses can form in the groin and leave deep scars.

Chapped skin

Sore, cracked, rough skin on areas that have been repeatedly wet, inadequately dried, or exposed to the cold. The hands and face (particularly the lips) are the most commonly affected areas.

Chapping occurs when the skin becomes excessively dry due to lack, or removal, of the natural oils that help keep it supple. This tends to happen in cold weather because the oil-secreting glands produce less oil. Repeated washing or wetting removes the oils.

A chalazion on the lower lid
Many small chalazions disappear spontaneously. Larger ones may require surgery.

Chapped skin can often be prevented by using protective gloves or *barrier creams* and by drying the skin carefully. Lanolin-based hand cream or face cream usually helps skin that is already chapped.

Character disorders

See *Personality disorders*.

Charcoal

A form of carbon. Charcoal is used as an adsorbent agent in the emergency treatment of some types of poisoning and drug overdose.

Charcot-Marie-Tooth disease

An inherited muscle-wasting disease that mainly affects the legs. (See *Peroneal muscular atrophy*.)

Charcot's joint

A joint damaged by injuries that have gone unnoticed because of loss of sensation affecting the joint. (See *Neuropathic joint*.)

Checkup

See *Examination, physical*.

Cheilitis

Inflammation, cracking, and dryness of the lips. Cheilitis can be caused by ill-fitting dentures, a local infection, allergy to cosmetics, too much sunbathing, or deficiency of riboflavin (vitamin B_2). In riboflavin deficiency, the corners of the mouth are chiefly affected. Until the underlying problem is remedied, a soothing skin cream will relieve the soreness.

Chelating agents

Chemicals used in the treatment of poisoning by metals such as lead, arsenic, and mercury. Chelating

C

PROCEDURE FOR A CESAREAN SECTION

A cesarean section allows delivery of a baby through a horizontal or vertical cut in the abdominal and uterine walls. The mother is given epidural anesthesia, so that she remains conscious during the procedure, or general anesthesia.

HOW IT IS DONE

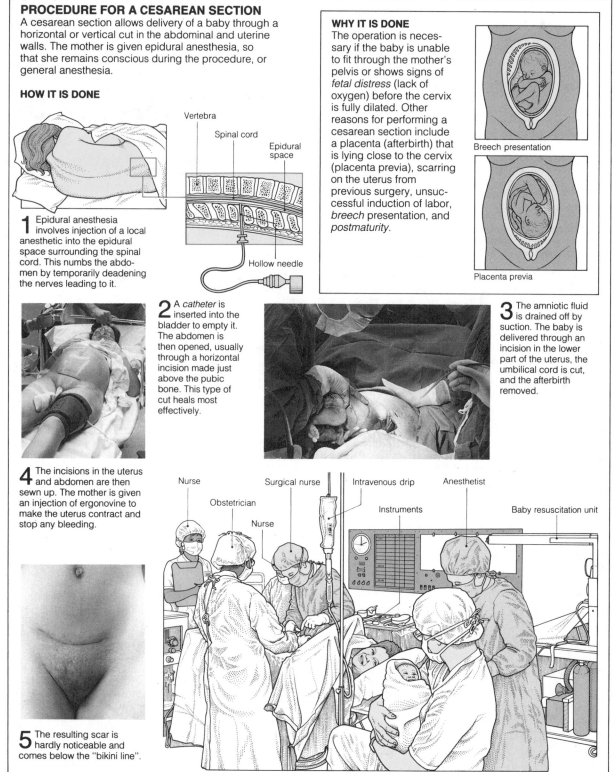

Vertebra

Spinal cord

Epidural space

Hollow needle

1 Epidural anesthesia involves injection of a local anesthetic into the epidural space surrounding the spinal cord. This numbs the abdomen by temporarily deadening the nerves leading to it.

2 A *catheter* is inserted into the bladder to empty it. The abdomen is then opened, usually through a horizontal incision made just above the pubic bone. This type of cut heals most effectively.

4 The incisions in the uterus and abdomen are then sewn up. The mother is given an injection of ergonovine to make the uterus contract and stop any bleeding.

5 The resulting scar is hardly noticeable and comes below the "bikini line".

WHY IT IS DONE

The operation is necessary if the baby is unable to fit through the mother's pelvis or shows signs of *fetal distress* (lack of oxygen) before the cervix is fully dilated. Other reasons for performing a cesarean section include a placenta (afterbirth) that is lying close to the cervix (placenta previa), scarring on the uterus from previous surgery, unsuccessful induction of labor, *breech* presentation, and *postmaturity*.

Breech presentation

Placenta previa

3 The amniotic fluid is drained off by suction. The baby is delivered through an incision in the lower part of the uterus, the umbilical cord is cut, and the afterbirth removed.

Nurse

Obstetrician

Nurse

Surgical nurse

Intravenous drip

Instruments

Anesthetist

Baby resuscitation unit

agents act by combining with these metals to form less poisonous substances. *Penicillamine* is a commonly used chelating agent.

Chemonucleolysis
The injection of the enzyme chymopapain into a prolapsed intervertebral disk (see *Disk prolapse*) that is pressing on spinal nerve roots, causing *sciatica*. The enzyme dissolves the soft center of the disk, causing it to shrink, thus relieving pressure. The procedure attracted initial enthusiasm but now seems to be less popular.

Chemotherapy
The treatment of infection or cancer by drugs that act selectively on the cause of the disorder. Drugs used in chemotherapy may also have substantial effects on normal tissue.

Infections are treated by *antibiotic drugs*, which may be bactericidal (killing bacteria) or bacteriostatic (stopping further bacterial growth and allowing the body's immune system to take over and destroy the bacteria). In the same way, *anticancer drugs* act either by destroying tumor cells or by stopping them from multiplying.

One problem with chemotherapy is that natural selection leads to the emergence of resistant bacteria or cells. This effect is minimized by the discriminatory use of antibiotics, and, in cancer chemotherapy, by giving several different types of anticancer drugs simultaneously.

A further problem with cancer chemotherapy is that the drugs act on all rapidly dividing cells, not just tumor cells. Thus, they may affect the bone marrow, the intestinal lining, the hair follicles, the ovaries and testes, and the mouth, sometimes causing severe side effects. Antibiotic drugs act selectively on bacterial cells, which have a different structure from human cells. Antibiotic chemotherapy therefore has generally less serious side effects than cancer chemotherapy.

Chenodeoxycholic acid
A chemical in *bile* that reduces the amount of *cholesterol* released by the *liver* into the bile.

Chenodeoxycholic acid is sometimes prescribed as a treatment for small *gallstones* if they contain mainly cholesterol and no calcium. Treatment takes several months, during which time progress is monitored by *X rays* or *ultrasound scanning* of the *gallbladder*. Chenodeoxycholic acid may cause diarrhea and, rarely, liver damage. It

DIAGNOSING CHEST PAIN
To make an accurate diagnosis of the underlying cause, it is important for the patient to describe the location, quality (e.g., burning, pressing, or sharp), severity, and duration of the pain, any factors that relieve it or make it worse, and any other symptoms, such as breathing difficulty. In addition, the physician will perform a physical examination, including listening to chest sounds with a stethoscope and feeling for areas of tenderness in the chest wall. He or she may also arrange for other diagnostic procedures to be carried out.

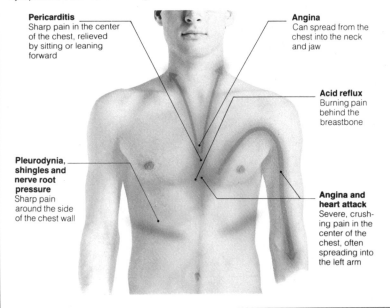

Pericarditis
Sharp pain in the center of the chest, relieved by sitting or leaning forward

Angina
Can spread from the chest into the neck and jaw

Acid reflux
Burning pain behind the breastbone

Pleurodynia, shingles and nerve root pressure
Sharp pain around the side of the chest wall

Angina and heart attack
Severe, crushing pain in the center of the chest, often spreading into the left arm

should not be taken during pregnancy lest it adversely affect the fetus.

Chest
The upper part of the trunk. Known technically as the *thorax*, the chest extends from the base of the neck down to the *diaphragm*.

Chest pain
Chest pain usually does not have a serious cause, although occasionally it may be a symptom of a disorder that requires medical attention. The pain may occur in the chest wall (in the skin, the underlying muscles, or the ribs) or in an organ within the chest.
CAUSES
The most common causes of pain in the chest wall are a strained muscle (which usually follows exercise) or an injury, such as bruising or a broken rib (due to a blow, fall, or other accident).

Pressure on a nerve root attached to the spinal cord may result in a sharp pain that travels to the front of the chest. This pain may be caused by *osteoarthritis* of, or injury to, the vertebrae, or, more rarely, a *disk prolapse*.

Pain in the side of the chest may be due to *pleurodynia* (inflammation of the muscles between the ribs and the diaphragm associated with a viral infection).

The viral infection *herpes zoster* (shingles) may cause pain in the chest wall. The pain, which is severe, runs along the course of a nerve and is followed by a rash of blisters in the *dermatome* (the area of skin supplied by that particular nerve).

In *Tietze's syndrome*, inflammation at the junctions of the rib cartilages causes pain on the front of the chest wall which increases with movements of the chest.

Within the chest, pain may be caused by *pleurisy* (inflammation of the pleurae, the membranes surrounding the lungs and covering the inner surface of the chest wall). The pleurisy itself may be brought on by *bronchitis*, *pneumonia*, or, rarely, by *pulmonary embolism* (a blood clot lodged in an artery in the lungs). The pain of pleurisy is worse when the sufferer breathes in.

Malignant tumors of the lung (see

CHEST PAIN Pain anywhere between the neck and the bottom of the rib-cage that may be dull and persistent, stabbing, burning, or crushing.

C

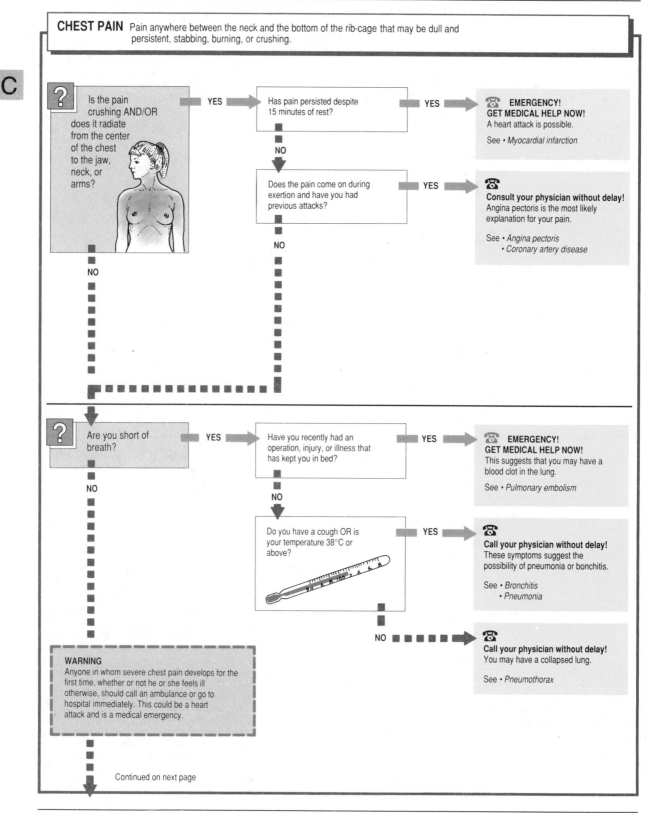

Is the pain crushing AND/OR does it radiate from the center of the chest to the jaw, neck, or arms?

YES → Has pain persisted despite 15 minutes of rest?

YES → ☎ **EMERGENCY! GET MEDICAL HELP NOW!** A heart attack is possible.

See • *Myocardial infarction*

NO

Does the pain come on during exertion and have you had previous attacks?

YES → ☎ **Consult your physician without delay!** Angina pectoris is the most likely explanation for your pain.

See • *Angina pectoris* • *Coronary artery disease*

NO

NO

Are you short of breath?

YES → Have you recently had an operation, injury, or illness that has kept you in bed?

YES → ☎ **EMERGENCY! GET MEDICAL HELP NOW!** This suggests that you may have a blood clot in the lung.

See • *Pulmonary embolism*

NO

NO

Do you have a cough OR is your temperature 38°C or above?

YES → ☎ **Call your physician without delay!** These symptoms suggest the possibility of pneumonia or bonchitis.

See • *Bronchitis* • *Pneumonia*

NO → ☎ **Call your physician without delay!** You may have a collapsed lung.

See • *Pneumothorax*

WARNING
Anyone in whom severe chest pain develops for the first time, whether or not he or she feels ill otherwise, should call an ambulance or go to hospital immediately. This could be a heart attack and is a medical emergency.

Continued on next page

C

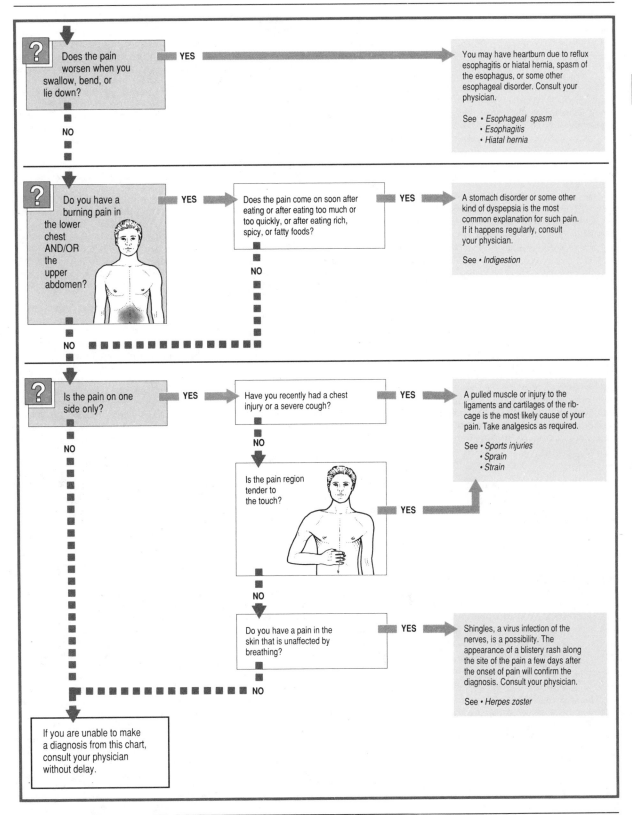

Does the pain worsen when you swallow, bend, or lie down?

YES → You may have heartburn due to reflux esophagitis or hiatal hernia, spasm of the esophagus, or some other esophageal disorder. Consult your physician.

See • *Esophageal spasm*
• *Esophagitis*
• *Hiatal hernia*

NO

Do you have a burning pain in the lower chest AND/OR the upper abdomen?

YES → Does the pain come on soon after eating or after eating too much or too quickly, or after eating rich, spicy, or fatty foods?

YES → A stomach disorder or some other kind of dyspepsia is the most common explanation for such pain. If it happens regularly, consult your physician.

See • *Indigestion*

NO

NO

Is the pain on one side only?

YES → Have you recently had a chest injury or a severe cough?

YES → A pulled muscle or injury to the ligaments and cartilages of the rib-cage is the most likely cause of your pain. Take analgesics as required.

See • *Sports injuries*
• *Sprain*
• *Strain*

NO

Is the pain region tender to the touch?

YES →

NO

Do you have a pain in the skin that is unaffected by breathing?

YES → Shingles, a virus infection of the nerves, is a possibility. The appearance of a blistery rash along the site of the pain a few days after the onset of pain will confirm the diagnosis. Consult your physician.

See • *Herpes zoster*

NO

NO

If you are unable to make a diagnosis from this chart, consult your physician without delay.

C

Lung cancer; Mesothelioma) may cause pain as they grow and press on the pleura and ribs.

Acid reflux (regurgitation of acid stomach fluid into the esophagus) may lead to heartburn, a burning pain behind the sternum. Heartburn may also be a symptom of *hiatal hernia*.

Various heart disorders can cause chest pain. Most common of these is *angina pectoris*, which is due to the heart muscle receiving too little blood (and therefore oxygen), commonly as a result of *coronary artery disease*. The pain, which resembles that of severe indigestion or of a heavy weight pressing on the chest, is felt in the center of the chest and may spread outward to the throat, jaw, or arms (usually the left one). It usually occurs when the work load of the heart muscle is increased by exertion, and is relieved by rest.

Myocardial infarction (damage to the heart muscle due to an inadequate blood supply) produces pain in the same areas as angina but the pain is more severe and persistent.

The pain of acute *pericarditis* (inflammation of the membrane that surrounds the heart) is also felt in the center of the chest and it may be severe enough to resemble the pain of a heart attack. It can often be relieved by leaning forward. Acute pericarditis is rare and tends to occur in young adults after or with a viral infection.

Mitral valve prolapse has been associated with many symptoms, including chest pain. The chest pain may be sharp and left-sided.

Chest pain may also be a result of anxiety and emotional stress. (See *Hyperventilation; Panic attack*.)

INVESTIGATION AND TREATMENT

Chest pain not associated with a trivial cause (such as bruising from a minor injury) should receive medical attention. Whether or not emergency treatment is necessary depends on the type and location of the pain and on the accompanying symptoms.

The treatment of chest pain depends on the underlying cause. For example, antibiotics may be prescribed for chest pain caused by pneumonia, and surgery may be necessary for the treatment of a malignant lung tumor or for some cases of coronary artery disease. (See also *Chest pain* symptom chart on preceding pages.)

Chest X ray

One of the most frequently performed medical tests, usually carried out to examine the heart or lungs. The proce-

dure is simple, quick, and painless, and is normally performed on an outpatient basis. Mobile equipment means that it can also be used (although somewhat less accurately) at the bedside of patients in hospital, and in patients' homes.

WHY IT IS DONE

Chest X rays are usually used to confirm a diagnosis in patients suspected of having a heart disorder, such as enlargement of a heart chamber, or a lung disease, such as tuberculosis or lung cancer.

HOW IT IS DONE

The X ray stand holds a film in a large, flat cassette positioned at chest level. The patient stands between the film and the X ray machine, facing the film cassette with the chest touching it and the chin projecting over the top. The hands are placed on the hips and the elbows swung forward, to move the shoulder blades to the side so that they do not obscure the lungs. A lead apron or screen protects the lower half of the body from radiation.

The patient takes (and holds) a deep breath while the technician operates equipment that passes X rays for a fraction of a second through the upper trunk from the back. The resultant X-ray picture provides an image not only of the heart and lungs but of major blood vessels, bones, and joints. (See also *X rays*.)

Cheyne-Stokes respiration

An abnormal pattern of breathing in which the rate and depth of respiration vary rhythmically. Deep, rapid breathing gradually becomes slower and shallower until breathing actually stops for some 10 to 20 seconds. Respiration then resumes, with deep, rapid breathing, and the cycle repeats itself. Each cycle lasts a few minutes.

Cheyne-Stokes respiration may be caused by disease or malfunctioning of the part of the brain that controls breathing (as occurs in some cases of *stroke, head injury, metabolic disorder*, or drug overdose). It may also occur as a result of *heart failure* and in some healthy people at high altitudes, especially during sleep.

Chickenpox

A common and mild infectious disease of childhood, characterized by a rash and slight fever. It is sometimes called varicella. Chickenpox is rare in adults; when it does occur it usually takes a more severe form.

INCIDENCE AND CAUSE

Throughout the world, most people

have had chickenpox by the age of 10. The disease is caused by the varicella-zoster virus. Although an attack confers lifelong immunity, the virus remains dormant within nerve tissues after the attack and may reappear later in life to cause *herpes zoster* (shingles).

The virus is spread from person to person in airborne droplets. Patients are highly infectious from about two days before the rash appears until about a week after.

In most children, chickenpox is no more than an inconvenience. However, adults who have never had the disease should avoid it by staying away from children with chickenpox and also from anyone with shingles. Women in the final stage of pregnancy should be particularly careful, since the disease may be serious in pregnancy and the newborn child may develop a severe attack.

SYMPTOMS

Two to three weeks after infection, a rash appears behind the ears, in the armpits, on the trunk, upper arms, and legs, inside the mouth, and sometimes in the trachea (windpipe) and bronchial tubes, causing a dry cough. The rash comes in crops appearing after 12 to 48 hours and consists of clusters of small, red, itchy spots that become fluid-filled blisters, 2 to 3 mm in diameter, within a few hours. After several days the blisters dry out and form scabs. Children usually have only a slightly raised temperature, but an adult may have severe *pneumonia* with breathing difficulties and fever. Those taking *immunosuppressant drugs* are more susceptible to a severe form of the disease. Rarely, *encephalitis* (inflammation of the brain) occurs as a complication.

DIAGNOSIS AND TREATMENT

Diagnosis is usually obvious from a simple examination of the patient. In most cases, rest is all that is needed for a complete recovery, which usually takes place within 10 days in children, but over a longer period in adults.

Acetaminophen can be taken to reduce fever, and *calamine* lotion relieves the itchiness of the rash. In severe cases, *acyclovir* (an antiviral drug) may be prescribed for the patient, but it must be used early in the course of the disease.

Children should be discouraged from scratching the blisters, which could lead to secondary bacterial infection and so to scarring (keeping the child's nails short is a good idea).

Specific antivaricella-zoster *immunoglobulin* has been used to prevent outbreaks in nurseries. Experimental *vaccines* have been tried but so far their use has been confined to high-risk groups such as children on treatment for leukemia.

Chigoe

 A painful, itchy, pea-sized swelling caused by a sand flea (also called the jigger or burrowing flea). When stepped on, the flea penetrates into the skin of the feet, under the toenails, or between the toes.

The chigoe flea lives in sandy soil only in Africa and tropical America. The burrowing fleas are pregnant females, which lay their eggs under the skin.

Avoidance involves wearing shoes or sandals outdoors in tropical countries (this also protects against *hookworms*). In the event of a suspected chigoe infestation, consult a physician. Chigoe fleas should be removed with a sterile needle and the wounds treated with an antiseptic.

Chilblain

An itchy, purple-red swelling, usually on a toe or finger, caused by excessive constriction (narrowing) of small blood vessels below the surface of the skin in cold weather.

Chilblains are most common in the young and the elderly, and women are more susceptible than men. Chilblains generally heal without treatment; talcum powder may partially relieve itching. People susceptible to chilblains can help prevent them by keeping their feet and hands warm in cold weather.

Child abuse

Any form of physical or emotional mistreatment or mismanagement of a child, by acts or omissions that cause actual or potential harm to the child's health, well-being or development, or expose the child to unnecessary risk or suffering. Child abuse includes the use of a child for sexual purposes.

Cases of child abuse today are coming to light with increasing frequency, probably not just because such abuse may be more widespread, but also because there is a greater awareness of the problem. Nurses, physicians, teachers, and other professionals who deal with children are now legally required to report child abuse cases that come to their attention.

Child abuse occurs at all levels of society. The problem appears to be more common in lower socioeco-

nomic groups, possibly because of the greater stress on unsupported families with poor living standards. However, child abuse may be less easily recognized in higher socioeconomic groups.

The person injuring the child is usually a parent, but may be a stepparent, a parental friend or lover, a guardian, or a sibling.

CAUSES

Being deprived or ill-treated when young seems to predispose people to abuse their own children by repeating the pattern of their own experience. This is particularly likely if the abused people have become parents at an early age, when they are too immature and inexperienced to cope with the stress and demands made on them by a young child. *Alcohol dependence, drug dependence,* or emotional disturbances are other causative factors, since they may lessen a parent's self-control.

A child born following an unwanted pregnancy may be at increased risk of abuse, as may a child whose *bonding* relationship with the mother was disturbed at birth.

Children under 3 years old are at greatest risk of physical abuse or emotional abuse because they are very demanding and are not old enough to be reasoned with.

PHYSICAL ABUSE

Physical injury is the most readily recognized form of abuse. Its incidence has been estimated at 6 percent, but most experts in the field think it is much higher. Physical abuse covers a wide range of behaviors from failure to adequately protect a child from risks and hazards to excessive or extreme discipline.

Inflicting injury on a child is most often an impulsive act, the result of a sudden loss of temper. Infants and toddlers may be picked up and shaken vigorously, which can damage the eyes and rupture blood vessels in the brain, and eventually cause severe brain damage. Slaps or punches are usually delivered to the head, resulting in black eyes and other facial bruises, cuts on the inner lip, and bone fractures.

Some injuries are inflicted deliberately as mistaken or unnecessarily severe acts of discipline. For example, a parent may try to teach a child not to play with fire by burning the child with a cigarette. Such injuries present different characteristics from injuries that occur accidentally and may reveal to a pediatrician or other examiner that, whatever the reason given for

them by the parents, deliberate infliction is the real cause.

Premeditated, repeated physical assault is rare. When it does occur, it is a sign that a parent is severely disturbed and that the risks to the child are grave. These types of assault can lead to multiple fractures, damage to internal organs, and even to death. Such abuse is sometimes accompanied by deliberate neglect, with no attempt made to feed or clothe the child adequately.

Physical abuse may also take the form of giving drugs to a child—for example, to sedate an overactive toddler or sometimes to poison a child deliberately. Addictive drugs are also sometimes given, with obvious risks.

A child with serious injuries may be admitted to hospital for full examination. The Children's Aid Society (CAS), with legal and police cooperation, can intervene to assess the situation in an effort to protect the child and ensure his or her safety. The CAS may obtain a court order, if it deems this necessary, and remove the child from the home.

The child's interests remain paramount, but the parents, who may be under great stress, should be treated sympathetically.

EMOTIONAL ABUSE OR NEGLECT

Neglect of physical and emotional needs, such as love, stimulation, and guidance, is another form of abuse which courts have recognized only more recently. Such abuse is often unintentional, arising from the parents' lack of understanding of their child's needs. The parents may themselves be emotionally disturbed and require psychiatric help.

Indications that a child is being emotionally abused include failure to thrive, slow development, poor learning ability, and lack of normal emotional responses. Emotionally deprived children are often insecure, have poor self-esteem, and find it difficult to relate to others.

The diagnosis is usually confirmed when the child begins to improve in terms of health, growth, and development after appropriate intervention. Management of the situation is aimed at the family as a whole and is the same as for physical abuse.

SEXUAL ABUSE

Sexual abuse can be defined as the use of a child for the sexual gratification of an adult. Sexual abuse of children has been increasingly recognized in recent years. Most frequently, sexual abuse occurs within the family; usually the victim is a girl, although adolescent boys may also be at risk. Sexual exploitation of both sexes occurs in pornography and prostitution.

Most cases of sexual abuse consist of a father, close relative, or family friend taking advantage of a girl's affection to obtain sexual gratification from her. This form of abuse is usually secretive, because of the man's awareness of the gravity of the offense, and is morally coercive, because of the power he holds over the girl.

Sexual abuse may come to light because of an obvious complaint from the child, a relative, or friend, or the child may display disturbed behavior or have symptoms of a *sexually transmitted disease*. Police, psychiatrists, and social workers usually cooperate in managing the problem, the main aims being to prevent further sexual abuse and to rehabilitate the child through therapy.

Childbed fever

See *Puerperal fever*.

Childbirth

The process by which an infant moves from the uterus to the outside world. Childbirth normally occurs at between 38 and 42 weeks' gestation (pregnancy), timed from the mother's last normal menstrual period.

For most women in developed countries, who receive proper medical care during pregnancy (see *Prenatal care*) and delivery, childbirth presents no serious problems. In developing countries, however, the number of women who die from childbirth remains high (see *Maternal mortality*).

Specialized equipment and the availability of *blood transfusions* and *antibiotic drugs* have made childbirth much safer for mother and baby. However, increased concern among women that childbirth has become overmechanized in many hospitals has led to the popularity of "natural childbirth," which advocates the avoidance of unnecessary medical intervention. Many hospitals now recognize the right of women to choose the type of birth they would like, provided their wishes are compatible with safety. Women are encouraged to make "birth plans" with their obstetricians and to discuss matters such as possible methods of pain relief and preferred positions during delivery.

ONSET OF LABOR

It is often difficult to know when labor has started. During the last three months of pregnancy the uterus starts to contract in preparation for the birth, and these *Braxton Hicks' contractions* may be mistaken for the start of labor. However, when contractions become progressively more painful, regular, and at shorter intervals, then labor has probably started. Two other events may also happen. The mucous plug that has blocked the cervical canal during pregnancy may be expelled as a bloody discharge. This is called a "show" and means that the cervix is beginning to stretch. Rupture of the membranes that surround the amniotic fluid in which the baby floats may occur at any time up to delivery. The leakage of amniotic fluid, called "breaking of the waters," varies from woman to woman. It may be a slow trickle of fluid from the vagina, or it may be a sudden gush.

STAGES OF LABOR

Labor is divided into three stages (see illustrated box on facing page for details). The first stage covers the period from the onset of labor until the woman's cervix is fully dilated. The second stage lasts from full dilatation of the cervix until delivery of the baby. The third stage lasts from delivery of the baby until the placenta (afterbirth) has been expelled.

Childbirth, complications of

Difficulties and complications occurring after the onset of labor. These complications may be associated with the mother or the baby, or both. Some are potentially life-threatening, particularly to the baby, because they may impair its oxygen supply and cause brain damage (see *Fetal distress*).

MATERNAL PROBLEMS

If contractions begin, or if the membranes rupture, before 37 weeks' gestation, premature labor may occur, with the risk of delivery of a small, immature baby who may not be developed adequately to survive (see *Prematurity*). Drugs such as salbutamol or ritodrine can sometimes stop premature labor. However, if the gestation is more than 34 weeks and hospital conditions are suitable, or if other complications are present, it may be safer to allow labor to progress. Premature rupture of the membranes can also lead to infection in the uterus; the baby must be delivered as soon as possible and the infection treated with *antibiotic drugs*.

Slow progress early in a normal labor is most often the result of failure of the cervix to dilate, usually due to inadequate contractions of the uterine muscles. This problem is often treated by giving intravenous infusions of synthetic *oxytocin* to augment the naturally occurring oxytocin that causes the muscles of the uterus to contract during labor.

The mother may tire during a long labor so that she is unable to push strongly enough, or the muscular contractions of the uterus may be ineffective; in these cases, *forceps delivery*, *vacuum extraction*, or even *cesarean section* may be required.

A major hazard in childbirth is blood loss. Bleeding before labor (*antepartum hemorrhage*) or during labor (intrapartum hemorrhage) may be due to premature separation of the placenta from the wall of the uterus. Less commonly, it arises because of a condition called *placenta previa* in which the placenta lies over the cervical opening instead of being attached to the uterine wall.

Blood loss after the delivery (*postpartum hemorrhage*) is usually due either to failure of the uterus to contract normally after the birth or to retention of part of the placenta. With blood transfusions now a relatively commonplace procedure, complications from hemorrhage have decreased dramatically in the last 40 years.

In rare instances, women suffer from *eclampsia* (convulsions associated with raised blood pressure) during or just prior to the onset of labor. If eclampsia occurs, it is treated by giving *anticonvulsant drugs* and oxygen, and by inducing labor or performing a cesarean section.

FETAL PROBLEMS

If the baby is in a *malposition* (not lying in the normal head-down position in the uterus), vaginal delivery may be difficult or impossible. A baby in the breech position (bottom downward) can be delivered vaginally, although delivery by cesarean section may be preferable (see *Breech delivery*). A baby lying horizontally is always delivered by cesarean section because the arm and shoulder usually become jammed in the pelvis.

Multiple pregnancies (see *Pregnancy, multiple*) may be a problem during delivery because it is often difficult to predict the position of the second or subsequent babies. It is also more likely that such babies will be born prematurely.

FETAL-MATERNAL PROBLEMS

Sometimes the mother's pelvis is too small in proportion to the baby's head (a condition known as cephalopelvic disproportion), making vaginal deliv-

STAGES OF BIRTH

At the onset of labor, painful and regular contractions begin and the cervix starts to dilate. The mother is usually examined vaginally every two to four hours to assess the extent of dilation. The duration of labor depends on several factors, but primarily on whether it is a first or subsequent baby. *Fetal heart monitoring* is often performed, and the frequency, strength, and duration of the mother's contractions are recorded. During the second stage contractions become stronger and the woman feels the urge to push; however, she is advised to push only during a contraction. Once delivered, the baby is usually placed on the mother's abdomen, but may first be warmed, dried, and checked by a physician.

ELECTRONIC FETAL MONITORING

This may be carried out if the fetus is at risk, or as a routine procedure. The detecting device is linked to a monitoring machine.

Printout

Fetal heart rate

Uterine contractions

Detecting devices

Here, the baby's heartbeat is picked up by a metal plate strapped to the mother's abdomen (lower belt). A plate beneath the upper belt detects the mother's contractions.

An alternative method is to attach to the baby's head an electrode linked to the monitor by a wire led through the mother's vagina.

THE FIRST STAGE

With the first contractions, the normally thick, tough cervix becomes thinned and softened and is gradually pulled up until it becomes effaced (merged with the walls of the uterus). The cervix then begins to dilate (open) with each contraction. It is fully dilated when the opening is approximately 10 cm in diameter. This stage can take 12 hours or more for first babies, but only a few hours for subsequent babies.

Uterus

Cervix

The head emerges
At this point, an episiotomy is sometimes performed to prevent tissues from tearing.

THE SECOND STAGE

As the baby's head descends, it reaches the pelvic floor muscles, which cause the head to rotate until eventually the baby's chin is pointing down to the woman's rectum. As the baby is pushed farther down, the anus and perineum (the area between the genitalia and anus) begin to bulge out, and soon the baby's head can be seen at the opening of the vagina. As the head emerges, the perineal tissues are stretched very thin; sometimes it is necessary to perform an *episiotomy* to prevent the tissues from tearing. As soon as the baby's head emerges, it turns so that it is once more in line with the baby's body; the physician usually helps this rotation.

With the next few contractions, first one shoulder and then the other is delivered; then the rest of the baby slides out. After delivery, the umbilical cord is clamped and cut.

Delivery of the baby
Once both shoulders are out, the rest of the baby emerges easily.

THE THIRD STAGE

Within three to 10 minutes after the baby's birth, the placenta (afterbirth) is usually expelled. Drugs such as ergonovine or oxytocin may be used to aid in its expulsion, or the placenta may have to be manually removed by an obstetrician. Any tears or incisions are cleaned and stitched. This may be done while the mother holds her baby.

Placenta

Umbilical cord

Placenta being delivered
The placenta is usually expelled a few minutes after the baby's birth.

FIRST AID: EMERGENCY CHILDBIRTH

PREPARING FOR THE BIRTH

1 Summon medical help and reassure the mother. Stay calm—most births are normal and natural.

2 Wash hands and scrub nails under running water. Do not dry them. Wash hands frequently during the birth. Make sure everything you use is clean: bedding, sheets, towels, and cloths.

3 Prepare a flat surface, using a clean sheet or towel, a plastic sheet, or fresh newspaper.

4 Prop the mother up with pillows. Her legs should be bent and apart, and the feet flat.

WARNING
DO NOT attempt to delay the birth by crossing the mother's legs or pushing in the baby's head. This is very harmful.

YOU WILL NEED
- Sterilized scissors (boil for 10 minutes and wrap in clean cloth).
- Clean pieces of string, boot laces, or strips of cloth about 22 cm long for tying the cord.
- Container in case the mother vomits.
- Container or plastic bag for the afterbirth (which must be taken to a physician for examination).
- Sanitary towels or clean cloth to place over the mother's vagina after the birth.
- Cradle (or a box or drawer) and soft blanket for the baby.

1 As the baby's head emerges, support it with cupped hands. If a membrane covers the face, tear it with your hands and remove quickly. If the cord is looped around the neck, ease it gently over the head. DO NOT touch the baby's head until it is out.

2 Support the shoulders as they emerge. One appears first, the second follows easily if you carefully raise the head. DO NOT pull on the baby's head.

3 Support the body as it comes out. Using a clean cloth, wipe away any mucus or blood from the baby's mouth.

4 If the baby fails to breathe immediately, hold the head lower than the body to drain mucus away. DO NOT slap the baby on the back. Blow hard on the chest or tap the soles of the feet. If these methods fail, start *artificial respiration*.

5 When the cord has stopped pulsating, tie it firmly once 15 to 20 cm away from the baby and again 5 to 10 cm away. Cut between the ties with sterilized scissors. Wrap the baby and place him or her on the mother's abdomen.

6 The afterbirth is delivered within 10 minutes. To help control blood flow, place a hand on the mother's abdomen and gently massage the uterus every few minutes until it feels firm. DO NOT pull on the cord to deliver the afterbirth.

ery impossible or hazardous. In these cases, delivery by cesarean section is usually necessary.

Childbirth, natural

The avoidance of unnecessary medical intervention during the delivery of a baby, especially the use of relaxation techniques as a means of coping with pain and minimizing the use of drugs during labor.

Natural childbirth techniques are taught by a number of organizations. Classes are taught by obstetricians, midwives, or other qualified childbirth educators. Pregnant women and their partners usually attend classes during the last three months of the pregnancy. Involvement of the partner is an important feature of the natural childbirth method.

The primary purpose of the classes is to teach relaxation techniques, often using breathing exercises, to help women cope with the pain of uterine contractions. Relaxation techniques help a mother to be aware of muscle tension and to relax during labor. Involvement of the woman's partner helps him to provide full encouragement and support during labor.

The classes also supply information about female anatomy, the physiology of pregnancy, fetal development, labor, delivery, and the postnatal period. Other topics (such as nutrition, breast-feeding, and parental skills) are also covered.

Child development

Children acquire physical, mental, and social skills in well-recognized stages called developmental milestones. Although there is wide variation in the rate at which each child progresses, most children develop certain skills by a predictable age (see illustrated box overleaf).

FACTORS AFFECTING DEVELOPMENT

A child becomes capable of developing certain skills only as his or her nervous system matures. The time taken for maturity to develop is determined genetically for each individual and modified by environmental factors in the uterus and after birth. For instance, girls often begin to walk and/or talk at an earlier age than boys. Premature children miss out on some growing time in the uterus; the time they take to progress should be calculated from the full-term pregnancy date, not the actual date of birth.

Sight and hearing are both crucial to a child's general developmental progress; any defect will affect the child's ability to watch, listen, learn, and imitate. Intelligence also affects a child's development, especially in the acquisition of speech and the ability to coordinate muscles for precise movements, such as holding a pencil.

The home environment plays an important part in developing the child's potential for certain skills. Speaking to and playing with children is essential for language development and for practicing new physical skills. Introducing children to other children at the age of 2 or 3 years provides them with plenty of stimulation.

HOW A CHILD DEVELOPS SKILLS

Reflex actions present at birth (see *Reflex, primitive*) gradually disappear as the child learns to perform voluntary actions and develops sufficient muscle strength and control to perform them. Often, the child's actions progress from seemingly unconnected movements to the ability to control part of his or her body. In most children, development begins with control of the head and progresses down the body until control of the arms, trunk, and legs is attained. Walking is achieved in numerous stages, from lying with the head raised, to sitting unsupported, crawling, standing unsupported, toddling, and, finally, walking unaided.

A baby begins to develop hand-eye coordination from birth. He or she watches objects, learns to focus and judge distances, and develops the connection of seeing and doing by watching his or her hands. Both hand-eye and body-limb coordination can be encouraged in an older child (by practicing ball games, for example).

At birth, a child communicates his or her needs by crying. Once vision and hearing are sufficiently developed, a child watches the parent's mouth intently to learn how to smile and listens to the parent speaking before attempting to imitate sounds. A child is able to concentrate on learning only one skill at a time, often forgetting a recently mastered skill that will appear again some time in the future.

DEVELOPMENTAL MILESTONES

When assessing the development of a child, specialists in child development look at abilities in four main areas: locomotion; hearing and speech; vision and fine movement; and social behavior and play. All children acquire skills in much the same order—for example, a child will not stand before learning to sit. The rate at which these skills are acquired varies enormously; a more detailed professional investigation is necessary only if a child's progress is significantly slower than average or if the parent is concerned for some other reason (see *Developmental delay*).

Child guidance

A multidisciplinary diagnosis and advice team service for a child who is suffering from emotional or *behavioral problems*. These may include poor school performance, disruptive or

C

PAIN RELIEF IN LABOR AND DELIVERY

Method	Why given	Possible effects on baby
Narcotic analgesics	Routine pain relief during labor	Less responsive at birth; respiratory problems, particularly in premature babies
Epidural	Routine pain relief during labor and childbirth, forceps delivery, and cesarean section	Brief drop in fetal heart rate; fetal monitoring is recommended during and after the procedure
Paracervical block	Pain relief during active labor (after the fetal head is engaged)	Drop in fetal heart rate; respiratory problems
Pudendal block	Forceps delivery	None
Local anesthetic into perineum	Forceps delivery, episiotomy, and repair of perineal tear	None
General anesthesia	Cesarean section	Reduced responsiveness at birth; respiratory problems, particularly in premature babies

CHILD DEVELOPMENT

LOCOMOTION

By 6 months, babies lift up their heads and chests and roll from front to back and from back to front. They can sit up with support, bounce up and down, and bear weight on their legs if supported.

9-month-old children try to crawl, sit without support, pull themselves up to standing or sitting positions, and step purposefully on alternate feet if supported.

1-year-old children crawl on hands and knees, walk around furniture (holding on), and may walk alone or with one hand held.

At 18 months, children can walk well with feet closer together, can stoop to pick up objects, run with care, walk upstairs with one hand held, and crawl backward downstairs.

VISION AND FINE MOVEMENT

By 6 months, babies look intently at everything and everybody. They follow moving objects with their eyes and reach out for objects with one or both hands. Objects are transferred from hand to hand and brought to the mouth.

9-month-olds are visually very alert. Grasp involves mostly the index and middle fingers. They can manipulate objects with both hands, but have difficulty voluntarily releasing grasped objects.

1-year-old children can grasp small objects well and release grasped objects easily. Both hands are used equally. They can hold a block in each hand and bang the blocks together.

At 18 months, children can build a tower of three blocks (when shown), enjoy turning pages of a book, can grip a crayon, scribble, and make dots. They may use one hand more than the other.

HEARING, UNDERSTANDING, AND SPEECH

By 6 months, babies turn their heads to locate sources of sound and have begun to understand the tone of their mother's voice. They enjoy making vowel sounds and tuneful noises. They laugh, chuckle, and squeal.

9-month-olds listen to sounds and understand "no" and other words. They babble in long strings (making sounds such as ba-ba, da-da, ma-ma) and start using sound to attract attention. (Deaf babies' utterances are monotonous and do not develop in complexity.)

1-year-old children turn when they hear their own names. They have some understanding of how other people feel, know what most household objects are used for, may babble meaningfully to themselves, and may say two or three words.

At 18 months, children comprehend short communications spoken directly to them, but do not understand the difference between statements, commands, and questions. Vocabulary may contain six to 20 words.

SOCIAL BEHAVIOR AND PLAY

6-month-olds enjoy looking at their images in mirrors and playing peekaboo games. They can grasp objects and also shake, bang, and otherwise manipulate them. However, they will not look for objects that are shown and then hidden. They are shy with strangers.

9-month-olds look for objects that are shown and then hidden, thus showing the beginnings of memory. They imitate hand clapping, wave bye-bye, and show great determination in getting objects. They continue to be shy with strangers.

1-year-old children spend less time putting objects in their mouths and more time releasing objects—throwing them, dropping them, putting them in boxes. They play pat-a-cake and like to be around a familiar adult to whom they demonstrate affection.

At 18 months, children actively explore their homes. They enjoy putting things in and taking things out of boxes and looking at picture books. They use spoons and cups and can take off their shoes and socks. They are also determined, impetuous, selfish, and cannot be reasoned with. They alternate between clinging to a familiar adult and struggling to break free.

C

LOCOMOTION

2-year-olds climb furniture and walk up and down stairs (with two feet to each step).

3-year-olds can climb with agility, throw and kick balls, ride tricycles, and run around corners.

4-year-olds walk up and down stairs with one foot on each step, and can stand, walk, and run on tiptoe.

5-year-olds can stand and hop on one foot, and are skillful in rolling, sliding, and swinging.

VISION AND FINE MOVEMENT

2-year-olds can build towers of six or seven blocks, can unscrew a lid, and show a definite right- or left-handedness.

3-year-olds hold crayons with an adult grasp and can undo buttons, but may need help buttoning them up. Their handedness is clearly established.

4-year-olds hold a pencil with a mature grasp, can copy simple letters (i.e., O,T,H, or V), and can build a tower of more than 10 blocks.

5-year-olds can match 10 or 12 colors, can copy many more letters, and can draw the full body of a person with a recognizable head and facial features.

HEARING, UNDERSTANDING, AND SPEECH

2-year-olds begin to listen to general conversation. They obey simple instructions and can use 50 or more words meaningfully. They constantly talk to themselves and can put two or more words together to communicate.

3-year-olds listen to general conversation and enjoy nursery stories. They understand the difference between statements, commands, and questions. They have large vocabularies and speak clearly in sentences, but there may be some errors.

4-year-olds can repeat softly spoken words at a distance of 1 m. They speak fluently and with correct grammar, and can provide their full names, ages, and addresses. They tell long stories, confusing fact and fantasy.

5-year-olds enjoy reciting rhymes, telling stories, and having books read to them.

SOCIAL BEHAVIOR AND PLAY

2-year-olds ask the names of everything and enjoy participating in nursery rhymes and songs. They ask for food and drink and indicate toilet needs. They begin to play with toys more imaginatively, though they may not like to share them. They are constantly demanding and will throw tantrums if their desires are thwarted.

3-year-olds constantly ask questions. They can dress and undress and eat with a fork and spoon. They are dry and clean during the day and sometimes at night. Three-year-olds can play with toys imaginatively and will share with others. They can be reasoned with and have fewer tantrums. They are also more affectionate to younger siblings.

4-year-olds continue to ask questions constantly. They are more independent and skillful in dressing, undressing, eating, and washing. They need to play with other children and can share with others. They can understand past, present, and future.

5-year-olds ask the meaning of abstract words. They like to build complex structures out of bricks or other objects. They continue in imaginative and dramatic play. They enjoy companionship and understand the need for rules and fair play. They have an understanding of time and are generally sensible, restrained, and independent.

C

withdrawn behavior at school or at home, aggressive or violent acts, breaking the law, or *drug abuse.*

SOURCES OF HELP

Trained professionals from a number of disciplines offer help to such children and their families. A physician will arrange referral to the most appropriate team for assessment and, possibly, therapy.

Psychiatrists are medical physicians with a special interest and training in the field of mental problems. Their techniques may range from *psychotherapy* to treatment with drugs. The latter are rarely used.

Clinical and educational *psychologists* are nonmedical specialists whose main role is diagnosis and assessment by means of intelligence and personality tests. They may also assess a child's progress during treatment. Many clinical psychologists also provide psychotherapy.

Psychiatric social workers are also nonmedical specialists. They are specially trained to deal with family problems and relationships within the family. In some instances they may be given legal responsibility for children who have severe personality or family problems.

These specialists often work closely together, either in hospital pediatric departments, schools, or special child-guidance clinics.

HOW IT IS DONE

Various methods of assessment and therapy may be employed, depending on the age of the child and the particular problem involved. For young children, *play therapy* may be used for diagnosis, by observing the child's behavior during play, and also for therapy, by providing an environment in which the child can express his or her emotions freely.

For older children, *counseling* or psychotherapy may be tried. For the child who has fallen behind in schoolwork or is thought to have a learning disability, examination of intellectual performance may be required before corrective action is taken.

Group therapy may be used as a means of helping older children. Various interactions develop within a group and, under the guidance of a professionally qualified group leader, these interactions can be examined and discussed to help children gain insight into their problems.

Family therapy may be used in cases where there are conflicts and difficulties between the child and one or both parents.

Chill

A shivering attack accompanied by chattering teeth, pale skin, goose pimples, and feeling cold. Chill frequently precedes a *fever*. Repeated or severe shivering suggests serious illness and a physician should be consulted.

Chinese medicine

Most of the various techniques of traditional Chinese medicine are based on the theory that there is a universal life-force, called chi, which manifests itself in the body as two complementary qualities known as yin and yang. According to traditional beliefs, the vigorous yang and restraining yin must be balanced, and the chi must flow evenly for good health. An imbalance in the yin and yang and disruption of the flow of chi in the body produce illness.

The traditional Chinese treatments therefore aim to restore the yin-yang balance and normalize the flow of chi. To achieve this aim various techniques have evolved over the centuries, notably *acupressure, acupuncture,* Chinese *herbalism,* and *t'ai chi.*

In general, these treatments are incompatible with orthodox Western medicine and most physicians do not recommend them. However, some techniques may help when standard treatment has not been effective.

Chinese restaurant syndrome

A short-lived illness that some people develop after eating food containing *monosodium glutamate* (MSG). Only about 5 percent of the population is susceptible to it.

Monosodium glutamate is present naturally in some foods, such as soya beans and some types of seaweed, that are frequently used in Chinese cooking. The substance is also used as a flavor-enhancing *food additive* in many types of "fast foods."

SYMPTOMS AND PREVENTION

The most common symptoms, which usually occur within three hours of a meal, are pain in the neck and chest, palpitations of the heart, feeling hot, and headache. Nausea, dizziness, and other symptoms have also been reported, and some people compare Chinese restaurant syndrome to the effects of migraine.

The symptoms pass and have no long-term effects. Affected people should avoid food containing MSG as an additive.

Chiropody

See *Podiatry.*

Chiropractic

A healing profession based on the theory that disease and pain are due to abnormal nerve function secondary to improper relationships between the nerves and the joints, especially in the spinal column. Chiropractors attempt to restore or maintain health by *manipulation,* primarily of the spinal column and pelvis.

Some physicians believe that a trained manipulator can relieve certain types of back pain, but the medical profession does not accept that there is a scientific basis for chiropractic in the treatment of diseases such as heart disease, diabetes, and cancer.

Chlamydial infections

Chlamydiae are a group of microorganisms, intermediate in size between bacteria and viruses, that cause various infectious diseases in humans and animals (particularly birds). Like viruses, chlamydiae can multiply only by first invading the cells of another life-form; otherwise, they behave more like bacteria than viruses and are susceptible to treatment with antibiotic drugs.

Two main species of chlamydiae cause disease in humans. Different strains of CHLAMYDIA TRACHOMATIS cause various types of genital, eye, and lymph node infections. CHLAMYDIA PSITTACI mainly affects birds, but is occasionally spread to humans to cause a lung infection.

CHLAMYDIA TRACHOMATIS INFECTIONS

GENITAL INFECTIONS In the tropics, strains of CHLAMYDIA TRACHOMATIS cause the sexually transmitted disease *lymphogranuloma venereum.*

In developed countries, by far the most important impact of CHLAMYDIA TRACHOMATIS is as a cause of *nonspecific urethritis* (NSU). This is the most common sexually transmitted disease in Canada; CHLAMYDIA TRACHOMATIS can be isolated from the urethras of at least 50 per cent of men with NSU and is also present in the genital tracts of about 20 per cent of women attending clinics for sexually transmitted diseases.

In men, nonspecific urethritis may cause a discharge from the penis and complications such as swelling of the testes, a condition which, if untreated, may lead to infertility. In women, however, the equivalent condition, nonspecific genital infection (NSGI), is usually symptomless, but may lead to *salpingitis* (inflammation of the fallopian tubes) which may cause the victim to become infertile.

Treatment is with *antibiotic drugs*, such as *tetracycline* or *erythromycin*, and is usually rapidly successful. Treatment of sexual partners is advisable to prevent reinfection.

EYE INFECTIONS A child born to a woman with a chlamydial infection of the cervix may acquire an acute eye infection called neonatal *ophthalmia*.

In parts of Africa and Asia, usually where hygiene is poor, certain strains of CHLAMYDIA TRACHOMATIS cause *trachoma*. This serious eye disease is the main cause of blindness worldwide.

CHLAMYDIA PSITTACI INFECTION
The only disease that can be caused by CHLAMYDIA PSITTACI in humans is a type of pneumonia called *psittacosis*. It is a rare infection, usually contracted from parrots, parakeets, pigeons, or poultry. The disease can be treated with antibiotic drugs but is sometimes fatal in elderly and debilitated patients.

Chloasma
A condition, also called melasma, in which blotches of pale brown skin pigmentation appear on the forehead, cheeks, and nose.

Chloasma sometimes develops during pregnancy. In some cases, the spots merge, forming the so-called "mask of pregnancy." More rarely, chloasma occurs in women who have been taking oral contraceptives or around the time of menopause.

The pigmentation is aggravated by sunlight. It usually fades gradually, but may be permanent or recur in successive pregnancies. There is no treatment, although avoiding direct sunlight and changing the brand of oral contraceptive (if appropriate) may help.

Chloral hydrate
One of the oldest *sleeping drugs* in use today. Chloral hydrate is mainly used as a short-term treatment for insomnia, especially in the elderly.

Chlorambucil
An *anticancer drug* used to treat some types of cancer, including *Hodgkin's disease* and cancer of the ovary.

Chloramphenicol
An *antibiotic drug* widely prescribed in the form of eye-drops or ointment to treat *conjunctivitis* caused by a bacterial infection.

Chloramphenicol tablets or injections carry a risk of causing aplastic *anemia* (inability of the bone marrow to produce blood cells) and are used only

to treat serious infections that are resistant to safer types of antibiotics.

Chlorate poisoning
Toxic effects caused by chemicals present in some defoliant weed killers.

Swallowing of chlorates can cause kidney and liver damage, corrosion of the intestine, and methemoglobinemia (a chemical change in the blood pigment *hemoglobin*). Symptoms of poisoning include ulceration in the mouth, abdominal pain, and diarrhea. Even small doses can prove fatal, especially in children, and medical help should be obtained immediately if poisoning is suspected.

Weed killers that are spilled on the skin or into the eyes should be washed off with plenty of water.

Chlordiazepoxide
A *benzodiazepine* drug used mainly to treat anxiety, but also in the management of alcohol withdrawal.

Chlorhexidine
A type of disinfectant. Chlorhexidine is widely used to cleanse the skin before surgery or before a blood sample is taken. It is also used to wash out the bladder as a treatment for *urinary tract infection* in people who have a permanent urinary *catheter*.

Chlorhexidine occasionally causes skin irritation; bladder irrigation with a concentrated solution may cause hematuria (blood in the urine).

Chlorine
A poisonous, yellowish-green gas with very powerful bleaching and disinfecting properties. If inhaled in even very small amounts, chlorine gas is highly irritating to the lungs; inhalation of large amounts is rapidly fatal.

Chloroform
A colorless liquid producing a vapor that acts as a general anesthetic when inhaled. Because it caused a high incidence of liver damage and heart problems it has been replaced in operating rooms by safer drugs.

Chloroform is still occasionally used in some countries as an emergency anesthetic for major first aid or field surgery. It is also sometimes used as a flavoring and preservative for other medicines, although research has indicated that it may be carcinogenic.

Chloroquine
A drug used in the prevention and treatment of *malaria* and occasionally as an *antirheumatic drug*.

When taken to prevent malaria, chloroquine is usually prescribed with other drugs because some strains of malaria parasite are now resistant to it. Chloroquine remains the main treatment for acute attacks of malaria.

Chloroquine is also used to treat *rheumatoid arthritis* and *lupus erythematosus* that have not responded to treatment with other drugs.

Possible side effects include nausea, headache, diarrhea, rashes, and abdominal pain. Since long-term treatment (as for rheumatoid arthritis) can damage the retina, causing blurred vision and sometimes even blindness, regular eye tests are usually carried out to detect early changes.

Chlorpheniramine
An *antihistamine drug* used in the treatment of allergies such as allergic *rhinitis* (hay fever), allergic *conjunctivitis*, *urticaria* (hives), and *angioedema* (allergic facial swelling). Chlorpheniramine is also an ingredient of some over-the-counter *cold remedies*.

Chlorpromazine

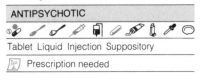

ANTIPSYCHOTIC

Tablet Liquid Injection Suppository

Prescription needed

The first *antipsychotic drug* to be marketed. Introduced in the early 1950s, it remains one of the most widely used drugs of this group. It is also sometimes used as an *antiemetic drug*.

WHY IT IS USED
Chlorpromazine is used primarily in the treatment of schizophrenia, mania, and other disorders in which confused or abnormal behavior may occur. It does not cure the underlying disorder, but does relieve particular symptoms. Chlorpromazine reduces delusional and hallucinatory experiences, which are the major features of psychotic illness. It may also help to reduce the irritability and overactivity that are characteristic of manic illnesses.

Chlorpromazine is also used in the treatment of nausea and vomiting, especially if caused by drug treatment, radiation therapy, or anesthesia.

POSSIBLE ADVERSE EFFECTS
Chlorpromazine sometimes produces serious side effects, including *parkinsonism* (a movement disorder), slow reactions, and blurred vision. It may also cause *photosensitivity* (increased sensitivity of the skin to light).

C

Chlorpropamide

A drug used to treat noninsulin-dependent *diabetes mellitus*. (See *Hypoglycemics, oral*.)

Chlorthalidone

A powerful, long-acting thiazide *diuretic*. Because it helps remove excess salt and water from the body, it is used to treat *edema* and *hypertension*. Because it also reduces the amount of calcium in the urine, it may be used to treat kidney stones.

Chlorthalidone depletes potassium, and may cause cardiac *arrhythmias*. For this reason, it is usually given with a potassium supplement.

Choking

Partial or complete inability to breathe due to an obstruction of the airway, usually by food, drink, or an inhaled or swallowed foreign body. If the blockage is only partial, the choking person can usually inhale enough air to cough out the obstruction. If the airway is completely blocked, the person will be unable to breathe and, unless the blockage is cleared, he or she will die of suffocation. (See *First Aid* boxes on this and facing pages.)

CAUSES

Choking is caused by blockage of any part of the airway—the pharynx (throat), larynx (voice box), trachea (windpipe), or bronchi (air passages from the trachea into the lungs). Most cases of choking occur when food or drink "goes down the wrong way," that is, when it enters the trachea and bronchi instead of passing from the pharynx into the esophagus. Although this can be alarming, it is normally corrected by coughing.

Obstruction by something that partially blocks the airway is more serious. In adults the cause is usually a fishbone or a piece of meat. In children, who are more vulnerable to this type of choking because their airways are narrower, the obstruction is often a peanut or small plaything, such as a bead. Less commonly, choking may be due to inhaling vomit.

TREATMENT

Emergency medical help should be summoned if the obstruction cannot be cleared. The doctor will probably try to clear the blockage manually; if this fails, an emergency *tracheostomy* (making an incision into the trachea and inserting a tube through it into the lungs) will be performed. When the airway has been restored, the physician can use a laryngoscope, bronchoscope, or esophagoscope (viewing

FIRST AID: CHOKING

CONSCIOUS VICTIM

1 A person clutching the throat may be choking. Encourage the victim to cough up the obstruction. If this fails, and the victim can no longer speak or cough, use the method below.

2 Clasp the victim, placing one clenched fist just under the sternum (breastbone) and grasping the fist with the other hand. Then make a quick, hard, thrusting movement inward and upward.

UNCONSCIOUS VICTIM

1 Straddle the victim. Place the heel of one hand on the victim's abdomen, slightly above the navel; place your other hand on top, fingers interlaced. With elbows straight, press in with a quick upward thrust. Repeat 6 to 10 times.

2 If this fails, try to remove the obstruction with your index finger. If the victim is still unconscious, summon emergency help. If breathing has stopped, start *artificial respiration*.

tubes through which instruments can be passed) to locate and clear the obstruction (see *Bronchoscopy*; *Esophagoscopy*; *Laryngoscopy*).

Cholangiocarcinoma

A malignant growth in one of the *bile ducts* that carry bile from the liver and gallbladder to the small intestine. Very rare in North America, the disease is more common in certain parts of Africa and Asia. The cause of the cancer is unknown. The main symptoms of cholangiocarcinoma are *jaundice* and weight loss.

Cholangiography

A procedure that enables the *bile ducts* to be seen on X-ray film after filling them with a contrast medium (a substance opaque to X rays).

WHY IT IS DONE

Cholangiography is used when people who have had their gallbladders removed are suspected of having biliary stones. Biliary stones are similar to gallstones, but they form in the bile ducts instead of the gallbladder. Cholangiography is usually employed as a follow-up to *ultrasound scanning* if this has failed to establish the presence of stones.

Cholangiography is also performed during a *cholecystectomy* (operation to remove the gallbladder) to ensure that no stones have been left behind in the bile ducts. Cholangiography is also useful for diagnosing narrowing or tumors of the bile ducts.

HOW IT IS DONE

The contrast medium may be injected slowly into a vein, in which case the

C

FIRST AID: CHOKING

INFANT

Straddle the baby over your arm with the head lower than the trunk, supporting the head by holding the baby's jaw. Deliver four quick but light back blows between the shoulder blades.

If this fails, turn the infant on his or her back, place two fingers in the center of the chest; make sure you do not touch the sternum. Press inward rapidly four times.

---

liver will excrete it several hours later in bile into the ducts. More satisfactory images can be obtained by injecting the contrast medium directly into the ducts.

This may be done either through an endoscope (a flexible viewing instrument) passed into the ducts via the mouth, stomach, and duodenum (see *ERCP*), or by means of a long, fine needle inserted through the abdomen into the liver. Once the ducts have filled, X-ray pictures are taken and any stones are apparent.

Cholangitis
Inflammation of the common bile duct (see *Biliary system*). There are two types: acute ascending cholangitis and sclerosing cholangitis.

ACUTE ASCENDING CHOLANGITIS
This type is usually due to bacterial infection of the duct and its content of bile. It generally results from blockage of the duct—by a gallstone, tumor, following surgery, or, in some parts of the world, by entry of a worm or fluke into the duct (see *Bile duct obstruction*). The infection moves up the duct and may affect the liver.

The main symptoms are recurrent bouts of jaundice, abdominal pain, and chills and fever. Attacks may vary from mild episodes to a severe, life-threatening illness with *septicemia* (spread and multiplication of bacteria in the bloodstream) and *kidney failure* from toxins circulating in the blood.

The infection is usually diagnosed from the patient's symptoms, although investigations such as *liver function tests* and *ultrasound scanning* may also be carried out.

Mild cases are treated with *antibiotic drugs* and a high intake of fluids. In severe cases, if there is no improvement within 24 hours, the infected material is drained from the bile duct by surgery or endoscopy.

Once the patient has recovered, the cause of the blockage must be determined and appropriate treatment of the cause of the obstruction provided (see *Bile duct obstruction*).

SCLEROSING CHOLANGITIS
In this rare condition, all the bile ducts, within and outside the liver, become narrowed. Sclerosing cholangitis leads to *cholestasis* (stagnation of bile in the liver), chronic jaundice, and itching of the skin due to excess levels of the bile pigment bilirubin in the blood and skin. The liver is progressively damaged.

No treatment is available other than the possibility of a *liver transplant*. The drug *cholestyramine* may be prescribed to relieve itching.

Chole-
A prefix that means relating to the bile or the biliary system, as in cholelithiasis (the formation of stones in the biliary system).

Cholecalciferol
An alternative name for vitamin D_3 (see *Vitamin D*).

Cholecystectomy
Surgery to remove the gallbladder.

WHY IT IS DONE
Cholecystectomy is usually performed to deal with the presence in the gallbladder of troublesome *gallstones*, often because they are causing recurrent attacks of *biliary colic*. Many surgeons advocate cholecystectomy at an early stage to treat acute *cholecystitis* (inflammation of the gallbladder). Emergency cholecystectomy is occasionally required to treat perforation (rupture) of the gallbladder or *empyema* (an accumulation of pus). Many gastroenterologists believe that it is unnecessary to remove a gallbladder that contains stones unless the stones are causing symptoms.

HOW IT IS DONE
The procedure for the operation is shown in the illustrated box on page 270. Simple cholecystectomy takes almost one hour, but duct exploration may add considerably to this time. Most patients are out of hospital within five to seven days.

RISKS AND OUTLOOK
The chief risk is inadvertent damage to the common bile duct. Severe inflammation sometimes obscures the anatomy and the surgeon may decide it is safer to perform a cholecystostomy (removal of gallstones by opening but not removing the gallbladder).

The outcome of cholecystectomy operations is generally good—symptoms are relieved completely in 90 percent of patients. About three weeks should be allowed for recovery from the operation. Loss of the gallbladder has little adverse effect on the digestive system.

Cholecystitis
Inflammation of the gallbladder, causing severe abdominal pain. There are two types: acute and chronic.

CAUSES
Acute cholecystitis is almost always caused by a *gallstone* obstructing the outlet (cystic duct) from the gallbladder. The trapped bile becomes concentrated by absorption of its water content and causes chemical irritation of the gallbladder walls; this is followed by bacterial infection of the stagnating bile.

Repeated mild attacks of acute cholecystitis can lead to chronic cholecystitis, in which the gallbladder walls thicken and the gallbladder shrinks and ceases to store bile. Medical opinions differ on whether chronic cholecystitis produces recognizable symptoms that justify surgery.

SYMPTOMS AND COMPLICATIONS
The main symptom of acute cholecystitis is severe constant pain in the right side of the abdomen, just under the ribs, which worsens on movement. The pain is accompanied by fever and, occasionally, *jaundice*.

C

PROCEDURE FOR CHOLECYSTECTOMY

If simple removal of the gallbladder is performed, it will take approximately an hour. However, more extensive exploration of the ducts may prolong the procedure.

With the patient under general anesthesia, an incision is made under the rib cage on the right-hand side; the cut may be vertical, horizontal, or oblique, according to the patient's build.

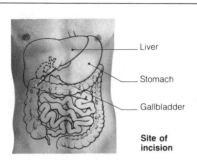

Liver

Stomach

Gallbladder

Site of incision

1 Gallstones, as shown by an ultrasound scan or by a cholecystogram (X-ray image of the gallbladder), such as the one above, increase in prevalence with age.

2 After an incision has been made, the liver is pulled up to expose the gallbladder. The thin membrane covering it is incised so that the cystic duct and artery can be identified.

3 The artery to the gallbladder and the cystic duct leading from it are tied and cut, and the gallbladder is removed. If the person has jaundice, X rays are taken to ensure that there are no stones in the common bile duct. If the X ray reveals the presence of stones, they are removed.

4 Drains are placed under the liver (and in the bile duct if it was opened) and the abdominal incision is closed. The two drains are removed, respectively, 48 hours and eight to 10 days later, after another X ray shows there are no more stones.

In some cases complications develop. These complications may include a form of *empyema* (in which the gallbladder fills with pus) or *peritonitis* (inflammation of the membrane that lines the abdominal cavity) if the gallbladder bursts.

In either case, the patient is extremely ill and requires urgent surgical treatment.

The ill-defined gastrointestinal symptoms attributed to chronic cholecystitis are indigestion, vague pains in the upper abdomen, nausea, and belching. These symptoms may be aggravated by eating fatty food.

DIAGNOSIS AND TREATMENT

A physician makes a provisional diagnosis of acute cholecystitis by listening to a description of the symptoms and by performing a physical examination. The patient is usually admitted to hospital at once and given *analgesic drugs* (painkillers), *antibiotic drugs*, and an *intravenous infusion* to provide nutrients and fluid. *Ultrasound scanning* or *radionuclide scanning* may be used to make a firm diagnosis and exclude other possible causes of *abdominal pain*, such as a duodenal ulcer or pancreatitis.

Acute cholecystitis usually subsides without urgent surgery but, to prevent recurrences, most patients are advised to have a *cholecystectomy* (surgical removal of the gallbladder). This operation can be performed either during the initial attack or after an interval of several weeks. Cholecystectomy is usually recommended for chronic cholecystitis although the results are less certain.

Cholecystography

An X-ray procedure for examining the gallbladder and common bile duct after they have been filled with a contrast medium (a substance opaque to X rays). The main use of the technique is to detect gallstones, usually as a follow-up procedure to *ultrasound scanning* if this test has failed to enable a definite diagnosis to be made. Cholecystography is not usually the procedure chosen first to study the gallbladder and is now performed much less often than formerly.

HOW IT IS DONE

The patient swallows tablets containing a contrast medium, which, after about 12 hours, is excreted by the liver into the bile. The opaque bile is stored by the gallbladder, which then shows up when X-ray pictures are taken. Gallstones, which do not absorb the contrast medium, appear on the X-ray film as "holes."

Cholera

An infection of the small intestine caused by the comma-shaped bacterium *VIBRIO CHOLERAE*. Cholera results in profuse watery diarrhea, which in severe untreated cases can lead to rapid dehydration and death. Infection is always acquired by swallowing contaminated food or water.

HISTORY, CAUSE, AND INCIDENCE

Cholera has been known for centuries in northeast India, where outbreaks of the disease occur regularly. In the 19th century, with the opening up of world trade routes and the increase in Muslim and Hindu pilgrimages, cholera spread throughout the world, causing millions of deaths in epidemics.

During the first half of the 20th century the disease was confined to Asia, but since 1961 a new pandemic (worldwide epidemic) has spread from Indonesia to much of the rest of Asia, Africa, the Mediterranean, and the Gulf Coast of North America.

A few cases of cholera occur in Canada in most years, mainly among travelers who have returned from visits to Asia or Africa.

SYMPTOMS

Cholera starts suddenly, between one and five days after infection, with diarrhea, often accompanied by vomiting. More than 500 ml of fluid may be lost each hour in the diarrhea and, if not replaced, this loss of fluid may cause death within only a few hours. The fluid loss is brought about by the action of a toxin produced by the cholera bacterium that greatly increases the passage of fluid from the bloodstream into the large and small intestines.

TREATMENT

Cholera is treated by replacing the lost fluid with drinks of water containing the correct proportions of various salts and sugar (see *Rehydration therapy*). However, if dehydration develops despite fluid replacement by mouth, the patient may be given extra fluid by means of *intravenous infusion*. *Antibiotic drugs*, especially *tetracycline*, can shorten the period of diarrhea and infectiousness.

With adequate rehydration, patients usually make a full recovery. However, in major epidemics following natural disasters, there may be insufficient supplies of clean water or so many people may be affected that few are left to nurse the sick.

PREVENTION

Worldwide, cholera is controlled by improving sanitation—in particular by ensuring that sewage is not allowed to contaminate water supplies that will later be used for drinking. Travelers to cholera-infected areas should restrict themselves to water boiled before drinking or to bottled drinks from reliable sources.

A vaccine that provides some protection against the disease is advisable when traveling to Africa and to the Middle and Far East. The protection it gives is short-lived (six months) and precautions still must be taken with drinking water. Usually, no country insists that travelers arriving directly from Europe or North America have a cholera vaccination certificate, but regulations change from time to time, and a certificate is sometimes required if travel has been via a cholera-infected area. International travelers should therefore check vaccination requirements before departure.

Cholestasis

Stagnation of *bile* in the small *bile ducts* within the liver, which leads to a characteristic type of *jaundice* and to liver disease. The obstruction to the flow of bile may be intrahepatic (within the liver) or extrahepatic (in the bile ducts outside the liver).

CAUSES

Intrahepatic cholestasis may occur as a result of viral *hepatitis* (inflammation of the liver) or as a side effect of a number of drugs.

The bile ducts outside the liver can become blocked or constricted for various reasons, including gallstones or tumors (see *Bile duct obstruction*); rarely, the ducts are absent from birth (see *Biliary atresia*).

TREATMENT

In the case of viral hepatitis, there is no specific treatment; the flow of bile improves gradually as the liver inflammation resolves. Drug-induced cholestasis usually disappears if use of the causative drug is stopped.

Extrahepatic bile duct obstruction and biliary atresia can often be treated surgically to ensure a free passage of bile from the liver to the duodenum.

Cholesteatoma

A rare but serious condition in which skin cells proliferate and debris collects within the middle ear.

Cholesteatoma usually occurs as a result of a long-standing *otitis media* (middle ear infection) together with a defect in the eardrum (see *Eardrum, perforated*). In such cases, skin may grow inward from the ear canal into the middle ear. If the cholesteatoma continues untreated, it may grow and damage the small bones in the middle ear and surrounding bony structures.

Cholesteatoma requires surgical removal either through the eardrum or by *mastoidectomy* (excision of the mastoid bone behind the ear together with the cholesteatoma). If there is residual deafness, reconstructive surgery may be performed; alternatively, a hearing-aid may be required.

Cholesterol

Chemically a *lipid*, cholesterol is an important constituent of body cells. It is also involved in the formation of *hormones* and bile salts and in the transport of fats in the bloodstream to tissues throughout the body. Most cholesterol in the blood is made by the liver from a wide variety of foods, but especially from saturated *fats*. However, a small amount of cholesterol is absorbed directly from cholesterol-rich foods, such as eggs and dairy products.

Both cholesterol and fats (triglycerides) are transported around the body in the form of *lipoproteins*. These are particles with a core, made up of cholesterol and triglycerides and an outer wrapping of *phospholipids* and apoproteins ("carrier" proteins).

CHOLESTEROL-RELATED DISEASES

The level of cholesterol in the blood—which can be measured by analysis of a blood sample—is influenced by diet, heredity, and metabolic diseases such as *diabetes mellitus*. There is overwhelming evidence that a high blood cholesterol level increases the risk of developing *atherosclerosis* (accumulation of fatty deposits on the inner lining of arteries), and with it the risk of *coronary artery disease* or *stroke*.

Recent research has shown that the risk of developing atherosclerosis can be assessed more accurately by measuring the proportions of different types of lipoproteins in the blood. In general, cholesterol in the blood in the form of high-density lipoproteins (HDLs) seems to protect against arterial disease; conversely, cholesterol in the form of low-density lipoproteins (LDLs) or very low-density lipoproteins (VLDLs) is a risk factor.

A group of metabolic disorders, the *hyperlipidemias*, cause abnormally high levels of lipids in the blood; people with these disorders are more susceptible to heart disease and stroke than normal. Such people may need treatment with low-fat diets and drugs to lower their lipid levels. People with relatives who have had a heart attack or stroke before the age of 50 should have their blood checked.

Cholestyramine

A *lipid-lowering drug* used to treat some types of *hyperlipidemia* (high levels of fat in the blood). Cholestyramine reduces the amount of *bile* salts reabsorbed into the blood from the small intestine. By reducing the level of bile salts in the circulation, cholestyramine increases the need for the liver to convert *cholesterol* into bile salts, thereby reducing high levels of cholesterol in the blood.

Cholestyramine is also used to treat diarrhea caused by abnormal digestion of fats, a feature of disorders such as *Crohn's disease*.

C

Chondritis

Inflammation of a *cartilage*, usually caused by mechanical pressure, stress, or injury. Costochondritis is a form of chondritis affecting the cartilage between the ribs and the sternum (breastbone). This causes tenderness over the sternum and pain if pressure is exerted on the ribs at the front of the chest. Chondritis affecting the cartilage lining the hip and knee joints may eventually lead to *osteoarthritis*.

Chondro-

A prefix that denotes a relationship to *cartilage*, as in chondroblast, a cell that forms cartilage.

Chondromalacia patellae

A painful disorder of the knee, also known as anterior knee pain. The condition most commonly affects adolescents, in which the cartilage directly behind the patella (kneecap) is damaged. When, rarely, it occurs in adults, the condition is known as retropatellar arthritis.

CAUSE

The cause is uncertain. One theory is that certain knee injuries or activities in which the knee is bent for long periods (e.g., horse riding) weaken the inner part of the quadriceps (main thigh muscle). As a result of this weakness, the patella is tilted when the knee is straightened; instead of sliding smoothly across the lower end of the femur (thighbone) it rubs against it, roughening the smooth cartilage that covers both bones.

SYMPTOMS AND DIAGNOSIS

Pain is felt when the knee is straightened and is particularly bad when using stairs. After examination, the physician may order *X rays*, but these do not normally show any specific signs and their main purpose is to exclude other possibilities.

TREATMENT AND OUTLOOK

Analgesic drugs (painkillers) may be given to relieve tenderness in the knee. In many cases, the condition improves without further treatment. If symptoms persist, treatment consists of strengthening the inner part of the quadriceps by exercises or electrical stimulation, which usually clears up the problem. If pain still persists, it may indicate considerable damage to the cartilage; surgery may be necessary to alter the angle of the patella permanently, thus preventing further friction on the cartilage. In rare severe cases, it is necessary to remove the patella—an operation that hinders mobility surprisingly little.

Chondromatosis

A condition in which multiple benign tumors, called chondromas, arise within bones. The tumors consist of cartilage cells and most commonly develop in the bones of the hand.

Usually the tumors cause no symptoms, but occasionally they lead to thinning of the lining of the bone and a resultant fracture, which may occur without any causative injury.

Chondrosarcoma

A cancerous growth of cartilage that can develop within a bone or on its surface, occurring most commonly within large bones, such as the femur (thighbone), tibia (shin), and humerus (upper arm bone). Chondrosarcoma is one of the more common types of primary *bone cancer*; overall, however, the incidence of bone cancers in the population is low.

Chondrosarcoma usually occurs in middle age and may develop from a benign tumor (see *Chondromatosis; Dyschondroplasia*) or from a previously normal area of bone. It causes pain, swelling, and, occasionally, tenderness. X rays show an abnormal area of bone. The tumor grows slowly and does not spread elsewhere until its later stages, so amputation of the bone above the tumor usually results in a permanent cure.

Chondrosarcoma is different from an *osteosarcoma* (cancer of bone cells), which has usually spread to other parts of the body (e.g., the lungs) before it causes any symptoms.

Chordee

Abnormal curvature of the penis, usually downward. Chordee most often occurs in males with *hypospadias*, a birth defect in which the urethral opening lies on the underside of the penis instead of at the tip. Corrective surgery is usually performed when the child is between 1 and 3 years old. Untreated chordee may make sexual intercourse very difficult.

Chorea

A condition characterized by irregular, rapid, jerky movements, usually affecting the face, limbs, and trunk. These movements are involuntary and, unlike *tics*, they are not predictable, but occur at random. Sometimes they resemble fragments of coordinated movements. Chorea disappears in sleep. Chorea is sometimes combined with athetosis (continuous writhing movements), a condition known as *choreoathetosis*.

TYPES AND CAUSES

Chorea arises from disease or disturbance of structures deep within the brain, in particular the paired nerve cell groups called the *basal ganglia*. Chorea is a feature of *Huntington's chorea* and *Sydenham's chorea*. It may also occur in pregnancy, when it is called chorea gravidarum. Chorea may be a side effect of certain drugs, including *oral contraceptives*, drugs used to treat some psychiatric disorders, and drugs used to treat *Parkinson's disease*; the choreic movements usually disappear when the drug is withdrawn.

TREATMENT

If chorea has occurred as a drug side effect, the drug may be withdrawn and a substitute prescribed. If there is an underlying disease, the physician may prescribe a drug that inhibits the nervous system pathways concerned with movement.

Choreoathetosis

A condition that is characterized by uncontrollable movements of the limbs, face, and trunk, which combine the jerky, rapid fidgeting movements characteristic of *chorea* and the slower, continuous writhing movements of *athetosis*.

Choreoathetosis may occur in children with *cerebral palsy* or as a side effect of certain drugs.

Choriocarcinoma

A rare malignant tumor that develops from the *placenta* in the uterus. It is a type of trophoblastic tumor (a tumor derived from cells in the placental attachment of the fertilized ovum to the wall of the uterus).

INCIDENCE AND CAUSES

Choriocarcinoma occurs in about one in 20,000 pregnancies, usually as a complication of a *hydatidiform mole* (a benign tumor of the trophoblast). Much less frequently, choriocarcinoma follows an abortion; very rarely, it develops after a normal pregnancy. Occasionally, the tumor may not develop until months or even years after the pregnancy.

If untreated, the tumor invades and destroys the walls of the uterus and may spread to the vagina and vulva. Distant spread may occur to the liver, lungs, brain, and bones.

SYMPTOMS

The tumor may become apparent because of persistent bleeding from the vagina after an abortion or for more than eight weeks after childbirth. There may be no early symptoms, the disease being suspected and diagnosed only after the cancer has spread to the lungs, causing symptoms such as breathlessness and coughing up of blood, or to the brain, producing mental changes.

DIAGNOSIS

Successful treatment depends upon diagnosing the disease at an early stage. Diagnostic tests include *ultrasound scanning* and measurement of the blood and urine levels of human chorionic gonadotrophin (HCG), a hormone normally produced by the placenta. Abnormally high levels of HCG are found in patients with trophoblastic diseases.

Women who have had a hydatidiform mole must have regular examinations for at least two years after it has been removed to check that there are no signs of choriocarcinoma.

TREATMENT

Treatment of choriocarcinoma is with *anticancer drugs*, especially *methotrexate*. *Hysterectomy* (surgical removal of the uterus) may be necessary if persistent bleeding occurs despite drug treatment. The use of anticancer drugs has dramatically reduced the mortality from this once highly lethal cancer. Nowadays, if the tumor is detected early, nearly all patients should be cured.

Chorion

One of the two membranes that surround the *embryo*. The chorion lies outside the *amnion* and develops into the *placenta*. Chorionic tissue may be removed for prenatal diagnosis (see *Chorionic villus sampling*).

Chorionic villus sampling

A method of diagnosing abnormalities in a fetus in which a small sample of chorionic tissue is taken from the edge of the placenta and analyzed in the laboratory. Chorionic villus sampling (CVS) is usually performed in the first three months of the pregnancy; it may also be performed in the middle months of pregnancy.

Chorionic villus sampling is a possible alternative to *amniocentesis* in some cases. Chorionic villus sampling can be performed earlier in the pregnancy than amniocentesis. It also has the advantage that the results of *chromosome analysis* are available sooner after the test.

WHY IT IS DONE

The procedure is usually performed to determine whether a pregnant woman who has a family history of—or who is otherwise at increased risk of having a child with—a chromo-

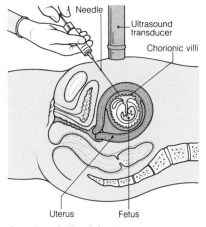

Sampling via the abdomen
A few chorionic villi are sucked through a hollow needle from the placenta.

somal disorder, such as *Down's syndrome*, or a genetic disease, such as *thalassemia*, is carrying a child affected by the condition.

Because the test can also identify the sex of the fetus, it can be performed on a woman who is a known carrier of a sex-linked disease (such as the bleeding disorder *hemophilia*) in order to predict the child's chance of having the disease.

HOW IT IS DONE

Chorionic villus sampling is an outpatient procedure. In some cases the woman is sedated before the sample is taken. The procedure takes about half an hour to complete.

The most common method of performing the test is to introduce a cannula (hollow tube), with a syringe attached, through the vagina and into the uterus. The cannula is directed using *ultrasound scanning* or an *endoscope* (a viewing tube with a light and lens attached). The syringe is used to suck a few chorionic villi (minute fingerlike projections) from the fetal side of the placenta. The chorionic villi are genetically identical to the fetus.

An alternative method is to insert a hollow needle through the abdominal wall and into the uterus, under ultrasound guidance, and withdraw some villi through the needle.

After removal, the villi are transferred to the laboratory. The cells are grown in an appropriate *culture* medium to allow *chromosome analysis* to be carried out.

RESULTS

If the test reveals genetic abnormalities in the fetus, the parents may choose to terminate the pregnancy (see *Abortion, induced*).

RISKS

Chorionic villus sampling occasionally causes complications, such as perforation of the amniotic sac (the membrane that encloses the fetus), bleeding, and infection. The test itself seems to increase the risk of pregnancy loss by 1 to 2 percent above the usual miscarriage rate of 3 to 4 percent in all pregnancies at this stage. As the procedure becomes more routine, it is hoped that risks will decline.

The main advantage of CVS lies in providing the woman with the choice of having an abortion in the first three months of pregnancy rather than facing the increased health risks and emotional strain of a late abortion (as is the case when amniocentesis is employed).

Choroid

A layer of tissue containing many blood vessels that lies at the back of the *eye* behind the retina. Pigment between the blood vessels is visible through an *ophthalmoscope* (see *Eye, examination of*). The choroidal vessels supply nutrients and oxygen to the light-sensitive cells in the retina and to surrounding tissues in the eye.

Choroiditis

Inflammation of the *choroid*. Choroiditis may occur on its own or as part of a generalized inflammation affecting the whole eye. It is commonly caused

STRUCTURE OF CHOROID
The choroid thickens around the lens to form the ciliary body. Ciliary muscles found between it and the lens contract to control the lens' shape.

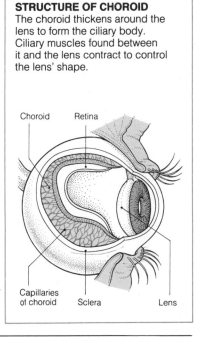

by infections such as *toxocariasis* or *toxoplasmosis*, more rarely by *sarcoidosis*, *syphilis*, and *histoplasmosis*, or may have no obvious cause.

Treatment may include *corticosteroid drugs* for the inflammation, and *antibiotic drugs* for any causative infection.

Christian Science

A religious movement founded by Mary Baker Eddy. Following a near-fatal accident in 1862, she supposedly was healed after reading one of the New Testament healing miracles. Eddy devoted the rest of her life to spreading the ideas of Christian Science. Strict Christian Scientists reject orthodox medicine and will, for example, refuse to allow themselves or members of their families to receive blood transfusions, opting to die rather than break the faith.

Christmas disease

A rare type of *bleeding disorder* caused by a defect in the blood coagulation mechanism (see *Blood clotting*). Christmas disease has very similar features to another bleeding disorder, *hemophilia*, and is sometimes called hemophilia B. It is named after a man named Christmas, the first patient in whom the disease was shown to be distinct from hemophilia, and was first described in 1952.

Both Christmas disease and hemophilia are *genetic disorders* in which there is deficient production of one of the proteins in blood. In Christmas disease the deficiency is of a protein called factor IX, while in hemophilia the deficiency is of factor VIII.

Chromium

A metallic element, which is essential for life because of its vital role in the activities of several *enzymes* (substances that promote biochemical reactions in the body). Chromium is required only in minute amounts (see *Trace elements*); chromium deficiency is unknown.

In excess, chromium is toxic, although poisoning is rare. Chromium produces inflammation of the skin and, if inhaled, damages the nose. People exposed to certain chromium fumes also have an increased risk of developing *lung cancer*.

Chromosomal abnormalities

Variations from normal in the number or structure of *chromosomes* contained within a person's cells. In most cases, the chromosomal abnormality is present in all the cells; it may have any-

thing from a lethal to virtually no effect, depending on the particular type of abnormality.

INCIDENCE AND CAUSES

About one in every 200 babies born alive has a chromosomal abnormality. Among fetuses that have been spontaneously aborted, about one in two has such an abnormality; this suggests that most chromosomal abnormalities are incompatible with life and that those seen in babies born alive are generally the less serious ones.

The cause in most cases is some fault in the process of chromosome division, either during the formation of the egg or sperm, or during the first few divisions of the fertilized egg. Occasionally, one of the parents has an abnormal arrangement of his or her own chromosomes.

TYPES

A complete extra set of chromosomes per cell is called polyploidy and is lethal. Other chromosomal abnormalities can be classified according to whether they involve the 44 autosomes or the two sex chromosomes (see *Chromosomes*). Abnormalities affecting the autosomes are slightly less common than abnormalities of the sex chromosomes, but tend to produce more serious and widespread effects.

AUTOSOMAL ABNORMALITIES

An extra autosome means that one of the 22 pairs of autosomes occurs in triplicate instead of as a pair—a phenomenon called *trisomy*. The most common trisomy, occurring in about one in 650 live births, is *Down's syndrome*; it is due to the presence of three chromosomes labeled number 21. Other trisomies are rare and usually cause multiple physical defects and death soon after birth. All trisomies are more common with advancing maternal age.

Sometimes, a part of a chromosome is missing (for instance, in *cri du chat syndrome*) or an extra bit is present and joined to another chromosome.

All these autosomal abnormalities, as well as causing physical defects of varying severity, tend to cause mental retardation as well.

Occasionally, a person has a normal chromosomal complement, but part of one chromosome is not in its proper position; instead, it is joined to another chromosome—a phenomenon called *translocation*. The person is normal, but some of his or her children may suffer from an abnormality through inheriting too much or too little chromosomal material.

SEX CHROMOSOME ABNORMALITIES

About one girl in 2,500 is born with only one X chromosome in her cells instead of two—a condition known as *Turner's syndrome*. The chromosome annotation for this defect is 45 XO (meaning 45 chromosomes, including a single X chromosome), compared with the normal female chromosome annotation of 46 XX (meaning 46 chromosomes, including two X chromosomes). Turner's syndrome causes characteristic physical abnormalities, defective female sexual development, and infertility.

All other sex chromosome abnormalities involve extra chromosomes. A boy born with one or more extra X chromosomes has *Klinefelter's syndrome*. The annotation for this is usually 47 XXY or 48 XXXY. Klinefelter's syndrome occurs in about one in 500 male births, although it is often not diagnosed until puberty. The condition causes defective male sexual development, infertility, and, in some cases, mild mental retardation.

Some women are born with an extra X chromosome (47 XXX) and men with an extra Y chromosome (47 XYY). These people are usually normal physically, but may have an increased risk of mild mental retardation and perhaps psychological problems. The extra chromosome is not recognized unless it is sought out.

DIAGNOSIS AND TREATMENT

Abnormalities are diagnosed by *chromosome analysis*, which is now possible early in pregnancy using *chorionic villus sampling*. Because of the fundamental nature of chromosomal abnormalities—affecting every one of a person's cells—no "cure" is possible. Many disorders caused by autosomal chromosome defects result in early death. Others, including Down's syndrome, are compatible with the survival of a physically and mentally handicapped individual. Children and adults with Down's syndrome, although handicapped, can usually integrate well into the community. Hormonal or surgical treatment, or both, can help correct some of the developmental defects of Klinefelter's and Turner's syndromes.

Anyone with a child or other member of the family with a chromosomal abnormality should obtain *genetic counseling* to establish the risk of his or her future children being affected and also to discuss other considerations of family planning. Fortunately, the risk of an abnormality recurring within a family is usually low.

Chromosome analysis

Study of the chromosomal material in an adult's, child's, or unborn baby's cells to discover whether a *chromosomal abnormality* is present or to establish its nature.

WHY IT IS DONE

Certain fetuses have a higher-than-average chance of being born with a chromosomal abnormality, particularly if the mother is 35 years or older, if she has previously had a child with a chromosomal defect, or if either the mother or father carries a defect or *translocation* (rearrangement) of his or her chromosomes.

In such cases, the parents are usually offered, at around the 16th week of pregnancy, chromosome analysis of cells that can be obtained from the fetus by a technique called *amniocentesis*. If no abnormality is found, the test spares the parents months of needless anxiety.

Some centers offer an alternative, *chorionic villus sampling*, which may have greater risks (regarding loss of the fetus). However, this procedure can be carried out as early as eight weeks into pregnancy. This permits a much earlier and safer abortion, should one be chosen.

Chromosome analysis is also carried out when a baby is stillborn, or is born with physical abnormalities that suggest a chromosome defect. The analysis clarifies the nature and type of defect, which in turn will affect the genetic and other counseling given to the parents.

Analysis of a person's sex chromosomes may also be carried out for any of the following reasons: establishing the chromosomal sex of a child in cases where the genitals have an ambiguous appearance (see *Genitalia, ambiguous*); confirming or excluding the diagnosis of sex chromosome abnormalities such as *Turner's syndrome* and *Klinefelter's syndrome*; or the investigation of *infertility*.

Chromosomes

Threadlike structures present within the nuclei of cells. Chromosomes carry the inherited, genetic information that directs the activities of cells and, thus, the growth and functioning of the entire body.

All the cells of any one person (with the exception of egg or sperm cells) ordinarily carry precisely the same chromosomal material. This is because everyone develops, by a process of cell division, from a single, fertilized egg cell and, with each cell division, the chromosomal material originally present in the fertilized egg is faithfully copied. A rare exception to this rule is seen in people with *mosaicism*, in which some of a person's cells contain one set of chromosomal material and other cells contain a slightly different set.

Although most chromosomal material is the same for everyone, certain parts differ from one person to another; these differences make each person (with the exception of identical twins) unique. Chromosomes determine physical characteristics, such as sex, hair texture and color, skin and eye color, nose shape, height, and (probably to a lesser extent) mental abilities and personality.

Each chromosome contains up to several thousand *genes* (hereditary units) arranged in single file along its length. A single gene is responsible for just one small aspect of body chemistry (e.g., the synthesis of a particular enzyme).

STRUCTURE AND NUMBERS

Chemically, a chromosome consists of an extremely long chain of the hereditary substance *DNA* (deoxyribonucleic acid) along with a coating of protein. This combination of DNA and protein is called chromatin. The sequence of chemical units, or bases, in the DNA provides the coded instructions for cellular activities.

PROCEDURE FOR CHROMOSOME ANALYSIS

1 Fetal cells are obtained by amniocentesis or by chorionic villus sampling, or white blood cells are obtained from the blood of the baby, child, or adult being tested.

2 These cells are suspended in a medium containing substances that encourage the cells to divide. Chemicals are then added that stop the cells from dividing at a stage where their chromosome content is most easily visible.

3 The cells are spread on a microscope slide and stained, then a selected few (in which the chromosomes are clearly visible and well separated) have their nuclei photographed or are closely examined through a high-power microscope.

4 The chromosomes are matched up and arranged into the 22 pairs of autosomes together with the sex chromosomes. Study of these reveals any abnormalities.

Male   Female

Each cell contains the chemical machinery for decoding these instructions (see *Genetic code; Nucleic acids*).

Although DNA chains are relatively enormous (compared, for example, with a molecule of water), their long, filamentous shape means that chromosomes cannot normally be seen in cell nuclei, even with the aid of a powerful microscope. But, shortly before any cell divides, its DNA molecules contract (probably by forming into tight coils) and, if cell division is chemically halted and the cell stained with a dye, the chromosomes can be seen with a microscope as dark rods in the nucleus, a few thousandths of a millimetre long.

This technique has shown that human cells (with the exception of egg and sperm cells) normally contain 46 chromosomes consisting of 23 pairs.

AUTOSOMAL AND SEX CHROMOSOMES

Of the 23 pairs of chromosomes, 22 are the same in both sexes and are called autosomal chromosomes. The two members of a pair cannot be told apart under the microscope—being alike in their length, the position of their centromeres (constrictions at a point along their lengths), and in other aspects—but at the molecular level they differ slightly, in particular in the sequence of chemical bases in their DNA. One member of each pair is derived originally from a person's mother and the other from the father.

The remaining two chromosomes are called sex chromosomes. In females they form a pair and are called X chromosomes. Again, they look alike but differ slightly at the molecular level. In males, however, the two sex chromosomes are completely different. One is an X chromosome, but the other is a much shorter chromosome called the Y chromosome. The Y chromosome is believed to provide all the information for the development of male sexual characteristics. In its absence, the female pattern of development occurs.

As with the autosomal chromosomes, one of a person's sex chromosomes (an X) has come originally from the ovum of the mother and the other (an X in girls and a Y in boys) has come from the sperm of the father.

CHROMOSOME DIVISION

When a cell divides, its components are duplicated into the two offspring cells; this applies also to the chromosomes. Shortly before division, the DNA in each chromosome is copied. This means that, when the chromosomes are viewed just before division,

they appear not as single but as double rods, conjoined in the region of their centromeres. This gives all 46 chromosomes (not just the sex chromosomes) an X-shaped appearance in the nuclei. As the normal cell division proceeds—a process known as *mitosis*—these duplicated chromosomes are pulled apart, dividing at the centromeres, so that each daughter cell receives a single copy of each of the usual 46 chromosomes.

When egg or sperm cells are formed (a process known as *meiosis*) there are two important departures from the normal process of chromosome division. First, after the DNA has been copied, but before division takes place, some sections of chromosomal material are exchanged between the two members of all the paired chromosomes. This helps ensure that each of a person's eggs or sperm contains a different combination of chromosomal material—and explains why all brothers and sisters (except identical twins) have a unique appearance.

The second difference is that, because eggs and sperm receive only 23 chromosomes, their formation requires two consecutive divisions—a first one in which the 46 duplicated chromosomes in the parent cell are split into two groups of 23, followed by a second division in which the 23 duplicated chromosomes in each daughter cell are pulled apart. Thus, the original parent cell gives rise to four separate egg or sperm cells.

DISORDERS

Defective chromosome division during the formation of eggs and sperm—or more rarely during the first few divisions of a fertilized egg—can lead to various *chromosomal abnormalities*. Their precise nature can be investigated by *chromosome analysis*.

Chronic

A term describing a disorder or set of symptoms that has persisted for a long time. In some disorders, such as chronic active *hepatitis*, the time is specified as six months or longer.

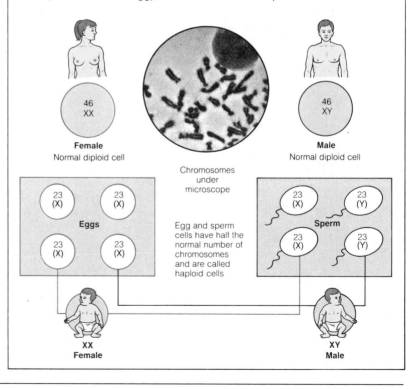

EGG AND SPERM CELLS

These differ from other body cells in that they contain only 23 chromosomes—one from each of the 22 autosome pairs plus an X chromosome (in the case of an egg) and either an X or a Y (in the case of a sperm). Because they have only half the normal complement, they are said to be haploid, while other cells are called diploid.

46
XX

Female
Normal diploid cell

46
XY

Male
Normal diploid cell

Chromosomes under microscope

23
(X)

23
(X)

Eggs

23
(X)

23
(X)

Egg and sperm cells have half the normal number of chromosomes and are called haploid cells

23
(X)

23
(Y)

Sperm

23
(X)

23
(Y)

XX
Female

XY
Male

Chronic disorders are usually contrasted with acute ones (of sudden onset and short in duration). In addition to the difference in duration between the two, the term acute suggests the presence of symptoms such as high fever, severe pain, or breathlessness, with a rapid change in the patient's condition from one day to the next. By contrast, a person with a chronic infection shows little change in symptoms from day to day and may be able, with some difficulty, to carry out his or her daily activities.

A person with a chronic disease may experience an acute exacerbation (flare-up) of symptoms. Also, people who have had an acute illness such as a *stroke*, or who have been injured in an accident, may be left with permanent disabilities, but their condition is not chronic. A chronic disorder implies a continuing disease process with progressive deterioration (sometimes despite treatment).

Chronic fatigue syndrome
See *Myalgic encephalomyelitis*.

Chronic obstructive lung disease
See *Lung disease, chronic obstructive*.

Cimetidine

ULCER HEALING
Tablet Liquid Injection
📋 Prescription needed

An H₂-*receptor antagonist* used as an *ulcer-healing drug*. Introduced in 1976, cimetidine reduces the secretion of hydrochloric acid in the stomach and, by doing so, promotes healing of gastric and duodenal ulcers (see *Peptic ulcer*) and reduces *esophagitis* (inflammation of the esophagus).

Cimetidine usually relieves symptoms within one to two weeks and heals an ulcer in more than 75 percent of cases after one to two months. Once the ulcer has healed, a maintenance dose of cimetidine is often prescribed; without such treatment the chance of an ulcer recurring is high.

There is a slight risk that cimetidine may temporarily relieve the symptoms of *stomach cancer* in its early stages, and delay the diagnosis. Cimetidine is therefore usually prescribed for no longer than two months unless investigations, such as *gastroscopy* and *barium X-ray examinations*, have ruled out the possibility of cancer.

Most chromosomes have a constriction called a centromere that divides them into long and short "arms"

Appearance of chromosomes
This is the appearance just after a chromosome has copied itself. The two copies are joined at the centromere.

POSSIBLE ADVERSE EFFECTS
Cimetidine interferes with the breaking down by the liver of certain drugs, such as *anticoagulant drugs* and *anticonvulsant drugs*. Some people taking cimetidine suffer from confusion, dizziness, and headaches; these adverse effects usually disappear when the drug is stopped.

Circadian rhythms
Any biological pattern based on a cycle approximately 24 hours long, also called a diurnal rhythm. (See also *Biorhythms*.)

Circulation, disorders of
Conditions affecting the flow of blood from the heart around the body. (See *Arteries, disorders of*; *Capillary*; *Veins, disorders of*.)

Circulatory system
The *heart* and blood vessels, which together are responsible for maintaining a continuous flow of blood throughout the body. Also called the cardiovascular system, the circulatory system provides all body tissues with a regular supply of oxygen and nutrients, and carries away carbon dioxide and other waste products.

STRUCTURE AND FUNCTION
The circulatory system consists of two main parts: the systemic circulation, which comprises the blood supply to the entire body except the lungs, and the pulmonary circulation to the lungs, which is responsible for reoxygenating the blood (see the illustrated box overleaf).

The systemic circulation begins at the left side of the heart, where the left atrium receives oxygen-rich blood from the pulmonary circulation. The blood is ejected from the left atrium to the left ventricle, a powerful pump that sends the blood out through the *aorta*, the body's main artery. Other arteries branching off the aorta carry the blood all over the body, into the

arterioles (small arteries) that supply the various organs. The arterioles branch further into a network of capillaries. These extremely fine blood vessels have thin walls to allow oxygen and other nutrients to pass easily from the blood into the tissues, and carbon dioxide and other wastes to pass in the opposite direction.

The capillaries deliver the deoxygenated blood into venules (small veins), which join to form veins. These carry the blood into the *venae cavae*, the body's two main veins, which then return the blood to the right atrium of the heart.

From the right atrium, the blood enters the pulmonary circulation. It passes to the right ventricle, which pumps the blood through the pulmonary artery to the lungs. Here, carbon dioxide passes out of the blood, and oxygen enters. The reoxygenated blood then returns through the pulmonary veins to the left atrium of the heart, where it re-enters the systemic circulation.

Within the systemic circulation there is a bypass to the liver called the portal circulation. Capillaries carrying nutrient-rich blood from the stomach, intestine, and other digestive organs join to form venules which, in turn, meet to form veins. These then merge to form the portal vein, which conveys the blood to veins, venules, and capillaries in the liver. Nutrients pass from the capillaries into the liver cells for processing and storage or re-entry into the general circulation, and the blood continues to rejoin the main systemic circulation via the inferior vena cava.

On its journey from the heart to the tissues, blood is forced along the arteries at high pressure. However, on the return journey through the veins and back to the heart, the blood is at low pressure. It is kept moving by the muscles in the arms and legs compressing the walls of the veins, and by valves in the veins preventing the blood from flowing backward. (See also *Lymphatic system*; *Respiration*.)

Circumcision
Removal of the foreskin of the penis. Circumcision may be performed on newborn male babies for religious reasons. It may also be carried out on older children or on adults.

WHY IT IS DONE
Circumcision is a religious ritual practised for many centuries by Jews and Muslims. In some countries it is also routinely carried out for reasons of

C

CIRCULATORY SYSTEM

The heart and blood vessels create a continuous flow of blood around the body to provide tissues with oxygen and nutrients. The system also removes waste products. The systemic circulation deals with the supply of blood to all parts except the lungs; the pulmonary system reoxygenates the blood.

Resin cast of coronary arteries
Shown (left) is a cast of the arrangement of blood vessels that supply the heart muscle. The larger vessels are the coronary arteries; these branch off the root of the aorta, the massive artery that receives oxygenated blood from the heart. The coronary arteries and their branches supply blood and oxygen to all parts of the heart muscle.

SYSTEMIC CIRCULATION

Internal carotid artery
External carotid artery
Subclavian artery
Aorta
Pulmonary vein
Heart
Brachial artery
Superior mesenteric artery
Inferior vena cava
Radial artery
Iliac vein
Femoral artery
Peroneal artery

Internal jugular vein
Subclavian vein
Femoral vein
Great saphenous vein
Small saphenous vein

Key
Oxygenated blood
Deoxygenated blood

PULMONARY CIRCULATION

Trachea
Superior vena cava
Right atrium
Right ventricle
Inferior vena cava
Aorta
Left ventricle
Alveoli
Lung
Aorta
Left atrium

Blood is pumped by the left side of the heart, via arteries, to the body, where it gives up oxygen. It then drains, via the venae cavae, to the right side, is pumped to the lungs, receives oxygen from the alveoli, and returns to the left side.

CAPILLARY NETWORK

All tissues contain a network of tiny blood capillaries. Blood enters these from the arterioles and is drained by venules.

Artery   Arteriole   Capillary bed   Venule   Vein

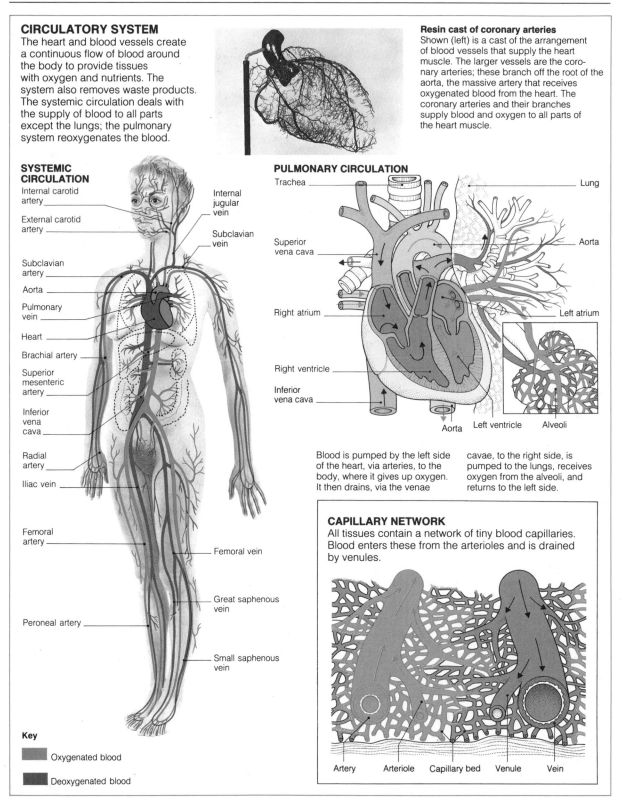

hygiene (because circumcision prevents the accumulation of secretions under the foreskin).

Medical reasons for circumcision include a foreskin that is tight (see *Phimosis*) causing ballooning on urination, or recurrent attacks of *balanitis* (infection under the foreskin due to retained secretions). The foreskin may also be removed because it is tight and painful during intercourse, or because of attacks of paraphimosis (painful compression of the shaft of the penis by a retracted foreskin).

HOW IT IS DONE

In newborn babies, circumcision can be done using a local anesthetic; in older children and adults, general anesthesia is used. The operation consists of carefully cutting away the inner and outer layers of the foreskin and then stitching the raw edges together. A dressing is not usually required. The patient can usually return home the same day.

Circumcision, female

Removal of all or parts of the clitoris, labia majora, and labia minora, sometimes combined with narrowing of the entrance to the vagina. The operation is common in parts of Africa. In the early 1980s it was estimated that more than 84 million women in 30 countries had been circumcised.

There is absolutely no valid medical purpose for the procedure. Circumcision may cause retention of urine, injuries during sexual intercourse, and may also lead to loss of sexual desire and other psychological problems. Childbirth is likely to be made more hazardous.

Efforts to end the practice completely have met with little success in some countries.

Cirrhosis

A disease of the *liver* caused by chronic damage to its cells. Bands of *fibrosis* (internal scarring) break up the normal structure of the liver. The surviving cells multiply to form regeneration nodules (islands of living cells separated by scar tissue). Because these nodules are inadequately supplied with blood, liver function is gradually impaired—for example, the liver no longer effectively removes toxic substances from the blood (see *Liver failure*). In addition, the distortion and fibrosis of the liver leads to *portal hypertension* (high blood pressure in the veins from the intestines and spleen to the liver), which can cause serious complications.

INCIDENCE AND CAUSES

In Canada, about 3,000 deaths a year are attributed to alcohol consumption. About 75 percent of these deaths are a direct result of chronic liver disease and cirrhosis.

Heavy alcohol consumption is the most common cause of cirrhosis in developed countries. The risk is related to the amount of alcohol consumed rather than the type, and women are more susceptible to the condition than men (see *Alcohol*).

Hepatitis (inflammation of the liver) can lead to cirrhosis. Chronic viral hepatitis (particularly that caused by the hepatitis B virus) is the most common cause of cirrhosis in the Middle and Far East and Africa (see *Hepatitis, viral*). A special pattern of liver inflammation called chronic active hepatitis is usually present before the cirrhosis develops (see *Hepatitis, chronic active*). Autoimmune chronic active hepatitis, with similar liver changes but with no obvious viral infection, occurs in developed countries.

Rarer causes of cirrhosis include diseases and defects of the *bile ducts*, which can cause primary or secondary *biliary cirrhosis*; *hemochromatosis*, in which increased iron absorption occurs; *Wilson's disease*, in which there is an increase in copper absorption; *cystic fibrosis*, in which the bile ducts become obstructed by sticky mucus; and "cardiac cirrhosis," in which *heart failure* has led to long-standing congestion of blood in the liver.

SYMPTOMS AND SIGNS

There may be no symptoms of cirrhosis; the disease may not be discovered until a routine medical examination or blood test is performed for some other reason. The most common symptoms are mild *jaundice*, *edema* (fluid collection in the tissues), mental confusion, and vomiting of blood. Examination may detect enlargement of the liver and spleen.

In men, enlargement of the breasts and loss of body hair are thought to be due to an abnormality in the sex hormone balance caused by liver failure associated with cirrhosis.

COMPLICATIONS

Cirrhosis may lead to various complications, any of which may be the first sign of the condition. *Ascites* (collection of fluid in the abdominal cavity) can occur because of low protein levels in the blood and high blood pressure in the veins leading to the liver. The high pressure in these veins also leads to *esophageal varices* (enlarged veins in the wall of the esoph-

agus), which can rupture, causing vomiting of blood. *Confusion* and *coma* can result from the accumulation of toxic materials poisonous to the brain that would normally be processed and detoxified by a healthy liver. *Hepatoma* is a primary cancer of liver cells that may complicate any form of cirrhosis.

DIAGNOSIS

Although the symptoms and signs of cirrhosis, or the results of *liver function tests*, may suggest cirrhosis of the liver, the diagnosis is usually confirmed by *liver biopsy* (removal of a sample of tissue for microscopic analysis), which may also show features that point to the underlying cause. Special blood tests and *cholangiography* (X rays of the bile ducts) may be performed to exclude the rarer causes.

TREATMENT

The cirrhotic process itself can be treated by slowing the process that is causing liver cell damage. Abstinence from alcohol can lead to substantial improvement. In some cases, specific treatment for the underlying cause may be available.

Ascites may be controlled by giving *diuretic drugs* and sometimes by reducing salt intake. Bleeding esophageal varices can be obliterated by injecting them with a sclerosant solution (a liquid that blocks off the affected veins) via a gastroscope (see *Gastroscopy*). The pressure in the veins can be reduced by using a *shunt* operation to divert the blood supply away from the engorged, dilated veins.

Confusion can usually be improved by measures that reduce the level of toxic waste products and other poisonous substances circulating in the blood. Such measures may include reducing the protein intake in the diet and giving *antibiotic drugs* to reduce the number of bacteria in the intestines. In some cases, however, a *liver transplant* may offer the only chance of a long-term cure.

Cisplatin

An *anticancer drug* that is used especially to treat certain cancers of the testis and ovary. Cisplatin can be used on its own or in combination with other anticancer drugs.

Clap

A slang term for the sexually transmitted infection *gonorrhea*.

Claudication

A cramplike pain in one or both legs that develops on walking and may eventually cause a limp.

C

The usual cause of claudication is blockage or narrowing of arteries in the legs due to *atherosclerosis* (see *Peripheral vascular disease*). Patients typically find that they have to stop walking after a particular distance because of pain in the calves. After a short rest, they may be able to resume walking. This is called intermittent claudication.

A rarer cause is spinal stenosis (narrowing of the canal carrying the spinal cord), causing pressure on nerve roots that pass into either leg.

Claustrophobia

Intense fear of being in enclosed spaces, such as elevators or small rooms, or of being in crowded areas. Claustrophobia may originate from a previous bad experience involving an enclosed space (such as being locked in a cupboard). *Behavior therapy* is the usual form of treatment.

Clavicle

The medical name for the collarbone. There are two such bones, both slightly curved, and they join the top of the sternum (breastbone) to the scapula (shoulder blade). The clavicles support the arms and transmit forces from the arms to the central skeleton.

The ligaments that link each clavicle to the sternum and scapula are very strong, which explains why the clavicle is rarely dislocated but frequently broken. Most fractures occur as a result of a fall onto the shoulder or an outstretched arm. When the clavicle is broken, the arm tends to sag and must be supported by a *sling* and a figure-

of-eight bandage to keep the broken ends of the clavicle together until the fracture has healed. Healing is usually complete within three weeks.

Clawfoot

A deformity of the foot, also known as pes cavus, in which there is an exaggerated arch and turning under of the tips of the toes. The disorder may be present from birth or may result from disturbance or damage to the nerve or blood supply to the muscles of the foot.

The condition can be helped by using a molded insole in the shoe to redistribute body weight evenly over the foot. Occasionally, surgical cutting of a tendon on the underside of the foot may be performed in an attempt to flatten the foot.

Clawhand

A deformity of the hand in which the fingers are permanently curled. Clawhand is caused by an injury to the ulnar nerve, which controls some of the muscles involved in hand and finger movements.

Treatment includes repair of the damaged nerve, if possible. Otherwise, symptoms may be relieved by using splints to hold the fingers straight or by surgical cutting of a tendon in the wrist to allow the fingers to straighten.

Clawtoe

A deformity of one or more toes. The end of an affected toe bends downward so that the toe curls under itself. The cause is unknown. A painful corn may develop on the tip of the toe or over the top of the bent joint.

Protective pads can sometimes relieve excessive pressure from footwear. In severe cases, surgical treatment of the toe may be needed.

Cleft lip and palate

Cleft lip is a vertical, usually off-center split in the upper lip that may be a small notch or may extend up to the nose. In some cases the upper gum is also cleft or notched, and the nose is crooked. Although cleft lip is also sometimes known as hare lip, this term properly refers only to a midline cleft lip, which is extremely rare.

Cleft palate is a gap that most commonly runs along the midline of the palate (the roof of the mouth that separates the mouth from the nasal cavity). The cleft may extend from the back of the palate forward to behind the teeth and allow open communica-

tion with the nasal cavity. Many people with cleft palate are partially deaf and may have other *birth defects*. In some cases the lip or palate is cleft on both sides.

Cleft lip and palate are present from birth, occurring either singly or together. About one in 500 babies is born with one or both deformities. Of every nine affected babies, two have only a cleft lip, three have only a cleft palate, and four have both. Inheritance is complicated but one third of those affected have relatives with one or both deformities.

DIAGNOSIS AND TREATMENT

All babies should be routinely examined for cleft lip and cleft palate immediately after birth. Babies with a cleft lip can breast-feed, but those with a cleft palate must be bottle-fed using a special teat.

Surgery, usually at about 3 months, can repair a cleft lip so that it looks almost normal, and there are rarely any speech defects. A cleft palate is usually repaired when the baby is about 1 year old; in some cases, further operations, dental management, and speech therapy are also necessary.

Clergyman's knee

Inflammation of the bursa (fluid-filled sac) that acts as a cushion at the pressure point over the tibial tubercle (the bony prominence below the knee). The inflammation is caused by prolonged kneeling. (See *Bursitis*.)

Climacteric

The *menopause*, which indicates the end of menstruation (and thus fertility) in the female. Strictly speaking, the "menopause" refers to the last menstrual period and the "climacteric" refers to the interval of time—months or years—during which symptoms may occur due to falling levels of female sex hormones.

Clindamycin

An *antibiotic drug*. Clindamycin has severe side effects and is used only to treat serious infections that do not respond to other antibiotic drugs.

Clitoridectomy

An operation to remove the clitoris (see *Circumcision, female*).

Clitoris

Part of the female genitalia. A small, sensitive, erectile organ, the clitoris is located just below the pubic bone and is partly enclosed within the folds of

LOCATION OF CLAVICLE

The two slightly curved bones join the top of the sternum to the shoulders and help support the arms.

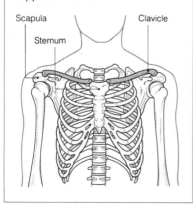

Scapula

Clavicle

Sternum

C

LOCATION OF CLITORIS

The clitoris is a small, sensitive, erectile organ located just below the pubic bone, partly enclosed within the labia.

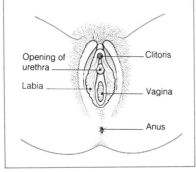

the *labia*. The clitoris is richly supplied with nerves and blood vessels. During sexual stimulation, the clitoris swells and becomes more sensitive.

Clofibrate

A *lipid-lowering drug* that reduces high levels of *cholesterol* and triglycerides (see *Fats and oils*) in the blood. Clofibrate is sometimes used to treat certain types of *hyperlipidemia*.

Clomiphene

A drug used to treat female *infertility* caused by failure to ovulate. Multiple births may occur.

HOW IT WORKS

Normal *ovulation* (the release of a ripened egg from one of the ovaries) is stimulated by the action of two *gonadotropins* (follicle-stimulating hormone and luteinizing hormone) released from the *pituitary gland*. This secretion is stimulated by chemicals released by the *hypothalamus*.

Failure to ovulate, one of the most common causes of infertility, is usually due to an abnormally low production of these gonadotropins. Clomiphene works by blocking the action of *estrogen hormones* in the hypothalamus. Estrogens normally reduce the output of gonadotropins from the pituitary gland. As a result, the production of gonadotropins is increased and sometimes ovulation is stimulated. Occasionally, clomiphene must be given with gonadotropins before ovulation will occur.

POSSIBLE ADVERSE EFFECTS

Minor side effects include hot flashes, nausea, headache, breast tenderness, and, occasionally, blurred vision. All usually improve when the dose is reduced or if a gonadotropin is also taken. Between 5 and 15 percent of the women who take clomiphene develop *ovarian cysts*. These cysts shrink when the dose is reduced.

Clomipramine

A tricyclic *antidepressant drug* used mainly as a long-term treatment for *depression*. Clomipramine is less sedating than many other antidepressants and is particularly useful when depression is associated with irrational fears and obsessive behavior.

Possible adverse effects include dry mouth, blurred vision, and constipation. If an overdose is taken, clomipramine may cause dangerously abnormal heart rhythms and coma.

Clonazepam

A *benzodiazepine drug* mainly used as an *anticonvulsant drug* to prevent and treat epileptic seizures. Clonazepam is particularly effective in preventing petit mal attacks in children. Possible adverse effects include drowsiness, dizziness, fatigue, and irritability.

Clone

An exact copy. In medicine the term usually refers to one of three main types: clones of cells, clones of genes, and clones of organisms.

Clones of cells are all descended from one original cell. Many types of cancer are thought to be cellular clones derived from one abnormal cell. Monoclonal antibodies (substances obtained from a clone of cells) have been used to identify certain types of cancer and infection (see *Antibody, monoclonal*).

Clones of genes are duplicates of a single gene. Gene cloning is a valuable research tool, because once several copies of a gene have been made the gene can be studied in detail.

Clones of organisms can be produced by removing the nuclei from cells of one individual and transplanting them into the egg cell of another individual. When these eggs mature into living plants or animals, they are all identical as they contain only the genes of the donor nuclei. To date, this process has been successful only with simple organisms.

Clonidine

An *antihypertensive drug* (a drug used to treat high blood pressure). Clonidine works by reducing nerve impulses from the brain to the heart and circulatory system.

When clonidine is given in high doses, sudden stopping of the drug or missed doses may lead to a dangerous rise in blood pressure. Rarely, an unexpected rise in blood pressure develops when clonidine is given with a *beta-blocker drug*.

Other possible adverse effects, more common in patients on high dosages, include drowsiness, dizziness, dry mouth, and constipation. Such effects often decrease with continued treatment or may require a reduction in dose.

Clonus

An abnormal response of a *muscle* to stretching. Muscles normally respond to being stretched by contracting once and then relaxing. In clonus, stretching sets off a rapid series of muscle contractions.

Clonus is a sign of damage to nerve fibers that carry impulses from the motor cortex within the *cerebrum* of the brain to a particular muscle. One typical example of clonus is called ankle clonus. A physician may demonstrate this in the course of an examination by forcibly jerking the front of the foot upward, thus stretching the muscles of the calf, which are then triggered into a series of rhythmical contractions. Clonic muscle contractions are also a feature of seizures in grand mal *epilepsy*.

Clorazepate

A *benzodiazepine* drug commonly used to treat anxiety and nervousness. It can cause dizziness and drowsiness, and can be habit-forming if used over long periods.

Clotrimazole

A drug used to treat yeast and fungal infections, especially *candidiasis* (thrush). (See *Antifungal drugs*.)

Clove oil

A colorless or pale yellow oil distilled from the dried flower buds of EUGENIA CARYOPHYLLUS. Clove oil is sometimes used to relieve abdominal pain due to *flatulence*, but its main use today is in flavoring pharmaceuticals. Applied externally, clove oil is germicidal and mildly analgesic (painkilling). It is also used as a domestic remedy for toothache, but repeated application may damage the gums.

Cloxacillin

A penicillin-type antibiotic used to treat infections with staphylococcal bacteria. (See *Penicillin drugs*.)

C

Clubbing

Thickening and broadening of the tips of the fingers and toes, usually with increased curving of the fingernails and toenails.

Clubbing is associated with certain chronic lung diseases, including *bronchiectasis*, *lung cancer*, fibrosing *alveolitis*, and lung *abscess*; and with heart abnormalities that result in *cyanosis* (bluish complexion due to lack of oxygen in the blood). Clubbing is also occasionally associated with the inflammatory bowel diseases *Crohn's disease* or *ulcerative colitis*. Rarely, clubbing may be inherited, in which case it is not a sign of any disease.

Clubfoot

A deformity of the foot, present from birth. (See *Talipes*.)

CMA

See *Canadian Medical Association*.

CNS

An abbreviation for *central nervous system* (the brain and spinal cord).

CNS stimulants

Drugs that increase mental alertness. (See *Stimulant drugs*.)

Coagulation, blood

The main mechanism by which blood clots (solidifies). Coagulation involves a complex series of reactions in the blood plasma (the fluid part of blood as distinct from the blood cells). The end result of this process is the formation of an insoluble substance called fibrin, which provides much of the framework for a blood clot. (See also *Blood clotting*.)

Coal tar

A thick, black, sticky substance distilled from coal. Coal tar is a common ingredient of ointments and some medicinal shampoos. These preparations, which often also contain *antiseptics* and *corticosteroid drugs*, are prescribed for skin and scalp conditions such as *psoriasis* and some forms of *dermatitis* and *eczema*.

Coarctation of the aorta

An abnormality, present from birth, in which there is a localized narrowing of the aorta (the large artery that supplies blood from the left side of the heart to the rest of the body).

The narrowing occurs in the part of the aorta that supplies blood to the lower part of the body, including the legs; blood supply to the upper part of the body is not affected. In order to compensate for the reduction in blood supply to the lower part of the body, the heart works harder, causing *hypertension* (abnormally high blood pressure) in the upper part of the body, while the blood pressure in the legs is normal or low.

The cause is unknown. Coarctation of the aorta occurs in about 10 percent of babies born with heart defects (see *Heart disease, congenital*), or in about one in 3,500 of all babies.

SYMPTOMS AND DIAGNOSIS

The symptoms often first appear in early childhood and depend on the degree of abnormality of the blood pressure. Symptoms may include headache, weakness after exercise, cold legs, and, rarely, breathing difficulty and swelling of the legs due to *heart failure*.

A physical examination of the child usually reveals the following abnormalities associated with the defect: a murmur (abnormal heart sound), weak or absent pulses in the groin, lack of synchronization between groin and wrist pulses, and higher blood pressure in the arms than in the legs. The diagnosis is confirmed by X rays of the chest that show bulging of the aorta on either side of the narrowed segment, among other abnormalities.

TREATMENT AND OUTLOOK

Surgery is necessary to prevent progressive hypertension, even when there are no symptoms. The narrowed segment of the aorta is removed and the two ends rejoined. The operation is usually performed between the ages of 4 and 8. Despite successful repair of the aorta, high blood pressure may persist, requiring drug treatment to lower it.

Cobalamin

A cobalt-containing complex molecule that forms part of *vitamin B₁₂*.

Cobalt

A metallic element and a constituent of *vitamin B₁₂*. Radioactive cobalt is used in *radiation therapy*.

Cocaine

A drug obtained from the leaves of *ERYTHROXYLON COCA* and similar plant species indigenous to parts of South America.

WHY IT IS USED

Cocaine was once used as a local anesthetic (see *Anesthesia, local*), mainly for minor surgical procedures on the eye, ear, nose, or throat. It is sometimes sprayed onto the back of the throat before examination of the lungs or stomach with an *endoscope*. Because of its potential for abuse, cocaine has largely been replaced by other local anesthetics.

The onset of anesthesia is rapid and the effects last for about one hour. Cocaine also constricts blood vessels, helping to localize its effect. However, some cocaine is usually absorbed into the bloodstream; this may interfere with the action of chemical *neurotransmitters* in the brain, producing feelings of euphoria and increased energy.

ABUSE

The effects of cocaine on the brain have led to its abuse. Regular inhaling of the drug can damage the lining of the nose. Continued use can lead to psychological dependence (see *Drug dependence*), and *psychosis* may develop if high doses are taken. Overdose can cause seizures and *cardiac arrest*. "Crack," a purified form of cocaine, produces a more rapid and intense reaction that also wears off very quickly; it has caused deaths due to adverse effects on the heart. (See also *Drug abuse*.)

Cocci

Spherically shaped *bacteria* that cause various infections (see *Staphylococcal infections*; *Streptococcal infections*).

Coccygodynia

A pain in the region of the *coccyx*. Coccygodynia is usually caused by a fall in which the base of the spine strikes a hard surface. It may also be caused by prolonged pressure on the coccyx due, for example, to habitual slouching in a chair or to use of the *lithotomy position* during childbirth. Occasionally, coccygodynia may occur for no obvious reason.

Treatment may include the application of heat, injections of a local anesthetic, and manipulation, but these measures are not always successful. The pain usually eases in time with or without treatment. In very rare cases of persistent, incapacitating pain, surgical removal of the coccyx may be considered.

Coccyx

A small triangular bone at the base of the *spine*. The coccyx consists of four tiny bones that are fused together; it is all that remains of the tailbone structure of our evolutionary ancestors.

Together with a much larger bone called the *sacrum*, which lies above it, the coccyx forms the back section of the *pelvis*—a bowl-shaped, bony structure

C

ANATOMY OF COCCYX
The coccyx consists of four fused bones at the base of the spine. With the sacrum, it forms the back of the pelvis.

Four bones of coccyx fused together

that provides protection to lower abdominal organs such as the uterus and bladder and supports the upper body.

There is very little relative movement between the coccyx and sacrum. Later in life, the coccyx and sacrum commonly fuse together.

Cochlea
The spiral-shaped organ in the inner *ear* that transforms sound vibrations into nerve impulses for transmission to the brain.

Cochlear implant
A device for treating severe deafness that consists of one or more electrodes surgically implanted inside or outside the *cochlea* in the inner ear. Unlike a *hearing aid*, which amplifies sounds, the implant receives and passes on electrical signals. It cannot restore normal hearing but may allow a greater understanding of speech.

WHY IT IS DONE
In rare cases, damage to structures in the cochlea (through disease, injury, or drug poisoning) is so great and the resultant deafness so profound that a hearing aid serves no useful purpose. If some nerve fibers have survived, it is sometimes possible to stimulate them electrically by an implant.

HOW IT IS DONE
One or more tiny electrodes are implanted either inside or outside the cochlea. At the same time, a miniature receiver is implanted under the skin, either behind the ear or in the lower part of the chest. A wire connecting the electrodes to the receiver is also implanted at this time.

Directly over the implanted receiver, the patient wears an external transmitter, which is connected to a sound processor and a microphone.

OUTLOOK
In general, an implant enables the user to hear the rhythms of speech, and sometimes also the intonation of the voice. Understanding obtained through lipreading is increased, and the deaf person is able to converse more effectively.

However, the usefulness of an implant for any particular person cannot be reliably predicted, and, in this respect, the technique is considered to be experimental. Some patients are greatly helped by the implant and can understand and repeat simple words without needing to lipread. Others find that their comprehension of lipreading is increased. However, a final group are not helped at all by the implant, either because the signal is poor, an electrical fault occurs, or an infection develops and the implant has to be removed.

Codeine

ANALGESIC ANTIDIARRHEAL
COUGH REMEDIES

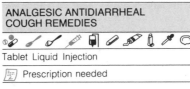

Tablet Liquid Injection

Prescription needed

A narcotic *analgesic drug* (painkiller), derived from the opium poppy plant, in use since the early 1900s. It is not as strong as some other narcotic analgesics and is often used in combination with other analgesic drugs. In Canada, a pharmacist may supply without prescription compounds containing a limited proportion of codeine.

WHY IT IS USED
Codeine is most useful in the relief of mild to moderate pain. It is also used as a *cough remedy*, because it suppresses the part of the brain that triggers coughing, and as an *antidiarrheal drug*, because it slows down muscle contractions in the intestinal wall.

POSSIBLE ADVERSE EFFECTS
Codeine may cause dizziness and drowsiness, especially if taken with alcohol. When taken over a long period, codeine may cause constipation and be habit-forming.

Cod-liver oil
A pale yellow oil obtained from the liver of fresh cod. Cod-liver oil is a valuable source of *vitamin A* and *vitamin D*. Before vitamin drops became

Electrodes implanted in cochlea

Subcutaneous fat

Receiver coil

Signals

Transmitter coil

Microphone (sometimes set into an ear mold)

Skin

Speech processor

How a cochlear implant works
Sounds picked up by the microphone are converted into electronic signals by the processor and relayed to the external transmitter, which sends them through the skin to the receiver. The waves then travel along the wire to the electrodes in the cochlea.

common, cod-liver oil was often given to children as a dietary supplement to ensure the healthy development of bones and skin. Excessive use may be dangerous.

Cognitive-behavioral therapy
A method of treating mental disorders based on the idea that the way we perceive the world and ourselves (our cognitions) influences our emotions and behavior.

A person suffering from *depression* may believe that all undesirable events are due to his or her behavior and that all desirable events are due to chance. The therapist shows the patient that these interpretations may be false, suggests more positive ways of thinking, and encourages the patient to try out these new ideas during his or her everyday activities.

Because cognitive-behavioral therapy is based on the manner in which

C

each person relates to the environment, it allows treatment to be more specifically tailored to the individual's needs than do more traditional forms of *behavior therapy*.

Coil
Any of the various types of intrauterine contraceptive device (see *IUD*).

Coitus
Sexual intercourse (from the Latin word for a going together).

Coitus interruptus
The contraceptive technique in which the male partner withdraws his penis from the vagina before ejaculation occurs. This technique is not reliable as a contraceptive method, because sperm may sometimes be released before orgasm occurs. Coitus interruptus has been blamed for *psychosexual dysfunction* in both men and women. (See also *Contraception*.)

Colchicine
A drug extracted from the autumn crocus flower. Colchicine has been in use since the 19th century as a treatment for *gout*. Although it has now been mainly superseded by newer drugs (because it causes many side effects), colchicine continues to be used both as a treatment for acute attacks of gout and to reduce the frequency of attacks.

Cold, common
A viral infection that causes inflammation of the mucous membranes lining the nose and throat, resulting in a stuffy, runny nose and sometimes also a sore throat, headache, and other discomfort.

CAUSES
Almost 200 viruses, all broadly similar in their effects, are known to cause colds. The most common belong to one of two groups—the rhinoviruses and the coronaviruses.

Most colds are contracted by breathing in virus-containing droplets that have been sneezed or coughed into the atmosphere or by rubbing the eyes or nose with fingers that have picked up a virus by hand-to-hand contact or by handling contaminated objects, such as hand towels.

INCIDENCE
Almost everyone occasionally gets a cold. The incidence is highest among schoolchildren (who may have as many as 10 colds a year) and declines with increasing age. On average, a young adult has two or three colds per

year, an elderly person has one or none at all. The reason for this is that children at school are exposed to a host of different viruses to which they have not yet become immune and which they pass to one another. Adults gradually build up immunity against a wide variety of viruses responsible for colds.

Colds are most frequent in winter, probably because people tend to spend more time during these months crowded together indoors.

SYMPTOMS
Most colds are what are popularly known as head colds—that is, infections confined to the nose and throat. The first symptoms are often a tickle in the throat, a watery discharge from the nose, and sneezing. In some cases the discharge may thicken and become yellow or green. Other symptoms may develop—watering eyes, a slight fever, a sore throat, a cough, aching muscles and bones, headache, listlessness, and chills.

In some cases, infection spreads and causes *laryngitis*, *tracheitis* (inflammation of the trachea or windpipe), acute *bronchitis*, *sinusitis*, or *otitis media* (inflammation of the middle ear). In these cases, a more serious secondary bacterial infection may follow.

Colds can also aggravate existing respiratory disorders, such as *asthma*, chronic bronchitis, and chronic ear infections. They may also reactivate dormant HERPES SIMPLEX virus, causing *cold sores*.

TREATMENT
A physician should be consulted only if a cold fails to clear up within a week or so, if the infection has spread beyond the nose or throat, or if the cold has aggravated a chronic chest infection or ear disorder. If a secondary bacterial infection is suspected, *antibiotic drugs* may be given.

PREVENTION
Many people believe there are ways of preventing colds—by avoiding cold drafts and dampness, for instance, or by taking large quantities of vitamin C—but there is no scientific evidence that any such measures work.

OUTLOOK
The search to find a cure for the common cold continues. In volunteer experiments, the drug *interferon* has proved effective in preventing and reducing the severity of colds, but has caused local inflammation. Another area of research involves the use of synthetic *antigens* (substances that stimulate the immune system to produce antibodies).

Cold injury
Localized tissue damage caused by chilling—as distinct from *hypothermia*, which refers to generalized chilling; the two may occur together.

The most serious form of cold injury is *frostbite*, a hazard of very cold, dry conditions. The frostbitten area of skin and flesh is frozen, hard, and white; it may be caused by exposure to the cold air sometimes coupled with restriction of the blood supply to the affected area.

Immersion foot is another type of cold injury, occurring when the legs and feet have been cold and damp for many hours or days, and blood supply to the feet has been restricted by tight-fitting footwear.

In established frostbite and immersion foot, the main risk is that blood flow will be slowed so much that the tissues will die, leading to *gangrene* (tissue death). Treatment may take several months.

Less serious forms of cold injury include *chilblains*, caused by rapid rewarming of the skin after being out in cold weather, and *chapped skin* of the lips, nose, and hands from exposure to cold, windy conditions.

Cold remedies
Preparations for the relief of symptoms of the common cold. Many different preparations are available over-the-counter. The main ingredient is usually a mild *analgesic drug* (painkiller), such as *acetaminophen* or *ASA*, which helps to relieve aches and pains. Other common ingredients include *antihistamine drugs* and *decongestant drugs*, which help to reduce nasal congestion, and *caffeine*, which acts as a mild stimulant. *Vitamin C* is frequently included in cold relief products, but there is no evidence that it speeds recovery.

Cold sore
A small skin blister, usually around the mouth, caused by the HERPES SIMPLEX virus. Usually, several blisters occur together in a cluster.

CAUSE AND INCIDENCE
The strain of the virus usually responsible for cold sores is called HSV1 (HERPES SIMPLEX virus type 1). Most people—perhaps as many as 90 percent worldwide—are infected by HSV1 at some time in their lives. The first attack may pass unnoticed or may cause an illness resembling influenza and painful ulcers in the mouth and on the lips—a condition called gingivostomatitis.

Subsequently, the virus lies dormant in nerve cells, but in some people it is occasionally reactivated, causing cold sores. Such sores tend to recur when a person with the virus is exposed to hot sunshine or a cold wind, is suffering from a common cold or other infection, or is feeling run down; women seem more likely to develop cold sores around the time of their menstrual periods. Some people are afflicted regularly throughout the year. Prolonged attacks can occur in people with an underlying disease that affects their immunity to infection, or in those taking *immunosuppressant drugs* (transplant or cancer patients, for example.)

SYMPTOMS
An outbreak is often preceded by a telltale tingling in the lips. The blisters are small at first but soon enlarge, sometimes causing itching, irritation, and soreness. Within a few days they burst and become encrusted. Most disappear within a week.

TREATMENT
If cold sores are particularly troublesome, a physician may prescribe *idoxuridine* paint or the antiviral drug *acyclovir* (in tablet or cream form) to soothe them. Both treatments are most effective if given as early as possible after symptoms develop.

No effective preventive treatment is available, although some people find that applying a lip salve before exposure to the sun does help prevent outbreaks. (See also *Herpes simplex*.)

Colectomy
The surgical removal of part or all of the *colon* (the major part of the large intestine).

WHY IT IS DONE
A partial colectomy may be performed to relieve severe cases of *diverticular disease* or to remove either a malignant tumor in the colon or a narrowed part of the intestine that is obstructing the passage of feces.

A total colectomy is carried out in cases of *ulcerative colitis* that cannot be controlled with drugs; in cases of long-standing ulcerative colitis in which *colonoscopy* (examination of the colon through a viewing instrument) suggests there may be a hidden malignancy; and in cases of familial *polyposis coli*, a rare condition in which potentially malignant growths stud the lining of the colon.

HOW IT IS DONE
In a partial colectomy, the diseased section of the colon is removed and the two ends of the severed colon are joined together; they fuse in a matter of weeks. A temporary *colostomy* (which allows the discharge of feces from the large intestine through an artificial opening in the abdominal wall) may also be required. The temporary colostomy is closed when the rejoined colon has healed.

In a total colectomy the whole of the large intestine is removed; the rectum (last part of the large intestine) may be removed or left in place. If the rectum is removed, an *ileostomy* (similar to a colostomy, but involving the small instead of the large intestine) is performed. If the rectum is left in place, the ileum (the last part of the small intestine) may be joined directly to it.

RECOVERY PERIOD
The patient is usually in hospital for eight to 12 days. After discharge, it may take up to two months or so at home to recover from the operation. A patient with an ileostomy or colostomy should receive training—before leaving hospital and preferably from a specialist nurse—on caring for the opening in the abdomen.

OUTLOOK
The bowel usually functions normally after most partial colectomies. If a large section of the colon has been removed, or if the ileum has been joined directly to the rectum, the greatly reduced ability of the intestines to absorb water from the feces can cause diarrhea. *Antidiarrheal drugs*, such as *codeine*, *loperamide*, or *diphenoxylate*, may be required.

Colic
A severe, spasmodic pain that occurs in waves of increasing intensity, reaches a peak, and then abates for a short time before returning. The intermittent increase in pain occurs when the affected part of the body contracts.

Colic in a bile duct (see *Biliary colic*) or in the urinary tract (see *Renal colic*) is often the result of obstruction by a stone. Intestinal colic may be due to obstruction of the intestine (see *Intestine, obstruction of*), to intestinal infections, or simply to intestinal gas. (See also *Colic, infantile*.)

Colic, infantile
Episodes during which an infant, who is otherwise completely well, is irritable, cries or screams excessively, and draws up the legs.

CAUSES AND INCIDENCE
Infantile colic is thought to be due to spasm in the intestines, although there is no proof of this, and the cause of the presumed spasm is unknown.

The condition is common, occurring in approximately one in 10 babies. It often first appears around the third or fourth week of life. Usually it clears up without treatment by the age of 12 weeks, hence the popular name "three-month colic." The condition is harmless, although it can be highly distressing to a tired parent.

SYMPTOMS
The baby cries or screams incessantly, draws up the legs toward the stomach in a characteristic position, may become red in the face, and may pass wind. Episodes of colic tend to be worse in the evenings and do not respond to the usual means of comforting the infant, such as feeding, cuddling, or diaper changing.

If the baby seems to be ill between the bouts of colic, is failing to gain weight satisfactorily, or has diarrhea, constipation, or a fever, a physician should be consulted because the baby may have a more serious underlying problem.

TREATMENT
No treatment is usually required. *Antispasmodic drugs* have sometimes been given for infantile colic in the past, but these drugs are not now generally recommended for babies under 6 months old.

Parents may find that it helps to distract the baby by diaper changing, cuddling, or bathing. The baby may be soothed by rhythmic activities such as being taken for a car ride, being rocked, or being placed facedown on a lap while his or her back is stroked. Other possibly helpful measures include using white noise (e.g., radio static) in the baby's room, applying warmth (e.g., from a warm facecloth) to the baby's abdomen, carrying the baby in a front sling, or giving the baby a pacifier.

Parental anxiety is likely to make the baby even more irritable, and parents should do their best to avoid becoming overtired.

Colistin
One of the polymyxin group of *antibiotic drugs*. Colistin is used only to treat severe infections that are resistant to other antibiotics, as there is a risk that it may damage the kidneys and nerve tissue.

Colitis
Inflammation of the *colon* (part of the large intestine) causing diarrhea, usually with blood and mucus. Other symptoms may include abdominal pain and fever.

C

CAUSES

Colitis may be due to infection by various different types of microorganism, such as *CAMPYLOBACTER* and *shigella* bacteria, viruses, or amebae.

Antibiotic drugs may sometimes provoke a form of colitis. Prolonged use of antibiotics commonly has a direct irritative effect on the colon. In some cases, antibiotics cause colitis by killing some types of bacteria that normally live in the intestine and allowing the proliferation of *CLOSTRIDIUM DIFFICILE* bacteria, which produce a toxin that irritates the colon.

Ischemia (impairment of blood supply) of the intestinal wall is a very rare cause of colitis in the elderly. Intestinal ischemia is usually due to *atherosclerosis* (accumulation of fatty deposits on the inner lining of arteries).

Colitis is a feature of *ulcerative colitis* and *Crohn's disease*, which are serious intestinal disorders of unknown origin that most commonly start in young adulthood.

Other disorders that can cause symptoms similar to those of colitis include *proctitis* (inflammation of the rectum), *diverticulitis* (inflammation of pouches in the colon), or cancer of the colon (see *Colon, cancer of*).

DIAGNOSIS

A physician may suspect colitis if severe diarrhea, with or without blood or mucus, persists for more than five days despite eating no solid foods and restricting the diet to clear fluids (such as water, tea, or clear soups). The physician will then usually send a sample of feces to a laboratory to be examined for the presence of microorganisms.

If no infection is found, *sigmoidoscopy* (inspection of the rectum and colon with a viewing instrument) or *colonoscopy* (inspection of the colon with a viewing instrument) may be performed to look for any inflammation or ulceration of the lining. A *biopsy* (removal of a sample of tissue for microscopic analysis) of inflamed areas or ulcers may be performed to look for the changes of ulcerative colitis or Crohn's disease. A barium enema (see *Barium X-ray examinations*) may be performed to look for any areas of narrowing or severe inflammation in the colon.

TREATMENT

When colitis is caused by an infection it usually gets better without any special treatment. However, campylobacter infections are sometimes treated with the antibiotic drug *erythromycin*, amebic infections with *metronidazole*,

and clostridium infections with metronidazole or *vancomycin*.

Colitis caused by ischemia is treated by surgical excision of the diseased section of colon.

Crohn's disease and ulcerative colitis are treated with *corticosteroid drugs*, with other drugs such as *sulfasalazine*, or by a special diet and vitamin supplements. Surgery does not cure these diseases and is reserved for the treatment of complications.

Collagen

A tough, fibrous *protein*. Collagen is the body's major structural protein, forming an important part of *tendons*, *bones*, and *connective tissues*. Because of its tough, insoluble nature, collagen helps hold together the cells and tissues of the body.

Collagen diseases

Two groups of diseases are referred to as collagen diseases—true collagen diseases and connective tissue diseases. True collagen diseases are uncommon, usually inherited, and due to faulty formation of *collagen* fibers. Features of true collagen diseases include thin, slack skin, and poor wound healing.

Connective tissue diseases are types of *autoimmune disorder* (in which a person's *immune system* reacts against his or her own organs or tissues). Autoimmune disorders often affect blood vessels and, as a result, produce secondary damage in connective tissues. Diseases of this type are sometimes called collagen vascular diseases. They include *rheumatoid arthritis*, systemic *lupus erythematosus*, *polyarteritis nodosa*, *scleroderma*, and *dermatomyositis*.

Collarbone

The common name for the *clavicle*.

Collar, orthopedic

A device worn to treat neck pain or instability. There are two basic types of orthopedic collar: soft collars, usually made of foam, and stiff collars, usually made of foam reinforced with plastic.

A soft collar can provide pain relief by limiting movement of the neck, by transferring some of the weight of the head from the neck to the chest, and by providing local warmth. Stiff collars may be used to provide support when a fractured neck has almost healed or when the cervical vertebrae (neck bones) have become unstable for some other reason.

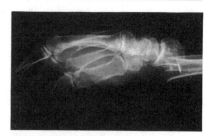

X ray of Colles' fracture
The wrist has been pushed back over the broken bone. This gives a classic "dinner fork" appearance when viewed from the side.

Colles' fracture

A break in the *radius* (one of the lower arm bones) just above the wrist, usually caused by a fall.

In a Colles' fracture the wrist and hand are displaced backward, resulting in restriction of movement and severe pain and swelling. Colles' fracture is the most common type of fracture in people over 40.

CAUSES

Colles' fracture usually occurs when someone stumbles when walking or slips on an icy pavement and puts out a hand to lessen the impact of the fall. Such a fall rarely produces a fracture in a young person, but it may be enough to break a bone weakened by *osteoporosis*, an invariable feature of aging. When a young person suffers a Colles' fracture, it is usually the result of a more violent injury and often extends to the wrist joint itself.

TREATMENT AND OUTLOOK

The two ends of the broken bone are usually manipulated back into position, under a local or a general anesthetic, and a plaster *cast* is applied. Healing usually takes up to six weeks. When the cast is removed, the wrist may be stiff and exercise may be needed to restore its flexibility.

Minor deformity of the wrist may result from Colles' fracture, but movement of the hand and wrist usually returns to normal. In cases where the injury was extensive, however, there is an increased likelihood that arthritis will develop.

Colloid

A state of matter similar to a suspension. A typical suspension—milk, for example—consists of insoluble particles of a substance suspended in a liquid. These particles are large and heavy enough to be separable from the liquid by centrifugation (spinning at high speed). A colloid is basically the same, except that its particles are significantly smaller and lighter than those of a suspension; they can be separated from the remaining part of the colloid only by ultracentrifugation (spinning at extremely high speed).

In medicine, colloid preparations containing *plasma proteins* (proteins in the fluid portion of blood) or certain complex carbohydrate molecules may be given to treat *shock*. Such colloid preparations are called plasma expanders. Colloids containing gold or technetium are used in some *radioisotope scanning* techniques.

The term colloid is also used to refer to the protein-containing material that fills the follicles of the *thyroid gland*.

Colon

The major part of the large intestine. The colon is a segmented tube, about 1.3 m long and 6.5 cm wide, that forms a large loop in the abdomen. Its segments, known as haustrations, give it an irregular outline.

The colon consists of four sections: the ascending, transverse, descending, and sigmoid colon. The first part, the ascending colon, starts at the *cecum*, in the lower right-hand side of the abdomen, and extends up to a sharp bend just below the liver. This point, called the hepatic flexure,

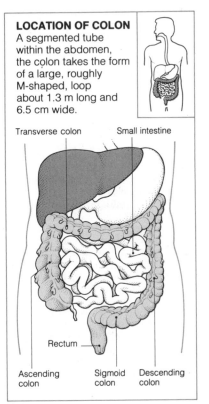

LOCATION OF COLON
A segmented tube within the abdomen, the colon takes the form of a large, roughly M-shaped, loop about 1.3 m long and 6.5 cm wide.

Transverse colon   Small intestine

Rectum

Ascending colon   Sigmoid colon   Descending colon

marks the beginning of the transverse colon, which loops across the abdomen, passing below the stomach to the spleen on the left-hand side of the abdomen. Here, there is a sharp downward bend (called the splenic flexure) that marks the start of the descending colon. From this point, the descending colon passes down the left side to approximately the brim of the pelvis, where it adopts an S-shaped course of variable length (the sigmoid colon) and finally connects with the *rectum* at the lower left-hand side of the abdomen.

STRUCTURE

The colon is a muscular tube with a lubricated inner lining. Its walls have four layers. The outermost layer, called the serous coat, is a tough, fibrous membrane with a smooth outer surface. This membrane protects the colon from damage when intestinal movements cause it to rub against the abdominal wall.

The next layer consists of three bands of longitudinal muscles and an inner band of circular muscles. Rhythmic contractions and relaxations of these muscles (*peristalsis*) squeeze the intestinal contents through the colon. (See illustrated box on *Peristalsis*.)

Inside the muscular layer is the third layer, the submucous coat. It consists of *connective tissue*, blood vessels, and lymphatic vessels.

The innermost layer is the mucous coat, which contains numerous tubular glands. These glands produce large amounts of mucus to lubricate the passage of digested material through the colon. Unlike the small intestine, the mucous coat of the colon (and the rest of the large intestine) is not folded into *villi* (tiny, finger-like projections).

FUNCTION

The functions of the colon are, principally, to absorb water (and also a small amount of mineral salts) from the digested material passing through the colon and to concentrate indigestible waste for expulsion as *feces*.

When the intestinal contents enter the colon, digestion has been completed and the material is in the form of a liquid. As this liquid passes through the colon, the water and salts it contains are absorbed into the blood vessels in the submucous coat. By the time the intestinal contents pass out of the colon into the rectum, almost all the water has been absorbed and the contents are in the form of feces. (See also *Digestive system*; *Intestine* disorders box.)

Colon, cancer of

A malignant tumor of the *colon* (the major part of the large intestine). The colon is one of the most common of all cancer sites. In Canada, about 7,400 males and 7,200 females are diagnosed with cancers of the colon and rectum each year.

These cancers account for about 11 percent of all cancer deaths.

CAUSES

Cancer of the colon has no single cause; there are a number of possible contributory factors.

The higher incidence of cancer of the colon in Western countries suggests an environmental, probably dietary, factor. It is thought that a high-meat, high-fat, and low-fiber diet encourages the production and concentration of *carcinogens*.

There is also thought to be a genetic factor. Brothers, sisters, and children of people suffering from cancer of the colon are more likely than average to acquire the disease later in life.

Cancer of the colon frequently occurs in association with some other diseases of the colon, such as *ulcerative colitis* and familial *polyposis*.

SYMPTOMS

An inexplicable change in bowel movements (either constipation or diarrhea) lasting for 10 days or so may be one of the first symptoms of cancer of the colon.

Blood mixed in the feces (as opposed to the blood from *hemorrhoids*, which usually coats the feces) is another important warning signal. However, if the cancer is high up in the colon, blood can be detected only by chemical tests.

There may be pain and tenderness in the lower abdomen. Sometimes, however, there are no symptoms until the cancer grows so big that the intestine becomes obstructed (see *Intestine, obstruction of*) or perforates (ruptures).

DIAGNOSIS AND TREATMENT

Tests on feces, *barium X-ray examinations*, *sigmoidoscopy* (inspection of the colon and rectum with a viewing instrument), and *colonoscopy* (inspection of the colon with a viewing instrument) may be carried out.

Treatment depends on the stage of development of the cancer, but, in most cases, a partial *colectomy* (removal of part of the colon) is performed. The diseased tissue and a small amount of surrounding normal tissue are removed and the cut ends are sewn together to reestablish the channel. If the disease is extensive, surgery may not be possible.

C

The long-term prospects vary according to the stage the disease has reached when it is discovered. More than 50 percent of patients survive in good health for at least five years after a colectomy. Nonsurgical treatments merely arrest the growth and spread of the cancer and are not curative. The earlier the tumor is detected, the greater the chances of a full recovery after treatment. Anyone over the age of 50 who experiences an inexplicable change in bowel movements should see a physician without delay. (See also *Rectum, cancer of*.)

Colon, disorders of
See *Intestine* disorders box.

Colon, irritable
See *Irritable bowel syndrome*.

Colonoscopy
Examination of the inside of the *colon* (the major part of the large intestine) by means of a long, flexible, fiber-optic viewing instrument called a colonoscope (see *Endoscopy*).

WHY IT IS DONE
Colonoscopy is used to investigate symptoms (such as bleeding from the bowel) and to look for disorders of the colon, such as colitis, polyps (small, benign, grapelike growths), and cancer. Attachments at the end of the instrument enable the physician to take biopsy specimens (small samples of tissue or cells for microscopic analysis), or to remove polyps.

HOW IT IS DONE
The patient takes *laxative drugs* for one or two days before the examination to empty the colon of feces. Because the procedure causes slight discomfort, the patient is lightly sedated beforehand. The colonoscope is passed into the colon through the anus and guided along the length of the colon, which the operator examines through a viewing lens. A complete examination of the entire colon can take from 10 minutes to a couple of hours.

Colon, spastic
See *Irritable bowel syndrome*.

Color blindness
See *Color vision deficiency*.

Color vision
The ability to discriminate different parts of the color spectrum (see illustrated box on facing page). Color vision probably evolved as an aid to finding or catching food.

THE COLOR SPECTRUM
Light perceived by the human eye consists of electromagnetic radiation (energy waves) with wavelengths between about 400 and 700 nanometres (a nanometre is a millionth of a millimetre).

Going from the short to the long end of this spectrum, different wavelengths produce the sensations of violet, indigo, blue, green, yellow, orange, and red when they impinge upon the retina of the eye and stimulate nerve signals, which are processed in the rear of the brain.

Light consisting of a single wavelength—pure spectral color—is rare in nature. The light reflected or emitted by most objects consists of a complex mixture of many different wavelengths, known as a spectral mixture. White light consists of a fairly uniform mixture of all wavelengths of the visible spectrum. The number of possible spectral mixtures is infinite, and a major task of the retina and brain is to sort and interpret the information available in order to produce a usefully large but finite number of perceivable colors (estimated at several million).

CONE FUNCTION
The light-sensitive cells in the retina are of two main types, rods and cones. Of these types, the rods vary little in their response to different light wavelengths, and thus play little, if any, part in color vision. The cone cells, of which there are roughly 4 million to 7 million per eye, play the major part and are more concentrated within a central area of the retina called the macula lutea; about 25,000 of the cones are in the fovea in the center of this area. Consequently, color vision is most accurate for objects viewed directly and is poor at the periphery of vision. Color perception also requires a minimum level of total available light—below this level, only the rods respond, and everything is seen as shades of gray. When light impinges upon a cone, it causes a structural change in pigment contained within the cone, which in turn causes the cone to emit an electrical impulse. Light of any wavelength and of sufficient intensity, in general, causes all cones to respond to some extent, but any single cone responds better (i.e., produces impulses more frequently) to certain wavelengths than others. Overall, it has been found that there are probably three classes of cone, responding maximally to light wavelengths of 445, 535, and

570 nanometres. Any particular light wavelength produces a unique overall pattern of response from all the cones together, and consequently any two wavelengths produce different patterns of response.

This offers some explanation of how the retina distinguishes light of different wavelengths, but gives few clues as to how information about complex mixtures of wavelengths is sorted, transmitted to the brain, and interpreted. The retina seems to contain other cells that receive, analyze, and compare the signals coming from several classes of cone. Further integration of the signals is accomplished as they are carried to the brain, where additional processing occurs, allowing for the perception of color. (See also *Color vision deficiency*; *Eye*; *Perception*; *Vision*.)

Color vision deficiency
Any abnormality of the *color vision* system that causes difficulty distinguishing between certain colors. Such deficiencies are of various types and differ markedly in degree. Mild forms of deficiency, which are by far the most common, allow vision that is completely adequate for most everyday purposes.

True "color blindness" (monochromatism), in which the world is seen only in shades of black, white, and gray, is extremely rare.

CAUSES AND TYPES
Most cases of color vision deficiency are caused by an inherited defect of the light-sensitive pigment in one or more classes of cone cell in the retina and/or an abnormality or reduced number of the cone cells themselves. Acquired color vision deficiency may result from certain retinal and optic nerve diseases or from injury.

The two common types of hereditary color vision deficiency are reduced discrimination of light wavelengths within the middle (green) and long (red) parts of the visible spectrum. In the more severe cases, a person with green deficiency (deuteranopia) has great difficulty distinguishing oranges, greens, brown, and pale reds. For a person with severe red deficiency (protanopia) all reds are markedly dulled. These inherited defects are usually sex-linked (see *Genetic disorders*), i.e., the majority of those affected are male, although women may carry the defect and pass it on to some of their children.

A further very small group have a blue deficiency, called tritanopia, which may be inherited or due to the toxic effects of poisons or drugs on, or degenerative processes of, the retina or optic nerve.

INCIDENCE

Among white people of European origin, about 8 percent of males and less than 1 percent of females have either green or red deficiency. The prevalence is generally lower in people of Asian origin and even lower among black people. The prevalence of both blue deficiency and monochromatism may be as low as one affected person per 100,000.

SYMPTOMS

Most people with defective color vision have no reason to suspect there is anything abnormal about the way they see, because they have no ready access to how other people see the world and because most cases are mild and do not interfere with everyday activities. Most cases come to light only when a person is noticed making mistakes with color discrimination, such as confusing close shades of colors, or when the person's color vision is tested.

DIAGNOSIS AND MEASUREMENT

Color vision is commonly tested, generally by means of special color plates under daylight conditions, during childhood or before admission to occupations for which good color discrimination is needed.

COLOR VISION

Light, consisting of radiation of various wavelengths, is focused on the retina, where light-sensitive rod and cone cells are stimulated to emit nerve impulses. Some initial processing of this "signaling" occurs in the ganglion cells of the retina, before impulses pass to the brain via the optic nerve.

Location of color-sensitive cells
Light passes through the whole thickness of the retina before striking the rods and cones. Color vision depends mainly on the cones, concentrated in a region of the retina called the fovea.

Color response of cones
There are three classes of cone, and the graph shows how these vary in their response to the light spectrum. One class responds best to light of long wavelengths (red-sensitive cones), one to short wavelengths (blue-sensitive), and one to intermediate wavelengths (green-sensitive).

Response to white light
White light consists of a mixture of all wavelengths (colors), so it stimulates all three classes of cone to signal equally. This pattern of response produces the sensation of whiteness in the brain.

Response to red light
Light with a long wavelength (red light) produces a strong response from red-sensitive cones, a weak response from blue-sensitive cones, and an intermediate response from green-sensitive cones. This pattern of signaling is interpreted as the color red in the brain.

Key
G Green-sensitive
R Red-sensitive
B Blue-sensitive

More complicated testing may also be used. The anomaloscope shines a variable mixture of green and red lights, and the person is asked to adjust the mixture until it appears the same as a fixed yellow light. If the adjusted mixture looks far too red or too green to someone with normal vision, the subject of the test is color defective. The severity of the defect is also measurable in this way.

OUTLOOK

People with the common, inherited, types of color vision deficiency retain the defect for life. It could be important for them to know about the abnormality, especially if they are considering an occupation that depends on color discrimination: a person who is severely color deficient could be dangerous in certain jobs, such as that of pilot, train engineer, or electrician. Mild color vision deficiencies, however, rarely cause trouble.

Colostomy

An operation in which part of the *colon* (major part of the large intestine) is brought through an incision in the abdominal wall and formed into an artificial opening to allow the discharge of feces into a lightweight bag attached to the skin. The colostomy may be temporary or permanent.

WHY IT IS DONE

In a severely ill patient, a temporary colostomy may be carried out as an emergency measure to deal with an obstruction or perforation in the large intestine that is preventing the patient from passing feces. The colostomy is made above the obstruction and, by allowing the feces to discharge, enables the patient to become well enough to undergo a partial *colectomy* (an operation to remove part of the large intestine) to remove the obstruction. A temporary colostomy may also be performed at the same time as a colectomy in order to allow the colon to heal without feces passing through it. Temporary colostomies are closed when the rejoined colon has healed.

A permanent colostomy is needed if all or part of the rectum or anus must be removed (e.g., to treat cancer of the rectum), making normal defecation impossible.

RECOVERY PERIOD

For two or three days after the operation the patient is fed intravenously. He or she is then given a light diet and begins to pass feces through the stoma (artificial opening) into a lightweight bag that is attached by adhesive seals to the skin around the stoma. After a bowel movement, the bag is exchanged for a new one.

During this period the patient should receive advice and training from a specialist stoma care nurse on how to look after the stoma and on how to change the colostomy bag.

After leaving hospital, the patient usually needs to convalesce for several weeks before returning to normal activities. The stoma care nurse will make visits to check progress.

OUTLOOK

A person with a colostomy may eventually establish an almost normal bowel routine. The bowel usually discharges feces into the bag once or twice a day; the bag is then changed.

A person with a colostomy can expect to lead a normal life after he or she has fully recovered from the operation. There are usually no complications. Occasional problems, such as prolapse (protrusion) of part of the colon through the abdominal opening, or blockage to the passage of feces due to narrowing of the stoma, can usually be treated surgically.

Colostrum

The thick, yellowish fluid produced by a mother's breasts during the first few days after childbirth. Colostrum is replaced by mature breast milk about four to five days after birth. Compared with mature breast milk, colostrum contains less fat and sugar, and more minerals and protein. It has a high content of *lymphocytes* (white blood cells) and *immunoglobulins*, which help protect the baby from infection.

Colposcopy

Visual inspection of a woman's *cervix* (neck of the uterus) and *vagina* under illuminated magnification. The procedure is performed with a colposcope, a viewing instrument using a series of lenses to give different degrees of magnification.

WHY IT IS DONE

Colposcopy is performed to recognize or exclude the presence of any areas of precancerous tissue or early cancer in the cervix (see *Cervix, cancer of*). In most cases, the gynecologist has been alerted by an abnormal *cervical smear test*, by smears that repeatedly show

---

PROCEDURE FOR COLOSTOMY

An incision is made in the abdominal wall and either a small loop of the colon or (if the rectum and anus have been removed) the severed end of the colon is pulled through. If a loop of the colon is used, an opening is made in it large enough for the feces to pass through. The edges of this opening or the edges of the severed end of the colon are stitched to the skin at the edge of the abdominal incision to create a stoma (artificial opening).

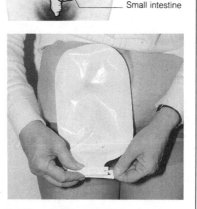

Large intestine

Possible sites of colostomy openings

Small intestine

Diseased part of rectum removed

Open end of bowel brought through to skin surface

Position of colostomy bag
The bag is attached to the skin around the stoma by adhesive seals. After a bowel movement, a new bag is attached.

---

inflammation or infection, or by an abnormal appearance of the cervix during visual inspection at the time of a vaginal examination.

HOW IT IS DONE

Colposcopy is a painless procedure requiring no anesthetic. With the woman in the lithotomy position (lying on her back with legs apart and supported), the vagina and cervix are exposed using a speculum (an instrument that widens the opening and separates the walls of the vagina). The exposed tissues are first wiped with a dry sponge; the area is then washed with a solution of either dilute acetic acid or saline. The tissues are visually inspected under magnification to identify any suspicious-looking areas.

The applied solution causes any precancerous areas to show up either white (instead of their natural pink state) or with a characteristic surface pattern due to abnormal blood vessels. Once any such areas are seen, a *biopsy* sample of the tissue can be obtained.

If the biopsy sample shows cells typical of severe dysplasia (abnormal growth) or an early cancer, treatment is required. If the whole of the abnormal area can be seen during colposcopy, the abnormal tissue can be destroyed by *diathermy, cryosurgery*, or *laser treatment*. If any of the abnormal area is within the cervical canal and therefore out of sight of the colposcope, a *cone biopsy* (removal of a conical section of the cervix for inspection) is needed.

Coma

A state of unconsciousness and unresponsiveness distinguishable from *sleep* in that the person does not respond to external stimuli (e.g., shouting or pinching) or to internal stimuli (e.g., a full bladder).

CAUSES

Coma results from disturbance or damage to areas of the brain involved in conscious activity or the maintenance of consciousness—in particular, parts of the *cerebrum* (the main mass of the brain), upper parts of the *brain stem*, and central regions of the brain, especially the *limbic system*.

The damage may be the result of a *head injury*, or of an abnormality such as a *brain tumor, brain abscess*, or *intracerebral hemorrhage*; all are shown by *brain imaging* techniques.

More often, there has been an accumulation of poisonous substances that intoxicate brain tissues (due to a drug overdose, advanced liver or kidney disease, acute alcoholic intoxication, or in uncontrolled *diabetes mellitus*) or there has been impairment of blood flow to some brain areas, leading to cerebral *hypoxia* (lack of oxygen). *Encephalitis* (inflammation of the brain) and *meningitis* (inflammation of the brain's protective coverings) can also cause coma.

SYMPTOMS

Varying depths of coma are recognized. In less severe forms, the person may respond to stimulation by uttering a few words or perhaps moving an arm. In severe cases, the person fails to respond in this way to repeated vigorous stimuli. However, even deeply comatose patients may show some automatic responses—they continue to breathe unaided, may cough, yawn, blink, and show roving eye movements, indicating that the lower brain stem, which controls these responses, is still functioning.

Measurement of variations in the depth of coma is important in assessment and treatment. Variations can be recorded by systems that classify the coma according to the person's verbal behavior, the movements he or she makes, and the state of the eyes (whether open, shut, or roving).

A person may remain alive for many years in a state of deep coma provided the brain stem is still functioning (and also provided he or she receives appropriate nursing care). If the lower brain stem is damaged or diseased, the vital functions of coughing, swallowing, and breathing are impaired and artificial ventilation and maintenance of the circulation may be needed to maintain life. Complete irreversible loss of brain stem function leads to death (see *Brain death*).

Combination drug

A preparation that contains more than one active, therapeutic substance. The antibiotic co-trimoxazole, which contains sulfamethoxazole and trimethoprim, is one such example.

Comedo

Another name for a *blackhead*.

Commensal

A usually harmless bacterium or other organism that normally lives in or on the body. Occasionally, commensals may cause disease, especially in people with impaired immunity.

Commode

A portable chair that contains a removable toilet bowl in its seat. Commodes are useful for patients who are not confined to bed but who are not mobile enough to use the toilet.

Communicable disease

Any disease caused by a microorganism or parasite that can be transmitted (directly or indirectly) from one person or animal to another. (See also *Contagious; Infectious disease*.)

Compartment syndrome

A painful cramp caused by compression of a group of muscles within a confined space. An example is tibial compartment syndrome, affecting the muscles on the outer side of the shin.

Compartment syndrome may occur if muscles have become enlarged as a result of intensive training or injury. During exercise, blood flow into muscles increases and the muscles expand slightly. In compartment syndrome, the muscles are compressed, causing cramps due to obstruction of the blood flow through the muscles. Exercise-induced cramps usually disappear when the exercise is stopped. Severe cases may require treatment by *fasciotomy* surgery to improve blood flow and prevent development of a permanent *contracture* (deformity caused by shrinkage of tissues).

Compensation neurosis

Psychological reaction to injury affected by the prospect of financial compensation, also called accident or "traumatic" neurosis.

Symptoms vary, but headache, dizzy spells, loss of concentration, anxiety, and mild depression are common, as are neurological symptoms, such as pain and tingling in the legs or numbness in the affected part. Symptoms do not depend necessarily on the severity of the injury.

Some specialists consider the neurosis to be a genuine and persistent psychiatric reaction; others insist it is an attempt, conscious or unconscious, to manipulate the situation for profit. Repeated medical assessments, legal wrangling, and contradictory experts make this one of the most difficult areas of psychiatric diagnosis. Backing the idea of a genuine organic disorder, recent studies have shown that some people's symptoms persisted even after a satisfactory settlement of their insurance claims.

Complement

A group of proteins in *blood* plasma. Complement is an important part of the *immune system*, destroying foreign cells. The complement system is usually activated by reactions between antigens and antibodies.

Complex

A term meaning a group or combination of related items. In medicine it is used, for example, to refer to a combination of signs and symptoms forming a syndrome (as in *Eisenmenger complex*) or to a collection of substances that share a similar structure or function (as in *vitamin B complex*).

In psychology, a complex is a group of unconscious ideas, beliefs, and memories that have great emotional importance. The term was first used by Sigmund Freud and Carl Jung to sum up psychological states deriving from experiences and relationships in childhood. The *Oedipus complex* is an important example, affecting all levels of adult behavior and attitudes.

Compliance

The degree to which patients follow medical advice. Research suggests that the degree of compliance is generally greater among patients who are provided with adequate information. For example, patients are more likely to comply with a drug treatment if they know whether the drug is likely to produce side effects or interact adversely with their other medications and under what circumstances it should be discontinued.

Complication

A condition that results from a preceding disorder or from the treatment of that disorder. For example, in a case of *appendicitis*, the inflamed appendix may rupture, spreading infection throughout the abdominal cavity and causing a serious complication called *peritonitis*. The childhood condition *mumps* occasionally has complications that may be serious, particularly *encephalitis* (inflammation of the brain) or *orchitis* (inflammation of the testes). Recovery from an operation may be complicated by *wound infection*.

Compos mentis

Latin for "of sound mind."

Compress

A pad of lint or linen applied, under pressure, to an area of skin, and held in place by a bandage. The pad may be soaked in ice-cold water or wrapped around ice to provide a cold compress for reducing pain, swelling, and bleeding under the skin after an injury (see *Ice pack*).

Compresses that have been soaked in hot water increase the circulation and are useful for bringing boils to a head. A dry compress may be used to stop bleeding from a wound (see *Bleeding* first-aid box) or may be smeared with medication to help treat an infected area of skin.

Compression syndrome

A collection of symptoms caused by pressure on a nerve that supplies the muscles in a particular area of the body and carries sensations from that area. The symptoms may include numbness, tingling, discomfort, and muscle weakness. The best known is *carpal tunnel syndrome* (which affects the hand), caused by pressure on the median nerve as it passes under a ligament in the wrist.

Compulsive behavior

See *Obsessive-compulsive disorder*.

Computed tomography

Another name for *CT scanning*.

Computer-aided diagnosis

The physician makes a diagnosis by considering the patient's symptoms and medical history, examining the patient, and, when necessary, making use of special tests and procedures. The computer has made possible many new investigative procedures, such as *CT scanning* and *MRI* (see *Imaging techniques*). It can also be used to aid diagnosis in the following ways.

PROBABILITY-BASED SYSTEMS

With probability-based systems the computer is used to store vast quantities of information involving cases of many different disorders. For example, it may be programmed with the details of thousands of cases of stomach pain—giving, for each patient, the exact type, location, and duration of the pain, accompanying symptoms, and the relevant medical history, together with the eventual diagnosis. A physician confronted with a new case of stomach pain can enter the details into the computer, which, in a matter of seconds, will compare them with those already stored in its memory. It will then print out a list of the most likely diagnoses.

Although such computers are currently used in comparatively few hospitals, they are proving valuable in the treatment of people isolated from medical services, such as oil-rig crews or deep-sea divers. If someone becomes ill, the computer may be used to diagnose whether the case is

an emergency requiring the person to be transported to a hospital.

PATTERN-RECOGNITION SYSTEMS

Computers can also be programmed to recognize and interpret visual data. One example is the examination of cells under a microscope. The computer has the ability to recognize abnormal cells. This could be of great future significance in certain types of *blood count* (e.g., a differential white blood cell count) and also in *cervical smear tests*, in which cells taken from the cervix are examined under a microscope for early signs of cancer. At present, each of the millions of smears taken annually needs examination by a laboratory technician, who can check only a comparatively small number per day.

Conception

The *fertilization* of a woman's *ovum* (egg) by a man's *sperm*, followed about five days later by implantation of the resultant blastocyst in the lining of the uterus, thus starting a *pregnancy*. (See also *Contraception*.)

Concussion

Brief unconsciousness, usually lasting only a few seconds, that follows a violent blow to the head or neck. The loss of consciousness is due to disturbance of the electrical activity in the brain, and in most cases is not associated with any damage. Nevertheless, concussion should always be reported to a physician because of the possibility of serious consequences.

Among the more common causes of concussion are traffic accidents, sports injuries, falls, industrial accidents, and blows received in fights.

SYMPTOMS AND TREATMENT

Common symptoms immediately following concussion include confusion, inability to remember events immediately before the injury, dizziness, blurred vision, and vomiting. The more prolonged the period of unconsciousness, the more severe and persistent symptoms tend to be.

Repeated concussion—as happens, for example, to some boxers—can damage the brain and cause the "punch-drunk" syndrome: slow thinking, impaired concentration, and slurred speech.

Anyone who has been knocked out should see a physician, who will usually advise 24 hours of bed rest, either in hospital or at home, under observation. The person should not drive a car or play any sport during this time. If new symptoms develop, such as drowsiness, difficulty breathing, repeated vomiting, or visual disturbances, they should be reported to the physician immediately since they could signify damage to part of the brain or an *extradural hemorrhage* (bleeding between the skull and the outside of the brain).

The initial symptoms usually start to clear within a few days. If they fail to do so, medical opinion should be sought again, at which time the physician may wish to have the condition investigated further. (See also *Head injury*.)

Conditioning

The formation of a specific response or type of behavior to a specific stimulus in the environment. Theories of conditioning are based largely on the work of the Russian physiologist Ivan Pavlov and the American psychologist B. F. Skinner.

TYPES

CLASSICAL CONDITIONING If a stimulus that consistently produces a particular response is paired repeatedly with a second stimulus (which would not itself produce the response), the second stimulus (the conditioned stimulus) will eventually produce the response even without the presence of the first stimulus (the unconditioned stimulus).

Classical conditioning was described by Pavlov, who demonstrated the phenomenon in dogs. He noted that food (the unconditioned stimulus) caused dogs to salivate (the unconditioned response). He found that if a bell (the conditioned stimulus) was rung immediately before the food was presented to the dog, the dog would eventually produce the conditioned response of salivating when it heard the bell alone, without any food being presented.

Pavlov noted that a conditioned response to a specific conditioned stimulus would also occur in response to a similar conditioned stimulus. Thus, a dog conditioned to salivate when shown a round object would also salivate, although not as much, when shown an elliptical one. He also found that the conditioned response would eventually fade unless reinforced by occasional pairing of the conditioned with the unconditioned stimulus.

OPERANT CONDITIONING The central concept of this type of conditioning is that behavior can be modified by a system of rewards and/or punishments.

Much of the early work in this field was done by B. F. Skinner, who demonstrated the phenomenon in laboratory animals. Skinner placed a hungry rat in a box. It moved randomly about the cage, but occasionally accidentally pawed a lever, which released a pellet of food. Eventually the rat learned that the action of pressing the lever led to the reward of food. Thus the rat became conditioned to press the lever whenever it wanted food.

EFFECTS

Many behavioral psychologists believe that all behavior is learned by a process of conditioning. They regard some psychiatric problems as inappropriate behavior patterns that have been learned through conditioning. Treatment for these disorders can also be based on the principles of conditioning, which can be used to modify inappropriate behavior patterns (see *Behavior therapy*).

Condom

A barrier method of contraception in the form of a thin latex rubber or plastic sheath placed over the penis before intercourse. In addition to their contraceptive effect, condoms provide both partners with some degree of protection against the sexual transmission of disease. (See *Contraception, barrier methods of*.)

Conduct disorders

A group of behavioral disturbances, occurring in childhood or adolescence, in which the individual persistently and repetitively violates the rights and privileges of others. These violations may include vandalism, arson, assault, and robbery, as well as less aggressive forms of behavior such as truancy, substance abuse, and persistent lying. (See also *Adolescence; Behavioral problems in children*.)

Condyloma acuminatum

See *Warts, genital*.

Cone biopsy

A surgical technique in which a conical or cylindrical section of the lower part of the *cervix* (neck of the uterus) is removed.

WHY IT IS DONE

A cone biopsy is performed if a woman has had an abnormal *cervical smear test* or a series of abnormal smears, and if visual inspection of the cervix by *colposcopy* has failed to delineate the exact area of cancer or a precancerous condition (see *Cervix, cancer of*). Sometimes a cone biopsy is performed if a smear test suggests the presence of cancer, but colposcopy has failed to detect any abnormality on the outer surface of the cervix or at the entrance to the canal. In the latter cases there may be a precancerous area or cancer confined to the cervical canal, out of sight of the colposcope.

Cone biopsy can now be accomplished by *laser treatment* or by *cryosurgery*. (See also illustrated box on biopsy of the *Cervix*.)

Confabulation

The use of a fictional story to make up for gaps in memory. Confabulation differs from lying in that it is motivated by the need to make sense of one's past rather than by a desire to deceive a listener. The phenomenon occurs most commonly in chronic alcoholics suffering from *Wernicke-Korsakoff syndrome*. It also occurs in some people with head injuries.

Confidentiality

The ethical principle that a physician does not disclose to others information given in confidence by a patient. This concept was introduced by the ancient Greek physician Hippocrates and has been adopted by medical associations in all countries.

The physician's responsibility for maintaining confidential records has become more difficult with modern trends in medical practice. Clinics and health centers may have scores of medical and ancillary staff with access to records. In hospitals with computerized records, thousands of staff members may have such access. To prevent breaches in confidentiality, everyone working in a medical setting is expected to understand and respect the code of confidentiality. Some computer systems make it possible to render the sensitive sections of medical records secure.

The patient's consent to disclosure is required before a physician may give confidential information to an employer, insurance company, or lawyer. When required by law to disclose confidential information, a physician (unlike a lawyer) does not have any "privilege" that allows refusal. A physician who persists in refusal is in contempt of court.

Physicians who treat children are expected to discuss their findings with the parents. As children mature, a point is reached at which their confidences merit the same respect as those of adult patients. In general, physicians believe that they should respect a child's request for confidentiality.

293

C

Most legal systems require physicians to override confidentiality in certain circumstances. For example, they are required to notify specified infectious diseases; if patients with certain of these diseases refuse treatment, the health authorities may be informed so that treatment or isolation may be imposed by law. Physicians are also generally required to notify the police if they treat gunshot wounds or know of other serious crimes.

Physicians who breach confidentiality without legal justification may be sued and damages may be awarded against them. They may also be brought before the ethical committee of their professional body, which may have the right to suspend or cancel their legal right to practice.

Confusion
A disorganized mental state in which the abilities to remember, think clearly, and reason are impaired.

TYPES AND CAUSES
Confusion can be acute or chronic. Acute confusion can arise as a symptom of *delirium*, in which the activity of the brain is affected by fever, drugs, poisons, or injury. Elderly people are particularly prone to acute confusional states from these causes, and especially from certain drugs (e.g., *antianxiety drugs* or *alcohol*).

Chronic confusion is often associated with *alcohol dependence*, long-term use of antianxiety drugs, and certain organic (physically based) mental disorders. Chronic confusion is a feature of *dementia*, a brain disorder commonly caused by the progressive degeneration and death of brain cells.

SYMPTOMS AND SIGNS
People who are acutely confused are temporarily unable to organize their thoughts. They may also suffer from terrifying hallucinations and may behave in a violent and abusive manner. Few people are able to recollect the period of confusion once it has passed.

Chronic confusion is generally noticeable by features such as absent-mindedness, poor short-term memory, and a tendency for the sufferer to repeat himself or herself. Chronically confused people may also become depressed and frustrated, but they are less likely to become aggressive or violent. Many of the conditions responsible for chronic confusion tend to be slowly progressive.

DIAGNOSIS AND TREATMENT
The cause of a person's confusion can often be diagnosed from a detailed description of the symptoms (often from a relative) and a general physical examination of the patient. In some cases, further tests may be necessary for an accurate diagnosis.

Treatment varies a great deal, depending on the underlying cause, and can often produce a marked improvement. *Sedative drugs* may be of benefit to some people who are acutely confused. Drugs are of little help to elderly chronically confused patients, for whom skilled, supervised care is the most important aspect of treatment.

Congenital
A term that means "present at birth." Thus, a congenital abnormality may have been inherited from the parents, may have occurred as the result of damage or infection in the uterus, or may have occurred at the time of birth. Congenital abnormalities are often also called *birth defects*.

Note that "congenital" does not mean the same as "hereditary." Not all congenital abnormalities are inherited, and many hereditary diseases (such as *Huntington's chorea*) are not apparent at birth.

Diseases and disorders that are neither congenital nor inherited but which are caused by external factors—for example, infection, injury or poisoning—are termed "acquired."

Congestion
A term that usually refers to the accumulation of an excessive amount of blood, *tissue fluid*, or *lymph* in part of the body.

A major cause of congestion is an increase in the flow of blood to a particular area of the body, as occurs in inflammation. Another possible cause of congestion is reduced drainage of blood from the affected area, as can occur in *heart failure*, in venous disorders such as *varicose veins*, and in *lymphatic disorders*.

In *nasal congestion*, inflammation of the nasal lining is accompanied by an increase in mucus production.

Congestive heart failure
See *Heart failure*.

Conjunctiva
The transparent membrane covering the sclera (white of the eye) and lining the inside of the eyelids. Cells in the conjunctiva produce a fluid (similar to tears) that lubricates the lids and the cornea. Blood vessels within the conjunctiva are normally invisible to the naked eye, but become engorged in *conjunctivitis* and other inflammatory conditions.

Conjunctivitis
Inflammation of the conjunctiva, causing redness, discomfort, and a discharge from the affected eye. Conjunctivitis is very common: at least one person in 50 who visit a physician does so because of this complaint.

CAUSES AND TYPES
The common causes are infections (especially in children) and allergy (more common in adults).

INFECTIVE CONJUNCTIVITIS Most conjunctival infections are caused by bacteria (e.g., staphylococci), which are spread by hand-to-eye contact, or by viruses associated with a cold, sore throat, or illness such as *measles*. Viral conjunctivitis sometimes occurs in epidemics, spreading rapidly through schools and other groups.

Newborn babies occasionally develop conjunctivitis soon after birth, a condition known as neonatal *ophthalmia*. This condition results from the spread of infection from the mother's cervix during birth and may be caused by various microorganisms, including those responsible for *gonorrhea*, genital *herpes*, or *chlamydial infection*. The infection may spread to the entire eye and can cause blindness.

Keratoconjunctivitis is an inflammation of both the conjunctiva and the cornea; it is often due to a viral infection. *Trachoma* is a serious form of conjunctivitis; it is caused by a type of chlamydial infection that is most common in tropical countries.

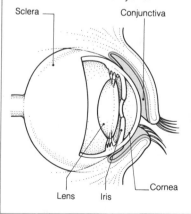

LOCATION OF CONJUNCTIVA
This transparent membrane covers the white of the eye and lines the inside of the eyelids.

Sclera

Conjunctiva

Lens

Iris

Cornea

ALLERGIC CONJUNCTIVITIS An allergic response of the conjunctiva may be provoked by a variety of substances, including cosmetics (such as mascara), contact lens cleaning solutions, and pollen.

SYMPTOMS

All types of conjunctivitis cause redness, irritation, itching, discharge, and occasionally photophobia (abnormal sensitivity to bright light). In infective conjunctivitis the discharge contains pus and may cause the eyelids to be stuck together in the morning. In allergic conjunctivitis the discharge is clear, and the eyelids are often swollen.

DIAGNOSIS

Diagnosis is made from the appearance of the eye. If an infection is suspected, swabs may be taken to find out the causative organism, especially in a newborn baby when an exact diagnosis may be needed.

TREATMENT

Warm water is used to wash away the discharge and remove any crusts on the eyelids.

Suspected infections are treated with eye drops or ointment containing an *antibiotic drug* (such as *chloramphenicol*). Viral conjunctivitis tends to get better without treatment.

Allergic conjunctivitis may be relieved by the use of eye drops containing an *antihistamine drug*. Occasionally, eye drops containing a *corticosteroid drug* may be prescribed provided that there is definitely no accompanying infection (which could be worsened by a corticosteroid).

Connective tissue

The material that holds together the various structures of the body. Some structures are made up of connective tissue, notably *tendons* and *cartilage*. Connective tissue also forms the matrix (ground substance) of *bone* and the nonmuscular structures of *arteries* and *veins*.

Connective tissue diseases

See *Collagen diseases*.

Conn's syndrome

A disorder caused by the secretion of excessive amounts of the hormone aldosterone by a benign tumor of one of the adrenal glands. (See also *Aldosteronism*.)

Consciousness

An awareness of self and surroundings, so that a person knows what he or she is doing and intends to do. The awareness is dependent on sensations (especially visual and auditory), memories, and experiences.

Such awareness requires intact brain function, particularly within the *cerebrum* (the main mass of the brain) and the reticular system in the *brain stem*. The content of consciousness relies heavily on the functions of the cerebrum—for example, on memory and the interpretation of sensations—while wakefulness is linked with the reticular system.

Although a person may be conscious, a great deal that goes on within the brain is still below the level of consciousness. In psychological terms this activity is referred to as *subconscious* activity.

Disturbance of consciousness leads to impaired attention, concentration, and understanding. Thought processes become slowed and memory fails. There appears to be a lack of direction to thoughts and actions. Although patients can be stimulated to respond, their responses are faulty. As the level of arousal deteriorates, the person may eventually pass into a state of *stupor* and then *coma*.

Consent

The legal term describing a patient's agreement to a physician performing an operation, arranging a drug treatment, or carrying out diagnostic tests. Physicians should be sure that patients consent to all diagnostic procedures and treatments. This consent must be given voluntarily, after the physician has presented facts any reasonable person in the patient's position would want to know before agreeing to or rejecting the proposed procedure. The physician must explain (without being asked to do so) the possible risks and benefits of the procedure, and any reasonable alternative procedures, and he or she must do so in language the patient can understand. The explanation should include information on the risks of surgical complications or death, and the possible side effects of all medications. If the patient is incompetent, the physician has a duty to obtain consent from a duly recognized substitute decision maker.

In obtaining consent for a patient's participation in a research project, the patient must be told (without having to ask and in language the patient can understand) whatever a reasonable person in the patient's position would want to know. The patient must be competent. In addition to those requirements of voluntary, informed and competent consent, patients must be told the purpose of the study and that they are free to withdraw from it at any time without compromising their treatment. Consent to a research procedure is invalid if any pressure to consent was put on the patient.

WITHHOLDING CONSENT

Children or people with serious mental disorders cannot give consent, but consent can be given on their behalf by parents or relatives. There have been several instances in Canada where the courts have intervened to overrule a parent's decision to withhold consent to vital treatment for a child.

Parents may consent to a child's participation in research only if possible harm to the child is minimal.

Constipation

The infrequent or difficult passing of hard, dry *feces*. In most cases constipation is harmless, but occasionally it may be a symptom of an underlying disorder, especially if it is of recent onset in an adult over 40. Many people worry that they do not move their bowels often enough, but, in fact, regularity and comfort of bowel action are more important than frequency. However, any persistent change in the pattern of bowel movements should be investigated by a physician to rule out the possibility of a serious disorder.

CAUSES

The most common cause of constipation in developed countries is insufficient *fiber* in the diet. Fiber, which is found in foods such as whole-grain bread, fresh fruit, and vegetables, provides the bulk that the muscles of the *colon* (the major part of the large intestine) need to stimulate propulsion of the feces.

Lack of regular bowel-moving habits is another cause of constipation. This may be the result of poor toilet-training in childhood or of repeatedly ignoring the urge to move the bowels. In the elderly the latter is sometimes due to immobility. Another cause of constipation in some elderly people is weakness of the muscles of the abdomen and the pelvic floor, which prevents adequate pressure when attempting to move the bowels. In people suffering from *hemorrhoids* (piles) or an *anal fissure* (a crack in the skin around the anus), the pain experienced on passing feces can be severe enough to inhibit the initiation of bowel movements.

C

C

CONSTIPATION Infrequent or difficult passing of hard bowel movements.

Have you always tended to suffer from constipation?

YES ▶ Do you often resist the urge to move your bowels because you are too busy?

YES ▶ This can lead to an eventual loss of normal bowel reflexes. You should try to reestablish a regular habit by always going to the bathroom when you feel the urge.

NO

NO ▼ Have you used laxatives regularly for a long time?

YES ▶ Overuse of laxatives can eventually make your bowel inactive. Stop taking the laxatives and try adding bran and extra fruit to your diet instead.

See • *Laxative drugs*

NO

Dietary fiber
This should be an essential part of everyone's diet because it provides bulk to help the large intestine carry away body wastes. Not only does it help prevent constipation and certain diseases of the large intestine but it may also help lower the level of fats in the body.

Your constipation is probably due to a lack of fluid, fruits, vegetables, and whole-grain cereals in your diet. Increase your intake. If no improvement results, consult your physician.

See • *Fiber, dietary*

Has defecation become painful?

YES ▶ A tear in the lining of the anus or hemorrhoids may cause such pain. Consult your physician.

See • *Anal fissure*
• *Hemorrhoids*

NO

Do you have lower abdominal pain?

YES ▶ Have you had similar episodes of pain and constipation for many years?

YES ▶ You probably have an irritable bowel. Consult your physician.

See • *Irritable bowel syndrome*

NO

☎
Consult your physician without delay!
An irritable bowel or diverticular disease (pouches in the walls of the large intestine) may cause such symptoms. However, the slight possibility of intestinal cancer must also be ruled out.

See • *Diverticular disease*
• *Intestine, cancer of*
• *Irritable bowel syndrome*

Fiber-rich foods
Fruit, leafy vegetables, potato skins, whole-grain bread and cereals, dried peas and beans, and bran are all examples of high-fiber foods.

NO

Continued on next page

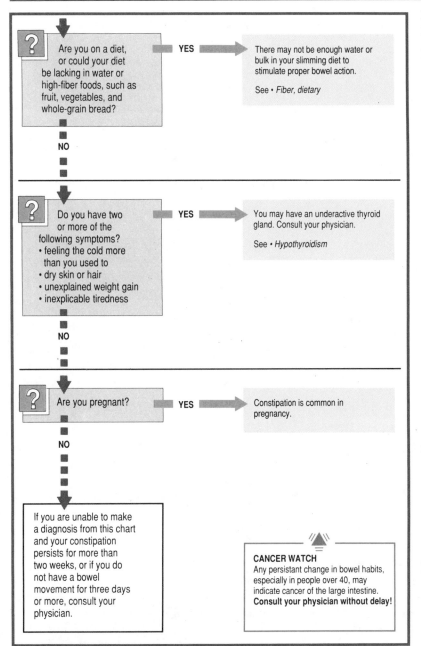

Are you on a diet, or could your diet be lacking in water or high-fiber foods, such as fruit, vegetables, and whole-grain bread?

YES → There may not be enough water or bulk in your slimming diet to stimulate proper bowel action.

See • *Fiber, dietary*

NO

Do you have two or more of the following symptoms?
• feeling the cold more than you used to
• dry skin or hair
• unexplained weight gain
• inexplicable tiredness

YES → You may have an underactive thyroid gland. Consult your physician.

See • *Hypothyroidism*

NO

Are you pregnant?

YES → Constipation is common in pregnancy.

NO

If you are unable to make a diagnosis from this chart and your constipation persists for more than two weeks, or if you do not have a bowel movement for three days or more, consult your physician.

CANCER WATCH
Any persistant change in bowel habits, especially in people over 40, may indicate cancer of the large intestine. **Consult your physician without delay!**

In *irritable bowel syndrome*, the person may experience intermittent constipation, sometimes alternating with diarrhea. In *hypothyroidism*, colonic contractions slow down and result in chronic constipation. Narrowing of part of the colon—due to *diverticular disease* or cancer (see *Colon, cancer of*), for example—is another possible cause of constipation.

A physician usually investigates the condition by obtaining a detailed case history, carrying out a physical examination, and arranging for special tests.

TREATMENT
Prolonged use of *laxative drugs* can impair the normal functioning of the colon, and their use should generally be avoided except in cases where straining to pass feces will aggravate another existing condition, such as hemorrhoids.

Constipation can usually be cured by a few self-help measures—estab-

lishing a regular routine for using the toilet, acting on any urge to move the bowels, increasing the amount of fiber in the diet, and drinking more fluids. If constipation continues despite these measures, medical advice should be obtained.

A physician should also be consulted if constipation occurs after years of normal bowel habits, or if it is accompanied by blood in the feces, pain on moving the bowels, loss of a sense of well-being, or weight loss.

Constriction
A narrowed area, or the process of narrowing, as of the pupil.

Contact lenses
Very thin, shell-like, transparent disks fitted on the *cornea* (the transparent outer coating of the eye) to correct defective *vision*. Contact lenses alter the power of the cornea by replacing the existing outer surface with a plastic surface that is curved to compensate for the visual defect.

Leonardo da Vinci in 1508 was the first to describe the possibility of using contact lenses. The first lens was made by Eugen Frick in 1887; it was made of glass and covered the entire front surface of the eye. The conventional small hard lens made of transparent plastic was first introduced in the 1940s and many millions have been used since.

WHY THEY ARE USED
Contact lenses can correct most of the defects in vision for which glasses are prescribed and can correct some conditions that glasses cannot.

Vanity and convenience account for most contact-lens wear. Unlike glasses, contact lenses are almost undetectable when worn, and generally do not fall off, nor mist up.

Contact lenses are useful for some people with particular optical problems or medical conditions. For people with extreme *myopia* (nearsightedness) or who have had cataracts removed, contact lenses may be preferable to glasses because glasses can produce considerable distortion of vision in these cases. Contact lenses can also be useful for hiding scars on the surface of the cornea. Patients with irregular corneas (such as may follow corneal disease, corneal injury, corneal ulceration, or corneal grafting) may be helped by contact lenses.

TYPES
HARD PLASTIC LENSES These give good optical vision, are long-lasting and durable (possibly five years or more of

C

use), inexpensive, and easy to maintain. However, they are sometimes difficult to tolerate and occasionally fall out; severe pain can result if grit gets into the eye and under the lens. When the lenses are removed after prolonged wear, vision with glasses may be temporarily blurred.

HARD, GAS-PERMEABLE LENSES Introduced in the early 1980s, these have the same visual qualities as hard plastic lenses, but are more comfortable and easier to get used to because they allow oxygen to pass through the lens to the eye. However, they are less durable (possibly giving up to five years of wear) and more expensive.

SOFT LENSES Also called hydrophilic (having a strong affinity for water) lenses, these are the most comfortable because of their high water content, which can range from 38 to 80 percent. They are usually easy to wear from the beginning, can be worn for long periods, and are ideal for occasional use since the eye generally tolerates them for short periods of time despite infrequent wearing. Soft lenses can correct myopia and *hypermetropia* (farsightedness). They cannot correct much *astigmatism* because, being flexible, they mold themselves to the shape of the eye, and thus cannot correct the irregularly shaped cornea that is the cause of this condition. Other drawbacks of soft lenses include fragility, a relatively short life (12 to 18 months), more complicated maintenance, and a higher price than hard lenses. Extremely thin, specially designed soft lenses with a high water content can be worn for periods of up to one month. These "extended-wear" contact lenses may increase the risks and dangers of infection.

SPECIAL LENSES Rigid, scleral lenses, which cover the whole of the front of the eye, are used to hide eyes disfigured by injury or disease. Hard or soft bifocal contact lenses can be produced, but can be difficult to fit, and vision may not be satisfactory.

Toric contact lenses (lenses of uneven surface curvature) are a type of soft lens used to correct high degrees of astigmatism; such lenses can be made in all materials.

CARE
Basic care procedures are shown in the illustrated box. Periodic follow-up examinations are needed to ensure that the lenses continue to fit correctly and are not harming the eyes.

PROBLEMS
A few people are unable to wear contact lenses because they have particu-

CARE AND INSERTION OF CONTACT LENSES

Hard lenses may require several solutions, one for cleaning, one for wetting, and possibly one for storage. If used, the storage solution is washed off before lens insertion. The wetting solution is used before inserting a lens in the eye.

Care of soft lenses is more complicated. Because the lenses are permeable and absorb any chemi-cals they come in contact with, the solutions must be weaker. Disinfection with a chemical or heating system is required to prevent contamination and infection. Two or three solutions may be necessary, but intermittent cleaning with a third system, such as an enzyme tablet or an oxidizing agent, is also required to remove mucus and protein.

Tear layer
Cornea
Lens
Contact lens
Hard lens
Soft lens

1 Wash your hands thoroughly under running water and carefully rinse off all traces of soap.

2 If you like, use a rubber sucker to remove a hard lens from its container. Rinse the lens thoroughly.

Inverted lens

3 Place the lens on your index finger. If it is a soft lens, make sure that it has not turned inside out. If it has, you will see an out-turned rim.

4 Keep both eyes open, hold the upper lid open, and look straight ahead or at the lens as you bring it up to your eye.

5 Place the lens on your eye. Look downward and then release the lid. If necessary, the lens may be centered by gently massaging the eyelid (the photograph on the right shows a hard lens correctly positioned).

larly sensitive eyes, difficult optical requirements, or poor personal hygiene habits.

Lenses can irritate the eye because of dryness due to problems with tear production, which may be inadequate, especially in older people.

Hard plastic contact lenses may cause abrasion of the cornea if they are worn for too long. Symptoms are pain and excessive tear production. Covering the affected eye with a patch and/or applying eye drops containing *antibiotic drugs* usually clear up symptoms within 24 hours.

Some people who wear soft lenses develop sensitivity of the eyes and lids either to the maintenance solutions or to altered mucus. Symptoms include decreased lens tolerance, stinging, increased lens movement, increased mucus, and redness of the conjunctiva. An affected person must generally stop wearing contact lenses for several months and then start again with new lenses and a different type of maintenance solution.

Other problems that may occur with any type of contact lens are infections, redness of the eye, and unexpected changes in the eye itself. Contact lens wear should be stopped and an eye examination arranged if the eyes become red or infected, if vision is blurred, or if the lenses become uncomfortable.

Contact tracing
A service, provided by clinics treating *sexually transmitted diseases* (STDs), that aims to control their spread.

WHY IT IS DONE
If a person is diagnosed as having an STD, it may be possible to identify from whom it was caught and to whom it may have been passed on. If these contacts are encouraged to have an examination and to receive treatment if necessary, the spread of the disease can be reduced. Contacts may be infected although they may have no obvious symptoms.

Contact tracing is also sometimes undertaken for infections such as tuberculosis, meningitis, and some imported tropical diseases.

HOW IT IS DONE
At clinics involved in the treatment of sexually transmitted infections, trained health workers interview patients after their diagnosis to explain the nature of the disease, its mode of transmission, and the complications that might occur if the disease is left untreated. Patients are also given printed leaflets, which they are

recommended to give to their contacts, and which advise the contacts of the need for treatment.

Contagious
A term describing a disease that can be transferred from one person to another by ordinary social contact, such as by sharing a home or workplace. All contagious diseases, such as the common cold, chickenpox, or measles, are infectious, but many *infectious diseases*, such as typhoid, syphilis, or AIDS, are not contagious (being spread by other means of transmission, such as contamination of food or water by infected human excreta, by sexual contact, or by contaminated blood).

Contraception
The control of fertility to prevent *pregnancy*. Contraception can be achieved by various methods, which work by preventing the formation of ova (eggs) by the woman, stopping sperm from meeting an ovum in the fallopian tube (thus preventing fertilization), or preventing a fertilized ovum from implanting in the lining of the uterus.

METHODS
Contraception may be achieved or attempted in the following ways: by total abstinence from *sexual intercourse*; by methods involving periodic abstinence from intercourse (see *Contraception, natural methods of*); by *coitus interruptus*; by barrier methods, including the use of condoms, diaphragms, cervical caps, spermicides, and contraceptive sponges (see *Contraception, barrier methods of*); by hormonal methods, including the use of *oral contraceptives*, implants, and injections (see *Contraceptives, injectable*); by intrauterine devices (see *IUDs*); by postcoital methods (see *Contraception, postcoital*); or by sterilization of the male (see *Vasectomy*) or female (see *Sterilization, female*).

Breast-feeding was once considered to be a method of contraception because frequent suckling causes changes in the hormone levels in the body that can prevent ovulation. The unreliability of the effect on ovulation is, however, too great for breast-feeding to be considered a contraceptive method today.

MEASURING CONTRACEPTIVE EFFECTIVENESS
Contraceptives are measured not so much by their effectiveness as by their failure rate. The failure rate is the rate of pregnancies per 100 woman-years of use (i.e., the number of pregnancies among 100 women using the method

for one year, or 50 using it for two years). The lower the failure rate, the more effective and useful the contraceptive. Failure rates do not take into account the fact that failures are more likely in the first year of use, while the woman is getting used to the method.

There are two ways of defining contraceptive effectiveness: theoretical, or "method," effectiveness; and "use" effectiveness (i.e., the effectiveness in actual use).

THEORETICAL (METHOD) EFFECTIVENESS This is the effectiveness of a particular contraceptive method when used exactly as prescribed by the manufacturers, the physician, or the clinic. Theoretical failure rates are usually much lower than the failure rates of contraceptives in actual use.

USE EFFECTIVENESS This measures the effectiveness of the method under all circumstances. It takes into account pregnancies resulting from incorrect use (for example, forgetting to take the pill or not putting on a condom correctly). Use effectiveness is almost always markedly lower than theoretical effectiveness in "user-dependent" methods, such as barriers. With "nonuser-dependent" methods, such as IUDs and sterilization, there is less of a difference.

RISKS INVOLVED IN CONTRACEPTIVE METHODS Risks vary a great deal depending on the method. Perhaps the greatest risk in all cases is failure of the contraceptive method, which can lead to unwanted pregnancy and all that this entails (such as an elective *abortion*, possible danger to the health or life of the mother, or danger to the health of any existing children).

Risks inherent in contraceptives themselves must also be weighed against the benefits. Hormonal contraceptives are linked with *cardiovascular disease*, particularly in women over 35 who smoke, and there is some evidence of a link with *breast cancer* in women under the age of 35. IUDs may be associated with an increase in *pelvic inflammatory disease*, particularly in women who have more than one sex partner; and sterilization carries the risks of a surgical operation.

CONTRACEPTIVE RESEARCH New forms continue to be investigated although the constraints of licensing authorities, the great cost, and the paucity of funds have slowed the pace. However, a few of the promising lines of research are as follows.

HORMONAL CONTRACEPTION New forms of hormonal contraception include the use of *luteinizing hormone-releasing hor-*

mone (a hormone that regulates the release of other hormones that control the ovulatory cycle), which may be given as a nasal spray.

STEROIDAL VAGINAL RINGS Made of silicone-rubber containing a progestogen, these are at an advanced stage of development. They are inserted into the vagina where they release the progestogen, which acts directly on the reproductive organs.

PINPOINTING OVULATION Various methods to determine the exact time of ovulation continue to be researched; this would be of great help in improving natural methods of contraception.

VACCINES These are being studied, but still present problems. Vaccines are being developed against sperm, against the outer coat of the ovum, and against the hormone that helps maintain a pregnancy.

THE MALE PILL This continues to be researched, but so far without much practical progress. The main problem is that the testes are continually producing millions of sperm, while the ovaries have a definite number of ova present at birth and release only one each month—making suppression of ovulation simpler than suppression of sperm production.

Contraception, barrier methods of

The use of a device and/or chemical to block or otherwise stop sperm from reaching the ovum, thus preventing fertilization and pregnancy. Barrier contraceptives include the condom (placed over the erect penis); and the diaphragm, the cervical cap, and the contraceptive sponge, which are all positioned within the vagina. Spermicides are recommended in combination with barrier devices for maximum protection.

Barrier methods, especially condoms, are advisable for people with more than one sex partner because they help to prevent the sexual transmission of diseases such as AIDS and hepatitis B.

TYPES

CONDOM A sheath of fine, latex rubber or plastic, about 17 cm long, usually lubricated for ease of application. A condom normally has a teat at its end to hold ejaculated sperm. Condoms are available over-the-counter in various sizes, colors, and textures; also, some types are precoated with spermicide.

A condom should be carefully rolled on to the erect penis before intercourse. The tip of the condom should be squeezed as it is rolled on,

so that no air is trapped in the end (trapped air may lead to bursting of the condom when ejaculation occurs). The rim of the condom should be held close to the penis when it is withdrawn from the vagina, which should occur after orgasm but before the erection subsides.

DIAPHRAGM This is a hemispherical dome of thin rubber with a metal spring in the rim. It fits diagonally across the front wall of the vagina, with the top part of the rim up behind the cervix (neck of the uterus) and the opposite edge of the rim resting on the ledge above the pubic bone. Diaphragms are available in a range of sizes and must be properly fitted, the size and type being determined by each individual's anatomy.

A diaphragm must be used with a spermicidal agent and be left in place for six hours after intercourse. Without disturbing the diaphragm, additional spermicide should be used if intercourse is repeated within the six-hour period.

CERVICAL CAP Smaller and more rigid than the diaphragm, this latex rubber device fits tightly over the cervix (rather than covering the vaginal vault), where it is held in place by suction. There are three types: the cervical cap, which is thimble-shaped; the vault cap, which is bowl-shaped; and the vimule cap, which combines features of both the cervical and vault caps. Caps are often used by women who cannot use diaphragms because of anatomical changes, such as prolapse of the uterus or of the front wall of the vagina. As with the diaphragm, a cap must be properly fitted and used with a spermicide.

CONTRACEPTIVE SPONGE This device is a disposable circular polyurethane foam sponge about 5 cm in diameter that is impregnated with spermicide. The sponge incorporates a loop for easy removal. Before being inserted high into the vagina, the sponge should be moistened with water to activate the spermicide. It should be left in position for at least six hours after intercourse. Contraceptive sponges have been available in Canada since 1990.

SPERMICIDE A wide range of spermicides is available, including aerosol foams, creams, jellies, pessaries, soluble plastic film, or foaming tablets, which are placed in the vagina as near to the cervix as possible. Some preparations are recommended for use with a condom, diaphragm, or cap. Others are intended to be used alone;

they are inserted into the vagina using a syringelike applicator. Some spermicides should not be used with rubber barrier devices.

Spermicides should be applied shortly before intercourse; a fresh application is needed when intercourse is repeated or prolonged. Spermicides must be used in accordance with the manufacturer's instructions because the length of time for which they remain effective varies. They should not be washed away until six to eight hours after intercourse.

EFFECTIVENESS

If used consistently and correctly, employing both mechanical and chemical means, barrier methods can be highly effective in preventing conception. Failure rates in actual use vary between four and seven pregnancies per 100 woman-years of use for the male condom, diaphragm, or contraceptive cap; nine to 16 pregnancies per 100 woman-years of use for the contraceptive sponge; and 20 to 40 pregnancies per 100 woman-years of use for spermicides used alone. (See Contraception for the definition of woman-years.)

Contraception, hormonal methods of

The use by women of synthetic progestogens, frequently combined with synthetic estrogens, to prevent pregnancy. The best-known form of hormonal contraception is the contraceptive pill (see Oral contraceptives). Contraceptive hormones can also be administered in the form of contraceptive implants or injectables, but at the time of writing these had not yet been approved for sale in Canada (see Contraceptives, injectable).

Hormonal methods of contraception work by suppressing ovulation in most (although not all) menstrual cycles, and by acting on the cervical mucus to make it thick and impenetrable to sperm. They also cause thinning of the endometrium (lining of the uterus).

Contraception, natural methods of

Periodic abstinence from sexual intercourse to avoid conception. All natural methods of contraception attempt to pinpoint the fertile period around the time of ovulation, so that intercourse can be avoided on the days when fertilization might occur.

Natural methods of contraception need great motivation on the part of the couple, with a strong commitment

C

METHODS OF CONTRACEPTION

Contraception may follow natural, barrier, hormonal and postcoital methods. Sterilization interferes with part of the reproductive system to render the individual infertile. (At the time of writing, hormonal implants were not available in North America.)

Hormonal method

Pill

Mini-pill

Pill

The pill
Prevents ovulation, changes the cervical mucus to prevent sperm penetration, or alters the uterine lining to prevent implantation.

Hormonal implant
Capsules containing a pro-gestogen are inserted into the arm, where they release progestogen into the blood.

Barrier method

Spermicidal foam and gel

Condom

Sponge

Diaphragm plus spermicide

Caps

Diaphragm in position
Held in place over the cervix by means of a coiled metal spring in its rim, the diaphragm prevents sperm from reaching the cervix.

IUDs

The condom
A tube-shaped piece of latex rubber that usually has a teat to hold ejaculate. It should be used with spermicide, examined for holes before use, and have all air squeezed out of the tip to prevent bursting. The rim should be held during withdrawal to stop the condom from slipping off.

IUD in position
A small piece of molded plastic with string attached, sometimes with copper or a female hormone added. The IUD is worn in the uterus.

STERILIZATION

Offers an almost completely safe and reliable form of birth control. It is usually irreversible. It has no effect on the production of sex hormones, so a man produces sperm-free semen and a woman produces normal eggs.

Male sterilization (vasectomy)
The vas deferens on each side is cut so that sperm cannot pass from testes to penis.

Female sterilization
Two cuts are made below the navel, and a laparo-scope is inserted. An attachment to this is used to seal off the tube ends.

Mucosal and temperature methods
The temperature method involves charting the woman's temperature to ascertain whether ovulation has taken place. The mucosal method involves studying the cervical mucus throughout the woman's menstrual cycle.

to abstain from intercourse when there could be a possibility of pregnancy. They are the only forms of contraception permitted by the Roman Catholic church.

TYPES

CALENDAR METHOD This is the oldest method of natural contraception. The calendar method attempts to predict a woman's fertile period with reference to the length of her menstrual cycle, making the assumption that ovulation occurs 14 days before menstruation. Because of its high failure rate, this method has now been largely superseded by other natural methods of contraception.

TEMPERATURE METHOD Also known as the basal body temperature method, this method makes use of the fact that a woman's body temperature is higher in the second half of the menstrual cycle, after ovulation has taken place. The temperature should be taken at the same time each day (normally first thing in the morning), using a special ovulation thermometer marked in fractions of degrees. Intercourse is not considered safe until there has been a sustained temperature rise for at least three days.

CERVICAL MUCUS METHOD This method attempts to pinpoint the fertile period by observing and charting the amount and appearance of the mucus secreted by the cervix (neck of the uterus) during the menstrual cycle. Menstruation is followed by "dry" days when the mucus forms a thick plug that blocks the cervix. The mucus then becomes thick and viscid and appears at the vulva. At about the time of ovulation it turns thin, watery, elastic and slippery, and flows more easily. A few days after ovulation it begins to become thick and viscid again, and this state lasts until the start of the next menstrual period.

Using the cervical mucus method, intercourse should be avoided from the first appearance of mucus after the dry days until four days after the last appearance of the thin, watery mucus that occurs around the time of ovulation.

SYMPTOTHERMAL METHOD This method of contraception combines the temperature and the cervical mucus methods. Intercourse is permitted during the dry days after menstruation, but must stop as soon as mucus is felt. Intercourse can be resumed only when both the sustained rise in temperature and the four-day period after the last appearance of thin, watery mucus have taken place.

FAILURE RATES OF CONTRACEPTIVE METHODS

Method	Pregnancies
Sterilization (male or female)	0.05
Combined oral contraceptive	0.5
Injectable contraceptives	1.5
Progestogen-only pill	2.5
IUD	2.5
Condom plus spermicide	2.5
Diaphragm/cap plus spermicide	2.5
Natural methods (overall)	10.0
Spermicide alone	25.0
Coitus interruptus	25.0
No contraception	80.0

Pregnancies 0 10 20 30 40 50 60 70 80 90 100

The chart shows the approximate number of pregnancies that can be expected if 100 couples use a given contraceptive method, or none at all, for one year.

SIDE EFFECTS

Once the techniques have been mastered and a woman can observe and chart the necessary changes, there are no provable side effects. There is, however, a supposition that a higher incidence of miscarriages or birth defects could occur among pregnancies that result from a failure of these methods because of the fertilization of so-called "aged" ova by "aged" sperm. This supposition has been neither completely proved nor disproved.

Contraception, postcoital

An attempt to prevent pregnancy following unprotected sexual intercourse. Postcoital contraception is normally used only in exceptional circumstances and must be provided soon after intercourse. Methods are not 100 percent effective, so women are advised to have a pregnancy test a month after treatment.

TYPES

There are two main types of postcoital contraception: use of *oral contraceptives* (sometimes known as the "morning-after pill") and use of an *IUD* (coil).

ORAL CONTRACEPTIVES These must be started not later than 72 hours after unprotected intercourse. The most common method is to give two high-dose oral contraceptive pills as soon as possible, followed by a further two pills 12 hours later. Treatment sometimes causes nausea and vomiting, and an *antiemetic drug* may be needed at the same time.

IUD For use as a postcoital method of contraception, an IUD must be inserted within five days of unprotected intercourse.

Contraception, withdrawal method of

See *Coitus interruptus*.

Contraceptive

Any agent that diminishes the likelihood of conception. Contraceptives can be hormonal (such as oral contraceptives), chemical (such as spermicides), or mechanical (such as condoms). (See also *Contraception*.)

Contraceptive implant

A hormonal method of contraception in which long-acting contraceptive drugs are inserted under the skin. Contraceptive implants consist of small capsules containing a *progestogen drug*. The implants remain active for several years, steadily releasing progestogen into the bloodstream. Fertility returns soon after the implants are removed.

Contraceptive implants are very effective and may be suitable for women who want long-term protection against pregnancy and who are unable to use *oral contraceptives* or an *IUD*. Contraceptive implants had not been approved by either Health and Welfare Canada or the U.S. Food and Drug Administration at the time of writing. (See also *Contraception, hormonal methods of*.)

Contraceptives, injectable

A hormonal method of contraception in which long-acting *progestogen drugs* are given by injection. Injectable contraceptives are administered every two or three months.

Injectable contraceptives may be suitable for women who want long-term protection against pregnancy and who are unable, or who do not want, to use *oral contraceptives* or an *IUD.* Injectable contraceptives are extremely effective, with a failure rate of only two per 100 woman-years (see *Contraception* for the definition of woman-years).

Side effects may be troublesome, especially during the first few months of use. There may be menstrual disturbances, such as heavy or scanty periods, irregular periods, or amenorrhea (absence of periods). Other possible side effects include weight gain, headaches, and nausea. Even if side effects are severe, there is no way of neutralizing the activity of injectable contraceptives once administered. The drug must run its normal two-to-three-month course. The return of fertility may be delayed for some time after injections are discontinued. Health and Welfare Canada had not approved injectable contraceptives when this book was written.

Contractions, uterine
The spasms of rhythmic, squeezing muscular activity that affect the walls of the *uterus* during *childbirth.* These true labor contractions differ from *Braxton Hicks' contractions,* which are milder contractions that are often noticeable during the last few weeks of pregnancy. True contractions are characterized by the discomfort they cause, by their regularity, and by the fact that they increase in strength and frequency from the start of the first stage of labor.

Contracture
A deformity caused by shrinkage of tissue in the skin, muscles, or tendons. Contractures may restrict the movement of joints.

Skin contractures commonly occur as a result of scarring following extensive burns. Other types of contracture may be caused by inflammation and shrinkage of *connective tissues* (materials that surround body structures and hold them together).

Examples include *Dupuytren's contracture,* which affects tendons and fibrous tissue in the hand, and *Volkmann's contracture,* in which muscle fibers in the arm are damaged, usually by reduced blood supply following an injury.

Contraindication
Any factor in a patient's condition that makes it unwise to pursue a certain line of treatment—such as drug therapy or surgery.

Controlled trial
A method of testing the value of a treatment—such as a new drug—or comparing the effectiveness of different treatments.

WHY IT IS DONE
The effectiveness of a treatment cannot accurately be assessed simply by administering it to a group of sick people and seeing if their conditions improve. With many illnesses, a significant proportion of patients tend to get better even if the treatment they are given is useless. Reasons for this phenomenon include the healing properties of time, the psychological reassurance of the physician, and the fact that both the patient and physician believe the treatment will work (the so-called *placebo* effect). A controlled trial is a scientific attempt to unravel the true effect of a treatment from the psychological side benefits of "being treated."

HOW IT IS DONE
In a typical controlled drug trial, a sample of patients with the illness that the drug is thought to cure is randomly split into two groups. It is checked that the groups are well matched in age, sex, social class, etc. One group is given a normal course of the drug—for example, a pill to be taken every day. The other patients—called the control group—are given an identical course of treatment, except that their pills are "dummy," or placebo, tablets, containing none of the drug being tested, but only an inert substance such as starch. Alternatively, the control group may be given a well-established drug treatment but with the drug disguised to appear identical to the test drug.

After a predetermined period, the two groups are assessed medically. If the improvement in the illness has been significantly greater in the patients given the test drug over those given the dummy tablets, this suggests that the drug does have a real curative effect. Any benefits (or side effects) of treatment separate from the pharmacological effects of the drug have been accounted for (or "controlled") by the use of identical treatment regimens for the two groups.

To be of any use, controlled trials must be conducted "blind"—that is, the patients do not know whether they are receiving the real or the dummy treatment. In a further refinement—the "double-blind" controlled trial—neither the patients nor the physicians who assess them know who is receiving which treatment. The results of trials require detailed and careful statistical analysis before any conclusions can be drawn.

Contusion
Damage to the skin and underlying tissues from a blunt injury such as a fall; the skin may be grazed and the tissues bruised.

Convalescence
The recovery period following an illness or a surgical operation during which the patient regains strength before returning to normal activities. The convalescent period can vary from one or two days (following an infection such as influenza or tonsillitis) to several weeks (following a heart attack or a major operation). Special convalescent homes were formerly popular for patients of all ages, but today such homes are generally reserved for the elderly.

Conversion disorder
A psychological disorder in which it is thought that painful emotions are repressed and unconsciously converted into physical symptoms. The repressed idea is expressed symbolically by the particular bodily symptom. For instance, a paralyzed right arm may represent guilt over an injury that the patient, using that arm, inflicted on another person; mutism may represent sexual guilt, the mouth symbolizing the vagina.

This disorder serves mainly to relieve anxiety, but the sufferer may also "benefit" by gaining sympathy and avoiding responsibility. Such symptoms may also be part of other psychiatric or organic disorders.

Treatment requires *psychotherapy* involving exploration of the person's history and childhood experiences.

Convulsion
See *Seizure.*

Convulsion, febrile
Twitching or jerking of the limbs with loss of consciousness occurring in a child after a rapid rise in temperature. Febrile convulsions are common; about one child in 20 has one or more attacks. The seizures tend to run in families, are usually not serious, and occur mainly in children between 6 months and 5 years old.

CAUSES AND SYMPTOMS
Febrile convulsions are caused by an immaturity of the temperature-lowering mechanism in the brain, allowing the temperature to rise too rapidly in

response to an infection, commonly measles, *roseola infantum*, *influenza*, or an upper respiratory tract infection, such as *pharyngitis*, *tonsillitis* or *otitis media* (inflammation of the middle ear). The sudden rise in temperature excites the brain cells, causing them to discharge impulses to the muscles, which then contract. There is no underlying brain defect; seizures triggered by fever are distinct from those triggered by *meningitis* or *encephalitis*, which are infections of the central nervous system.

The child loses consciousness and his or her arms and legs twitch uncontrollably for a few minutes. After regaining consciousness, the child may be drowsy.

TREATMENT

During a seizure, objects that could be harmful should be moved out of the child's way. Biting the tongue is rare and no attempt should be made to prevent this happening by wedging the mouth open (which can cause cuts and broken teeth). Once the seizure is over, the child should be placed in the *recovery position*. Every effort should be made to lower the temperature by sponging the child's face and body with lukewarm water, and by using a fan (if one is available).

If the child has not had a seizure before, a physician should be consulted; if the seizure lasts for more than five minutes, an ambulance should be called. In some cases, investigative tests, such as a *lumbar puncture*, are performed to determine whether the seizure has a serious cause, such as *meningitis*. Drug treatment with *diazepam* or *paraldehyde* may be given to control the seizure or to avert further episodes. Treatment may also be given for an underlying infection.

PREVENTION

If an infectious illness develops in a susceptible child, parents can often prevent seizures from occurring by reducing the child's temperature. *Acetaminophen* should be given at the first signs of fever and repeated every four to six hours as necessary; you should give the full dose for the child's weight as instructed on the package. Most of the child's clothing should be removed, and he or she should be cooled by sponging the face and body with lukewarm water and also by using a fan if possible.

Most children who have febrile convulsions are completely normal and suffer no ill effects from the attacks. A second seizure occurs in about 30 to 40 percent of cases, usually within the following six months. In most children, the risk of developing *epilepsy* (recurrent seizures) is very small. However, recurrences are more likely if a child has a preexisting abnormality of the brain or nervous system, if the first febrile convulsion was limited to only part of the body (e.g., one side) or was prolonged (longer than 15 minutes), and if there are family members with epilepsy. Children with all of these factors have about a one in 10 chance of developing epilepsy.

Cooley's anemia

A term formerly used to refer to the blood disorder beta *thalassemia* major in which two defective genes are inherited—one from each parent.

Copper

A metallic element that forms an essential part of several *enzymes* (substances that promote biochemical reactions in the body). Copper is needed by the body only in minute amounts (see *Trace elements*); deficiency is very uncommon.

Copper poisoning is rare, occurring mainly in people who drink homemade alcohol distilled using copper tubing. Symptoms of poisoning include nausea, vomiting, and diarrhea. Copper excess may also result from *Wilson's disease*, a rare inherited disorder of copper metabolism.

Cordotomy

An operation to divide bundles of nerve fibers within the *spinal cord*.

Cordotomy is performed to relieve persistent pain that has not responded to treatment with strong *analgesic drugs* (painkillers) or *TENS* (transcutaneous electrical nerve stimulation). In theory, cordotomy can treat pain anywhere in the body, depending on the part of the cord that is operated on. In practice, however, it is often difficult to locate precisely the nerves responsible for pain in the upper part of the body, and the operation is most frequently performed for pain in the lower trunk and legs, usually on patients with cancer.

Corn

A small area of thickened skin on a toe, caused by the pressure of a tight-fitting shoe. People with high foot arches are affected most, because the arch increases the pressure on the tips of the toes when walking.

If a corn is painful, the obvious solution is to change to shoes that fit more

Cross section of corn

- Epidermis
- Plug of keratin (dead skin cells)
- Dermis
- Nerve
- Subcutaneous fat

comfortably; the corn should then gradually disappear. A spongy ring or corn pad—available in various sizes at pharmacies—can be placed over the corn to ease pressure. If the corn persists, a podiatrist can remedy the problem by paring away the thickened skin with a scalpel.

Cornea

The front part of the tough outer shell of the eyeball. The cornea is transparent and is shaped like a thin-walled cap or dome. It is about 12 mm in diameter, less than 1 mm thick, and has a convex front surface like the front of a camera lens. (See illustration on facing page).

At its circumference the cornea joins the sclera (white of the eye), which is easily seen. The cornea itself, being transparent, is less obvious. The black pupil and the colored iris are visible beneath it.

The cornea performs two main functions: it helps focus light rays on to the retina at the back of the eye and it protects the front of the eye. To warn of possible damage, the cornea's surface is extremely sensitive, and small scratches and foreign bodies are thus very painful.

The cornea must be kept moist (by tears) in order to remain healthy. This function is performed by the lacrimal gland and the mucus-secreting and fluid-secreting cells in the eyelids and conjunctiva (the thin lining of the rest of the surface of the eye and the inside of the eyelids).

The endothelial cells (the cells that form the inner cell layer of the cornea) in adults cannot reproduce themselves. If they are severely damaged, there may be permanent corneal clouding, because one of the functions of the cell is to pump excess water out of the cornea to keep it transparent.

C

Corneal abrasion

A scratch or defect in the epithelium (outer layer) of the cornea. The abrasion may be caused by a small, sharp particle in the eye (see *Eye, foreign body in*) or by an injury (e.g., by a twig).

Corneal abrasions usually heal quickly but may meanwhile cause severe pain and photophobia (abnormal sensitivity to bright light) and increased production of tears.

Pain may be relieved by covering the eye with a patch, by *analgesic drugs* (painkillers), and, if the eye muscles go into spasm, by eye drops containing cycloplegic drugs (drugs that paralyze the ciliary muscles in the eye). Eye drops containing *antibiotic drugs* are usually also given to prevent any risk of bacterial infection, which could cause serious corneal ulceration, abscess, or even blindness.

Corneal abrasions usually heal completely within a few days, but (rarely) they may recur, probably because the new epithelium fails to stick properly to the underlying tissue. Patching the eye, application of bland ointments, and even prescription of a soft "bandage" contact lens may be tried.

Corneal graft

The surgical transplantation of corneal tissue. Most corneal grafts are homografts, in which tissue is taken from a human donor and put into the eye of a recipient with a corneal disorder. A much smaller number are autografts, in which a person's cornea is simply repositioned—for example, it may be rotated to a position in which the effect of a scar on the corneal surface is lessened. Donor corneal tissues can now be stored for days for future use. An "eye bank" handles the donor corneas.

WHY IT IS DONE

A corneal graft is carried out when a patient has an eye with good visual potential (most of the eye is healthy)

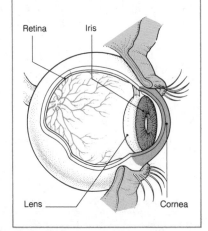

LOCATION OF CORNEA
The cornea is a transparent thin-walled dome forming the front of the eyeball. It consists of five layers of differing thickness.

Retina Iris

Lens Cornea

DISORDERS OF THE CORNEA

The cornea is a living structure, much like very specialized skin, and is prone to many disorders.

CONGENITAL DEFECTS

These are rare. Microcornea (smaller than normal) or megalocornea (bigger than normal) may occur in one or both eyes. In *buphthalmos*, or "ox-eye", the entire eyeball is distended from *glaucoma* (raised pressure in the eye). This often leads to haziness of the cornea.

INJURY

Trauma to the cornea is common and is usually minor, a frequent occurrence being a *corneal abrasion* (scratch) caused by a particle in the eye or by overuse of contact lenses. An abrasion may become infected and progress to a *corneal ulcer*. Penetrating corneal injuries can cause scarring with loss of transparency, which may lead to severe impairment of vision.

Chemical injuries to the cornea can result from acid or alkali splashes, the latter being the more serious. All contact with corrosive substances is dangerous, and immediate flushing of the eye with large volumes of water is essential if sight is to be saved.

The term *keratopathy* can be applied to any corneal disorder, but is also used more specifically for certain types of corneal damage.

Actinic keratopathy is damage to the outer layer of the cornea by ultraviolet light. Exposure keratopathy is the damage done to a cornea deprived of the normal protection afforded by the tear film and the blink reflex.

INFLAMMATION

Keratitis means inflammation of the cornea. However, because the cornea contains no blood vessels, true inflammatory reactions are uncommon.

INFECTION

The cornea can be infected by viruses, bacteria, and fungi. Some of these cause ulceration, which may lead to penetration. *Herpes simplex* is especially dangerous.

NUTRITIONAL DISORDERS

Keratomalacia is the result of vitamin A deficiency and is common in severely undernourished children. The cornea becomes soft and often perforates. Keratomalacia is a major cause of blindness in some tropical countries.

DEGENERATION

Degenerative conditions occur mainly in the elderly, and are more common in previously damaged eyes. Corneal changes include calcium deposition, thinning, and spontaneous ulceration.

OTHER DISORDERS

Keratoconjunctivitis sicca (dry eye) occurs when the tear film is inadequate. This is a feature of *Sjögren's syndrome*, the *Stevens-Johnson syndrome*, and various rheumatic disorders. Corneal dystrophies are inborn errors of corneal structure or function that may appear at various ages and may lead to opacification. One form of dystrophy is *keratoconus*, in which the cornea thins and bulges forward into a conical shape. Edema (fluid accumulation) of the cornea occurs when the endothelium (inner layer) fails to prevent the internal fluid of the eye from entering the cornea, so impairing vision.

INVESTIGATION

Corneal disorders are examined under high magnification, using a slit-lamp microscope. In the majority of cases, the appearance of the various conditions is characteristic and diagnosis is straightforward. Corneal ulcers may require gentle scraping so that samples can be obtained for viral, bacterial, or fungal *culture* in the pathology laboratory.

but with substantially impaired vision caused by a cornea that is scarred or clouded (see *Cornea* disorders box).

HOW IT IS DONE

The patient is given a general or a local anesthetic. The diseased area of the cornea is then cut out and replaced with a similarly shaped piece of donor tissue, which is fastened in place with stitches. Most corneal grafts are full-thickness but if the back part of the cornea is healthy, the cornea is sometimes split, with only the front, diseased part removed and replaced.

OUTLOOK

The success rate for corneal grafts is high, but depends on the type of corneal disorder (certain corneal problems have lower transplant success rates than others). Generally, however, corneal grafts have a much better chance of success than other types of transplant. This is because the healthy cornea has no blood vessels, so there is less access for the white blood cells, which bring about rejection of donor tissue. Matching certain features of the donor's and recipient's immune systems (see *Histocompatibility antigens*) has also improved the success rate of corneal grafts. Unlike the recipients of other transplants, who get antirejection treatments for life, there is usually no need for the recipient of a corneal graft to receive *immunosuppressant drugs* to lessen the chance of rejection.

Corneal transplant

See *Corneal graft*.

Corneal ulcer

A break, erosion, or open sore in the outer layer of the *cornea*, sometimes extending into the underlying stroma (middle layer).

CAUSES

The most common cause is a *corneal abrasion* (scratch), but an ulcer may also be produced by chemical damage, or by infection with various bacteria, fungi, or viruses (particularly with the *herpes simplex* virus or the virus that causes *herpes zoster*).

Certain eye conditions may make an ulcer more likely—for example, *keratoconjunctivitis sicca* (dry eye), eyelid deformities such as *entropion* or *ectropion*, or diminished sensation in the cornea, which more easily permits injury to occur.

SYMPTOMS, DIAGNOSIS, AND TREATMENT

Corneal ulcers are very painful, though chronic ones may become less so. They are easily recognized by a physician who introduces some fluorescein dye into the eye and shines a blue light on it; the fluorescein fills the ulcer and reflects back green light.

Superficial, noninfectious ulcers caused by mechanical injury usually heal quickly. If an infection is suspected, swabs will be taken to identify the causative microorganism and the physician will then prescribe suitable drug treatment. Sometimes, a predisposing eye condition may need to be treated in addition to the ulcer. Noninfectious ulcers that fail to heal quickly sometimes respond to a "bandage" contact lens or to *tarsorrhaphy* (temporary joining of the eyelids).

Coronary

Strictly, a term used to describe any structure that encircles like a crown (from "corona," the Latin word for crown). In practice, the term usually refers to the coronary arteries that encircle and supply the heart. In popular usage, coronary often means a *coronary thrombosis* or a *myocardial infarction* (heart attack).

Coronary artery bypass

An operation to circumvent narrowed or blocked coronary arteries by grafting on additional blood vessels to transmit blood flow.

When a coronary artery is narrowed or blocked the function of the heart muscle it supplies is impaired. A bypass operation reestablishes blood flow to a part of the heart that is receiving insufficient blood supply. A new artery (usually a leg vein) is placed between the *aorta* and the coronary artery beyond the point of blockage. This new artery is called a bypass graft.

Usually, symptoms of coronary artery disease—*angina* or heart failure—can be controlled by drugs, weight loss (if appropriate), not smoking, and adopting a sensible diet and life-style. If this fails to relieve the symptoms, surgical treatment will be considered. When the disease is localized to one or two segments of artery, it may be possible to relieve blockages by balloon angioplasty. However, in cases not responding to treatment by drugs, bypass surgery may be recommended in preference to angioplasty.

HOW IT IS DONE

Definite sites of blockage must be identified using *angiography* (an X-ray technique). The operation is done under general anesthesia, requires two surgeons and specially trained technicians. It lasts up to five hours. As many as four grafts may be installed in a single operation. The heart is temporarily stopped, and the circulation maintained with a *heart-lung machine*, a pump outside the body that adds oxygen to the blood and keeps it circulating. The procedure is described in the *Coronary artery bypass* box on the facing page.

RECOVERY PERIOD

After a coronary artery bypass the patient spends two to four days in an intensive care unit, where his or her heart and other bodily functions can be carefully monitored. Hospital stay altogether is generally seven to 10 days, and return to work is usually possible after about 12 weeks.

OUTLOOK

When candidates are appropriately selected, coronary bypass surgery offers the patient another chance to feel well again and to return to a normal life. In about one sixth of the cases operated on so far, blockage recurs in the grafts within seven years, and a second operation is required.

Coronary artery disease

Damage to, or malfunction of, the heart caused by narrowing or blockage of the coronary arteries, which supply blood to the heart muscle. The two most common features of coronary artery disease are *angina pectoris* (chest pain caused by insufficient blood supply to the heart muscle) and acute *myocardial infarction* (heart attack).

INCIDENCE

Although this extremely common disorder is a leading cause of death, the death rate from coronary artery disease has decreased some 40 percent in the last 20 years. Part of this decline is thought to be due to better medical treatment of *hypertension* (raised blood pressure), one of the causes of coronary artery disease, and part is due to improved surgical treatment of narrowed coronary arteries. Also, emergency treatment of heart attacks has improved, and people are adopting a less heart-disease-prone life-style by taking more exercise, eating a healthier diet, and smoking less.

CAUSES

The symptoms of coronary artery disease are caused by reduction in the blood flow to the heart muscle. The coronary arteries are first narrowed and may eventually be blocked by plaques (patches) of atheroma (cholesterol-rich fatty deposits) which can cause *atherosclerosis*. Further narrowing or blockage may be caused by thrombi (blood clots) formed on the roughened surface of the plaques.

C

CORONARY ARTERY BYPASS

In Canada, more than 15,500 open heart operations are done each year; 70 percent of these are coronary bypass operations. On properly selected patients, the operation gives rapid relief of angina and some types of heart failure.

HOW IT IS DONE

Coronary artery bypass is a major procedure, requiring two surgeons and lasting up to five hours.

1 The first surgeon makes an incision down the center of the patient's chest. The heart is then exposed by opening the pericardium.

Site of incision

2 Simultaneously, several incisions are made in the leg, and a length of vein is removed.

3 Before any incisions are made in the coronary arteries, the patient is connected to a heart-lung machine. This takes over the function of the heart and lungs while the surgeon repairs the heart.

Heart-lung machine

4 A section of the vein taken from the leg is then sewn to the aorta and to a point below the blockage. If several arteries are blocked, they can be bypassed by using other sections from the same leg vein, or an arterial graft may be taken from the chest.

5 The heart-lung machine is disconnected, allowing blood to flow back into the coronary arteries.

WHY IT IS DONE

Narrowed coronary arteries are unable to supply the heart muscle with a sufficient amount of blood; as a result, it becomes starved of oxygen. This may cause angina (chest pain) or heart tissue damage. By attaching lengths of a vein taken from the leg (or in some cases a length of mammary artery) to the aorta and to a point below the blockages, the narrowed or blocked sections can be bypassed.

Before the operation

Diseased coronary artery

Affected area

Coronary arteries

After the operation

Bypass

First surgeon prepares heart for bypass

Second surgeon removes vein from leg

Anesthetist

Oxygenated blood from heart-lung machine

Superior vena cava (tied off)

Deoxygenated blood to heart-lung machine

Inferior vena cava (tied off)

Pericardium

Aorta

Bypass

Coronary arteries

6 Finally, the breastbone is wired together, and pericardium and chest are sewn up.

Atherosclerosis has many inter-related causes, including smoking, lack of exercise, being overweight, and having a raised blood cholesterol level (which itself is linked in part with a diet rich in dairy and animal fats). Other important factors include a genetic predisposition and diseases such as *diabetes mellitus* and hypertension.

The importance of personality traits, behavior, and stress as causes of coronary artery disease is still disputed. Some doctors believe that heart attacks are more frequent in people with "type A" personalities. Such individuals are always in a hurry, checking the time, impatient with delays, and interrupting colleagues in mid-sentence—but they are also doers and achievers.

There is some evidence that heart attacks occur more frequently in people who are depressed after the death of a relative, loss of a job, or some other adverse life event. However, the medical consensus is that these psychological and behavioral factors are less important than physical and life-style factors—smoking, unhealthy diet, high blood pressure, and lack of exercise.

SYMPTOMS

In its early stages, atherosclerosis of the coronary arteries is symptomless. The first symptom is usually either angina pectoris or a heart attack.

The pain of angina pectoris is typically brought on by exertion and relieved by rest. The pain is a dull ache in the middle of the chest or a feeling of pressure that may spread up to the neck or down the arms (the left arm more commonly than the right). In some cases the pain occurs only in an arm or in the neck. The characteristic pain comes on predictably after a certain amount of exertion—after walking halfway up the stairs, for instance—and disappears after resting for a minute or so.

Angina occurs when the heart muscle is working hard and getting too little blood for the amount of effort being expended. If the blood supply to part of the muscle is cut off completely by a blood clot or spasm in one of the coronary arteries (a coronary thrombosis), the result is an acute myocardial infarction (a heart attack)—death of a portion of the heart muscle. The main symptom is intense chest pain of the same type as angina, but not relieved by rest and not necessarily brought on by effort; in addition the victim may become cold, sweat profusely, feel weak and nauseated, or even lose consciousness

as the pumping action of the heart is weakened and shock ensues.

Angina and myocardial infarction may lead to disturbances in the electrical conduction system of the heart with resulting *arrhythmias* (heartbeat abnormalities) ranging from *ectopic beats* (misplaced beats) to *tachycardia* (rapid beats) and *ventricular fibrillation* (ineffective fluttering of the heart muscle). The latter causes rapid loss of consciousness and is fatal if not treated within a few minutes.

DIAGNOSIS AND INVESTIGATION

A myocardial infarction may produce such clear-cut symptoms that the diagnosis is in no doubt. Confirmatory tests may include *ECG* (electrocardiography) and measurement of the level of substances called cardiac enzymes released into the blood by damaged muscle. The conditions of patients who have intermittent attacks of angina are usually assessed by ECG both at rest and during exercise (see *Cardiac stress test*).

When the angina is persistent, severe, changing in quality, or of recent onset, the patient's condition is assessed by various *heart imaging* techniques. These imaging procedures, such as coronary *angiography* (injection of a radiopaque substance into the arteries followed by X ray), give the physician detailed, precise data on the extent of the narrowing of the coronary arteries and on any damage to the heart muscle. The data helps in determining whether medical or surgical treatment is the best choice.

TREATMENT

Angina may be relieved by a range of drugs that improve blood flow through the coronary arteries and/or reduce the work load on the heart during exercise. These drugs include

glyceryl trinitrate and other *nitrate drugs, beta-blockers, calcium channel blockers,* and *vasodilator drugs.* Arrhythmias are commonly treated with beta-blockers, calcium channel blockers, and specific *antiarrhythmic drugs.* If the heart's pumping action is weak, it may sometimes be improved by vasodilators or *digoxin.*

If drug treatment fails to relieve the symptoms, or if investigation shows extensive narrowing of the coronary arteries, blood flow may be improved by *coronary artery bypass* surgery (in which a vein graft is used to circumvent the narrowed segment). If the disease is localized to one or two segments of artery, it may be possible to relieve blockages using balloon *angioplasty* (a technique by which a narrowed segment of artery is stretched by a small balloon).

A heart attack is usually treated initially in a hospital *coronary care unit.* Treatment may be given with *thrombolytic drugs* in an attempt to dissolve the blood clot in the coronary artery, the affected artery may be widened by angioplasty or may be immediately bypassed by surgery, or treatment may simply be aimed at allowing the heart to recover by a natural process of healing.

OUTLOOK AND PREVENTION

Coronary artery disease is a disease of middle to old age, but its foundations are laid in the teens and early adult life. The chances of developing the disease can be considerably reduced by an "anticoronary" life-style. The person who has never smoked, exercises regularly, is the correct weight, has normal blood pressure, and eats a prudent diet is unlikely to develop symptoms of coronary artery disease until late in life.

RATES OF NEW CASES OF CORONARY HEART DISEASE IN CANADA

Rate (per 100,000)   Female •••   Male •••

A combination of healthier living and better treatment of heart disease has led to a dramatic decline in new cases. The death rate, too, has decreased some 40 percent in the last 20 years. In Canada the disease reached its highest levels in the late 1960s.

Even when symptoms develop, treatment can do a great deal to halt their progression. Studies of patients treated by coronary bypass surgery for disease affecting all the major coronary arteries have shown that 80 to 90 percent are still alive five years after the operation. Survival is even better among those with less extensive disease; they can usually be treated with drugs. Survival is substantially improved in patients who give up cigarette smoking.

Coronary care unit
A small ward, specially staffed and equipped for the care of acutely ill patients who are suspected of being in the process of suffering, or who have suffered, a *myocardial infarction* (heart attack). In the unit, patients are kept under close surveillance and given immediate treatment if a complication such as *cardiac arrest* (cessation of heartbeat), *arrhythmia* (irregular or very rapid or slow heartbeat), or *heart failure* occurs.

A coronary care unit usually holds only five to 10 people, and the ratio of specially trained nurses to patients is high: one-to-one or one-to-two. The ward is equipped with monitoring equipment that provides a continuous record of each patient's heart rhythm, respiratory rate, and blood pressure, and contains specialized equipment for providing treatment, such as *defibrillation* (a technique for restoring normal heart rhythm) and *ventilation* (machine-assisted breathing) to help the patient breathe.

Coronary heart disease
Disease of the arteries that supply blood to the heart muscle, causing damage to, or malfunction of, the heart. (See *Coronary artery disease*.)

Coronary thrombosis
Narrowing or blockage of one of the coronary arteries (which supply blood to the heart muscle) by a thrombus (blood clot). This causes a section of the heart muscle to die because it has been deprived of oxygen.

Coronary thrombosis is one of the main processes involved in *coronary artery disease*, the major cause of death in Canada. Sudden blockage of a coronary artery causes an acute *myocardial infarction* (death of a portion of heart muscle). The terms coronary thrombosis and myocardial infarction thus tend to be used interchangeably, but the latter is the more precise medical term for heart attack.

Coroner
A public official, who may or may not be a physician, appointed to inquire into the cause of an unexpected or accidental death, or one that occurs under suspicious circumstances. (See *Autopsy*.)

Corporate practice
A corporation or management company formed under provincial law by a number of physicians who want to receive provincial Medicare payments as a group and to practice medicine as a group.

Cor pulmonale
Enlargement and strain of the right side of the heart due to chronic lung disease. Damage to the lungs increases resistance to blood flow from the heart through the branches of the pulmonary artery and causes pulmonary hypertension (increased pressure in the pulmonary artery). The resultant 'back pressure' strain on the heart may eventually cause right-sided heart failure with *edema* (fluid collection in the tissues). (See *Pulmonary hypertension*.)

Corpuscle
Any minute body or cell, particularly red and white *blood cells* or certain types of nerve endings.

Corset
A device worn around the trunk to treat *back pain* and spinal injuries or deformities (see *Spine* disorders box).

Soft corsets, usually made of cotton fabric stiffened with plastic or metal, have straps enabling them to be tightened. Most commonly prescribed for back pain, corsets work in the same way as the belts worn by weight-lifters—by increasing pressure on the abdomen they take the weight of the trunk off the lower spine. They also restrict painful movements and help keep the back warm.

Rigid corsets are made of plaster or lightweight plastic and must be molded to the body. They are used to immobilize and support a spinal column that has become unstable through injury, or to help correct faulty alignment of the spine, as occurs in *scoliosis* (spinal curvature).

Cortex
The outer layer of certain organs, such as the brain, kidneys, or adrenal glands. The innermost region of some organs and other body structures is called the *medulla*.

Corticosteroid drugs

COMMON DRUGS

Beclomethasone Betamethasone Cortisone Dexamethasone Fludrocortisone Hydrocortisone Prednisolone Prednisone

C

> **WARNING**
> Sudden withdrawal of corticosteroid drugs may cause serious illness or death. Always inform a physician if you are taking or have recently taken corticosteroids.

A group of drugs similar to the natural corticosteroid hormones produced by the cortex of the *adrenal glands*.

WHY THEY ARE USED
Corticosteroid drugs have a wide variety of uses. They are prescribed as hormone replacement therapy to patients with an inadequate level of natural corticosteroids caused by *Addison's disease*, following surgical removal of the adrenal glands, or when the *pituitary gland* has been destroyed by disease, surgery or irradiation.

Corticosteroid drugs are used in the treatment of inflammatory intestinal disorders, such as *Crohn's disease* and *ulcerative colitis*. *Temporal arteritis* needs urgent treatment with corticosteroids to reduce inflammation in the artery leading to the retina and so prevent blindness.

Other disorders that often improve with corticosteroid treatment include *asthma*, *rheumatoid arthritis*, *eczema*, *iritis* (inflammation of the iris), and

Spinal corset
Most often prescribed for back pain, this type of corset is usually made of cotton stiffened with metal or plastic.

C

allergic *rhinitis* (hay fever). The injection of corticosteroids around an inflamed tendon or joint may relieve pain in disorders such as *tennis elbow* and *arthritis*.

Corticosteroid drugs are also used to suppress the immune system to prevent rejection of a transplanted organ (see *Transplant surgery*) and in the treatment of some types of cancer, such as a *lymphoma* or *leukemia*.

POSSIBLE ADVERSE EFFECTS

The incidence and severity of any adverse effects depends on the dosage, the form in which the drug is given, and the duration of treatment.

Adverse effects are uncommon when corticosteroids are given in the form of a cream or by inhaler because only small amounts are absorbed into the bloodstream. Corticosteroid tablets taken in high doses for long periods may cause *edema* (accumulation of fluid in tissues), *hypertension* (high blood pressure), *diabetes mellitus*, *peptic ulcer*, *Cushing's syndrome*, *hirsutism* (excessive hairiness), inhibited growth in children, and, in rare cases, *cataract* or *psychosis*. High doses of corticosteroid drugs also increase susceptibility to infection by impairing the body's *immune system*.

Long-term treatment with corticosteroid drugs suppresses production of *ACTH* (adrenocorticotrophic hormone) by the pituitary gland, which in turn suppresses production of corticosteroid hormones by the adrenal glands. Sudden withdrawal of the drugs may lead to *adrenal failure*, which may result in collapse, coma, and even death.

Corticosteroid hormones

A group of hormones produced by the *adrenal glands* that control the body's use of nutrients and the excretion of salts and water in the urine.

Corticotropin

An alternative name for *ACTH* (adrenocorticotropic hormone).

Cortisone

A synthetic *corticosteroid drug* used to reduce inflammation in severe allergic, rheumatic, and connective tissue diseases. It is also used as a replacement hormone in *Addison's disease*, in which there is a corticosteroid hormone deficiency, and after removal of the *adrenal glands*.

Coryza

A term for the nasal symptoms of the common cold (see *Cold, common*).

Cosmetic dentistry

Procedures to improve the appearance of the teeth. In many cases, these treatments are also necessary to restore or prevent further damage to the teeth and/or gums.

Teeth that are out of alignment can become decayed because the bite is incorrect (see *Malocclusion*) and because the teeth are hard to keep clean. Such teeth can be moved into proper position by fitting an *orthodontic appliance* (brace). Correction is usually best carried out during childhood, when the teeth and jaws are still growing and developing, but can also be performed in adults.

The main use of a *crown* is to restore normal tooth structure and thus prevent further damage when a tooth is severely decayed or has been broken. However, crowns can also be fitted primarily for cosmetic reasons when a front tooth is damaged or discolored; in this case a porcelain crown is fitted to match the color of the natural teeth.

Bonding is a relatively new technique that has a wide range of cosmetic uses. It can be used to treat chipped or malformed teeth, to close small gaps between front teeth, or to cover stained or discolored teeth. In some cases it can be used instead of a crown for front teeth.

Teeth that have become discolored because the pulp is dead or has been removed may be treated by bleaching (see *Bleaching, dental*).

Cosmetic surgery

An operation performed primarily to improve appearance rather than to improve function or to cure disease.

WHY IT IS DONE

Cosmetic surgery can improve appearance in a number of ways. Skin blemishes can be removed, and the appearance of an unsightly scar improved. The shape and size of the nose, chin, jaw, or breasts can be altered. Excess skin and fat, and any unsightly creases or marks that come with age or loss of weight, can be removed from the eyelids, face, breasts, or stomach.

An individual's expectations of the benefits of cosmetic surgery are often too great, however. Cosmetic surgery will not produce a dramatic change in personality or cure depression that a person attributes to his or her appearance. Nor can it reproduce an exact replica of someone else's features. Some procedures (such as *face-lifts* and *hair transplants*) may need to be repeated over the years; other procedures (such as *body contour surgery*) may result in uneven residual fat and unattractive scarring. Anyone contemplating cosmetic surgery should first discuss the operation in detail with his or her physician.

Costalgia

Pain around the chest due to damage to a rib or to one of the intercostal nerves (which run beneath the ribs). A

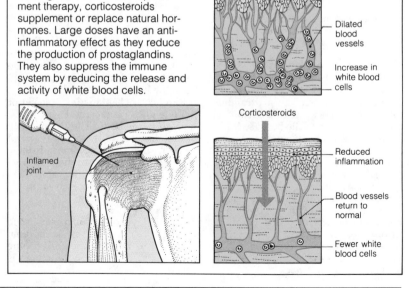

HOW CORTICOSTEROIDS WORK

When given as hormone replacement therapy, corticosteroids supplement or replace natural hormones. Large doses have an anti-inflammatory effect as they reduce the production of prostaglandins. They also suppress the immune system by reducing the release and activity of white blood cells.

Inflamed skin

Dilated blood vessels

Increase in white blood cells

Inflamed joint

Corticosteroids

Reduced inflammation

Blood vessels return to normal

Fewer white blood cells

C

TYPES OF COSMETIC SURGERY

There are various different cosmetic surgery procedures, some of the more commonly performed of which are shown below. The different procedures vary in the permanency of their results and in the likelihood of achieving a satisfactory appearance.

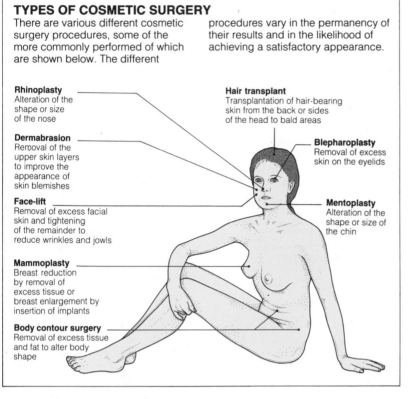

Rhinoplasty
Alteration of the shape or size of the nose

Dermabrasion
Removal of the upper skin layers to improve the appearance of skin blemishes

Face-lift
Removal of excess facial skin and tightening of the remainder to reduce wrinkles and jowls

Mammoplasty
Breast reduction by removal of excess tissue or breast enlargement by insertion of implants

Body contour surgery
Removal of excess tissue and fat to alter body shape

Hair transplant
Transplantation of hair-bearing skin from the back or sides of the head to bald areas

Blepharoplasty
Removal of excess skin on the eyelids

Mentoplasty
Alteration of the shape or size of the chin

broken rib produces pain and tenderness over the affected part of the rib cage. The pain is made worse by deep breathing and often persists for several weeks after the original injury.

Damage to one of the intercostal nerves is most commonly a result of an attack of the viral infection *herpes zoster* (shingles). The pain is difficult to treat successfully and tends to persist for several months or longer.

Co-trimoxazole

An *antibacterial drug* that contains trimethoprim and sulfamethoxazole. Co-trimoxazole is commonly prescribed for the prevention and treatment of urinary tract infections, and the treatment of infections of the respiratory tract, gastrointestinal tract, skin, and ear. It is also used to treat prostatitis, gonorrhea, and pneumocystis pneumonia.

Possible adverse effects include nausea, vomiting, sore tongue, rash, and, in rare cases, blood disorders and jaundice.

Cough

A reflex action to try to clear the airways of mucus, sputum (phlegm), a foreign body, or other irritants or blockages. A cough is said to be productive when it brings up mucus or sputum, and unproductive, or dry, when it does not.

CAUSES
Many coughs are due to irritation of the airways by dust, smoke, or gases, or by mucus dripping from the back of the nose. Another common cause of coughs is inflammation of the upper respiratory tract, usually due to a viral infection (see *Cold, common; Laryngitis; Pharyngitis; Tracheitis*).

In a child, inflammation of the upper respiratory tract can cause narrowing of the airways, leading to *croup* (a condition that is characterized by hoarseness, noisy breathing, and a barking cough) and breathing difficulty. Infection with the bacterium BORDETELLA PERTUSSIS produces the characteristic cough of *pertussis* (whooping cough).

Bronchitis (inflammation of the bronchi, the air passages into the lungs) produces thick mucus and sputum and causes severe coughing. The disorder may be brought on by an infection, but often occurs as a result of smoking (see *Cough, smoker's*). In *bronchiectasis* (distortion or widening of the bronchi), a large amount of infected sputum accumulates in the bronchi, making the sufferer cough persistently in an attempt to bring up the sputum, which may be associated with bleeding.

Bronchospasm (temporary narrowing of the bronchi) causes a dry cough that is usually worse at night. It is a feature of *asthma*, but may also be due to infection or an allergic reaction.

The damage to lung tissues caused by *pneumonia* (inflammation of the lungs) results in a painful productive cough. Damage to the lungs brought about by pulmonary *edema* (accumulation of fluid in the lungs) produces a cough that is dry at first, but which later may bring up frothy, blood-stained sputum. The cough associated with viral bronchitis and viral pneumonia is often dry and persistent, and may interrupt sleep.

Various chronic lung infections, notably *tuberculosis*, may cause a cough. Many *pneumoconioses* (dust diseases of the lungs) also cause a cough, which is usually accompanied by shortness of breath.

An inhaled foreign object, such as a peanut, that lodges in the larynx causes violent coughing to relieve *choking*. If the object travels further down and blocks a bronchus, inflammation and mucus will be produced at the site of obstruction, leading to a persistent cough.

Lung cancer and, less commonly, other tumors of the air passages usually first cause a mild cough and then a more severe one that may produce blood-stained sputum.

Sometimes, especially in children, coughing develops as a nervous reaction to stress.

SELF-HELP
In some cases, a dry cough may be relieved by sucking throat lozenges or by drinking warm, soothing drinks, such as honey and water. If these are ineffective, narcotic *cough remedies* help to relieve symptoms and may be particularly useful at bedtime to permit sleep.

Productive coughing is the body's way of unblocking airways that are obstructed by mucus or sputum and, in such cases, cough suppressants should be avoided because they can do more harm than good. An expectorant cough medication and/or drinking lots of fluids can help to loosen mucus or sputum if there is difficulty coughing it up.

A physician should be consulted if any cough persists for more than a week, if the cough is severe, or if it is

C

COUGH A noisy expulsion of air from the lungs that may produce sputum (phlegm) or be "dry."

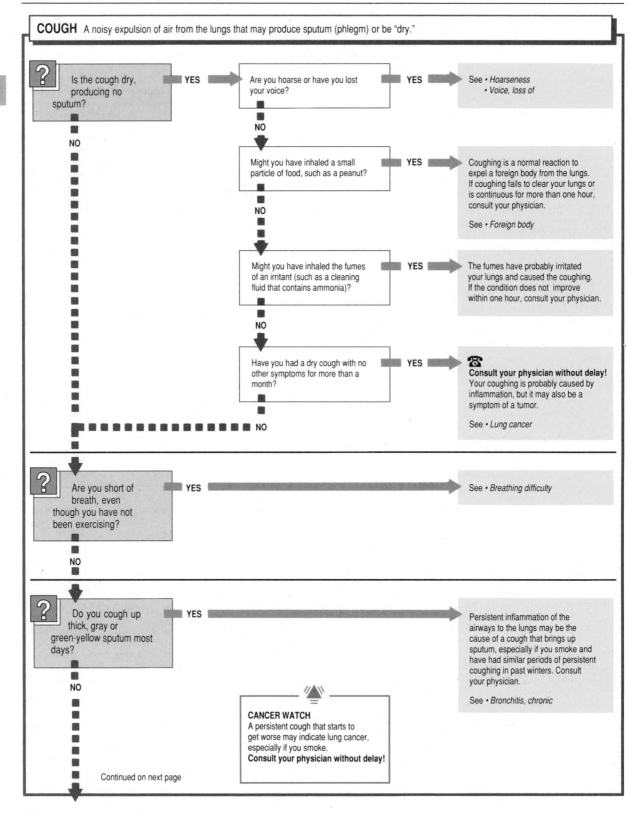

? Is the cough dry, producing no sputum?

YES → Are you hoarse or have you lost your voice? **YES** → See • *Hoarseness* • *Voice, loss of*

NO ↓

Might you have inhaled a small particle of food, such as a peanut? **YES** → Coughing is a normal reaction to expel a foreign body from the lungs. If coughing fails to clear your lungs or is continuous for more than one hour, consult your physician.

See • *Foreign body*

NO ↓

Might you have inhaled the fumes of an irritant (such as a cleaning fluid that contains ammonia)? **YES** → The fumes have probably irritated your lungs and caused the coughing. If the condition does not improve within one hour, consult your physician.

NO ↓

Have you had a dry cough with no other symptoms for more than a month? **YES** → ☎ **Consult your physician without delay!** Your coughing is probably caused by inflammation, but it may also be a symptom of a tumor.

See • *Lung cancer*

NO

NO ↓

? Are you short of breath, even though you have not been exercising?

YES → See • *Breathing difficulty*

NO ↓

? Do you cough up thick, gray or green-yellow sputum most days?

YES → Persistent inflammation of the airways to the lungs may be the cause of a cough that brings up sputum, especially if you smoke and have had similar periods of persistent coughing in past winters. Consult your physician.

See • *Bronchitis, chronic*

NO ↓

CANCER WATCH
A persistent cough that starts to get worse may indicate lung cancer, especially if you smoke.
Consult your physician without delay!

Continued on next page

Have you had your cough for several weeks or months AND has it been getting more severe?

YES

☎

Consult your physician without delay!
Asthma or chronic bronchitis may be the cause of your symptoms, but the possibility of tuberculosis or lung cancer also exists.

See • *Asthma*
• *Bronchitis*
• *Lung cancer*
• *Tuberculosis*

NO

Of recent origin – within the past week.

Is your temperature 38°C or above?

YES → Are you breathless? **YES**

☎

Call your physician without delay!
These symptoms suggest that you may have pneumonia.

See • *Pneumonia*

NO

You may have acute bronchitis or a viral infection. Treat the fever. If there is no improvement in 24 to 48 hours, consult your physician.

See • *Fever*

NO

Do you have a runny nose AND/OR a sore throat?

YES

You probably have a cold. Take analgesics and gargle with salt water.

See • *Cold, common*

NO

If you are unable to make a diagnosis from this chart, consult your physician.

C

---

accompanied by symptoms such as chest pain, green sputum and cough-ed-up blood, or if the patient has breathing difficulty.

TREATMENT
Treatment depends on the underlying disorder that is causing the cough. For example, an *antibiotic drug* may be given for a bacterial infection; a *bronchodilator drug* and/or a *corticosteroid drug* for asthma; *breathing exercises* and *postural drainage* (lying in a position that allows mucus to drain from the bronchi) for bronchiectasis and chronic bronchitis; and surgery or *radiation therapy* for cancer.

Coughing up blood
Known medically as hemoptysis, coughing up blood is due to rupture of a blood vessel in the airways, lungs, nose, or throat.

Coughed-up blood may be in the form of bright red or rusty brown streaks or clots in or on the sputum (phlegm), a pinkish froth, or, more rarely, pure blood. The form it takes depends as much on the size of the ruptured blood vessel as on the underlying cause. Coughing up blood should not be confused with blood in the mouth, which is usually due to a nosebleed or to bleeding gums.

Because of the possibility of a serious underlying disorder, all cases of coughing up blood require medical assessment.

CAUSES
Any disorder that causes a persistent *cough* can produce hemoptysis by putting strain on the blood vessels in the airways.

The most common cause of coughing up blood is an infection—such as *pneumonia*, *bronchitis*, or *tuberculosis*—in which inflammation of the bronchi (airways into the lungs) and alveoli (air sacs) damages a blood-vessel wall. Similarly, in *bronchiectasis* the bronchi become enlarged and distorted, which can lead to rupture of a blood vessel and coughing up blood.

Another cause of coughing up blood is congestion in, and subsequent rupture of, blood vessels within the lungs. Congestion can be due to *heart failure*, *mitral stenosis* (narrowing of the mitral valve in the heart), or *pulmonary embolism* (blood clot lodged in an artery in the lungs).

A malignant tumor can lead to coughing up blood by eroding the wall of a blood vessel in the larynx (voice box), bronchi, or alveoli.

INVESTIGATION AND TREATMENT

A *chest X ray* may be carried out. Anyone who smokes, who is older than 40, whose chest X rays are abnormal, or who has coughed up blood more than once may require *bronchoscopy*, a diagnostic procedure in which a flexible viewing instrument is passed into the lungs. In about one third of cases, however, no underlying cause is found.

Treatment depends on the cause, but may include *antibiotic drugs*, *anticoagulant drugs*, and *diuretic drugs*.

Cough remedies

COMMON DRUGS

Expectorants
Guiafenesin

Cough suppressants
Antihistamines Codeine Dextromethorphan

A bewildering variety of over-the-counter medications is available. The majority of *cough* remedies consist of a syrupy base to which various active ingredients and flavorings are added.

Two main groups of drugs are used: expectorants, intended for coughs that are producing sputum (phlegm), and cough suppressants, intended for dry coughs. It is important to select the correct type of medication—a cough suppressant taken for a sputum-producing cough may interfere with the coughing up of sputum and delay recovery.

HOW THEY WORK

Expectorants "loosen" a cough by stimulating the production of watery secretions in the lungs. Some expectorants also have a mucolytic action (a direct effect on the sputum that makes it less sticky).

Cough suppressants act on the part of the brain that controls the coughing reflex. Drugs with this effect include some *antihistamine drugs* and the narcotic analgesic drug *codeine*.

POSSIBLE ADVERSE EFFECTS

All cough suppressants have a sedative effect and may cause drowsiness. Using cough remedies to alleviate the symptoms of a persistent cough may delay diagnosis of a serious disorder.

Cough, smoker's

A recurrent cough that is very common among smokers, particularly heavy smokers and those who have smoked for a long time. In many cases, the sufferer becomes accustomed to his or her cough and regards it as normal.

Usually, coughing is triggered by the accumulation of thick sputum (phlegm) in the airways (a feature of chronic *bronchitis*), which is caused by inflammation of the airways due to smoking. There is no such thing as a "normal" cough.

TREATMENT

Stopping smoking usually stops the persistent cough, although this does not happen immediately. In general, the longer the person has been smoking, the longer the cough will persist after giving up.

Because of the association between smoking and *lung cancer*, it is essential for a smoker to seek medical advice about his or her cough, particularly if there is any change in its frequency or character. (See also *Tobacco smoking*.)

Counseling

Advice and psychological support given by a health professional and usually aimed at helping a person cope with a particular problem (for example, bereavement or cancer treatment). A more general exploration of a person's feelings and attitudes, not aimed at one particular problem, is sometimes included in the definition.

WHY IT IS DONE

Counseling can help people with problems at school, work, or within the family; provide advice on medical problems, family planning, abortion, and sexual and marital problems; help people deal with drinking and drug problems; and provide support during various life crises.

Physicians may use a counseling style when interviewing a patient whose medical problem is complicated by personal circumstances, or when the patient's reason for consulting the physician is not clear.

HOW IT IS DONE

Some counseling, especially for genetic disorders (see *Genetic counseling*) or the treatment of cancer, consists mainly of providing personalized

information in a setting in which the patient, or client, is encouraged to ask questions and express any doubts and uncertainties.

Techniques used in psychotherapeutic counseling are essentially similar. The counselor encourages the individual to make statements about his or her feelings, experiences, and problems. These statements can then be discussed and explored for inconsistencies as a means of helping the individual develop a greater and more realistic understanding of his or her problems.

Usually, counseling is a one-to-one activity. However, in some situations, such as *sex therapy*, representatives of a particular point of view or gender model may take part (for example, one male and one female counselor). This is termed co-counseling. Counseling may also occur in small groups. (See also *Child guidance*; *Family therapy*; *Marriage guidance*; *Psychotherapy*.)

Cowpox

An infection caused by the VACCINIA virus, which usually affects cows.

An attack of cowpox used to confer immunity against *smallpox* (now extinct) because the viruses responsible for the two diseases were very similar. This fact was the basis of smallpox vaccination. Vaccinia virus, which gave its name to "vaccination," continued to be used as smallpox vaccine until smallpox was eradicated in the 1970s.

Coxa vara

A deformity of the hip in which the angle between the neck and head (ball) of the femur (thigh bone) and the shaft of the femur is reduced, causing shortening of the leg and a limp.

CAUSES

The most common cause of coxa vara is injury—either a fracture of the neck of the femur or, during adolescence, injury to the developing part of the head of the bone. The deformity can also occur if the bone tissue in the neck of the femur is soft instead of firm, so that it bends under the weight of the body. This softening may be congenital (present at birth) or it may be the result of a bone disorder such as *rickets* or *Paget's disease*.

SYMPTOMS, DIAGNOSIS, AND TREATMENT

The symptoms are pain and stiffness in the hip and difficulty in walking. The disorder is diagnosed by X rays, which reveal the deformity.

Treatment depends on the underlying condition. In some cases, an oper-

C

ation may be performed to cut the deformed part of the bone and reposition the two ends at the correct angle (see *Osteotomy*). This usually eases the condition so that the patient can walk with only minor discomfort.

Crab lice
See *Pubic lice*.

Cradle cap
A condition common in babies in which thick, yellow scales occur in patches over the scalp. Cradle cap is harmless if the scalp skin does not become infected. The condition tends to recur.

Cradle cap is a form of seborrheic *dermatitis*, which may also occur on the face, neck, behind the ears, and in the diaper area. The skin in these areas may look red and inflamed.

TREATMENT
Cradle cap is best treated by daily use of a mild, antidandruff shampoo.

Alternatively, warm olive oil or mineral oil may be rubbed into the baby's scalp and left on overnight to loosen and soften the scales, which can then be gently washed off the following day. This procedure may need to be repeated for several days until all the scales have been washed off.

The baby's hair should be brushed daily using a clean soft-bristled brush. This will also help loosen the scales.

If the condition seems to be worsening or if the skin looks inflamed, a physician should be consulted. A mild ointment containing an *antibiotic drug* and a *corticosteroid drug* may be prescribed for use until the condition improves.

Cramp
Painful spasm in a muscle caused by excessive and prolonged contraction of the muscle fibers. Cramps are a common occurrence and usually last only a few moments.

Appearance of cradle cap
Most prevalent between 3 and 9 months of age, it is not clear why cradle cap occurs, but it is not a result of poor hygiene.

Cramps often occur during or immediately after exercise because of a buildup of lactic acid and other chemicals in the muscles (caused by increased muscular activity) and small areas of muscle-fiber damage.

FUNCTIONS OF CRANIAL NERVES
Some cranial nerves are principally concerned with delivering sensory information from organs, such as the ears, nose, and eyes, to the brain. Others carry messages that move the tongue, eyes, and facial (and other) muscles, or stimulate glands such as the salivary glands. A few have both sensory and motor functions. One of the nerves—the 10th cranial, or *vagus nerve*—is one of the most important components of the *parasympathetic nervous system*, which is concerned with maintaining the rhythmic automatic function of the internal body machinery. It has branches to all the main digestive organs, the heart, and the lungs.

C

Cramps can also occur during any repetitive movement, such as writing (see *Cramp, writer's*), or through sitting or lying in an awkward position. Anything that causes profuse sweating, such as a fever, very hot weather, or prolonged exercise, can lead to cramps in resting muscles; the loss of sodium salts in the sweat disrupts muscle cell activity.

Cramps at night usually have no known cause. In some cases, night cramps may be due to *peripheral vascular disease* (narrowing of blood vessels in the legs).

TREATMENT

Cramp can be relieved by massaging or stretching the muscles involved. If cramps occur regularly at night, your doctor may prescribe a drug containing calcium or quinine, which can help prevent painful recurrences.

If cramps persist for longer than about an hour, they are likely to be due to a more serious condition and medical attention should be sought immediately.

Cramp, writer's

Painful spasm in the muscles of the hand, which makes writing or typing impossible. In most cases the muscles in the hand are still able to perform other tasks, indicating that the problem may be psychological in origin. However, despite this theory, writer's cramp does not respond to psychotherapy. Drug treatment has also been found to have little effect. Writer's cramp sometimes improves if the hand is rested for a few months, but often the problem is permanent. Occasionally the other hand becomes affected.

Cranial nerves

Twelve pairs of nerves that emerge directly from the brain—as opposed to the *spinal nerves*, which connect with the spinal cord. All but two of the cranial nerve pairs connect with nuclei in the *brain stem* (the lowest section of the brain). The other two (the olfactory and optic nerves) link directly with parts of the *cerebrum*. All the nerves emerge through various openings in the cranium (skull surrounding the brain); many then soon divide into several major branches.

Craniopharyngioma

A tumor of the pituitary gland. Craniopharyngioma is very rare, with 25 to 50 cases in Canada each year. More than half of those affected are under 20 years old.

Symptoms include headaches, vomiting, defective vision, stunted growth, and failure of sexual development. If untreated, a craniopharyngioma may result in permanent brain damage.

Craniopharyngiomas are identified by *brain imaging* techniques and are usually removed surgically.

Craniosynostosis

The premature closure of one or more of the joints (known as synostoses or *sutures*) between the curved, flattened bones of the *skull* (cranium); also called craniostenosis.

Craniosynostosis is three times more common in boys than in girls. It may occur before birth, and one third of those affected have other *birth defects*. It also may occur in an otherwise healthy baby, or in a baby affected by another disorder such as rickets. The condition occasionally runs in families.

If all of the skull joints are involved, the growing infant's brain may be compressed and the pressure inside the skull may increase. If the abnormality is localized, the head may be deformed.

DIAGNOSIS AND TREATMENT

The diagnosis is made from the outward appearance of the skull and from skull *X rays* or *CT scanning*. If the brain is compressed, treatment must be undertaken to prevent brain damage. An operation is performed to separate the skull bones by cutting away the fused edges and separating the bony plates.

Craniotomy

Removal of part of the skull to carry out an operation on the brain, such as for the removal of a sample of tissue for analysis, removal of a tumor, or drainage of an abscess or blood clot.

After the operation, the bone is replaced and the membranes, muscle, and skin are sewn back into position. Following successful surgery, the patient can usually leave hospital within a week. He or she will

PROCEDURE FOR CRANIOTOMY
Before the operation, all or part of the patient's scalp is shaved. After a general anesthetic has been given, layers of skin, muscle, and membrane are cut away from the skull at the planned operation site and the bone is cut with a saw. The lid of bone is then either lifted back on a hinge of muscle or removed completely. The dura (the outer membrane lining the brain) is then opened to reveal the inner membranes and the brain.

Burr holes
A series of burr holes is made. They must be very close together if the bone is thick.

Burr
Skull
Dura
Brain

Brain

Skin hinged back

Flap of skull hinged back

Gigli's saw
The cuts between the burr holes are made using Gigli's saw, which is passed between the burr holes using a malleable saw guide.

Burr hole   Gigli's saw

generally experience mild headaches for a time, but little real pain.

Cranium
The part of the *skull* around the brain.

Cream
A thick, semisolid preparation used to apply medications to the skin for therapeutic or prophylactic (preventive) purposes. Creams are useful in the treatment of dry skin conditions because their high water content gives them a moisturizing effect.

Creatinine clearance
See *Kidney function tests*.

Crepitus
The grating sound heard, and the sensation felt, when two rough surfaces rub together. Crepitus may be experienced when the ends of a broken bone rub against each other, or in *osteoarthritis* when the cartilage that covers the bony surfaces of a joint has worn away and the roughened areas of the joint grind against each other. The sound is usually loud enough to be heard by the naked ear. Fainter sounds, audible through a *stethoscope*, are produced in the lung as a result of inflammation—due to pneumonia, for example.

The term crepitus is also used to describe the sounds made when an area of air under the skin (see *Emphysema, surgical*) or gas *gangrene* (gas within infected tissues) is pressed.

Cretinism
A *congenital* condition characterized by mental retardation, stunted growth, and coarse facial features in infants. Cretinism results from insufficient or absent production of thyroxine (a *thyroid hormone*) by the thyroid gland at birth.

A routine test performed on all newborn infants reveals symptoms of cretinism. A complete cure is possible by means of replacement therapy with thyroxine provided the condition is recognized early. (See also *Hypothyroidism*.)

Creutzfeldt-Jakob disease
A very rare degenerative condition of the brain thought to be due to a slow virus (one that causes no signs of disease until many years after the original infection).

In most instances, no source of infection is discovered. However, rarely, infection has been linked with brain surgery when instruments contaminated by the virus have been used, with transplant of an infected cornea, and with treatment with growth hormone extracted from pituitary glands after death (current growth hormone preparations are products of genetic engineering and carry no risk).

The condition causes progressive *dementia* and *myoclonus* (sudden muscular contractions). Muscular coordination diminishes, the intellect and personality deteriorate, and blindness may develop. As the disease progresses, the power of speech is lost and the body becomes rigid. There is no treatment and death usually occurs within three to 12 months of onset.

Crib death
See *Sudden infant death syndrome*.

Cri du chat syndrome
A *congenital* condition characterized by a catlike cry due to a small larynx. Mental handicap, poor brain development, a small head, an unusual rounded face with small jaw and wide spacing between the eyes, a low birth weight, and shortness of stature are other typical features.

Cri du chat syndrome is rare and is the result of a *chromosomal abnormality*; a portion of one particular chromosome is missing in each of the affected individual's cells. No treatment is possible. The child needs special care and schooling if he or she survives infancy. (See also *Genetic counseling*.)

Crisis
A term that describes a turning point in the course of a disease (marking the onset of either recovery or deterioration), an emergency, or a distressing time of emotional difficulty (such as divorce, or a serious illness or death in the family). In medicine, the term was in common use before the advent of antibiotics when patients who had lobar *pneumonia* would be watched for the crisis.

Crisis intervention
The provision of immediate advice or help to people with acute personal or sociomedical problems.

Many voluntary organizations have been established to help people in crisis. Help may also be available at walk-in centers or social services departments. In addition to other crisis services, these centers may offer *counseling*, usually with the aim of helping clients cope with crises rather than of providing longer-term help.

Critical
A term used to mean seriously ill, or to describe a crucial state of illness from which it is uncertain whether the patient will recover.

Crohn's disease
A chronic inflammatory disease that can affect any part of the gastrointestinal tract from the mouth to the anus. Crohn's disease may cause pain, fever, diarrhea, and loss of weight.

The most common site of inflammation is the terminal ileum (the end of the small intestine where it joins the large intestine). The intestinal wall becomes extremely thick due to continued chronic inflammation, and deep, penetrating ulcers may form. The disease tends to be patchy; areas of the intestine that lie between diseased sections may appear to be normal, but even these areas are usually mildly affected.

CAUSES AND INCIDENCE
The cause is unknown. It may represent an abnormal allergic reaction or may be an exaggerated response to an infectious agent, such as a bacterium or a virus. There is a slight genetic predisposition (inherited tendency) to develop the disease.

The incidence of Crohn's disease in North America varies between three and six new cases per year per 100,000 population. The incidence in most developed countries seems to have increased over the last 30 years. A person may be affected by the disease at any age, but the peak periods are adolescence and early adulthood and after the age of 60.

SYMPTOMS
In young people, the ileum is usually involved, and the disease causes spasms of pain in the abdomen, diarrhea, and chronic sickness due to loss of appetite, anemia, and weight loss. The ability of the small intestine to absorb food is reduced. In the elderly, it is more common for the disease to affect the rectum and cause rectal bleeding. In both groups, the disease may also affect the anus, resulting in chronic abscesses, deep fissures (cracks), and fistulas (abnormal passageways).

Crohn's disease can also affect the colon (the major part of the large intestine), causing bloody diarrhea. In rare cases, the disease also affects the mouth, esophagus, stomach, and duodenum (the upper part of the small intestine).

Complications may affect the intestines or may develop elsewhere. The

C

thickening of the intestinal wall may narrow the inside of the intestine so much that an obstruction occurs.

About 30 percent of patients with Crohn's disease develop a fistula. Internal fistulas may form between loops of intestine. External fistulas from the intestine to the skin of the abdomen or the skin surrounding the anus may follow a surgical operation (or the rupture of an abscess) and may cause leakage of feces onto the skin.

Abscesses (pus-filled pockets of infection) form in about 20 percent of patients. Many of these abscesses occur around the anus, but some occur within the abdomen.

Complications in other parts of the body may include inflammation of various parts of the eye, severe arthritis affecting various joints of the body, *ankylosing spondylitis* (an inflammation of the spine), and skin disorders (including *eczema*).

DIAGNOSIS

If the symptoms suggest Crohn's disease, a physical examination may reveal tender abdominal swellings that indicate thickening of the intestinal walls. *Sigmoidoscopy* (examination of the sigmoid colon and rectum with a viewing instrument) may confirm the disease's presence in the rectum. X rays using barium meals or barium enemas (see *Barium X-ray examinations*) will show thickened loops of intestine with deep fissures.

It may be difficult to differentiate between Crohn's disease that affects the colon and *ulcerative colitis*, an inflammatory bowel disease that is limited to the large intestine, but *colonoscopy* (examination of the colon using a flexible viewing instrument) and *biopsy* (removal of a sample of tissue for microscopic examination) may help with diagnosis in doubtful cases. In addition, blood tests may show evidence of protein deficiency or *anemia*.

TREATMENT

Sulfasalazine may be given by mouth to try to control the inflammatory process and *corticosteroid drugs* may be given by mouth or as enemas. Patients suffering from severe acute attacks may require admission to hospital for blood transfusion, intravenous feeding, and intravenous administration of corticosteroid drugs. The severity of the disease fluctuates widely, and patients are usually under long-term medical supervision.

Some patients find that particular foods exacerbate their symptoms. Others may benefit from a high-vitamin, low-fiber diet.

A surgical operation to remove damaged portions of the intestine may be needed to treat chronic obstruction or blood loss. If the small intestine is involved, the surgeon will remove as little of the intestine as possible, seeking only to remove the most affected parts since the surgery is not curative.

If the large intestine is involved, surgery may involve removal of narrowed obstructing segments.

Emergency surgery may sometimes be required to deal with an abscess. Simple drainage of an abscess will produce an external fistula, but occasionally the patient is too ill for any further treatment. Surgery may also occasionally be required for obstruction, perforation (rupture), or severe bleeding.

OUTLOOK

The disease is chronic and the symptoms fluctuate over many years, eventually subsiding in some patients. Many patients require surgical treatment at some stage to deal with complications of the disease. The recurrence rate after surgery is high, although recurrences may be delayed for many years.

Some patients in whom the disease is localized remain in normal health indefinitely and seem to be cured. There is no predisposition to intestinal cancer.

Crossbite

A type of *malocclusion* in which some or all of the lower front teeth overlap the upper front teeth. In a normal bite, the reverse is true.

Cross-eye

A type of *strabismus* (squint) in which one of the eyes turns inward relative to the other.

Cross-matching

A procedure used to determine compatibility between the blood of a person who requires a *blood transfusion* and that of a blood donor.

Red blood cells from the donor are mixed with serum from the recipient, and red blood cells from the recipient are mixed with serum from the donor. After a short time, the mixtures are examined on a glass slide under a microscope. Grouping together of the red cells to form a small clump indicates the presence of antibodies in the serum, showing that the blood is not compatible. If no clumping occurs, the donor's blood may be safely transfused to the recipient.

Appearance of cross-eye
Many cases of cross-eye can be corrected to improve appearance and vision.

Croup

A term meaning a harsh sound, applied to a condition due to narrowing and inflammation of the airways in infants and young children. Croup causes hoarseness, stridor (a grunting noise during breathing), and a barking cough. It is very common in children up to the age of about 4 years. In older children and adults, the airways are wider and the cartilage in the wall is stiffer, so that the effect of any swelling or inflammation is less marked.

CAUSES

Croup may be caused by a viral or bacterial infection that affects the larynx (voice box), the epiglottis which covers the larynx (see *Epiglottitis*), or the trachea (windpipe). Infectious croup tends to occur in winter. Other causes include *diphtheria*, *allergy*, spasm caused by deficient *calcium* in the blood, and the inhalation of a *foreign body*, such as a peanut.

TREATMENT

Most cases are mild and pass quickly. A parent should remain calm and comfort the child; once soothed, the child will be able to breathe more easily. Providing a warm mist for the child to inhale (e.g., by using a room humidifier or sitting in the bathroom with the shower running) may also help.

If a child is distressed and you are concerned, you should call your physician. If the child is struggling to breathe or turns blue, medical help should be obtained immediately. The child should be taken to hospital where he or she may be given humidified oxygen in a tent. If breathing is seriously obstructed, treatment involves either the passage of a tube down the throat or an operation called a *tracheostomy*, in which a tube is passed into the throat through the neck to bypass the obstruction. In either case, the tube can usually be removed within a few days and complete recovery takes place after a few more days.

Crowding, dental
See *Overcrowding, dental*.

Crown, dental
An artificial replacement for the crown of a tooth (the part above the gum) that has become decayed, discolored, or broken. A porcelain crown is usually used on front teeth because of its similarity in color to natural teeth, but back teeth require the greater strength of a crown made from gold or from porcelain fused to metal.

Cruciate ligaments
Two ligaments in the knee that pass over each other to form a cross (hence their name, from the Latin word "crux," meaning cross). The ligaments form connections between the femur (thigh bone) and tibia (shin) inside the knee joint.

The role of the cruciate ligaments is to prevent overbending and overstraightening at the knee joint. Consequently, if these ligaments are torn, the knee joint becomes unstable and may cause pain.

Crush syndrome
Damage to a large amount of body muscle—most commonly as a result of a serious road traffic accident—causing *kidney failure*. Protein pigments released into the bloodstream from the damaged muscles temporarily impair the functioning of the kidney. As a result, some substances normally excreted in the urine build up to toxic levels in the blood. Without treatment the kidney failure may be fatal but treatment by *dialysis* gives the kidneys a chance to recover their function.

Crutch palsy
Weakness or paralysis of muscles in the wrist, fingers, and thumb due to pressure under the arm affecting the nerves that supply these muscles. Such pressure may be caused by a crutch pressing tightly under the arm—hence the name.

A crutch will cause crutch palsy only if it is too tall for the individual and is used for prolonged walking. A crutch should fit comfortably under the arm when standing upright, with the hand taking much of the weight.

Crutch palsy can also occur if a person falls asleep with one arm over the back of a chair so that the top of the chair presses into the armpit. Often this occurs after a bout of drinking, giving the disorder its common name of Saturday night palsy.

Symptoms usually improve without treatment because damage to the nerves is only temporary. In rare cases, exercises are needed to strengthen the wrist and fingers.

Crying in infants
Occasional crying in a baby is normal. It is the baby's only means of communicating a need. Only when the baby is inconsolable or the crying is unusual in any way should it be regarded as signifying a problem.

CAUSES
Crying in infants is a response to needs or discomforts, such as hunger, thirst, a wet or soiled diaper, tiredness, interrupted sleep, a desire to be comforted, feeling hot or cold, boredom, or separation from parents. Most healthy babies stop crying when their needs are attended to.

Persistent crying, when it is not due to a persistently ignored or unrecognized need, may be a baby's reaction to the overwrought state of a parent. In a minority of cases, crying may be due to illness, commonly an ear or throat infection, or a viral fever. Persistent crying may indicate maltreatment (see *Child abuse*).

TREATMENT
A crying baby should always be attended to. The idea that attending to a crying infant is "giving in" is wrong. Persistent lack of attention is believed to have an adverse effect on emotional development in later life.

If a baby continues to cry after a feed and a change of diaper, parents should make sure that their child is not uncomfortable or too hot or cold, and should try to comfort the baby. A baby sling can be used to provide continuous physical contact. The baby may also prefer being propped up in a chair rather than lying flat, so that he or she can look around.

HOW CROWNS ARE FITTED
The tooth is filed to form a peg over which the replacement is fitted. An impression of the peg and natural tooth is taken and a replica made. Using this as a model, the crown is constructed.

Cast full crown

Porcelain fused to metal crown

Porcelain jacket crown

Three-quarter crown

1 A cracked, heavily filled, or broken tooth can be replaced by a crown.

2 The remaining part of the tooth is shaped to receive the crown.

3 The crown, a hollow shell, is fitted over the shaped tooth and cemented in place.

POST CROWNS
If the natural tooth is heavily decayed or has been weakened, a post crown is fitted.

Tooth root

Damaged tooth

1 This tooth is so decayed that a retaining peg cannot be fashioned.

2 The natural crown of the tooth is completely removed.

Tooth trimmed

Gold post in root canal

Crown

3 A post is cemented into the root canal and the crown is cemented over the post.

C

Parents should try to get as much sleep as possible, and should put aside at least one period during the day for relaxation. If the baby cries at night, parents should take turns attending to him or her.

Medical advice is usually necessary only if a baby cries persistently despite all attempts to soothe him or her, if a normally quiet baby starts to cry a lot, if a baby also has diarrhea, vomiting, fever, or seems unwell, or if a baby cries only weakly or not at all. Parents should not attribute these more serious symptoms to teething or colic without first consulting their physician.

Cryo-
A prefix meaning ice-cold. It is often used to indicate that a procedure uses freezing or low temperatures.

Cryopreservation
The preservation of living cells by freezing. The technique is used chiefly to store human eggs, sperm, and blood for later use.

WHY IT IS DONE
If a woman is infertile because of blocked fallopian tubes, eggs can be removed from her ovaries and then frozen and stored until they can be used for *in vitro fertilization*.

Treatment of cancer by means of radiation therapy or chemotherapy carries the slight risk of damaging sperm. If the man wants to retain the option of future fatherhood, a sample of his sperm is collected before treatment begins and frozen for possible later use in *artificial insemination*. Sperm from donors can also be frozen and used later to enable a woman whose husband is infertile to bear a child.

Plasma and blood belonging to rare blood groups can be preserved by freezing and stored in a blood bank for long periods until needed.

HOW IT IS DONE
The cells to be preserved are first immersed in a fluid, usually glycerol. Glycerol enters and surrounds the cells so that they are protected from the normally destructive effect of freezing. The temperature is progressively lowered as the concentration of protecting fluid is increased until the final storage temperature of about −180°C is reached.

OUTLOOK
Apart from widespread cryopreservation of cells, there has also been some success with freezing and reusing small areas of tissue, such as the cornea and portions of skin. This has led to experimental work on the possibility (as yet unfulfilled) of cryopreservation of major organs, such as the heart, liver, and kidneys, taken from people who have recently died, for transplantation. This would enable transplants to be carried out on a normal surgical time scale rather than as a race against time.

Cryosurgery
The use of temperatures below freezing to destroy tissue. The term is also applied to the use of cold during surgery to produce adhesion between an instrument and body tissue. Cryosurgery has been in common use only for the past decade; in many cases it is proving to be a useful alternative to more traditional forms of surgery or radiation therapy.

WHY IT IS DONE
Because cryosurgery causes only minimal scarring, it is particularly valuable for dealing with malignant tumors in the cervix and in major organs, such as the liver or intestines, in which heavy scarring can block vital openings or channels.

Cryosurgery is a good method for operating on tiny structures in the eye, and has proved particularly useful in *cataract surgery* and for treating *retinal detachment*.

Cryosurgery is also a common technique for removing *warts*, *skin tags*, some birthmarks, and certain types of skin cancer, such as *basal cell carcinoma*. *Hemorrhoids* (piles) and other anal disorders can be treated rapidly and effectively.

HOW IT IS DONE
Treatment of an internal tumor with cryosurgery is a major operation requiring a general anesthetic. The growth is destroyed in one of two ways—by applying a metal probe cooled to the temperature of liquid nitrogen (about −160°C), or by spraying it with liquid nitrogen.

Cryosurgery on the skin and for hemorrhoids is usually performed on an outpatient basis. The procedure, using a cooled metal probe, is virtually painless because the extreme cold paralyzes the nerves in the skin. After treatment, a blister develops, which may weep for a few days before healing. Although there is little scarring, the treated area may show up as a patch of paler skin.

Cryotherapy
The use of cold or freezing in treatment. (See also *Cryosurgery*.)

Cryptococcosis
A rare infection caused by inhaling the fungus *CRYPTOCOCCUS NEOFORMANS*. This fungus is found throughout the world, especially in soil contaminated with pigeon droppings. Infection with the fungus may cause *meningitis* (inflammation of the coverings of the brain and spinal cord) or granular growths in the lungs, skin, or elsewhere. Most, but not all, cases occur in people whose resistance to infection has been drastically lowered by diseases such as *AIDS* and *Hodgkin's disease* or by treatment with *immunosuppressant drugs*.

SYMPTOMS
Meningitis is the most usual, and serious, form that the illness takes. Symptoms include headache, stiffness in the neck, fever, drowsiness, blurred vision, and a staggering gait. If the infection is not treated, it may end in coma and death. When the disease attacks the lungs it causes chest pain and a cough, sometimes with sputum (phlegm); there may also be a skin rash of ulcerating spots.

DIAGNOSIS AND TREATMENT
Cryptococcal meningitis is diagnosed from a sample of fluid drawn from the spine. An X ray may be needed to detect any damage to the lungs, and laboratory examination of the sputum, lung *biopsy* (removal of a sample of tissue for microscopic analysis), and *bronchoscopy* (inspection of the bronchi with a viewing instrument) may be needed.

Most cases in which only the lungs have been infected need no treatment. When the meninges have been affected, a combination of *amphotericin B* and another *antifungal drug*, flucytosine, is usually given for about six weeks. Although these drugs are usually effective, relapses can occur.

Cryptorchidism
A developmental disorder of male infants in which the testes fail to descend normally into the scrotum. (See *Testis, undescended*.)

Cryptosporidiosis
A type of diarrheal infection caused by *protozoa*. Cryptosporidiosis may be spread from person to person, or from domestic animals (especially calves) to people. The disease is most common in children but also occurs in male homosexuals.

The main symptom is usually an attack of watery diarrhea that lasts about a week. There may also be fever, nausea, and abdominal pain. The infection may be much more severe in people whose *immune system* is suppressed, especially those with *AIDS*.

Diagnosis is confirmed by microscopic examination of a sample of feces. Treatment, other than *rehydration therapy*, is not usually necessary, except in immunosuppressed patients.

CT scanning

A diagnostic technique in which the combined use of a computer and *X rays* passed through the body at different angles produces clear cross-sectional images ("slices") of the tissue being examined. CT (computed tomography) scanning—also known as CAT (computed axial tomography) scanning or whole body scanning—provides clearer and more detailed information than X rays used by themselves. CT scanning also has the advantage of tending to minimize the amount of radiation exposure.

WHY IT IS DONE

The first CT scanner, which came into operation in 1972, was developed to study the brain. Since then, CT brain scanning has revolutionized the diagnosis and treatment of tumors, abscesses, and hemorrhages in the brain, as well as strokes and head injuries. These once required tests, such as *angiography* and ventriculography (an outmoded technique for imaging the ventricles of the brain), that were not only difficult to perform, lengthy, and not always clear-cut in their findings, but also entailed some risk to the patient. CT scanning, on the other hand, is simple, quick, accurate, and involves only modest exposure to radiation (see box below).

As well as being essential for the study of the brain, CT scanning is invaluable in investigating disease of any part of the trunk. It is particularly useful for locating and imaging tumors, and for facilitating needle *biopsy* (removal of a sample of tissue via a needle).

RESULTS

Using the information produced by the scanner, a computer constructs cross-sectional images of the tissue under examination. These images, when displayed on a TV screen, reveal soft tissues (including tumors) more clearly than normal X-ray pictures. The images are particularly valuable in brain scans due to their sharp definition of the ventricles (fluid-filled spaces).

The images can be manipulated electronically to provide the best view of the area of interest, and adjacent two-dimensional "slices" can be reconstructed to produce three-dimensional representations as well as images in different planes.

Culture

A growth of bacteria or other microorganisms, cells, or tissues cultivated artificially in the laboratory.

WHY IT IS DONE

Microorganisms are collected and cultivated to enable the cause of an infection to be accurately diagnosed. Cultivation produces larger numbers of microorganisms in a form suitable for further tests.

C

PERFORMING A CT SCAN

CT scanning combines the use of a computer and X rays passed through the body at different angles to produce clear cross-sectional images of areas of body tissue. Before the scan is carried out, a contrast medium may be injected to make blood vessels, organs, or abnormalities show up more clearly; a drink of contrast medium may be given to highlight loops of intestine.

1 The patient lies on a table that can be moved up or down to allow easy transfer and accurate positioning within the machine.

A central sliding cradle in the table moves the patient, at a controllable rate, into the machine

The machine can be tilted in either direction to allow precise areas to be X-rayed

2 A great number of X-ray beams, each of low dosage and lasting only a fraction of a second, are passed through the body at different angles as the scanner rotates around the patient.

Right kidney

Spinal cord

Spine

Rib

Abnormal left kidney

Cysts

Cysts

Gas in stomach   Liver

3 The amount of X rays absorbed by different tissues is recorded by detectors in the scanner and transformed by a computer into an image, which is interpreted by a radiologist.

C

Healthy cells are cultured to diagnose various disorders prenatally and for studying chromosomes. Human tissues, such as skin, may be cultured to produce larger amounts for use in grafting. Other tissues, notably human *amnion* and monkey kidney, are cultivated to provide a medium in which viruses can be grown and identified in the laboratory; viruses will multiply only within living cells.

HOW IT IS DONE

MICROORGANISMS The type of specimen collected from the patient depends on the suspected site of infection. For example, a throat swab is taken if a streptococcal throat infection is suspected, a urine specimen is collected if urinary tract infection is thought likely, a sputum sample if respiratory infection is suspected, or a feces sample if gastrointestinal infection is suspected. Likewise, a blood sample is cultured if the blood is thought to be infected. Bacteria, fungi, and, occasionally, viruses may be cultured directly from the blood.

The specimen is collected in a sterile container and is incubated at body temperature in a carefully chosen culture medium. Liquid or solid culture media, usually agar gel or meat-based broth, are used for culturing bacteria. These media contain various nutrients chosen for the particular needs of the organism suspected of causing the infection; the media may also contain ingredients to discourage the growth of other organisms.

Any bacteria present will multiply to form visible colonies. The type of bacteria can be identified by noting the appearance of the colony, by chemical tests, and by examining the bacteria under the microscope. Bacterial cultures can be tested with various antibiotics to determine which antibiotic may be the most effective against a particular infection.

CELLS AND TISSUES For the diagnosis of prenatal abnormalities, cells are collected by *amniocentesis* or by *chorionic villus sampling*. Cells for studying chromosomes (see *Chromosome analysis*) are cultured from white blood cells or cells gathered from the inside of the cheek. Cells and tissues to be used for analysis, for growing viruses, or for grafting are cultured in a small amount of fluid containing nutrients essential for their growth.

Cupping

An ancient form of treatment used to draw blood to the surface of the skin. Although cupping fell out of favor during the development of modern medicine, it is still used in folk healing in some countries, China and Turkey, for example. Common conditions treated include bronchitis, asthma, and musculoskeletal pains.

A small vessel—commonly a glass jar, animal horn, ceramic vessel, or a bamboo tube with a closed end—is applied to the skin and heated. When it cools and the air inside contracts, a partial vacuum is created, causing the skin to be sucked into the vessel, producing a rounded area of inflammation. Believers think that the inflammatory response is therapeutic.

Curare

An extract from the bark and juices of various trees which has been used for centuries by South American Indians as an arrow poison. The principal active ingredient is tubocurarine, a drug that inhibits muscle contractions by interfering with the action of *acetylcholine*, a *neurotransmitter* (chemical released from nerve endings). Curare kills by causing widespread muscle paralysis in the victim.

Cure

To treat successfully; that is, to restore to normal health after an illness. The term usually means the complete disappearance of a disease rather than just a halt in its progress. Any medication or therapy used in the treatment of an illness may also be called a cure.

In general, infections may be cured, as may some tumors. By contrast, chronic conditions, such as *osteoarthritis*, or endocrine deficiency diseases, such as *hypothyroidism* (underactivity of the thyroid gland), are never cured but instead undergo remission or are controlled with long-term hormone treatment.

Curet

A spoon-shaped surgical instrument for scraping away material or tissue from an organ, cavity, or surface.

Curettage

The use of a sharp-edged, spoon-shaped surgical instrument called a curet to scrape abnormal tissue, or tissue for analysis, from the lining of a body cavity or from the skin. Curettage is commonly used to remove infected material from an abscess, to scrape tissue from the lining of the uterus as part of a *D and C* (dilatation and curettage) operation, and to remove small growths from the skin. (See also *Curettage, dental*.)

Curettage, dental

The scraping of the wall of a cavity or other surface with a dental *curet* (a narrow, spoon-shaped, scaling instrument). It is one method used in the treatment of simple periodontal pockets occurring in *periodontitis*. The curet is used to remove the lining of the periodontal pocket as well as diseased tissue from the lateral surfaces of the root. This enables the healthy, underlying tissue to reattach itself to the root surface.

Curling's ulcer

A type of *stress ulcer* (a disruption in the lining of the stomach or duodenum following any severe injury, infection, or shock) that occurs specifically in people who have suffered extensive skin burns. Ulcers develop about 24 hours after the burns and are usually small and multiple. Diagnosis and treatment are as for other types of stress ulcer.

Cushing's syndrome

A hormonal disorder caused by an abnormally high level of corticosteroid hormones in the bloodstream. The excess may be caused by overactivity of the *adrenal glands*, which normally produce corticosteroid hormones, or by prolonged administration of *corticosteroid drugs*. Cushing's syndrome can occur at any age, but is most common in middle age.

CAUSES AND INCIDENCE

Most cases of Cushing's syndrome today are caused by prolonged use of corticosteroid drugs, which are widely used to treat inflammatory conditions such as *rheumatoid arthritis*, *inflammatory bowel disease*, and *asthma*. Such cases are usually mild; the patient is often described as having cushingoid features rather than Cushing's syndrome.

Cushing's syndrome is sometimes produced directly by an *adrenal tumor* that causes excessive secretion of corticosteroids. The condition may also be caused indirectly by overactivity of the *pituitary gland*, often due to a *pituitary tumor*. The pituitary gland controls the activity of the adrenal glands by producing a hormone called ACTH (adrenocorticotropic hormone); this stimulates the cortex (outer part) of the adrenal glands to grow and secrete excess corticosteroids. Cases caused by pituitary overactivity (sometimes called Cushing's disease) are much more common in women.

Some lung cancers and various other tumors may also lead to Cushing's syndrome by secreting ACTH and thus leading to excess secretion of corticosteroids by the adrenal glands. This cause of Cushing's syndrome is more common in men.

SYMPTOMS

People with Cushing's syndrome have a characteristic appearance. The face appears round ("moon-faced") and red, the trunk tends to become obese with a humped upper back, and the limbs become wasted. Acne develops and purple stretch marks may appear on the abdomen, thighs, and breasts. The skin is thin and bruises easily. The bones become weakened by *osteoporosis* and are more likely to fracture. Women may become increasingly hairy. Affected people are more susceptible to infection and may suffer from *peptic ulcers*.

Mental changes often occur, causing *depression*, *paranoia*, or sometimes *euphoria*. *Insomnia* may be a problem. Patients may develop *hypertension* (high blood pressure) and *edema* (fluid collection in the tissues). About one fifth of patients develop *diabetes mellitus*. In children, Cushing's syndrome may suppress growth.

DIAGNOSIS

Anyone suspected of having Cushing's syndrome should be examined by an endocrinologist. Confirmation of the diagnosis may require measurement of ACTH levels in the blood and of corticosteroid levels in the blood and urine. *CT scanning* of the adrenal and pituitary glands may be performed to look for abnormalities.

TREATMENT

If corticosteroid drugs are the cause, Cushing's syndrome will usually disappear if the dose of drugs is gradually reduced.

If the cause is shown to be a tumor or overgrowth of an adrenal gland, the gland is removed surgically. If the cause is a pituitary tumor, the gland is removed surgically or the tumor is shrunk by irradiation and medication. Patients subsequently need hormone replacement therapy to compensate for lack of production of adrenal and pituitary hormones.

Cusp, dental

One of the protrusions on the grinding surface of a tooth (see *Teeth*).

Cutaneous

A term meaning relating to the skin.

Cutdown

The creation of a small incision in the skin over a vein in order to gain access

to the vein. A physician may perform a cutdown if a vein cannot be identified through the patient's skin when it is necessary to take blood or to give intravenous fluid.

CVS

See *Chorionic villus sampling*.

Cyanide

Any of a group of substances that contain a carbon atom and a nitrogen atom bound together by a triple chemical bond. Most cyanides are highly poisonous due to their ability to block a specific *enzyme* (cytochrome oxidase) which plays an essential role in the uptake of oxygen by cells. This blocking action deprives cells of the ability to utilize oxygen, which, in turn, produces a rapid progression of symptoms from breathlessness, through paralysis and unconsciousness, to death.

Because of their toxicity, the use of cyanides in industry (such as in electroplating, "case hardening," gold mining, and polymer manufacture) is carefully controlled. Hydrogen cyanide is used to kill rodents and to fumigate buildings. It has also been used in gas chambers in the United States. Certain other cyanides are powerful eye irritants and are used in some tear gases.

Cyanocobalamin

A name for *vitamin B$_{12}$*.

Cyanosis

A bluish coloration of the skin and mucous membranes (such as the lining of the mouth) due to too much deoxygenated *hemoglobin* in the blood. Cyanosis is generally most obvious in the beds of the fingernails and toenails, and on the lips and tongue.

Cyanosis is most commonly due to slow blood flow through the skin in low temperatures (the familiar sign of turning blue with cold). In such cases, where no other symptoms are present, cyanosis does not indicate a serious underlying disease.

In other cases, cyanosis requires medical investigation as it may be a sign of a serious disorder. Cyanosis of the fingers and toes even in relatively warm conditions may indicate poor peripheral blood circulation (see *Peripheral vascular disease*). Cyanosis may also be a sign of a heart or lung disorder, such as *heart failure*, a heart disorder present at birth (see *Heart disease, congenital*), lung damage, or *pulmonary edema* (fluid in the lungs).

Cyclobenzaprine

A *muscle relaxant* drug chemically similar to the tricyclic *antidepressant* drugs. It is mainly used to treat painful muscle spasm caused by injury.

Cyclophosphamide

An *anticancer drug* used mainly in the treatment of *Hodgkin's disease* and *leukemia*, often in combination with other anticancer drugs. Cyclophosphamide is also useful as an *immunosuppressant drug*, helping prevent rejection of a transplanted organ by modifying the body's natural defenses against foreign cells. Cyclophosphamide is also used occasionally to treat certain connective tissue diseases such as severe systemic *lupus erythematosus*.

Possible adverse effects are as for other anticancer drugs; there may also be a severe form of *cystitis*.

Cycloplegia

Paralysis of the ciliary muscle of the *eye*. Cycloplegia impedes *accommodation* (the process by which the shape of the lens adjusts to focus light rays from near objects onto the retina).

Cycloplegia may be induced by drugs, known as cycloplegic drugs, to facilitate examination of the eye.

Cyclosporine

An *immunosuppressant drug* that suppresses the body's natural defenses against abnormal cells. Cyclosporine was introduced in 1984.

WHY IT IS USED

Cyclosporine's immunosuppressant action is of particular use following *transplant surgery*, when the body may start to reject the transplanted organ unless the immune system is damped down. Cyclosporine is now widely used following many different types of transplant surgery, including heart, kidney, bone marrow, liver, and pancreas transplants. Its use has considerably reduced the risk of tissue rejection and also the need for large doses of *corticosteroid drugs*. Cyclosporine may need to be taken in oral form for an indefinite period following transplant surgery.

POSSIBLE ADVERSE EFFECTS

Because cyclosporine reduces the effectiveness of the immune system, people being treated with this drug have an increased susceptibility to infection. Any flulike illness or localized infection requires immediate treatment by a physician.

Swelling of the gums and increased hair growth are fairly common side effects. Cyclosporine has also been

C

C

found to cause kidney damage in some people. Regular monitoring of kidney function is therefore necessary for people being given this drug. If signs of kidney damage, such as proteinuria (protein in the urine), are detected, the dose of cyclosporine may need to be reduced or another drug substituted.

Cyclothymia

A personality characteristic typified by marked changes of mood. Cyclothymic individuals may change, for no apparent reason, from being cheerful, energetic, and sociable to being gloomy, listless, and withdrawn. Mood swings may last for days or months and may follow a regular pattern. Sometimes there are periods of relatively normal behavior.

Cyclothymia resembles *manic-depressive illness* in some respects but the mood swings of cyclothymia are less severe; in some cases there is a family history of manic-depressive illness. People with cyclothymia who are predominently "high" may have successful careers; others may resort to episodes of heavy drinking or difficult behavior.

Cyproterone acetate

A synthetic hormone that blocks the action of *androgen hormones* (male sex hormones) and has effects similar to those of *progesterone hormone* (a female sex hormone).

Cyproterone acetate is used in the treatment of cancer of the prostate (see *Prostate, cancer of*). It is also occasionally used to reduce male sex drive. Cyproterone acetate may be prescribed in combination with an *estrogen drug* to treat women with severe acne or excessive hair growth.

Possible adverse effects, which usually diminish as treatment continues, include breast tenderness and weight gain.

Cyst

An abnormal lump or swelling, filled with fluid or semisolid material, that may occur in any body organ or tissue.

Many different processes cause the development of cysts. Some types, such as *sebaceous cysts* in the skin, result from blockage of the ducts leading from fluid-forming glands. Others, such as *ovarian cysts* or *Baker's cysts*, form as a result of abnormal activity or growth of a fluid-forming tissue when there is no means for the fluid to escape. Cysts may also form around parasites in diseases such as

hydatid disease or *amebiasis*. A *dermoid cyst* is a type of skin cyst that may contain particles of hair follicles, sweat glands, nerves, and teeth.

Cysts are usually harmless in themselves but may sometimes disrupt the function of the tissues in which they grow; in some cases this may necessitate surgical removal of the cyst.

Cyst-/cysto-

Prefixes that denote the bladder, as in *cystitis* (inflammation of the bladder) and *cystoscopy* (endoscopic examination of the bladder).

Cystectomy

Surgical removal of the bladder. Cystectomy must be followed by the creation of an alternative passageway for the expulsion of urine, usually via a specially constructed channel emerg-

ing in a stoma (mouth-like opening) in the lower abdomen (see *Urinary diversion*). Cystectomy is a means of treating cancer of the bladder (see *Bladder tumors*).

HOW IT IS DONE

Before undergoing surgery, cystectomy patients are advised to discuss the operation and its consequences with their physicians and with an enterostomy (stoma care) technician.

The basic steps in the procedure are shown in the illustrated box below. Cystectomy is accompanied by removal of the prostate gland and seminal vesicles in men, and by removal of the uterus, ovaries, and fallopian tubes in women.

OUTLOOK

Patients need to adapt to wearing an external pouch for the collection of urine and to learn about care of the

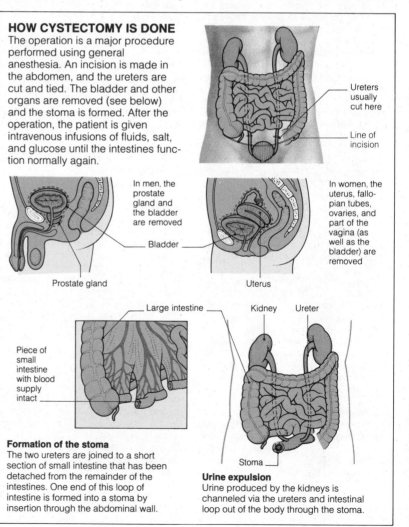

HOW CYSTECTOMY IS DONE
The operation is a major procedure performed using general anesthesia. An incision is made in the abdomen, and the ureters are cut and tied. The bladder and other organs are removed (see below) and the stoma is formed. After the operation, the patient is given intravenous infusions of fluids, salt, and glucose until the intestines function normally again.

Ureters usually cut here

Line of incision

In men, the prostate gland and the bladder are removed

Bladder

Prostate gland

In women, the uterus, fallopian tubes, ovaries, and part of the vagina (as well as the bladder) are removed

Uterus

Large intestine

Piece of small intestine with blood supply intact

Kidney   Ureter

Stoma

Formation of the stoma
The two ureters are joined to a short section of small intestine that has been detached from the remainder of the intestines. One end of this loop of intestine is formed into a stoma by insertion through the abdominal wall.

Urine expulsion
Urine produced by the kidneys is channeled via the ureters and intestinal loop out of the body through the stoma.

stoma. Many patients are able to return to an active and healthy life.

Removal of the reproductive organs with the bladder results in infertility. Cystectomy also usually causes impotence in men (due to damage to nerve tracts involved in penile erection).

Cysticercosis

An infection characterized by the presence, in tissues such as the muscle and brain, of cysts formed by the larval stage of the pork *tapeworm*. Cysticercosis is very rare in developed countries, but relatively common in certain developing countries.

Cystic fibrosis

An inherited disease, present from birth, characterized by a tendency to chronic lung infections and an inability to absorb fats and other nutrients from food. The disease is also called "mucoviscidosis" because the main feature is secretion of viscid (sticky) mucus which is unable to lubricate and flow freely in the nose, throat, airways, and intestines.

When cystic fibrosis (CF) was first identified in the 1930s, before effective *antibiotic drugs* were available, almost all sufferers died in early childhood. More recently, however, and particularly since 1975, the outlook has changed dramatically. With more advanced methods of diagnosis and treatment, including the use of a wide range of antibiotics, more than two thirds of CF sufferers now survive into adult life, although few of them are in perfect health. But despite the improved outlook CF remains a serious and potentially fatal disorder.

CAUSES AND INCIDENCE

CF is caused by a defective *gene*. The defect is of the recessive type, which means that a person must inherit it in a double dose (one gene from each parent) before any outward abnormality is apparent (see *Genetic disorders*). People who inherit the defective gene in a single dose (from one parent only) are called "carriers"; they are usually unaware of the fact and have no symptoms.

Among Western Europeans and white North Americans, about one person in 22 is such a "carrier." The chance that both members of any (random) procreating white couple are carriers is roughly one in 500. In this event, each of their children has a one in four chance of inheriting the defective gene from both parents and of being born with CF. The incidence of the disease is thus about one per 2,000

live births. The incidence in Jewish, Asian, and African populations is much lower.

The mechanism by which the gene defect leads to the features of CF is unknown. It is known, however, that certain glands do not function properly. Most seriously, the glands in the lining of the bronchial tubes produce thick mucus, which predisposes the person to chronic lung infections. Another malfunction is poor or absent secretion of the pancreatic enzymes, which are involved in the breakdown of fats and their absorption from the intestines; this causes malnutrition. Sweat glands are also affected and secrete excessive amounts of sodium chloride (common salt).

SYMPTOMS AND SIGNS

The pattern of development of the disease, and the severity of its features, varies considerably among individuals. Hence, although the disease is sometimes obvious soon after birth, in other cases it escapes detection for months or years.

In a typical case, the child passes unformed feces that are pale, oily, and foul-smelling, and in some cases he or she may fail to thrive. In many cases, the child's growth is stunted. The child also suffers from recurrent upper respiratory tract and chest infections, causing constant coughing and breathlessness. Without early diagnosis and treatment, *pneumonia, bronchiectasis,* and *bronchitis* develop, and the lungs become damaged.

Infertility occurs in the majority of male sufferers and some affected females. Some otherwise healthy adult males have been diagnosed as having CF after attending an infertility clinic. *Heatstroke* and collapse may occur in hot climates due to the excessive loss of salt in the sweat.

DIAGNOSIS AND TREATMENT

Suspicious symptoms should be reported to a physician as soon as they are noticed because the sooner intensive *physiotherapy* and treatment with appropriate antibiotic drugs is started, the less lung damage will be caused by chest infections. Once cystic fibrosis is suspected, the diagnosis is easily confirmed or refuted by simple laboratory tests, including a sweat test.

Confirmation of the diagnosis and supervision of treatment is best carried out from a special center staffed by pediatricians, nurses, and physiotherapists who have a particular knowledge of the disease.

To enable food to be properly digested, *pancreatin* (a replacement pan-

creatic enzyme preparation) must be taken with meals. The diet needs to be rich in calories and proteins, and a vitamin supplement is often prescribed. These measures bring about weight gain and more normal feces.

AFFECTED FAMILIES

The parents of a child with CF must assume that any subsequent child has a one in four chance of being born with the disease. Unaffected siblings of affected people have a two in three chance of being "carriers," creating problems if they are thinking of co-parenting with someone who also has CF in the family.

Recent research has succeeded in establishing the location of the gene that causes CF on *chromosome* number 7. Biochemical "markers" near to the gene have also been identified. It is now therefore possible to detect the carrier state and also to test for CF before birth.

The following service is offered to parents who already have a CF child and are contemplating a further pregnancy. First, it is established whether both parents are definitely carriers through tests to see whether markers for the defective gene are present. If the markers are present, then between eight and 10 weeks into pregnancy, fetal cells obtained by *chorionic villus sampling* are analyzed to see if the markers of CF are present. Alternatively, chemical tests on cells obtained by *amniocentesis* (at 17 or 18 weeks of pregnancy) can indicate whether or not the child will have CF. The parents may choose to terminate the pregnancy if the fetus is affected.

OUTLOOK

The highly specialized treatment given to CF sufferers today provides them with a much better quality of life than was formerly possible. Even so, most suffer permanent lung damage and have a considerably shortened life expectancy. Some sufferers have been treated by a *heart-lung transplant*, while others have been given only a *lung transplant*; the results so far are very encouraging.

Cystitis

Inflammation of the inner lining of the *bladder*, usually caused by a bacterial infection. Anything that obstructs the voiding of urine from the bladder, or leads to incomplete voiding of urine, tends to encourage infection; stagnant urine in the bladder or urethra (the tube leading from the bladder to the exterior) provides a good breeding ground for bacteria.

C

C

INCIDENCE AND CAUSES

In women, cystitis is common because the urethra is short, making it easier for infective agents to pass from the urethral opening up into the bladder. The bacteria may come from the vagina or from the intestine via the anus. Most women have cystitis at some time. A *calculus* (stone) in the bladder, a *bladder tumor*, or a *urethral stricture* increases the risk of infection.

In men, cystitis is rare (because of the longer urethra) and usually occurs only in the presence of an obstruction, which in most cases is due to an enlarged *prostate gland* compressing the urethra where it leaves the bladder. Less commonly, the obstruction is due to a urethral stricture.

In children, cystitis is often due to a structural abnormality of the ureters (tubes that carry urine from the kidneys to the bladder) at the point at which they enter the bladder, allowing reflux (backward flow) of urine into the ureters when the bladder muscle contracts. This leads to incomplete voiding of urine and to subsequent infection.

Another possible source of infection is the introduction of a catheter (drainage tube) into the bladder—a procedure used to drain urine in a variety of circumstances (see *Catheterization, urinary*), including the treatment of incontinence and urinary retention. Diabetics are particularly susceptible to urinary tract infections.

SYMPTOMS

The main symptom of cystitis in both sexes is a frequent urge to pass urine, with only a small amount of urine passed each time. Passing urine is accompanied by pain, which is usually of a burning or stinging nature. Sometimes, the urine is foul smelling or contains blood. There may be a fever and occasionally chills and continuous discomfort in the lower abdomen. Children may have no urinary symptoms but may develop a fever or cry when passing urine.

DIAGNOSIS

The diagnosis of a urinary infection can be confirmed by examining a sample of urine under the microscope, looking for pus cells, and by growing bacteria in a *culture*. When no infection is found in someone with symptoms of cystitis, the diagnosis may be *urethritis* (inflammation of the urethra), bacterial *prostatitis* (in men only), or *urethral syndrome* (in women only), in which the cause is thought, in some people, to be trauma to the urethra from sexual activity.

TREATMENT

People with symptoms of cystitis should drink large quantities of fluids to help flush out the bladder (which should be emptied completely every time urine is passed) and should keep the urine alkaline by taking a teaspoon of sodium bicarbonate in water every six hours. Women who are prone to cystitis should empty the bladder as soon as possible after intercourse.

If an infection is present, *antibiotic drugs* are prescribed to destroy the bacteria and prevent the infection from spreading to cause *pyelonephritis* (infection of the kidneys).

In many cases, the physician will start the patient on a course of antibiotics, especially when there are pus cells in the urine, before waiting for the result of the urine culture. The physician will then check the results of the culture in order to confirm the presence of an infection and to check the sensitivity of the bacteria to various antibiotics.

Prompt treatment of cystitis with antibiotic drugs usually settles the infection within 24 hours. More tests are performed on any man or child who has cystitis, and on women who suffer from recurrent infection. (See also *Urinary tract infection*.)

Cystocele

A swelling at the front and top of the vagina formed where the bladder pushes against weakened tissues in the vaginal wall. Weakened tissues may be associated with descent of the uterus from its normal position down into the vagina (see *Uterus, prolapse of*).

A cystocele may not cause symptoms, but occasionally the urethra (through which urine drains from the bladder to the exterior) is pulled out of position. This may cause stress *incontinence* (leakage of urine on coughing, lifting, or sneezing) or the bladder may not empty completely when urine is passed. The urine remaining in the bladder may then become infected, causing frequent and painful urination (see *Cystitis*).

Exercises to strengthen the pelvic floor muscles (which support the bladder, uterus, and other pelvic organs) may help relieve the symptoms (see *Pelvic floor exercises*). In many cases, surgery is needed to lift and tighten the tissues at the front of the vagina.

Cystometry

A procedure carried out to provide information about normal bladder function and about abnormalities either of the nerves supplying the bladder or of the bladder muscle itself. Cystometry measures changes in pressure as the bladder fills. It also shows the total bladder capacity and detects any residual urine after the bladder has fully contracted.

WHY IT IS DONE

Cystometry is used to investigate urinary *incontinence* or poor bladder emptying caused by damage to the bladder muscles (following childbirth or pelvic surgery, for example) or to disruption of the nerve control of these muscles (as in *Parkinson's disease* or *diabetes mellitus*).

HOW IT IS DONE

The examination, which takes about 20 minutes, is performed by a urologist or a trained urological technician. It is usually done on an outpatient basis and no anesthetic is required. A catheter (flexible tube) and a probe for measuring pressure are inserted into the bladder and sometimes the rectum. The bladder is gradually filled with water or carbon dioxide and a series of pressure readings is taken.

Cystoscopy

The examination of the *urethra* and *bladder* cavity using a cystoscope (viewing instrument inserted up the urethra). Modern cystoscopes have a metal sheath with interchangeable lenses, allowing a viewing angle ranging from zero to 120 degrees.

WHY IT IS DONE

Cystoscopes have both diagnostic and therapeutic uses. Diagnostic uses include inspection of the bladder cavity for calculi (stones), *bladder tumors*, and sites of bleeding and infection, as well as the obtaining of individual urine samples from the *ureters* to look for the presence of infection or tumor cells. It is also possible to inject radiopaque dye into the ureters via the cystoscope, allowing the taking of X rays to investigate the site of any obstruction to the flow of urine. This procedure is known as retrograde pyelography (see *Urography*).

Many diseases of the urethra and bladder lend themselves to treatment via the cystoscope. For example, bladder tumors can be removed, analyzed under the microscope, and treated with diathermy or laser; calculi can be crushed or removed with basket forceps from the bladder or ureter; and

stents (narrow tubes) can be inserted into a ureter to relieve any obstruction (see illustration below).

Cystostomy

The surgical creation of a hole in the bladder. A cystostomy is usually performed to drain urine when the introduction of a *catheter* (flexible tube) into the bladder via the urethra is inadvisable or impossible.

Cystourethrography, micturating

An X-ray procedure for studying a person's bladder while he or she is passing urine. Micturating cystourethrography is most commonly performed on young children who have had urinary infections. The technique allows detection of reflux of urine (backflow of urine up the *ureters*) as the bladder contracts. In severe cases, reflux leads to repeated infection and possible kidney damage.

-cyte

The suffix that denotes a cell. A *leukocyte* is a white blood cell; an *erythrocyte* is a red blood cell.

Cyto-

The prefix used to describe a relationship to a cell, as in *cytology*, the study of cells.

Cytology

The study of individual cells, as distinct from *histology* (the study of

groups of cells forming a tissue). The main application of cytology in medicine is to detect abnormal cells; it is thus used extensively to diagnose cancer. Cytology is becoming more important in *prenatal screening* for certain fetal abnormalities. A cytologist is a specialist in this field.

APPLICATIONS

The best known use of cytology is screening for cancer of the cervix, a procedure known as a *cervical smear*, or *Pap smear*, test. A scraping of cells from the cervix and vagina is examined under a microscope; if the cells show precancerous changes, the woman's condition can be observed and she can be treated before cancer develops.

Cytology is also used to confirm (or exclude) the diagnosis of other cancers. Coughing up of blood may be due to lung cancer, but a cytological examination of cells in a sample of sputum (phlegm) will help determine whether or not cancer is actually the cause. Similarly, cytology is valuable in detecting recurrent tumors in people who have already been treated for cancer. It is used particularly in cases of bladder cancer, in which tumors tend to recur after the original cancer has been successfully treated. Regular urinary cytology can detect any recurrent tumors at an early stage. Cytology may be helpful in determining the cause of conditions such as *pleural effusion* (fluid in the pleural cavity around the lungs) and *ascites* (fluid in the abdominal cavity). Examination of cells in a sample of fluid usually indicates whether the condition is caused by cancer or an infection.

Fine needle aspiration *biopsy* of internal organs is growing as a method of diagnosis that utilizes cytology. A needle is guided to the organ (often with the help of *ultrasound* or *CT scanning*) and a sample taken for examination. The procedure may eliminate the need for surgical biopsy or a major operation.

The other major application of cytology is in various screening techniques for the early detection of fetal abnormalities such as Down's syndrome. The most widely used of these techniques is *amniocentesis*, in which a sample of the fluid that surrounds the fetus is removed and the cells in the fluid are examined for abnormalities. *Chorionic villus sampling* is a newer technique that can be performed earlier in the pregnancy. Usually, the cells must be cultured before an analysis can be made.

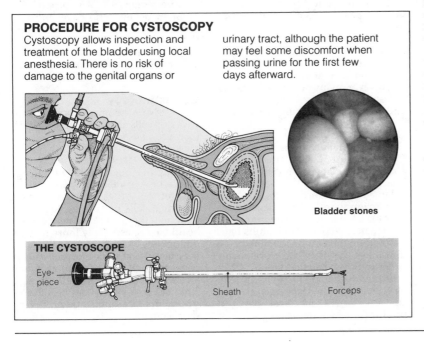

PROCEDURE FOR CYSTOSCOPY

Cystoscopy allows inspection and treatment of the bladder using local anesthesia. There is no risk of damage to the genital organs or

urinary tract, although the patient may feel some discomfort when passing urine for the first few days afterward.

Bladder stones

THE CYSTOSCOPE

Eye-piece

Sheath

Forceps

C

CYTOLOGY METHODS

Cells for cytological examination are obtained in several ways, depending on the part of the body being investigated. Recent improvements in imaging techniques have made it possible to collect cells from previously inaccessible sites. If the cytologist can make a definite diagnosis from a cell sample removed from a tumor using a very fine needle, the patient may be spared an exploratory operation.

Cells from the cervix
These are scraped away with a spatula.

Cells from the respiratory tract or esophagus
These are usually obtained by using an *endoscope* and small brush or suction tube.

Cells from body fluids
These are obtained either by passing the fluid through a filter or by centrifugation.

Aspiration biopsy
A very fine needle can be accurately passed into a suspected tumor and a biopsy sample of cells removed.

EXAMINATION UNDER THE MICROSCOPE

The cells are smeared on a microscope slide and stained with dyes. The cytologist then examines them, looking for abnormalities of size or shape in the cells or their nuclei. The smears are then graded—as normal, as displaying abnormalities, or as showing malignant cells.

Normal cells in cervical smear

Smear showing abnormal cells

Smear showing malignant cells

MODERN DEVELOPMENTS

Various cytological techniques are being developed to improve the ability to detect abnormal cells. Cells aspirated from various organs or tissues, as well as cells from cervical smears, can be studied further by the technique of *flow cytometry* (which uses a laser beam to scan cells and produce an image of the cells' DNA contents, thus differentiating between benign and malignant cells).

The use of monoclonal antibodies—highly specific proteins that react with only one particular type of protein on the surface of a cell (see *Antibody, monoclonal*)—makes it easier to detect small numbers of abnormal cells in the midst of many normal ones, thereby improving the sensitivity of cytological tests for cancer.

A refinement of this particular technique involves labeling the monoclonal antibodies with special fluorescent stains, which make the antibodies stand out clearly against a dark background.

Other modern techniques have made it possible to detect abnormalities in *chromosomes* and even in individual *genes*. Such procedures have a potentially wide application for prenatal screening for genetic disorders and chromosomal abnormalities.

However, many of these techniques are still in the developmental stage and are not yet generally available.

Cytomegalovirus

One of the family of *herpes* viruses. Cytomegalovirus has the unique effect of causing the cells that it infects to take on a characteristic enlarged appearance.

Infection with the cytomegalovirus (CMV) is extremely common. Approximately 80 percent of adults have *antibodies* to the virus in their blood (an indication that they have previously been infected by the virus). CMV infection may cause an illness resembling infectious *mononucleosis* (glandular fever), but in most cases it produces no symptoms.

More serious CMV infections can occur in people who have impaired immunity, such as the elderly and those with *AIDS*. A pregnant woman can transmit the CMV virus to her unborn child, which could cause malformations and brain damage.

Cytopathology

The study of the microscopic appearances of cells in health and disease. (See also *Cytology*.)

Cytotoxic drugs

A group of drugs that kill or damage cells; a type of *anticancer drug*.

Cytotoxic drugs primarily affect abnormal cells but during long-term treatment they can also damage or kill healthy cells, especially those that are multiplying rapidly. For example, they may affect noncancerous cells in bone marrow, causing anemia and increasing susceptibility to infection. Such adverse effects can be offset if treatments are spread over several short courses.

Dacryocystitis

Inflammation of the tear sac, which lies between the inside corner of the eyelids and the nose.

CAUSES

Dacryocystitis usually results from blockage of the duct that carries tears from the tear sac to the nose. Inflammation may be followed by bacterial infection of fluid trapped in the tear sac. In infants, the tear duct may fail to develop normally. In adults, the cause of the duct blockage is usually unknown. Rarely, it follows an injury; more often, it follows inflammation in the nasal region.

Mechanism of dacryocystitis
Inflammation of the tear sac occurs when the duct that carries tears from the tear sac becomes blocked.

SYMPTOMS

Usually only one eye is affected. There may be pain, redness, and swelling in the area between the inner corner of the eyelids and the nose. Occasionally, pus discharges from the inner corner. Prior to infection in the tear sac, the only symptom may be a watery eye due to obstruction of the duct.

TREATMENT

Irrigation can sometimes clear the obstruction. A *cannula* (fine tube) is introduced into one of the drainage openings into the tear duct and saline flushed through it. Antibiotic eye drops or ointment are prescribed to treat infection. In infants, massage of the tear sac can empty the sac and sometimes clear a blockage.

If irrigation and antibiotics fail to clear up the symptoms, a dacryocystorhinostomy (surgery to drain the tear sac into the nose) can be performed. In the infirm and elderly, if recurrent infection is a problem, the tear sac may be removed.

Danazol

A drug used in the treatment of *endometriosis* (a condition in which fragments of the tissue that normally lines the uterus occur elsewhere in the pelvic cavity), fibrocystic breast disease (breast tenderness and lumpiness that worsen before menstruation), and *menorrhagia* (heavy periods).

HOW IT WORKS

Danazol suppresses the release of *gonadotrophin hormones* (pituitary hormones that stimulate activity in the ovaries). This reduces the production and release of estrogen from the ovaries. The change in hormone levels usually prevents ovulation and results in irregularity or complete absence of menstruation.

Danazol is usually administered in courses lasting a few months. The disorder may recur after treatment has been discontinued.

POSSIBLE ADVERSE EFFECTS

Adverse effects may include nausea, dizziness, rash, back pain, weight gain, and flushing. Pregnancy should be avoided while taking (and shortly after taking) danazol because the drug can cause masculine characteristics in a female fetus.

D and C

A gynecological procedure in which the endometrium (lining of the uterus) is scraped away. D and C is an abbreviation for dilatation and curettage. The procedure is commonly used to diagnose the cause of and to treat *menorrhagia* (heavy menstrual bleeding) and other disorders of the *uterus*. D and C is also used as a means of terminating a pregnancy (see *Abortion, induced*) and may sometimes be carried out following a *miscarriage*.

HOW IT IS DONE

D and C is usually carried out under general anesthesia. The cervix is dilated (stretched open) so that a *curet* (a spoon-shaped surgical instrument) can be inserted into the uterus to scrape away the endometrium. The scrapings may then be examined under the microscope to assess the condition of the uterus.

RESULTS

Removal of the endometrium causes no side-effects and it may be beneficial if the lining has thickened, causing heavy periods. The endometrium soon grows again during the menstrual cycle (see *Menstruation*).

Procedure for D and C
The vagina is dilated with a speculum, the cervix is dilated, and a curet is inserted into the uterus to scrape away the endometrium.

Dander

Minute scales shed from an animal's skin, hair, or feathers. Both humans and pets produce such scales, which float in the air or settle on a surface, making up a large proportion of household dust. Human *dandruff* is a type of dander, except that the scales produced by the scalp are relatively large and easily visible.

Some people are allergic to animal dander and develop symptoms of allergic *rhinitis* (hay fever) or *asthma* if they breathe in the scales.

Dandruff

A common, harmless, but irritating condition in which dead skin is shed from the scalp, often producing unsightly white flakes in the hair and on the collar and shoulders of clothes. The usual cause of the condition is seborrheic *dermatitis*, an itchy, scaly rash on the scalp, which may also occur on the face, chest, and back.

The hair should be shampooed frequently with an antidandruff shampoo. If this fails, a physician may prescribe a cream or lotion containing a *corticosteroid drug* to be applied to the scalp or a cream containing an *anti-*

fungal drug, which sometimes helps (even though dandruff is not a fungal infection). Whatever the type of treatment, dandruff usually requires constant control.

Dantrolene

A *muscle-relaxant drug* used to relieve muscle spasm caused by *spinal injury,* *stroke,* or neurological disorders such as *cerebral palsy* or *multiple sclerosis.* Dantrolene does not cure the underlying disorder, but often leads to a gradual improvement in mobility.

POSSIBLE ADVERSE EFFECTS
Dantrolene acts predominantly on the muscles rather than on the nervous system; consequently, it causes less sedation than many other muscle-relaxant drugs. Alcohol should be avoided during treatment, however, because it increases the sedative effect. Dantrolene may cause diarrhea, muscle weakness, and, rarely, liver damage. In rare cases, dantrolene may also cause a skin rash on exposure to sunlight. Exposure to the sun should therefore be avoided during treatment.

Dapsone

An *antibacterial drug* used in the treatment of *Hansen's disease* (leprosy) and *dermatitis herpetiformis,* a rare disorder of the skin.

Dapsone may cause nausea, vomiting, and, rarely, damage to the liver, red blood cells, and nerves. During long-term treatment, blood tests are carried out regularly to monitor liver function and the number of red cells in the blood.

Daydreaming

Conjuring up pleasant or exciting images or situations in one's mind during waking hours. Everyone daydreams to some extent, but it may be more common during unhappy or stressful periods in a person's life.

Children and teenagers may spend a considerable amount of time daydreaming. In general, this is not a cause for concern unless schoolwork and/or relationships suffer, in which case it may be advisable to seek professional help.

DDT

The generally used abbreviation for the insecticide dichloro-diphenyl-tri-chloro-ethane. Developed in Switzerland in the early 1940s, DDT was much more effective than earlier insecticides and it became an important weapon against insect-transmit-ted diseases, particularly in hot climates. A disadvantage of DDT is that some insects have become resistant to its toxic effects. Moreover, this resistance is genetically determined, so that a DDT-resistant insect may pass the resistance on to its offspring. (See also *Pesticides.*)

Deafness

Complete or partial inability to hear. Total deafness is rare and is usually congenital (present from birth). Partial deafness, ranging from mild to severe, is most commonly the result of an ear disease, injury, or degeneration of the hearing mechanism with age.

All deafness is either conductive or sensorineural. Conductive deafness results from faulty propagation of sound from the outer to the inner ear, usually as a result of damage to the eardrum or the three connected bones in the middle ear—the malleus, incus, and stapes. In sensorineural deafness, sounds that reach the inner ear fail to be transmitted to the brain because of damage to the structures within the inner ear or damage to the acoustic nerve, which connects the inner ear to the brain.

CAUSES
CONDUCTIVE DEAFNESS In an adult, the most common cause of conductive deafness is *earwax* blocking the outer ear canal. Less commonly, *otosclerosis* (in which the stapes loses its normal mobility) may be responsible. In a child, *otitis media* (middle ear infection) and collection of sticky fluid in the middle ear (see *Glue ear*) are by far the most common causes of this type of deafness.

Rarely, conductive deafness can be caused by *barotrauma* (damage to the eardrum or middle ear due to sudden pressure changes in an aircraft or under water) or by a perforated eardrum (see *Eardrum, perforated*) following injury, a middle ear infection, or surgery on the ear.

SENSORINEURAL DEAFNESS Defects of the inner ear are sometimes congenital, due to an inherited fault in a chromosome, to *birth injury,* or to damage to the developing fetus—for example, as the result of the mother having had *rubella* (German measles) during pregnancy. Damage to the inner ear may also occur soon after birth as the result of severe *jaundice.*

Sensorineural deafness that develops in later life can be caused by damage to the cochlea and/or labyrinth due to prolonged exposure to loud noise, to *Meniere's disease,* to certain drugs (such as *streptomycin*), or to some viral infections. The cochlea and labyrinth also degenerate naturally with old age, resulting in *presbycusis.*

Damage to the acoustic nerve may be the result of an *acoustic neuroma* (a benign tumor on the nerve). As the acoustic neuroma enlarges, it causes increasing deafness.

INCIDENCE
Deafness at birth is sensorineural and incurable. Such deafness is rare, occurring in only about one in 1,000 babies. Deafness that develops in young children is usually conductive and curable. Some degree of hearing loss due to middle ear infections is common in children starting school, but its prevalence is decreasing because of better treatment. About 4 percent of the adult Canadian population suffers from significant conductive deafness. The hearing mechanism gradually degenerates with age, and approximately 20 percent of the population over 65 has a significant hearing disability.

SYMPTOMS, SIGNS, AND DIAGNOSIS
A baby suffering from congenital deafness fails to respond to sounds, and, although crying is often normal, he or she does not babble or make the other baby noises that usually precede speech. These symptoms may be first noticed by a parent. In a young child, a physician will conduct *hearing tests* during the child's regular checkups to detect any hearing loss, which is usually due to glue ear.

In an adult who has started to become deaf, sounds heard are not only quieter than before but are also distorted and less clear, high tones are less audible than low ones, the sounds "s", "f", and "z" are not heard, and speech may be difficult to understand if there is background noise. Deafness in one ear may be noticed only when that ear alone is used (for example, when the sufferer uses the affected ear when on the telephone).

Deafness may be accompanied by *tinnitus* (noises in the ear) and *vertigo* (dizziness and loss of balance). It sometimes causes confusion, *paranoia,* and auditory *hallucinations,* and can lead to withdrawal and *depression.*

Examination of the ear with an *otoscope* (a viewing instrument with a light attached) can show if the outer ear canal is obstructed by wax, or if the eardrum is inflamed, perforated, or has fluid behind it.

To determine whether deafness is conductive or sensorineural, hearing tests are carried out.

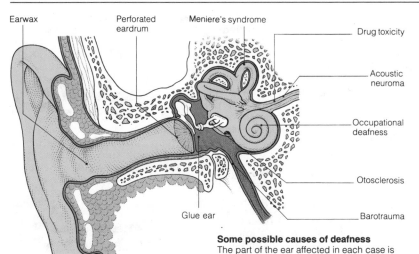

Earwax | Perforated eardrum | Meniere's syndrome

Drug toxicity

Acoustic neuroma

Occupational deafness

Otosclerosis

Glue ear

Barotrauma

Some possible causes of deafness
The part of the ear affected in each case is shown. Some of the problems (e.g., earwax) cause conductive deafness; others (e.g., drug toxicity) cause sensorineural deafness.

TREATMENT

Children born deaf need special instruction if they are to learn to speak. The process is a long and difficult one, but eventually many children can communicate effectively, often with sign language.

Conductive deafness in children due to glue ear is treated by an operation to drain the fluid from the middle ear through a hole in the eardrum (see *Myringotomy*). While awaiting surgery, a child should sit at the front of the classroom to hear as much as possible.

When conductive deafness is caused by wax in the ear, a physician or nurse can remove the wax by syringing the ear with warm water.

A perforated eardrum is usually allowed to heal of its own accord, but, if it has not done so after two or three months, a surgical repair, called *tympanoplasty*, is often carried out.

Conductive deafness due to otosclerosis is usually treated by *stapedectomy*, a surgical procedure in which the fixed stapes is replaced with an artificial substitute.

Hearing aids are sometimes used to lessen deafness caused by otosclerosis, in which case the hearing aid may take the form of a bone-conducting device that transmits sound to the inner ear through a vibrating pad touching the bone behind the ear. The main use of hearing aids, however, is in treating sensorineural deafness, which cannot be cured because the structures of the inner ear are too delicate to allow surgery to be performed on them. The hearing aids used in

these cases increase the volume of sound reaching the inner ear by means of an amplifier and an earphone that fits into the outer ear.

A new development in the treatment of sensorineural deafness is the *cochlear implant*, in which electrodes that can receive sound signals are implanted in the inner ear. To the present, however, it has achieved only limited success.

Lipreading is an invaluable aid for all deaf people, whatever the type and severity of their deafness. People addressing a deaf person should remember to face him or her and not shout, which only distorts sounds.

Various household aids, such as an amplifier for the earpiece of a telephone, are readily available. (See also *Ear; Hearing*.)

Death

Permanent cessation of all vital functions; the end of life. The classic indicators of death are the permanent cessation of the function of the heart and lungs and in the overwhelming majority of cases these remain the criteria by which a physician diagnoses and certifies death.

During the 1960s, however, medical technology advanced to the stage where artificial (machine-assisted) maintenance of breathing and heartbeat became possible in cases where the lungs and heart would otherwise have stopped functioning due to gross structural brain damage. This prompted a reexamination of concepts of death and the development of criteria for the diagnosis of *brain death*.

This is defined as the irreversible cessation of all functions of the entire brain, including the brain stem.

An individual can thus now be certified legally dead if there is either irreversible cessation of circulatory and respiratory functions or if the criteria for brain death are satisfied.

DIAGNOSIS OF DEATH

The determination of death is considered to be a medical diagnosis. However, physicians are expected to exercise their medical judgment within a defined legal framework.

The diagnosis of death under normal circumstances, when the individual is not on a *ventilator* (breathing machine), is based on absence of spontaneous breathing, absence of heartbeat, and on the pupils being dilated (wide open) and unresponsive to light.

The criteria for diagnosing brain death are based on the determination of the irreversible cessation of brain function. There must be clear evidence of irreversible damage to the brain; persistent deep coma; no attempts at breathing when the patient is taken off the ventilator; and absence of brain stem function (e.g., no response of the pupils to light, no grimacing in response to painful stimuli, and no involuntary blink when the surface of the eye is touched). The guidelines warn that this assessment might not be reliable if the patient is intoxicated, has a very low body temperature, or is in shock.

An *EEG* showing absence of electrical activity in the brain's cerebrum is not required, but sometimes provides useful confirmatory evidence of brain death diagnosed by the above criteria. (See also *Death, sudden; Mortality*.)

Death, sudden

Death that occurs unexpectedly in a person who previously seemed to be healthy and who had not complained of any symptoms of illness (deaths due to *accidents* are excluded).

The most common cause of sudden death in adults is *cardiac arrest*. People older than about 35 who die from cardiac arrest are frequently found at *autopsy* (postmortem examination) to have had *coronary artery disease*, and may have died as a result of *myocardial infarction* (heart attack) or cardiac *arrhythmia* (irregularity of heartbeat); younger victims are often found to have had an undiagnosed congenital heart abnormality.

Sudden death may also occur in people suffering from unsuspected

D

myocarditis, *stroke*, or *pneumonia*. Other less common causes include *anaphylactic shock*, *asthma*, and *suicide*.

To reduce the risk of sudden death from heart disease, any person about to begin an exercise program after a period of inactivity should consult a physician for a checkup, especially if exertion causes chest pain, breathlessness, extreme fatigue, or palpitations, or if he or she is overweight, smokes, or has a family history of coronary artery disease.

In infants (mainly up to 1 year old), death that occurs without warning is called *sudden infant death syndrome* (SIDS) or crib death. The causes of SIDS are unknown, although there are several theories.

Cases of sudden death must be reported to the police, who decide whether or not an autopsy should be performed.

Debility
Generalized weakness and lack of energy. Debility may be caused by a physical disorder (such as *anemia*) or by a psychological disorder (such as *depression*).

Debridement
Surgical removal of foreign material and/or dead, damaged, or infected tissue from a wound or burn to expose healthy tissue. Such treatment promotes healthy healing of badly damaged skin, muscle, and other tissue.

Decalcification, dental
The dissolving of minerals in a tooth. Dental decalcification is the first stage of tooth decay. It is caused by the bacteria in *plaque* acting on refined carbohydrates (mainly sugar) in food to produce acid. After prolonged or numerous exposures, the acid causes changes on the surface of the tooth. The decalcified area can be seen as a chalky white patch when the plaque is brushed away. The process is partly reversible at this stage if a mineralizing solution is applied.

If the decalcification penetrates the enamel, it spreads along the junction between the enamel and dentin, and then into the dentin. Lack of professional treatment at this stage will permit bacteria to enter the pulp. Further destruction of dentin will then be caused by bacterial enzymes, and the pulp, once infected, may die. (See also *Caries, dental.*)

Decay, dental
See *Caries, dental*.

Decerebrate
The state of being without a functioning *cerebrum* (the cerebral hemispheres and associated structures), which is the main controlling part of the brain. This situation occurs when the *brain stem* (the upward extension of the spinal cord) is severed, which effectively isolates the cerebrum.

Deciduous teeth
See *Primary teeth*.

Decompression sickness
A hazard of divers (both recreational and professional) and of others who work in or breathe compressed air or other gas mixtures. It is also known as the "bends" and was formerly known as caisson disease. Decompression sickness results from the formation of gas bubbles in the diver's tissues during ascent from depth.

CAUSES AND INCIDENCE
The amount of gas that can be held dissolved in a tissue (such as blood or body fat) increases with pressure (i.e., as a diver descends underwater) and decreases when the pressure is released. At depth, divers accumulate large quantities of inert gas in their tissues from the high-pressure gas mixture they breathe (see *Scuba-diving medicine*); if air is being breathed (as is usual for recreational divers), the main inert gas is nitrogen.

When the diver ascends, pressure falls and the gas can no longer be held within the tissues; if the pressure reduction is rapid, the gas may form bubbles—just as bubbles form in a bottle of beer when the cap is flipped off. The bubbles may block blood vessels, causing various symptoms.

Trained divers and industrial compressed air workers avoid problems by allowing the excess gas that has built up in their tissues to escape slowly via the blood into their lungs during controlled, very slow ascent or release of pressure.

SYMPTOMS
Symptoms may appear any time within 24 hours after a dive. Common symptoms include skin itching and mottling, and severe pains in and around the larger joints, particularly the shoulders and knees. Symptoms of impairment of the nervous system (such as leg weakness, visual disturbances, or problems with balance) are particularly serious, as is a painful, tight feeling across the chest, which may indicate the presence of bubbles in the vessels that supply the heart and in the circulation to the lungs.

Pressure increased (descent)

Inert gas dissolved in tissue fluids and blood

Pressure reduced (ascent)

Bubbles form in blood vessels and tissues

Bubble blocking blood vessel

How decompression occurs
On ascent, pressure is reduced rapidly and the gas may form bubbles that may, in turn, cause symptoms. Divers avoid this by ascending slowly.

TREATMENT
Any diver with the symptoms described should be transported immediately to, and placed inside, a decompression chamber. Pressure within the chamber is raised by pumping in air; this causes the bubbles within the diver's tissues to redissolve, and the symptoms to disappear. Subsequently, the pressure in the chamber is slowly reduced, allowing the excess gas to escape safely via the blood and lungs.

OUTLOOK
If treated promptly by decompression, most divers with the "bends" make a full recovery. However, in serious, untreated cases, there may be long-term complications such as partial paralysis. Repeated episodes lead to degenerative disorders of the bones and joints.

Decompression, spinal canal
A surgical procedure to relieve pressure on the spinal cord or on a nerve root emerging from the cord.

WHY IT IS DONE
Pressure on the spinal cord may be due to a *disk prolapse*, to a tumor (in most cases benign) of the membranes surrounding the cord or of the cord itself, to a narrow spinal canal, which may be present from birth or caused by *osteoarthritis*, or to fracture of the vertebrae after an accident. Any of

these conditions can cause weakness or paralysis of the limbs and loss of bladder control.

HOW IT IS DONE

To treat major disk prolapses and tumors, a *laminectomy* (removal of the bony arches of one or more vertebrae) to expose the affected part of the cord or nerve roots must be performed. Severely prolapsed disks are cut away and affected nerve roots are freed from surrounding tissues. Sometimes a surgeon may approach the spinal cord from the front.

When pressure is being caused by a tumor or abscess in a vertebra, the affected section of bone is removed. If a large portion of bone is removed, bone grafting is carried out at the end of the operation.

RECOVERY PERIOD

Confinement to bed in a flat position is necessary initially, with measures taken to prevent *bedsores* and *physiotherapy* given to keep the leg muscles strong. Usually a patient can get up within a few days. Heavy lifting must be avoided for several weeks.

OUTLOOK

Recovery of movement, sensation, and bladder control, and achievement of pain relief after treatment depend on the severity and duration of the pressure before the operation, the success of the surgery in relieving the pressure, and whether damage was sustained by the cord and nerves during the operation.

Decongestant drugs

COMMON DRUGS

Oxymetazoline Phenylephrine Phenylpropanolamine Pseudoephedrine Xylometazoline

---

WARNING
Symptoms worsen when, after several days of treatment, decongestants are suddenly withdrawn. Use only in low doses for a short time.

Drugs used to relieve *nasal congestion*. Small amounts of these drugs are present in many over-the-counter *cold remedies*, which are available in tablet or nose drop form. Decongestant drugs are commonly used in the treatment of upper *respiratory tract infections*, especially in patients susceptible to *otitis media* (middle ear infection) or *sinusitis* (sinus infection).

POSSIBLE ADVERSE EFFECTS

Taken by mouth, decongestant drugs may cause tremor and palpitations;

THE ACTION OF DECONGESTANTS

Decongestants work by narrowing blood vessels in the membranes that line the nose. This action reduces swelling, inflammation, and the amount of mucus produced by the nasal lining.

Enlarged blood vessel

Swollen nasal lining

Constricted blood vessel

Less mucus

Reduced swelling

Mucus

Nasal passage

Congested nasal lining
When blood vessels enlarge in response to infection or irritation, increased amounts of fluid pass into the lining, which swells and produces more mucus.

Effect of decongestants
Chemicals stimulate constriction of the blood vessels in the nasal lining, which reduces swelling, mucus production, and nasal congestion.

---

they are therefore not usually prescribed if a person has heart disease. In the form of nose drops, only small amounts are absorbed into the blood and adverse effects are unlikely.

If decongestant nose drops are taken for several days and then stopped, congestion frequently recurs and may be worse than that for which the drug was taken. For this reason, decongestants should be taken for as short a time as possible.

Decubitus ulcer

See *Bedsores*.

Defecation

The expulsion of *feces* from the body via the anus.

Defense mechanisms

Techniques used by the mind in order to cope with unpleasant or unwelcome events, experiences, impulses, or emotions.

For example, death of a relative normally provokes grief and/or anger. One defense against these emotions may be repression—refusing to recognize these feelings and appearing to be unaffected by the event. Another reaction is denial—carrying on as though the relative is still alive.

A person who feels guilty about hating his or her father may transfer this hate to another person or turn the bad feelings toward himself or herself.

Disturbing impulses may take the opposite form in conscious thought. For instance, a person with strong sexual feelings may be excessively prudish or inhibited. The body's defense mechanisms against infection are described under *immune system*.

Defensive medicine

The practice of ordering diagnostic tests and carrying out certain procedures primarily to protect the physician against a charge of malpractice.

Defibrillation

A technique in which a brief electric shock is administered to the heart, usually via two metal plates placed on the wall of the chest. It is also called cardioversion. The technique is performed to treat some types of *arrhythmia* (irregular or rapid heartbeat). The sudden burst of electricity through the heart converts *fibrillation* (rapid, uncoordinated heartbeat) or *tachycardia* (rapid heartbeat) back into a normal, regular heartbeat. Occasionally a drug, such as lidocaine, is injected into a vein before the procedure to try to stabilize the heart rhythm.

Defibrillation can be carried out as an emergency procedure to treat *ventricular fibrillation*, which most commonly starts after a *myocardial infarction* (heart attack). It may also be used to treat an arrhythmia that has lasted several hours or days.

D

Defoliant poisoning

The toxic effects of chemicals that are applied to plants to kill them by causing their leaves to drop off. Commonly used as weedkillers, defoliants are poisonous if swallowed. Therefore they should always be kept in clearly labeled containers and stored out of children's reach. The most widely used defoliant weedkillers are sodium chlorate, potassium chlorate (see *Chlorate poisoning*), and *paraquat*.

Another well-known group of defoliants are the phenoxy herbicides which may be contaminated with dioxin, a substance that is highly toxic to humans. One such herbicide (known as Agent Orange) was used by US forces in the Vietnam war. There have been claims that Agent Orange (due to its dioxin content) caused nerve and other disorders in many Vietnam veterans, Vietnamese civilians and others exposed to it (as well as birth defects in their children), but toxicologists are divided as to the extent of these long-term effects.

Deformity

Any malformation or distortion of part of the body. Deformities may be *congenital* (present from birth) or they may be acquired as a result of injury, disease, disorder, or disuse.

Most congenital deformities are relatively rare. Among the more common are clubfoot (*talipes*) and *cleft lip and palate*.

Injuries that can cause deformity include burns, torn muscles, broken bones, and dislocated joints. Among the various diseases and disorders that may cause deformity are infections, such as *tuberculosis* and *Hansen's disease* (leprosy); damage to or disorders of nerves, such as paralysis of the facial nerves; some deficiency diseases, such as *rickets*; and a condition of unknown cause called *Paget's disease* of the bone.

Disuse of a part of the body—as a result of being bedridden or confined to a wheelchair, for example—can lead to deformity through stiffening and *contracture* (shortening) of unused muscles or tendons.

Many deformities can be corrected by *plastic surgery*, various orthopedic techniques (including surgery), exercise, or by a combination of these methods. For example, cleft lip and palate are now treated by surgery during childhood. It is often possible to prevent a deformity due to disuse by ensuring that the patient gets regular exercise.

Degeneration

Physical and/or chemical changes in cells, tissues, or organs that reduce their efficiency. Degeneration is a feature of aging and may also be due to a disease process. Other known causes include injury, reduced blood supply, poisoning (by alcohol, for example), or a diet deficient in a specific vitamin. (See also *Degenerative disorders*.)

Degenerative disorders

A term for a range of conditions in which there is progressive impairment of both the structure and function of part of the body. This definition excludes diseases caused by infection, inflammation, altered immune responses, chemical or physical damage, or malignant change. Many of the features of aging, such as wrinkling, are due to degenerative changes in body tissues, but, in degenerative disorders, the changes come on earlier in life, are more rapid, and typically affect some organs and not others.

Microscopic examination of an organ affected by degenerative disease often shows that the number of specialized cells or structures is reduced and that their place has been taken by *connective tissue* or scar tissue.

Some diseases that were once thought to be degenerative disorders later proved to be due to slow viruses (for example, *Creutzfeldt-Jakob disease*). *Parkinsonism* (a disorder that shares the symptoms of *Parkinson's disease*) may be traceable to poisoning—with carbon monoxide or with MPTP, an impurity formed during the illegal manufacture of one of the many *designer drugs*. Future research may identify specific infective or environmental causes for other disorders that are now thought to be degenerative.

NERVOUS SYSTEM

Among degenerative disorders affecting the nervous system the most common is *Alzheimer's disease*, the main cause of presenile and senile *dementia*. In *Huntington's chorea*, dementia is combined with disorders of movement. Here, susceptibility to the degenerative changes in the brain is due to an abnormality in a single gene; the disease is transmitted from one generation to the next in a dominant pattern of inheritance (see *Genetic disorders*). In Parkinson's disease and in degenerative disorders that affect the *cerebellum*, abnormalities of movement are the main features. In *motor neuron diseases*, including *Werdnig-Hoffmann disease*, the prime symptom is muscular weakness.

EYES

Blindness in early adult life can be caused by a condition called Leber's *optic atrophy*, which is due to loss of nerve cells in the retina. *Retinitis pigmentosa*, another retinal degeneration, can cause blindness in childhood, but some vision may be preserved until late middle age. Both disorders have a genetic basis. By contrast, senile *macular degeneration* is not an inherited condition and rarely develops before the age of 60.

JOINTS

The most familiar degenerative disorder is *osteoarthritis*, also sometimes known as degenerative joint disease. Susceptibility to the condition seems to run in families; it also develops in sports enthusiasts and manual workers who have repeatedly damaged their joints. The prime features of osteoarthritis are thinning and destruction of the cartilage covering the surfaces of the joints, and overgrowth and distortion of the bone around affected joints.

ARTERIES

Some hardening of the arteries seems to be a feature of aging. In some individuals, however, the degenerative changes in the muscle coat of these blood vessels are unusually severe and calcium deposits may be seen on X-ray films (as in Monckeberg's sclerosis, a type of *arteriosclerosis*).

MUSCLES

Degeneration of muscles occurs in a group of genetic disorders, known as *muscular dystrophies*, which cause distinctive patterns of muscular weakness and are sometimes associated with increased muscle bulk.

Deglutition

The medical term for *swallowing*.

Dehiscence

The splitting open of a partly healed wound; the term is most commonly used to refer to the splitting open of a surgical incision that has been closed with sutures or clips.

Dehydration

A condition in which a person's water content has fallen to a dangerously low level. Water accounts for about 60 percent of a man's weight and 50 percent of a woman's, and the total water content must be kept within fairly narrow limits for healthy functioning of cells and tissues (see *Water*).

The concentration of mineral salts and other substances dissolved in the body's fluids must also be kept within a narrow range. In many cases of dehydration, the body's salt content, in addition to the water content, has been depleted.

CAUSES

Normally, dehydration is prevented by the sensation of thirst, which encourages a person to drink when the body is short of water. This mechanism may fail because water is not available or because of high losses of water from the body.

Even in a temperate climate, a minimum of 1.5 litres of water is lost by an adult every 24 hours through the skin via perspiration, from the lungs into the air, and in the urine to rid the body of waste products. Severe dehydration is likely to develop within a few days if no water is taken. In a hot climate, an extra 2 to 5 litres of water may be lost in sweat every day, or up to 10 litres a day in someone doing hard physical work. In central Canada, the sudden onset of hot summer weather may expose runners or those doing heavy work to unexpected and severe dehydration.

Large amounts of water may also be lost in vomit or diarrhea, particularly if the diarrhea is profuse and watery (as in *cholera*) or in the urine of anyone with uncontrolled *diabetes mellitus, diabetes insipidus,* and some types of *kidney failure*. In all these cases, the thirst sensation may not encourage sufficient water intake to balance the losses.

Babies tend to become dehydrated more rapidly than adults because their normal water loss per hour makes up a much higher proportion of their water content.

SYMPTOMS AND SIGNS

Symptoms and signs of water depletion include severe thirst, dry lips and tongue, an increase in heart rate and breathing rate, dizziness, confusion, and eventual coma. The skin looks dry and loses its elasticity. Any urine passed is small in quantity and dark colored. If there is also salt depletion (usually as a result of heavy sweating, vomiting, or diarrhea), additional symptoms may include lethargy, headaches, cramps, and pallor.

PREVENTION

When living in a hot climate, or when suffering from a fever, vomiting, or diarrhea, the simplest rule is to drink enough water to produce urine that is consistently pale. For most people, this often means drinking well beyond the point of thirst (possibly 0.5 litre of water every hour during the heat of the day).

Salt losses from heavy sweating need to be replaced either in the diet or by adding a quarter of a teaspoon of table salt to each 0.5 litre of drinking water. Bottled mineral water can help maintain the intake of salts. For vomiting and diarrhea, *rehydration therapy* is needed; special salt and glucose rehydration mixtures can be purchased from drugstores. Children are particularly susceptible to severe dehydration by diarrhea and it is worth taking a supply of these mixtures if planning a visit to a warm country with small children.

TREATMENT

Once dehydration has developed, fluid and salt replacement may be required at a far faster rate than that needed simply to prevent dehydration. In severe cases of dehydration, fluids must be given intravenously. The water/salt balance has to be carefully monitored by blood tests and adjusted if necessary.

Déjà vu

French for "already seen." A sense of having already experienced an event that is happening at the moment. Déjà vu is a common phenomenon that has never been properly explained. Some people believe that it is due to an unconscious emotional response caused by similarities between the current event and some past experience. Others believe that a neurological "short circuit" results in the experience registering in the memory before reaching consciousness. Frequent occurrence of déjà vu may sometimes be a symptom of *temporal lobe epilepsy.*

Delinquency

Antisocial or criminal behavior in someone aged 17 or younger. The term is often used to describe behavior such as playing truant, running away from home, drinking alcohol, or *drug abuse.*

Delinquency is probably caused by a combination of factors—social, psychological, and biological—but relatively few young offenders suffer from a definite mental disorder or mental retardation.

Child guidance or *family therapy* may be recommended for young offenders and their families. Persistent offenders are sometimes sent to group homes or detention centers.

Delirium

A state of acute mental confusion, commonly brought on by physical ill-

ness. The symptoms are those of disordered brain function, and vary according to personality, environment, and the severity of illness. Failure to understand events or remember what has been happening, increased anxiety, physical restlessness, and sudden swings of mood occur as delirium worsens. At its most severe, the patient may hallucinate, suffer from *illusions* (for example, seeing nurses as threatening monsters), lapse into a terrified panic, and resort to shouting and violence. Usually the symptoms are worse at night, because of sleep disturbance and the fact that darkness and quiet make visual illusions more likely.

CAUSES

While any severe illness may underlie this state, high fever and disturbances of body chemistry are commonly present. Children and older people are most susceptible, particularly after major surgery or when there is a pre-existing brain disturbance such as *dementia.*

Drugs, various poisons, and alcohol are common precipitants.

TREATMENT

Treatment is of the underlying physical disorder, with appropriate nursing to reduce anxiety. Suitable lighting, calm and clear communication, appropriate seclusion, and known, trusted attendants are all important. Particular attention must be paid to fluids and nutrition, but *tranquilizer drugs* (such as *haloperidol* or *thioridazine*) are sometimes necessary to reduce the physical restlessness. The control of infection by *antibiotic drugs* has made delirium much rarer than formerly.

Delirium tremens

A state of confusion accompanied by trembling and vivid *hallucinations.* It usually arises in chronic alcoholics after withdrawal or abstinence from alcohol, often following admission to hospital with an injury or for a surgical operation.

SYMPTOMS AND SIGNS

In the early stages, symptoms include restlessness, agitation, trembling, and sleeplessness. Overactivity of the *sympathetic nervous system* causes a rapid heartbeat, fever, dilation (widening) of the pupils, and profuse sweating that may lead to dehydration. Confusion follows, with visual and sometimes auditory hallucinations, and the patient appears terrified. Convulsions may also occur. Symptoms usually subside within three days.

D

TREATMENT

Treatment consists of rest, rehydration, and sedation in hospital. *Sedative drugs* used include *chlorpromazine*, *chlordiazepoxide*, or chlormethiazole. The physician may order that injections of vitamins, particularly of thiamine (see *Vitamin B complex*), be given, because some of the features of delirium tremens seem to be linked with thiamine deficiency (see *Wernicke-Korsakoff syndrome*).

Delivery

Expulsion or extraction of a baby from the mother's uterus. In most cases the baby lies lengthwise in the uterus with its head facing downward and is delivered head first through the vaginal opening by a combination of uterine contractions and maternal effort at the end of the second stage of labor (see *Childbirth*).

If the baby is lying in an abnormal position (see *Breech delivery; Malpresentation*), if uterine contractions are weak, or if there is disproportion between the size of the baby's head and the mother's pelvis, a *forceps delivery* or *vacuum extraction* may be required; these are called operative deliveries. In some cases, vaginal delivery is impossible or potentially dangerous to the mother or the baby, and *cesarean section* is necessary.

Deltoid

The triangular muscle of the shoulder region that forms the rounded flesh of the outer part of the upper arm, and passes up and over the shoulder joint. The wide end of the muscle is attached to the scapula (shoulder blade) and the clavicle (collarbone). The muscle fibers converge to form the apex of the triangle, which is attached to the humerus (upper-arm bone) about halfway down its length.

The central, strongest part of the muscle raises the arm sideways. The front and back parts of the muscle twist the arm.

Delusion

A fixed, irrational idea not shared by others and not responding to reasoned argument. The central idea in a paranoid delusion involves persecution or jealousy. For instance, a person may believe that he or she is being poisoned or that a partner is persistently unfaithful (see *Paranoia*). A person who is suffering from delusions of grandeur may believe, for example, that he or she is Napoleon or the Queen.

LOCATION OF THE DELTOID
The deltoid muscle of the shoulder region forms the rounded, outer part of the upper arm and is attached to the scapula and clavicle.

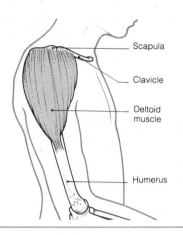

Scapula

Clavicle

Deltoid muscle

Humerus

Persistent delusions are a sign of serious mental illness, notably *schizophrenia* and *manic-depressive illness*. (See also *Hallucination; Illusion*.)

Dementia

A general decline in all areas of mental ability. Dementia is usually due to brain disease and is progressive, the most obvious feature being decreasing intellectual ability.

INCIDENCE

Dementia is the great health problem of modern developed societies, since long life is creating an increasing proportion of elderly citizens. Some 10 percent of those aged over 65 and 20 percent of those aged over 75 are affected to some degree by dementia.

CAUSES

Traditionally, dementing illnesses were divided into presenile (under 65 years of age at onset) and senile (over 65 years). This is now regarded as an artificial division, although treatable causes are more common in the younger age group. Such causes include *head injury, brain tumor, encephalitis, myxedema, syphilis,* pernicious *anemia,* and *alcohol dependence.* However, only some 10 percent of cases are due to one of these "reversible" illnesses.

In the majority of cases, dementia is due to *cerebrovascular disease,* including *strokes,* or to *Alzheimer's disease.* Cerebrovascular disease is often due to narrowed or blocked arteries in the brain and can sometimes be helped by treatment of *hypertension* (high blood

pressure) or heart disease. However, recurrent loss of blood supply to the brain usually results in a deterioration that characteristically occurs gradually but in steplike stages. Alzheimer's disease, in which there is gradual loss of brain cells and shrinkage of the brain substance, is at present completely irreversible.

SYMPTOMS

The person with dementia may not remember recent events, may become easily lost in a familiar neighborhood, may fail to grasp what is going on, and may become confused over days and dates. These symptoms tend to come on gradually and may not be noticed at first. People also tend to cover up their problems by *confabulation* (making up stories to fill the gaps in their memories). Sudden emotional outbursts or embarrassing behavior (such as urinating in public) may be the first obvious signs of the condition.

Commonly, the person's failures in judgment result in the magnification of his or her unpleasant personality traits; families may have to endure unreasonable demands, accusations, pilfering, and even physical assault. *Paranoia, depression,* and psychotic *delusions* may occur as the disease worsens. Irritability or anxiety, of which the patient retains some awareness, gives way to a shallow indifference toward all feelings. Personal habits deteriorate, clothes and possessions become soiled and dirty, and speech becomes incoherent. Demented individuals may then need total nursing care for feeding, toilet, and physical activities.

TREATMENT

While appropriate treatment of certain illnesses is effective in arresting decline (such as surgery for a brain tumor or thyroid hormone replacement for myxedema), management of the most common Alzheimer-type illness is based on the treatment of symptoms. The patient should be kept clean and well nourished in comfortable surroundings with good nursing care. *Sedative drugs* will be given for obvious restlessness or paranoid beliefs. These measures can help ease the distress for both patient and family. Timing of a transfer to suitable hospital or custodial care must be sensitively organized.

Research into medication to alleviate memory loss and intellectual decline has shown some promise, but no truly effective treatment is yet available. Several experimental drugs

D

that increase the amount of the chemical *acetylcholine* in the brain have produced remissions in some patients in clinical trials but these drugs also have serious side effects.

Dementia praecox
An outdated term for severe *schizophrenia*, especially that developing in adolescence or early adulthood.

De Morgan's spots
Harmless red or purple raised spots in the skin, about 2 mm across, which usually affect middle-aged or elderly people. De Morgan's spots are also called cherry spots or cherry angiomas and consist of a cluster of minute blood vessels. With increasing age they become more numerous but do not increase in size. The spots are of no significance, although they may bleed if injured.

Demyelination
Breakdown of the fatty sheaths that surround and electrically insulate nerve fibers. The sheaths provide nutrients to the nerve fibers and are vital to the passage of electrical impulses along them. Demyelination "short-circuits" the functioning of the nerve, causing loss of sensation, coordination, and power in specific areas of the body. The affected nerves may be within the central nervous system (CNS), comprising the brain and spinal cord, or may be part of the peripheral nervous system, which links the CNS to the body's sense receptors, muscles, glands, and organs.

Patches of demyelination are the prime feature of *multiple sclerosis*, a

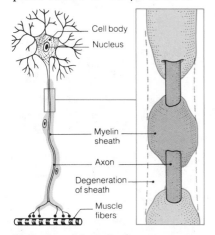

Cell body
Nucleus

Myelin
sheath

Axon

Degeneration
of sheath

Muscle
fibers

Mechanism of demyelination
The fatty myelin sheaths that surround and insulate nerve fibers break down, causing the affected nerves to "short-circuit."

disease with symptoms that include blurred vision, muscle weakness, and loss of coordination. The cause of the demyelination is not known. In many cases, attacks of demyelination alternate with periods of partial or complete recovery of nerve function.

Encephalomyelitis is a rare disorder in which there is inflammation of nerve cells within the CNS and sometimes areas of demyelination. It may be due to a viral infection or very rarely to an allergiclike reaction following immunization.

Dendritic ulcer
A type of *corneal ulcer* characterized by threadlike extensions that branch out in various directions from the center. The ulcer is commonly caused by infection of the cornea by the *herpes simplex* virus.

Dengue
A tropical disease caused by a virus spread by the mosquito *AEDES AEGYPTI*. It occurs in Southeast Asia, the Pacific region, parts of Africa, South and Central America, and the Caribbean. There have also been occasional outbreaks in Mexico, Puerto Rico, and the US Virgin Islands.

Symptoms and signs appear five to eight days after a bite by an infected mosquito and include fever, headache, rash, and severe joint and muscle pains. These symptoms often subside after about three days, recur a few days later, and then subside again. Serious complications are uncommon. Full recovery may take several weeks. The symptoms of severe muscle and bone pain that are associated with the disease have led to the alternative name of breakbone fever.

No specific treatment is available for dengue, although *analgesic drugs* (painkillers) may relieve symptoms. No vaccine is available at present; avoidance involves personal protection against mosquito bites in areas where the disease is prevalent (see *Insect bites*).

Densitometry
The measurement of bone density, as determined by the concentration of calcified material.
WHY IT IS DONE
Densitometry is used to confirm the presence of *osteoporosis* (wasting away of bone substance) or to diagnose *rickets* in young children. It is also useful in assessing the response of these conditions to treatment.

HOW IT IS DONE
The most accurate way to measure bone density is by analyzing the weight and content of a bone *biopsy* sample. However, this technique is time-consuming and requires an operation to remove the sample. *CT scanning* provides detailed pictures of internal bone structure, which enable changes in bone density to be seen.

A relatively new densitometry technique is single or dual photon absorption, in which the pattern of absorption of a beam (or beams) of radiation as it passes through the bone is analyzed on an electronic counter. The dual photon method is used to evaluate the mineral content of the type of bone found in the vertebrae and most other bones where fractures from osteoporosis occur.

Density
The "compactness" of a substance, defined as its mass per unit volume. Because of the close relationship between mass and weight (a mass achieves weight when acted on by gravity) the densities of substances can be compared directly by weighing standard volumes of them under the same gravitational conditions. For instance, a cubic centimetre of lead always weighs much more than a cubic centimetre of wood at the earth's surface; lead is therefore denser than wood. In radiology, the term density relates to the amount of radiation absorbed by the structure being X-rayed. Bone, which absorbs radiation well, appears white on X-ray film. By contrast, a lung, which contains mostly air, absorbs very little radiation and appears dark on film. The same holds true in *CT scanning*. (See also *Specific gravity*.)

Dental emergencies
Injuries or disorders of the teeth and gums that require immediate treatment because of severe pain and/or because delay could lead to poor healing or complications.

A tooth that has become avulsed (completely dislodged from its socket) should be gently washed, reimplanted as rapidly as possible (see *Reimplantation, dental*), and then immobilized with a splint. The success rate is about 90 percent if the tooth is out of its socket for 30 minutes or less and the patient is young. An extruded tooth (one that is partly dislodged from its socket) should be manipulated back into the socket within a few minutes of the injury.

D

A direct blow to a tooth may cause a fracture (see *Fracture, dental*). Sometimes a blow hard enough to fracture teeth may also fracture the jaw; the fractured parts may need to be wired together to allow them to heal (see *Wiring of the jaw*).

Toothache may be so severe that eating and sleeping are disturbed. Temporary pain relief can be gained by placing a sedative dressing in the tooth until the cause of the pain can be treated. The most severe dental pain is usually caused by an abscess (infection). This is treated either by *antibiotic drugs* to reduce the swelling, or by draining the abscess (see *Abscess, dental*), followed by endodontic treatment. Swelling, pain, and inflammation may also occur around an impacted or erupting wisdom tooth, and the jaw may become stiff and difficult to open. This requires immediate treatment to prevent the infection from spreading (see *Impaction, dental*).

Vincent's disease (see *Gingivitis, acute ulcerative*) comes on suddenly and causes pain, inflammation, ulceration, and bleeding of the gums. It is a destructive condition, and professional treatment should be sought as quickly as possible.

Dental examination
Examination of the mouth, gums, and teeth by a dentist. A dental examination may be performed as a routine check at least once a year or as part of the assessment of the condition of a person complaining of a symptom.
WHY IT IS DONE
Routine examinations enable dental caries (tooth decay) and diseases of the gums and mouth to be detected and treated at an early stage before they cause serious damage. The examinations also allow the efficiency of *oral hygiene* to be checked.

It is particularly important for children to have their teeth examined regularly by a dentist so that the replacement of primary teeth by permanent teeth can be monitored. If any problems occur, such as crowding, the dentist can refer the child for *orthodontic* treatment at the correct stage.
HOW IT IS DONE
Before the examination, the dentist or dental hygienist usually asks about the patient's general health, especially if it is the person's first visit or the first visit for a long time. Understanding the person's general health is important since it can affect the type of treatment that is recommended. A person

with a heart valve disorder, for example, may be under increased risk of contracting bacterial *endocarditis* after extraction of a tooth or any other dental treatment. Particular care is also needed when treating people with *diabetes mellitus* or people who have had *hepatitis*. The dentist should also ask about any drugs the patient is taking; people taking certain drugs can react badly to anesthesia. The dentist also needs to know whether the patient is allergic to any drugs.

If a patient is complaining of pain, the dentist will inquire when the pain was first noticed and whether it is continuous or intermittent.

The dentist begins by noting the general appearance of the patient and by examining the face and neck externally. The face is inspected for puffiness that might indicate a dental *abscess* and the neck for swollen lymph glands, which may be caused by an infection of the mouth or teeth. The dentist may also feel the *temporomandibular joint* (jaw joint) for any abnormal movements.

The dentist next examines the patient's bite and the teeth as a whole, noting any tilted, rotated, overlapping, or missing teeth and observing points of contact between teeth, and the presence of any excessive movement in a tooth when the patient makes chewing movements.

Using a mirror to see the backs of the teeth and into the back of the mouth, the dentist then examines individual teeth, using a metal instrument to probe for cavities or chips. Fillings and crowns are inspected for fit, jagged edges, and signs of erosion or cracks. If teeth are missing, the alveolus (bone that surrounds and supports the teeth) is examined for signs of abnormality, especially if the patient is to be fitted with a prosthodontic appliance, such as a dental *bridge*. If the patient wears a *denture*, this is checked to make sure that it still fits properly.

The gums and inside of the mouth are examined for signs of disease. Gums that are red, puffy, or receding or that bleed easily when touched

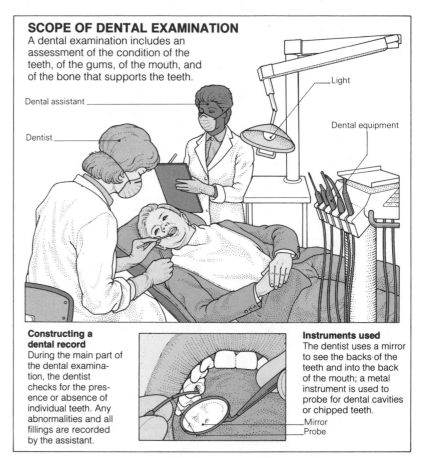

SCOPE OF DENTAL EXAMINATION
A dental examination includes an assessment of the condition of the teeth, of the gums, of the mouth, and of the bone that supports the teeth.

Dental assistant

Dentist

Light

Dental equipment

Constructing a dental record
During the main part of the dental examination, the dentist checks for the presence or absence of individual teeth. Any abnormalities and all fillings are recorded by the assistant.

Instruments used
The dentist uses a mirror to see the backs of the teeth and into the back of the mouth; a metal instrument is used to probe for dental cavities or chipped teeth.
Mirror
Probe

with the probe may indicate *gingivitis* or *periodontitis*. White discoloration of the inside of the mouth may signify *candidiasis* or *leukoplakia*.

Finally, the dentist assesses the accumulation of plaque and calculus on the teeth; this indicates the efficiency of the patient's oral hygiene. *Dental X rays* are an integral part of the examination in some 95 percent of new patients.

Dental extraction
See *Tooth extraction*.

Dental X ray
An image of the teeth and jaws that provides information essential for detecting, diagnosing, and treating conditions that can threaten oral and general health. The part to be imaged is placed between a tube emitting *X rays* and a photographic film. Because X rays are unable to pass easily through hard tissue (such as teeth and bone), a shadow of the teeth and bone is seen on the film.

WHY IT IS DONE
X rays can reveal disorders of the teeth and surrounding tissues that a dentist would not see during a normal visual examination of the mouth. Small caries (areas of decay), abscesses, cysts, tumors, and other disorders can be detected and treated before obvious signs and symptoms have developed, thereby avoiding long-term

damage. Early identification of problems, such as impacted teeth, allows treatment to be carefully planned and carried out at an early stage.

RISKS
The amount of radiation received from dental X rays is extremely small, and the risk of any harmful effects is negligible. However, a woman who is, or suspects she may be, pregnant should tell her dentist, who may postpone X rays until after the pregnancy, or will cover her abdomen with a leaded apron (which blocks X rays).

Dentifrice
A paste, powder, or gel used with a toothbrush to clean the teeth. Although brushing without a dentifrice removes food debris and some dental *plaque*, a slightly abrasive dentifrice is needed to remove the remaining plaque and the pellicle (a thin film formed from saliva).

A dentifrice contains the following: a mild abrasive—usually an insoluble salt, such as dicalcium phosphate; synthetic detergents; binding and moistening agents; thickening agents; flavorings; and colorings. Most dentifrices also contain *fluoride*, use of which has resulted in a dramatic drop in the incidence of dental *caries*.

Various desensitizing dentifrices are available for use on teeth that are sensitive because of exposed dentin near the gum margin.

Dentin
Hard tissue surrounding the pulp of a tooth (see *Teeth*).

Dentistry
The science or profession concerned with the teeth and their supporting structures. Dentistry involves the prevention, diagnosis, and treatment of disease, injury, or malformation of the teeth, gums, and jaws. The majority of dentists work in general dental practice; others practice in a specialized branch of dentistry.

Dentists in general practice undertake all aspects of dental care, including cleaning teeth, filling cavities, extracting teeth, correcting problems with tooth alignment, and fitting crowns, bridges, and dentures. They also check for cancer of the mouth, perform cosmetic procedures (such as bonding), and give general advice on how to care for the teeth and gums.

Dentists in general practice may refer patients to a consultant in one of the specialized branches of dentistry. *Orthodontics* concerns the moving of improperly aligned teeth to improve function and appearance. *Prosthetics* concerns the provision of bridgework and dentures to replace missing teeth and the provision of substitutes for missing oral tissues. Two branches specialize in the treatment of diseases: *endodontics* involves the treatment of diseases of the pulp, while *periodontics*

TYPES OF DENTAL X RAY
There are three different types of X ray. Each is useful for revealing particular problems.

Bite-wing X rays
These X rays show the crowns of the teeth. They are useful for detecting areas of decay between teeth and changes in bone caused by periodontal (gum) disease. The film is in a holder with a central tab onto which the patient bites.

Periapical X rays
These X rays give detailed pictures of whole teeth and the surrounding gums and bone. They show unerupted or impacted teeth, root fractures, abscesses, cysts, tumors, and the characteristic bone patterns of some skeletal diseases. The film, in a protective casing, is placed in the patient's mouth and is held in position behind the teeth to be X-rayed.

Panoramic X rays
These X rays show all the teeth and surrounding structures on one large film. They are invaluable for finding unerupted or impacted teeth, cysts, jaw fractures, or tumors. Pictures are recorded continuously onto film as the camera swings around from one side of the jaw to the other.

involves the treatment of disorders that damage the supporting structures of the teeth, such as the gums.

Dental hygienists are qualified to carry out scaling (the removal of calculus from the teeth) and to demonstrate methods of keeping the teeth and gums healthy (see *Oral hygiene*).

Dentition

The characteristics of a person's *teeth*, including the number and arrangement in the jaw. The term is also used to describe the *eruption of teeth*.

Denture

An appliance that replaces missing natural teeth. A denture consists of an acrylic (tough plastic) and/or metal base mounted with acrylic or porcelain teeth. A natural appearance is achieved by choosing artificial teeth of the size, color, and shape that closely resemble the original teeth and that blend with the contours of the face.

FITTING

The dentist takes impressions of the upper and lower gums. The impressions are removed from the mouth and allowed to harden. Models are then made by pouring plaster of Paris into the hardened impressions. Denture baseplates created from these models will fit the mouth accurately, but, to ensure that the bite will be correct when the artificial teeth are positioned, the dentist must also record the relationship of the upper and lower jaw. This is done by having the patient bite onto wax-rimmed plates (bite blocks) that can be trimmed to indicate the correct relative positions of the jaws.

Using the bite blocks as a guide, a temporary denture with the teeth waxed into position is then produced. The patient tries it on so that the dentist can make adjustments to the position or choice of teeth. When the dentist and patient are satisfied with the bite and appearance, the wax is replaced by acrylic, and the finished, polished dentures are fitted at the patient's next visit.

Additional visits may be needed to ease any part of the baseplate that is uncomfortable.

Dentures fitted immediately after tooth extraction usually require extra visits so that adjustments to the fit can be made as the tissues heal. Often a new acrylic lining is fused to the existing baseplate after healing is complete. Sometimes a soft lining (made of impression material) is inserted temporarily to minimize pain.

TYPES OF DENTURES

Partial dentures	Partial dentures are used when only some teeth are missing. They fill unsightly gaps, make chewing easier, maintain clear speech, and keep the remaining teeth in position. Teeth on either side of a gap may tip (making cleaning more difficult) or drift (placing unnatural stress on the	tissues of the mouth). Partial dentures are held in place by metal clasps that grip adjacent teeth or by clasps combined with metal rests (extensions of the denture plate that rest on the tooth surface).
Full dentures	Full dentures are needed when there are no teeth left in the mouth. They stay in place by resting on the gum ridges and, in the case of upper dentures, by	suction. Fitting is usually delayed for several months after extraction of teeth to allow the gums to shrink and change shape as they heal.
Immediate dentures	Immediate dentures are fitted immediately after extraction of teeth. They protect the gum and control bleeding from extraction sites. Since a toothless period is avoided, they are particularly useful	for replacing front teeth. However, they can be expensive and require follow-up visits for refitting or relining so that they fit comfortably.

Deodorant

A substance that removes unpleasant odors, especially body odors. Deodorants may contain *antiseptics* to destroy bacteria, perfume to mask odors, and *antiperspirants* to reduce the production of sweat. Deodorant preparations are a useful aid against body odor caused by decomposition of sweat by bacteria on the skin.

People who have had a *colostomy* or an *ileostomy* can reduce odor by taking deodorant drugs, such as bismuth, by mouth and by putting deodorant liquids into the stoma bags.

Deoxyribonucleic acid

See *DNA*; *Nucleic acids*.

Dependence

Psychological or physical reliance on persons or drugs. An infant is naturally dependent on parents, but, as he or she grows, dependence normally wanes. Some adults never become fully independent and make excessive demands for love, admiration, and help from others.

Alcohol and drugs (such as opiates, amphetamines, and tranquilizers) may induce physical or emotional dependence. A person who is dependent may develop physical symptoms (such as sweating and abdominal pains) or emotional distress if deprived of the drug. The pattern of dependence varies with the drug and with the individual. (See also *Alcohol dependence; Drug dependence*.)

Depersonalization

A state of feeling unreal, in which there is a sense of detachment from self and surroundings. Depersonalization is frequently accompanied by *derealization*, in which the world is experienced as unreal. Depersonalization, which is rarely serious, usually comes on suddenly and may last for moments or for hours.

Depersonalization may sometimes occur in people who are otherwise perfectly healthy, especially if they are tired or worried. More often, depersonalization occurs in people with *anxiety disorders*, especially when *hyperventilation* takes place during a *panic attack*. Other causes of depersonalization include drugs (such as *LSD* or *marijuana*), *migraine*, and *temporal lobe epilepsy*.

Depilatory

A chemical hair remover, such as barium sulfide, in the form of a cream or paste. Depilatories are used to remove hair for cosmetic reasons and also in treating *hirsutism*.

HOW THEY WORK

Depilatories dissolve hair at the surface of the skin. They do not affect the hair root and therefore do not permanently remove the hair.

POSSIBLE ADVERSE EFFECTS

Depilatories may cause an irritant reaction, with inflammation and swelling. It is advisable to test them first on a small area of skin (they are not usually recommended for use on the face). Depilatories should not be used after a hot bath or shower. Heat increases blood flow to the skin and opens skin pores, thus increasing the amount of chemical that is absorbed into the body.

Depot injection

An intramuscular (into a muscle) injection of a drug that is specially formulated to give a slow, steady release of its active chemicals into the bloodstream. Depot injections usually contain a much higher dose than that normally given by injection. Release of the drug is slowed by the inclusion of substances such as oil or wax. The release of the active drug can be made to last for hours, days, or weeks, depending on the formulation.

A depot injection is useful for patients who may not take their medication correctly. A depot injection also prevents the necessity of giving a series of injections over a short period. Examples of drugs given by depot injection include *corticosteroid drugs* and *antipsychotic drugs*.

Disadvantages of this type of injection include side effects caused by the uneven release of the drug into the bloodstream and prolonged adverse reactions caused by the long-acting nature of the treatment.

Depression

Feelings of sadness, hopelessness, pessimism, and a general loss of interest in life, combined with a sense of reduced emotional well-being. Most people experience these feelings occasionally, in many cases as a normal response to a particular event. For example, it is natural to feel depressed when a close relative dies. However, if the depression occurs without any apparent cause, deepens, and persists, it may be a symptom of any of a wide range of psychiatric illnesses. When a person's behavior and physical state are also affected, it then becomes part of a true depressive illness.

SYMPTOMS

Symptoms vary with the severity of the illness. In a person with mild depression, the main symptoms are anxiety and a variable mood. Sometimes he or she has fits of crying that occur for no apparent reason. A person with more serious depression may suffer from loss of appetite, difficulty in sleeping, loss of interest and enjoyment in social activities, feelings of tiredness, and loss of concentration. Movement and thinking may become slowed; in some cases,

however, the opposite occurs, and the person becomes extremely anxious and agitated. Severely depressed people may have thoughts of death and/or *suicide*, and feelings of guilt or worthlessness. In extreme cases, they may have *hallucinations* or *delusions* (believing, for example, that someone is poisoning them).

Intensity of symptoms often varies with the time of day. Most depressed people feel slightly better as the day progresses, but in some people the symptoms are worst at night. As a depressive illness progresses, the symptoms become more and more prominent. Finally, the person may become totally withdrawn and spend most of the time huddled in bed.

CAUSES

Usually, a true depressive illness has no single obvious cause. It may be triggered by certain physical illnesses (such as a viral infection), by hormonal disorders (such as *hypothyroidism*), or by hormonal changes after childbirth (see *Postnatal depression*). Some drugs, including *oral contraceptives* and *sleeping drugs*, are contributing factors. If the depression is part of a *manic-depressive illness*, inheritance may play a part, since this illness tends to run in families.

Some people become depressed during the winter months of most years (see *Seasonal affective disorder syndrome*) probably in response to the long hours of darkness.

Aside from these biological causes, social and psychological factors may play a part. Lack of a satisfactory mother-child relationship may lead to depression in later life (see *Bonding*), especially when it is combined with difficult social circumstances. For example, a woman whose mother died early in her life may be particularly vulnerable if she has to cope with bringing up a child on her own. Depression may also be related to the number of disturbing events or changes in a person's life.

INCIDENCE

Depression is the most common serious psychiatric illness. Some 10 to 15 percent of people suffer from it at some time in their lives, especially the milder forms. The more severe manic-depressive type affects only about 1 to 2 percent of depressed people, but the incidence of all forms of the illness increases with age. This may be due to social isolation, failing mental powers, and physical illness.

Depression appears to be more common in women, with about one in

six seeking help for depression at some time in their lives (as opposed to only one in nine men). This may be a true difference or may result from the fact that women are more prepared to visit physicians for their depressive symptoms while men may be more likely to resort to alcohol, violence, or other expressions of discontent.

TREATMENT

There are three main forms of treatment for depression, depending on the type and severity of the illness.

Psychotherapy, whether individual or in a group, is most useful for those whose personality and life experiences are the main causes of their illness. Many types of therapy are available, such as an informal, purely practical approach to problem-solving, or the more structured approaches of *cognitive-behavioral therapy* and *psychoanalysis*.

Drug treatment is used for people with predominantly physical symptoms. *Antidepressant drugs* are usually effective in more than two thirds of these patients, provided the drugs are taken in a sufficient dosage over a long enough period of time.

ECT (electroconvulsive therapy), which is given under a general anesthetic, is usually reserved for treating severely depressed people, especially if they are suffering from delusions or have failed to respond to other forms of treatment. ECT is effective and safe, and may be lifesaving; the only side effect may be mild, temporary memory impairment. Trials have demonstrated that ECT relieves severe depression faster than drugs.

OUTLOOK

Although depressive illness is a common cause of distress and social problems, the outlook is good for most sufferers, provided they are given appropriate treatment and advice. The main risk is suicide. In Canada the rate of suicide is about 14 per 100,000 population; at least 80 percent of these deaths are related to depression. Although data from all parts of the country are not reported consistently, many studies have shown that the rate of suicide in the native population is much higher than among nonnative Canadians. It has been estimated at 34 per 100,000 in the native population overall, and 170 per 100,000 for Indian males aged 20-24.

Many people suffering from depression do not require hospitalization and make a good recovery. People with severe and prolonged depression (especially the elderly)

D

may require continuous treatment and may be socially handicapped. However, spontaneous recovery is possible after many years of illness.

Derangement

An outdated term for severe mental disorder. It was first used in the 19th century to describe the idea of an orderly mind that had become "disarranged." Today, the term derangement is usually applied to wild, disturbed behavior rather than to a specific mental state.

The term derangement also applies to disorders of the ligaments in the knee joint (i.e., internal derangement of the knee).

Derealization

Feeling that the world has become unreal. It usually occurs with *depersonalization* and shares the sudden onset, symptoms, and causes of that condition. Sufferers commonly describe the feeling as "looking at the world through a glass screen". Derealization may be caused by excessive tiredness, *hallucinogenic drugs*, or disordered brain function.

Dermabrasion

Removal of the surface layer of the skin by high-speed sanding to improve the appearance of scars, such as those of *acne*, or remove tattoos. The skin is numbed with a local anesthetic and the surface is removed by a spinning abrasive wheel. Healing takes about two weeks and the full effect of the treatment is apparent after two months.

Dermatitis

Inflammation of the skin, sometimes due to an allergy but in many cases occurring without any known cause. Many types of dermatitis are better known as *eczema* (for example, atopic, discoid, infantile, and hand eczema).

Apart from eczemas, the three main forms of skin inflammation are seborrheic dermatitis, contact dermatitis, and photodermatitis.

SEBORRHEIC DERMATITIS

This is a red, scaly, itchy rash that develops on the face (particularly the nose and eyebrows), scalp, chest, and back. On the scalp it is the most common cause of *dandruff*. The rash often develops during times of stress, but its exact cause is unknown. Generally, the treatment of dermatitis must be tailored to each case. Applying *corticosteroid drugs* and/or drugs to kill microorganisms is often helpful. It is important to avoid scratching affected areas or exposing them to irritating substances such as detergents.

CONTACT DERMATITIS

In this type of dermatitis, the rash is a reaction to some substance that comes in contact with the skin. The reaction may result from a direct toxic effect of the substance or it may be an allergic response.

Among the more common causes of the reaction are detergents (including traces left in washed clothes), nickel (e.g., in watch straps, bracelets, necklaces, and the fastenings of underclothes), chemicals (e.g., in rubber gloves and condoms), certain plants (e.g., ragweed), certain cosmetics, and some medications in the form of creams, lotions, or drops.

The type of rash varies considerably according to the substance causing it, but it is often itchy, and may flake or blister; distribution of the rash corresponds to the skin area that has been in contact with the causative substance. Rashes may be treated with corticosteroid medications.

If the causative substance is not known, it may be possible to identify it by a patch test (see *Skin tests*).

Contact dermatitis
Reaction to the nickel in a watch strap produced the itchy, blistering rash on the inside of the wrist shown above.

PHOTODERMATITIS

This type of dermatitis occurs in people whose skin is abnormally sensitive to light. In the most common form of photodermatitis, a cluster of spots or blisters develops on any part of the body exposed to the sun (see *Photosensitivity*).

Dermatitis artefacta

Any self-induced skin condition. Dermatitis artefacta may range from a mild scratch self-inflicted by someone under stress to severe and extensive mutilation by a psychologically disturbed person.

The skin damage may take any form—ulcers, blisters, or scratches. The damage often has a symmetrical or bizarre pattern and, to the trained eye, does not resemble that seen in any skin disease.

Dermatitis herpetiformis

A chronic skin disease in which clusters of tiny, red, intensely itchy blisters occur in a symmetrical pattern on various parts of the body, most commonly the back, elbows, knees, buttocks, and scalp.

The disease usually develops in adult life and is believed to be related to *celiac disease*, a condition in which the small intestine is allergic to gluten, a constituent of wheat and certain other cereals. One of the symptoms of celiac disease is chronic diarrhea, which also occurs in some people with dermatitis herpetiformis. Both conditions often improve after treatment with a gluten-free diet.

Dermatographia

See *Dermographism*.

Dermatology

The branch of medicine concerned with the *skin* and the disorders that affect it. Also included in this specialty are the hair and nails, together with their various disorders. Problems include everything from wrinkles, warts, and hair loss to acne, athlete's foot, and skin cancer. Skin diseases are relatively common, accounting for about 15 percent of all illnesses.

Diagnostic techniques used in dermatology include *skin biopsy* (removal of a sample of tissue for microscopic analysis). Methods of treatment include drug therapy, surgery, and the destruction of unwanted growths by *cryosurgery* (freezing), *electrocautery* (burning), *laser treatment*, and *radiation therapy*.

Dermatopathology is the study of the microscopic appearance of diseased skin tissue.

Dermatome

An area of skin supplied with nerves from one spinal root (see *Nervous system*). The entire surface of the body is an interlocking mosaic of dermatomes, the pattern of which is very similar from one person to another.

Loss of sensation in a dermatome signifies damage to a particular nerve root, the most usual cause of which is a *disk prolapse*. The rash in *herpes zoster* (shingles) is usually confined to one dermatome.

Dermatome, surgical

A surgical instrument for cutting variable thicknesses of skin for use in skin grafting. Types include a drum dermatome, for removal of skin pieces of a precise thickness, and an electric dermatome, which can remove long strips of skin.

Dermatomyositis

A rare, sometimes fatal, disease in which the muscles and skin become inflamed, causing muscle weakness.

CAUSES AND INCIDENCE

The disorder belongs to a group of illnesses called the *autoimmune disorders*, in which, for reasons that are not fully understood, the *immune system* (body's defenses against disease) starts attacking the body's own tissues. Dermatomyositis is sometimes associated with underlying cancer of an internal organ. Two thirds of people suffering from dermatomyositis are middle-aged women.

SYMPTOMS

The first sign is often a red rash on the bridge of the nose and cheeks, followed by a purple discoloration on the eyelids and sometimes a red rash on the knees, knuckles, and elbows. Muscles then start to become weak, stiff, and painful, particularly those in the shoulders and pelvis where the limbs join the trunk. The skin over the affected muscles feels thicker than normal. Sometimes the muscle pains precede the rash. The sufferer may also experience bouts of nausea, weight loss, and fever.

DIAGNOSIS AND TREATMENT

The diagnosis is confirmed by blood tests, *EMG* (electromyography) to detect the electrical activity of muscles, and a skin or muscle *biopsy* (removal of a small piece of tissue for microscopic analysis).

Treatment is with *corticosteroid drugs* and/or *immunosuppressant drugs* (to reduce the inflammation) and *physiotherapy* (to prevent muscles from scarring and shrinking as they heal).

OUTLOOK

In about 50 percent of cases, full recovery occurs after a few years. In about 30 percent, the disease is persistent, causing muscle weakness. In the remaining 20 percent, it eventually affects the lungs and other organs and may be fatal.

Dermatophyte infections

A group of common fungal infections affecting the skin, hair, and nails, also known as *tinea* and, popularly, as ringworm.

Dermographism

Greater than normal sensitivity of the skin to mechanical irritation, to the extent that firm stroking leads to the appearance of itchy wheals (raised areas), which are slightly darker than the surrounding skin. Dermographism means "writing on the skin," and it is sometimes possible with a few finger strokes to write visible words on a sufferer's back.

Dermographism is a form of *urticaria* (hives) and is most common among fair-skinned people with a tendency to allergic conditions such as *eczema*.

Dermoid cyst

A benign tumor with a cell structure similar to that of skin, and containing hairs, sweat glands, and sebaceous glands. Dermoid cysts may also contain fragments of cartilage, bone, and even teeth. The cysts may occur in various parts of the body.

Dermoid cysts account for about 10 percent of all ovarian tumors. Ovarian dermoid cysts range in size from a few millimetres to 10 or more centimetres in diameter. They may cause discomfort and abdominal swelling, but only rarely do they become malignant (cancerous).

Dermoid cysts in the skin most commonly occur on the head or neck, causing a small painless swelling. This type of dermoid cyst is usually congenital (present from birth) and contains only skin structures.

Surgical removal of dermoid cysts is recommended in most cases. (See also *Teratoma*.)

Appearance of dermoid cyst on head
The growth is firm, painless, and has an inner cavity that contains a fatty substance and sometimes hair, teeth, and bony material.

Dermoid tumor

See *Dermoid cyst*.

DES

See *Diethylstilbestrol*.

Desensitization

A technique, used in *behavior therapy* for treating *phobias*, in which the patient is gradually exposed to the cause of the fear.

Desensitization, allergy

See *Hyposensitization*.

Designer drugs

A group of illegally produced chemicals that mimic the effects of specific drugs of abuse. Made in illicit laboratories, these drugs are cheap to produce and thus undercut the street prices of drugs such as *LSD* and *amphetamine drugs*.

Designer drugs are often made in such a way that their structures are subtly different from those of the drugs they imitate. As a result, these drugs may circumvent laws controlling the manufacture and distribution of drugs in some countries.

TYPES

Designer drugs can be divided into three major groups: those derived from narcotic *analgesic drugs* (painkillers) such as meperidine and fentanyl; drugs that mimic amphetamines; and variants of phencyclidine (PCP, also called *Angel dust*), a *hallucinogenic drug* originally used in animal anesthesia.

POSSIBLE ADVERSE EFFECTS

Designer drugs are highly potent. Some derivatives of fentanyl, for example, are between 20 and 2,000 times more powerful than *morphine*; this has led to a high incidence of death due to *drug poisoning*.

Amphetamine derivatives cause brain damage at doses only slightly higher than those required for a stimulant effect. Although they have been abused as aphrodisiacs, amphetamine derivatives commonly impair orgasm in both men and women and may prevent erection.

Many designer drugs contain impurities. For example, a substance known as MPTP, contained within a meperidine derivative, has caused permanent brain damage resulting in *parkinsonism*. Phencyclidine variants often cause seizures and psychosis.

Desipramine

A slow-acting tricyclic *antidepressant* useful in severe prolonged depression. Desipramine is less sedating than other antidepressants, and is likely to have minor side effects, but an overdose of this drug can cause cardiac *arrhythmias*.

D

Desmoid tumor

A growth, usually in the abdominal wall. The tumor is hard, with a well-defined edge.

Desmoid tumors occur most frequently in women who have had children. Stretching or bruising of the abdominal muscle fibers during pregnancy may be a factor in their development. Desmoid tumors may also arise at the sites of old surgical incisions in the abdomen or elsewhere in the body, and they are often regarded as overgrowths of scar tissue.

Surgical removal is the usual treatment, although recurrence of the growth at the same site is common.

Detergent poisoning

The toxic effects that occur as a result of swallowing the cleaning agents in shampoos, laundry powders, and cleaning liquids. Detergent poisoning causes vomiting, diarrhea, and a swollen abdomen. Victims should drink large quantities of fluids to dilute the detergent.

Development

The process of growth and change by which an individual matures physically, mentally, emotionally, and socially. Development takes place in the following major phases: during the first two months of pregnancy (see *Embryo*); to a lesser extent, during the rest of pregnancy (see *Fetus*); during the first five years of life (see *Child development*); and during *puberty* and *adolescence*.

Developmental delay

A term used when a baby or young child has not achieved new abilities within the normal time range and has a pattern of behavior that is behind what is appropriate for his or her age.

Development is an increase in abilities—physical, mental, emotional, and social—and is a well-orchestrated process, with new abilities and new patterns of behavior appearing at given ages, while existing patterns of behavior change and sometimes disappear (see *Child development*).

Delays may be of varying severity and may affect any or all of the major areas of human achievement (i.e., development of the ability to walk upright, of fine hand-eye coordination, of listening, language, and speech, and of social interaction). Developmental delay is not a term used for slow increase in physical size (see *Growth; Short stature*) or for late appearance of sexual characteristics (see *Puberty; Puberty, delayed*). The term is not usually applied to children over the age of 5.

In general, the child who is slow in one or two aspects of development and is of average or perhaps advanced ability in others needs to be distinguished from the child who is delayed in most aspects. When there is a significant delay in a few aspects, there may be a specific (although often not obvious) disability such as a visual or hearing impairment, which, if adequately treated, may allow the child to catch up. Children who are developmentally delayed in most aspects usually have a more generalized problem—for example, lack of adequate stimulation and teaching at home or a slowness to learn because of limited intellectual abilities.

CAUSES

Some important causes of generalized developmental delay are shown in the accompanying table. It is important to remember that a child born prematurely will reach most developmental milestones later than other children. Parents should take into account how old the baby would be if he or she had been born at the normal time rather than prematurely. Causes of delay in specific areas are as follows.

WALKING AND MOVEMENT SKILLS There is an enormous time range within which most children learn to walk; most begin between the ages of 9 and 15 months, but a child who crawls fast and efficiently may delay longer.

In most late walkers, no serious cause is found. Late walking is an inherited feature in some families and is probably due to delayed maturation of the nervous system. Such children learn to walk a few months later than other children, and from then on usually develop new skills at a normal rate. Other children develop slightly unusual patterns of locomotion—for example, creeping on their abdomens or shuffling on their bottoms. These traits also tend to run in families. Such children may miss out on the crawling stage. They eventually stand and walk and from then on follow the normal developmental sequence in all other developmental aspects.

A more specific reason for delayed walking and other skills is weakness of the leg muscles and other muscles. This can occur in boys with *muscular dystrophy* and in children with *spina bifida. Cerebral palsy* is a disorder that affects all aspects of motor development; it may cause slowness and difficulty in gaining control of the head,

neck, and back muscles during the first few months of life, as well as delay in sitting and walking.

HAND-EYE COORDINATION Any defect of vision or of the nerves and muscles used to control fine finger movements may be a cause of delayed manipulative skills. However, the most common cause is not a specific abnormality but lack of experience; stimulation and encouragement are extremely important in the acquisition of these skills. If a child has only large toys to play with and is not encouraged to use the small finger muscles, skills involving these muscles will be delayed. Similarly, if a child is left lying down for most of the time instead of in a sitting position, the hands will not be in the correct position to acquire certain skills.

RESPONSE TO SOUND If a child is unresponsive to sound it may be due to *deafness*. However, children who are not talked to may show a lack of interest in the human voice, although they may respond normally to other sounds. Children exposed continually to a great deal of noise may show little interest in sound.

A rare cause of unresponsiveness to the human voice is *autism*. An affected child can hear normally but shows little interest in human contact of any kind. Although unresponsive to human voices, autistic children often become obsessively interested in particular sound-producing toys.

SPEECH AND LANGUAGE The most important cause of delayed speech is a hearing problem. Another common cause is lack of stimulation (when parents do not talk to the child sufficiently). In other cases (more commonly in boys than girls), delayed speech runs in families. Twins are often late talkers, perhaps because they may receive less individual parental attention. Some twins develop a private language that includes idiosyncratic words and nonverbal communication.

Children exposed to two or more languages may show signs of speech delay and may confuse the languages. However, many children become naturally bilingual or trilingual.

Any generalized difficulty with muscle control can affect speech production; muscle control can be a particular difficulty in children with *cerebral palsy*. Damage to, or structural defects of, the speech muscles, larynx (voice box), or mouth may also cause speech difficulties, as may any disorder affecting the speech area of the brain (see *Aphasia; Dysarthria; Dysphonia; Speech disorders*).

BLADDER AND BOWEL CONTROL Children vary enormously in the age at which control of bowel and bladder function is acquired. Usually bowel function is acquired first. Delay in bladder control is much more common than delayed bowel control. (See *Encopresis; Enuresis; Soiling*.)

ASSESSMENT
In many instances, the parents are the first to notice that their child is not acquiring new skills at the same rate as his or her peers. A physician should be consulted. Problems are sometimes detected during one of the developmental checks that are carried out routinely in child and well-baby clinics. These checks are performed by family physicians, pediatricians, or other health professionals at varying ages, but usually at birth, 6 weeks, 6 to 8 months, 12 to 15 months, 2 years, 3 years, and 5 years.

If developmental delay is discovered, the first step is to establish the cause by undertaking a full assessment. This examination usually includes hearing and vision testing, a full physical examination, and thorough developmental assessment. Further investigation is arranged as necessary. It may include referral to a pediatrician, neurologist, psychologist, speech therapist, occupational therapist, or physiotherapist.

TREATMENT
Once the severity of the delay and the probable cause have been discovered, the appropriate treatment can be arranged. In many cases, the parents can be reassured that there is no serious abnormality and that their child can be expected to develop normally without any specific treatment. Sometimes advice is given regarding suitable toys and other forms of education and stimulation.

Treatment may include a course of *speech therapy* or *family therapy*, or provision of *glasses* or a *hearing aid*. In some cases it is felt that the child's best interests are served by admission to a special school or unit for children with specific difficulties—for example, a school for physically handicapped children, or a language unit.

Whatever the cause of the developmental delay, children can be helped to achieve their full potential by the provision of appropriate therapy. Parents are often of prime importance in providing this help.

Deviation, sexual

A form of sexual behavior in which intercourse between adults is not the final aim. Instead, the man (deviation is rare in women) achieves erection and orgasm in other ways, such as by being whipped or wearing women's clothes. Forms of sexual deviation include *exhibitionism, fetishism, frottage, necrophilia, pedophilia, sadomasochism,* and *transvestism*.

Dexamethasone

A *corticosteroid drug* prescribed as a nasal spray to relieve *nasal congestion* caused by allergic *rhinitis* (hay fever) and as eye drops in the treatment of *iritis* (inflammation of the iris). Dexamethasone is given in tablet form to treat severe cases of *asthma* and to reduce inflammation of the brain due to *head injury, stroke,* or a *brain tumor*. Occasionally, dexamethasone may be injected into an inflamed joint to relieve pain and stiffness caused, for example, by *osteoarthritis*.

POSSIBLE ADVERSE EFFECTS
Dexamethasone in the form of a nasal spray or eye drops may cause minor local side effects, such as nosebleed or eye irritation. When prescribed for a prolonged period or in high doses, dexamethasone tablets may cause the adverse effects common to the corticosteroid group of drugs.

Dextroamphetamine

A central nervous system stimulant (see *Amphetamine drugs; Stimulant drugs*). Dextroamphetamine is used to treat *narcolepsy* (a rare condition characterized by excessive sleepiness). Paradoxically, it is also used to treat children with *hyperactivity*, although the reason it helps in this condition is not known.

Dextroamphetamine is no longer recommended as an *appetite suppressant* for people trying to lose weight.

ABUSE
Because of its stimulant properties, dextroamphetamine has become a drug of abuse, one of a group commonly referred to as "uppers." If use is prolonged, the stimulant effects lessen and a higher dose must be taken to produce the desired effect. In an overdose, dextroamphetamine can cause seizures and hypertension (high blood pressure).

Dextrocardia

A rare condition, present from birth, in which the heart is situated in, and points toward, the right-hand side of the chest instead of the left. The heart may also, but not necessarily, be malformed. Sometimes, the position of the abdominal organs is also reversed, so that the liver is on the left-hand side and the stomach on the right. When all organs are on the opposite side of the body from where they are customarily found, the condition is known as *situs inversus*.

Abnormal position   Normal position

Heart positions
In dextrocardia, the heart is situated in, and points toward, the right-hand side of the chest instead of the left.

The cause of dextrocardia is unknown. No treatment is necessary unless the heart is malformed, in which case surgery to correct the malformation may be required.

Dextromethorphan

A cough suppressant available over-the-counter as an ingredient in a number of *cough remedies*.

Dextrose

Another name for *glucose*, one of the monosaccharide sugars. Dextrose is absorbed from digested *carbohydrates* through the intestinal wall into the bloodstream. It is also available in the form of tablets, as an injection for use in the emergency treatment of *hypoglycemia* (low blood sugar level), and as a component of infusion fluids used for intravenous feeding (see *Feeding, artificial*).

Diabetes, bronze

Another name for *hemochromatosis*, a rare disease in which excessive amounts of iron are deposited in tissues such as the liver, pancreas, and skin. Its name comes from the bronze skin coloration and *diabetes mellitus* that usually develop in sufferers.

Diabetes insipidus

A rare condition that is characterized by polyuria (the passing of large quantities of dilute urine) and polydipsia (excessive thirst) to compensate. These symptoms also occur, in a milder form, early in *diabetes mellitus*, a much more common disease that in all other respects is different from diabetes insipidus.

CAUSES

Diabetes insipidus usually results from a failure of the *pituitary gland* to secrete *ADH* (antidiuretic hormone). Normally, this hormone reduces the amount of water passed by the *kidneys* into the urine. Diseases of the pituitary gland, including damage from injury or a tumor, can cause failure of ADH secretion. Diabetes insipidus may follow brain surgery and may be temporary in such cases.

In rare cases, the disease is due to failure of the kidneys to respond to normal levels of ADH, when it is called nephrogenic diabetes insipidus. This type of the disease is usually congenital (present from birth), but may result from kidney disease or from certain drugs.

SYMPTOMS, DIAGNOSIS, AND TREATMENT

A person with diabetes insipidus may pass between 5 and 20 litres of urine every 24 hours—provided this output is matched by a similar intake of water. If water is unobtainable or withheld, *dehydration* may occur, leading to confusion, stupor, and coma.

Diabetes insipidus is usually treated with synthetic ADH, given in the form of a nasal spray. ADH is ineffective for people with nephrogenic diabetes insipidus; in such cases, treatment consists of a combination of a low-sodium diet and, paradoxically, thiazide *diuretic drugs*.

Diabetes mellitus

A disorder caused by insufficient or absent production of the hormone *insulin* by the *pancreas*. Insulin is an important hormone responsible for the absorption of glucose into cells for their energy needs and into the liver and fat cells for storage. If there is a deficiency of insulin, the level of glucose in the blood becomes abnormally high, causing polyuria (the passing of large quantities of urine) and polydipsia (excessive thirst). The body's inability to store or use glucose causes weight loss, hunger, and fatigue. Diabetes mellitus also results in disordered *lipid* (fat) metabolism and accelerated degeneration of small blood vessels.

Apart from the symptoms of thirst and polyuria, the disease has nothing in common with the much rarer disorder *diabetes insipidus*.

There are two principal types of diabetes mellitus. Insulin-dependent (type I) diabetes, the more severe form, usually first appears in young people under the age of 35 and most commonly between the ages of 10 and 16. It develops rapidly. The insulin-secreting cells in the pancreas are destroyed, probably as a result of an *immune response* after a viral infection, and insulin production ceases almost completely. Without regular injections of insulin, the sufferer lapses into a coma and dies.

The other main type, non-insulin-dependent (type II) diabetes, is usually of gradual onset and develops mainly in people over 40. In many cases it is discovered only during a routine medical examination. Insulin is produced, but not enough to meet the body's needs, especially when the person is overweight. Often the body is resistant to the effects of insulin. In most cases, insulin-replacement injections are not required; instead, a combination of dietary measures, weight reduction, and oral medication keeps the condition under control.

CAUSES AND INCIDENCE

Diabetes mellitus tends to run in families. However, of those who inherit the genes responsible for the insulin-dependent form, only a small proportion eventually develop the disease. In these cases, the disorder is thought to be the delayed result of a viral infection that damaged the pancreas several years earlier.

In the case of non-insulin-dependent diabetes, a greater proportion of the people who are predisposed to the disease by heredity actually go on to develop the disease.

Although obesity is the primary factor that leads to the unmasking of latent diabetes, other causes that may uncover or aggravate diabetes are certain illnesses (among them *pancreatitis* and *thyrotoxicosis*), certain drugs (including some *corticosteroid drugs* and *diuretic drugs*), infections, and pregnancy (see *Diabetic pregnancy*).

In Canada, about two persons in 1,000 develop insulin-dependent diabetes. The number with non-insulin-dependent diabetes is probably much greater, but is difficult to estimate since different diagnostic criteria are used for the disease and the course of the condition is quite variable.

DIAGNOSIS

A physician who suspects diabetes mellitus in a patient can often obtain confirmation by testing a sample of urine for its glucose level. Further confirmation is obtained when significantly high glucose levels are found in blood samples following an overnight fast or from samples taken two hours after a meal. Glucose-tolerance tests are sometimes required.

TREATMENT

The aims of treatment are to prolong life, to relieve symptoms, and to prevent long-term complications. Success depends on keeping the level of blood glucose as near normal as possible through maintenance of normal weight, regular physical activity, careful dietary management, and, if necessary, injections of insulin.

In people with insulin-dependent diabetes, treatment consists of regular self-injections—between one and four times a day—with insulin (either obtained from animals or of a human type synthesized by *genetic engineering*). In addition, the person must follow a diet in which carbohydrate intake is regulated and spread out over the day according to a consistent timetable. By these means, marked fluctuations in the glucose levels in the blood can be avoided.

Disturbances in the careful balance between insulin and glucose intake can result in *hyperglycemia* (too much glucose in the blood), causing the symptoms of the untreated disease, or *hypoglycemia* (too little glucose in the blood), which can cause weakness, confusion, dizziness, sweating, and even seizures and unconsciousness. To help prevent this, people with either type of diabetes mellitus are advised to monitor their blood and/or urine glucose levels regularly with do-it-yourself testing kits (see illustrated box below). As a precaution against an attack of hypoglycemia, insulin-dependent diabetics need to carry some sugar or glucose with them at all times.

For difficult-to-control diabetes, an insulin pump is an alternative treatment for those who are willing to monitor their blood glucose levels carefully. Insulin is continuously infused from a refillable pump through a needle implanted in the skin. In some people, however, control is no better than that from multiple daily injections.

In non-insulin-dependent diabetes, because the pancreas does produce some insulin, the disorder can often be controlled by dietary means alone (regulating the carbohydrate intake with meals spaced out over the day). This not only lowers the blood glucose level, but also reduces weight. If diet fails to lower the glucose level suffi-

ciently, *hypoglycemic* tablets (oral anti-diabetic drugs that stimulate the pancreas to produce more insulin) may be prescribed, although these are ineffective unless dietary restrictions are observed.

All people with diabetes need regular advice from their physicians so that any complications can be detected and treated at an early stage. Diabetics should wear or carry information identifying them as diabetics in case of an emergency.

COMPLICATIONS

Complications eventually develop in a large number of diabetics. These complications tend to be more likely if the diabetes has not been well controlled, but they can occur even if there has

D

LIVING WITH DIABETES MELLITUS

As the level of glucose in the blood rises, the volume of urine required to carry it out of the body is increased, causing not only a frequent need to urinate but also constant thirst. The high levels of sugar in the blood and urine impair the body's ability to fight infection, leading to urinary tract infections (such as *cystitis* and *pyelonephritis*), vaginal yeast infections (*candidiasis*), and recurrent skin infections.

Because the body's cells are starved of glucose, the sufferer feels weak and fatigued. The cells are able to obtain some energy from the breakdown of stored fat, resulting in weight loss. However, the chemical processes involved in this breakdown of fat are defective (especially in insulin-dependent diabetics) leading to the production of acids and substances known as ketones, which can cause coma and sometimes death.

Other possible symptoms of undiagnosed diabetes include blurred vision, boils, increased appetite, and tingling and numbness in the hands and feet.

Symptoms develop in all untreated insulin-dependent diabetics, but symptoms develop in only one third of those who have the non-insulin-dependent type. There are many people suffering from a mild form of the disease who are unaware of it. The disease is often diagnosed only after complications of the diabetes have been detected.

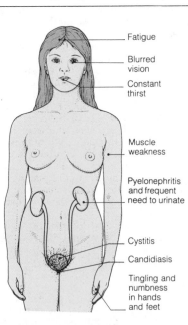

- Fatigue
- Blurred vision
- Constant thirst
- Muscle weakness
- Pyelonephritis and frequent need to urinate
- Cystitis
- Candidiasis
- Tingling and numbness in hands and feet

Testing urine for glucose
Urine can be tested for glucose by means of a chemically impregnated strip dipped into a sample of urine. The resulting color change in the strip is compared with a chart to indicate the glucose level.

Direct testing of blood glucose
A pricking device is used to obtain blood, which is spread on a chemically coated strip. The strip is inserted into an instrument that reads the blood glucose.

DEVICES FOR INJECTING INSULIN

Insulin can be injected using a disposable syringe and needle or a pen with refill cartridges (below), or it may be infused continuously from a portable pump (right).

- Insulin pen
- Spare needles
- Refill cartridge
- Cannula
- Pump

Insulin pen
This device is useful if multiple daily injections are needed.

Portable pump
The pump infuses insulin by way of a cannula inserted through the skin.

D

been good control. Complications include *retinopathy* (damage to the retina, the light-sensitive area at the back of the eye, and the blood vessels serving it) which may need laser treatment to prevent blindness, peripheral *neuropathy* (damage to nerve fibers), and *nephropathy* (kidney damage) which occasionally requires dialysis and/or a kidney transplant. Ulcers on the feet, which in severe cases can develop into *gangrene*, are another risk, but with good foot care they can usually be prevented.

Diabetics also have a higher-than-average risk of *atherosclerosis* (accumulation of fatty deposits on the inner lining of arteries), *hypertension* (high blood pressure), other *cardiovascular disorders*, and *cataracts* (opacities in the lens of the eye).

There are, however, people who have lived full and active lives with diabetes mellitus for 50 years or more with few complications.

OUTLOOK

With modern treatment and sensible self-monitoring, almost all diabetics can look forward to a normal life span. The life expectancy of people who have well-regulated, insulin-dependent diabetes is little different from that of nondiabetics. Those with the non-insulin-dependent illness have a slightly reduced life expectancy because of circulatory and heart disorders; however, these disorders were often already present when the diabetes was diagnosed.

Diabetic pregnancy

Special precautions are necessary for pregnant women with preexisting *diabetes mellitus*, and also for those women who develop diabetes during pregnancy (a condition known as gestational diabetes).

PREEXISTING DIABETES

Nearly all women with established diabetes mellitus can have a normal pregnancy, provided the diabetes is well controlled throughout. It is important to plan the pregnancy and to make sure that the blood glucose level is under particularly good control before and at the time of conception; otherwise there is a slightly increased chance of the baby being malformed. (No special precautions are needed by a diabetic man planning to become a father.) If control is poor during the pregnancy, there may be an increase in the amount of glucose reaching the baby (which makes the baby grow faster than normal) and this may cause difficulties at birth.

Conversely, the growth of infants of diabetic mothers may be stunted; these babies may have complications in the days immediately after birth.

GESTATIONAL DIABETES

Gestational diabetes is most often detected in the second half of pregnancy, when increased glucose appears in the urine or the baby is found to be bigger than expected when a physician examines the mother's abdomen (although these findings do not always mean the mother is diabetic). It appears that the mother does not produce enough insulin to keep the blood glucose levels normal during the pregnancy. Some obstetricians now screen for diabetes at 26 weeks. True gestational diabetes disappears with the delivery of the baby, but can be a sign of future diabetes in up to three quarters of these mothers.

CARE

Diabetic pregnancies must be supervised at hospital prenatal clinics. Some hospitals offer pre-pregnancy clinics for those with established diabetes to help women achieve good control before conception. At many hospitals, the care of diabetic women in pregnancy is shared between an obstetrician and a physician who is a specialist in diabetes. Stringent control over blood glucose levels, especially toward the end of pregnancy, is the key. If there are complications or the baby is large, early delivery may be considered.

The chances that the baby of a diabetic parent will become diabetic are about one in 100 and, if both parents are diabetic, about one in 20.

Diagnosis

The determination by a physician of the nature and cause of a person's problem. Usually this entails identifying both the disease process—pneumonia or cirrhosis of the liver, for example—and the agent responsible, such as pneumonia due to legionnaires' disease, or cirrhosis due to alcohol. Diagnosis is part science and part art; an experienced physician relies not only on his or her scientific knowledge and experience, but also on intuition to recognize the pattern of an illness and establish a diagnosis.

THE MEDICAL HISTORY

The patient's own account of his or her illness is perhaps the most important part of the diagnostic procedure. This history provides vital clues, which can then be augmented by questions from the physician in an exchange that may last some 20 to 30

minutes in a complex case or if the physician has not previously seen the patient. What the physician is looking for is a pattern of symptoms that is strongly suggestive of a single disease. For example, the features of a migraine headache, duodenal ulcer, enlarged prostate gland, or angina pectoris are often unmistakable.

In some circumstances the physician may not attempt to reach a final diagnosis. If a patient has had a sore throat for only 48 hours, the physician may be content to treat the condition symptomatically, while awaiting the results of a throat culture or other tests. However, when symptoms have been more prolonged, the physician will want to reach at least a provisional diagnosis before beginning treatment, partly because any treatment is likely to affect the symptoms and thus make diagnosis difficult.

EXAMINATION AND TESTS

Tests may be ordered after a physical examination and the formation of a provisional diagnosis.

Confirmation of a diagnosis may be obtained in a variety of ways, including tissue biopsy, culture of microorganisms, or finding the cause by surgery. If specific treatment (either with drugs or by surgery) relieves the symptoms and cures the patient, the diagnosis is likely to have been correct—although it is also possible that the patient may have recovered spontaneously and the treatment may simply have coincided with the time of recovery. Alternatively, if the patient dies, a pathologist can usually, but not always, determine by postmortem examination what the disease process was (see *Autopsy*).

Dialysis

A technique used to remove waste products from the blood and excess fluid from the body as a treatment for *kidney failure*.

WHY IT IS DONE

The main function of the kidneys is the maintenance of *electrolyte* and water balance and the excretion of waste products. One fifth of the blood pumped by the heart goes to the kidneys; the kidneys filter approximately 1,500 litres of blood daily. From this volume of blood, the kidney reabsorbs important elements, such as sodium, potassium, calcium, amino acids, glucose, and water. The kidneys excrete, as urine, the nitrogenous waste of protein breakdown known as urea, as well as other excess minerals, toxins, and drugs.

STEPS IN DIAGNOSING A CONDITION

A physician may go through several steps to ascertain the cause of a person's problem. The medical history, physical examination, and tests may prove vital clues. A physician usually makes at least a provisional diagnosis before beginning any treatment because treatment can mask symptoms, making the physician's task of establishing an exact diagnosis more difficult.

Taking the medical history

Perhaps the most important part of the diagnostic procedure is the patient's own account of his or her illness—the medical history. "Listen to the patients, they are telling you their diagnosis" is the traditional teaching given to medical students. Many physicians believe that the medical history provides the strongest basis for ascertaining a diagnosis. The added information derived from the physical examination is small, but, at times, critical.

Conducting a physical examination

After the medical history has been obtained, the physician has in mind a short list of probable diagnoses. A physical examination helps shorten the list. The physician is then left with a differential diagnosis. A differential diagnosis is a group of possible diseases that could account for the patterns of symptoms and signs (i.e., physical findings, such as enlargements of lymph nodes or tenderness in a specific region of the abdomen).

Ordering special tests

Next, based on his or her working diagnosis the physician may order a series of laboratory tests on the blood (and sometimes the urine) and may also arrange for diagnostic imaging of suspect organs by techniques such as *ultrasound scanning, X rays,* *CT scanning, MRI,* or *radionuclide scanning.* The results of these tests either confirm the physician's working diagnosis or narrow the possibilities so the physician may be confident that he or she has found the correct diagnosis.

Using a computer

Physicians today also use computer systems and algorithms to help reach a diagnosis. Both approaches rely on analysis of large numbers of patient records to quantify probabilities and to devise an orderly series of questions—a decision tree. The main purpose of computer assistance is to remind the physician of the full range of possible diagnoses of a particular set of symptoms, thereby making it less likely that any possibility will be overlooked. It remains the task of the physician to integrate the facts and decide upon a diagnosis.

In people whose kidneys have been damaged, this process may fail—either suddenly (in acute kidney failure) or gradually (in the chronic form of the disease). Wastes start to accumulate in the blood, with harmful, sometimes even life-threatening, effects. In severe cases, the function of the kidneys must be taken over by the artificial means of dialysis. In cases of acute kidney failure, dialysis continues until the kidneys recover and start functioning normally again. However, in chronic kidney failure, patients may need to undergo dialysis for the rest of their lives or until they can be given a *kidney transplant*. Dialysis therapy may not always be appropriate if kidney failure is part of an otherwise rapidly fatal disorder.

HOW IT IS DONE

There are two methods of dialysis. Hemodialysis, which filters out wastes by passing blood through an artificial kidney machine, was pioneered early in the 1940s. Peritoneal dialysis, which makes use of a natural filtering membrane within the body's abdomen (the peritoneum), was developed in the early 1970s.

In most cases, hemodialysis is performed in outpatient dialysis centers by specially trained nurses, but many patients now undergoing dialysis carry it out themselves with a kidney machine installed at home.

Peritoneal dialysis may be performed in a hospital, but an increasing number of patients are now able, once the catheter has been inserted into the abdomen, to carry out the dialysis themselves at home, a procedure known as continuous ambulatory peritoneal dialysis (CAPD). In Canada, the number of patients maintained on dialysis is steadily increasing. In 1990, there were an estimated 6,000 such patients; two thirds of them were on hemodialysis, the remainder on peritoneal dialysis.

For patients with chronic kidney failure, hemodialysis needs to be carried out several times a week. In the treatment of acute kidney failure, the process is carried out more intensively over a period of days or weeks until the kidneys are working normally again. Complications may include weakening of the bones (see *Osteomalacia; Osteodystrophy*), *anemia,* infections, and *pericarditis.* Complications of peritoneal dialysis are the same as for hemodialysis, plus *peritonitis.*

OUTLOOK

Long-term dialysis enables people who would once have died from chronic kidney failure to live relatively normal lives. Their diet and fluid intake may need to be restricted somewhat and they may not feel completely well. However, many do return to full or part-time employment. Since the patient's health is invariably affected in the long run, many physicians feel that dialysis should be replaced with a kidney transplant, which, if successful, can restore general health dramatically.

D

PROCEDURE FOR DIALYSIS

There are two methods of removing wastes from the blood and excess fluid from the body when the kidneys have failed. The first, hemodialysis, may also be used as emergency treatment in some cases of poisoning or drug overdose. It makes use of an artificial kidney (or "kidney machine") and can be carried out at home. Peritoneal dialysis, also done in the home, requires an abdominal incision (which is performed in the hospital).

HOW HEMODIALYSIS IS DONE

1 Access to the bloodstream for dialysis is obtained by a shunt or an *arteriovenous fistula* connecting an artery to a vein.

Vein   Artery   Shunt sewn into blood vessel

2 A needle connected to plastic tubing passes blood to the artificial kidney and back to the patient. The artificial kidney consists of many layers of special membrane.

Artificial kidney machine

Blood out of kidney machine

Machine that prepares dialysate

Blood into kidney machine

Dialysate to and from kidney machine

4 The dialysate is discarded and the purified blood is returned to the patient. Each session lasts two to six hours.

WHY IT IS DONE

In people with damaged kidneys, the process of maintaining the balance of electrolytes and water, and of excreting waste products, may fail, causing harmful, if not life-threatening, effects. Dialysis can take over the function of the kidneys until they start working normally again. Or dialysis can function for the kidneys for the rest of a seriously affected person's life if a kidney transplant is not performed.

Diseased kidney
The kidney at right was removed from a person with adult polycystic kidney disease—one of many disorders that may damage kidney function to the extent that dialysis is needed.

3 The membrane separates the patient's blood from a special fluid called dialysate. Wastes, toxic molecules, and excess fluid pass from the blood into the dialysate.

Blood cell

Artificial membrane

Dialysate

Waste chemicals

Shunt

HOW PERITONEAL DIALYSIS IS DONE

1 A small abdominal incision is made (using a local anesthetic); a catheter is inserted through it into the peritoneal cavity. Dialysate from a bag attached to the catheter passes into the cavity, where it is left for several hours.

Spinal column

Catheter

Fluid

Bag   Bladder

Blood cell

Fluid   Peritoneal   Capillary
membrane wall

2 Waste products and excess water from the blood vessels lining the peritoneal cavity seep through the peritoneal membrane into the cavity and mix with the dialysate. The fluid is then allowed to drain out (by the release of a clamp) through the catheter and into the empty dialysate bag.

3 The bag is discarded and replaced with a bag containing fresh dialysate. The procedure, which takes about an hour, can be performed during the day or overnight.

Diamorphine

A synthetic, narcotic *analgesic drug* (painkiller) which is similar to *morphine*. Diamorphine is an alternative name for heroin and is used medically to relieve severe pain caused by injury, surgery, myocardial infarction (heart attack), and painful chronic diseases, such as cancer. It is also used to relieve distress in acute heart failure, and is occasionally used as a cough suppressant when other remedies have been ineffective.

Because of the risk of dependence, diamorphine is prescribed with caution. Other adverse effects include nausea, vomiting, and constipation. (See also *Heroin abuse*.)

Diaper rash

A common condition affecting babies with otherwise healthy skin. Diaper rash results from skin irritation by substances contained in the feces or urine. Friction from rough diapers and prolonged wetting also play a part. Babies vary in their susceptibility to diaper rash. In some babies, diaper rash may be the first indication of sensitive skin and future skin problems, such as *eczema*.

TREATMENT AND OUTLOOK

Prevention is better than cure in most health-related issues and this is especially true of diaper rash. The aim is to keep the baby's skin dry for as long as possible. A breast-fed newborn passes urine about 20 times each day and has a bowel movement after each feeding, so keeping the skin dry for lengthy periods presents a major practical problem. Change diapers frequently and, after each change, apply a water-repellent emollient. Ideally, the diaper should be left off for an hour or so each day.

Cloth diapers should be well rinsed and kept soft. Sometimes an ointment containing a mild *corticosteroid drug* needs to be prescribed to suppress the inflammation. It is often prescribed in combination with an antifungal drug to kill any thrush organisms that are present (see *Candidiasis*).

Diaphragm, contraceptive

The most commonly used female barrier method of contraception, in the form of a hemispherical dome of thin rubber with a metal spring in the rim. The diaphragm is individually fitted. (See *Contraception, barrier methods*.)

Diaphragm muscle

The dome-shaped sheet of muscle that separates the thorax (chest) from the abdomen. The diaphragm is attached to the spine, ribs, and sternum (breastbone).

The diaphragm plays a vital role in breathing. For air to be drawn into the lungs, the muscle fibers of the diaphragm contract, thereby pulling the whole diaphragm downward. This action enlarges the chest, and air passes into the lungs to fill the increased space. (See also *Breathing*.)

Diarrhea

Increased fluidity, frequency, or volume of bowel movements, as compared to the usual pattern for a particular person. Diarrhea itself is not a disorder but is a symptom of an underlying problem.

Acute diarrhea affects almost everybody from time to time—usually as a result of eating contaminated food or drinking contaminated water. These attacks normally clear up within a day or two with or without treatment. Chronic diarrhea may be the result of a serious intestinal disorder and requires investigation by a physician.

Diarrhea can be very serious in infants because of the risk of severe, potentially fatal, *dehydration*. Elderly people are also at risk of dehydration as a consequence of diarrhea.

DIARRHEA IN ADULTS

Normally, the *colon* (the major part of the large intestine) absorbs much of the water from the liquid food residues that pass through it, producing semisolid *feces*. However, if the intestinal contents pass through the colon too quickly, or if the small intestine is inflamed and secretes fluid into the fecal material, diarrhea may result.

CAUSES Acute diarrhea starts abruptly and usually lasts from a few hours to two or three days. The most common cause is *food poisoning*. Diarrhea that affects two or more people within six hours of them sharing a meal usually indicates that the food has been contaminated by toxins from STAPHYLOCOCCUS bacteria. Toxins from CLOSTRIDIUM bacteria cause diarrhea within six to 12 hours after eating. If diarrhea develops 12 to 48 hours after eating, it may be due to contamination by bacteria such as SALMONELLA or CAMPYLOBACTER, or by a virus such as the rotavirus or Norwalk virus. Infective *gastroenteritis* may also be acquired as a result of droplet infection, with adenoviruses or echovi-

ANATOMY OF THE DIAPHRAGM

The diaphragm is attached to the spine, the lower pairs of ribs, and the lower end of the sternum (breastbone). The muscle fibers of the diaphragm converge on the central tendon, a thick, flat plate of dense fibers. There are openings in the diaphragm for the esophagus, phrenic nerve (which controls diaphragm movements and hence breathing), and the aorta and vena cava blood vessels.

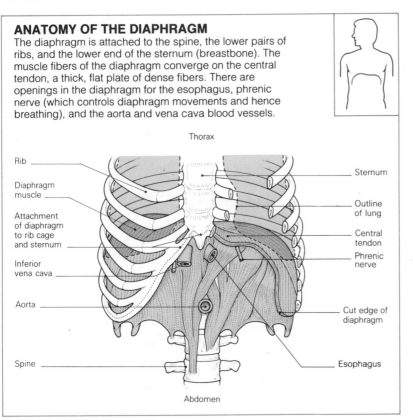

Thorax

Rib

Diaphragm muscle

Attachment of diaphragm to rib cage and sternum

Inferior vena cava

Aorta

Spine

Sternum

Outline of lung

Central tendon

Phrenic nerve

Cut edge of diaphragm

Esophagus

Abdomen

D

DIARRHEA Frequent passing of unusually loose bowel movements.

? Have you had other attacks of diarrhea during the past few weeks?

YES → Do the attacks occur when you are under emotional stress?

YES → Stress can often cause diarrhea. However, if you also have bouts of cramping abdominal pain and alternating constipation and diarrhea, consult your physician.

See • *Anxiety*
 • *Diverticular disease*
 • *Intestine, cancer of*
 • *Irritable bowel syndrome*

NO ↓

NO ↓

Have you been having bouts of lower abdominal pain?

YES → See • *Abdominal pain*

WARNING
A child who has diarrhea may be seriously ill if he or she has any one of the following danger signs:
• continuous abdominal pain for six hours or more
• repeated vomiting for more than 12 hours
• refusal to drink
• sunken eyes
• passing no urine for six hours or more
Call your physician now!

NO ↓

☎
Consult your physician without delay!
A persistent change in bowel habit should always be investigated to rule out the slight possibility of cancer.

See • *Intestine, cancer of*

? Is there blood in your bowel movements?

YES →

☎
Consult your physician without delay!
Raw, inflamed areas may have developed along the intestines or at the anus. Bloody diarrhea may also be due to infection. This is especially likely if you have recently returned from abroad; dysentery may be a possibility.

See • *Dysentery*
 • *Ulcerative colitis*

NO ↓

? Have you felt sick or been vomiting AND/OR is your temperature 38°C or above?

YES → Inflammation of the digestive tract as a result of infection or food poisoning is probable. Consult your physician.

See • *Gastroenteritis*

NO ↓

? Have you recently started to take any medicines?

YES → Sensitivity to certain drugs may cause diarrhea. If you feel that drugs you are taking may be causing your problems, consult your physician.

NO ↓ Continued on next page

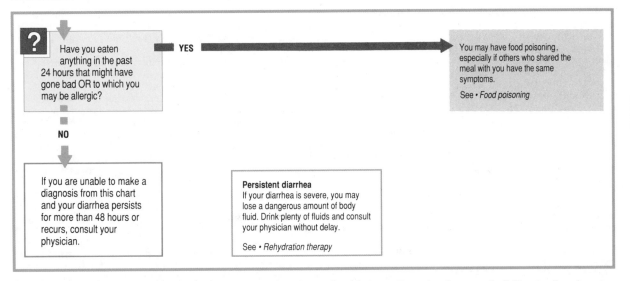

? Have you eaten anything in the past 24 hours that might have gone bad OR to which you may be allergic?

YES You may have food poisoning, especially if others who shared the meal with you have the same symptoms.

See • *Food poisoning*

NO

If you are unable to make a diagnosis from this chart and your diarrhea persists for more than 48 hours or recurs, consult your physician.

Persistent diarrhea
If your diarrhea is severe, you may lose a dangerous amount of body fluid. Drink plenty of fluids and consult your physician without delay.

See • *Rehydration therapy*

ruses, for example. Acute diarrhea may be caused by interference with the intestinal flora (harmless bacteria in the intestine) as a result of travel to a country where these bacteria are of a different type.

Other causes of acute diarrhea include anxiety and, less commonly, *shigellosis* (bacillary dysentery), *typhoid fever* and *paratyphoid fever*, drug toxicity, *food allergy*, and *food intolerance*. In the case of shigellosis and amebic dysentery (see *Amebiasis*), there may be blood in the feces.

Chronic diarrhea generally takes the form of repeated attacks of acute diarrhea. Causes include *Crohn's disease*, *ulcerative colitis*, *diverticular disease*, cancer of the colon (see *Colon, cancer of*), *thyrotoxicosis*, and *irritable bowel syndrome*. In all of these conditions, except thyrotoxicosis and irritable bowel syndrome, the bowel movements may contain blood.

TREATMENT The water and electrolytes (salts) lost during a severe attack of diarrhea need to be replaced to prevent dehydration. It is possible to buy ready-prepared powders of electrolyte mixtures to be added to a specific amount of water. Half a litre of the oral rehydration liquid should be drunk every hour, and no solid food eaten, until the diarrhea subsides. Alternatively it is possible to make up an oral rehydration solution: dissolve one teaspoon of salt and eight teaspoons of sugar (which helps the intestine absorb the water and salt) in one litre of water.

It is important to be accurate with the quantities as too much salt may cause further dehydration.

Antidiarrheal drugs should generally not be taken to treat attacks of diarrhea resulting from infection because they may prolong the illness. However, they may be useful if the diarrhea is disabling or if it is associated with abdominal pain. Examples are *codeine* phosphate, *diphenoxylate* and *loperamide*.

Diarrhea that recurs, persists for more than a week, or is accompanied by blood in the bowel movements requires investigation by a physician to discover the underlying cause. In addition to taking the patient's case history, the physician will probably arrange for a *culture* of the feces to determine whether or not infection is the underlying cause. If it is not, other tests may be carried out, such as a barium enema or meal (see *Barium X-ray examinations*), *sigmoidoscopy*, and a *biopsy* of the rectum. These tests enable the physician to discover the underlying cause of the diarrhea; treatment will be for that cause.

DIARRHEA IN INFANTS
Most cases of diarrhea in infants are acute and carry the risk of rapid dehydration (especially when accompanied by vomiting). Dehydration can be fatal unless countered quickly.

CAUSES The most common cause is gastroenteritis resulting from a viral infection. Babies who are entirely breast-fed are less likely to contract the illness than those who have been bottle-fed. Viral gastroenteritis can damage the lining of the small intestine, thereby impairing its ability to absorb nutrients, and can cause a temporary deficiency of the enzyme lactase. The latter may lead to lactose

intolerance (inability to absorb sugar from milk), which may produce secondary diarrhea that can last for several weeks.

TREATMENT An infant with diarrhea should not be fed milk. He or she should be given an electrolyte mixture (obtainable from a pharmacist) to replace lost water and salts.

If the diarrhea clears up within 24 hours, milk can be gradually reintroduced over a 24-hour period. The first feeding should consist of one part milk to three parts water, the second of equal parts of milk and water, the third of three parts milk to one part water, and the fourth of undiluted milk.

If the diarrhea persists for more than 48 hours, a physician should be consulted.

A physician should be called urgently if the infant shows signs of dehydration at any stage during the illness. Signs of dehydration include drowsiness, unresponsiveness, prolonged crying, loose skin, glazed eyes, a depressed *fontanelle* at the front of the head, and a dry, sticky mouth and tongue.

Diastole

The period in the heartbeat cycle when the heart muscle is at rest; it alternates with the period of muscular contraction (*systole*).

Diathermy

The production of heat in a part of the body using high-frequency electric currents or microwaves. The heat generated can be used to increase blood flow and to reduce deep-seated pain

D

in rheumatic and arthritic conditions. By using large currents, enough heat can be produced to destroy tumors and diseased parts without causing bleeding. A diathermy knife is an instrument used by surgeons to coagulate bleeding vessels or to separate tissues without causing them to bleed (see *Electrocoagulation*).

Diathesis

A predisposition toward certain disorders. For example, a bleeding diathesis is present when a *bleeding disorder* (such as hemophilia) makes a person susceptible to prolonged bleeding after an injury. A diathesis may be inherited or may be acquired as a result of an illness.

Diazepam

BENZODIAZEPINE ANTICONVULSANT MUSCLE RELAXANT
Tablet Capsule Injection Rectal suppository
Prescription needed

One of the best known and most widely used *benzodiazepine drugs*. Diazepam is used mainly to treat *anxiety* and *insomnia*. It is also prescribed as a *muscle-relaxant drug* (for example, to treat spasm of the back muscles), and as an *anticonvulsant drug* in the emergency treatment of *epilepsy*. Diazepam is also commonly used to treat the symptoms of alcohol withdrawal.

POSSIBLE ADVERSE EFFECTS
Diazepam may cause drowsiness, dizziness, and confusion; driving and hazardous work should therefore be avoided. Alcohol increases the sedative effect of the drug and should be avoided during the use of diazepam.

Like other drugs in this group, diazepam can be habit-forming if taken regularly, and its effect may diminish with prolonged use. Individuals who have taken diazepam regularly for more than two weeks should never stop their treatment suddenly. Instead, they should gradually decrease the dose under medical supervision to avoid withdrawal symptoms (which may include anxiety, sweating, and, in rare circumstances following large doses, seizures).

Diclofenac

A *non-steroidal anti-inflammatory drug* used for symptomatic relief of pain due to various types of arthritis. Common side effects are gastrointestinal distress, headache, and dizziness.

Dicumarol

An *anticoagulant drug* used primarily to prevent or treat venous *thrombosis*. Like all anticoagulants, blood levels of the drug have to be monitored by frequent *blood-clotting tests*.

Dicyclomine

An *antispasmodic drug* used to relieve abdominal pain in *irritable bowel syndrome* and infantile *colic*. Dicyclomine may cause dry mouth, blurred vision, and constipation.

Dienestrol

An *estrogen drug* used in the form of a cream to treat atrophic *vaginitis* (dryness of the vagina), which commonly occurs after the *menopause*.

Diet

See *Nutrition*.

Diet and disease

Until comparatively recently, medical concern about diet in developed countries was focused on dietary deficiencies in the poor. Today, however, deficiency diseases are very rare in developed countries (except in alcohol-ics, in people with malabsorptive intestinal disorders, and in people on extremely restricted diets). Instead, the pendulum has swung the other way, and many common disorders are due partly to overconsumption of certain types of food.

In poorer developing countries, dietary deficiencies remain a major problem. In these countries, starvation or malnutrition may result in *marasmus* or *kwashiorkor* in children. Specific vitamin deficiencies in childhood may cause *rickets* or blindness due to *keratomalacia*; lack of certain vitamins in adult life may lead to *beriberi*, *pellagra*, or *scurvy*.

FATS
Virtually all people in developed countries have some degree of *atherosclerosis* (narrowing of arteries by deposits of fatty material), which can lead to cardiovascular diseases (such as *coronary artery disease, stroke*, and *peripheral vascular disease*). A major cause of atherosclerosis is a high level of the chemical *cholesterol* in the blood which most nutritionists attribute to diets that are high in saturated *fats*, which are found in high-fat meats and

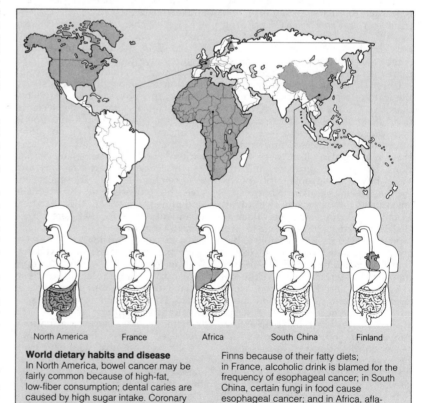

World dietary habits and disease
In North America, bowel cancer may be fairly common because of high-fat, low-fiber consumption; dental caries are caused by high sugar intake. Coronary artery disease is common among Finns because of their fatty diets; in France, alcoholic drink is blamed for the frequency of esophageal cancer; in South China, certain fungi in food cause esophageal cancer; and in Africa, aflatoxins may cause liver cancer.

North America   France   Africa   South China   Finland

dairy products. The disease is much less common in countries (such as Japan) in which fat in the diet is minimal and mostly unsaturated.

CALORIES

Obesity places a person at greater risk of acquiring serious disorders, such as *diabetes mellitus*, coronary artery disease, stroke, and *osteoarthritis*. The cause is simply an excess intake of *calories* (units of energy). It is estimated that about one third of the populations of developed countries is overweight (10 percent or more above the accepted range of weight for a given height) and a small proportion of these is obese (20 percent or more above the range).

ALCOHOL

Overconsumption of *alcohol* can lead to *cirrhosis* of the liver, brain damage (see *Wernicke-Korsakoff syndrome*), peripheral *neuritis*, and *cardiomyopathy*, and has been linked with *pancreatitis*, esophageal cancer (see *Esophagus, cancer of*), and many other disorders. People with *alcohol dependence* tend to become malnourished.

FIBER

The part played by diet in digestive disorders is less clear than its contribution to cardiovascular disease and obesity, but there is evidence suggesting that lack of fiber may be an important factor in some illnesses. Fiber—found in foods such as whole-grain bread and vegetables—provides bulk to enable the large intestine to work effectively and also helps regulate the absorption of nutrients in the small intestine. Lack of dietary fiber has been implicated in a number of intestinal disorders such as *diverticular disease*, chronic *constipation*, and *hemorrhoids*.

SALT

In developed countries, *hypertension* (high blood pressure) is far more prevalent than in developing countries. One theory is that some people are genetically susceptible to develop high blood pressure in middle age if they consume too much salt. For this reason, some nutritionists consider it prudent not to have a high salt intake.

DIET AND CANCER

Comparisons of the patterns of cancer in different countries suggest that diet may be an important factor. A high intake of fat (and possibly of meat) has been linked with cancer of the bowel (see *Colon, cancer of*) and *Breast cancer*. Moldy foods are known to cause cancer of the esophagus and *liver cancer*, and research groups are examining many other associations.

GOOD DIETARY HABITS

Eat fresh rather than preserved, packaged, or convenience foods.

Eat plenty of vegetables and fruit. When raw or lightly cooked, they retain a higher nutritional value.

Eat whole-grain products, including whole-grain bread.

Cut down consumption of red meat; instead, eat fish, poultry, and legumes.

Keep the fat content of your diet low and use polyunsaturated fats and vegetable oils rather than saturated fats.

Cut down on sugar in all foods.

When choosing filling foods, eat potatoes in their skins, pasta, or rice.

FOOD ALLERGIES

It is fashionable to ascribe a great deal of illness to food allergy, but in fact the numbers of people in whom disease can definitely be traced to this factor are small. They include those who suffer from *celiac disease*, as the result of an intolerance to gluten, a protein in cereals; some migraine sufferers, in whom food such as chocolate or red wine produces an attack; and people who develop a rash after eating shellfish or soft fruit (see *Urticaria*). Some attacks of *asthma* and *eczema* may be due to an allergy to eggs and dairy products; an allergy to food additives, such as colorings, may be a factor in eczema and *irritable bowel syndrome*. Some physicians believe that allergy to food additives is a major cause of behavioral disorders, such as *hyperactivity* in children, but research suggests that this association is rare.

Treatment for self-diagnosed food allergy should always be supervised by a physician. It is a time-consuming process in which suspected items in the diet are excluded one at a time.

A PRUDENT DIET

Although the connection between certain types of food and disease has not been proved in all cases, enough evidence exists to indicate that it is wise to make sure your diet is low in fats and sugar and high in fiber. The fats and sugar should be replaced with starchy foods and cereals. (See also *Nutritional disorders*.)

Dietetics

The application of nutritional science to the maintenance or restoration of health. Dietetics involves not only a detailed knowledge of the composition of foods, the effects of cooking and processing, and dietary requirements, but also psychological aspects, such as eating habits (see *Nutrition*).

Diethylstilbestrol

A drug that mimics the natural estrogen hormone *estradiol*; it may be used to replace or supplement estrogen when natural hormone production is abnormal.

WHY IT IS USED

Diethlystilbestrol (DES) is used to treat the symptoms of *hypogonadism* (underdeveloped ovaries), symptoms of the *menopause* (such as hot flashes and sweating), and atrophic *vaginitis* (dryness of the vagina), which is common after the *menopause*.

DES is sometimes prescribed in high doses as a postcoital contraceptive (see *Contraception, postcoital*). It is also useful in the treatment of prostate cancer. It was formerly used as a treatment for threatened miscarriage, but this use has been abandoned as a result of evidence that vaginal cancer may develop many years later in daughters of women who took DES.

POSSIBLE ADVERSE EFFECTS

Side effects are as for other estrogen drugs. DES should not be taken during pregnancy.

Differentiation

The process by which the cells of the early *embryo*, which are almost identical and have not yet taken on any particular function, gradually diversify to form the distinct tissues and organs of the more developed embryo.

In cancer terminology, the word means the degree to which the microscopic appearance of a tissue resembles normal tissue.

Diffusion

The spread of a substance (by movement of its molecules) in a fluid from an area of high concentration to one of lower concentration, thus producing a uniform concentration throughout.

Diflunisal

A *nonsteroidal anti-inflammatory drug* (NSAID) used to relieve joint pain and stiffness in *osteoarthritis*, *rheumatoid arthritis*, and other types of arthritis. It is also prescribed to treat back pain, sprains, and strains. Occasionally, it is prescribed to ease pain after a minor

D

THE DIGESTIVE PROCESS

Digestion starts when food enters the mouth. It continues as the food is propelled through the digestive tract by waves of muscular contractions (peristalsis). The digestive process also involves other organs (the salivary glands, liver, gallbladder, and pancreas), which produce enzymes and acids that help break down the food.

ACTION OF DIGESTIVE AGENTS

Agent or enzyme (where produced)	Digestive action
Amylase (mouth and pancreas)	Converts starch (a form of carbohydrate) to maltose
Sucrase, maltase, and lactase (pancreas and small intestine)	Break down vegetable and milk sugars into glucose, fructose, and galactose
Hydrochloric acid (stomach) Pepsin (stomach) Trypsin (pancreas) Peptidase (small intestine)	Assist in the breakdown of proteins into polypeptides, peptides, and amino acids
Lipase (pancreas) Bile salts and acids (liver—stored in the gallbladder)	Break down fats into glycerol and fatty acids

TIME SCALE

The approximate period food spends in each part of the digestive system is shown below.

Mouth
1 minute

Esophagus
10 seconds

Stomach
2–4 hours

Small intestine
1–6 hours

Large intestine
10 hours—several days

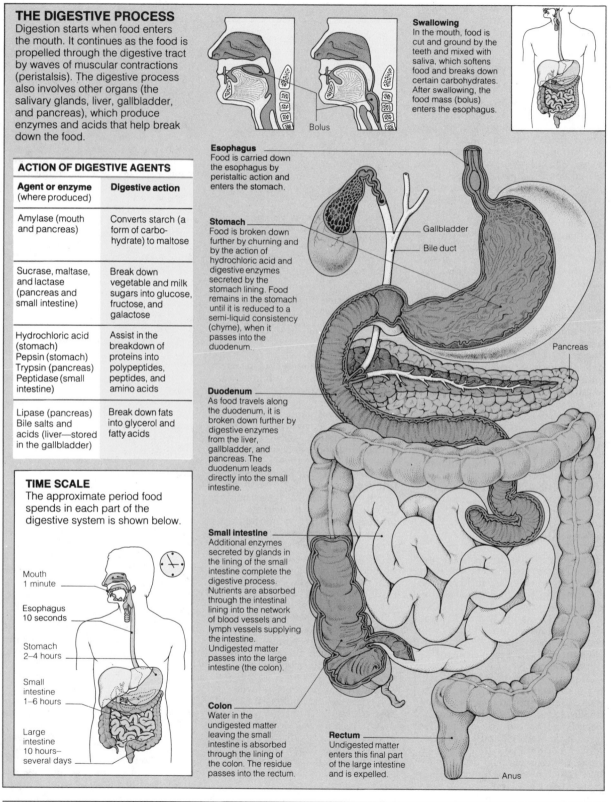

Bolus

Swallowing
In the mouth, food is cut and ground by the teeth and mixed with saliva, which softens food and breaks down certain carbohydrates. After swallowing, the food mass (bolus) enters the esophagus.

Esophagus
Food is carried down the esophagus by peristaltic action and enters the stomach.

Stomach
Food is broken down further by churning and by the action of hydrochloric acid and digestive enzymes secreted by the stomach lining. Food remains in the stomach until it is reduced to a semi-liquid consistency (chyme), when it passes into the duodenum.

Gallbladder

Bile duct

Pancreas

Duodenum
As food travels along the duodenum, it is broken down further by digestive enzymes from the liver, gallbladder, and pancreas. The duodenum leads directly into the small intestine.

Small intestine
Additional enzymes secreted by glands in the lining of the small intestine complete the digestive process. Nutrients are absorbed through the intestinal lining into the network of blood vessels and lymph vessels supplying the intestine. Undigested matter passes into the large intestine (the colon).

Colon
Water in the undigested matter leaving the small intestine is absorbed through the lining of the colon. The residue passes into the rectum.

Rectum
Undigested matter enters this final part of the large intestine and is expelled.

Anus

operation or dental treatment. Diflunisal may cause nausea, indigestion, diarrhea, and a rash.

Digestive system

The group of organs that breaks down food into simple chemical components that the body can absorb and use for energy and for building and repairing cells and tissues.

The digestive system consists of the digestive tract (also known as the alimentary tract or alimentary canal) and various associated organs. The digestive tract is basically a tube through which food passes; it consists of the *mouth*, *pharynx* (throat), *esophagus* (gullet), *stomach*, *intestines* (the small intestine, comprising the *duodenum*, *jejunum*, and *ileum*, and the large intestine, comprising the *cecum*, *colon*, and *rectum*), and the *anus*.

The associated digestive organs—such as the *salivary glands*, *liver*, and *pancreas*—secrete digestive juices that break down food as it passes through the tract.

Food and the products of digestion are moved through the intestine, from the throat to the rectum, by *peristalsis* (waves of muscular contractions of the intestinal wall).

THE DIGESTIVE PROCESS

The human diet is made up of foods consisting of nutrients and energy sources (*vitamins*, *minerals*, *carbohydrates*, *proteins*, and *fats*), residues (mainly vegetable *fiber*), and water. Most vitamins and minerals are absorbed into the bloodstream without change. However, before other nutrients can be absorbed into the bloodstream, they must be broken down by digestive agents into simpler substances with smaller molecules.

Part of food breakdown is physical, performed by the teeth, which cut and chew food, and the stomach, which churns it. The rest of the process is chemical, performed by the action of *enzymes*, acids, and salts.

Carbohydrates, which are provided mainly by starchy and sugary foods, are the body's principal source of energy. The digestive process eventually converts all carbohydrates (except those that make up dietary fiber) to three simple forms of sugar: glucose, fructose, and galactose.

Proteins, which are found in abundance in meat, fish, eggs, cheese, peas, beans, and lentils, are essential for the growth, replacement, and repair of cells. Proteins are broken down into *polypeptides*, *peptides*, and *amino acids*.

Fats (also known as lipids), which are found in meat and dairy products, and also in oily plant foods such as peanuts and avocados, provide energy and some of the materials for cell building and maintenance. They are broken down into *glycerol*, glycerides, and *fatty acids*.

The digestive process begins in the mouth, where the teeth chop food and the salivary glands secrete saliva, which lubricates the food and contains enzymes that begin to break down carbohydrates. The mouth also contains sensory nerves, in the taste buds on the tongue. The tongue manipulates food in the mouth and forms it into small balls (called boli) for easy swallowing.

From the mouth, food passes into the pharynx, which then pushes it into the esophagus. The esophagus does not contribute to the breakdown or absorption of food products; its sole function is to squeeze food down into the stomach. In the stomach, food is mixed with hydrochloric acid and pepsin produced in the stomach lining; these help break down proteins. The stomach also breaks down food mechanically by its continual churning action. When the food has been converted to a semi-liquid consistency, it passes into the duodenum.

The liver produces bile salts and acids, which are stored in the gallbladder and then released into the duodenum. These salts and acids help break down fats. The pancreas also releases digestive juices into the duodenum, and these juices contain enzymes that further break down carbohydrates, fats, and proteins. The final breakdown stages are completed in the small intestine, carried out by enzymes produced by glands in the lining of the intestine.

As the broken down products of digestion pass through the small intestine, they are absorbed by its thin lining and pass either into the bloodstream or into the lymphatic system.

Finally, the food residue passes into the large intestine, where much of the water it contains is absorbed by the lining of the colon. Undigested matter is then expelled as feces.

DISORDERS

Some digestive system disorders disrupt the digestive process, either because they obstruct the passage of food, or because they interfere with the breakdown or absorption of nutrients. Other conditions have little effect on the digestion of nutrients but produce gastrointestinal symptoms.

Digestive system disorders result from various causes, including birth defects, inherited biochemical disorders, parasitic infections, and chronic allergic conditions. (See also disorder boxes for *Mouth, Esophagus, Stomach, Liver, Gallbladder, Pancreas,* and *Intestine.*)

Digitalis drugs

A group of drugs extracted from plants belonging to the foxglove family and used to treat heart conditions. The most commonly used drugs in this group are *digoxin* and *digitoxin*.

Digital subtraction angiography

See *Angiography*.

Digitoxin

DIGITALIS		
Tablet	Liquid	Injection
Prescription needed		

A *digitalis drug*. Digitoxin is used to treat *heart failure* (reduced pumping efficiency) and certain types of *arrhythmia* (irregular heartbeat). Digitoxin is usually prescribed as an alternative to *digoxin* for patients with kidney disease.

Digoxin

The most widely used of the *digitalis drugs*. Digoxin is used in the treatment of *heart failure* (reduced pumping efficiency) and certain types of *arrhythmia* (irregular heartbeat), such as *atrial fibrillation* (a rapid, irregular beating of the heart muscle).

HOW IT WORKS

Digoxin increases the force of heart muscle contractions, making the heart work more efficiently. It also slows down abnormally rapid impulses as they pass between the atria (upper chambers of the heart) to the ventricles (main chambers of the heart), which allows the ventricles time to fill up with blood and empty normally with each contraction.

POSSIBLE ADVERSE EFFECTS

If digoxin is to be effective, the dose must be just below that of a toxic dose. The patient must therefore be given regular blood tests to ascertain the digoxin level. An excessive dose may cause loss of appetite, nausea, vomiting, and headache. Digoxin occasionally disrupts the normal heartbeat, causing *heart block* (an abnormally slow rate of contraction).

D

D

Adverse effects are more likely if the potassium level in the body is low. Patients who are also taking *diuretic drugs* (and therefore are more likely to become deficient in potassium) are given regular blood tests to monitor potassium levels.

Because digoxin is removed from the body mainly in the urine, patients with kidney disease are usually given *digitoxin* as an alternative drug because of the risk of a buildup of toxic levels of digoxin.

Dilatation

A condition in which a body cavity, tube, or opening is enlarged or stretched due to normal physiological processes or because of disease.

The term dilatation also refers to procedures for achieving such enlargement, as in dilatation and curettage.

Dilatation and curettage

See *D and C*.

Dilation

A term that is sometimes used as an alternative to *dilatation*.

Dilator

An instrument for stretching and enlarging a narrowed body cavity, tube, or opening.

Diltiazem

A *calcium channel blocker* used in the treatment of *hypertension* (high blood pressure) and *angina pectoris* (chest pain due to impaired blood supply to heart muscle). Taken regularly, diltiazem reduces the frequency of angina attacks, but acts too slowly to relieve pain in an acute attack.

Diltiazem may cause headache, appetite loss, nausea, constipation, and swelling of the ankles.

Dimenhydrinate

An antihistamine especially effective against nausea and vomiting that occurs in conjunction with *vertigo*, or because of pregnancy, or as a result of radiation treatments. Like other antihistamines, it can cause drowsiness.

Dioxin

The name of a group of chemicals that are among the most highly toxic substances known. They are contaminants of some defoliant weedkillers (see *Agent Orange* and *Defoliant poisoning*). Dioxins have also been detected in minute traces in some bleached paper products.

Diphenhydramine

An *antihistamine drug* that is used to treat various allergic disorders, such as *urticaria* (hives) and allergic *rhinitis* (hay fever).

Diphenhydramine is also prescribed as an *antiemetic drug* to relieve nausea and vomiting in pregnancy and to prevent *motion sickness*. It is used as an ingredient in some *cough remedies* because of its cough-suppressant effect.

POSSIBLE ADVERSE EFFECTS

Diphenhydramine quite often causes drowsiness and, because of its sedative effect, has occasionally been used to treat *insomnia*. Driving and hazardous work should be avoided if the drug is causing sedation. Other possible side effects include dry mouth and blurred vision.

Diphenoxylate

An *antidiarrheal drug* chemically related to the narcotic *analgesic drugs* (painkillers). Diphenoxylate works by reducing the contractions of the muscles in the walls of the intestine, thus slowing down the frequency of bowel movements.

POSSIBLE ADVERSE EFFECTS

In normal doses, drowsiness and abdominal pain occur in rare instances. When taken in high doses, diphenoxylate produces euphoria due to its narcotic ingredient. Adding *atropine* to the preparation prevents abuse; a dose high enough to produce euphoria causes unpleasant side effects, such as dry mouth, flushing, blurred vision, and vomiting.

Diphtheria

An acute bacterial illness that causes a sore throat, fever, and, sometimes, more serious or even fatal complications. Diphtheria was one of the most important causes of childhood death worldwide until the 1930s. Since then, mass immunization has made it extremely rare in developed countries. Diphtheria is still a hazard in some developing countries and is a risk for nonimmunized travelers to such countries.

CAUSES AND INCIDENCE

Diphtheria is caused by the bacillus *CORYNEBACTERIUM DIPHTHERIAE*. It may live in the skin or in the nose of a person immune to the disease or, during an infection, may multiply in the throat or skin. Serious complications are caused by a toxin released by the bacterium into the blood.

In Canada, only about 5 to 10 cases of diphtheria are reported each year.

SYMPTOMS

When a nonimmune person is infected by the bacterium, it usually multiplies in the throat, giving rise to a membrane that appears over the tonsils and may spread over the palate or downward to the larynx (voice box) and trachea (windpipe). This may cause breathing difficulties and a husky voice. Other symptoms include enlarged lymph nodes in the neck, an increased heart rate, and mild fever. Sometimes, infection is confined to the skin, where it may cause no more than a few yellow spots or sores with an appearance similar to *impetigo*.

Life-threatening symptoms develop only in nonimmune people and are caused by the bacterial toxin. Occasionally, victims collapse and die within a day or so of developing throat symptoms. More often they are recovering from this condition when *heart failure* or paralysis of the throat or limbs develops. These later complications can occur up to seven weeks after onset of infection in the throat. If victims survive the disease they make a complete recovery.

PREVENTION

The *DPT vaccine* (against diphtheria, pertussis, and tetanus) is given routinely in three spaced doses during the first year of life. The practice of immunizing against diphtheria must continue, despite the extreme rarity of the disease in developed countries, because carriers may bring the infection from countries where the disease is more common; if large numbers of children were not immune, there could be an epidemic.

Those traveling to developing countries who are in doubt as to whether or not they were immunized against diphtheria as children should have their immune status checked. People who are not immune should be vaccinated.

Spread of effective immunization programs to all countries could eradicate diphtheria (as smallpox has been eradicated), although this possibility is not envisaged at present.

TREATMENT

Penicillin drugs kill diphtheria organisms in the throat but are ineffective against the toxin in the blood. If diphtheria is suspected, an *antitoxin* (derived from the blood of immunized horses) must be given as soon as possible in addition to penicillin. If severe breathing difficulties develop in a patient, a *tracheostomy* (surgical introduction of a breathing tube into the windpipe) may be necessary.

PHYSICAL AIDS FOR THE DISABLED

A variety of articles exist that are specially designed or adapted to assist disabled people in performing everyday activities. Aids include prostheses, supports, and mobility aids that enable disabled people to function more efficiently, as well as equipment designed to help them perform specific tasks more easily.

Devices that help vision, hearing, and movement improve the ability of disabled people to cope with all aspects of everyday life. Such devices include walking frames, glasses, hearing aids, artificial limbs, corsets, and wheelchairs. Ventilators, home dialysis, and artificial feeding devices are life-sustaining aids.

There are various household aids available that can help people cook, feed themselves, wash, dress, use the toilet, and get in and out of beds and chairs. Specially designed furniture and other devices can help disabled parents care for their children. Sexual aids can facilitate an active sex life.

Faucet turner
A device that helps grip and turn faucets.

Tongs
Extending tongs to pick up dropped items. Closes up to fit in pocket or handbag.

Bottle opener
A small hand-held device designed to grip and open small bottle tops.

Cutlery
A range of knives, forks, and spoons with thick, molded handles for easy manipulating.

Toothpaste extruder
A wall-mounted device that dispenses toothpaste with minimal finger pressure.

Scissors
Self-opening scissors with easy-grip handles.

"A" frame
A lightweight walking frame that doubles as a seat and can be folded flat.

Victims are kept in isolation until no diphtheria bacilli can be detected in the nose and throat (by swabs taken on six consecutive days).

Diplopia
The medical term for *double vision*.

Dipsomania
A form of *alcohol dependence* in which periods of excessive drinking and craving for drink alternate with periods of relative sobriety.

Dipyridamole
A drug that reduces the stickiness of platelets in the *blood* and thus helps prevent the formation of abnormal blood clots within arteries.

Dipyridamole is used together with *ASA* or *warfarin* to prevent the formation of clots following *heart valve surgery*. It may also be given to people who have recently had a *myocardial infarction* (heart attack) or undergone *coronary artery bypass* surgery. Dipyridamole may also reduce the frequency of *transient ischemic attacks* (symptoms of stroke lasting less than 24 hours).

Possible adverse effects include headache, flushing, and dizziness.

Disability
A measurable physical or mental loss or impairment, which may be temporary or permanent.

A distinction may be made between disability and *handicap*, defining disability as the physical disorder (e.g., muscle weakness or blindness) and handicap as the extent to which a disorder impairs normal functioning. Thus two people with the same disability may suffer different degrees of handicap because one person manages to cope with everyday living better than the other. In practice, however, the distinction between disability and handicap is vague and the two terms are often used interchangeably. (See also illustrated box showing aids for the disabled; *Rehabilitation*.)

Discharge
A visible emission of fluid from an orifice or a break in the skin (such as a wound or burst boil). Discharge may be a normal occurrence, such as some types of *vaginal discharge*, or may be due to infection or inflammation, such as occurs in *rhinitis* (inflammation of the lining of the nose), *urethritis* (infection of the urethra), and *proctitis* (infection of the rectum).

Disclosing agents
Dyes that make the *plaque* deposits on teeth more visible so that they can be

D

Plaque revealed by disclosing agent
Bacteria, mucus, and food debris build up quickly as plaque if teeth are not brushed and flossed regularly.

seen and removed. When giving information about *oral hygiene*, a dentist or dental hygienist may apply a disclosing solution to the teeth to show the presence of harmful dental plaque and pellicle (a film formed from saliva), and to demonstrate an effective method of tooth cleaning.

Discolored teeth

Teeth tend naturally to darken with age. The red pulp tissue in the center of the tooth, which makes young teeth look bright, gradually recedes while at the same time more dentin is laid down around it, resulting in the tooth's dull yellow color.

Both the tooth's surface and its internal structures are liable to be stained by a variety of substances introduced into the mouth or carried by the blood supply.

Extrinsic stains, which are those found on the tooth's surface, are common, but are usually easily removed by polishing and can be prevented by regular tooth cleaning. However, intrinsic stains, those within the tooth's substance, are permanent. Many stains, both extrinsic and intrinsic, can be covered or diminished with cosmetic dental procedures, such as *bonding* and *bleaching*.

EXTRINSIC NONMETALLIC STAINS

BROWNISH-BLACK DEPOSIT Smoking tobacco or chewing betel nuts can lead to staining due to accumulation of tars and resins. The discoloration may be worse on the inside surfaces of the teeth.

BLACK STAIN A firmly attached black or brown line, close to and following the contour of the gum, usually on the inside surfaces of the upper back teeth. More common in children, it is thought to be due to pigment-producing bacteria.

GREEN STAIN A heavy, "furry," grayish-green stain, firmly attached close to the gum, usually on the front surfaces of the upper front teeth. It is most commonly found in children and may be due to staining of remnants of developmental membrane by color-producing bacteria.

DULL YELLOW STAIN This may be due to discoloration of *plaque* by dyes in foodstuffs; it is easily removed.

BROWN SPOTS Dark areas near the gum line may be due to areas of thinned enamel becoming stained by tea or other foods. Brown coloration may also result if the areas become remineralized (i.e., if the enamel is built up again through deposition of calcium and phosphate from saliva).

ORANGE-RED STAIN This may be caused by pigment-producing bacteria; it is easily removed.

STAINED DENTIN With advancing age, the full thickness of enamel may be worn away in parts and the dentin becomes stained by dyes in foods.

EXTRINSIC METALLIC STAINS

Stains of this type may follow the use of medicines containing metallic salts. Iron-containing liquids stain the teeth brown. Inhalation of metallic dust by metal workers (prior to stringent safety measures) caused accumulation of metals in the plaque. Brass, copper, lead, bronze, and other copper alloys caused a bluish-green stain, iron produced brown staining, and mercury led to black staining.

INTRINSIC STAINS

BLACK TEETH Teeth may darken following the death of the pulp or the removal of the pulp during *root canal treatment*. Darkening is caused by the decomposition of red blood cells that pass from damaged blood vessels in the pulp into the dentin.

TETRACYCLINE STAINING The antibiotic *tetracycline* causes discoloration of primary or permanent teeth. Which teeth are affected depends on the stage of tooth development, the amount taken, and the type of tetracycline prescribed. Tetracycline given to a pregnant woman often causes discoloration of her child's teeth. If mildly affected, the teeth will appear yellow but, if severely affected, they will be brown or blue-violet.

After the age of 7 years, discoloration is less likely to occur, because all the crowns of the important teeth are already formed.

FLUOROSIS Mottling of the tooth enamel occurs if excessive amounts of fluoride are taken during development of the enamel (see *Fluorosis*).

OTHER CAUSES *Hepatitis* during infancy may cause yellow-brown discoloration of the primary teeth due to the inclusion of bile pigments in the developing teeth. The teeth of children with *congenital* malformation of the *bile ducts* may be similarly affected. Congenital erythropoietic *porphyria* (a rare inherited disorder) causes reddish-brown or purple discoloration.

Disinfectants

Substances that kill microorganisms and thus prevent infection. The term is usually applied to strong chemicals that are harmful to human tissue and so are used to decontaminate inanimate objects, such as items of medical equipment. Decontaminants that are safe for human tissue are known as *antiseptics*.

Disk, intervertebral

A flat, circular, platelike structure containing *cartilage* which lines the joints between adjacent *vertebrae* (bones) in the *spine*.

Each intervertebral disk is composed of a hard, outer layer and a soft, jellylike core. The material acts as a shock absorber to cushion the vertebrae during movements of the spine, and to minimize jarring when jumping or running.

With increasing age, intervertebral disks may wear out, becoming less supple and more susceptible to damage from injury. One of the most common forms of damage is a *disk prolapse*, in which part of the disk's soft center bulges out through a weak area in the hard, outer layer. This may compress a spinal nerve root and produce symptoms, such as muscle weakness and/or pain in the back and leg.

Diskography

A diagnostic technique in which a contrast medium visible on *X-ray* films is injected into an invertebral disk, one of the shock-absorbing structures between adjacent *vertebrae* (bones of the *spine*).

WHY IT IS DONE

Diskography is one of the methods used to diagnose *disk prolapse*. Ordinary X-ray films fail to show the disks, which appear on the film only as spaces between the vertebrae.

HOW IT IS DONE

The patient is given a local anesthetic. A long thin needle is passed, under X-ray guidance, through the skin into the disk so that the contrast medium can be injected into the disk. X-ray pictures are then taken. Occasionally the site of the injection is sore afterward, but the pain usually disappears fairly quickly.

RESULTS
The image obtained provides only a rough outline of the disk, but reveals clearly any leakage of contrast medium if the disk is ruptured. In some people the rupture may be due to small tears in the disk rather than to a prolapse. If the procedure causes pain in the spine, and sciatica (pain down the back of a leg) or arm pain, there is a strong possibility that there is a disk prolapse.

Because of its relative imprecision, diskography is of more limited use than *CT scanning* or *myelography.*

Disk prolapse
A common, painful disorder of the *spine,* in which an invertebral *disk* ruptures and part of its pulpy core protrudes, causing painful and at times disabling pressure on a nerve.

About 95 percent of disk prolapses occur in the lower back, but they can affect any part of the back or the neck.

CAUSES AND INCIDENCE
Although a prolapsed disk may sometimes be caused by a sudden strenuous action (such as lifting a heavy weight), it usually develops gradually as a result of degeneration of the disks with age. People between the ages of 30 and 40 are the most likely victims. Over the age of 30, disks start to dehydrate and become less resilient but, after 40, extra fibrous tissue forms around them, increasing their stability. Disk prolapses are slightly more common in men than in women, and their incidence is higher in people who spend long periods sitting without a break.

DIAGNOSIS
Many other disorders may cause back and leg pain or neck and arm pain, and various tests may be needed to arrive at a firm diagnosis. After the physician has examined the spine and tested movement and reflexes in the affected arm or leg, he or she may arrange for tests, including the following: *X rays, CT scanning, myelography* (X ray after injection of a radiopaque substance around the spinal cord), *diskography* (X ray after injection of a radiopaque substance into a disk), and *EMG* (tests of electrical activity in the muscles).

If a certain nerve root is suspected of being compressed, a local anesthetic may be injected into its lining; if this relieves the pain, the location of the trouble is confirmed.

SYMPTOMS AND TREATMENT OF DISK PROLAPSE

A prolapsed disk in the lower back causes low back pain and, if the sciatic nerve root is compressed, *sciatica* (pain running down the back of the leg from the buttock to the ankle), sometimes accompanied by numbness and tingling. Low back pain and sciatica are usually aggravated by coughing, sneezing, bending, and sitting for long periods. Prolonged pressure on the sciatic nerve can lead to weakness in the muscles of the leg.

A prolapsed disk in the neck causes neck pain, stiffness, and, if the root of a nerve that is in the arm is compressed, tingling and weakness in that arm and hand.

In rare cases, pressure is exerted on the spinal cord itself, sometimes leading to paralysis of the legs and loss of bladder or bowel control.

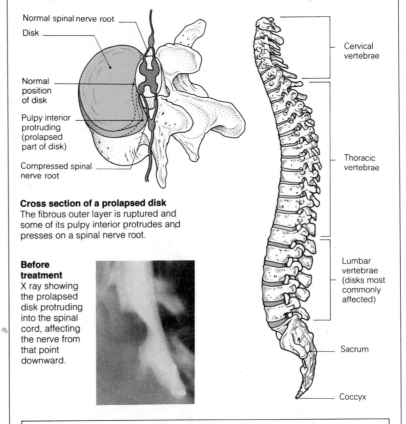

Normal spinal nerve root
Disk
Normal position of disk
Pulpy interior protruding (prolapsed part of disk)
Compressed spinal nerve root

Cervical vertebrae
Thoracic vertebrae
Lumbar vertebrae (disks most commonly affected)
Sacrum
Coccyx

Cross section of a prolapsed disk
The fibrous outer layer is ruptured and some of its pulpy interior protrudes and presses on a spinal nerve root.

Before treatment
X ray showing the prolapsed disk protruding into the spinal cord, affecting the nerve from that point downward.

TREATMENT
Disk prolapse often responds to bed rest (lying flat on the back on a firm mattress for a few weeks) and analgesics; later, a supportive collar or corset and special exercises are helpful. If these measures fail and the nerve root compression is producing muscle weakness, an operation may relieve the pressure (see *Decompression, spinal canal*).

Shoulders, hips, and ankles should be aligned to ease pressure on spine

D

TREATMENT
In most cases, symptoms are relieved by bed rest and a variety of other measures (see box on previous page). However, if the pain is persistent, if muscle function is impaired, or if bladder or bowel functions are impaired, surgical techniques, such as decompression of the spinal canal (see *Decompression, spinal canal*) or *chemonucleolysis* may be necessary.

Disk, slipped
See *Disk prolapse*.

Dislocation, joint
Complete displacement of the two bones in a joint so that they are no longer in contact, usually as a result of injury. (Displacement that leaves the bones in partial contact is called *subluxation*.) Dislocation is usually accompanied by tearing of the joint ligaments and damage to the joint capsule (the membrane that encases the joint); it is the tearing that makes the injury so painful. Injury severe enough to cause dislocation often also causes fracture of one or both of the bones involved.

SYMPTOMS AND COMPLICATIONS
Dislocation restricts or prevents the movement of the joint and is usually accompanied by severe pain. The joint looks misshapen and soon swells. In some cases, dislocation is followed by complications. For example, dislocation of the spinal vertebrae resulting from a severe back injury can damage the spinal cord, sometimes causing paralysis below the point of injury. Dislocation of the shoulder or hip joint can damage major nerves in the arm or leg, which again sometimes results in paralysis.

Rarely, the tissue around a dislocated joint, usually the shoulder, becomes so weakened that after the joint has mended only minimal pressure causes another dislocation.

TREATMENT
FIRST AID A person without medical qualifications should not attempt to manipulate the joint back into position because of the risk of seriously damaging nerves around the joint or making an accompanying fracture worse. A *splint* or, in the case of a dislocated shoulder, a *sling* should be applied to prevent movement of the joint. The victim should not take any food or drink because a general anesthetic will probably be required when the bones are reset.

PROFESSIONAL The joint is usually first X-rayed to see whether a fracture is present. Then the bones are manipulated back into their proper position as quickly as possible, or, when manipulation is not feasible, an operation may be performed to reset them. After either procedure, the joint is usually immobilized by means of a splint or plaster cast to allow it to heal without disturbance. Recurrent dislocation is treated by surgery to shorten and tighten the ligaments of the joint, thus strengthening it.

Disopyramide
An *antiarrhythmic drug* used to treat abnormally rapid heartbeat, such as may occur after a *myocardial infarction* (heart attack). Disopyramide reduces the force of heart muscle contraction and, as a result, may occasionally aggravate preexisting *heart failure*. Other possible adverse effects of the drug include dry mouth, constipation, and blurred vision.

Disorientation
Confusion as to time, place, or personal identity. The experience is similar to being awakened from a deep sleep. The disoriented person's speech and behavior tend to be muddled, and he or she is often unable to answer simple questions about time, date, present location, name, or address.

Disorientation is usually caused by *head injury*, *intoxication*, or a chronic brain disorder, such as *dementia*. It may occasionally be due to *somatization disorder* (a psychological illness). (See also *Confusion; Delirium*.)

Displacement activity
The transference of feelings from one object or person to another. This is usually a conscious act, performed to obtain emotional relief in a manner that will not cause harm to oneself or to another person. For example, a person who is angry may hit a wall or throw something rather than risk harming someone else.

Displacement is regarded as an unconscious *defense mechanism*, by some psychotherapists. Disturbing or unwelcome feelings are prevented from entering consciousness by being transferred to another person or object. An understanding of this unconscious process is an important part of the interpretation of a patient's dreams during *psychoanalysis*.

Dissociative disorders
A group of psychological illnesses in which a particular mental function becomes cut off from the mind as a whole. Although the process of dissociation is common in everyday life (e.g., not hearing what is said because of concentration on another task), it can lead to serious problems. A common type of dissociative disorder is hysterical amnesia. The affected person is unable to remember personal history, but can still speak, read, and learn new material (see *Hysteria*). Other forms of this disorder are *fugue, depersonalization*, and *multiple personality*. (See also *Conversion disorder*.)

Distal
A term describing a part of the body that is further away from another part with respect to a central point of reference, such as the trunk. For example, the fingers are distal to the arm with the trunk as the reference point. The opposite of distal is *proximal*.

Disulfiram
A drug that acts as a deterrent to drinking *alcohol*. Disulfiram is prescribed for people who request help for *alcohol dependence*. It is usually combined with a counseling program.

HOW IT WORKS
Alcohol is normally converted in the liver to acetaldehyde, which in turn is broken down to form acetic acid. Disulfiram slows down the breakdown of acetaldehyde, resulting in an increased level of this toxic substance which causes flushing, headache, nausea, dizziness, and palpitations. These unpleasant symptoms usually start within an hour of drinking alcohol and can last for several hours.

POSSIBLE ADVERSE EFFECTS
Drowsiness and a metallic or garlic taste in the mouth frequently occur, but usually disappear within a few days. Large amounts of alcohol taken during treatment can cause unconsciousness, so anyone taking disulfiram should carry a card to that effect.

Dithranol
See *Anthralin*.

Diuretic drugs

COMMON DRUGS

Thiazide
Bendroflumethiazide Chlorthalidone Hydrochlorothiazide

Loop
Ethacrynic acid Furosemide

Potassium-sparing
Amiloride Spironolactone Triamterene

A group of drugs that help remove excess water from the body by increasing the amount lost as *urine*. All diuretics act on the kidneys, the organs that govern the body's water content.

TYPES

The various types of diuretic drug differ markedly in their speed and mode of action.

THIAZIDE DIURETICS These diuretics cause moderate diuresis (increased urine production) and are suitable for prolonged use.

LOOP DIURETICS So called because they act on the region of the kidneys called Henle's loop, these are fast-acting, powerful drugs, especially when given by injection. Loop diuretics are particularly useful as an emergency treatment for *heart failure*.

POTASSIUM-SPARING DIURETICS These are often used along with thiazide and loop diuretics, both of which may cause potassium deficiency.

CARBONIC ANHYDRASE INHIBITORS Drugs that block the action of carbonic anhydrase (an enzyme that affects the amount of bicarbonate ions in the blood); these diuretic drugs cause moderate diuresis but are effective only for short periods.

OSMOTIC DIURETICS These are powerful diuretics that are used to maintain urine production after serious injury or major surgery.

WHY THEY ARE USED

By increasing the production of urine, diuretic drugs reduce the amount of water in the circulation and thus reduce the *edema* (fluid retention in tissues) that causes breathlessness and ankle swelling in *heart failure*, *nephrotic syndrome* (a kidney disorder), and *cirrhosis* of the liver. Diuretics can also relieve bloating and breast tenderness in *premenstrual syndrome*.

Diuretic drugs lower the blood pressure and are therefore used in the treatment of *hypertension* (high blood pressure). Carbonic anhydrase inhibitors are sometimes used to treat *glaucoma* (abnormally high fluid pressure in the eyeball).

POSSIBLE ADVERSE EFFECTS

Diuretic drugs may cause chemical imbalances in the blood, most commonly hypokalemia (low levels of potassium in the blood). Symptoms of this condition include weakness, confusion, and palpitations. Treatment usually consists of a course of potassium supplements or a potassium-sparing diuretic drug. A diet rich in potassium (containing plenty of fruits and vegetables) may be helpful.

Some diuretic drugs may raise the level of uric acid in the blood, and thus increase the risk of *gout*. Certain types of diuretics increase the blood sugar level, an effect that can cause or aggravate *diabetes mellitus*.

Diurnal rhythms

A biological pattern based on a daily cycle; also called *circadian rhythms*. (See also *Biorhythms*.)

Diverticula

Small sacs or pouches that protrude externally from the wall of a hollow organ (such as the colon or the esophagus). Diverticula are thought to be caused by pressure forcing the lining of the organ through areas of weakness in the wall. The presence of diverticula in the walls of the intestines is the characteristic feature of *diverticular disease*.

Diverticular disease

The presence of small externally protruding sacs or pouches known as *diverticula* in the wall of the intestines and any symptoms or complications caused by their presence.

Diverticula may form in any part of the intestine but usually affect the lower part of the *colon* (the major section of the large intestine). The cause is not conclusively established, but diverticula are thought to arise when pressure forces the lining of the colon through areas of weakness in the intestinal wall.

The term *diverticulosis* merely signifies the presence of diverticula in the intestine. *Diverticulitis* is a complication produced by inflammation due to obstruction and, occasionally, perforation (formation of a hole) in one or more diverticula.

Diverticulitis

Inflammation of *diverticula* in the intestine, particularly in the *colon*. It is a form of *diverticular disease* and a complication of *diverticulosis*.

Diverticulitis is associated with perforation (rupture) of diverticula and may lead to the formation of abscesses in the tissue around the colon. In exceptional circumstances, perforation may lead to *peritonitis* (inflammation of the lining of the abdomen). Bleeding of the intestinal wall may occur. Other complications of diverticulitis include the development of a stricture (narrowed section) in the intestine, or

---

HOW DIURETICS WORK

The normal filtration process of the kidneys (which takes place in the tubules) removes water, salts (mainly potassium and sodium), and waste products from the bloodstream. Most of the salts and water are returned to the bloodstream, but certain amounts are expelled from the body along with the waste products in the urine.

Diuretic drugs interfere with this normal kidney action. Osmotic, loop, and thiazide diuretics reduce the amount of sodium and water taken back into the blood, thus increasing urine volume. Other diuretics increase blood flow through the kidneys and thus the amount of water they filter and expel in the urine.

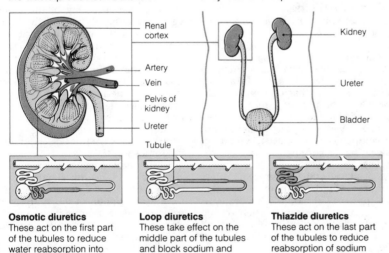

Renal cortex
Artery
Vein
Pelvis of kidney
Ureter
Tubule

Kidney
Ureter
Bladder

Osmotic diuretics
These act on the first part of the tubules to reduce water reabsorption into the bloodstream.

Loop diuretics
These take effect on the middle part of the tubules and block sodium and chloride reabsorption.

Thiazide diuretics
These act on the last part of the tubules to reduce reabsorption of sodium into the bloodstream.

D

of a *fistula*, an abnormal channel that connects the affected part of the intestine to another part of the intestine or to the bladder or vagina.

SYMPTOMS AND SIGNS

Diverticulitis may cause fever, vomiting, abdominal pain, and rigidity of the abdomen over the area of the intestine involved. An abscess may be felt as a tender lump when a physician examines the abdomen. Intestinal hemorrhage may produce bleeding from the rectum.

TREATMENT

Diverticulitis usually subsides with bed rest and *antibiotic drugs*. In severe cases, a liquid diet or *intravenous infusion* may be required. Surgical treatment may be needed if perforation causes a large abscess or peritonitis, if bleeding cannot be controlled, or if a stricture develops. In most cases requiring surgery, the diseased section of the intestine is removed and the remaining sections are joined together.

Some patients are given a temporary *colostomy* (an operation in which part of the colon is brought to the abdominal wall to form an opening for the discharge of feces).

Diverticulosis

The presence of *diverticula* in the intestine, particularly in the *colon*. Diverticulosis is a form of *diverticular disease*. Complications, which are uncommon, include intestinal hemorrhage and *diverticulitis*.

CAUSES AND INCIDENCE

Lack of adequate dietary fiber (see *Fiber, dietary*) is believed to play an important role in the development of diverticulosis. The incidence of the condition increases with age: it is rare before the age of 20 but is found in more than half of all people in North America and Western Europe who are 80 years of age or older. In developing countries, however, diverticulosis is very rare.

SYMPTOMS

Symptoms occur in only 20 percent of patients with diverticulosis and usually result from spasm or cramp of the intestinal muscle near diverticula.

Many patients have symptoms of *irritable bowel syndrome*, which may coexist with diverticulosis. In such patients, symptoms include a bloated sensation, episodes of pain in the lower abdomen, and changes in bowel habits (constipation, diarrhea, or alternating attacks of both).

Intestinal hemorrhage may produce bleeding from the rectum.

X ray showing diverticulosis
In this X ray, taken after a barium meal, the bright, winding tube is the patient's colon. The knobs on its outer surface are diverticula.

DIAGNOSIS

Diverticula of the colon are easily diagnosed by *barium X-ray examination* or by *colonoscopy* (inspection of the colon with a flexible viewing instrument). A physician should also investigate the possibility of cancer of the large intestine (see *Colon, cancer of; Rectum, cancer of*) in patients with symptoms of diverticulosis; tumors developing in affected areas may be difficult to diagnose.

TREATMENT

In patients with muscle spasms that cause cramps, a high fiber diet, fiber supplements, and *antispasmodic drugs* may relieve symptoms. A high fiber diet has also been shown to reduce the incidence of complications. Bleeding from diverticula usually subsides without treatment, but occasionally requires surgical treatment such as that for diverticulitis. Otherwise, surgery is rarely necessary.

Diving medicine

See *Scuba-diving medicine; Decompression sickness*.

Dizziness

A sensation of unsteadiness and lightheadedness. Dizziness may be a mild, brief symptom that occurs by itself, or it may be part of a more severe, prolonged attack of *vertigo* (characterized by a spinning sensation) accompanied by nausea, vomiting, sweating, or fainting.

CAUSES

Most attacks of dizziness are harmless and are caused by a momentary fall in the pressure of blood to the brain, as can occur, for example, when getting up quickly from a sitting or lying position (a phenomenon called *postural hypotension*). Postural hypotension is more common in the elderly and in people taking *antihypertensive drugs* to

treat high blood pressure. Similar symptoms may result from a temporary, partial blockage in the arteries that supply the brain—a *transient ischemic attack* (symptoms of stroke lasting less than 24 hours).

Other causes of dizziness include tiredness, stress, fever, *anemia, heart block* (impairment of electrical activity within the heart muscle, causing slow, uncoordinated beating of the individual heart chambers), *hypoglycemia* (low blood sugar level), and *subdural hemorrhage* (bleeding between the outer two membranes that cover the brain).

Dizziness as part of vertigo is usually due to a disorder of the inner ear, the *acoustic nerve*, or the *brain stem*.

The principal disorders of the inner ear that can cause dizziness and vertigo are *labyrinthitis* and *Ménière's disease*. In labyrinthitis, the labyrinth (the fluid-filled canals in the inner ear which play a vital role in balance) becomes inflamed, usually as a result of a viral infection. In severe cases, any movement of the head causes vomiting and fainting. In Meniere's disease (a degenerative disease of the inner ear), the dizziness and vertigo are often associated with *deafness* and *tinnitus* (noises in the ear).

Disorders of the acoustic nerve are relatively rare causes of dizziness and vertigo. They include *acoustic neuroma* and cases of *meningitis* in which the acoustic nerve is affected.

Disorders of the brain stem that can cause dizziness and vertigo include *migraine* that involves blood vessels in the brain stem; *brain tumors* that press on the brain stem; and *vertebrobasilar insufficiency* (narrowing of the blood vessels that supply part of the brain stem). Vertebrobasilar insufficiency, which is often due to *cervical osteoarthritis* (arthritis of the neck region of the spine), produces pain and dizziness on turning the head or moving the neck.

DIAGNOSIS AND TREATMENT

Brief episodes of mild dizziness usually clear up after taking a few deep breaths, or, if this fails, after resting for a short time.

Severe, prolonged, or recurrent dizziness should be investigated by a physician, who will make a diagnosis from a description of the symptoms, from a physical examination, and, in some cases, from the results of further diagnostic tests.

Treatment, when necessary, depends on the underlying cause. For example, certain cases of dizziness

DIZZINESS A sense of being dazed and unsteady sometimes accompanied by a sensation of spinning.

D

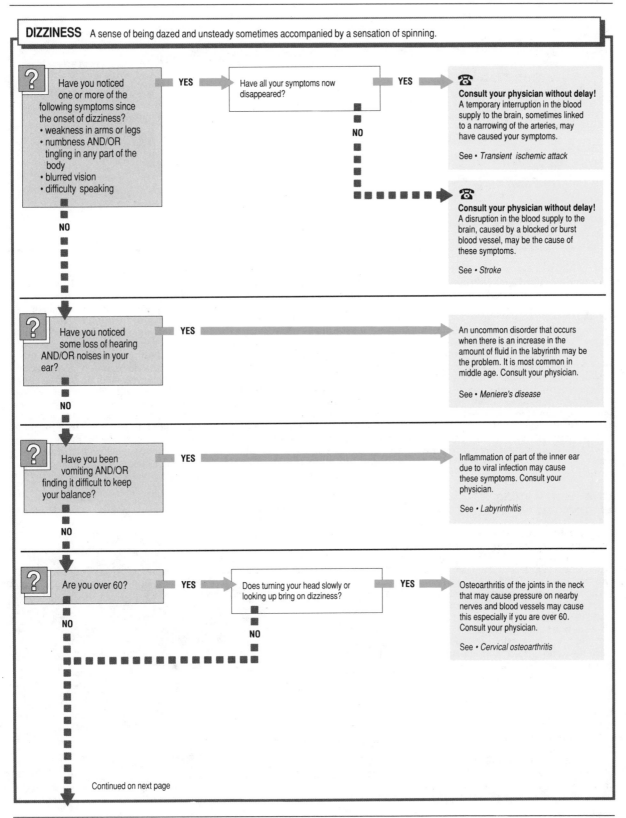

Have you noticed one or more of the following symptoms since the onset of dizziness?
• weakness in arms or legs
• numbness AND/OR tingling in any part of the body
• blurred vision
• difficulty speaking

YES → Have all your symptoms now disappeared?

YES → ☎ **Consult your physician without delay!** A temporary interruption in the blood supply to the brain, sometimes linked to a narrowing of the arteries, may have caused your symptoms.

See • *Transient ischemic attack*

NO → ☎ **Consult your physician without delay!** A disruption in the blood supply to the brain, caused by a blocked or burst blood vessel, may be the cause of these symptoms.

See • *Stroke*

NO

Have you noticed some loss of hearing AND/OR noises in your ear?

YES → An uncommon disorder that occurs when there is an increase in the amount of fluid in the labyrinth may be the problem. It is most common in middle age. Consult your physician.

See • *Meniere's disease*

NO

Have you been vomiting AND/OR finding it difficult to keep your balance?

YES → Inflammation of part of the inner ear due to viral infection may cause these symptoms. Consult your physician.

See • *Labyrinthitis*

NO

Are you over 60?

YES → Does turning your head slowly or looking up bring on dizziness?

YES → Osteoarthritis of the joints in the neck that may cause pressure on nearby nerves and blood vessels may cause this especially if you are over 60. Consult your physician.

See • *Cervical osteoarthritis*

NO

NO

Continued on next page

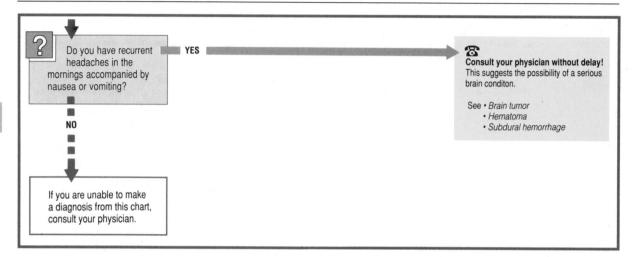

Do you have recurrent headaches in the mornings accompanied by nausea or vomiting?

YES

☎ **Consult your physician without delay!**
This suggests the possibility of a serious brain conditon.

See • *Brain tumor*
• *Hematoma*
• *Subdural hemorrhage*

NO

If you are unable to make a diagnosis from this chart, consult your physician.

and vertigo due to a disorder of the inner ear may be treated with *antiemetic drugs* or with *antihistamine drugs*.

DNA

The commonly used abbreviation for deoxyribonucleic acid, the principal molecule carrying genetic information in almost all organisms; the exceptions are certain viruses that use *RNA* (ribonucleic acid) to carry genetic information. DNA is found in the *chromosomes* of cells; its double-helix structure allows the chromosomes to be copied exactly during the process of cell division. (See also *Nucleic acids*.)

DNA fingerprinting
See *Genetic fingerprinting*.

Dogs, diseases from
A number of infectious or parasitic diseases may be acquired from contact with dogs. Such diseases may be caused by viruses, bacteria, fungi, protozoa, worms, insects, or mites.

Dogs and humans share various parasites. Many of these parasites show a marked preference for dogs, but may accidentally transfer to humans who stroke a dog's fur or touch contaminated feces.

Overall, diseases contracted from dogs, especially the more serious ones, are uncommon and must be looked at together with the psychological benefits and pleasure that owners derive from their pets.

SPECIFIC DISEASES
The most serious disease that can be caught from a dog is *rabies*, usually transmitted by a bite. Dog bites can also cause serious bleeding and shock.

Two potentially serious, although rare, diseases caused by the ingestion of worm eggs from dogs are *toxocariasis* and *hydatid disease*. Toxocariasis is mainly an infection of children. The passage of worm larvae through the body can cause allergic symptoms, such as *asthma*, and, rarely, a larva may lodge in an eye and cause blindness. Hydatid disease can lead to the harmful presence of cysts in the liver, lungs, brain, or elsewhere. Usually, however, sheep, not people, pick up the infection and then reinfect dogs.

In the tropics, walking barefoot on sand or soil previously contaminated with dog feces can lead to infection with dog *hookworms*.

Bites from dog *fleas* are an occasional nuisance. The fleas inhabit places in a house where the dog habitually rests and, if the dog is absent, may jump onto humans for a meal. *Ticks* and *mites* from dogs, including a canine version of the *scabies* mite, are other common problems. The fungi that cause *tinea* (ringworm) infections cause progressive hair loss in dogs and can be caught by humans.

Some people become allergic to animal *dander* (tiny scales derived from fur or skin and present in household dust) and have such symptoms as asthma or *urticaria* (hives) when a dog is in the house. (See also *Cats, diseases from; Zoonoses*.)

Ticks and fleas
Ticks may transfer from a dog's fur; fleas inhabit the pet's resting places and can cause irritating bites.

Worms and eggs
Worm eggs in dog feces are a more serious danger than adult worms.

Transmission of infection
Transmission from feces occurs when a person (often a child) directly handles a dog's feces or anus (or contaminates his or her fingers with fecal material from the soil or from the dog's fur) and transfers infective

Dander
Tiny scales from dog fur (known as dander) may cause an allergic reaction if they are inhaled.

organisms to his or her mouth. Infection can also occur from eating food that has been contaminated with dog feces. Other means of transferring infection are through saliva and direct contact with an infected dog.

D

Domperidone

An *antiemetic drug* used to relieve the nausea and vomiting that occurs in some gastrointestinal disorders or during treatment with *anticancer drugs* or *radiation therapy*. Adverse effects of the drug, which are rare, may include breast enlargement and secretion of milk from the breast.

Donor

A person who provides blood for transfusion, tissues or organs for transplantation, or semen for artificial insemination.

Many individuals carry donor cards to indicate that they have bequeathed all or parts of their bodies to be used, should they die unexpectedly, for the treatment of others. The bequest may also be made by the next of kin at the time of death.

Donors should be free of cancer (other than primary brain cancer), should be free of serious infection (such as hepatitis B), and should not carry HIV (the AIDS virus). Organs are usually taken from people between the ages of 3 and 65.

In general, organs for transplantation must be removed within a few hours of *brain death*, and before or immediately after the heartbeat has stopped. An organ is used only if it is completely healthy.

In about one third of kidney transplants, the kidney is provided by a living donor. The living volunteer is usually a sibling or parent whose body tissues match well on the basis of *tissue typing*. Tests are performed to make sure that both kidneys are healthy before one is removed for transplantation. A healthy donor's life is not shortened because the remaining kidney grows to compensate for the kidney that has been removed.

Suitable related donors whose tissue types match may also provide bone marrow for transplantation and sometimes skin for grafting. (See also *Artificial insemination; Blood donation; Bone marrow transplant; Organ donation; Transplant surgery*.)

Do not resuscitate

If a patient has a severe, progressive, and irreversible disease, a physician may write an order to the hospital staff not to carry out heroic measures to reestablish heartbeats or respiration, should either of them cease. Such an order can only be written at the request of the patient, or, if the patient is not competent, at the request of the next of kin.

COMMONLY DONATED BODY PARTS

The organs that are most frequently donated are kidneys, corneas, heart, lungs, liver, and pancreas.

Blood for transfusion and semen for artificial insemination are also given by donors.

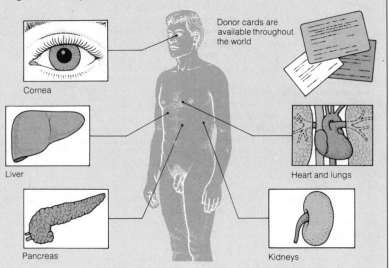

Donor cards are available throughout the world

Cornea

Liver

Pancreas

Heart and lungs

Kidneys

Dopamine

A *neurotransmitter* (chemical released from nerve endings) found in the brain and around some blood vessels. Dopamine blocks activity in specific nerves and is important in the control of body movements. A deficiency of dopamine in the *basal ganglia* (groups of nerve cells deep within the brain) causes *Parkinson's disease*.

Synthetic dopamine is injected as an emergency treatment for shock caused by a *myocardial infarction* (heart attack) or *septicemia* (blood infection) and as a treatment for severe *heart failure* that has not responded to other drugs. Dopamine increases the efficiency of the heartbeat and helps return the blood pressure to normal.

Doppler effect

A change in the frequency with which waves from a given source reach an observer when the source is in rapid motion with respect to the observer.

When a fast-moving train blows its whistle as it passes through a station, a person standing on the platform hears an apparent increase in pitch (frequency) as the train approaches and then a lowering of pitch as the train passes and is moving away. In fact, the whistle gives off a constant pitch, but it seems to rise and then fall to the person on the platform because the wavelengths of the sound from the approaching train are progres-

sively foreshortened whereas the wavelengths from the receding train are stretched. This change in the perceived frequency of sound as a result of movement is called the Doppler effect or Doppler shift.

The Doppler effect is utilized in various medical *ultrasound scanning* techniques. In these techniques, an emitter sends out pulses of ultrasound (inaudible high-frequency sound) of a specific frequency. When these pulses bounce off a moving object—blood flowing through a blood vessel or the beating heart of a fetus in the uterus, for example—the frequency of the echoes is changed from that of the emitted sound (the Doppler effect in action). A special sensor detects the frequency changes and, for the examples above, converts this data into information about how fast the blood is flowing, for example, or the rate at which the fetal heart is beating.

Doppler ultrasound techniques are also used to measure blood pressure in superficial blood vessels and to detect air bubbles in *dialysis* and *heart-lung machines*.

Dorsal

Relating to the back, located on or near the back, or describing the uppermost part of a body structure when a person is lying facedown. For example, dorsalgia is pain in the back, and the dorsal part of the hand is the back of the hand. In human anatomy, the term dorsal means the same as posterior. The opposite of dorsal is *ventral* (anterior or front).

Dose

A term used to refer to the amount of a drug taken at a particular time, or to the amount of radiation an individual is exposed to during one session of *radiation therapy*.

DRUG DOSE

The dose of a drug can be expressed in several ways: in terms of the weight of its active substance, usually in milligrams; in terms of the volume of liquid to be drunk, usually in millilitres; or in terms of its biological activity potential (its effects on body tissues as calculated in a laboratory), a value usually given in units or international units.

It is not possible to compare the effects of two different drugs from the same group on the body simply by comparing the size of the doses. This is because some drugs are "stronger" (more potent) than others, just as various alcoholic drinks differ in their alcohol content.

RADIATION DOSE

The dose of radiation received during a session of radiation therapy is expressed in units called rads or grays (see *Radiation units* box). These units are a measure of the amount of radiation absorbed by body tissues. Different types of body tissue are able to absorb different amounts of energy from the same beam of radiation.

Double-blind

A type of *controlled trial*—the aim of which is to test the effectiveness of a treatment or to compare the benefits of different treatments. Double-blind trials differ from other types of controlled trials in that neither the patients taking part nor the physicians who assess the treatments know which patients are receiving which treatment. This eliminates any conscious or unconscious expectations (on the part of the patients and physicians) about which treatment will be most effective, which might affect the results of the trial.

For example, a new drug and an older, standard treatment might be compared by having the two drugs made up (by a person who otherwise takes no part in the trial) in identical capsules and giving them to different groups of patients on a random selection (chance) basis. The patients are later examined by one or more physicians. Only after all assessments have been made is the identity of the drug that was given to each patient revealed—usually by the person who originally prepared the capsules.

Double vision

The seeing of two instead of one visual image of a single object, also known as diplopia. This condition should not be confused with *blurred vision*.

CAUSES

Double vision is usually a symptom of a squint (a deviation or malalignment of the two eyes), although not all types of squint produce double vision. Paralytic squint is a type that commonly causes double vision; in this type, movement of the patient's eye in a particular direction is impaired due to paralysis of one or more of the eye muscles. Tilting or turning the head can sometimes overcome the double vision.

A tumor in the eyelid pressing on the front of the eyeball may cause temporary image separation by distorting the shape of the front of the eye and thus causing a slight displacement in the path of light rays entering that eye (and thus variation in the points at which they are focused on the retina). A tumor or blood clot behind the eye that prevents the normal movement of the eyeball may also be a cause of double vision.

In endocrine-related *exophthalmos*, protrusion of the eyeballs is the result of an underlying hormonal disorder. In exophthalmos, double vision results from swelling and weakness of the eye muscles, causing abnormal alignment and motion of the eyes.

Rarely, double vision arises because of an abnormality within the eye. For example, *lens dislocation* may cause some light rays to pass through the lens and others to pass around it, thereby causing separate images to fall on the retina.

Example of double vision
Two images, rather than a single image, are seen. Prompt investigation by a physician is required.

A child with a squint that may be causing double vision should be seen by a physician for diagnosis and treatment. Without treatment in early childhood, squint can lead to *amblyopia* (lazy eye).

The onset of double vision in adult life needs immediate investigation to exclude the possibility of a tumor, aneurysm, and/or nervous system abnormality. The double vision could be a symptom of a serious underlying disorder that requires prompt medical attention. Treatment depends on the cause.

Douche

Introduction of water and/or a cleansing agent into the vagina using equipment consisting of a bag and tubing with a nozzle attached.

In the past, douches were used by some women after sexual intercourse to cleanse the vagina and to try to prevent conception. They were also used by women who were worried about having excessive or offensive vaginal discharge. Douches were sometimes recommended to treat vaginal infections and were also used after vaginal repair operations.

Today, physicians rarely recommend douches for any reason. Douching is unnecessary for purposes of hygiene because the vagina is normally slightly acidic and cleans itself. As a method of *contraception*, douching is completely ineffective. Furthermore, use of a douche can be harmful, because it may introduce infection into the vagina or may spread an existing vaginal infection into the uterus or fallopian tubes.

Down's syndrome

A *chromosomal abnormality* resulting in mental handicap and a characteristic physical appearance. Down's syndrome was originally named "mongolism" because it was thought that the facial features of affected children resembled those of Mongolians. The term "mongolism" is no longer used by the medical profession.

CAUSES

The cause of Down's syndrome remained a mystery until 1959, when researchers discovered that each of the body cells of people with Down's syndrome has one too many chromosomes—47 instead of the normal 46. Because the extra chromosome is number 21 (affected individuals have three, instead of two, number 21 chromosomes), the disorder is also called trisomy 21.

There are several possible reasons for the chromosomal abnormality. In most cases it is the result of a failure of the two chromosomes numbered 21 in a parent cell to go into separate daughter cells during the first stage of sperm or egg cell formation (see *Chromosomes*). Some eggs or sperm are therefore formed with an extra number 21 chromosome and, if one of these takes part in fertilization, the resulting baby will also have the extra chromosome. This type of abnormality is particularly likely if the mother is aged over 35, suggesting that defective egg formation, rather than sperm formation, is usually at fault.

A less common cause is a chromosomal abnormality in either parent, known as a *translocation*, in which part of one of the parent's own number 21 chromosomes has joined with another chromosome. The parent is unaffected except for the high risk of having children with Down's syndrome. The chromosomal translocation may be familial, and relatives who are at risk of having an affected child should be tested by a blood sample for *chromosome analysis*.

INCIDENCE
About one in 650 babies born is affected by Down's syndrome. The incidence of affected fetuses rises steeply with increased maternal age to about one in 40 among mothers aged over 40. Pregnant women aged over 35, and those who have already had a child with Down's syndrome, are usually offered chromosome analysis of the fetus' cells by *amniocentesis* or *chorionic villus sampling*. Current research is looking at several chemical blood tests which may be used to screen all pregnant women for the condition.

SYMPTOMS
Most people with Down's syndrome have eyes that slope up at the outer corners and folds of skin on either side of the nose that cover the inner corners of the eye. The face and features are small, the tongue is large and tends to protrude, the head has a flattened back, and the hands are typically short and broad. The degree of mental handicap varies. A Down's syndrome child's IQ may be anywhere from 30 to 80. Virtually all affected children are capable of a limited amount of learning, including in some cases the ability to read. Down's syndrome children are usually affectionate, friendly, and cheerful, and they get along well with other members of the family.

Typical features
The eyes slope upward at the outer corners and the inner corners are covered, the facial features are small, and the tongue is large and tends to stick out. The back of the head is usually flat.

Inward-curving finger
— Single transverse crease

Down's syndrome

Normal

About one quarter of Down's syndrome children have a heart defect at birth (see *Heart disease, congenital*). They also have a higher-than-average incidence of intestinal *atresia* (narrowing at some point in the intestines), congenital *deafness*, and acute *leukemia*. Children with Down's syndrome are especially susceptible to repeated ear infections. Potential instability of joints in the neck make certain types of physical activity inadvisable. For unknown reasons, *atherosclerosis* (narrowing of arteries by deposits of fatty material), which leads to an increased risk of heart disease, tends to develop early in adults affected by Down's syndrome.

DIAGNOSIS
Because of the distinctive physical features, Down's syndrome is usually recognized soon after birth. The diagnosis is confirmed by a count of the chromosomes in white blood cells taken from a blood sample (see *Chromosome analysis*).

TREATMENT
There is no cure for the mental handicap, but Down's syndrome children can make the most of their capabilities through constant educational and environmental stimulation. Institutional care is sometimes necessary, but affected children are generally happiest in a sympathetic home environment. It is possible to alter the facial appearance by plastic surgery.

OUTLOOK
Until recently (less than a generation ago) most Down's syndrome children did not survive beyond their teens because of the high incidence of defects present from birth as well as their susceptibility to infection. Advances in medical and surgical techniques, together with improved long-term care facilities, have extended the life expectancy of sufferers from Down's syndrome, although they still tend not to survive beyond early middle age.

Doxepin
A tricyclic *antidepressant* useful in treating major depressive episodes. Doxepin has a stronger sedative effect than other antidepressants; this may be helpful if the patient has difficulty sleeping.

Doxorubicin
An *anticancer drug*, given by injection, usually in combination with other anticancer drugs. Doxorubicin is used to treat a variety of cancers, including *leukemia*, *Hodgkin's disease*, and *lung cancer*.

Doxycycline
A *tetracycline drug*. Doxycycline has been found to be more effective than most other tetracycline antibiotics in the treatment of chronic *prostatitis* (inflammation of the prostate), *pelvic inflammatory disease*, and attacks of chest infection in chronic *bronchitis*. Doxycycline is also used to treat severe attacks of traveler's diarrhea (see *Gastroenteritis*).

Because its action lasts longer than that of some other tetracyclines, doxycycline needs to be taken only once or twice a day.

Possible adverse effects—nausea and indigestion, for example—can be reduced by taking doxycycline with food; absorption of doxycycline, unlike that of many other tetracyclines, is not impaired if the drug is taken with food.

DPT vaccination
An injection that provides immunity against *diphtheria*, *pertussis* (whooping cough), and *tetanus*; also known as triple vaccine.

HOW IT IS DONE
DPT vaccine is given as a course of three injections at around the ages of 3, 5, and 9 months. The precise age at which the injections are given is variable. A booster dose of diphtheria and tetanus vaccine is given at nursery or

elementary school entry age. In Canada, almost all children are vaccinated before the age of 7.

WHY IT IS DONE

DPT vaccination causes the body to produce *antibodies* against diphtheria, pertussis, and tetanus infections. The vaccine does not provide complete immunity to diphtheria, but it does reduce the risk of serious illness with the infection. An adult exposed to a case of diphtheria and who has not had DPT in the past 10 years should receive a booster dose of the diphtheria component of the vaccine.

The pertussis vaccine does not provide absolute protection, but children who have been immunized suffer from only a mild version of the disease and are unlikely to become seriously ill, whereas the disease can be fatal in unimmunized children. The protection gradually wanes, so adults can get the infection. In adults, the disease is mild, but adults can infect unimmunized children.

Protection against tetanus is not permanent; it needs to be "boosted" with another shot every 10 years or at the time of any dirty, penetrating injury if vaccination has not been performed within the last five years.

RISKS

In the cases of diphtheria and tetanus, the life-threatening feature of the infection is a toxin (poison) produced by the bacteria. The vaccine contains toxoids—modified versions of the diphtheria and tetanus toxins—that stimulate the formation of antibodies. Because the toxoids are chemicals, not organisms, reactions to them are rare.

Pertussis vaccine consists of killed bacteria, which stimulate the formation of antibodies. It is more likely than the other components of the vaccine to provoke a reaction and commonly causes slight fever and some irritability for a couple of days after the vaccination. More serious reactions are *seizures* (convulsions) and an allergic reaction that may lead to breathing difficulty and *shock*. Such serious reactions are rare, and permanent damage from the vaccine is even rarer.

Physicians are now agreed that for most children, the benefits of DPT vaccination outweigh the minimal risk from the vaccine. Vaccination should be postponed if the child has a feverish illness. The pertussis element of the vaccine should not be given to children who have previously had a severe reaction to the vaccine, or to those who have certain nervous system disorders such as *epilepsy*.

Drain, surgical

An appliance inserted into a body cavity or wound to release air or to permit drainage.

TYPES

The simplest drains are soft rubber tubes that pass from a body cavity into a dressing. More sophisticated drains are wide-bore tubes that connect to a collection bag or bottle. A valve prevents air or fluid from passing back into the body. Another type, corrugated drains, have a series of curved ridges to help collect fluid from a wound. Suction drains consist of a thin tube with many small holes to help collect fluid or air, which is drawn into a vacuum bottle. Suction can also be applied to a drain by means of a vacuum pump. A T-shaped drain is used to remove bile from the biliary system after surgery.

Dream analysis

The interpretation of a person's dreams as part of *psychoanalysis* or *psychotherapy*. First developed by Sigmund Freud, the technique is based on the idea that a person's repressed feelings and thoughts are revealed in dreams, but in a disguised manner. The therapist unravels the significance of the dream by using a knowledge of the patient's character to interpret symbols, and by asking the patient for any associations suggested by the dream.

Dreaming

Mental activity that takes place during *sleep*. Evidence strongly suggests that dreaming occurs only during periods of REM (rapid eye movement) sleep, which last for about 20 minutes and occur four or five times a night.

PHYSIOLOGY

Although arguments about the exact function of dreams persist, the physiological aspects of dreams are well understood. By using an *EEG* to record the electrical activity of the brain, it is possible to describe various phases of sleep in terms of their different electrical patterns. Compared to other phases, the REM phase is active, as if the sleeper were awake but drowsy. Blood flow and brain temperature increase and there are sudden changes in heart rate and blood pressure. All this may indicate that the brain is restoring itself for further activity.

Dreaming can be seen as a parallel process in which the mental impressions, feelings, and ideas that have been taken in during the day are

TYPES OF DRAINS

Wide-bore drain

Corrugated drain

Perforated drain

T-shaped drain

sorted out. The content of dreams therefore closely represents the day's preoccupations—with the ideas and memories distorted by the lack of a conscious and awake mind.

People roused during periods of REM sleep report especially vivid dreams, but those who wake normally after normal dream activity has ended may not remember dreaming at all.

SIGNIFICANCE

As a proportion of total sleep, REM sleep is much greater in young babies and after head injury. This suggests that REM sleep may have an important role in promoting brain activity. Whether or not dreams have an important psychological role is more controversial. Depriving people of their dreams by constantly waking them during REM phases was once thought to cause severe psychological disorders, but this is now less generally accepted. Some *hypnotic drugs* suppress REM sleep without causing obvious psychological harm.

Dressings

Protective coverings for *wounds*. Dressings are placed directly onto wounds and may be used to control *bleeding*, to absorb secretions, or to prevent contamination by bacteria or foreign material such as dirt.

Dressings should be large enough to cover a wound completely. They should be sterile so that they do not introduce bacteria that could cause infection. A dressing should also be absorbent in order to prevent the accumulation of sweat; otherwise, the skin around the wound becomes moist and soft, thus encouraging infection. Unless a wound needs regular cleaning, dressings should be left undisturbed. Wounds should be covered for as short a time as possible.

APPLYING A DRESSING

The basic procedure for applying a dressing is shown in the illustrated box below.

TYPES

ADHESIVE BANDAGES Available in a range of sizes, these consist of absorbent pads held in place by waterproof adhesive backings. They are commonly used to protect small wounds, such as cuts and abrasions, but may also be used to cover surgical wounds.

GAUZE Usually applied in layers, gauze is made of cotton or a synthetic mate-rial and is used to cover larger wounds. It is held in place by a bandage or a length of adhesive tape. The gauze is usually applied dry, but ribbon gauze, soaked in a substance that promotes healing, may be used for packing deep wounds. Prepacked, sterile, unmedicated dressings consist of layers of fine gauze and a pad of absorbent cotton attached to a roller bandage.

NONSTICK DRESSINGS These dressings consist of a nonadherent contact layer of perforated polyethylene or viscose with an impregnated gauze pad back-ing. Such dressings do not adhere to wounds and can be removed without disturbing newly formed tissue.

IMPROVISED DRESSINGS In an emergency, almost any clean, dry, and absorbent material (e.g., a handkerchief or piece of sheeting) may be used to cover a wound if a sterile dressing is not avail-able. Cottonwool or other fibrous materials should not be used because the fibers may become embedded in the wound.

Dressler's syndrome

An uncommon condition, also called postinfarction syndrome, that may occur after a *myocardial infarction* (heart attack) or after heart surgery. The con-dition is characterized by fever, chest pain, *pericarditis* (inflammation of the membrane surrounding the heart), and *pleurisy* (inflammation of the membrane surrounding the lungs).

Dressler's syndrome is thought to be an *autoimmune disorder*. The body's immune system produces *antibodies* (proteins with a defensive role) which are directed against the damaged areas of heart muscle.

The features of the condition first appear any time between a few days and several weeks after a myocardial infarction or heart surgery. The diag-nosis is confirmed by detecting specif-ic antibodies in the blood. Treatment with *ASA* usually clears the condition, although, in some more severe cases, treatment with *corticosteroid drugs* is needed.

Dribbling

A term commonly used to denote involuntary leakage of urine (see *Incontinence, urinary*) or of saliva from the mouth.

Dribbling of saliva, also known as drooling, is normal behavior in infants up to the age of about 12 months. Dribbling of saliva in an adult may simply be due to poorly fitting den-tures or may be the result of facial paralysis, *dementia*, or another serious disorder of the nervous system, most commonly *Parkinson's disease*. Drib-bling of saliva may also be caused by obstruction to swallowing.

Drip

See *Intravenous infusion.*

Drop attack

A brief disturbance affecting the ner-vous system, causing a person to fall suddenly to the ground without warning. Unlike in *fainting*, the per-son may not lose consciousness, but injuries can occur to the hands, face, or knees as a result of the fall.

CAUSES AND INCIDENCE

Although drop attacks can affect all age groups, elderly women are the most commonly affected. The causes are not fully understood, although in some cases there may be a fall in blood flow to nerve centers in the *brain stem*.

FIRST AID: DRESSINGS

1 Remove outer protective wrapping, being careful not to touch the gauze. If possible, wash your hands before touching the unwrapped dressing. Then hold the dressing, gauze-side down, over the wound.

Assorted dressings
In addition to sterile dressings, plain gauze and a variety of adhesive bandages can be used.

2 Wind the short end of the bandage once around the arm and dressing. Bandage firmly (not tightly) and cover the gauze pad.

3 Secure by tying the bandage ends over the gauze pad using a reef, or square, knot (left end over right end, and under; right end over left end, and under).

D

Occasionally, elderly men may experience a drop attack while passing urine or while standing. Lowered blood pressure or an abrupt alteration in heart rhythm may be involved; it is advisable for a man who has previously had an attack to sit down while urinating.

Another rare cause of drop attacks is a block in the flow of cerebrospinal fluid around the brain, usually in patients with a type of *hydrocephalus*. Also sometimes described as drop attacks are akinetic seizures (a rare form of *epilepsy*), in which the sufferer falls suddenly to the ground and briefly loses consciousness but does not have muscular spasms.

TREATMENT
There is no treatment for drop attacks in the elderly. Akinetic seizures respond to *anticonvulsant drugs*.

Dropsy
An outmoded term for generalized *edema* (fluid collection in body tissues). In the past, many people were certified dead "due to dropsy," which, however, is not a disease in itself, but merely a sign of malfunction in the body (especially congestive *heart failure* or kidney disease).

Drowning
Death caused by suffocation and *hypoxia* (lack of oxygen) associated with immersion in a fluid.

In about four fifths of drownings the person has inhaled liquid into the lungs; in the other fifth, no liquid has entered the lungs—a condition called dry drowning (see *Drowning, dry*). People who are resuscitated after prolonged immersion are said to be victims of "near drowning."

INCIDENCE AND CAUSES
Drowning accounts for about 500 deaths a year in Canada. Many more are victims of near drowning. Worldwide, possibly as many as 200,000 people drown annually.

Many victims are competent swimmers who have failed to take into account factors such as tidal currents (or undertow) and have become tired, and then panicked. A relatively small number of victims are nonswimmers. Other drowning circumstances include floods, sinkings, immersion in very cold water after falling through ice, and infant drownings, which can occur in very shallow water. Even a few inches can be fatal.

Over one third of drowning victims have a significant amount of alcohol in their blood upon postmortem examination. Alcohol intoxication impairs judgment and at the same time reduces physical coordination—an extremely dangerous combination before swimming.

Some methods of minimizing the risks of a drowning accident are shown in the box below.

MECHANISM OF DROWNING
The thrashing movements that a panicking person makes at the surface of the water are incapable of keeping the body afloat, and the person begins taking in small amounts of water. Initially, automatic contraction of a muscle at the entrance to the windpipe—a mechanism called the laryngeal reflex—prevents water from entering the lungs and instead it enters the esophagus and stomach. However, the laryngeal reflex impairs breathing, which can quickly lead to hypoxia and to loss of consciousness.

If the person is buoyant at this point and floats face-up, his or her chances of survival are reasonable because the laryngeal reflex begins to relax and normal breathing may recommence.

FIRST AID AND TREATMENT
If a person is panicking at the surface of the water, he or she should be thrown any large item that will float. Ideally, the person in difficulties should be approached in a boat and reached out for. Approaching a panicky victim by swimming is extremely dangerous and may result in the deaths of both persons. Unless the victim is a child, unconscious, or injured, a swimming rescue without aids for towing or keeping the victim afloat should only be attempted by a person with adequate training. Even when the rescuer is trained in lifesaving, a rescue is safer and easier if the

---

DROWNING: RESCUE METHODS
Unless you are trained in lifesaving, or unless the victim is a child, is unconscious or is injured, never swim into a panicking swimmer's grasp: you may both drown. Extend something the victim can grasp—a life preserver, even a towel.

Reach or throw
If possible, reach out to the victim with a pole or throw out a buoyant object attached to a rope; a sturdy rope alone may be sufficient.

Rescuing from a boat
If the boat has a square stern, the victim should be brought in over the stern. Entry into a powerboat may be facilitated by bouncing the victim up and down in the water to gain momentum for a lift.

Swimming rescue
Use as a last resort. A panicky victim may have to be calmed before contact is made. Offer victim a buoyant object if possible. In an unaided tow, keep the victim's face above water.

MEASURES THAT MAY HELP PREVENT DROWNING ACCIDENTS

1 Never jump into deep water without ensuring that there is an easy and obvious method of exit.

2 Wear a life jacket or buoyancy device for all water sports (such as sailing and windsurfing).

3 Swim only in pools or from public beaches designated as safe and patrolled by lifeguards.

4 Do not drink alcohol before swimming or taking part in water sports of any kind.

5 Children should always be supervised when swimming and when they are taking baths.

6 Children should never walk on an iced-over pond or river unless the ice has first been tested by an adult.

rescuer tows out a buoyant object and offers it to the panicky victim before he or she can grab the rescuer. A victim who grasps the proffered object can either be urged to kick and thus stay afloat, or towed to shore.

An ambulance should be called and the person's medical condition assessed. If breathing and/or the pulse (felt in the neck) is absent, resuscitative measures should be started (see *Artificial respiration; Cardiopulmonary resuscitation*). These measures should be continued until an ambulance or physician has arrived.

Because of the operation of a primitive reflex, known as the "diving reflex," which preserves a minimal blood supply to the brain, victims can sometimes be resuscitated despite a long period of immersion in very cold water (which reduces the body's oxygen needs) and the initial appearance of being dead. In all cases of successful resuscitation, the person should be sent to a hospital for investigation and observation. Life-threatening symptoms may develop some hours after rescue, because water may have passed from the lungs into the blood and the lining of the lungs may have been damaged.

Drowning, dry

A form of *drowning* in which no fluid enters the lungs. About one fifth of fatal drowning cases are "dry." Victims of dry drowning have a particularly strong laryngeal reflex, which diverts water into the stomach instead of the lungs, but at the same time impairs breathing.

Drowsiness

A state of consciousness between full wakefulness and *sleep* or *unconsciousness*. Drowsiness is medically significant if it is abnormal, that is, if a person fails to awaken after being shaken, pinched, and shouted at, or wakes but almost immediately relapses into drowsiness.

Abnormal drowsiness may be the result of a *head injury*, high fever, *meningitis* (inflammation of the membranes that surround the brain and spinal cord), *uremia* (excess urea in the blood due to *kidney failure*), or *liver failure*. Alcohol or drugs may also produce this effect. In a person with *diabetes mellitus*, drowsiness may be due to *hypoglycemia* (low blood sugar), usually as a result of taking too much insulin, or to *hyperglycemia* (high blood sugar) due to inadequate control of the disorder.

Abnormal drowsiness should be treated as a medical emergency and professional help should be called immediately.

Drug

Any chemical substance that alters the function of one or more body organs or changes the process of a disease. Drugs include prescribed medicines, over-the-counter remedies, and substances, such as alcohol, tobacco, and drugs of abuse, that are used for nonmedical purposes. Many foods and drinks contain small quantities of substances classed as drugs—tea, coffee, and cola drinks, for example, all contain *caffeine*, which is both a *stimulant drug* and a *diuretic drug*.

Usually each drug is assigned three names: a detailed, descriptive chemical name; a shorter, generic name (see *Generic drug*) that has been officially approved; and a specific brand name chosen by the company that manufactures the drug.

Drugs are either licensed for prescription by a physician only or are over-the-counter preparations available at a pharmacy or supermarket.

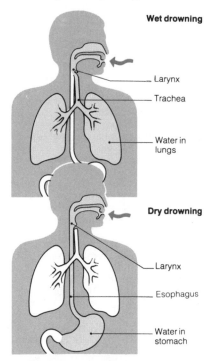

Wet drowning

— Larynx

— Trachea

— Water in lungs

Dry drowning

— Larynx

— Esophagus

— Water in stomach

Types of drowning
In four fifths of deaths due to drowning, the victim has inhaled liquid into his or her lungs. In the other fifth, no liquid is present in the lungs (dry drowning). In both cases, death is by suffocation.

SOURCES
Formerly, all drugs were naturally occurring substances extracted from animals, plants, and minerals. Today, most drugs are produced artificially in the laboratory, ensuring a purer preparation with a predictable potency (strength) that is safer for medical use. Some drugs, such as *insulin* and *growth hormone*, are now mainly synthesized by means of *genetic engineering* procedures.

New drugs are discovered in a number of ways: by screening a substance for different types of activity against a disease; by making alterations to the structure of an established drug; or, occasionally, by finding a new application for a drug that is being used for another condition.

CLASSIFICATION
A drug is classified in one of the following ways: first, according to its chemical makeup (a *corticosteroid drug*, for example); second, according to the disorder it treats (an *antihypertensive drug*, for example, is used to treat high blood pressure); or, third, according to its specific effect on the body (the effect of a diuretic drug, for example, is to produce diuresis, that is, to increase the volume of urine excreted).

EVALUATION
All new drugs are tested for their efficiency and safety. Tests usually go through three stages: laboratory trials on animals; laboratory trials on human volunteers; and, finally, clinical trials on patients.

If a drug meets standards of safety and efficacy, Health and Welfare Canada through its Health Promotion Branch (HPB) will authorize its sale in Canada. The HPB establishes standards of quality, purity of the preparation, and adequate labeling. The HPB and the manufacturer continue to evaluate a drug even after it has been widely prescribed, and if serious or frequent toxic effects are reported, the drug may be withdrawn or a warning issued. Provincial ministries of health also monitor the safety and distribution of drugs through special committees.

WHY DRUGS ARE USED
Drugs can be used in the treatment, prevention, or diagnosis of a disease. They are prescribed to relieve physical or mental symptoms, to replace a deficient natural substance (such as a *hormone*), or to stop the excessive production of a hormone or other body chemical. Some drugs are given to destroy foreign organisms, such as

D

bacteria or viruses. Others, known as *vaccines*, are given to stimulate the body's *immune system* (natural defenses) to form *antibodies*.

Antibiotic drugs, diuretic drugs, *analgesic drugs* (painkillers), and *tranquilizer drugs* are among the most commonly prescribed drugs. The most frequently used over-the-counter preparations include analgesics, *cough remedies*, *cold remedies*, *vitamin supplements*, and *tonics*.

HOW DRUGS WORK

Drugs act on cells in the body or the infecting organism by stimulating or blocking chemical reactions. In many cases, this action occurs because the drug mimics a chemical that occurs naturally in the body.

Some drugs act by binding (becoming attached) to a drug receptor (a specific site on the cell's surface that matches up with the chemical structure of the drug). This triggers a change in chemical activity within the cell. Other drugs work by being absorbed into the cell, where they affect the chemical processes directly.

Drugs may also have a *placebo* effect, which occurs as a result of the individual's expectations of the drug's action.

METHODS OF ADMINISTRATION

Drugs are given in different forms and in different ways (see table at right). These methods depend on many factors, including the severity of the illness, the part of the body being treated, the properties of the drug, and the speed and duration of action required.

ELIMINATION

Drugs taken by mouth that are not absorbed in the intestine are excreted in the feces. Drugs that have entered the bloodstream are eliminated via the kidneys, in the urine. Some drugs are broken down into inactive forms in the liver by *enzymes* before being eliminated.

COMPLIANCE

If drug treatment is to be beneficial, the full course must be taken as instructed by a physician. It is estimated that as many as two out of every five people who are prescribed a drug do not take it properly, if at all. Reasons for noncompliance include failure to understand instructions, fear of possible reactions, adverse effects, or simply not bothering to take the drug.

DRUG INTERACTIONS

Taking drugs together or in combination with food or alcohol may produce effects on the body that differ from

METHODS OF ADMINISTERING DRUGS

How taken		Action
By mouth		Drugs are digested and absorbed from the intestine in the same way as nutrients. How quickly the tablet or liquid works depends on how rapidly it is absorbed. This, in turn, depends on such factors as the drug's composition, how quickly the drug dissolves, and the effect of digestive juices on it.
By injection		Drugs given by injection have a very rapid effect. Injection is also used if digestive juices would destroy a drug.
As a cream, anal or vaginal suppository, pessary, nasal spray, or by inhaler		These drugs have a local effect on the parts of the body that are exposed to them as well as a systemic (generalized) effect if some of the drug is absorbed into the bloodstream from the site of application.

those occurring when a drug is taken on its own. Such drug interactions occur if chemicals in the different substances act on the same receptors or if one chemical alters the absorption, breakdown, or elimination of another.

Physicians commonly make use of interactions to increase the effectiveness of a treatment; combinations of drugs are often prescribed to treat infection, cancer, or hypertension (high blood pressure). Many interactions, however, are unplanned; they may reduce the benefit from a drug or increase its level in the blood and cause adverse effects.

Patients undergoing long-term drug treatment may be advised to carry cards that warn of potentially dangerous interactions from treatment that may be given during an emergency. Patients should tell their physicians about any other drugs they are taking to prevent interactions with drugs the physician may prescribe.

ADVERSE EFFECTS

Most drugs can produce adverse effects—harmful or unpleasant reactions that result from a normal dose of the drug. These adverse effects can be divided into predictable adverse reactions, which result from the chemical structure of the drug, and bizarre (unpredictable) reactions, which are unrelated to the drug's normal chemical effects on body cells.

Predictable adverse reactions are due to the difficulty in targeting a drug on a single organ. For example, *anticholinergic drugs* prescribed to relieve spasm in the intestine also cause blurred vision and dryness of the

mouth. Symptoms may wear off as the body adapts to the drug; otherwise, they usually are relieved by reducing the dose or increasing the interval between doses.

Any change in the absorption, breakdown, or elimination of a drug (caused, for example, by liver or kidney disease) that increases its concentration in the blood will increase the risk of predictable adverse effects.

Bizarre drug reactions may be due to a genetic disorder (for example, lack of a specific enzyme that usually inactivates the drug), an allergic reaction, or the formation of *antibodies* that damage tissue. Common side effects of this type include a rash, facial swelling, or jaundice. Occasionally, *anaphylactic shock* (a severe allergic reaction), characterized by breathing difficulty or collapse, may occur. Bizarre drug reactions usually make it necessary to withdraw the drug.

Many drugs cross the placenta and some adversely affect growth and development of the fetus. Most drugs pass into the breast milk of a nursing mother and some will have adverse effects on the baby.

A drug is useful only if its overall benefit to the patient outweighs the risk and severity of any adverse effects. Research on new drugs partly aims to discover preparations that act selectively on target organs to avoid unwanted effects on other tissues.

Drug abuse

The use of a drug for a purpose other than that for which it is normally prescribed or recommended. Among the many reasons for drug abuse are the desire to escape from reality or achieve a mystical experience, curiosity about a drug's effects, and the search for self-awareness.

Commonly abused drugs include *stimulant drugs*, such as *amphetamine drugs*; central nervous system depressants, such as *alcohol* and *barbiturate drugs*; *hallucinogenic drugs*, such as *LSD*; and *narcotic drugs*, such as *cocaine* and *heroin*. Certain types of drug are sometimes abused to improve performance in sports (see *Sports, drugs and*; *Steroids, anabolic*).

Problems resulting from drug abuse may arise from the adverse effects of the drug, from accidents during intoxication, and from the habit-forming potential of many drugs, which may lead to *drug dependence*.

Drug addiction
Physical or psychological dependence on a drug. (See *Drug dependence*.)

Drug benefit program
A government-funded social program to ensure that eligible persons receive essential medications. Drugs on a provincial list are dispensed by local pharmacies to identified participants. The cost is billed to the province.

Drug dependence
The compulsion to continue taking a drug, either to produce the desired effects that result from taking it, or to prevent the ill effects that occur when it is not taken.

TYPES
Drug dependence takes two forms: psychological and physical. A person is psychologically dependent if he or she experiences craving or emotional distress when the drug is withdrawn. In physical dependence the body has adapted to the presence of the drug, causing the symptoms and signs of *withdrawal syndrome* when the drug is withdrawn. Withdrawal is usually associated with severe physical and mental distress.

CAUSES AND INCIDENCE
Drug dependence develops as a result of regular and/or excessive use of a drug. Large numbers of people are dependent on *nicotine* in tobacco, on the *caffeine* in coffee and tea, and on *alcohol*. A significant proportion of the population is dependent on *tranquilizer drugs*.

Dependence develops most frequently with drugs that alter the individual's mood or behavior. The speed with which a drug acts on the body is another factor in the development of dependence. Intravenous drug abuse, for example, produces a rapid effect on the body, which reinforces the habit of injecting the drug.

Some people seem to be more susceptible to dependence than others. Factors that usually play a part include pressure from friends and associates, and environmental factors, such as poverty, unemployment, disrupted family life, and the availability of drugs. Hereditary factors may also play a part.

SYMPTOMS AND SIGNS
A mild withdrawal reaction may cause yawning, sneezing, a runny nose, watering eyes, and sweating. More severe reactions include diarrhea, vomiting, trembling, cramps, confusion, and, rarely, seizures and coma. These symptoms are usually relieved if the drug is taken again.

Withdrawal symptoms probably occur because the body has become adapted to the continuous presence of the drug, which reduces the release of certain natural chemicals (e.g., nicotine affects production of *epinephrine* and similar substances). When the drug is no longer taken or is withheld, the chemical deficiency is exposed.

COMPLICATIONS
Drug dependence may cause physical problems, such as lung and heart disease from tobacco smoking and liver disease from drinking excessive amounts of alcohol. Mental problems, such as anxiety and depression, are common during withdrawal. Dependence may also be associated with drug tolerance, in which an increasingly higher dose of the substance is needed to produce the desired effect.

Complications may occur as an indirect result of dependence. For example, people who inject a *narcotic drug* may become ill and die from *hepatitis* or *AIDS*, contracted as a result of introducing infection into the bloodstream via a dirty needle. In other cases, abusers may suffer from an overdose because of confusion about the dosage or because they take a purer, more potent preparation than they are used to. Social problems often result from the disruption of family life and from criminal acts carried out to pay for drugs.

TREATMENT
Controlled withdrawal programs are available in special centers and large hospitals. These programs usually offer supervised reductions in dose. Alternative, less harmful drugs may be given, as well as treatment for withdrawal symptoms. Social service agencies and support groups may provide follow-up care.

OUTLOOK
Successful treatment requires motivation on the part of the dependent person. Problems frequently recur when people return to the circumstances that originally gave rise to drug abuse and dependence.

Drug overdose
The taking of an excessive amount of a drug, which may cause toxic effects. (See *Drug poisoning*.)

Drug poisoning
The harmful effects on various organs of the body as a result of taking an excessive dose of a drug.

CAUSES AND INCIDENCE
Drug poisoning may be accidental or deliberate. Accidental poisoning is most common in young children under the age of 5 years who swallow colored tablets thinking they are candies. Child-resistant drug containers have helped reduce this risk. In adults, accidental poisoning usually occurs in elderly or confused people who are uncertain about their treatment and dosage requirements. Accidental poisoning may also occur during *drug abuse*.

Deliberate self-poisoning is usually unsuccessful and is done as a cry for help (see *Suicide*; *Suicide, attempted*). The drugs that are most commonly taken in overdose are *benzodiazepine drugs*, *antidepressant drugs*, *acetaminophen*, or *ASA*. Homicide may involve the administration of a drug by another person.

TREATMENT
In dealing with a drug overdose, first aid measures depend on the condition of the patient. If the patient is unconscious, ensure that the *airway* is clear and that there is normal breathing and a pulse before rolling the patient into the *recovery position* and summoning emergency help. If the person is not breathing, *artificial respiration* should be started.

Any individual who has taken a drug overdose and any child who has swallowed tablets that belong to someone else should be seen by a physician. It is important to identify the drugs which have been taken. Drug containers and any drugs that are near the victim may provide vital clues; save any you find. Call 911, your poison control center, or your local hospital emergency department for advice. If the victim is fully conscious, you may be advised to induce vomiting by sticking a finger down his or her throat or by giving an *emetic* if one is available.

Some drugs taken in excess may cause *hypothermia*; if this occurs, keep the victim warm with blankets.

Treatment in hospital may involve washing out the stomach using several litres of water passed down a tube through the mouth and esophagus (see *Lavage, gastric*). However, this procedure is effective only if it is performed within a few hours of taking the overdose.

Charcoal may be given by mouth in some cases to reduce the absorption of the drug from the intestine into the bloodstream. Increased production of urine may be induced by an *intravenous infusion* to speed up the elimination of the drug from the bloodstream; the infusion solution will be either acidic or alkaline depending on the drug taken.

Antidotes are available only for specific drugs. Such antidotes include *naloxone* (given to reverse breathing difficulty caused by *morphine*), methionine (given to reduce the formation of toxic substances from acetaminophen in the liver), and *chelating agents* such as deferoxamine (given to absorb and inactivate iron).

COMPLICATIONS
Drug poisoning may cause drowsiness and breathing difficulty (due to effects on the brain), irregular heartbeat, and, rarely, cardiac arrest, seizures, and kidney and liver damage. Monitoring of the heartbeat by *ECG* is usually carried out for the first 24 to 48 hours after poisoning with a drug that is known to have effects on the heart. *Antiarrhythmic drugs* are prescribed to treat any heartbeat irregularity as it develops. Seizures are treated with *anticonvulsant drugs*. In some serious cases, the patient requires artificial *ventilation* because of severe drug-induced breathing difficulty.

Blood tests to monitor liver function and careful monitoring of urine output are carried out if the drug is known to have any toxic effect on the liver or kidneys.

Dry eye
See *Keratoconjunctivitis sicca*.

Dry ice
Frozen *carbon dioxide*, also known as carbon dioxide snow. Unlike most substances, carbon dioxide changes directly from a gas to a solid when it is cooled, without first passing through

a liquid phase. In practice, dry ice is produced by allowing carbon dioxide gas stored under pressure to escape through a small nozzle. This rapid expansion cools the carbon dioxide to about −70ºC, and dry ice is formed as a powder. This powder is then compressed into cakes.

Dry ice is sometimes applied to the skin in *cryosurgery*, a freezing technique used, for example, to destroy *warts* and *nevi*.

Dry socket
Infection at the site of a recent tooth extraction, causing pain, bad breath, and an unpleasant taste. Dry socket is a complication of about 4 percent of extractions. It occurs most commonly when a blood clot fails to form in the tooth socket after a difficult extraction, such as removal of an impacted wisdom tooth (see *Impaction, dental*). Infection may also develop following a normal extraction if the blood clot becomes dislodged (for instance, because of excessive rinsing of the mouth). In some cases, the clot itself may become infected, or infection may already have been present before extraction. The inflamed socket appears dry, and exposed bone, which may be dead and fragmented, is often visible.

TREATMENT
The socket is gently irrigated to remove debris, and may then be coated with a soothing, anti-inflammatory paste, such as a mixture of zinc oxide and eugenol (oil of cloves). The infection usually begins to clear up within a few days. *Antibiotic drugs* may help prevent dry socket but are not usually effective once the condition is established.

DSM IIIR
The most recent edition of the "Diagnostic and Statistical Manual of Mental Disorders", published by the American Psychiatric Association in 1987. DSM IIIR provides criteria for classifying psychiatric illnesses and is widely accepted in other countries.

Dual personality
See *Multiple personality*.

Duct
A tube or a tubelike passage leading from a gland to allow the flow of fluids—for example, tears through the tear ducts.

Dumbness
See *Mutism*.

Dumping syndrome
Symptoms including sweating, faintness, and palpitations resulting from the rapid passage of food from the stomach into the upper intestine. Dumping syndrome mainly affects people who have had a partial or total *gastrectomy* (surgical removal of the stomach).

The symptoms may occur within about 30 minutes of eating (early dumping), or after 90 to 120 minutes (late dumping, usually due to low blood sugar and potassium levels). Some tense people may have symptoms of dumping even though their stomach is intact.

CAUSES
Gastric surgery interferes with the normal mechanism for emptying food from the stomach (see *Digestive system*). If a meal that is rich in carbohydrates is "dumped" too quickly from the stomach, the patient's upper intestine may swell and excessive amounts of certain hormones are released into the bloodstream. These excess hormones, combined with the intestinal swelling, cause the symptoms of early dumping.

As sugars are absorbed from the intestine, they rapidly increase the blood glucose level, causing an excess amount of *insulin* to be released. The abnormally high insulin level may in turn later lower the blood sugar level below normal, causing the symptoms of late dumping.

A person who has had a gastrectomy can avoid symptoms by eating frequent, small, dry meals that do not contain refined carbohydrates such as white sugar. Symptoms may also be prevented by lying down after a large meal. Drug treatment is not often successful, but adding *guar gum* to food to slow the emptying of the stomach and the absorption of sugars is sometimes effective.

Duodenal ulcer
A raw area in the wall of the *duodenum* (first part of the small intestine), caused by erosion of its inner surface lining. Duodenal ulcers and gastric ulcers (similar raw areas in the lining of the stomach) are also called *peptic ulcers* and have similar causes, symptoms, and treatment.

Duodenitis
Inflammation of the *duodenum* (first part of the small intestine). Duodenitis produces vague gastrointestinal symptoms and no physical signs. The cause is uncertain.

D

A diagnosis of duodenitis is made by *gastroscopy* (examination of the walls of the duodenum with a flexible viewing instrument passed through the esophagus, stomach, and pylorus). Gastroscopy shows a diffuse area of inflammation, with redness and swelling of cells in the duodenal lining and often bleeding after contact with the tip of the gastroscope. No direct link has yet been established between gastroscopic findings and the symptoms of duodenitis.

Treatment for duodenitis (which has not been proved to be effective) is similar to that for a duodenal ulcer (see *Peptic ulcer*).

Duodenum

The first part of the small intestine, extending from the pylorus (the muscular valve at the lower end of the stomach) to the ligament of Treitz, which marks the boundary between the duodenum and the jejunum (the second part of the small intestine).

Ducts from the pancreas, liver, and gallbladder feed into the duodenum through a small opening called the ampulla of Vater, which is surrounded by the sphincter of Oddi.

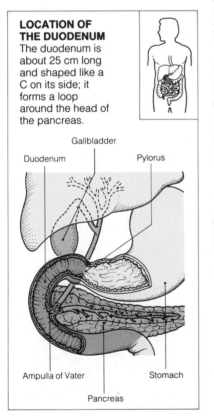

LOCATION OF THE DUODENUM
The duodenum is about 25 cm long and shaped like a C on its side; it forms a loop around the head of the pancreas.

Gallbladder
Duodenum
Pylorus
Ampulla of Vater
Stomach
Pancreas

Digestive enzymes in the pancreatic secretions and chemicals in the bile are released into the duodenum through this opening.

Dupuytren's contracture

A disorder of the hand in which one or more fingers become fixed in a bent position. In about half the cases, both hands are affected. The disorder is named after the French surgeon who first described it, Baron Guillaume Dupuytren (1777-1835).

CAUSES AND INCIDENCE
The cause is unclear. In most cases there is no apparent or known cause, although the condition is slightly more common in certain groups—for example, people whose work involves gripping tools, especially those that vibrate. The condition is a common feature in people with alcoholic liver *cirrhosis*. There is a slight tendency for the condition to run in families, although this does not necessarily mean it is inherited genetically. Men over 40 are most commonly affected.

SYMPTOMS AND SIGNS
The tissues under the skin in the palm of the hand become thickened and shortened, with tethering of the tendons that run into the fingers. A small, hard nodule forms on the palm of the hand and it spreads to form a band of hard tissue under the skin, with puckering of the skin itself. The affected fingers start to bend more and more over a period of months or years and cannot be pulled back straight.

TREATMENT
The only treatment is surgical and is performed when the deformity has become unsightly or has started to impede hand function. During surgery the bands of thickened tissue under the skin are cut and separated to free the tendons.

Dust diseases

A group of lung disorders caused by the inhalation, usually over several years at work, of dust particles which are absorbed into the lung tissues. There they may cause *fibrosis* (formation of scar tissue) and progressive lung damage with crippling symptoms.

The main symptoms are a cough and breathing difficulty. It may take at least 10 years of exposure to dusts containing coal, silica, talc, or asbestos before serious lung damage develops (see *Pneumoconiosis*).

Workers in relevant industries show considerable variation in their

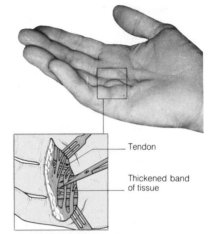

Tendon
Thickened band of tissue

Surgery for Dupuytren's contracture
Bands of tissue under the skin that have become thickened are cut and separated so that the tendons are freed.

susceptibility to dust disease. These people should be under regular medical supervision to ensure that any signs of disease are detected early and serious damage is thus prevented.

Dwarfism

See *Short stature*.

Dying, care of the

People who are near death should be given physical and psychological care that will make their final period of life as free from pain, discomfort, and emotional distress as possible.

Today, with good medical care, many deaths, even those from cancer, are pain-free and are associated with little physical discomfort. Emotional distress in the dying can be minimized if understanding and sensitivity are shown by the people who care for them. Caregivers may include physicians and other medical professionals, counselors, social workers, clergy, family, and friends. Family and friends should realize that caring for a dying person may cause them great emotional strain. They may also feel guilty because they are unable to do more for the dying person. They, too, may benefit from counseling.

TALKING ABOUT DEATH
Over the last 20 years it has become more common for physicians to tell dying people, particularly cancer patients, the facts relating to their diagnoses. Generally, if a person can discuss the likely outcome of his or her illness and can prepare for death, then dying itself is eased. However, there are people who prefer not to know or

who block out the knowledge. The wishes of the patient should be paramount; these wishes may not always be clear and those caring for the patient need considerable perception and understanding. Careful probing may be necessary to ascertain how much a dying person really wants to be told.

Sometimes, even though the dying person has made it clear that he or she would prefer to talk about death, family members feel unable to do so. This may make the patient feel very isolated. Sometimes, a dying person may find it easier to talk to someone who is not a relative. Specially trained people, such as counselors or members of the clergy, may be able to help promote communication between patient and family.

PHYSICAL CARE

For most dying people, pain is often the most feared problem. Today, however, virtually all pain can be relieved by the use of analgesic drugs (painkillers). Regular, low doses of drugs are given so that pain never builds up and the patient remains alert. Powerful narcotic analgesics, such as morphine and other opiates, are commonly given to relieve severe pain in dying people.

When analgesic drugs are not adequate, other methods may be necessary. These include *nerve blocks* (in which a nerve carrying pain from the body to the brain is interrupted by an injection or surgery), *cordotomy* (severing of nerve fibers in the spinal cord), and *TENS* (transcutaneous electrical nerve stimulation), which is less likely to be effective if narcotic analgesics have been used.

Physical symptoms other than pain may also cause distress. Nausea and vomiting may be a problem when the liver or kidneys have ceased to function adequately. A combination of two or three drugs may occasionally control symptoms. An obstruction in the esophagus can cause vomiting and difficulty in swallowing and may need to be relieved by an operation or by *laser treatment* through an *endoscope*. Another common problem in the dying is breathlessness, which may be relieved by morphine.

The patient may develop aches or become stiff from being in bed. Comfort can be improved by keeping the patient as active as possible.

Toward the end, the dying person may become restless and may suffer from breathing difficulty due to *heart failure* or *pneumonia*. These symptoms

can be relieved by medication and by placing the patient in a more comfortable position.

PSYCHOLOGICAL CARE

Emotional care is at least as important as the relief of pain. Many people feel anger or depression at the thought of dying; feelings of guilt or regret over the past are also common emotional responses. Ultimately, however, given loving, caring support from family, friends, and others, most terminally ill people come to terms with the thought of death. Sometimes *antidepressant drugs* are prescribed to relieve severe depression.

A great cause of anxiety and worry may be fear of a painful end. Patients should be reassured that adequate pain relief will be maintained at all times and that even when death is very close they need not fear suffering. Most people sink into unconsciousness just before the end and die "in their sleep."

Fear of dependency and loss of dignity may also cause worry. The dying person should be allowed to participate as much as possible in discussions about family matters and decisions regarding the future.

Preparing for death may include practical matters, such as writing a will, or less tangible things such as saying "sorry," "thank you," or "goodbye." Confession and reassurance from a priest or spiritual counselor are also important for some people. Perhaps the most pressing need for the terminally ill person is communication. Relatives, friends, and caregivers must be willing to share the dying person's concerns.

HOME OR HOSPITAL?

The treatment of most types of cancer requires hospital facilities at some time. However, once an illness has a foreseeable end, many terminally ill people prefer to return home; many families also choose to care for a dying relative at home. Few terminally ill patients require complicated nursing for a prolonged period, and the sort of loving understanding and emotional care needed may be best provided at home. At home, too, the dying person can maintain some dignity and independence, avoid isolation, and participate in family life. By contrast, a hospital is better equipped to deal with acute illness.

HOSPICES

Hospices are small units, sometimes linked to a general hospital, that have been established specifically to care for the dying and their families. The

number of hospices has grown considerably during the last few years. Hospital routine is generally absent; instead, the efforts of the hospice staff, who are specially trained in terminal care, are directed toward the relief of physical and emotional pain. Basic to the hospice philosophy is the idea that dying people and their families need help, care, and understanding. It has been argued that a dying person might find the sight of other people dying depressing, but it has been found that most people who die in a hospice are reassured by seeing for themselves that death occurs peacefully. (See also *Terminal care*.)

Dys-

A prefix meaning abnormal, difficult, painful, or faulty, as in dysuria (pain on passing urine).

Dysarthria

A *speech disorder* caused by disease or damage to the physical apparatus of speech, or to nerve pathways controlling this apparatus.

Dysarthria differs from *aphasia* (a type of language disorder that affects speech) in that dysarthric patients have nothing wrong with the language center in the brain. They are able to formulate, select, and write out words and sentences grammatically; it is only vocal expression that causes problems. *Dysphonia* is a speech disability with a more restricted meaning than dysarthria, referring only to defects of sound production caused by some disease or damage to the larynx (voice box).

CAUSES

Dysarthria is a common feature of many degenerative conditions affecting the nervous system, such as *multiple sclerosis, Parkinson's disease,* and *Huntington's chorea*. It also affects some children who have *cerebral palsy*. Dysarthria may result from a *stroke, brain tumor,* or an isolated defect or damage to a particular nerve (such as the hypoglossal nerve that controls movements of the tongue).

Structural defects of the mouth, as often occur in cases of *cleft lip and palate*, or even ill-fitting dentures, may also affect speech.

TREATMENT

There is no specific treatment for dysarthria. In some cases, drug or surgical treatment of the underlying disease or structural defect may restore the ability to speak clearly. In other instances, patients may benefit from *speech therapy*.

D

Dyschondroplasia

A rare disorder, also called multiple enchondromatosis, present from birth and characterized by the presence of multiple tumors of cartilaginous tissue within the bones of a limb. Dyschondroplasia is caused by a failure of normal bone development from cartilage. The bones of an affected limb are shortened, resulting in deformity. Rarely, a tumor may become cancerous (see *Chondrosarcoma*).

Dysentery

A severe infection of the intestines, causing diarrhea (often mixed with blood, pus, and mucus) and abdominal pain. The person may spend hours straining on the toilet, producing little but bloodstained watery mucus.

There are two distinct forms of dysentery. *Shigellosis*, also called bacillary dysentery, is caused by infection with any of a group of bacteria called SHIGELLA. The diarrhea starts suddenly and is watery; sometimes *toxemia* (the presence of bacterial toxins in the blood) develops. *Amebic dysentery* is caused by the protozoan (single-celled) parasite ENTAMOEBA HISTOLYTICA. This form starts more gradually and often persists.

The main risk with dysentery is *dehydration* caused by the diarrhea.

Dyskinesia

Abnormal muscular movements caused by a brain disorder. Uncontrollable twitching, jerking, or writhing movements cannot be suppressed and may impair the performance of voluntary movements. The disorder may involve the whole body or may be restricted to a group of muscles.

Different types of dyskinesia include *chorea* (mainly jerking movements), *athetosis* (writhing movements), *choreoathetosis* (a combined form), *tics* (repetitive fidgets), *tremors*, and *myoclonus* (muscle spasms).

Dyskinesia may result from brain damage at birth or may be a side effect of certain drugs, particularly some *antipsychotic drugs* or the antiemetic *metoclopramide*. The affected brain region is a group of linked nerve centers (the *extrapyramidal system*), which includes the *basal ganglia*.

Dyskinesia due to drugs often disappears when drug use is stopped. Otherwise, dyskinesia is difficult to treat. Drugs such as tetrabenazine may help reduce chorea, but often a physician must prescribe several drugs in turn before one (if any) is effective. (See also *Parkinsonism*.)

Prevalence of amebic dysentery
Amebic dysentery is most prevalent in countries where standards of hygiene are low. The photograph shows a magnified sample of ENTAMOEBA HISTOLYTICA.

Dyslexia

A specific reading disability characterized by difficulty in coping with written symbols. The term is not used to describe other types of reading difficulty, such as problems arising from brain damage or mental handicap, or from speech or visual defects.

Dyslexia does not include reading problems caused by educational or social neglect.

CAUSES AND INCIDENCE

Emotional disturbance, minor visual defects, and failure to "train" the brain have all been suggested as possible causes of dyslexia, but there is now good evidence that a specific, sometimes inherited, neurological disorder underlies true dyslexia. Some 90 percent of people with dyslexia are male.

SYMPTOMS

The key feature of dyslexia is that in other respects a child with dyslexia has completely normal intelligence. Thus, his or her attainment of reading skills lags far behind other scholastic abilities and overall IQ. Usually, the child can read numbers or musical notes much more easily than words.

Furthermore, while many young children tend to reverse letters and words (for example, writing or reading p for q, b for d, was for saw, no for on), the majority soon correct such errors. Dyslexic children continue to confuse these symbols. Letters are transposed (as in pest for step) and spelling errors are common. These children may even be unable to read words they can spell correctly. Writ-

ing from dictation may be difficult even though most dyslexic children can copy sentences.

TREATMENT

It is important to recognize the problem early to avoid any added frustrations. Specific remedial teaching can help the child develop "tricks" to overcome the deficit, and avoidance of pressure from parents combined with praise for what the child can do is equally important. Given appropriate support and training, sufferers can usually overcome their difficulties, and develop successful careers.

Dysmenorrhea

Pain or discomfort during or just before a menstrual period. Most teenage girls and young women suffer to some degree from what is called primary dysmenorrhea. This usually starts two or three years after *menstruation* begins, once ovulation is established. The problem often diminishes after the age of about 25 and is rare following childbirth.

Dysmenorrhea is known to be associated with the hormonal changes that occur during a period, but the exact mechanism of the link between them remains uncertain. One possibility is that dysmenorrhea is due to excessive production of, or undue sensitivity to, *prostaglandins*, the hormonelike substances that stimulate muscular spasm of the uterus.

Secondary dysmenorrhea begins in adult life and is due to an underlying disorder, such as *endometriosis* or *pelvic inflammatory disease*.

Either type of dysmenorrhea may or may not be accompanied by *premenstrual syndrome* (a bloated feeling, irritability, depression, and other changes that commonly occur in the days preceding menstruation).

SYMPTOMS

Dysmenorrhea is typically felt as cramplike pain or discomfort in the lower abdomen, which may come and go in waves. There may also be a dull ache in the lower back and, in some women, nausea and vomiting. In primary dysmenorrhea the pain starts shortly before a period and usually lasts for less than 12 hours. About 10 percent of women have symptoms severe enough to interfere with their work or leisure activities. In secondary dysmenorrhea the pain begins several days before a period and lasts until the period ends.

Mild primary dysmenorrhea is often relieved by *analgesic drugs* (painkillers), such as *ASA*, or *naproxen* (a prostaglandin inhibitor). Rest in bed with a heating pad or a hot-water bottle is a popular and sometimes effective remedy. If primary dysmenorrhea is severe, symptoms can usually be relieved by suppressing ovulation, with either *oral contraceptives* or other hormonal preparations.

Treatment of secondary dysmenorrhea depends on the cause.

Dyspareunia

The medical term for painful sexual intercourse. (See *Intercourse, painful*.)

Dyspepsia

The medical term for *indigestion*.

Dysphagia

The medical term for *swallowing difficulty*.

Dysphasia

A term sometimes used to describe a disturbance in the ability to select the words with which to speak and write (and/or to comprehend and read) caused by damage to regions of the brain concerned with speech and comprehension. (See also *Aphasia*.)

Dysphonia

Defective production of vocal sounds in *speech*, caused by disease or damage to the *larynx* (the voice box) or to the nerve supply to the laryngeal muscles. Dysphonia should be distinguished from *dysarthria* (in which speech is defective because of damage or disease to other body parts and nerve pathways involved in speech)

and from expressive *aphasia* (in which the ability to speak may be profoundly disturbed by damage to the speech center in the brain). (See also *Larynx* disorders box; *Speech disorders*.)

Dysplasia

Any abnormality of growth. The term applies to deformities in structures such as the skull (cranial dysplasia) and to abnormalities of single cells (cellular dysplasia). Abnormal cell features include the size, shape, and rate of multiplication of cells.

Dyspnea

The medical term for shortness of breath. (See *Breathing difficulty*.)

Dysrhythmia, cardiac

A medical term meaning disturbance of heart rhythm, sometimes used as an alternative to arrhythmia. (See *Arrhythmia, cardiac*.)

Dystocia

A term that means difficult or abnormal labor (see *Childbirth*). Dystocia may occur if the baby is very large, or if the mother's pelvis is abnormally shaped or too small for the baby to pass through. Other causes of dystocia include abnormal presentation of the baby (see *Malpresentation*), and ineffective uterine contractions. (See also *Childbirth, complications of*.)

Dystonia

Abnormal muscle rigidity, causing painful muscle spasms, unusually fixed postures, or strange movement patterns. Dystonia may affect a localized area of the body, or it may be more generalized.

Scoliosis due to dystonia
Injury to the back may result in dystonia and abnormal spasm of the back muscles, which, in turn, may lead to scoliosis (abnormal sideways curvature of the spine).

The most common types of localized dystonia are *torticollis* (painful neck spasm), and *scoliosis* (abnormal sideways curvature of the spine) caused by an injury to the back that produces muscle spasm.

More generalized dystonia occurs as a result of various neurological disorders, including *Parkinson's disease* and *stroke*, and may also be a feature of *schizophrenia*. Dystonia may be a side effect of *antipsychotic drugs*.

Dystonia is often difficult to treat but may respond to *anticholinergic drugs* or *benzodiazepine drugs*. In some cases *biofeedback training* may help. Dystonia of the eyelids, known as *blepharospasm*, can usually be treated successfully with injections of botulinum toxin, the agent responsible for *botulism*. The injections are effective for a few months and can be repeated as necessary.

Dystrophy

Any disorder in which the structure and normal activity of cells within a tissue have been disrupted by inadequate nutrition. The usual cause is poor circulation of blood through the tissue, but dystrophy can also be due to damage to nerves or to deficiency of a specific enzyme (catalytic protein) in the tissue.

In *muscular dystrophies*, muscle cells fail to develop normally, causing weakness and paralysis. In *leukodystrophies*, there is loss of the sheath surrounding nerves within the brain, causing various disturbances of sensation, movement, and intellect.

Corneal dystrophies are a rare, usually inherited, cause of blindness. In these conditions, cells lining the cornea are damaged and the eye's surface becomes opaque.

Dysuria

The medical term for pain, discomfort, or difficulty in passing urine. (See *Urination, painful*.)

E

Ear

The organ of hearing and balance. The ear consists of three parts: the outer ear, the middle ear, and the inner ear. The outer and middle ear are concerned primarily with the collection and transmission of sound. The inner ear is responsible for analyzing sound waves; it also contains the mechanism by which the body keeps its balance.

OUTER EAR

The outer ear consists of the pinna (also called the auricle), which is the visible part of the ear, composed of folds of skin and cartilage. The pinna leads into the ear canal (also called the meatus), which is 2.5 cm long in adults and closed at its inner end by the tympanic membrane (eardrum). The part of the canal nearest the outside is made of cartilage. The cartilage is covered with skin that produces wax, which, along with hair, traps dust and small foreign bodies.

The eardrum separates the outer ear from the middle ear. The eardrum is a thin, fibrous, circular membrane covered with a thin layer of skin. It vibrates in response to the changes in air pressure that constitute sound and works in conjunction with the other components of the middle ear.

MIDDLE EAR

The middle ear is a small cavity between the eardrum and the inner ear. It conducts sound to the inner ear by means of a chain of three tiny, linked, movable bones called ossicles. These bones link the eardrum to the oval window in the bony wall that forms the inner side of the middle ear cavity. The ossicles have names that describe their shapes. The malleus (hammer) is joined to the inside of the eardrum. The incus (anvil) has one broad joint with the malleus (which lies almost parallel to it) and a delicate joint to the third bone, the stapes (stirrup). The base of the stapes fills the oval window, which leads to the inner ear.

The middle ear is cut off from the outside by the eardrum, but it is not completely airtight; a ventilation passage, called the eustachian tube, runs forward and downward into the back of the nose. The eustachian tube is normally closed but opens by muscular contraction when we yawn or swallow.

The middle ear acts as a transformer, passing the vibrations of sound from the air outside (which is a thin medium) to the fluid in the inner ear (which is a thicker medium).

INNER EAR

The inner ear is an extremely intricate series of structures contained deep within the bones of the skull. It consists of a maze of winding passages, collectively known as the labyrinth. The front part, the cochlea, is a tube resembling a snail's shell and is concerned with hearing. (For a detailed discussion of how this system works, see *Hearing*.) The rear part (consisting of the saccule, utricle, and three semicircular canals) is concerned with *balance*. The semicircular canals are set at right angles to each other and are connected to a cavity known as the vestibule. The canals contain hair cells bathed in fluid. Some of these cells are sensitive to gravity and acceleration; others respond to the positions and movements of the head (i.e., side to side, up and down, or tilted). The information concerning posture or direction is registered by the relevant cells and conveyed by nerve fibers to the brain. (See also *Ear* disorders box.)

Earache

Pain in the ear, which may originate in the ear itself or may result from a disorder in a nearby structure. Earache is an extremely common symptom, especially in childhood.

CAUSES

The most frequent cause of earache is acute *otitis media* (infection of the middle ear), which occurs most commonly in young children. The pain is

---

ANATOMY OF THE EAR

The outer ear comprises the pinna and ear canal; the middle ear—the eardrum, malleus, incus, stapes, and eustachian tube; and the inner ear— the vestibule, semicircular canals, and cochlea. Sensory impulses from the inner ear pass to the brain via the vestibulocochlear nerve.

Pinna

Ear canal

Malleus

Incus

Stapes

Vestibulocochlear nerve

Semicircular canals

Vestibule

Eardrum

Cochlea

Eustachian tube

DISORDERS OF THE EAR

The ear is susceptible to a large variety of disorders, some of which can lead to *deafness*. *Vertigo* (dizziness associated with a disturbance of balance) may result from some disorders of the inner ear.

CONGENITAL DEFECTS

Very rarely, a baby is born with an absent or extremely narrowed external ear canal, and sometimes the small bones of the middle ear are deformed or absent. Occasionally, the pinna (external ear) is missing or distorted. *Rubella* (German measles) affecting a woman during the first three months of pregnancy can cause severe damage to the baby's hearing apparatus, leading to deafness. Most cases of congenital sensorineural deafness are genetic.

INFECTION

Infection is the most common cause of ear disorders. Infection may occur in the ear canal, leading to *otitis externa*, or may affect the middle ear, causing *otitis media*, which often leads to perforation of the eardrum (see *Eardrum, perforated*). Persistent *glue ear* (buildup of fluid within the middle ear), often due to infection, is the most common cause of hearing difficulties in children.

Middle ear infection can spread to cause *mastoiditis* (infection of the mastoid process, the bone behind the ear) or *brain abscess*, but these complications have become extremely rare since the introduction of antibiotics.

Virus infection of the inner ear may cause *labyrinthitis* with severe vertigo or sudden hearing loss, or both simultaneously.

INJURY

Cauliflower ear is the result of repeated injury to the pinna. Injury to the external ear canal and perforation of the eardrum can result from poking objects into the ear. A sudden blow, especially a slap, to the ear or a very loud noise may also perforate the eardrum. Prolonged exposure to loud noise or close proximity to a loud explosion can cause *tinnitus* (noises within the ear) and/or deafness. Pressure changes associated with flying or scuba diving can also cause minor damage and pain (see *Barotrauma*).

TUMORS

Tumors in the ear are rare, but occasionally a *basal cell carcinoma* (rodent ulcer) or a *squamous cell carcinoma* will affect the pinna. The latter may also involve the ear canal. Cancers of the middle and inner ears are extremely rare. *Acoustic neuroma* is a benign (nonmalignant), slow-growing tumor of the acoustic nerve that may press on structures within the ear to cause deafness, tinnitus, and imbalance. *Cholesteatoma*, a growing collection of skin cells and debris, is not a tumor, but may be equally dangerous.

OBSTRUCTION

Ear-canal obstruction is most often caused by dried *earwax*, but may also result from otitis externa. In children, a frequent cause is putting a foreign body into the ear (see *Ear, foreign body in*).

DEGENERATION

Deafness in many elderly people is due to *presbycusis*, deterioration of the hair cells in the cochlea.

POISONING/DRUGS

The inner ear is especially sensitive to damage by certain classes of drugs. The most important—the aminoglycoside *antibiotics* group—includes such drugs as neomycin and gentamicin. These drugs can cause damage to the cochlear hair cells, especially if used in high concentration and particularly in the presence of kidney disease, which can delay the excretion of the drugs from the body.

Other drugs that can damage ear function include quinine and the salicylates (including *ASA*) and the *diuretic drugs* furosemide, ethacrynic acid, and bumetanide.

OTHER DISORDERS

In *otosclerosis*, a hereditary condition, the base of one of the small bones in the middle ear becomes fixed, causing deafness. *Meniere's disease* is an uncommon disorder in which deafness, vertigo, and tinnitus result from the accumulation of fluid within the labyrinth in the inner ear.

INVESTIGATION

The function of hearing is investigated by various tuning-fork and audiometric *hearing tests*, which reveal different types and levels of hearing loss. The external ear canal and the eardrum may be examined with an *otoscope* and mirror; an otoscopic microscope may also be used.

The function of the balancing mechanism of the inner ear is investigated by observing *nystagmus* (jerky eye movements) when the head is placed in different positions or the whole body rotated, and when the ear is syringed with hot or cold water (*caloric tests*). These tests may be refined by *electronystagmography*.

likely to be severe and stabbing; there may also be loss of hearing and a raised temperature. If the eardrum bursts, the discharge of fluid may produce immediate relief from pain.

Another common cause of earache is *otitis externa* (inflammation of the outer ear canal), which is often caused by infection. Infection may affect the whole canal or it may be localized, sometimes taking the form of a boil or abscess. The earache may be accompanied by irritation in the ear canal, and by a discharge, and there may be slight hearing loss.

A much rarer cause of earache is *herpes zoster* infection, which causes blisters in the ear canal. The earache may persist for weeks or months after the infection has cleared up.

Intermittent earache may also occur in people with dental problems, *tonsillitis*, throat cancer (see *Pharynx, cancer of*), pain in the lower jaw or neck muscles, and other disorders affecting areas near the ear. Earache in such cases occurs because the ear and many nearby areas are supplied by the same nerves; the pain is said to be "referred" to the ear.

INVESTIGATION

After inspecting the outer ear, the physician will examine the ear canal and eardrum with an *otoscope* and, if necessary, a binocular microscope. The mouth, throat, and teeth are also examined. In some cases, X rays and other tests may need to be carried out (see *Ear, examination of*).

TREATMENT
Analgesic drugs may be given to relieve pain. Other treatment depends on the underlying cause of the earache. *Antibiotic drugs* may be prescribed for an infection. Pus in the outer ear may need to be aspirated (sucked out), usually as an outpatient procedure. Pus in the middle ear may require draining through a hole made in the eardrum, an operation known as *myringotomy*.

Ear, cauliflower
See *Cauliflower ear*.

Ear, discharge from
An emission of fluid from the ear, also known as otorrhea. The discharge may be watery or thick, clear or colored, odorless or foul-smelling, intermittent or continuous.

A discharge from the ear may be caused by infection of the outer ear (see *Otitis externa*). It is also commonly caused by perforation of the eardrum (see *Eardrum, perforated*), usually as a result of infection of the middle ear (see *Otitis media*). In very rare cases, following fracture of the skull (see *Skull, fracture of*), cerebrospinal fluid or blood may be discharged from the ear.

INVESTIGATION AND TREATMENT
Any discharge from the ear should be reported to a physician. A swab of the discharge will be taken and sent for laboratory analysis to identify the cause of any infection. *Hearing tests* may be performed.

X rays of the bones of the skull will be taken if there has been a *head injury* or if a serious type of middle ear infection is suspected.

Treatment depends on the cause and usually includes *antibiotic drugs*.

Eardrum, perforated
Rupture or erosion of the eardrum, usually as a result of infection. Perforation of the eardrum often causes brief, intense pain. There may be slight bleeding and a discharge from the ear (see *Ear, discharge from*).

Perforation of the eardrum usually leads to some reduction in hearing (although such an effect may be very slight).

CAUSES AND INCIDENCE
Most commonly, the eardrum is perforated as a result of a build up of pus in the middle ear due to uncontrolled acute *otitis media* (infection of the middle ear).

Perforation of the eardrum may also be associated with *cholesteatoma* (a chronic disease of the middle ear). Another less common cause of perforation is injury, such as may result from the insertion of a sharp object into the ear, a blow to the ear (usually a hard slap), a nearby explosion, *barotrauma* (pressure damage resulting from flying or diving), or a fracture to the base of the skull. Very rarely, perforation of the eardrum is caused by a tumor of the middle ear.

In some cases, a physician may deliberately puncture the eardrum to drain the middle ear (see *Myringotomy*).

Perforation of the eardrum was much more common before *antibiotic drugs* became widely available.

DIAGNOSIS
Diagnosis is confirmed by examination of the ear (see *Ear, examination of*). *Hearing tests* may be performed to assess any hearing loss.

TREATMENT
Anyone who suspects a perforated eardrum should cover the ear with a clean, dry pad (to prevent infection from entering the middle ear) and seek medical help. *Analgesic drugs* (painkillers) may be taken if required.

The physician will prescribe *antibiotic drugs* to treat, or sometimes to prevent, infection. Most perforations due to acute infection or injury heal quickly, usually within a month. If the perforation has failed to heal or close sufficiently within six months, a *myringoplasty* (an operation to repair the eardrum) may be performed.

Surgery is always necessary to treat perforation associated with the disorder cholesteatoma.

Ear, examination of
A physician will examine the ear to investigate the possible causes of the following symptoms: *earache*, discharge from the ear (see *Ear, discharge from*), hearing loss, a feeling of fullness in the ear, disturbance of *balance*, *tinnitus* (noises in the ear), or swollen or tender lymph nodes (see *Glands, swollen*) below or in front of the ear.

The physician can inspect only the pinna (the visible outer ear), the ear canal, and the eardrum. To investigate the middle and inner ears, more specialized tests are required.

HOW IT IS DONE
The physician begins by examining the pinna for any evidence of swelling, tenderness, ulceration, or deformity and examines the skin above and behind the ear for signs of previous surgery. To inspect the ear canal and eardrum, the physician usually uses an *otoscope* (a viewing instrument for examining the ear). If necessary, a more magnified, three-dimensional image can be obtained by using a binocular microscope.

To obtain images of the middle and inner ears, the physician may arrange for *X rays*, *tomography*, *CT scanning*, or *MRI* to be carried out. Hearing and balance may require assessment by means of *hearing tests*, *caloric tests*, and *electronystagmography*.

E

Ear, foreign body in
The external ear canal is a common location for foreign bodies. Children often insert small objects, such as peas or stones, into their ears and insects can fly or crawl into the ear.

TREATMENT
SMALL OBJECTS These must always be removed by a physician. Under no circumstances should removal ever be attempted by poking with cotton swabs; hairpins; or similar objects; these efforts usually drive the foreign object even farther into the ear canal.

FIRST AID: FOREIGN BODY IN EAR

DO NOT
- attempt to dislodge the object by probing. Small objects must be removed by a physician.
- pour liquid into the ear unless you are certain the object is an insect.

TO REMOVE AN INSECT

Tilt the victim's head so that the affected ear is facing upward. Pour lukewarm water into the ear and the insect may float to the surface. If this fails, call your physician.

The physician will remove the object either by *syringing* the ear or by grasping the object with a pair of fine-toothed forceps. A brief general anesthetic may be required if the object is impacted, as often occurs with organic foreign bodies, such as beans, which swell when moistened by ear secretions.

INSECTS An insect can sometimes be removed from the ear by getting the person to tilt his or her head so that the affected side is uppermost and then pouring olive oil or lukewarm water into the ear. If this is not successful, a physician will need to syringe the ear after killing the insect with chloroform or drowning it with oil. It is impossible for insects to penetrate to the brain.

Ear, nose, and throat surgery
See *Otorhinolaryngology*.

Ear piercing
Making a hole in the earlobe or, occasionally, another part of the external ear, to accommodate an earring. Ear piercing was once performed with a needle, but the risk of transmitting diseases through the use of unsterile needles caused this method to be replaced by a special ear-piercing gun.
HOW IT IS DONE
A local anesthetic is not necessary, since the procedure causes only minor discomfort. The earlobe is pierced by a stud, fired into it by the gun, which does not come into contact with the ear. The studs are of gold or gold-plate (cheaper metals can cause contact *dermatitis*), are kept sealed in a sterile pack before use, and are not handled during the procedure.

For six weeks after insertion, the studs must be cleaned regularly with hydrogen peroxide or rubbing alcohol to prevent infection; the studs are kept in the ears and turned twice daily to prevent the hole from closing.

Ears, pinning back of
See *Otoplasty*.

Earwax
A yellow or brown secretion, also known as cerumen, produced by glands in the outer ear canal. In most people, wax is produced in only small amounts, comes out on its own, and causes no trouble; in other people, so much wax forms that it regularly obstructs the canal.

Excess earwax may produce a sensation of fullness in the ear and, if the canal is blocked completely, partial deafness. These symptoms are made worse if water enters the ear and makes the wax swell. Prolonged blockage may also inflame the skin of the canal, causing irritation.
TREATMENT
Wax that causes blockage or irritation should be removed by a physician. A firm plug of wax can be removed using a ring probe, a right-angled hook, or *forceps*. If the wax is too soft for this, it can be softened further with oil and then flushed out with a syringe containing warm water (see *Syringing of ears*). If there is a possibility that the eardrum may be damaged, the physician will use suction instead of syringing.

A physician will sometimes suggest that a patient should soften his or her own earwax with mineral oil or hydrogen peroxide. Cotton swabs should never be used as they can push wax deep into the canal, making matters worse.

Ecchymosis
The medical term for a *bruise*.

ECG
The abbreviation for electrocardiogram, a record of the electrical impulses that immediately precede contraction of the heart muscle. The waves produced are known as the P,Q,R,S, and T waves.

An ECG is a useful means of diagnosing disorders of the heart, many of which produce deviations from normal electrical patterns. Among these disorders are *coronary artery disease, coronary thrombosis, pericarditis* (inflammation of the membrane surrounding the heart), *cardiomyopathy* (heart muscle disorders), *myocarditis* (inflammation of the heart muscle), and arrhythmias (see *Arrhythmia, cardiac*).

Echocardiography
A method of obtaining an image of the structure of the heart using *ultrasound* (inaudible, high-frequency sound waves). The sound waves are reflected differently by each part of the heart, resulting in a complex series of echoes which can be detected and displayed visually.
WHY IT IS DONE
Echocardiography is a major diagnostic technique used to detect structural, and some functional, abnormalities of the heart wall, the heart valves, and the heart's large blood vessels. Blood flow across valves is also measured.

The procedure is especially valuable for studying disorders of the heart valves. Abnormal opening and closing of the valves can be detected because they deviate from normal patterns of valve movement. Other diagnostic uses include detection of congenital heart disease (see *Heart disease, congenital*), various abnormalities of the large blood vessels, *cardiomyopathy* (heart muscle disorders), *aneurysms* (ballooning of the heart wall or the walls of blood vessels), *pericarditis* (inflammation of the membrane that surrounds the heart), and the presence of a blood clot within a heart chamber.
HOW IT IS DONE
Echocardiography is harmless and the patient feels nothing; it has the added advantage of producing recordings without having to place an instrument inside the patient's body.

The transducer (the instrument that sends out and receives sound signals) is placed on the chest in a position that allows its sound waves to reach the structures under investigation. The echoes are detected, amplified, and then displayed visually as a series of lines on an oscilloscope screen or a paper tape. This information is interpreted by cardiologists as a picture of the heart and its valves and the way they are working.

Echocardiography has recently become more sophisticated and methods have been developed that incorporate a moving transducer, or a set of transducers, attached to a computer. This allows a series of different views of the heart to be combined to produce a two-dimensional scan. When recorded on videotape, an easily recognizable picture of the activity of the interior of the heart can be seen.

Doppler echocardiography is a technique that allows the indirect measurement of the flow velocity of blood as it passes through the heart. This technique can be useful in the assessment of patients with congenital heart disease or with a heart valve disorder such as *aortic stenosis* or *mitral insufficiency*.

Echolalia
The compulsive repetition of what is spoken by another person. The tone and accent of the speaker are copied as well as the actual words. Echolalia may be a symptom of *schizophrenia* and sometimes occurs in people who suffer from *mental retardation* or from *autism*. Echolalia may be accompanied by echopraxia (imitating the behavior of another person).

THE ELECTROCARDIOGRAM (ECG)

Electrocardiography causes no discomfort. Electrodes connected to a recording machine are applied to the chest, wrists, and ankles. The machine displays the electrical activity in the heart as a trace on a moving graph or on a screen. Any abnormality is thus revealed to the physician. Normal and abnormal recordings are shown below.

An ECG can be taken at home, in the physician's office, or in the hospital; a 24-hour record can be obtained from a tape recorder worn by the patient.

Lead positions
Recordings are taken with a lead attached to these positions.

Portable electrocardiograph
A modern, lightweight, portable ECG machine. Leads from the machine are attached to the chest, wrists, and ankles using conducting jelly.

Printout

Normal rhythm
The heart chambers are contracting with regularity.

Ventricular fibrillation
Here, the contractions of the lower heart chambers are extremely irregular.

Complete heart block
The upper and lower heart chambers are beating independently.

Atrial fibrillation
Caused by the upper heart chambers beating fast and irregularly.

Normal ECG
This tracing shows the electrical activity preceding one normal heartbeat. The vertical axis shows the current flowing toward the recording lead. The rise at P occurs just before the atria (upper heart chambers) begin to contract, the QRS "spike" occurs just before the ventricles (lower chambers) begin to contract, and the rise at T occurs as the electrical potential returns to zero.

Eclampsia

A rare, serious condition of late pregnancy, labor, and the period following delivery. Eclampsia is characterized by seizures (convulsions) in the woman, sometimes followed by coma and death; eclampsia also threatens the life of the baby. The disorder occurs as a complication of moderate or severe (but not mild) *preeclampsia*, a condition of late pregnancy that is marked by *hypertension* (high blood pressure), *proteinuria* (protein in the urine), and *edema* (accumulation of fluid in the tissues).

CAUSES
In spite of intensive investigation, the cause of eclampsia and preeclampsia remains unknown. Eclampsia is thought to be caused by cerebral edema (accumulation of fluid in the brain tissue) consequent on preeclampsia. Preeclampsia was formerly thought to be due to a placental toxin (poison) but is now thought to be due to an abnormality in the *immune response* to the pregnancy.

Eclampsia occurs more commonly in women who have had little or no *prenatal care* because the development of preeclampsia in these women may go unrecognized and therefore untreated.

INCIDENCE
About half of all cases develop in late pregnancy, one third during labor, and the rest after delivery.

SYMPTOMS AND SIGNS
In eclampsia the symptoms that characterize severe preeclampsia are present. Before the onset of seizures, the woman may suffer from headache, confusion, blurred vision, and abdominal pain. The seizures consist of violent, rhythmic, jerking movements of the limbs caused by involuntary contraction of the muscles; there may also be breathing difficulty caused by constriction of the muscles of the larynx. The seizures may sometimes be followed by coma.

TREATMENT
The seizures are treated by ensuring that the woman can breathe properly (sometimes by inserting an *endotracheal tube* down her throat) and by giving *anticonvulsant drugs*, which prevent further seizures.

The baby's condition is monitored throughout. Rapid delivery (often by emergency *cesarean section*) is usually performed because the condition is likely to improve once the baby has been born.

OUTLOOK
In the past, many babies failed to survive eclampsia, because of lack of oxygen in the uterus. Nowadays, the outlook for the baby depends partly on the stage of pregnancy at which the condition occurs.

After delivery, the mother's blood pressure usually returns to normal within a week and proteinuria clears within six weeks. In a small number of cases, however, the woman develops serious complications before, during, or after delivery. These may include *heart failure, kidney failure, liver failure, intracerebral hemorrhage, pneumonia,* or *pulmonary edema.*

E

Econazole

An *antifungal drug*. Econazole is used in cream form to treat fungal skin infections (see *Athlete's foot; Tinea*), and in cream or pessary form to treat vaginal *candidiasis*.

This fast-working drug usually begins to act within two days. Skin irritation is a rare adverse effect.

ECT

The abbreviation for electroconvulsive therapy, which uses electric shocks to induce *seizures* as a treatment for severe *depression*. Anesthesia and *muscle-relaxant drugs* are used to minimize movements of the body during treatment and the effects of ECT are thus limited primarily to the brain.

WHY IT IS USED

ECT is now used almost exclusively to treat severe depressive illness that has become life-threatening because of accompanying weight loss and neglect. It is used less widely to treat *postpartum depression*, catatonic *schizophrenia*, and some cases of *mania* that have not responded to other treatments. ECT is not used to treat people with severe physical illness or those who have had a recent *myocardial infarction* (heart attack).

HOW IT IS DONE

The patient is given a general anesthetic and a muscle-relaxant drug before two padded electrodes are applied to the temple, one on each side or both on the same side. A controlled electric pulse is delivered to the electrodes from a small machine until a brain seizure occurs. The seizure is indicated by brief muscular rigidity, followed by twitching of the limbs and eyelids. Afterward, patients experience only mild discomfort similar to the discomfort felt after a minor dental operation.

Treatment usually consists of six to 12 seizures (two or three per week).

OUTLOOK

If a true brain seizure has been induced at each session, the patient's condition usually begins to improve by the third treatment, often dramatically. Temporary *amnesia* (memory loss) is a possible side effect. ECT usually relieves depression more rapidly than drug treatment.

Ectasia

A medical term meaning widening, usually used to refer to a disorder affecting a duct that carries secretions from a gland or organ. For example, mammary duct ectasia—a rare disorder that affects women mainly around the time of the menopause—is widening of the ducts that carry secretions from the tissues of the breast to the nipple.

-ectomy

A suffix denoting surgical removal. Tonsillectomy is surgical removal of the tonsils.

Ectoparasite

A parasite that lives in or on its host's skin and derives nourishment from the skin or by sucking the host's blood. Various *lice, ticks, mites*, and some types of *fungi* are occasional ectoparasites of humans. By contrast, endoparasites live inside the body.

Ectopic

A medical term used to describe a structure that occurs in an abnormal location or position, or an activity that occurs at an abnormal time.

Ectopic heartbeat

A contraction of the heart muscle that is out of the normal timed sequence. An ectopic heartbeat occurs shortly after a normal beat and is followed by a longer-than-usual interval.

Ectopic beats can occur in a heart that is otherwise functioning normally and may cause no symptoms. Multiple ectopic beats can sometimes cause *palpitations*.

After a *myocardial infarction* (heart attack), the occurrence of multiple ectopic beats is a sign of damage to the conduction system of the heart muscle. Multiple ectopic beats may lead to ventricular *fibrillation*, a rapid uncoordinated heartbeat that can cause collapse and death.

Multiple ectopic beats that are causing palpitations, or that occur after a myocardial infarction, are often treated with an *antiarrhythmic drug*. (See also *Arrhythmia, cardiac*.)

Ectopic pregnancy

A pregnancy that develops outside the uterus, most commonly in the *fallopian tube*, but sometimes in the ovary or, rarely, in the abdominal cavity or cervix. As the pregnancy develops, it may damage or rupture surrounding tissue, causing serious bleeding.

About one in every 200 pregnancies is ectopic. The condition creates a life-threatening situation that requires emergency treatment. More than 50 North American women die each year from ectopic pregnancies.

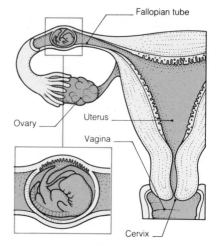

Location of an ectopic pregnancy
The pregnancy usually develops in the fallopian tube; occasionally it develops in the ovary, abdominal cavity, or cervix.

CAUSES

The fertilized ovum (egg) may become stuck in the fallopian tube if there is a *congenital* abnormality of the tube, or if the tube is damaged in any way. Damage may result from infection (see *Pelvic inflammatory disease*) or from surgery on the fallopian tubes.

A pregnancy that occurs following the failure of some methods of contraception has an increased risk of being ectopic. Ectopic pregnancy has been associated with use of an *IUD* (intrauterine contraceptive device), progesterone-only *oral contraceptives*, hormonal postcoital contraception (see *Contraception, postcoital*), and sterilization operations, especially if the fallopian tubes have been cauterized (see *Sterilization, female*).

SYMPTOMS AND SIGNS

Most ectopic pregnancies are discovered in the first two months, often before the woman realizes she is pregnant. In most cases a menstrual period is missed, but, in about 20 percent of affected women, menstruation occurs. Symptoms of ectopic pregnancy usually include severe pain in the lower abdomen and vaginal bleeding which may be mistaken for a period. Rupture or internal bleeding cause symptoms of *shock*—pallor, sweating, weakness, and faintness.

DIAGNOSIS AND TREATMENT

A *pregnancy test* may be performed but is often negative in this condition. *Ultrasound scanning* and a *laparoscopy* (examination of the abdominal cavity with a viewing instrument) may also be performed.

Once an ectopic pregnancy is confirmed, an operation is performed to remove the fetus (which is usually already dead), the placenta, and any damaged tissue at the site of the pregnancy. Any torn blood vessels are repaired and, if the fallopian tube cannot be repaired, it is removed. Many physicians prefer to remove the tube because of the risk of another ectopic pregnancy. If blood loss is severe, *blood transfusions* are needed.

OUTLOOK

It is still possible to have a normal pregnancy even if one fallopian tube has been removed, although the chances of conception are slightly reduced. Women with two damaged tubes may require *in vitro fertilization* to achieve an intrauterine pregnancy.

Ectropion

A turning outward of the eyelid so that the inner surface is exposed.

INCIDENCE AND CAUSES

Ectropion is most common in elderly people, usually affecting the lower lid and due to weakness of the muscle surrounding the eye.

The condition may also be caused by the contraction of scar tissue in the skin near either lid. Ectropion also often follows *facial palsy*, in which the muscles surrounding the eye (and other facial muscles on that side) are paralyzed.

The appearance of ectropion
An example of ectropion affecting the lower eyelid of one eye. The lid is turned outward to reveal the lining of its inner surface.

SYMPTOMS AND SIGNS

Even slight ectropion interferes with normal drainage of tears by distorting the opening of the tear duct. Chronic *conjunctivitis* may result, with redness, discomfort, and overflow of tears so that the skin becomes damp and inflamed. Constant wiping tends to pull the lid farther from the eye.

TREATMENT

Surgery to tighten the lid by removing a wedge of tissue is simple and effec-

tive in the early stages of ectropion. Plastic surgery using skin grafting may be needed if the condition is long-standing.

Eczema

An inflammation of the skin, usually causing itching and sometimes accompanied by scaling or blisters. Some forms of eczema are better known as *dermatitis* (such as seborrheic dermatitis, contact dermatitis, and photodermatitis). Eczema is sometimes caused by an *allergy*, but often occurs for no known reason.

TYPES

ATOPIC ECZEMA This chronic, superficial inflammation occurs in people who have an inherited tendency toward allergy. They, or members of their family, may also have other allergies, such as *asthma* or allergic *rhinitis* (hay fever).

Atopic eczema is common in babies and often appears between the ages of 2 months and 18 months. An intensely itchy rash occurs, usually on the face, in the inner creases of the elbows, and behind the knees. The skin often scales in these areas, and small red pimples may appear. As the baby scratches, the pimples begin to ooze and join to form large weeping areas. Infection may occur, particularly in the diaper area.

For mild cases, treatment consists of applying *emollients*, such as petroleum jelly, which help keep the skin in the infected area soft. In severe cases, ointments containing *corticosteroid drugs* may be prescribed, and *antibiotic drugs* may be given for infection. *Antihistamine drugs* may be prescribed to reduce itching, particularly if it keeps a baby awake at night. The baby should be prevented from becoming too hot, which aggravates the condition. Only cotton clothing should be in direct contact with the skin.

The condition often clears of its own accord as a child grows older, although it may come and go for several years. Most children outgrow atopic eczema by puberty.

NUMMULAR ECZEMA This type usually occurs in adults. The cause is unknown. Nummular eczema takes the form of circular, itchy, scaling patches anywhere on the skin, similar to *tinea* (ringworm), from which the eczema needs to be distinguished. Corticosteroid drugs may be applied to the affected skin to help reduce inflammation, although the disorder is persistent and often resistant to treatment.

Atopic eczema
An example of atopic eczema on the creases of the inner wrist, showing the characteristic pimples and raw, scaling skin. Because the rash is intensely itchy, scratching is usually inevitable and aggravates the condition.

HAND ECZEMA This type is usually a result of irritation by substances such as detergents and dishwashing liquid, but may occur for no ascertainable reason. Itchy blisters, up to about 2.5 cm across, develop, usually on the palms, and the hand may be covered with scales and cracks. Tests are performed to check for allergy.

Hand eczema usually improves if rubber gloves are worn over white cotton gloves when in contact with any irritants. The hands should be thoroughly patted dry after washing. An unscented hand cream should be applied several times a day. If severe, corticosteroids may be prescribed for the inflammation and antibiotics may be given for infection.

STASIS ECZEMA In people with varicose veins, the skin on the legs may become irritated, inflamed, and discolored. The most important factor is swelling of the legs, which may be controlled with compression bandages or stockings. Corticosteroid ointments may give temporary relief.

GENERAL TREATMENT

To reduce irritation and the likelihood of scratching, a soothing ointment should be applied to the affected areas, which should then be covered by a dressing to prevent scratching. Absorbent, nonirritating materials such as cotton should be worn next to the skin; irritating fabrics such as wool, silk, and rough synthetics should be avoided.

Edema

An abnormal accumulation of fluid in the body tissues. Edema may or may not be visible (as a swelling) and can be either localized (as after an injury) or generalized (as in *heart failure*). Generalized edema (also called anasarca) was formerly commonly known as dropsy.

E

WATER BALANCE IN THE BODY

Water accounts for roughly three fifths of body weight and is constantly exchanged between blood and tissues. Water is forced out of the capillaries (tiny blood vessels) and into the tissues by the pressure of blood being pumped around the body. By a reverse process, which depends on the water-drawing power of the proteins in the blood (see *Osmosis*), water is reabsorbed into the capillaries from the tissues.

These two mechanisms normally are in balance, keeping the levels of water in the blood and the tissues more or less constant.

Another factor involved in maintaining this balance is the action of the *kidneys*, which pass excess salt from the blood into the urine to be excreted from the body.

CAUSES OF EDEMA

Various disorders can interfere with these processes. Heart failure leads to blood congestion in the veins, creating backward pressure in the capillaries. This backward pressure overcomes osmotic pressure in the capillaries and thus causes more fluid than normal to be forced into the tissues at various places. Backward pressure can also be created by a tumor pressing on veins. The edema produced is confined to the area drained by the obstructed vein.

In *nephrotic syndrome*, an abnormal loss of protein from the blood reduces osmotic pressure and prevents enough fluid being drawn from the tissues into the blood. *Kidney failure* prevents salt being excreted from the body, allowing it to accumulate in the tissues and attract water to it.

Other disorders that can cause edema include *cirrhosis* of the liver, which leads to blood congestion in the veins of the liver, lowers blood protein (and therefore osmotic pressure), and causes salt retention. A deficiency of protein in the diet, as may occur in alcoholics, can also reduce osmotic pressure; edema in alcoholics may also be due to deficiency of thiamine (vitamin B$_1$), leading to *beriberi*.

Injury may cause edema by damaging capillaries and thus allowing fluid to leak out of them. In some instances, blockage of lymphatic vessels may result in *lymphedema*.

Edema may also be caused by certain drugs. These include *corticosteroid drugs*, *androgen drugs*, and high-estrogen *oral contraceptives*, which all act on the kidneys, causing a certain amount of salt retention.

Chronic edema
An example of chronic edema, showing the characteristic swelling and stretched, shiny skin. In this patient, the skin of the left leg is also ulcerated.

SYMPTOMS AND SIGNS

Until the excess fluid in the body increases by more than about 15 percent, edema may show itself only as an increase in weight. After that it is evident as a swelling, often in the lower part of the body (e.g., around the base of the spine and the ankles).

In severe cases, fluid accumulates in one or more of the large body cavities. For example, in *ascites*, fluid collects in the peritoneal cavity of the abdomen, causing abdominal swelling. In *pleural effusion*, fluid fills the pleural cavity of the lungs, resulting in breathing difficulty. In *pulmonary edema*, the air sacs of the lungs become waterlogged, causing breathing difficulty.

The presence of edema can be detected by pressing a finger into the swollen area. This action produces an indentation in the skin which slowly flattens out as the fluid seeps back.

TREATMENT

The aim is always to remedy the underlying cause of the edema. In many cases, however, the underlying cause is not remediable and the only treatment is to make the body excrete the excess fluid by increasing the output of urine by the kidneys. This is done by restricting dietary sodium and by the use of *diuretic drugs*, which may be needed indefinitely.

Edentulous

Without teeth, either because they have not yet grown or because they have fallen out or been removed.

EEG

The abbreviation for electroencephalogram. An EEG records the minute electrical impulses produced by the activity of the brain. The technique of electroencephalography was first used in medicine in 1928, although it had been known since the 19th century that electrical impulses could be recorded from animal brains.

WHY IT IS DONE

An EEG indicates, by the frequency of the recorded activity, the mental state of the subject—that is, whether he or she is alert, awake, or asleep. Also, by revealing characteristic wave patterns, the EEG can help in diagnosing certain conditions, especially *epilepsy* and certain types of *encephalitis*, *dementia*, and *brain tumor*.

Electroencephalography can also be used to monitor the condition of patients during surgery and to assess the depth of *anesthesia*. It is also used in determining *brain death*, but an EEG check is not required to make the determination.

Effusion

The escape of fluid through the walls of a blood vessel into a tissue or body cavity, often as a result of a vessel being inflamed or congested. For example, *pleural effusion*, a symptom of *heart failure*, occurs when raised blood pressure in the veins leads to fluid being forced out of the blood and through the walls of capillaries into the pleural cavity around the lungs.

Effusion, joint

The accumulation of fluid in a joint space, causing swelling, limitation of movement, and usually pain and tenderness of the affected area. A joint is enclosed by a capsule lined with a membrane called the synovium. This membrane normally secretes small amounts of fluid to lubricate the joint, but if it is damaged or inflamed (e.g., by *arthritis*) it produces excessive amounts of fluid.

Location of knee joint effusion
Excessive production and accumulation of fluid within a knee joint caused by injury or inflammation.

HOW ELECTROENCEPHALOGRAPHY IS DONE

A number of small electrodes are attached to the scalp. Shaving of the scalp is unnecessary. The electrodes are connected to an instrument that measures the brain's impulses in microvolts and amplifies them for recording purposes. The technique is painless, produces no side effects, and takes about 45 minutes. Recordings are taken with the subject at rest, with eyes open and then shut, during and after *hyperventilation*, and while looking at a flashing light. It is also helpful, especially when epilepsy is suspected, to record activity as the patient goes to sleep.

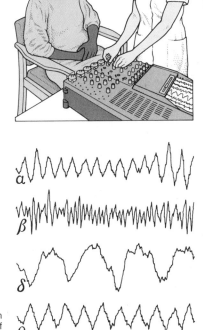

EEG wave patterns

Alpha waves
The prominent pattern of an awake, relaxed adult whose eyes are closed.

Beta waves
The lower, faster oscillation of a person who is concentrating on an external stimulus.

Delta waves
The typical pattern of sleep, but also found in young infants; rarely, they are caused by a brain tumor.

Theta waves
The dominant waves of young children. In adults, they may indicate an abnormality of the brain.

TREATMENT
Analgesic drugs (painkillers), *nonsteroidal anti-inflammatory drugs*, and injections of *corticosteroid drugs* help relieve pain and inflammation. The swelling can be reduced by rest, firm wrapping with a bandage, ice packs, and keeping the affected joint raised. In some cases, the fluid may need to be aspirated (drawn out) with a hypodermic needle and syringe. *Antibiotic drugs* may also be given if the cause is infective arthritis (also called septic arthritis). *Physiotherapy* may be necessary.

Egg
See *Ovum*.

Ego
The conscious sense of oneself, equivalent to "I." In Freudian *psychoanalytic theory*, this part of the personality maintains a balance between the primitive, unconscious instincts of the *id*, the controls of the *superego* (or conscience), and the demands of the outside world.

Ehlers-Danlos syndrome
An inherited disorder of *collagen*, the most important structural protein in the body. Affected individuals have abnormally stretchy, thin skin that bruises very easily. Wounds are slow to heal and leave paper-thin scars. Sufferers tend to bleed easily from the gums and digestive tract. The joints are exceptionally loose and are prone to recurrent dislocation.

Ehlers-Danlos syndrome is usually (although not always) inherited in an autosomal dominant pattern (see *Genetic disorders*). This means that many affected individuals have an affected parent; each of an affected person's children has a 50 percent chance of being affected.

There is no known specific treatment for Ehlers-Danlos syndrome, although unnecessary accidental injury, as may occur in contact sports such as hockey and soccer, should be avoided. The outlook for a normal life expectancy is good.

Eisenmenger complex
A condition affecting the heart and lungs in which a heart deformity leads to a buildup of pressure in the right side of the heart (see *Pulmonary hypertension*) that causes the abnormal flow of blood from the right side of the heart to the left side of the heart. Eisenmenger complex most often occurs in people with certain congenital heart defects (see *Heart disease, congenital*), such as uncorrected ventricular *septal defect*.

In people with Eisenmenger complex, deoxygenated blood in the right side of the heart is shunted through the defect into the left side of the heart and recirculated around the body, instead of being sent to the lungs to receive more oxygen. The resultant *hypoxia* (lack of oxygen in the blood) causes *cyanosis* (bluish discoloration of the skin), fainting, and breathing difficulty.

The diagnosis is confirmed by cardiac *catheterization* (the insertion under X-ray control of a thin tube into the patient's heart via a blood vessel) to measure pressure and the composition of *blood gases* within the four heart chambers.

Once Eisenmenger complex has developed, surgical correction of the original heart defect will not help. Drug treatment may help to control symptoms. Most affected people die in their 30s or 40s. A heart-lung transplant may offer new hope to severely disabled patients.

Ejaculation
The emission of *semen* from the penis at *orgasm*. Ejaculation is a reflex action that depends on regular and rhythmic pressure on the penis, usually during intercourse or masturbation. This stimulation acts on spinal nerves and triggers ejaculation.

Shortly before ejaculation the muscles around the epididymides (ducts where sperm are stored), the prostate gland, and the seminal vesicles contract rhythmically, forcing the sperm from the epididymides to move forward and mix with the secretions from the seminal vesicles and prostate. At ejaculation, this fluid is propelled through the urethra and out of the body.

Because both semen and urine leave the body by the same route, the bladder neck closes during ejaculation. This not only prevents ejaculate from going into the bladder but also stops urine from contaminating the semen. (See also *Reproductive system, male*.)

E

Ejaculation, disorders of

Conditions in which the normal process or timing of *ejaculation* is disrupted. Disorders of ejaculation are relatively common causes of unhappiness in relationships.

TYPES

PREMATURE EJACULATION In this disorder, ejaculation occurs before or very soon after penetration. Premature ejaculation is the most common sexual problem in men and is especially common in adolescents. Most adult men occasionally experience premature ejaculation, commonly because of overstimulation or anxiety about sexual performance. If premature ejaculation occurs frequently, the cause may be psychological. Sexual counseling and techniques for delaying ejaculation may help to alleviate the problem (see *Sex therapy*).

INHIBITED EJACULATION This is a rare condition in which erection is normal, or even prolonged, but ejaculation is abnormally delayed or does not occur at all. Inhibited ejaculation may be psychological in origin, in which case sexual counseling may help, or it may be a complication of another disorder, such as *diabetes mellitus* or the long-term effects of *alcohol dependence*. Inhibited ejaculation may also occur during treatment with certain drugs, such as some *antihypertensive drugs*.

RETROGRADE EJACULATION In this disorder, the valve at the base of the bladder fails to close during ejaculation. This forces the ejaculate back into the bladder. Retrograde ejaculation may occur as a result of a neurological disease, after surgery on the neck of the bladder, after *prostatectomy* (removal of the prostate gland), or after extensive pelvic surgery. There is no treatment, but intercourse with a full bladder can sometimes lead to normal ejaculation. (See also *Azoospermia*; *Psychosexual dysfunction*; *Sexual problems*.)

Elbow

The joint between the lower end of the *humerus* (upper-arm bone) and the upper ends of the radius and ulna (forearm bones). The elbow joint is stabilized by ligaments at the front, back, and sides. The elbow enables the arm to be bent and straightened, and the forearm to be rotated through almost 180 degrees around its long axis without more than slight movement of the upper arm.

DISORDERS

Disorders include *arthritis* and injuries to the joint and its surrounding muscles, tendons, and ligaments.

ANATOMY OF THE ELBOW

The elbow is a hinge joint between the lower end of the humerus and the upper ends of the radius and ulna. The biceps muscle bends and rotates the arm at the elbow.

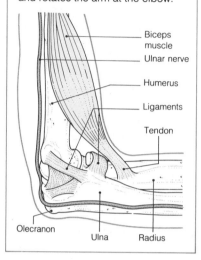

Biceps muscle
Ulnar nerve
Humerus
Ligaments
Tendon
Olecranon
Ulna
Radius

SOFT TISSUE INJURY AND INFLAMMATION Repetitive strain on the tendons of the forearm muscles at the points at which they attach to the elbow (at the bony outgrowths called epicondyles) can lead to an inflammation called *epicondylitis* at these points. The two main types of epicondylitis are *tennis elbow* and *golfer's elbow*. Alternatively, a *sprain* of the joint ligaments can occur, especially in children.

Olecranon *bursitis* occurs over the tip of the elbow in response to local irritation. Repeated overstraightening of the joint can cause damage to the cartilage that lines the joint. Strain on the joint produces an *effusion* (accumulation of fluid within the joint space) or traumatic *synovitis* (inflammation of the membrane that lines the joint capsule).

A sharp blow on the olecranon process (the bony tip of the elbow, also called the "funny bone") may impinge on the *ulnar nerve* as it passes in a groove in this area, causing temporary discomfort—a pins and needles sensation and lancing pains that shoot down the forearm into the fourth and fifth fingers.

FRACTURES A fall onto an outstretched hand or onto the tip of the elbow can lead to any of various types of fracture around or at the lower end of the humerus. Children may alternatively sustain an injury to the epiphyses (growing areas) at the ends of the

---

humerus, radius, or ulna. Dislocation of the elbow can occur at any age as a result of falling onto an outstretched hand; dislocations and fractures of the elbow frequently occur together.

ARTHRITIS *Osteoarthritis*, *rheumatoid arthritis*, and infective arthritis can affect the elbow joint.

Elderly, care of the

As people age they become prone to an increasing number of physical disorders and are more likely to suffer from loneliness and isolation. Efforts to stress personal pride and independence (along with appropriate medical care) can minimize physical and mental deterioration. Sensitive attention to psychological needs can help the elderly enjoy old age and can encourage them to feel that they are still useful members of society.

PHYSICAL CARE

Elderly people often ignore symptoms of illness, either because they do not want to be a nuisance to those caring for them or because they are afraid of being "put away" in a home. Some conditions, such as *hypothyroidism* (underactivity of the thyroid gland) and *anemia*, which is often due to a poor diet, cause a very gradual deterioration. Such deterioration may incorrectly be assumed to be a natural effect of old age, resulting in failure to diagnose actual medical conditions.

Failing vision and hearing are frequently regarded as inevitable features of old age, but in many cases surgical removal of a *cataract* or provision of a *hearing aid* can enable the individual to lead a more independent and active life.

To ensure that medical problems are detected early and treated, it is important that caregivers remain alert to the symptoms and signs of illness. In addition, all people over 65 years of age should have regular checkups.

PSYCHOLOGICAL CARE

Common causes of *depression* in the elderly are isolation, inactivity, and a feeling of not being wanted. Elderly people can be helped by making them part of family activities. Attending a day-care center or senior citizen club can provide contact with other people and the opportunity to develop new interests. *Dementia* (loss of normal brain function) becomes more common as a person ages and increases the level of supervision required.

DAY-TO-DAY CARE

Many elderly people prefer to live with their families, ideally in a separate section of the house, where they

PERCENTAGE OF CANADIANS AGED 65 AND OVER

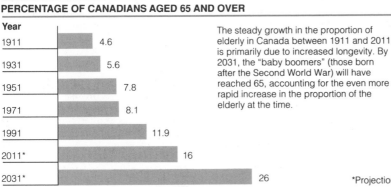

Year	
1911	4.6
1931	5.6
1951	7.8
1971	8.1
1991	11.9
2011*	16
2031*	26

*Projection

The steady growth in the proportion of elderly in Canada between 1911 and 2011 is primarily due to increased longevity. By 2031, the "baby boomers" (those born after the Second World War) will have reached 65, accounting for the even more rapid increase in the proportion of the elderly at the time.

can have some degree of independence. If this is not possible, they may be able to live near relatives so that help can be provided with daily activities, such as shopping, cooking, and laundry. Assistance with personal care may also be required.

While this type of arrangement may be ideal for the elderly person, the responsibility can be a great strain on other members of the family. Voluntary agencies can sometimes help by providing a daily meal or occasional domestic help.

The elderly person's home, or that part of the house set aside for his or her use, should be well heated in winter and cooled in summer to prevent *hypothermia* or *hyperthermia*; a high level of artificial illumination should be provided to make activities such as reading and sewing easier. The risk of falls can be reduced by ensuring that there are no loose rugs or slippery surfaces (see *Falls in the elderly*) and the person living alone can be provided with an alarm that enables him or her to summon help in an emergency.

Elective

A term used to describe a procedure, usually a surgical operation, that is not essential but can be performed at a chosen time. Because an elective procedure is not an emergency, it is often possible for the patient—in consultation with the physician—to select the most convenient time for the procedure. Elective surgery includes the correction of nonurgent medical conditions, such as *hemorrhoids* or a *hernia*, as well as some cosmetic procedures, such as *rhinoplasty*.

Electrical injury

Damage to the tissues caused by the passage of an electric current through the body and by its associated heat release.

The internal tissues of the body, being moist and salty, are good conductors of electricity. Dry skin provides a high resistance (several tens of thousands of ohms) to current flow, but moist skin has a low resistance (only a few thousand ohms) and thus allows a substantial current to flow into the body. Serious injury or death from domestic voltage levels is thus more likely in the presence of water. The danger of serious injury is increased if a person is "well-earthed" (i.e., in contact with a good conductor of electricity, such as a bath of water) and decreased if he or she is in a dry environment (especially if he or she is wearing rubber-soled shoes, which are poor electric conductors).

INCIDENCE

Electrical accidents in Canada cause 60 to 70 deaths each year. Many of these deaths occur in the home, as a result of handling a frayed electric cord or using an electrical appliance near water. Some deaths occur among workers in the electrical generating and construction industries as a result of contact with high voltages. Fewer than 10 Canadians die annually as a result of lightning accidents.

E

FIRST AID: ELECTRICAL INJURY

DO NOT
- attempt first aid until contact with the electric current has been broken
- touch the victim with anything wet

1 Pull the electric plug out. If this is impossible, stand on a dry object and push the victim away from the source using a dry broomstick.

2 If the victim is unconscious and not breathing, start *cardiopulmonary resuscitation*.

3 If the victim is breathing, place in the *recovery position*. Follow first aid advice for *burns* and *shock* until an ambulance arrives.

Many other Canadians are injured in electrical accidents every year, some seriously.

PHYSICAL EFFECTS

All except the mildest electric shocks may cause unconsciousness. The extent of tissue damage depends on the size and type of the current flowing through the body. Alternating current (AC) is more dangerous than direct current (DC) because it causes sustained muscle contractions, which, by preventing hand movement, may prevent the victim from releasing his or her grip on the source of the current.

A current as small as one tenth of an amp passing through the heart can bring about a fatal *arrhythmia* (disturbance of the heartbeat). This quantity is about the size of current passing through the filament of a very low-power bulb. The same current passing through the brain stem may cause the heart to stop beating and breathing to cease. Larger currents, generated by high voltages, may also cause charring of tissues, especially at points where the resistance is highest, usually where the current enters and exits from the body.

Electric shock treatment
See *ECT* (electroconvulsive therapy).

Electrocardiography
See *ECG*.

Electrocautery
A technique for destroying tissue by the application of heat produced by an electric current. Electrocautery can be used to remove certain skin blemishes, such as *warts*. (See also *Cauterization*; *Diathermy*; *Electrocoagulation*.)

Electrocoagulation
The use of high-frequency electric current to seal blood vessels by heat and thus stop bleeding. Electrocoagulation may be used during all forms of surgery to close freshly cut blood vessels. It is also used to destroy spider nevi and other kinds of abnormal blood vessel formations and to stop nosebleeds. The current is applied through a fine needle or, in surgery, may be delivered through a knife, enabling the surgeon to make bloodless incisions.

Electroconvulsive therapy
See *ECT*.

Electroencephalography
See *EEG*.

Electrolysis
Permanent removal of unwanted hair by means of short-wave electric current, which destroys the hairs' roots.

WHY IT IS DONE

Hair on the face and body can be removed temporarily by shaving or plucking, or by the use of depilatory creams, abrasives, or wax preparations. Electrolysis is the only means of permanent removal.

Before treatment a person should first ensure that the operator is fully trained; incompetent treatment can cause permanent disfigurement.

AREAS THAT CAN BE TREATED

With a few exceptions, electrolysis can be safely used on any part of the body where excessive hair is regarded as unsightly. Its use should be avoided on the lower margins of the eyebrows, where the skin above the eyelids is delicate and easily damaged, and it is questionable whether it should be used on the armpits because of a risk of bacterial infection. Electrolysis has no harmful effect on the breasts (where hair sometimes grows around the areola), or on the ability of mother or infant to breast-feed.

The legs are not well suited for electrolysis; treatment requires so many sessions that it is too time-consuming and expensive for most people.

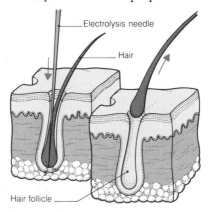

Electrolysis needle

Hair

Hair follicle

How electrolysis is done
To remove each hair, a fine needle is inserted into the follicle and a small electric current is passed through it. The current destroys the root of the hair, which is then pulled out. The procedure may cause some pain, but in skilled hands, it is harmless. If the treatment is successful, there should be no more hair growth from that follicle.

Electrolyte
A substance whose molecules dissociate (split) into its constituent *ions* (electrically charged particles) when dissolved or melted. For example,

sodium chloride (table salt) dissociates into positive sodium ions and negative chloride ions in water.

Electromyography
See *EMG*.

Electronystagmography
A method of recording the various types of *nystagmus* (abnormal jerky movements of the eye) to investigate their cause. Electrical changes caused by eye movements are picked up by electrodes placed near the eyes and are recorded on a graph for analysis.

Electrophoresis
The movement of electrically charged particles suspended in a *colloid* solution under the influence of an electric current. The direction, distance, and rate of movement vary according to factors such as the size, shape, and electrical charge of the particles.

Electrophoresis can be used to analyze mixtures of substances, particularly to identify different proteins in a mixture. For example, electrophoresis can be used to identify and quantify the various proteins in blood; furthermore, by comparing the results from a particular blood sample with normal values, it is possible to diagnose disorders such as *myeloma*, a tumor of the bone marrow that produces abnormally high levels of a specific *immunoglobulin* in the blood.

Elephantiasis
A disease found in the tropics, characterized by massive swellings of the legs, arms, and scrotum, with thickening and darkening of the overlying skin so that it resembles the skin of an elephant. Most elephantiasis is due to chronic lymphatic obstruction linked to *filariasis* (a worm infestation).

ELISA test
A laboratory blood test commonly used in the diagnosis of infectious diseases. ELISA stands for enzyme-linked immunosorbent assay. (See also *Immunoassay*.)

Elixir
A clear, sweetened liquid, often containing alcohol, that forms the basis for many liquid medicines, such as *cough remedies*.

Embolectomy
Surgical removal of an *embolus* (a fragment of material carried in the bloodstream) that has blocked a blood vessel (see *Embolism*).

The embolus may be removed during an operation performed under general anesthesia. An incision is made in the affected artery and the embolus aspirated (removed through a suction tube).

Alternatively, an embolus may be removed by a procedure known as balloon embolectomy, in which a *balloon catheter* is passed into the affected blood vessel. This procedure may be performed using local anesthesia.

Embolism

Blockage of an artery by a fragment of material traveling in the bloodstream. The particle causing the blockage is called an embolus and may consist of a blood clot, a bubble of air or other gas, a piece of tissue or tumor, a clump of bacteria, bone marrow, cholesterol, or fat, or any of various other substances.

TYPES

Blood clots are the most common type of embolus and in most cases have broken off from a larger clot that has formed elsewhere in the blood circulation. *Pulmonary embolism* is usually the result of a fragment breaking off from a deep vein *thrombosis* (a blood clot formed in a deep vein, usually in a leg) and being carried via the heart to block an artery supplying the lungs; this is a common cause of sudden, unexpected death. Similar blood clots may form on the lining of the heart after a *myocardial infarction* (heart attack) and then travel to the brain, resulting in a cerebral embolism, which is an important cause of *stroke*.

Air embolism, in which a small artery is blocked by an air bubble, is rare. Fat embolism, in which blood vessels are blocked by fat globules, is a possible complication of a major fracture of the arm or leg. Amniotic fluid embolism, in which some of the fluid that surrounds the baby in the uterus is forced into the mother's circulation, is a rare complication of late pregnancy.

SYMPTOMS

Factors that determine symptoms include the extent of blockage, the size and type of embolus, and the size, nature, and location of the affected blood vessel. In pulmonary embolism the sufferer feels faint and breathless, and has chest pains. If the embolus causes a *stroke*, the symptoms depend on which part of the brain is affected; it may, for example, cause inability to speak, inability to move a part of the body, loss of consciousness, or a disturbance of vision. In the small number of serious cases of fat embolism, the patient's heart rate and breathing rate rise dramatically, and there is restlessness and confusion accompanied by drowsiness.

TREATMENT

If a pulmonary or other severe type of embolism causes the person to collapse, emergency lifesaving procedures are carried out to maintain breathing and circulation. If the person survives, *embolectomy* (surgery to remove the blockage) may be possible. If surgery is not possible, *thrombolytic drugs* (drugs that dissolve blood clots) and *anticoagulant drugs* (drugs that prevent clot formation) may be administered.

OUTLOOK

In all severe types of embolism, survival depends on the success of resuscitation attempts, the importance of the vessel obstructed, and the speed with which blood flow is reestablished. If the source of the embolus is treated, the long-term prospects for the patient are good.

Embolization

Also called therapeutic embolism, the deliberate obstruction of a blood vessel to stop internal bleeding or to cut off blood flow to a tumor.

WHY IT IS DONE

Embolization is increasingly being performed to stop otherwise uncontrollable bleeding, particularly when the patient is too ill to undergo surgery. Among its uses are the control of bleeding from small vessels in the lining of the intestine, often due to a malformation of blood vessels (similar to a birthmark in the skin).

Using the technique to deprive a tumor of its blood supply has several effects. It can relieve the pain caused by the growth; it can cause the tumor to shrivel, making surgical removal easier; or it may stop the tumor from spreading. Embolization may be used to treat tumors that would be difficult to remove surgically, such as tumors in the liver. It is also used to treat certain vascular tumors on the face, such as *hemangiomas*, in preference to surgery that might leave unsightly scars.

HOW IT IS DONE

The procedure is usually carried out by a radiologist with the patient under a general anesthetic. The first step is to obtain an image of the blood vessel to be blocked and of the vessels leading to it. This image is obtained by means of *angiography*, an X-ray procedure in which a substance that is opaque to X rays is introduced into the blood vessels through a *catheter* (a flexible tube).

The catheter is then guided, by means of television monitoring, as

---

TYPES OF EMBOLISM

Embolisms are named after the part of the circulation affected or the embolus involved (e.g., a fat embolism is caused by fat globules, sometimes released from a bone fracture). When an embolus is released, it is carried through branches of an artery until it becomes lodged. Blood is prevented from reaching parts of the body beyond.

Embolism in the arm
This X ray of the upper arm was taken after the injection of contrast medium into the blood vessel. It shows, near the top, an embolus obstructing the normal flow of blood through one of the main arteries.

Cerebral embolism
A blockage of one of the arteries that supply blood to the brain; it is one of the most common causes of stroke.

Pulmonary embolism
A blockage of one of the arteries that supply blood to the lungs. This may cause chest pain, breathlessness, and sudden death.

Amniotic fluid embolism
The escape of some of the fluid that surrounds the baby in the uterus into the mother's circulation. This may cause blockage of an artery in one of her lungs.

Embolism in leg
An embolism may block one of the arteries that supply blood to the leg. Gangrene may occur below the blockage.

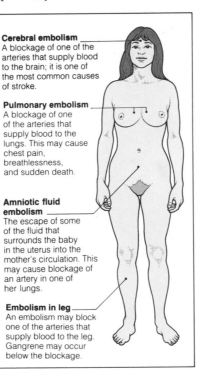

THE DEVELOPING EMBRYO

From the time of conception until the eighth week, the developing baby is known as an embryo. At conception, the fertilized egg consists of a single cell, the zygote, which contains genetic material from the sperm and the egg. The zygote divides several times to form a ball of cells, which then implants into the lining of the uterus. At the point of attachment, the outer layer of cells forms the placenta, while a group of cells within one area of the cell ball develops into the embryo. A sac filled with amniotic fluid forms around the embryo to protect it. As the embryo grows, it begins to form features and, by the fifth week, it has developed a recognizable head and limb buds.

Embryo at about six weeks
The embryo is floating in the amniotic sac. The smaller sac at left (the yolk sac) provides nourishment for the early embryo.

Passage to the uterus
The egg is fertilized in one of the fallopian tubes and is carried into the uterus, where it embeds in the uterine lining.

Fertilization of egg in fallopian tube

Ovary

Fertilized egg implants in uterine wall

Head

Notochord

Lower spine

Actual size:

Forebrain

Heart bulge

Umbilical cord

Tail

Actual size:

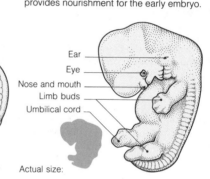

Ear

Eye

Nose and mouth

Limb buds

Umbilical cord

Actual size:

Three weeks
The embryo becomes pear-shaped, with a rounded head, pointed lower spine, and notochord running along its back.

Four weeks
The embryo becomes C-shaped and a tail is visible. The umbilical cord forms and the forebrain enlarges.

Six weeks
Eyes are visible and the mouth, nose, and ears are forming. The limbs grow rapidly from initial tiny buds.

INTERNAL ORGANS AT FIVE WEEKS

All the internal organs (such as the liver, pancreas, stomach, heart, lungs, kidneys, and sex organs) have begun to form by the fifth week. During this critical stage of development, the embryo is highly vulnerable to harmful substances consumed by the mother (such as alcohol and medication), which may cause birth defects.

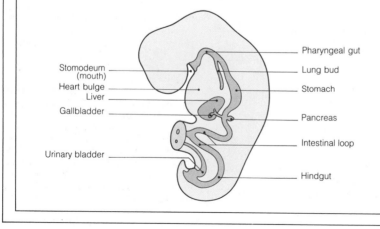

Stomodeum (mouth)

Heart bulge

Liver

Gallbladder

Urinary bladder

Pharyngeal gut

Lung bud

Stomach

Pancreas

Intestinal loop

Hindgut

Actual size:

Eight weeks
The face is more "human," the head is more upright, and the tail has gone. Limbs become jointed and digits appear.

close as possible to the vessel to be blocked, and the embolus that will block the blood vessel is released. Emboli are made of many materials, such as blood-clotting agents (e.g., fibrin), metal coils, silicone balloons, wool, and medicinal glue.

RISKS

There is always a risk that an embolus may lodge in the wrong blood vessel and cause problems; for example, an embolus that blocks a vessel in the brain may cause a *stroke*. The procedure is still being refined.

Embolus

A fragment of material that travels in the blood circulation and causes obstruction of an artery. An embolus is life-threatening if it blocks the flow of blood through a vital artery (see *Embolism*).

Embrocation

A medication rubbed into unbroken skin to relieve the muscular and joint pain of sprains and strains.

Embryo

The unborn child during the first eight weeks of its development following *conception*; for the rest of the pregnancy it is known as a *fetus*.

Development of the embryo (see illustrated box on facing page) is governed internally by *genes* inherited from the parents, and externally by factors such as the woman's diet and any drugs taken during pregnancy.

THE FIRST TWO WEEKS

The embryo develops from an egg that has been fertilized by a sperm (see *Fertilization*). It starts as a single cell—just large enough to be seen by the naked eye. As the fertilized egg travels along the tube to the uterus, the cell divides in two. These two new cells divide to form four cells. Cell divisions continue, each time doubling the number of cells. The cells form a spherical mass, in the center of which a hollow depression develops. Within the sphere, the cells then form into two very distinct groups: one makes up the wall lining the sphere; the other expands to form the embryo itself.

On about the sixth day the sphere of cells becomes attached to and then embedded in the lining of the uterus. At the site, the outer layer of cells obtains nourishment from the woman's blood; that part of the outer layer will later develop into the placenta.

Two bubbles form side by side within the cell mass. Between the bubbles a flat disk forms, consisting of layers of cells from which all the baby's tissues and organs will form. The amniotic sac develops around the growing embryo.

THE THIRD WEEK

Early in the third week, the disk of cells becomes pear-shaped. The head of the embryo forms at the rounded end and the lower spine at the pointed end. A group of cells develops along the back of the embryo to form the notochord, a rod of cells that constitutes the basis for the spine. From this time on, the embryo has two recognizable halves that develop more or less symmetrically. The notochord then furrows and the edges grow toward each other before fusing to form the neural tube. Later, the neural tube will develop into the brain and spinal cord.

THE FOURTH WEEK

During the fourth week the embryo becomes recognizable as a mammal. The back grows more rapidly than the front, giving the embryo a C-shape, and a tail becomes visible. Within the embryo, buds of tissue form that will later develop into the lungs, pancreas, liver, and gallbladder.

The neural tube extends toward the head of the embryo, where a broad fold becomes visible that eventually will grow into the brain. The developing ears first appear as pits. Rudimentary eyes develop in the form of stalks. The outer layers begin to form the limb buds and the branchial arches (folds of tissue) that are later to become the jaws and other structures in the neck.

Paired bulges appear on the sides of the neural tube that will become the cartilage, bone, and muscle of the back. On the front of the embryo, just beneath the head, a rudimentary heart develops in the form of a straight tube. As the branchial arches develop, the heart is pushed down into the chest. It is during this period that the embryo is at the greatest risk of birth defects caused by abnormal genetic or external factors (see *Birth defects*).

THE FIFTH WEEK

The external ears become visible, pits mark the position of the developing nose, the upper and lower jaws form, and the limb buds extend, becoming flattened at the end where the hands and feet will develop. The two folds of tissue meet at the front of the embryo and fuse to form the front wall of the chest and abdomen. The umbilical cord develops. Alcohol and other drugs consumed by the mother can be especially damaging now.

THE SIXTH TO EIGHTH WEEKS

The face becomes recognizably human, the neck forms, the trunk becomes less curved and the head more erect, the tail between the buttocks disappears, the limbs become jointed, and fingers and toes appear.

After eight weeks the embryo is about 2.5 cm long. Most of the internal organs have formed and all the external features are present.

Embryology

The study of the development and growth of the *embryo* and then the *fetus* from conception through the months of gestation until birth.

Embryology is an essential part of the medical student's training because it leads to a greater understanding of adult anatomy and of the way structural defects in the body may arise. For example, the occurrence of congenital heart defects, such as septal defects ("holes in the heart") and transposition of the main blood vessels, is easier to understand when the stages of fetal heart development have been explained.

Embryology was formerly based on the study of animal embryos and of dead human embryos at different stages of prenatal development. More recently, the nature of physical and chemical processes involved in embryo development has been established by examination of live embryos grown in the laboratory (see *Embryo, research on*).

Embryo, research on

Human *embryos* are grown for a few days (until the first two or three cell divisions have taken place) in specialized laboratories as part of one type of treatment for infertility (see *In vitro fertilization*). Physicians usually fertilize more eggs than they need for this procedure, since they do not know how many will "take" (begin the process of cell division and growth); the surplus embryos may then be frozen for use in later attempts at achieving a pregnancy.

Research on surplus embryos could be directed at improving the results of in vitro fertilization, at finding better methods of contraception, and at detecting genetic disorders at an early stage in pregnancy. However, in most countries, such research has been prohibited, or is not being carried out because the physicians concerned have agreed not to do so for ethical reasons.

Emergency

Any condition that requires urgent medical treatment, such as cardiac arrest (heart stoppage), or any procedure that must be performed immediately, such as *cardiopulmonary resuscitation*.

Physicians and nurses who work in hospital emergency departments are specially trained to deal with a broad range of injuries and conditions that require urgent medical attention.

Emesis

The medical term for *vomiting*.

Emetic

A substance that causes vomiting, used to treat some types of poisoning and drug overdose. Emetics work by stimulating the part of the brain that controls vomiting and/or by directly irritating the lining of the stomach.

The most widely used emetic is *ipecac*. Emetics should not be given to a person who is drowsy because he or she may inhale the vomit.

EMG

The abbreviation for electromyogram, a recording of the electrical activity in muscle. Electromyography takes 30 to 60 minutes to perform, depending on the number of muscles to be tested.

WHY IT IS DONE
An EMG can reveal the presence of muscle disorders, such as *muscular dystrophy*, or disorders in which the nerve supply to muscle is impaired, such as *neuropathy* or *radiculopathy*. In cases of nerve injury, the actual site of nerve damage can often be located.

HOW IT IS DONE
Electrical activity is measured during muscle contraction and when the muscles are at rest. To detect the electrical impulses, small disk electrodes are attached to the skin surface over the muscle. Alternatively, needle electrodes may be inserted into the muscle. The impulses are displayed on an oscilloscope screen and a permanent record can be made on film. Changes in the electrical wave patterns can be used in the diagnosis of certain nerve or muscle disorders.

EMI scanning

An obsolete term for *CT scanning*. EMI (Electrical and Musical Industries) developed the first commercially available CT scanner in 1972.

Emollient

A substance such as olive oil, lanolin, or petroleum jelly that has a soothing, softening effect when applied to the skin, eyes, or mucous membranes (e.g., the lining of the nose and mouth). By forming an oily film, emollients prevent the loss of water from these surfaces and therefore have a moisturizing effect. Emollients are used in creams, ointments, nasal sprays, and suppositories.

Emotional deprivation

Lack of sufficient loving attention and warm, trusting relationships during a child's early years, leading to difficulty in normal emotional development. Emotional deprivation may result if *bonding* does not occur in the early months of life, if a child is frequently separated from his or her parents for long periods during the first five years, or if parents cannot meet the child's emotional needs.

Children who are emotionally deprived may be impulsive, crave attention, cannot cope with frustration, and may be impaired in their intellectual development.

Emotional problems

A common term for a wide range of psychological difficulties. The problems may be due to upbringing, relationships, or psychiatric illness, but feelings of *anxiety* and *depression* generally predominate.

Empathy

The ability to partake in and understand the thoughts and feelings of another person by comparing them with one's own experiences. In *psychoanalysis* the therapist partly relies on empathy to establish a relationship with a patient.

Emphysema

A manifestation of chronic obstructive lung disease in which the alveoli (tiny air sacs) in the *lungs* become damaged. The disorder causes shortness of breath and in severe cases can lead to *respiratory failure* or *heart failure*.

CAUSES
In almost all cases, emphysema is caused by cigarette smoking. Atmospheric pollution is sometimes a predisposing factor. In rare instances, a predisposition to emphysema is inherited due to a deficiency of a chemical called alpha$_1$-antitrypsin in the lungs; the disease appears early in life, but its development is hastened and intensified by smoking.

The alveoli, of which there are many millions in each lung, are groups of air sacs at the end of bronchioles (tiny air passages). Through their thin walls, inhaled oxygen is passed into the bloodstream and carbon dioxide is removed from the capillaries to be breathed out. Tobacco smoke and other air pollutants are believed to cause emphysema by provoking the release of chemicals within the alveoli that damage the alveolar walls. Alpha$_1$-antitrypsin is thought to protect against this chemical damage; hence, people with a deficiency of this substance are particularly badly affected. The damage is slight at first, but in heavy smokers it becomes progressively worse, with the alveoli bursting and blending to form fewer, larger sacs with less surface area, and with consequent impairment of oxygen and carbon dioxide exchange. Over the years the lungs become less and less elastic, which further reduces their efficiency.

Eventually—sometimes after many years—the level of oxygen in the blood starts to fall, with either of two effects. In some cases *pulmonary hypertension* (raised blood pressure in the pulmonary artery) develops, leading to *cor pulmonale* (enlargement and strain on the right side of the heart) and, subsequently, *edema* (accumulation of fluid in the tissues), particularly in the lower legs. Other sufferers are able to compensate for oxygen deficiency to some extent by breathing faster. Why individuals react in one and not the other of these different ways is not known.

Emphysema is often accompanied by chronic *bronchitis*, also brought on by air pollutants and smoking.

SYMPTOMS AND SIGNS
Initially, and for a considerable time in mild cases, there may be no symptoms, but as the disease progresses it results in increasing shortness of breath. At first this may be noticed only when climbing stairs or steep inclines, but gradually it becomes more severe until eventually it occurs after only mild exercise or is present even at rest.

A sign of emphysema is a barrel-shaped chest associated with air being trapped in the outer part of the lungs. There may also be a chronic cough (caused by accompanying bronchitis) and a slight wheeze.

As the disease progresses, sufferers in whom cor pulmonale develops start to turn blue due to oxygen deficiency in the blood and their legs swell because of edema; these people are known as blue bloaters. Those who breathe rapidly and retain normal coloring are called pink puffers. Many people, however, show signs somewhere between these two extremes. As respiratory and/or heart failure develops, sufferers find it increasingly difficult to breathe.

DIAGNOSIS
The diagnosis is made from the patient's symptoms and signs, from a chest examination, and from various tests. A blood sample from an artery may be analyzed to measure the concentration of *blood gases* (oxygen and carbon dioxide). A venous blood sample may be analyzed to determine whether the disease is due to alpha$_1$-antitrypsin deficiency. *Chest X rays* are taken to exclude the possibility of another lung disease being responsible for the symptoms and to determine how great an area of the lungs has been affected. *Pulmonary function tests* are carried out to assess breathing capacity and the efficiency of the alveoli in exchanging gases.

TREATMENT
Because emphysema is incurable—lung tissue that has been damaged cannot be replaced—treatment can only control the disease. The patient must completely stop smoking to prevent further lung damage. Efficiency of remaining lung tissue may be improved in various ways. *Bronchodilator drugs* are given to widen the bronchioles. These drugs can be taken by means of a hand-held aerosol inhaler or an electrically operated *nebulizer* that produces a fine spray. Occasionally, *corticosteroid drugs*, taken by inhaler to reduce inflammation in the lungs, are also beneficial.

To treat edema, *diuretic drugs* may be given to reduce the volume of fluid in the body.

If the oxygen level of the blood falls considerably, *oxygen therapy* may be needed. Oxygen equipment may be available for use at home.

OUTLOOK
The course of the disease depends on how far it has progressed before the patient gives up smoking. If extensive areas of lung have been damaged or if cor pulmonale has developed, death occurs sooner or later from respiratory and/or heart failure.

Emphysema, surgical
The abnormal presence of air in tissues underlying the skin following injury or surgery. Surgical emphysema most often occurs as a complication of *pneumothorax* (the abnormal presence of air in the pleural cavity between the lung and the chest wall).

Empirical treatment
Treatment given because its effectiveness has been observed in previous, similar cases rather than because there is an understanding of the nature of the disorder and the way the treatment works. In the case of a *fever of unknown origin*, for example, a physician might prescribe antibiotic drugs on the basis of experience with similar cases.

Empyema
An accumulation of pus in a body cavity or in certain organs.

Pleural empyema occurs as a rare complication of a lung infection such as *pneumonia* or *pleurisy*; it may also develop after a severe injury to the chest that penetrates the pleural space. The main symptoms are chest pain, breathlessness, and fever. The diagnosis is confirmed by *chest X rays* and removal of a sample of pus for laboratory analysis. Treatment is by *aspiration* (removal of the pus by suction) and the injection of *antibiotic drugs*, or by an operation to open the infected cavity and drain the pus.

Empyema of the gallbladder may occur as a complication of *cholecystitis*, when it usually causes abdominal pain, fever, and sometimes jaundice. It is treated by *cholecystectomy* (surgical removal of the gallbladder).

Enalapril
An *ACE inhibitor drug* used in the treatment of *hypertension* (high blood pressure) and *heart failure* (reduced pumping efficiency of the heart). It may be given with a *diuretic drug*. Enalapril was introduced in 1986.

Enamel, dental
The hard outer layer of a tooth that covers and protects the inner structures (see *Teeth*).

Encephalins
An alternative spelling for *enkephalins*.

Encephalitis
Inflammation of the *brain*, usually caused by a viral infection. In many cases the *meninges* (the membranes that surround the brain) are also affected. An attack may be so mild that it is barely noticeable, but in most cases encephalitis is a serious and potentially life-threatening condition.

CAUSES AND INCIDENCE
The virus most commonly responsible for encephalitis is the *herpes simplex* virus type 1, which also causes cold sores. An increasing number of cases are caused by infection with *HIV* (human immunodeficiency virus), the organism responsible for *AIDS*. Rarely, the condition may be a complication of certain other viral infections, including such diseases as *measles* and *mumps*.

SYMPTOMS AND SIGNS
Encephalitis has variable effects but often starts with headache and fever, and progresses to hallucinations, confusion, paralysis of part or all of the body, and disturbances of behavior, speech, memory, and eye movement. There is a gradual loss of consciousness and sometimes coma. Epileptic seizures may also occur.

If as well as the brain the meninges are inflamed, the neck usually becomes stiff and the eyes become abnormally sensitive to light.

DIAGNOSIS
Diagnosis is based on symptoms, signs, and the results of *CT scanning* of the brain, an *EEG* (which records the electrical activity of the brain), and a *lumbar puncture* (taking a sample of cerebrospinal fluid from the spinal canal for analysis). Blood tests and, rarely, a brain *biopsy* (removal of a small sample of tissue for analysis) may also be required to confirm the diagnosis.

TREATMENT AND OUTLOOK
The antiviral drug *acyclovir*, administered by *intravenous infusion*, has proved an effective treatment for encephalitis caused by the herpes simplex virus, but when the disease results from other viral infections, there is at present no known effective treatment.

Depending on the cause of the encephalitis, some patients fail to recover, some are left with brain damage that results in mental impairment, behavioral disturbances, and persistent *epilepsy*, and others make a complete recovery.

Encephalitis lethargica
An epidemic form of encephalitis (inflammation of the brain). There have been no major outbreaks since the 1920s, although rare sporadic cases still occur. The symptoms are as for encephalitis, with additional lethargy and drowsiness.

About 40 percent of sufferers died during the major epidemics; of those who survived, many thereafter developed postencephalitic *parkinsonism*, a movement disorder marked by symptoms such as tremor, rigidity, immobility, and severely disturbed eye movements.

E

A small number of survivors from the post-World War I epidemics were still alive in the 1970s, when administration of a new antiparkinsonian drug, *levodopa*, brought a remarkable improvement in their conditions. However, after half a century of almost complete immobility, most sufferers were seemingly unable to cope with this "awakening," and lapsed back into their former torpid state.

Encephalomyelitis

Inflammation of the *brain* and *spinal cord*, resulting in damage to the *nervous system*. The condition occurs as a complication of about one in 1,000 cases of *measles*, developing a few days after the rash appears. Rarely, it may occur after other viral infections, such as *chickenpox*, *rubella* (German measles), or infectious *mononucleosis* (glandular fever), or it may follow vaccination against *rabies*. A related syndrome, *myalgic encephalomyelitis*, may cause muscular weakness, loss of energy, and poor health for months or years in some patients.

SYMPTOMS

Symptoms include fever, headache, drowsiness, confusion, epileptic seizures, partial paralysis or loss of sensation, and sometimes coma.

DIAGNOSIS AND TREATMENT

Diagnosis is as for *encephalitis*. Critically ill patients require careful nursing in a hospital. There is no cure for the disease, but *corticosteroid drugs* are given to reduce inflammation and *anticonvulsant drugs* are given to control epileptic seizures.

OUTLOOK

About 10 to 20 percent of patients die; those who recover may suffer permanent damage to the nervous system, causing mental retardation, *epilepsy*, paralysis, *hypopituitarism* (insufficiency of the pituitary gland), loss of sensation, or incontinence.

Encephalopathy

Any disease or disorder affecting the brain, especially chronic degenerative conditions (see *Brain* disorders box).

Wernicke's encephalopathy is a degenerative condition of the brain caused by a deficiency of thiamine (vitamin B_1); the condition is most common in alcoholics (see *Wernicke-Korsakoff syndrome*).

Hepatic encephalopathy is caused by the effect on the brain of toxic substances which have accumulated in the blood as a result of *liver failure*. Hepatic encephalopathy may cause

impaired consciousness, memory loss, personality change, tremors, seizures, stupor, and coma.

Bovine spongiform encephalopathy (BSE) is a new disorder contracted by cows from infected sheep or cattle tissue in their feed. The cause is probably a *slow virus*. BSE causes degeneration of the infected cow's brain and is fatal. Despite public fears, BSE is unlikely to be transmissible to humans.

Encopresis

A type of *soiling* in which children pass normal feces in unacceptable places after the age at which bowel control is normally achieved (usually when 2 to 3 years old).

Endarterectomy

An operation to remove the lining of an artery affected by *atherosclerosis* (narrowing by deposits of fatty material). Removing the diseased lining restores normal blood flow to the part of the body supplied by the artery.

WHY IT IS DONE

Endarterectomy is performed to treat *cerebrovascular disease* (in which there is a serious reduction of blood supply to the brain) or to treat *peripheral vascular disease* (in which blood supply to the limbs is impaired).

HOW IT IS DONE

Before surgery, the site of narrowing is located by means of an X-ray procedure called *angiography*, which requires a local anesthetic. For the operation itself the patient is given a general anesthetic.

Endarterectomy is a delicate procedure that may take several hours to perform. The artery is exposed, clamps are applied, an incision is made, and the diseased lining is removed along with any *thrombus* (blood clot) that has formed. The incision is closed with stitches.

RESULTS

New lining grows in the artery within a few weeks of surgery. The operation often brings about a considerable improvement in symptoms (for example, it can greatly reduce pain in the legs in peripheral vascular disease). The long-term effect is more limited, because narrowing of an artery is rarely confined to one site. When narrowing is widespread, *arterial reconstructive surgery* may have to be performed.

Endemic

A medical term applied to a disease or disorder that is constantly present in a particular region or a specific group of

people, in contrast to an *epidemic*, which is not generally present but occasionally affects a large number of people. *AIDS*, for example, has become endemic in central Africa and has also spread to many other parts of the world. The lung disease *pneumoconiosis* was formerly endemic in coal miners before government regulations enforced controls over safety levels of coal dust, the causative agent of the disease.

Endocarditis

Inflammation of the endocardium (internal lining of the heart), particularly of the heart valves, usually due to infection.

Endocarditis occurs most commonly in people whose endocardium has already been damaged (e.g., by congenital *heart disease* or by *rheumatic fever*), in people whose *immune system* has been suppressed by *anticancer drugs* or by *immunosuppressant drugs*, and in drug abusers who inject drugs intravenously. Endocarditis is also a rare feature of some types of cancer and of some *autoimmune disorders* (e.g., systemic *lupus erythematosus*).

CAUSES AND INCIDENCE

Endocarditis may be caused by bacteria, fungi, or other microorganisms. The microorganisms may be introduced into the bloodstream during cardiac surgery, particularly if artificial materials (e.g., a replacement valve) are inserted. The causative microorganisms may also be introduced during dental treatment (especially tooth extraction) and during surgical and investigative procedures performed on the gastrointestinal and genitourinary systems (e.g., examination of the bladder by *cystoscopy*). The microorganisms that cause endocarditis may also be introduced directly into the bloodstream on dirty needles.

People with an endocardium that is already damaged are particularly vulnerable to endocarditis because clots that form on the injured surface trap the causative microorganisms, which then multiply rapidly at the site of damage. Intravenous drug abusers are vulnerable to endocarditis, even if their hearts are healthy, because microorganisms from a dirty syringe or from unclean skin at the site of injection are injected and carried to the heart in the bloodstream. People with a suppressed immune system are vulnerable because they have a lowered resistance to infection, and organisms that would normally be harmless can lead to serious infection.

SYMPTOMS

Endocarditis may be subacute or acute. In the subacute form, the disease smolders undetected, sometimes for many months, during which time it causes serious damage to a heart valve. Symptoms are general and nonspecific; the sufferer may complain of fatigue and weakness, feverishness, night sweats, and vague aches and pains. On examination, the only evident abnormality may be a heart *murmur* that changes from time to time.

Acute endocarditis, which occurs less frequently, comes on suddenly. The patient suffers from severe chills, high fever, shortness of breath, and rapid or irregular heartbeat. The infection progresses quickly and may destroy the heart valves, leading to rapidly progressive heart failure (reduced pumping efficiency).

DIAGNOSIS AND TREATMENT

Any patient suspected of having endocarditis is given a thorough physical examination. Blood samples are taken and sent to the laboratory for analysis. *Cultures* of the blood are examined for bacteria or fungi, and the sensitivity of the organisms to different types of *antibiotic drug* is determined. Tests on the heart may include *ECG*, *echocardiography*, and *angiography*.

Patients are treated with high doses of antibiotic drugs, which are usually given intravenously. Drug treatment, which may last for as long as six weeks, is started in hospital and may be continued at home. *Heart valve surgery* may be needed to replace a valve that has been extensively damaged by infection or to replace an artificial valve. In some cases, heart valve replacement may need to be done as an emergency procedure.

PREVENTION AND OUTLOOK

People at risk of endocarditis because of a heart defect are prescribed antibiotic drugs before undergoing any procedure that runs a significant risk of introducing bacteria into the bloodstream. People at risk should also be aware of the warning signs of endocarditis and call a physician should they appear.

Before the introduction of antibiotic drugs, endocarditis was usually fatal. Today, treatment is successful in 65 to 80 percent of cases.

Endocrine gland

A gland that secretes *hormones* directly into the bloodstream rather than through a duct. Examples of endo-crine glands include the *thyroid gland, ovaries*, and *adrenal glands*, which release *thyroxine, estrogens*, and *hydrocortisone*, respectively. The endocrine glands in the body make up the *endocrine system*. (See also *Exocrine gland*.)

Endocrine system

A collection of glands that produce *hormones* (chemical substances necessary for normal body functioning). The various endocrine glands are shown in the illustrated box.

The hormones produced by the endocrine glands are responsible for numerous body processes, including growth, metabolism, sexual development and function, and response to stress. Any increase or decrease in the production of a specific hormone interferes with the process it controls.

Unlike *exocrine glands*, the secretions of which pass through ducts to local areas, endocrine glands are ductless and release their hormones directly into the bloodstream to be transported to organs and tissues throughout the body.

Endocrinology

The study of the *endocrine system*, including the investigation and treatment of its disorders. A physician who specializes in diseases and disorders of the endocrine glands and the hormones they secrete is called an endocrinologist.

The symptoms and signs of an endocrine disease, such as a *thyroid* disorder or *diabetes mellitus*, may lead a general practitioner to suspect such a disease, but confirmation usually requires referral to an endocrinologist for specialized tests, including measurement of the amounts of various hormones in the blood and urine.

Endodontics

The specialized branch of dentistry concerned with the causes, preven-

---

ENDOCRINE DISORDERS

In all endocrine disorders, there is either deficient or excess production of a hormone by a gland. Common causes of abnormal hormone production include a tumor or an autoimmune disease affecting a gland, or a disorder of the pituitary or the hypothalamus, which control many other glands. Abnormal hormone production often has a feedback effect on the secretion of trophic (stimulating) hormones by the pituitary and the hypothalamus—as in two of the examples shown. The blood levels of different hormones may need to be measured to pinpoint the cause of a disorder.

Thyrotoxicosis
This disorder is usually due to an autoimmune disease of the thyroid. Excess hormones cause the symptoms; the output of TSH and its hypothalamic-releasing hormone is reduced, but the thyroid continues to overproduce.

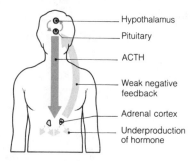

Addison's disease
Symptoms are caused by reduced hormone production by the defective adrenal cortices. Feedback is weak, so the pituitary pours out adrenocorticotropic hormone (ACTH), but it fails to stimulate the adrenals.

Cushing's disease
This disorder is caused by excess ACTH secretion by a pituitary tumor. This stimulates the adrenal cortices to make excess hydrocortisone, leading to the symptoms of the syndrome. Feedback fails to suppress ACTH secretion.

E

ENDOCRINE SYSTEM

The system consists of a collection of hormone-producing glands, many regulated by trophic (stimulating) hormones secreted by the pituitary. The pituitary is itself influenced by hormones secreted by the hypothalamus in the brain. Shown here are the principal glands with a note on the hormones they produce.

Pancreas

This gland secretes insulin and glucagon, which control the body's utilization of glucose.

Adrenal cortex

When stimulated by ACTH, the adrenal cortex produces hydrocortisone, which has widespread effects on metabolism; it also produces androgen hormones and aldosterone, which maintains blood pressure and the body's salt balance.

Ovaries

These produce the hormones estrogen and progesterone, which influence multiple aspects of female physiology. These processes are controlled by gonadotropic hormones secreted by the pituitary.

Pituitary gland

The pituitary gland secretes hormones that stimulate the adrenals, thyroid, pigment-producing skin cells, and gonads; it also secretes growth hormone, antidiuretic hormone, prolactin, and oxytocin.

Thyroid gland

This gland produces the hormones thyroxine, triiodothyronine, and calcitonin, which stimulate metabolism, body heat production, and bone growth. Thyroid activity is controlled by TSH, secreted by the pituitary.

Parathyroid glands

These glands secrete parathyroid hormone, which maintains the calcium level in the blood.

Testes

The testes produce testosterone in response to gonadotropins secreted by the pituitary. A combination of gonadotropins and testosterone stimulates sperm production and the development of other male characteristics.

CONTROL OF HORMONE PRODUCTION

Production of too much or too little hormone by a gland is prevented by feedback mechanisms. Variations in the blood level of the hormones are detected by the part of the brain known as the hypothalamus, which prompts the pituitary to modify its production of trophic (gland-stimulating) hormone accordingly.

1 The production of hormone by the target gland (in this illustration, the thyroid gland) and of trophic hormone by the pituitary gland is normal.

2 If hormone production by the target gland rises, the feedback effect causes less trophic hormone to be produced, which tends to return the situation to normal.

3 If hormone production by the target gland drops, the feedback lessens and more trophic hormone is produced, which tends to return the situation to normal.

tion, diagnosis, and treatment of disease and injury affecting the nerves and pulp in teeth and the periapical tissues in the gum. Common endodontic procedures are *root-canal treatment* and *pulpotomy*.

Endogenous

Arising within the body. For example, an endogenous infection may occur if bacteria from around the anus invade the urinary tract.

The term endogenous depression was formerly used of depression that was thought to be due to a chemical imbalance in the brain. Most disorders, however, are *exogenous* (caused by infections, poisoning, or injury).

In physiology the term describes the metabolism of substances in tissues or cells in the absence of nutrients.

Endometrial cancer

See *Uterus, cancer of.*

Endometriosis

A condition in which fragments of the *endometrium* (lining of the uterus) are located in other parts of the body, usually in the pelvic cavity.

Endometriosis is most prevalent in women aged 25 to 40 and may cause *infertility*. How it does this is not known, but about 10 to 15 percent of infertility patients have endometriosis and about 30 to 40 percent of women suffering from endometriosis are infertile.

The exact cause of endometriosis is uncertain, but in some cases it is thought to occur because fragments of the endometrium shed during *menstruation* do not leave the body with the menstrual flow. Instead, they travel up the fallopian tubes and into the pelvic cavity where they adhere to and grow on any pelvic organ.

These displaced patches of endometrium continue to respond to the menstrual cycle as if they were still inside the uterus, so each month they bleed. This blood cannot escape, however, and causes the formation of slowly growing cysts which may grow as large as a grapefruit. The growth and swelling of the cysts are responsible for much of the pain associated with endometriosis.

SYMPTOMS AND SIGNS

The symptoms of endometriosis vary widely, with abnormal or heavy menstrual bleeding being most common. There may be severe abdominal and/or lower back pain during menstruation, which is often most severe toward the end of a period. Other possible symptoms include dyspareunia (see *Intercourse, painful*) and digestive tract symptoms such as diarrhea, constipation, or painful defecation. In rare cases, rectal bleeding occurs at the time of the menstrual periods. In some cases, endometriosis causes no symptoms.

DIAGNOSIS AND TREATMENT

Laparoscopy (examination of the abdominal cavity with a viewing instrument) confirms the diagnosis.

Treatment depends on many factors, including the age and health of the patient, and the severity of the condition. Some cases are mild and require no treatment. In others, endometriosis is suppressed by pregnancy.

Drugs (including *danazol, progestogen drugs,* or the combined *oral contraceptive pill*) may be given to prevent menstruation. In severe cases, surgical removal of the cysts may be necessary in addition to drug therapy. A woman who does not want to have children or who is nearing the menopause may consider the possibility of having a *hysterectomy.*

Endometritis

Inflammation of the *endometrium* (uterine lining) due to infection. Endometritis is a feature of *pelvic inflammatory disease* (PID). It may also occur as a complication of abortion or childbirth, after the insertion of an *IUD,* or as the result of a *sexually transmitted disease.* Symptoms include fever, vaginal discharge, and lower abdominal pain. Treatment includes removing any foreign body (such as an IUD or retained placental tissue) and *antibiotic drugs.*

Endometrium

The lining of the inside of the *uterus.* The endometrium contains numerous glands and increases in thickness during the menstrual cycle until ovulation occurs. The surface layers are shed during *menstruation* if conception does not take place.

E

SITES OF ENDOMETRIOSIS

Fragments of the *endometrium* may travel from the uterus into the pelvic cavity via the fallopian tubes. They then implant on parts of the pelvic organs (such as the ovaries, vagina, cervix, bladder, and rectum). The patches of endometrium continue to respond to the menstrual cycle and bleed every month, causing the formation of painful cysts, which can be very small or may be as large as a grapefruit.

Severe endometriosis
The uterus, fallopian tubes, and ovaries shown above had large cysts around them due to endometriosis. Because the patient was nearing the menopause, the affected organs were surgically removed.

Fallopian tube

Uterus

Bladder

Vagina

Ovary

Rectum

Endorphins

A group of substances formed within the body that relieve pain. Endorphins have a similar chemical structure to *morphine* (it is because of this similarity that morphine has an analgesic effect).

In 1973 morphine was found to act at specific sites (called opiate receptors) in the brain, spinal cord, and at other nerve endings. This discovery led to the identification of small protein molecules produced by cells in the body that also act at opiate receptors; these morphinelike proteins were named endorphins (short for endogenous morphines).

Two other small proteins produced within the brain were originally considered to be examples of endorphins, but they have now been reclassified as *enkephalins* because they are released from different nerve endings.

FUNCTIONS

Since their discovery, endorphins have been found at several sites in the body (including the pancreas and testes) as well as in the nervous system. Research is being carried out to determine their full range of functions.

In addition to their analgesic effect, endorphins are thought also to be involved in controlling the body's response to stress, regulating contractions of the intestinal wall, and determining mood. They may also regulate the release of hormones from the pituitary gland, notably growth hormone and the *gonadotropin hormones* (which act on the ovaries or testes).

Addiction and *tolerance* to narcotic analgesics, such as morphine, are thought to be due to suppression of the body's production of endorphins; the withdrawal symptoms that occur when the effects of morphine wear off may be due to a lack of these natural analgesics. Conversely, acupuncture is thought to produce analgesia partly by stimulating the release of endorphins and enkephalins.

Endoscope

A tubelike viewing instrument, with lenses and a light source attached, that is inserted into a body cavity for the purpose of investigating and treating disorders. Some common types of endoscope and their uses are shown in the illustrated box on facing page.

Endoscopy

Examination of a body cavity by means of an *endoscope*, a tubelike instrument with viewing lenses, a steering mechanism and a light source attached, for purposes of diagnosis or treatment. Many procedures that formerly required a major surgical operation can now be performed much more simply by endoscopy. It is a safe procedure which can often be used without a general anesthetic.

Attempts to view the interior of the body through a rigid, lighted, telescopelike tube were made in the early 1900s, but endoscopy really began in the 1930s with the invention of a semiflexible gastroscope for viewing the stomach. In the 1960s, a second revolution came with the introduction of *fiber optics* (flexible bundles of glass or plastic fibers along which light is transmitted). This enabled more versatile instruments to be developed and led to the acceptance of endoscopy as a routine part of hospital medicine. A camera or video recorder can be used to make permanent records of the images that are seen through the endoscope.

USES

Endoscopy is a valuable aid in diagnosing disorders of the colon, stomach, bladder, lungs, or other organs, enabling the physician to study and photograph the relevant organ and to perform a *biopsy* (removal of a small piece of tissue for microscopic analysis). Because endoscopy can safely be repeated at frequent intervals, it is useful in assessing how well an ulcer of the stomach or duodenum is healing.

Endoscopy is valuable in the treatment of acute emergencies, such as bleeding from the stomach. It allows the cause and site of the bleeding to be identified and, in some cases, to be treated by *electrocoagulation* or *laser treatment*. Many minor disorders of the knee joint that formerly required a major operation can now be treated quickly and easily. Other uses include removal of polyps (small growths) and swallowed foreign bodies, local application of drugs, and sterilization operations for women. (See also *Arthroscopy; Bronchoscopy; Colonoscopy; Cystoscopy; ERCP; Gastroscopy; Laparoscopy; Laryngoscopy.*)

Endothelium

The layer of cells that lines the heart, blood vessels, and lymphatic ducts. The cells are squamous (thin and flat), providing a smooth surface that aids the flow of blood and lymph and helps prevent the formation of thrombi (blood clots). (See also *Epithelium*.)

Endotoxin

A poison produced by certain *bacteria* but not released until after the bacteria die; until then the toxin remains in the bacterial cell wall. Released endotoxins cause fever. They also make the walls of capillaries more permeable, causing fluid to leak into the surrounding tissue, sometimes resulting in a serious drop in blood pressure, a condition called endotoxic shock. (See also *Enterotoxin; Exotoxin*.)

Endotracheal tube

A tube passed through the nose or mouth into the trachea (windpipe), usually by an anesthetist. The endotracheal tube may be provided with an inflatable cuff at its lower end to give an airtight fit which prevents anything other than oxygen or anesthetic gases entering the lungs. The tube may be made of rubber or various types of plastic.

Endotracheal intubation is performed to ensure that a patient has a clear airway for the delivery of oxygen. It may be necessary if a patient is comatose, is undergoing anesthesia, or is unable to breathe properly because of a disorder affecting the lungs or airways. An endotracheal tube is used to deliver oxygen to the trachea during artificial *ventilation*.

Enema

A procedure in which fluid is passed into the rectum through a tube inserted into the anus. An enema may be performed as a treatment, to prepare the intestine for surgery, or as an aid to diagnosis.

WHY IT IS DONE

An enema may be given to clear the intestine of feces either to relieve constipation or in preparation for intestinal surgery. Soap and water were formerly used for this type of enema but today prepacked, small-volume enemas containing medication are used.

Enemas may also be used to administer medicine, such as *corticosteroid drugs* to relieve bleeding and inflammation in *ulcerative colitis* or, less commonly, salt solutions to treat severe *dehydration*.

A barium enema is used as an aid to the diagnosis of disorders of the large intestine (see *Barium X-ray examinations*).

HOW IT IS DONE

No anesthetic is needed, although the procedure may cause slight discomfort as the fluid stretches the intestine.

ENDOSCOPES

A typical flexible *fiberoptic* endoscope consists of a bundle of light-transmitting fibers. At one end is the head (featuring a viewing lens and steering device) and a power source. The tip has a light, a lens, and an outlet for air or water. Side channels enable attachments to be passed to the tip. In some endoscopes the tip may contain a camera that transmits a picture electronically to a screen.

A rigid endoscope is a straight, narrow viewing tube with a light source attached.

COMMON TYPES OF ENDOSCOPES

Instruments	Region	Nature
Cystoscope	Bladder	Rigid
Bronchoscope	Bronchi (main airways of the lungs)	Flexible or rigid
Gastroscope	Esophagus, stomach, and duodenum	Flexible
Colonoscope	Colon (large intestine)	Flexible
Laparoscope	Abdominal cavity	Rigid
Arthroscope	Knee joint	Rigid

E

Rigid endoscope

Light cable
Viewer
Handle

Power source
Water tubing
Handle

Tip

Flexible endoscope

Power source
Instrument attachment

Viewer
Steering mechanism
Tip

Endoscopic examination
The physician looks through the viewing lens and uses the handles to manipulate the attachments.

ATTACHMENTS

Various specialized attachments are available for use with the endoscope. They enable the physician to perform diagnostic and therapeutic procedures such as taking a biopsy specimen (a small piece of tissue for analysis).

Snare attachment
Grasping attachment
Lens
Light cable

Grasping forceps
Sharp-toothed forceps allow foreign bodies to be grasped firmly and removed.

Biopsy forceps
These are used for taking small samples of tissue for microscopic analysis.

Scissors
Tiny surgical scissors are used for cutting through tissue and removing small growths.

Brushes
Brush attachments are used to obtain cells for cytological examination.

Snare
This thin wire loop, through which an electric current is passed, is used to remove polyps.

Basket
A wire basket is sometimes used to trap and remove stones from the bile duct.

The patient lies on his or her side with hips raised on a pillow. A catheter (flexible tube) with a soft, well-lubricated tip, is gently inserted into the rectum and the enema fluid, warmed to prevent sudden contraction of the intestine, is slowly introduced through it.

Energy

The capacity to do work or effect a physical change; nutritionists now also refer to the fuel content of a food as its energy content.

There are many different forms of energy—including light, sound, heat, chemical, electrical, and kinetic (the energy possessed by an object by virtue of its motion)—and most of them play a role in the body. For instance, the retina converts light energy to electrical nerve impulses, thereby making vision possible. Muscles use chemical energy—obtained from food—to produce kinetic energy (movement) and heat.

Energy is measured in units called calories or joules. One calorie is defined as the amount of energy needed to raise the temperature of 1 g of water by 1°C; 1 calorie is equivalent to about 4.2 J (therefore, 1 J equals approximately 0.24 calorie). Because the calorie and the joule are very small, more practical units in dietetics are the kilocalorie (kcal) which is 1,000 calories, sometimes called simply a Calorie (C), and the kilojoule (1,000 joules, or 1 kJ).

TERMINOLOGY The total chemical energy in a food is gross energy. After an allowance is made for the approximately 5 percent that is not digested, the remainder is digestible energy. After allowing for loss in the urine (nitrogen compounds from proteins), the remainder is metabolizable energy (see *Metabolism*). *Carbohydrates* and *proteins* provide 4 kcal per gram; *fats* provide 9 kcal per gram.

In general, the energy liberated from the breakdown of *nutrients* is stored as chemical energy in the form of *ATP* (adenosine triphosphate) molecules. The energy in these molecules is then available to power processes that consume energy, such as muscle contraction or the building up of complex substances needed for repair and maintenance of body structures. Some body processes (muscle contraction, for instance) produce energy in the form of heat. A certain amount of this energy is needed to maintain body temperature, but any excess cannot be used and must leave the body by mechanisms such as radiation of heat from the skin or sweating.

Energy requirements

The amount of *energy* needed by a person for cell *metabolism*, muscular activity, and growth. This energy is provided by the breakdown of *carbohydrate, fat,* and *protein* in the diet and by stored nutrients in the liver, muscles and adipose tissue.

ENERGY EXPENDITURE
Energy is needed to keep the heart beating and the lungs functioning and to maintain body temperature. The rate at which these processes use energy is known as the basal metabolic rate (BMR). The BMR accounts for three quarters of the total daily expenditure of energy of the average sedentary person. Any form of movement increases energy expenditure above the BMR.

Additional energy is needed during growth to provide for extra body tissue. During pregnancy and lactation the mother's energy requirement increases because she must be able to meet the needs of the baby as well as her own.

When more energy is ingested as food than is spent, the surplus is stored and there is usually a gain in weight. When less is consumed than is spent, there is usually a loss of weight as the body stores are used up. (See also *Nutrition; Obesity.*)

Engagement

The descent of the head of the fetus into the mother's pelvis. In a woman's first pregnancy, engagement usually occurs by the 37th week but, in subsequent pregnancies, it may not occur until labor begins. Rarely, engagement may fail to occur—if, for example, the baby's position in the uterus is abnormal, the baby's head is too big for the mother's pelvis, or if there is *placenta previa* (abnormal position of the placenta across the opening of the uterus).

Engorgement

Overfilling of the breasts with milk. Engorgement is common a few days after childbirth, when the milk supply arrives quickly and forcibly (see *Breast-feeding*). The condition causes the breasts and nipples to become swollen and tender. This makes it not only painful for the mother to feed the baby but can make it very difficult for the baby to suck. Engorgement can make a woman more likely to suffer from *mastitis* (inflammation of the breast). The problem can be relieved by *expressing milk.*

Enkephalins

A group of small protein molecules produced in the brain and by nerve endings elsewhere in the body (in the digestive system and adrenal glands, for example). Enkephalins have an analgesic (painkilling) effect and are also thought to produce sedation, to affect mood, and to stimulate motivation.

Enkephalins were initially considered to be *endorphins* (endogenous morphines), but it has since been discovered that they are released by different nerve endings and that they differ slightly chemically.

Enophthalmos

A sinking inward of the eyeball. Enophthalmos is most commonly caused by fracture of the floor of the orbit (bony cavity making up the eye socket), or by shrinkage of the eye itself due to the formation of scar tissue following inflammation or injury.

Enteric-coated tablet

A form of drug preparation consisting of a tablet, the surface of which is covered with a substance that is resistant to the action of stomach juices. Enteric-coated tablets pass undissolved through the stomach into the small intestine, where the covering dissolves and the contents are absorbed.

Such tablets are used either when the drug might harm the stomach lining (as may occur with certain corticosteroid drugs, such as prednisone) or when the stomach juices may destroy the efficacy of the drug, as can happen with sulfasalazine.

The drawback of some enteric-coated tablets is that they may pass through the gastrointestinal tract without dissolving.

Enteric fever

An alternative name for either *typhoid fever* or *paratyphoid fever.*

Enteritis

Inflammation of the small intestine. Enteritis may result from infection, particularly *giardiasis* and *tuberculosis*, or from *Crohn's disease*, which is sometimes called regional enteritis. Enteritis usually causes diarrhea. (See also *Colitis; Gastroenteritis.*)

Enteritis, regional
Another name for *Crohn's disease*.

Enterobiasis
The medical term for infestation of the intestines by the small roundworm *ENTEROBIUS VERMICULARIS*. (See *Pinworm infestation*.)

Enterostomy
An operation in which a portion of small or large intestine is joined to another part of the gastrointestinal tract or to the abdominal wall. When part of the *colon* (large intestine) is brought through an incision in the abdominal wall to allow the discharge of feces into a bag attached to the skin, the operation is called a *colostomy*; when the ileum (last section of the small intestine) rather than the colon is used, the procedure is called an *ileostomy*.

Enterotoxin
A type of *toxin* (poison released by certain bacteria) that inflames the lining of the intestine, causing vomiting and diarrhea.

Staphylococcal *food poisoning* is caused by eating food contaminated with an enterotoxin produced by staphylococci bacteria; the toxin is resistant to heat and is therefore not destroyed by cooking. The bacteria themselves do not need to be alive or even present for this type of food poisoning to occur.

The severe intestinal purging that occurs in *cholera* is caused by an enterotoxin that is actually produced in the intestine by the cholera bacteria. (See also *Endotoxin*; *Exotoxin*.)

Entropion
A turning in of the margins of the *eyelids* so that the lashes rub against the *cornea* and the *conjunctiva*.

CAUSES
Entropion is sometimes congenital (present from birth), especially in fat babies. It is common in the elderly, when weakness of the muscles surrounding the lower part of the eye allows the lower lid plate to turn inward. Entropion of the upper or lower lid may be caused by scarring on the inner surface of the lid—for example, due to *trachoma*.

SYMPTOMS AND SIGNS
Entropion is often recognized by the sufferer or by his or her family. The lower lid margin is rolled inward so that the lashes are concealed, which sometimes irritates the conjunctiva.

When gentle pressure is applied with the fingertip over the lid, the margin pops out, revealing the lashes again.

COMPLICATIONS
In later life, entropion can cause irritation, conjunctivitis, or corneal ulceration. Untreated, persistent entropion may permanently damage the cornea and cause problems with vision and, in some people, blindness.

TREATMENT
Entropion in babies does not disturb the eye and nearly always disappears spontaneously within a few months. In the elderly or in sufferers from trachoma, surgery to correct the entropion prevents damage to the cornea.

ENT surgery
See *Otorhinolaryngology*.

Enuresis
The medical term for bed-wetting. Enuresis is a common phenomenon; about 10 percent of children still wet the bed at the age of 5 years, and many of these continue to do so until the age of 8 or 9. A slightly higher number of boys than girls are bed-wetters, and the problem tends to run in families.

CAUSES
In most cases, bed-wetting is due to slow maturation of nervous system functions concerned with bladder control. Occasionally it results from psychological stress. In a small number of bed-wetters, there is a specific physical cause—a structural abnormality of the *urinary tract* present from birth, *diabetes mellitus*, *urinary tract infection*, or a nervous system defect, such as *spina bifida* or spinal cord damage. In each of these cases, the child also has difficulty with daytime bladder control (see *Incontinence, urinary*).

INVESTIGATION
A physical examination, *urinalysis* (urine testing), and other procedures, such as *ultrasound scanning* and *urography* (X-ray imaging of the urinary tract), may be performed. *Cystometry* (a test of bladder function) is also occasionally carried out, usually only on older children who have daytime problems as well.

TREATMENT
In the absence of an ascertainable cause, or until the problem can be more fully investigated, treatment starts with training the child to pass urine regularly during the day. This helps the child to recognize when the bladder is full, even during sleep. Systems such as rewarding the child with a star on a chart for each dry night are often successful.

If such simple measures fail to work, a special nighttime alarm system may be recommended by the physician. The basic system consists of a pad, placed in the child's bed between the lower sheet and the mattress, that is sensitive to changes in humidity and triggers a loud alarm when urine is passed. Smaller alarms are now available that do not need pads under the sheet. The alarm awakens the child, who can then use the toilet. Eventually, the child wakes whenever urine is about to be passed. Alarms are said to be successful with over two thirds of bed-wetting children over 7 years old.

Other measures include getting the child to go to the toilet each night immediately before bed, and waking him or her to use the toilet two or three hours after going to bed. Some types of *antidepressant drugs* have also been used successfully, but many physicians do not prescribe them because the drugs generally cause side effects and are dangerous in overdose.

Parents should not punish a child for bed-wetting or focus undue attention on it, as this may only make the child more anxious and make the problem worse. The vast majority of bed-wetting children eventually become dry at night.

Environmental medicine
The study of the effects on health of different natural environmental factors, such as climate, altitude, sunlight, and the presence of various minerals. Working environments are studied separately (see *Occupational medicine*).

CLIMATE
There is convincing evidence that particular types of illness respond well to certain climates. For example, sufferers from chest disorders, such as chronic *bronchitis* and *asthma*, usually obtain some relief from their symptoms in a warm, relatively dry climate. Until the development of specific drug treatment in the 1940s, the prime treatment for pulmonary *tuberculosis* was to move the patient to a mountain sanatorium to enjoy the cool, clean, dry air.

ALTITUDE
Although mountainous regions have much less atmospheric pollution, they are not necessarily beneficial to health because air becomes thinner as altitude increases. Anyone with a chest disease who ascends quickly (over a matter of days) from sea level to 1,500 m may find that his or her

E

E

THE GROWING IMPORTANCE OF ENVIRONMENTAL MEDICINE

Large areas of the world are naturally hostile to humans and were, in the past, avoided. Today, exploitation of natural resources has lured people into these regions and has highlighted the importance of environmental medicine.

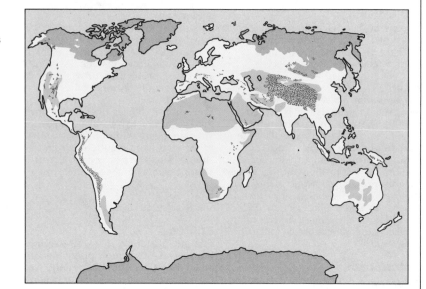

Key

Desert regions

Cold regions with average winter temperature below −23°C

Mountain regions above 3,000 m

---

breathing difficulty becomes worse. Above about 3,000 m, breathing becomes difficult even for healthy people. Rapid ascent from sea level to 3,600 m higher carries the risk of altitude sickness (see *Mountain sickness*), which can produce symptoms ranging from nausea and sleeplessness to coma or death. Only a few communities in the high Andes live permanently above that level but tourists climbing mountains in Africa and the Himalayas may develop altitude sickness.

Sustained living seems to be impossible above 6,000 m because at that level the blood cells increase to compensate for lack of oxygen. This strains the heart and causes a predisposition to thrombosis (abnormal blood clotting).

SUNLIGHT

White people who live in sunny climates may suffer ill effects from repeated exposure to sunlight, including wrinkling of the skin and an increased risk of skin cancers, such as *basal cell carcinoma* and malignant *melanoma*, and the precancerous condition solar *keratosis*.

MINERALS

Variations in the distribution of certain *minerals* in the environment are known to have an effect on health. For example, there is a slightly higher-than-average incidence of cancers in areas where the radioactive gas *radon* is emitted (from granitic rocks). In contrast, there is a lower-than-average incidence of *dental caries* in populations in regions where the water has a high *fluoride* content.

Enzyme

A protein that regulates the rate of a chemical reaction in the body. There are thousands of enzymes, each with a different chemical structure. It is this structure that determines the specific reaction regulated by an enzyme. To function properly, many enzymes need an additional component called a coenzyme, which is often derived from a *vitamin* or *mineral*.

Every cell in the body produces various enzymes; different sets of enzymes occur in different tissues, reflecting their specialized functions. For example, the *pancreas* produces the digestive enzymes lipase, protease, and amylase; among the numerous enzymes produced by the *liver* are some that metabolize drugs.

INDUCTION AND INHIBITION

Enzyme activity is influenced by many factors. Liver enzyme activity is increased by certain drugs, such as *barbiturate drugs*, which affect the rate at which other drugs are metabolized by the liver. This effect, known as enzyme induction, is responsible for many important drug interactions (see *Drug*).

Conversely, many drugs inhibit or block enzyme action. Some *antibiotic drugs* destroy bacteria by blocking bac-terial enzymes while leaving human ones unaffected. Similarly, some *anticancer drugs* work by blocking enzymes in tumor cells, affecting normal body cells to a lesser degree.

ENZYMES AND DISEASE

Measuring enzyme levels in the blood can be useful for diagnosing disorders of certain organs or tissues. For example, the level of heart enzymes is raised after a *myocardial infarction* (heart attack) because the damaged heart muscle cells release enzymes into the bloodstream; muscle enzyme levels are raised in *muscular dystrophy*; and liver enzymes—measured in *liver function tests*—may be raised as a result of certain liver disorders.

Many inherited metabolic disorders, such as *phenylketonuria, galactosemia*, and *G6PD deficiency*, are caused by defects in, or deficiencies of, specific enzymes.

ENZYMES AND TREATMENT

Enzymes can play a valuable role in treating certain diseases and disorders. Pancreatic enzymes may be given as digestive aids to patients with *malabsorption* related to pancreatic disease; enzymes that loosen sputum (phlegm) in the airways may be given to people with chronic lung disease; enzymes such as *streptokinase* and *tissue-plasminogen activator* are used to treat acute *thrombosis* (especially in the coronary arteries) and arterial *embolism* (especially pulmonary embolism). Papain from the fruit of the

HOW ENZYMES WORK

An enzyme is a protein that acts as a catalyst for a chemical change in the body—that is, it greatly speeds up the rate at which the change occurs. The change may be a small modification to the structure of a substrate (chemical) in a body tissue, the splitting of a substrate, or the joining of two substrates.

1 The shape of an enzyme determines its activity. It will combine only with a specific substrate that has molecules of a complementary shape.

2 When enzyme and substrate combine, their interaction causes a chemical change within the substrate—in this case, splitting it into two products.

3 After the reaction, the enzyme molecule is unchanged and can move on to combine with another substrate molecule and repeat the process.

papaw, a tree found mostly in the eastern United States, can be used in the dressing of wounds and ulcers because it dissolves dead tissue and coagulated blood and may thus reduce bruising and swelling.

Ependymoma

A rare type of *brain tumor* that occurs most often in children. It is a *glioma*, a tumor arising from the glial (supporting) cells within the nervous system. The symptoms, methods of diagnosis, and treatment of ependymomas are the same as for other types of brain tumor.

Ephedrine

A drug that stimulates the release of *norepinephrine* (a type of *neurotransmitter* released from nerve endings).

Ephedrine is prescribed as a *decongestant drug* to treat nasal congestion, and sometimes as a *bronchodilator drug* to treat asthma. Ephedrine eye drops relieve redness of the eye by narrowing blood vessels that have become widened in response to minor irritation. Occasional uses include the relief of motion sickness and of enuresis (bed-wetting) in children.

Epicanthic fold

A vertical fold of skin extending from the upper eyelid to the side of the nose. Epicanthic folds are a normal feature in Orientals but are rare in other races, except in babies, in whom they usually disappear as the nose develops. The folds, a feature of *Down's syndrome*, can be removed by minor cosmetic surgery.

Epicondylitis

A painful inflammation of an epicondyle, one of the bony prominences of the *elbow* at the lower end of the humerus (upper-arm bone). Various forearm muscles that bend or straighten the wrist or fingers are attached by *tendons* to the epicondyles. Overuse of these muscles can lead to epicondylitis due to repeated tugging of the tendons at their point of attachment to the bone.

Epicondylitis affecting the prominence on the outer side of the elbow, caused by overuse of the muscles that straighten the fingers and wrist, is called *tennis elbow*. When the prominence on the inner side of the elbow is affected, caused by overuse of muscles that bend the fingers and wrist, it is called *golfer's elbow*.

Epidemic

A medical term applied to a disease that for most of the time is rare in a community but that suddenly spreads rapidly to affect a large number of people. Epidemics of new strains of *influenza* are probably the most common, occurring periodically when the influenza virus changes to a form to which the population has no resistance. (See also *Endemic*.)

Epidemiology

The study of disease as it affects groups of people, as opposed to individuals. Originally, as its name suggests, epidemiology dealt mainly with epidemics of infectious diseases (such as cholera, plague, and influenza) and outbreaks of infections (such as gastroenteritis) associated with food poisoning. More recently, it has been applied to widespread noninfectious diseases, such as cancer and heart disease.

Members of a population (or, in comparative studies, populations) under study are carefully counted and defined in terms of each person's race, sex, age, occupation, social class, marital status, and the like. Then the *incidence* of the disorder (the number of new cases per week, month, or year) and its *prevalence* (the number of people with the disorder at any given time) are determined. These observations may be repeated at regular intervals to detect changes occurring over time. The result is an exact statistical record which often yields many valuable findings.

Groups that spend all their lives in one defined area often provide more useful information than very mobile populations whose environments change considerably over the course of their lives. For example, a high incidence of cancer of the esophagus has been studied among the inhabitants of one region of China and among other inhabitants of Iran. This incidence has been compared to similar groups in other regions of the countries; certain foods have been implicated.

COMPARATIVE EPIDEMIOLOGY

Comparative epidemiology is proving to be a most potent weapon in the attempt to understand better cancer, heart disease, and other widespread diseases that afflict people in developed countries today. Two or more groups are chosen—one having, the other not having, a characteristic that may affect the frequency of a disease. For example, in a study of the link between smoking and lung cancer, one group may consist of smokers and the other of nonsmokers; the proportion with cancer in each group is then calculated. In such cases, the epidemiologist is careful to make the two groups as nearly identical as possible in other respects, carefully matching such factors as age, sex, weight, and socioeconomic status.

Another approach is to compare a group of people having a certain disease, such as hypertension, with a control group of people without the condition but similar in other respects; the aim is to isolate identifying factors, such as obesity, which differ between the two groups.

The links discovered by comparative epidemiology—such as the correlation of a high level of fish oils in the diet and low prevalence of heart disease—do not demonstrate cause and effect. For example, epidemiologists have discovered that the prevalence of heart disease is high in countries in which most people have a car. This association obviously does not mean that owning a car causes heart disease, but because such ownership suggests a more sedentary lifestyle, the link reinforces the belief that lack of exercise increases the risk of heart disease.

Epidermolysis bullosa

A group of rare, inherited conditions in which blisters appear on the skin after minor damage. The disorder has a wide range of severity, from a type in which blisters form on the feet in hot weather, to a form in which there is widespread blistering and scarring.

CAUSES

The condition is caused by a genetic defect which may show either an autosomal dominant or an autosomal recessive pattern of inheritance (see *Genetic disorders*). It is diagnosed by means of a skin *biopsy* (removal of a small amount of skin for microscopic analysis).

OUTLOOK

No special treatment for the condition is available, although injury to the skin should be avoided and simple protective measures should be taken to prevent the rubbing of affected areas when blisters appear.

The outlook varies from a gradual improvement in mild cases to progressive serious disease in the most severe cases. Parents of affected children should obtain *genetic counseling* so that the risks of later children being affected can be calculated.

Epididymal cyst

A harmless swelling, usually painless, that may develop in the *epididymis*, located at the upper rear part of the testis. Small cysts are very common in men over the age of 40 and need no treatment. Rarely, they may become tender or may enlarge and become uncomfortable, in which case it may be necessary to have an operation to remove them surgically.

Epididymis

A long, coiled tube connecting the vasa efferentia (small tubes leading from the testis) to the vas deferens (the sperm duct leading to the urethra). Sperm cells produced in the testis pass slowly along the epididymis, maturing there until they are capable of fertilizing an egg. They are then stored in the seminal vesicles until *ejaculation* takes place.

Disorders affecting the epididymis include *epididymo-orchitis* (inflammation of the epididymis and testis) and *epididymal cysts* (fluid-filled swellings in the epididymis). Infection or injury can block the epididymis; if this occurs in both testes, infertility can result.

LOCATION OF THE EPIDIDYMIS
The epididymis runs along the back of the testis and links the vasa efferentia to the vas deferens.

Vas deferens

Vasa efferentia

Testis

Scrotum   Epididymis

Epididymitis

See *Epididymo-orchitis*.

Epididymo-orchitis

Acute inflammation of a *testis* and its associated *epididymis* (the coiled tube that carries sperm away from the testis). Epididymo-orchitis is characterized by severe pain and swelling at the back of the testis and is accompanied by swelling and redness of the *scrotum* in severe cases.

The inflammation is caused by infection. Often there is no obvious source of infection, but sometimes the

cause is a bacterial *urinary tract infection* that has spread via the vas deferens (sperm duct). In rare cases, epididymo-orchitis results from the spread of *tuberculosis*.

DIAGNOSIS

The symptoms of severe pain and swelling are similar to those of torsion of the testis, in which the testicular cord becomes twisted and blocks its own blood supply (see *Testis, torsion of*). An exploratory operation may be necessary to make a firm diagnosis and to save the testis. In some cases testicular scans may be helpful.

TREATMENT

Treatment is with *antibiotic drugs* and rest. If there is an underlying urinary tract infection, its cause is investigated. The tuberculous form of the disease usually responds to drugs used to treat other forms of tuberculosis. It may take several months for the testis to return to its normal size; in some cases, normal size is never regained. (See also *Orchitis*.)

Epidural anesthesia

A method of pain relief in which a local anesthetic is injected into the epidural space (the space around the membranes surrounding the spinal cord) in the middle and lower back to numb the nerves that supply the chest and the lower half of the body.

Epidural anesthesia is used to relieve pain during and after surgery, to relieve pain during *childbirth*, and in some cases to control cancer pain.

The anesthetic is usually introduced into the epidural space via a catheter (flexible, fine tube), which is left in place to allow further doses of anes-

Vertebra

Epidural space

Spinal cord

Hollow needle

Administering an epidural anesthetic
The anesthetic is injected into the epidural space (the region surrounding the spinal cord within the spinal canal).

thetic to be given as necessary. Epidural anesthesia may be combined with a light general anesthetic.

Epiglottis
The flap of cartilage lying behind the tongue and in front of the entrance to the *larynx* (voice box). At rest, the epiglottis is upright and allows air to pass through the larynx and into the rest of the respiratory system. During swallowing it folds back to cover the entrance to the larynx, preventing food and drink from being inhaled.

Epiglottitis
A rare but serious and sometimes fatal infection that mainly affects children between the ages of 2 and 6. Caused by the bacterium HEMOPHILUS INFLUENZAE, it results in sudden inflammation and swelling of the *epiglottis* (the flap of cartilage at the back of the tongue that closes off the *larynx* and *trachea* during swallowing). The swollen epiglottis obstructs breathing. If the condition is not recognized and treated promptly, it can cause death by suffocation.

SYMPTOMS
The illness comes on suddenly within a few hours. The child becomes feverish, develops stridor (noisy breathing), has difficulty swallowing, and drools because he or she cannot swallow saliva. Breathing becomes increasingly difficult and the child prefers to sit upright in an attempt to make breathing easier. Within a few hours of the onset of the illness, the child may develop cyanosis (bluish discoloration of the skin and mucous membranes) and become semiconscious due to lack of oxygen.

DIAGNOSIS
The symptoms and signs of epiglottitis resemble those of *croup*; expert assessment by an experienced pediatrician may be necessary to distinguish between them. For this reason, any child who becomes feverish and develops noisy breathing should be seen by a physician as soon as possible. If he or she suspects epiglottitis, the child will be admitted to hospital. In hospital, X rays of the neck are usually taken to help confirm the diagnosis.

TREATMENT
An *endotracheal tube* is usually passed through the nose or mouth and into the trachea in order to maintain breathing; artificial *ventilation* may be needed. Intravenous *antibiotic drugs* (usually *ampicillin* and/or *chloramphenicol*) are used to cure the infection.

With prompt treatment the outlook is good; recovery usually takes place within a week.

The H. INFLUENZAE bacterium is highly contagious; family members should be screened or treated with antibiotic drugs to prevent its spread.

Epilepsy
A tendency to recurrent seizures or temporary alteration in one or more brain functions.

Seizures are defined as transient neurological abnormalities caused by abnormal electrical activity in the brain. Human activities, thoughts, perceptions, ideas and emotions are normally the result of the regulated and orderly electrical excitation of nerve cells in the brain. During a seizure, a chaotic and unregulated electrical discharge occurs. In some cases, a stimulus such as a flashing light sets off this abnormal sequence, but often seizures appear without any obvious trigger.

Many people with epilepsy lead normal lives and have no symptoms between seizures. Some can tell when an attack is imminent as they experience an aura (a restless, irritable, or uncomfortable feeling) shortly before the attack.

CAUSES
Seizures are a symptom of brain dysfunction and, like symptoms in other parts of the body, can result from a wide variety of disease or injury. Seizures may occur in association with *head injury*, birth trauma, brain infection (such as *meningitis* or *encephalitis*), *brain tumor*, *stroke*, drug intoxication, drug or alcohol withdrawal, or a *metabolic disorder*. A tendency to seizures may develop for no obvious reason or it may be inherited.

FIRST AID: EPILEPTIC SEIZURE

DO NOT
- restrain the victim or place anything in the mouth
- attempt to move the victim unless he or she is in danger of further injury

1 Carefully loosen tight clothing around the neck.

2 When the attack is over, place the victim in the *recovery position* and allow him or her to regain consciousness.

INCIDENCE
About one person in 200 suffers from some form of recurrent seizures. The disorder usually starts in childhood or adolescence. However, many people outgrow epilepsy and do not require medication.

TYPES
Epileptic seizures can be classified into two broad groups—generalized and partial seizures.

The form a seizure takes depends on the part of the brain in which it arises and on how widely and rapidly it fans out from its point of origin.

Generalized seizures, which cause loss of consciousness, affect the whole body and may arise over a wide area of the brain. There are two main types of generalized seizure—grand mal and minor or absence (petit mal) seizures.

Partial seizures are usually caused by damage to a more limited area of the brain. Partial seizures are divided into simple seizures and complex seizures. In either of these types, the electrical disturbance may spread and affect the whole brain, causing a generalized seizure.

GRAND MAL During this type of generalized seizure the person falls down unconscious and the entire body stiffens and then twitches or jerks uncontrollably. There may be an initial cry; breathing is then absent or very irregular during the seizure. Following the seizure, the muscles relax, and bowel and bladder control may be lost. The person may feel confused and disoriented and perhaps have a headache; often he or she will want to sleep. These effects usually clear in several hours. The person usually has no memory of the event. Prolonged seizures, referred to as status epilepticus, can be fatal without emergency treatment.

MINOR SEIZURES (PETIT MAL) These brief seizures are sometimes called absences because they rarely last more than a minute and are marked by a sudden loss of consciousness without falling or major movements. They are much more prevalent in children than in adults, and may in some cases occur many times daily, interfering with schoolwork. Although the spells are often unnoticed, careful observation of the child may reveal minor movements, such as twitching of the fingers, blinking, and smacking of the lips. The child is usually unaware that he or she has had a seizure.

SIMPLE PARTIAL SEIZURES Consciousness is maintained in this type of partial seizure. An abnormal twitching

E

movement, tingling sensation, or even hallucination of smell, vision, or taste, occurs without warning and lasts several minutes.

Jacksonian epilepsy is a type in which twitching occurs and spreads slowly from one part of the body to another on the same side. Sufferers retain awareness during the event and can recall the details.

COMPLEX PARTIAL SEIZURES In this type of seizure, also known as *temporal lobe epilepsy*, conscious contact with the surroundings is lost. There may be abnormal behavior that is not easily recognized as being due to epilepsy. The sufferer becomes dazed and may not respond if addressed. Involuntary actions, such as fumbling with buttons or lip smacking, sometimes occur. These actions are called automatisms and (rarely) can take more bizarre forms. The person typically remembers little, if any, of the event.

PREVENTION
Many epileptics experience seizures at times of extreme fatigue or stress. Infectious illnesses, especially if fever is present, also lower the seizure threshold. By avoiding these situations and taking prescribed medication regularly, epileptics can reduce the frequency of seizures. Occasionally, epileptics discover a distracting technique that can abort a seizure once the aura has begun.

DIAGNOSIS
In making the diagnosis, the physician seeks as much information as possible about the attacks. Since patients frequently do not have recall, information may be obtained from witnesses.

After a complete examination of the nervous system, the physician usually orders an *EEG* to help with the diagnosis. It is important to realize that the EEG cannot always absolutely confirm or refute the diagnosis of seizures, and that the results must be weighed in the light of the person's symptoms and signs.

In some cases, an *ECG* (electrical monitoring of the heartbeat) is performed to exclude cardiac *arrhythmias* as a cause of loss of consciousness in an adult. *CT scanning* of the brain and *blood tests* may also be performed.

TREATMENT
Opinion is divided on whether a single seizure should be treated; physicians agree that people with recurrent seizures should take *anticonvulsant drugs*. Such drugs are the first line of treatment for epilepsy. In almost all cases, they lessen the frequency of sei-

zures, but may have unpleasant side effects, including drowsiness and impaired concentration. The physician will attempt to find the one drug that works best, but, with very severe epilepsy, a combination may be needed to control seizures. If no seizures occur for two to three years (depending on their cause), the physician may suggest reducing or stopping drug treatment.

Rarely, surgery may be considered if it is thought that a single area of brain damage (usually in the temporal lobe) is causing the seizures and if medication is ineffective.

OUTLOOK
If epilepsy develops during childhood and there is a definite family history of the disease, the chances are good that the problem will decrease after adolescence; it may even disappear altogether. However, seizure control is likely to be more difficult in temporal lobe epilepsy or if the disorder has been brought about by severe brain damage.

One third of those in whom epilepsy develops eventually grow out of the condition and experience no further seizures. Another third find that the seizures become less frequent in response to treatment. The conditions of the last third stay the same.

Sufferers from epilepsy are usually able to work, but the disorder may limit their choice of jobs. There are restrictions on obtaining a driving licence. It is advisable, unless the seizures are very well controlled, to avoid high-risk jobs involving heights or dangerous machinery and sports such as skiing. Many epileptics carry a special card, tag, or bracelet that states they have epilepsy. Epileptics are recommended to advise colleagues on what to do if a seizure occurs.

DEALING WITH AN EPILEPTIC SEIZURE
Most major epileptic seizures last only a minute or two and demand little of the bystander. All that is necessary is to let the attack run its course and to ensure that the person is in no physical danger and can breathe while he or she is unconscious.

The person should not be held down, nor should his or her movements be restrained. Any tight clothing around the neck should be loosened and something soft should be placed beneath the head. The mouth should not be forced open and no object should be wedged between the teeth. Once the convulsions have ceased, the victim should be put into the *recovery position*.

An ambulance should be called if the seizure continues for more than five minutes, if another seizure immediately follows the first one, or if consciousness is not regained a few minutes after the seizure ends.

Epiloia
See *Tuberous sclerosis*.

Epinephrine
A naturally occurring hormone, also called adrenaline, produced in the adrenal glands. Epinephrine has been produced synthetically as a drug since 1900.

Epinephrine is one of two chemicals (the other is *norepinephrine* or noradrenaline) released by the adrenal gland in response to signals from the sympathetic division of the *autonomic nervous system*. These signals are triggered by stress, exercise, or by an emotion such as fear.

Epinephrine increases the speed and force of the heartbeat and thereby the work that can be done by the heart. It widens the airways to improve breathing and narrows blood vessels in the skin and intestine so that an increased flow of blood reaches the muscles, allowing them to cope with the demands of exercise.

USE AS A DRUG
Epinephrine is sometimes given by injection as an emergency treatment for *cardiac arrest* (stopped heartbeat), *anaphylactic shock* (a severe allergic reaction) and the control of acute *asthma* attacks.

During surgery, it is occasionally injected into tissues to reduce bleeding. When combined with a local anesthetic, epinephrine prolongs the pain-deadening effect by slowing down the rate at which the anesthetic spreads into surrounding tissues.

Epinephrine eye drops are used to treat *glaucoma* and they are used during eye surgery because they reduce pressure in the eyeball. Epinephrine can also be used to stop nosebleeds and reduce *nasal congestion*.

POSSIBLE ADVERSE EFFECTS
Regular use of epinephrine as eye drops may cause a burning pain and, occasionally, blurred vision or pigment deposits on the eye's surface.

In nose-drop form, epinephrine may cause palpitations, restlessness, and anxiety; more recently developed *decongestant drugs* are now usually used to treat nasal congestion.

Epiphora
See *Watering eye*.

Epiphysis

Either of the two growing ends of the long bones (femur, tibia, fibula, ulna, radius, and humerus) of the limbs. The epiphysis is separated from the diaphysis (shaft of the bone) by a layer of cartilage, called the epiphyseal plate or growth plate.

During childhood and adolescence, bones grow as the result of *ossification*, a process in which cartilage cells multiply and absorb calcium to develop into bone. In this way, the cartilage in the ephiphyseal plate is gradually replaced by new bone.

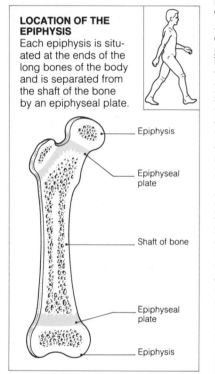

LOCATION OF THE EPIPHYSIS
Each epiphysis is situated at the ends of the long bones of the body and is separated from the shaft of the bone by an epiphyseal plate.

Epiphysis

Epiphyseal plate

Shaft of bone

Epiphyseal plate

Epiphysis

Epiphysis, slipped

See *Femoral epiphysis, slipped*.

Episcleritis

A localized patch of inflammation affecting the outermost layers of the *sclera* (the white of the eye) immediately under the *conjunctiva* (the transparent membrane covering the sclera).

Episcleritis usually occurs for no known reason and generally affects middle-aged men. It may be a complication of *rheumatoid arthritis*. The purplish patch of inflammation is oval, slightly raised, and less than 1 mm across. It may cause a deep, dull, aching pain that tends to be worse at night. During the day there may be *photophobia* (abnormal sensitivity of the eyes to light).

The condition usually disappears by itself within a week or two but may recur. Symptoms may be relieved by eye drops or ointment containing a *corticosteroid drug*.

Episiotomy

A surgical procedure in which an incision is made in the *perineum* (the tissue between the vagina and the anus) to facilitate the delivery of a baby. After delivery, the cut tissues are stitched back together.

WHY IT IS DONE
A large number of obstetricians advocate its use almost routinely on the grounds that a surgical cut will heal better than a tear, and that women who have had episiotomies will experience less trouble later in life from stretching of the vagina. Other obstetricians rarely perform episiotomies on the grounds that the naturally elastic vagina should not have to be cut to allow a normal delivery, and that small tears cause less damage and pain than an episiotomy.

If the perineum fails to stretch up over the baby's head and/or a large perineal tear looks likely, an episiotomy is advisable. It prevents a ragged tear that is more painful, more difficult to repair, and more commonly leads to complications. Episiotomy is usually necessary in a *forceps delivery*, because the instruments occupy additional space in the vagina, and in a *breech delivery*, in which there is little opportunity for gradual stretching of the perineal tissues by which it could be avoided.

An episiotomy is usually performed if the baby is suffering from *fetal distress* (the effects of receiving insufficient oxygen during labor), because episiotomy speeds delivery. An episiotomy is also usually performed to reduce pressure on the baby's head during a premature birth.

HOW IT IS DONE
As the baby's head descends through the maternal pelvis and begins to stretch the perineum, local anesthetic is injected into the area (unless the woman has already been given an anesthetic).

Scissors are used to make a cut extending from the back wall of the vagina through the perineal skin and muscles. This cut may be directed to the side of the anus (mediolateral) or in a direct vertical line with the anus (midline).

HOW IT IS REPAIRED
An episiotomy is usually repaired shortly after delivery of the baby. The woman lies on her back with her feet in stirrups. The perineum is thoroughly cleaned and more local anesthetic is injected if necessary. The vagina is then inspected to assess the size of the incision and to see whether further tears have occurred. The wound is repaired in layers, usually with absorbable sutures.

RECOVERY PERIOD
The woman can walk as soon as she wishes. Occasionally, *ice packs* and *analgesic drugs* are required. The perineum should be kept clean and care should be taken to avoid *constipation*. Absorbable sutures dissolve after about 10 days and thus do not require removal. In most cases, healing is straightforward. Discomfort in the region of the scar may be felt for some weeks.

Epispadias

A rare *congenital* abnormality in which the opening of the *urethra* is not in the glans (head) of the *penis*, but on the upper surface of the penis. The penis may also curve upward.

Surgery is carried out in infancy, using tissue from the foreskin to reconstruct the urethra and to create a penis that will allow satisfactory sexual intercourse in adult life. Sometimes more than one operation is needed to correct the condition. (See also *Hypospadias*.)

Epistaxis

The medical term for a *nosebleed*.

Epithelium

The cells, occurring in one or more layers, that cover the entire surface of the body and that line most of the hollow structures within it. (Structures that are not lined with epithelium are the blood vessels, lymph vessels, and the inside of the heart, which are lined with *endothelium*, and the chest and abdominal cavities, which are lined with *mesothelium*.)

Epithelium varies in cell type and thickness according to the function it performs. There are three basic cell shapes: squamous (thin and flat), cuboidal, and columnar. These structures may vary further. In the respiratory tract, for example, epithelial cells bear brushlike filaments called cilia that propel dust particles from inhaled air back up the bronchi and trachea.

Most internal organs lined with epithelium are covered with only one

E

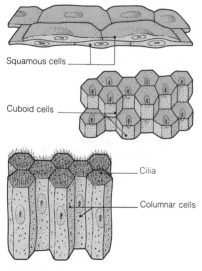

Types of epithelium
The cells of the epithelium vary in shape and size according to function. The three basic types are squamous, cuboidal, and columnar.

Squamous cells

Cuboid cells

Cilia

Columnar cells

layer of cells, but the skin, which is subjected to more trauma, consists of many layers with a dead outer layer of cells that is constantly being shed.

Epstein-Barr virus
A virus that causes infectious *mononucleosis*; the virus is also associated with *Burkitt's lymphoma* and cancer of the *nasopharynx*.

ERCP
The abbreviation for endoscopic retrograde cholangiopancreatography, an X-ray procedure for examining the *biliary system* and the pancreatic duct. ERCP is used mainly when *ultrasound scanning* or *CT scanning* fails to provide a sufficiently detailed image.
HOW IT IS DONE
ERCP is usually an outpatient procedure and takes 20 to 40 minutes. No food or drink is taken for eight hours before the examination. A *sedative drug* is usually given and a local anesthetic applied to the throat.

An *endoscope* (a flexible viewing tube with a lens and light attached) is passed down the esophagus, through the stomach, and into the *duodenum* (the upper part of the small intestine). The endoscope operator then passes a catheter (fine, flexible tube) through the endoscope into the ampulla of Vater (the opening in the duodenum that leads to the common bile duct and pancreatic duct). He or she then passes a radiopaque contrast medium (one that shows up on X-ray

film) through the catheter to fill the pancreatic duct and all the ducts of the biliary system. X-ray pictures are taken that show any abnormalities in the ducts.

If disease is detected, it can sometimes be treated at the same time. For example, stones obstructing the lower end of the common bile duct can be removed by using an attachment on the endoscope to widen the duct. If there is a suspected tumor at the ampulla, the endoscope can be used to perform a *biopsy* (removal of a small sample of tissue for analysis) or brushing of cells for cytological examination (see *Cytology*).

Erection
The hardness, swelling, and elevation of the *penis* that occurs in response to sexual arousal or physical stimulation. Erections are also common during sleep and may occur for no obvious reason in very young boys.

The penis contains three cylinders of erectile tissue with a network of blood vessels controlled by the spinal nerves. During an erection, the penis becomes filled with blood as the vessels dilate (widen) to allow increased blood flow. Muscles around the vessels contract and prevent blood from leaving, so maintaining the erection.

Erection, disorders of
Conditions in which the normal process of erection is disrupted. They include total or partial failure to attain or maintain erection (see *Impotence*), persistent erection without any sexual desire (see *Priapism*), and bowed erection (see *Chordee*).

Ergocalciferol
An alternative name for vitamin D₂ (see *Vitamin D*), also called calciferol.

Ergometer
A machine that measures the amount of physical work done and the body's response to a controlled amount of exercise. An ergometer makes continuous recordings, during and immediately after activity, of heart rate and rhythm (using an *ECG*), blood pressure, the rate of breathing, and the volume of oxygen taken up from the surrounding air.

The exercise, supervised by a physician, is done on a fixed bicycle, rowing machine, or treadmill, and the effort required is adjusted to suit the particular test being performed. In *fitness testing*, the exercise is vigorous enough to require maximum effort; in

a *cardiac stress test*, the exercise is adjusted to a level sufficient to produce a certain predetermined level of heart rate. The test is terminated if exercise causes symptoms such as chest pain or breathing difficulty.

Ergometrine
See *Ergonovine*.

Ergonovine
A drug given after *childbirth*, *miscarriage*, or *abortion* to control loss of blood from the uterus. Ergonovine is usually given in a single injection but tablets may also be needed in some cases. The drug works by causing the muscles of the uterus to contract, which compresses the blood vessels and thus reduces bleeding.

Ergot
A product of CLAVICEPS PURPUREA, a fungus that grows on rye and various other cereals. Ergot contains several *alkaloids* (nitrogen-containing substances) with medicinal and poisonous effects.

The most important drugs produced from ergot are *ergotamine*, used to treat migraine, and *ergonovine*, used to control blood loss from the uterus following childbirth, miscarriage, or abortion.

Before it was known that ergot was a poison, bread made with contaminated rye caused outbreaks of ergot poisoning. The effects included gangrene of the toes and fingers, seizures, mental disorders, and, in some cases, death.

Ergotamine
A drug used in the prevention and treatment of *migraine*. It works by constricting the dilated blood vessels surrounding the brain and is used as an alternative to *analgesic drugs* (painkillers).

Ergotamine is most effective if taken during the early warning stages of a migraine attack. Once the headache and nausea of migraine are present, it is less likely to be effective and may even increase the nausea.

Erosion, dental
Loss of enamel from the surface of a tooth as a result of attack by acids or other chemicals. The first sign of enamel loss is a dull, frosted appearance. As the condition progresses, smooth, shiny, shallow cavities form.

Erosion affecting the outer surfaces of the front teeth is most often caused by excessive consumption of citrus fruits, fruit juices, or carbonated drinks; it also sometimes occurs in people who use acid in industrial processes. Erosion mainly affecting the inner surfaces of the molar teeth may be caused by frequent regurgitation of acidic fluid—for example, in people suffering from *acid reflux* or *bulimia*.

Erosion may be combined with, and also accelerate, *abrasion* (mechanical wearing away of teeth) and attrition (wearing down of the chewing surfaces), leading to extensive damage to many teeth. (See also *Caries, dental*.)

Eroticism

The character and emotive nature of sexual excitement. The term derives from the ancient Greek for "desire," personified and deified as Eros. Sexual arousal may be stimulated by thoughts, by the touching of the erogenous zones (especially the mouth, breasts, genitals, and anus), or by a variety of other sensations (such as the look and feel of certain clothes, the scent of a perfume, or the sound of a piece of music).

In *psychoanalytic theory*, eroticism is contrasted with *narcissism* (self-love). Eroticism is a mature love that can be fulfilled only when the loved one is also satisfied. Narcissism is typical of immature personalities and is a love that merely wishes to satisfy itself.

Eruption

The process of breaking out or appearing, as of a skin rash or a new tooth.

Eruption of teeth

The process by which developing *teeth* move through the jaw and gum to project into the mouth.

DECIDUOUS DENTITION

Deciduous teeth (also called primary or milk teeth) usually begin to appear when a baby is about 6 months old. In most cases, the lower front teeth are the first to erupt. Occasionally, a baby is born with one or two teeth already visible. Other babies do not have any teeth visible until they are about 9 months old. All 20 deciduous teeth usually erupt by the time the child is 3 years old. Infants may suffer a mild general upset at the time of eruption (see *Teething*).

PERMANENT DENTITION

Permanent teeth (the secondary teeth) generally begin erupting when a child is 6 years old. The first permanent molars erupt toward the back of the mouth and appear in addition to, rather than replacing, the deciduous teeth. Children and parents are often unaware that these are permanent teeth.

The eruption of permanent teeth nearer the front of the mouth is preceded by reabsorption of the roots of the deciduous teeth, which become loose and detach. The succeeding permanent tooth emerges a few weeks after its deciduous predecessor is detached and falls out.

Wisdom teeth (the last molar teeth) usually erupt between the ages of 17 and 21, but in some people never appear. In others, wisdom teeth are impacted (blocked from erupting) because of insufficient space in the jawbone (see *Impaction, dental*).

Erysipelas

An infection, usually of the face, caused by streptococcal bacteria, which are thought to enter the skin through a small wound or sore. Young children and the elderly are most often affected.

The disorder starts abruptly with malaise, fever, headaches, and vomiting. Itchy, red patches appear on the face and spread across the cheeks and the bridge of the nose to form an inflamed area with raised edges. Within this area, pimples develop that first blister, then burst, and then crust over.

Treatment is with *penicillin drugs*, which usually clear the condition within a week. (See also *Cellulitis*.)

Erythema

A term meaning redness of the skin. Disorders of which skin redness is one feature include *erythema multiforme*,

E

TOOTH ERUPTION

The top diagrams show the approximate ages at which particular deciduous teeth usually appear. The ages at which specific types of permanent teeth usually appear are shown in the lower diagrams. Red denotes erupting teeth; gray denotes erupted deciduous teeth; white denotes erupted permanent teeth.

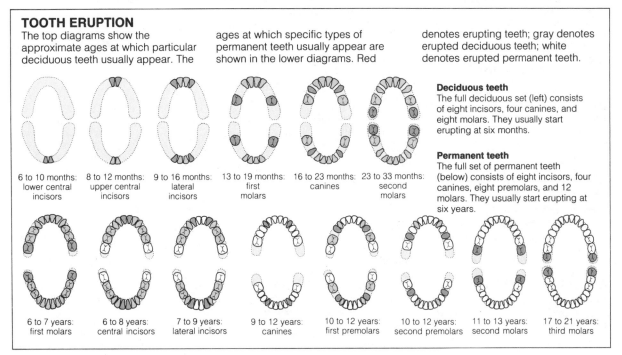

6 to 10 months: lower central incisors

8 to 12 months: upper central incisors

9 to 16 months: lateral incisors

13 to 19 months: first molars

16 to 23 months: canines

23 to 33 months: second molars

Deciduous teeth
The full deciduous set (left) consists of eight incisors, four canines, and eight molars. They usually start erupting at six months.

Permanent teeth
The full set of permanent teeth (below) consists of eight incisors, four canines, eight premolars, and 12 molars. They usually start erupting at six years.

6 to 7 years: first molars

6 to 8 years: central incisors

7 to 9 years: lateral incisors

9 to 12 years: canines

10 to 12 years: first premolars

10 to 12 years: second premolars

11 to 13 years: second molars

17 to 21 years: third molars

E

erythema nodosum, lupus erythematosus, erythema ab igne, and erythema infectiosum *(fifth disease).*

Erythema can have many causes, including *blushing, hot flashes, sunburn,* raised temperature, and inflammatory, infective, or allergic skin conditions such as *acne, dermatitis, eczema, erysipelas, rosacea,* and *urticaria* (hives).

Erythema ab igne
Red mottled skin that may also be dry and itchy, caused by exposure to strong direct heat. Erythema ab igne is most common in elderly women. It may occur on the shins, due to sitting too close to a fire, or on the abdomen, due to hugging a heating pad or a hot-water bottle.

Dryness and itching of the skin can often be relieved by an *emollient* (soothing cream). The redness usually fades in time, although it rarely disappears completely.

Erythema infectiosum
See *Fifth disease.*

Erythema multiforme
An acute inflammation of the skin, and sometimes of the internal mucous membranes (the thin moist tissue that lines bodily cavities), sometimes accompanied by generalized illness. Erythema multiforme means literally "skin redness of many varieties."

CAUSES AND INCIDENCE
The disease can occur as a reaction to certain drugs (including *penicillin drugs, sulfonamide drugs, salicylate drugs,* and *barbiturate drugs*), or may accompany certain viral infections (such as *herpes simplex* causing cold sores) or bacterial infections (such as *streptococcal infections* causing sore throat). Pregnancy, *vaccination,* and

The rash of erythema multiforme
The spots of this rash are usually itchy and have a bull's-eye appearance, with concentric rings of different shades of red around a pale center.

radiation therapy are other possible causes. However, half of all cases occur for no apparent reason. The disease is most common in children and young women.

SYMPTOMS
A symmetrical rash of red, often itchy spots, similar to the rash of measles, erupts on the limbs and sometimes on the face and the rest of the body. The spots may blister or may progress to form raised, red, pale-centered wheals—so-called target lesions. Those affected may have fever, sore throat, headache, and/or diarrhea.

In a severe form of erythema multiforme, called Stevens-Johnson syndrome, the mucous membranes of the mouth, eyes, and genitals become inflamed and ulcerated.

TREATMENT
If the treatment for some other disorder is believed to be the cause of the erythema, the treatment will be withdrawn. Any causative illness will be treated if possible. In some cases, *corticosteroid drugs* are given to reduce inflammation and irritation. Patients suffering from Stevens-Johnson syndrome are given *analgesic drugs* (painkillers), plenty of fluids (sometimes intravenously), *sedative drugs,* and sometimes corticosteroid drugs. Erythema multiforme usually clears within five to six weeks, although it may recur. Stevens-Johnson syndrome normally responds to treatment, but in some cases the patient may become seriously ill as a result of shock or inflammation within the body.

Erythema nodosum
A condition characterized by an eruption of red-purple swellings on the legs in association with another illness. It is most common between the ages of 20 and 50 and affects women more than men.

CAUSES AND INCIDENCE
The most common cause of erythema nodosum is a *streptococcal infection* of the throat, but the condition is also associated with other diseases, most commonly *tuberculosis* and *sarcoidosis,* and may occur as a reaction to certain drugs, including *sulfonamide drugs, penicillin drugs,* and *salicylate drugs.* In about one third of cases, no cause can be discovered.

SYMPTOMS
The swellings, which range from 1 to 10 cm in diameter, are shiny and tender and occur on the shins, thighs, and, less commonly, the arms. Joint and muscle pains and fever also usually occur.

TREATMENT
Effective treatment of any underlying condition clears the swellings. Bed rest, *analgesic drugs* (painkillers) and, occasionally, *corticosteroid drugs* may be necessary. The condition usually subsides within a month.

Erythrasma
A bacterial skin infection, caused by the organism CORYNEBACTERIUM, which affects the groin, armpits, and skin between the toes. Affected areas are raised above the rest of the skin and are irregularly shaped. On white skin, affected areas look red-brown; on dark skin, they may look either lighter or darker than the normal skin. There are usually no other symptoms. Erythrasma is more common in people with *diabetes mellitus.*

Erythrasma is diagnosed by inspecting the skin under a special light, called Wood's light, which shows up the affected areas as red fluorescent patches. The condition generally clears when treated with *erythromycin.*

Erythrocyte
Another name for a red blood cell. (See *Blood cells.*)

Erythroderma
See *Exfoliative dermatitis.*

Erythromycin

ANTIBIOTIC

Tablet Capsule Liquid Injection

Prescription needed

An *antibiotic drug* used to treat infections of the skin, chest, throat, and ears. Erythromycin is particularly useful in the treatment of *pertussis* (whooping cough) and *legionnaires' disease.* In children under 8 years old, erythromycin is a useful alternative to *tetracycline,* which can cause permanent staining of developing teeth.

Possible adverse effects include nausea, vomiting, abdominal pain, diarrhea, and an itchy rash.

Eschar
A scab on the surface of the skin formed to cover damage caused by a burn, abrasion, severe scratching, or some skin diseases and infections.

Esmarch's bandage
A broad, rubber bandage wrapped around the elevated limb of a patient

to force blood out of the blood vessels toward the heart; this enables surgery to be performed more easily in a blood-free area.

The Esmarch's bandage is wrapped from the toes or fingers upward, and a pneumatic (inflatable) tourniquet is then applied to the thigh or upper arm to stop blood from returning to the limb. The Esmarch's bandage is removed, leaving the inflated tourniquet in position during surgery.

Esophageal atresia

A rare *birth defect* caused by a failure of the esophagus to form correctly during embryonic development. A short section of the *esophagus* is absent, the part of the esophagus above the gap terminates in a pouch, and the lower part of the esophagus, projecting upward from the stomach, is also blind-ended.

In most cases of the condition there is also an abnormal channel, called a *tracheoesophageal fistula*, between one of the sections of esophagus and the trachea (windpipe). The incidence of esophageal atresia ranges from one in 1,000 to one in 3,000.

SYMPTOMS AND DIAGNOSIS
The diagnosis may be suspected even before birth if the mother is found to have *polyhydramnios* (excess amniotic fluid). The infant cannot swallow saliva or milk, and continuous drooling and regurgitation from the mouth occur. If there is an upper tracheo-esophageal fistula, milk may be sucked into the lungs; as a result, attempts at feeding provoke attacks of coughing and cyanosis (a blue-purple skin coloration).

A soft tube inserted into the nose can normally be passed down the esophagus; in cases of esophageal atresia, however, this will not be possible. The diagnosis is confirmed by a *chest X ray* taken after a *radiopaque* tube has been passed as far as possible down the esophagus.

TREATMENT
Swallowed saliva is sucked out via a tube, and the infant is artificially ventilated. Immediate surgery is necessary. Under a general anesthetic, the baby's chest is opened, the blind ends of the esophagus are joined and any tracheoesophageal fistula is closed.

Complications can be prevented by skilled nursing care. Some affected babies do not survive, especially if they are very small or if they also have severe heart disease. If the operation is successful, the baby will develop normally.

Esophageal dilatation

A procedure to stretch the *esophagus* after it has become narrowed by disease (see *Esophageal stricture*), which prevents normal swallowing. The usual cause of the narrowing is swelling and scarring from *esophagitis* (inflammation of the esophagus), but the narrowing may also be due to cancer (see *esophagus, cancer of*) or *achalasia* (inability of the muscles in the lower esophagus to relax).

HOW IT IS DONE
The patient must not eat for at least eight hours before the esophageal dilatation, which is usually carried out under sedation.

First, an *endoscope* (a fine, flexible viewing instrument) is passed through the mouth and down the esophagus to locate the obstruction. Stretching of the narrowed area is sometimes performed by passing a series of bougies (cylindrical rods with olive-shaped tips) over a guide wire passed down the esophagus. Increasingly commonly, stretching is now being performed by means of a *balloon catheter* (a fine tube with a balloon at the end), which is passed down the esophagus. After being inflated, the balloon is kept in position for three minutes and then deflated and withdrawn; the same procedure is repeated later with a larger balloon.

Esophageal diverticulum

A saclike outward protrusion of part of the wall of the *esophagus*.

TYPES
There are two types: a pharyngeal pouch (also called a Zenker's or pulsion diverticulum), and a mid-esophageal diverticulum (also called a traction diverticulum).

PHARYNGEAL POUCH This type is located at the top of the esophagus, at its entrance from the pharynx (throat). The pouch usually projects backward. The cause is a failure of the sphincter (circular muscle) at the entrance to the esophagus to relax during the act of swallowing, due to muscular incoordination. Instead, the sphincter resists the passage of food. As the powerful throat muscles used for swallowing work against this resistance, part of the lining of the esophagus is forced through the esophageal wall, thus forming the diverticulum.

Once the diverticulum is formed, it gradually enlarges, and food becomes trapped in it, causing irritation, difficulty in swallowing, *halitosis* (bad breath), and regurgitation. The diag-

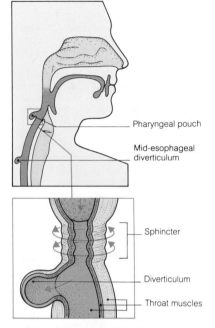

Pharyngeal pouch

Mid-esophageal diverticulum

Sphincter

Diverticulum

Throat muscles

Location of esophageal diverticulum
The pharyngeal pouch forms at the top of the esophagus as a reaction to the sphincter's failure to relax during swallowing. The usually symptomless mid-esophageal diverticulum is a pouch further down the esophagus.

nosis is confirmed by a barium swallow (see *Barium X-ray examinations*), and the diverticulum is treated by surgical removal. The sphincter muscle is partly cut at the same time to weaken it and prevent recurrence.

MID-ESOPHAGEAL DIVERTICULUM This disorder consists of a pouch formed further down the esophagus. It rarely causes symptoms and usually requires no treatment.

Esophageal spasm

Uncoordinated contractions of the muscles in the *esophagus*, which fail to propel food effectively down into the stomach. The contractions may be caused by some other esophageal disorder, such as reflux *esophagitis*, but in many cases they occur for no apparent reason. Women are affected more often than men. Pain is felt in the chest or upper abdomen and there is difficulty in swallowing. The symptoms are intermittent and do not worsen.

A barium swallow (see *Barium X-ray examinations*) will show the irregular contractions of the esophagus and, along with *endoscopy* (passage of a viewing instrument down the esophagus) and esophageal *manometry*, can

E

rule out the possibility of a more serious condition, such as a cancer. There is no specific treatment other than for an underlying cause.

Esophageal stricture

Narrowing of the *esophagus*, which may cause swallowing difficulty. Narrowing may be due to a cancer (see *Esophagus, cancer of*) or to any of numerous noncancerous causes. These include persistent reflux *esophagitis*, in which constant irritation from gastric acid causes inflammation and swelling followed by the formation of fibrous scar tissue and narrowing. Prolonged use of a *nasogastric tube* may inflame the esophagus, leading to a stricture, as may the accidental swallowing of a corrosive liquid.

The symptoms of a stricture are difficulty in swallowing, pain, weight loss, and regurgitation of food.

DIAGNOSIS AND TREATMENT

A barium swallow (see *Barium X-ray examinations*) shows a smooth narrowing of the esophagus. *Endoscopy* (passage of a viewing instrument down the esophagus) is used to look at the narrowed area, and a *biopsy* (removal of a sample of tissue for microscopic analysis) is performed to exclude the possibility of cancer.

In most cases, the narrowed area is widened by *esophageal dilatation*. In rare cases of very severe narrowing over a long segment of the esophagus (usually due to swallowing corrosives), the affected area may require surgical removal. A loop of colon may be substituted for the removed section, or the ends of the esophagus may be joined and the stomach brought up into the chest.

Patients who are too old or too frail for surgery may be treated by the insertion of a permanent pliable plastic tube through the narrowed area, or by the creation of a *gastrostomy* (a surgically produced opening in the stomach for a feeding tube).

Esophageal varices

Widened veins in the walls of the lower part of the *esophagus* and, in some cases, also in the upper part of the stomach. They develop as a consequence of *portal hypertension* (increased blood pressure in the portal vein due to liver disease). Blood passing from the intestines to the liver via the portal vein meets increased resistance and is diverted through the veins in the walls of the esophagus and stomach. The pressure causes the veins to balloon outward.

SYMPTOMS AND DIAGNOSIS

The affected veins are thin-walled and contain blood at high pressure; they may rupture, causing recurrent episodes of severe hematemesis (vomiting of blood) and melena (black feces). Most patients also have other symptoms of chronic liver disease.

Endoscopy (passage of a viewing instrument down the esophagus) or a barium swallow (see *Barium X-ray examinations*) shows the affected veins bulging from the esophageal walls.

TREATMENT

Acute bleeding may be controlled by means of a specially designed *balloon catheter*, which is passed into the esophagus and stomach; the balloon is inflated to press on the bleeding varices. Later, the varices may be treated with intravenous injection of synthetic *ADH* (vasopressin) and/or by injection of a sclerosant—a solution that clots the blood and permanently hardens and seals off the affected veins. Surgery may be performed to lower the pressure in the blood supply to the liver. Recurrent bleeding can sometimes be controlled by other drugs, such as *propranolol*.

Esophagitis

Inflammation of the *Esophagus*.

TYPES

The two main types are corrosive esophagitis, caused by swallowing caustic chemicals, and reflux esophagitis, caused by regurgitation of stomach contents into the esophagus.

CORROSIVE ESOPHAGITIS The severity of inflammation depends on the caustic chemical swallowed. Chemicals likely to cause very severe corrosive esophagitis include cleaning or disinfectant solutions. Immediately after swallowing such a chemical, there is severe pain with *shock* and swelling in the throat and mouth. Antidotes are of limited value and gastric lavage (washing out of the stomach) must be avoided as this may only increase the damage. Treatment consists mainly of reducing pain and providing nursing care until the esophagus heals.

REFLUX ESOPHAGITIS This is a very common condition. The main symptom is heartburn (a burning pain in the chest) which worsens on bending over. Symptoms may be worsened by alcohol, smoking, and obesity.

Reflux esophagitis is caused by poor function of the muscles of the lower esophagus, which permits reflux (regurgitation) of the stomach's acidic contents into the esophagus. Poor

function of the lower esophagus may be associated with a *hiatal hernia*, in which the top part of the stomach slides back and forth between the chest and the abdomen.

A less common alkaline form of esophagitis is caused by the presence of bile in the stomach, which may be a consequence of certain operations, such as partial *gastrectomy*. If the bile flows from the stomach into the esophagus, it causes inflammation of the esophagus, which tends to be severe and difficult to treat.

Barrett's esophagus is a complication of reflux esophagitis in which tissue normally found in the stomach lining occurs in the esophagus. This condition may lead to cancer.

DIAGNOSIS

A barium swallow (see *Barium X-ray examinations*) will show reflux of stomach contents, and *endoscopy* of the esophagus (passage of a viewing instrument down the esophagus) will show inflammation. In doubtful cases, special tests may be required. A

ANATOMY OF THE ESOPHAGUS
A muscular tube that propels food to the stomach from the throat. The upper and lower ends are bounded by sphincters—muscular valves that open to allow food to pass through.

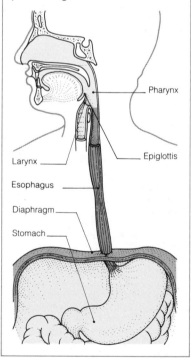

Pharynx

Epiglottis

Larynx

Esophagus

Diaphragm

Stomach

small tube may be swallowed and a probe positioned in the lower esophagus to record the acidity over a 24-hour period; alternatively, a dilute acid solution may be introduced into the stomach to see if it reproduces the symptoms.

TREATMENT
The treatment for most cases of persistent esophagitis is for the sufferer to change his or her diet and lifestyle—to reduce weight, avoid heavy meals, limit alcohol consumption, and stop smoking.

Antacid drugs may be taken to reduce the acidity of the stomach contents. Elevation of the head of the bed with blocks may be helpful. Sometimes, surgical treatment may be needed for a hiatal hernia.

Severe, chronic esophagitis of either type can cause an *esophageal stricture* (narrowing of the esophagus), which will require prolonged *esophageal dilatation* and/or extensive surgery.

Esophagoscopy
Examination of the *esophagus* by means of an *endoscope*, a thin, flexible viewing instrument with a light and lenses attached. (See *Gastroscopy*.)

Esophagus
The muscular tube that carries food from the throat to the stomach without interfering with the breakdown or absorption of food products.

STRUCTURE
The top end of the esophagus is the narrowest part of the entire digestive tract (see *Digestive system*) and is encircled by a sphincter (circular muscle) that is normally closed but can open to allow the passage of food. There is a similar sphincter at the point where the esophagus enters the stomach. The walls of the esophagus consist of strong muscle fibers arranged in bundles, some circular and others longitudinal. The inner lining of the esophagus consists of smooth, squamous epithelium (flattened cells).

FUNCTION
The esophagus acts as a conduit by which liquids and food are conveyed to the stomach and intestines for digestion. Food is propelled downward toward the stomach by *peristalsis* (powerful waves of contractions passing through the muscles in the esophageal wall). Gravity plays little part in getting food into the stomach, making it possible to drink while upside down. (See also *Swallowing*.)

Esophagus, cancer of
A malignant tumor of the *esophagus*, which ultimately causes difficulty in swallowing. Most esophageal cancers develop in the middle or lower sections of the esophagus.

CAUSES AND INCIDENCE
The causes of esophageal cancer are not fully understood, but smoking, a heavy consumption of alcohol, and drinking very hot drinks are thought to be risk factors.

The incidence varies throughout the world. About 800 cases are diagnosed in Canada each year, mainly in people over 50. The cancer is more common in men than in women and more common in black people than in white people. There is a particularly high incidence of esophageal cancer in parts of the Far East and Iran, where the cancer has been linked to chemicals in certain foods.

SYMPTOMS
Difficulty in swallowing is noticed first with solids and later with fluids (even saliva) and becomes progressively worse. If food cannot pass down the esophagus it is immediately regurgitated. Rapid weight loss occurs, but no pain develops until the cancer is well advanced. Re-

E

DISORDERS OF THE ESOPHAGUS

Despite its apparently simple structure, the esophagus is prone to a number of disorders, most of which lead to difficulty in, or completely prevent, swallowing and/or cause a pain in the chest.

CONGENITAL DEFECTS
Esophageal atresia is an absence from birth of a section of the esophagus, with the remaining sections ending in dead ends. It requires urgent surgical correction. Babies are also occasionally born with weblike constrictions of the esophagus. These are rarely serious enough to require treatment, but may, if necessary, be broken down with a rubber dilator.

INFECTION AND INFLAMMATION
Infections of the esophagus are uncommon, but may occur in severely immunosuppressed patients whose defenses against infection are weakened. The most common infections are *herpes simplex* virus infection or *candidiasis* (thrush) extending downward from the mouth. Both cause pain on swallowing.

Esophagitis (inflammation of the esophagus) is usually due to reflux of the contents of the stomach, causing heartburn (a burning sensation in the chest). A more severe form—corrosive esophagitis—can occur as a result of swallowing caustic chemicals. Either of these types of esophagitis may cause an *esophageal stricture*, with consequent difficulty in swallowing.

INJURY
Apart from the damaging effects of swallowing corrosive chemicals, the most common cause of injury to the esophagus is severe vomiting and retching, which can occasionally tear the esophageal lining (and result in bleeding) or in extreme cases lead to rupture. A hard, swallowed *foreign body* can also cause injury and sometimes perforation (formation of a hole) if it penetrates into the esophageal wall.

TUMORS
Tumors of the esophagus are not rare. The initial symptom is usually difficulty in swallowing. About 90 percent are malignant (see *Esophagus, cancer of*); the remainder are benign.

OTHER DISORDERS
An *esophageal diverticulum* is an outwardly protruding sac, usually at the top end of the esophagus, in which food may collect and cause halitosis (bad breath) and sometimes difficulty in swallowing. *Esophageal spasm* consists of uncontrollable contractions of the esophagus, which again may make swallowing difficult. In *achalasia*, the sphincter at the junction between the esophagus and stomach fails to relax to allow the passage of food, causing pain on swallowing and sometimes regurgitation of food. (See also *Swallowing difficulty*.)

INVESTIGATION
Esophageal disorders are investigated by barium swallow (see *Barium X-ray examinations*) and by *endoscopy*. Occasionally, a *biopsy* (tissue sample) may be taken for microscopic examination.

E

spiratory infections are common, because regurgitated fluid spills over into the trachea.

DIAGNOSIS

A barium swallow (see *Barium X-ray examinations*) can indicate the site and often the nature of the obstruction of the esophagus. Definite diagnosis is provided by examination of a *biopsy* sample (a small piece of tissue) obtained through an *endoscope* (viewing instrument) fitted with a tissue collecting attachment.

TREATMENT AND OUTLOOK

Esophagectomy (removal of the esophagus) provides the best hope of cure but is a major undertaking. Incisions are made in the abdomen, the chest, and sometimes the neck. Most of the esophagus is then removed and the stomach, or sometimes a portion of the colon, is pulled up into the chest and joined to the upper part of the esophagus.

For older patients who might not survive this operation, *radiation therapy*, sometimes combined with *anticancer drugs* (particularly cisplatin), can sometimes provide a significant regression of the cancer, relief from symptoms, and even an occasional cure. Some relief from starvation can also be achieved by intubation—the insertion of a rigid tube through the tumor to allow swallowing of liquid or semiliquid food, or by using a *laser treatment* to burn a passage through an obstructing tumor.

The overall outlook for esophageal cancer is poor, with only about 5 percent of patients surviving for five years; if the cancer is diagnosed early, the outlook is better.

Esotropia

A term for a convergent *squint*. One eye looks directly at an object while the other eye turns inward.

ESR

The abbreviation for erythrocyte sedimentation rate (i.e., the rate at which red blood cells sink toward the bottom of a test tube). Because the ESR is increased in certain disorders, it is a useful aid to diagnosis and can also be used to monitor the effect of treatment.

HOW IT IS DONE

Whole blood collected from the person on whom the test is being performed is mixed with anticoagulant (a chemical that prevents the blood from clotting) in a test tube and left undisturbed at a constant temperature for one hour.

The red blood cells, which can be seen as a dark red clump, settle toward the bottom of the tube, leaving the clear, straw-colored plasma at the top. The ESR is the number of millimetres the red cells fall in one hour.

RESULTS

The ESR is increased if the level of fibrinogen (a type of protein) in the blood is raised. Fibrinogen is raised in response to inflammation, especially when caused by infection or an *autoimmune disease*, such as *temporal arteritis*. The ESR is also increased if levels of *immunoglobulins* (another type of protein) are very high, as occurs in *multiple myeloma*.

Estradiol

The most important of the *estrogen hormones* (female sex hormones), essential for the healthy functioning of the reproductive system and for breast development.

In its synthetic form, estradiol is prescribed as a tablet to treat symptoms and complications of the *menopause* (see *Hormone replacement therapy*) and to stimulate sexual development in female *hypogonadism* (underdevelopment of the ovaries). It can be taken orally, given by injection, or be absorbed through the skin from a transdermal patch.

Estrogen drugs

COMMON DRUGS

*Dienestrol Diethylstilbestrol
Estradiol Estriol Ethinylestradiol*

WARNING
Tobacco smoking while taking estrogen drugs significantly increases the risk of abnormal blood clotting, which may cause myocardial infarction, pulmonary embolism, or stroke.

A group of drugs produced synthetically for use in *oral contraceptives* and to supplement or replace the naturally occurring *estrogen hormones* in the body. Estrogen drugs are often used in conjunction with *progestogen drugs*.

Estrogens suppress the production of *gonadotropin hormones* (hormones that stimulate cell activity in the *ovaries*). High doses of estrogens may be given as postcoital contraception (see *Contraception, postcoital*) because they prevent conception by blocking the effect of gonadotropins.

Synthetic estrogens are used to treat, and in some cases to prevent,

symptoms and disorders related to the *menopause*, including atrophic *vaginitis* (dryness of the vagina) and *osteoporosis* (decreased bone density).

Estrogens may also be used to treat certain forms of infertility, female *hypogonadism* (underdevelopment of the ovaries), menstrual disorders in which there is abnormal bleeding from the uterus, prostatic cancer (see *Prostate, cancer of*), and certain types of *breast cancer*.

POSSIBLE ADVERSE EFFECTS

Estrogen drugs may cause breast tenderness and enlargement, bloating, weight gain, nausea, reduced sex drive, depression, migraine, and bleeding between periods. Side effects often subside after two or three months, but, if they persist or are troublesome, a different estrogen drug may be prescribed. Vaginal creams containing estrogen should be used sparingly and usually only for a short time to reduce the risk of adverse effects throughout the body.

Estrogen drugs increase the risk of abnormal blood clotting and are therefore not recommended for people with a personal or family history of *stroke*, *pulmonary embolism*, or deep-vein *thrombosis*, or for people about to undergo surgery. Estrogen drugs may increase a person's susceptibility to *hypertension* (high blood pressure) and are not usually prescribed if a person has suffered from this disorder in the past. Estrogens should not be taken during pregnancy as they may adversely affect the fetus.

Estrogen hormones

A group of *hormones* (chemical messengers released by glands) essential for normal female sexual development and for the healthy functioning of the reproductive system. In women, they are produced mainly in the *ovaries*. Estrogen hormones are also formed in the *placenta* during pregnancy and, in both men and women, in small amounts in the *adrenal glands*. In men, estrogens have no known specific function.

Estrone

One of the *Estrogen hormones*.

ESWL

Extracorporeal shock wave lithotripsy. (See *Lithotripsy*.)

Ethambutol

A drug used in conjunction with other drugs in the treatment of *tuberculosis*. Ethambutol rarely causes side effects, although occasionally it may cause inflammation of the optic nerve, resulting in blurred vision.

Ethanol

The chemical name for the *alcohol* in alcoholic drinks; it is also called ethyl alcohol.

Ether

A colorless liquid that produces unconsciousness when inhaled. Ether (full name, diethyl ether) was the first general anesthetic. It was administered on a gauze mask placed over the patient's nose and mouth and was common until the 1930s. It is simple to administer and there is little risk of overdose, but its extreme inflammability led to its replacement by other, more powerful anesthetic agents (see *Anesthesia, general*) even though these require more skill on the part of the anesthetist.

Ethics, medical

Medical ethics covers all areas of the physician's conduct, but its primary focus is the physician-patient relationship, which is based on mutual trust. The physician's fundamental responsibilities to the patient under this relationship are (1) to preserve confidentiality, and (2) to respect the patient's autonomy (the right to make independent decisions). Medical ethics is also the basis for guidelines concerning physicians' responsibility to maintain proper standards of care, their participation in research, fee setting, relationships between referring physicians and consultants, and personal behavior.

The Canadian Medical Association Code of Ethics serves as a guideline for all provincial licensing bodies (Quebec has made slight modifications), which are responsible for investigating complaints and disciplining physicians. (See also *Consent*.)

Ethinylestradiol

A synthetic form of the female sex hormone estradiol. It is most commonly used in *oral contraceptives*, in which it is combined with a *progesterone drug*. Ethinylestradiol is also prescribed to stimulate sexual development in female *hypogonadism* (underdevelopment of the ovaries) and in the treatment of symptoms caused by the *menopause*, such as hot flashes and sweating (see *Hormone replacement therapy*). Ethinylestradiol is also used to treat menstrual disorders (see *Menstruation, disorders of*).

Ethosuximide

An *anticonvulsant drug* used to treat petit mal (a type of *epilepsy*). Ethosuximide is often prescribed in preference to other anticonvulsant drugs because, unlike some of them, it rarely causes drowsiness or liver damage. Ethosuximide may, however, cause nausea and vomiting and in rare cases affects the production of blood cells in the bone marrow and causes aplastic anemia (see *Anemia, aplastic*). Other types of epilepsy do not respond well to this drug.

Ethyl alcohol

Another name for ethanol, the *alcohol* in alcoholic drinks.

Ethyl chloride

A colorless, flammable liquid once used as a general anesthetic and now occasionally used as an *analgesic drug* (painkiller).

Applied to the skin as a spray, ethyl chloride quickly evaporates and, as a result, makes the skin feel so cold that any pain or irritation is reduced. It may be used to numb an area of skin before a minor surgical procedure, such as lancing a boil, and is sometimes used to alleviate the pain that arises from sprained or strained muscles or ligaments.

Ethyl chloride is also used in the treatment of *larva migrans*, a hookworm infection acquired from cats and dogs.

Etiology

The cause of a disease, or the study of the various factors involved in causing a disease.

For some cases of a particular disorder, a specific etiology can be identified: laboratory studies may show, for example, that an attack of diarrhea is due to a particular type of bacterium or virus. Other disorders have a multifactorial etiology: the causative factors of degenerative arthritis, for example, include genetic susceptibility, repeated joint injuries, and being overweight. However, many disorders, such as schizophrenia, are of unknown etiology.

Etretinate

A drug chemically related to *vitamin A* that is used in the treatment of severe *psoriasis*. Prescribed only under hospital supervision, etretinate is used when other drugs have failed to help. It works by reducing the production of keratin, the protein that forms the hard, outer layers of skin. Because of this action, etretinate is also occasionally used to treat other rare skin disorders that cause excessive skin thickening, such as *ichthyosis*.

Symptoms generally improve within four weeks of treatment and effects may persist for many months after therapy with the drug has been discontinued.

POSSIBLE ADVERSE EFFECTS
Etretinate can cause liver damage and a rise in blood fats; regular blood tests of liver function and fat levels are therefore usually carried out during treatment. Etretinate should never be taken during pregnancy because of the risk of damage to the developing fetus, and effective *contraception* must be continued for two years after stopping the drug. Blood should not be donated for one year after stopping.

Eucalyptus oil

A substance distilled from the leaves of eucalyptus trees. Eucalyptus oil is colorless, with an aromatic, camphorlike smell and a pungent, refreshing taste. The oil is used as a flavoring agent and—applied externally as a rub, inhaled as a vapor, or incorporated in tablets or pastilles—is also used in many proprietary remedies for coughs and colds. There is little evidence that eucalyptus oil has any curative properties, although it may relieve symptoms.

Eunuch

A man whose testes have been removed or destroyed so that he is sterile and lacks male hormones. The term was used especially to describe boys who were castrated before puberty to make them suitable for guarding harems.

A male who is castrated before puberty will have characteristic eunuchoid features: broad hips, narrow shoulders, and undeveloped male secondary *sexual characteristics* (i.e., he will have a small penis, a feminine distribution of body hair, and a high-pitched voice).

Euphoria

A state of confident well-being. Euphoria is a normal reaction to personal success. It can also be induced by drugs, including prolonged use of *corticosteroid drugs*.

Feelings of euphoria with no rational cause may be an indication of brain disease or damage caused by *head injury* (particularly damage to the frontal lobes), *dementia, brain tumors,* or *multiple sclerosis*.

E

ANATOMY OF THE EUSTACHIAN TUBE

The eustachian tube connects the middle ear with the back of the nose. The tube is divided into two separate parts: the first part runs within a bony canal and the second part is lined with cartilage.

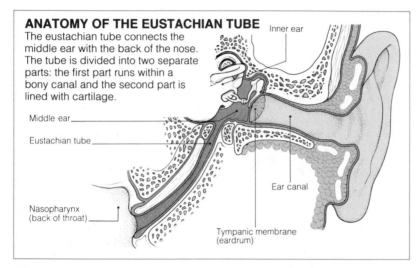

Inner ear

Middle ear

Eustachian tube

Nasopharynx
(back of throat)

Ear canal

Tympanic membrane
(eardrum)

Eustachian tube

The passage that connects each middle *ear* to the back of the nose.

STRUCTURE

The tube is about 36 mm long in an adult. From the middle ear it runs forward, downward, and inward; it ends in the space at the back of the nose just above the soft *palate* (part of the roof of the mouth). A smooth, moist, mucous membrane forms a lining within the tube.

FUNCTION

The eustachian tube acts as a drainage passage from the middle ear and maintains hearing by opening periodically to regulate air pressure. The lower end of the eustachian tube opens during swallowing and yawning, thus allowing air to flow up to the middle ear and equalizing air pressure on both sides of the eardrum.

If a change in external pressure is large and rapid, pressure may build up on one side of the eardrum, pushing it inward or outward; this is uncomfortable and dulls hearing. Most people have experienced this sensation in response to the increase in pressure that occurs when descending in a plane or going into a tunnel in a car or train. Symptoms can usually be relieved by swallowing hard.

DISORDERS

When a head cold blocks the eustachian tube, equalization cannot occur, which may cause severe pain. Because the displaced eardrum cannot vibrate properly, hearing may be temporarily impaired. A person with a blocked eustachian tube who is subjected to rapid changes in pressure may suffer from *barotrauma* (pressure damage to the eardrum or other structures).

Glue ear (accumulation of secretions in the middle ear) or chronic *otitis media* (middle ear infection) may occur if the eustachian tube becomes blocked, preventing adequate drainage from the middle ear. These conditions, which often cause partial hearing loss, are more common in children because their adenoids are larger and more likely to block the tube if they become infected. Children's eustachian tubes are also shorter, making it easier for bacteria to travel from infected areas in the throat to the middle ear.

Euthanasia

The act of killing a person painlessly to relieve his or her suffering. Even when requested by a patient with incurable disease, euthanasia (the literal meaning is "easy death") is against the law in most developed countries.

Euthanasia is distinct from non-intervention, which is the physician's recognition that a patient with an advanced or incurable disease has a right to refuse medical treatment.

Euthyroid

The term used to describe a person whose *thyroid gland* is functioning normally, or to describe a person who has been successfully treated for *hypothyroidism* (underactivity of the thyroid) or *hyperthyroidism* (overactivity of the thyroid) so that the gland functions normally.

Eversion

A turning outward. The term is commonly applied to a type of ankle injury or deformity in which the foot is turned outward.

Evoked responses

The tracing of electrical activity in the brain in response to a specific external stimulus. The responses are much smaller than the impulses recorded by an *EEG* and are a refinement of that technique. Evoked responses were first demonstrated in 1947. Today, with the increased sophistication of computerized electronic technology, evoked responses are a widely used diagnostic tool.

WHY IT IS DONE

The functioning of various sensory systems (e.g., sight, hearing, and touch) can be checked by this technique. The information obtained can reveal abnormalities in the system caused by inflammation, pressure from a tumor, or other disorders, and can confirm the diagnosis of *multiple sclerosis*. The test is extremely sensitive and can often pinpoint the location of a fault.

HOW IT IS DONE

The procedure is painless and usually takes 30 minutes to an hour. A set of small disk electrodes is attached to the scalp in the same way as for an EEG. The electrodes are attached to different parts of the scalp, depending on which sensory system is being tested. The output from the brain is linked to a computer, which produces a printout after a specific period of stimulation. Analysis is based on the time lapse between stimulus and response; the computer is used to extract this information from the background brain activity that shows up on an EEG.

For testing the visual system, a series of flashes from a stroboscopic light may be used. An example of a more demanding stimulus for the brain, which gives more consistent results, is a board made up of black and white squares constructed so that the colors alternate every second. To test hearing, the ears are subjected to different sounds. To test touch and pain sensations, small electrical stimuli are applied, for example, to a nerve at the wrist.

RESULTS

Testing of evoked responses does not necessarily give an unequivocal diagnosis and is used as a supplement to other tests of the nervous system (e.g., EEG or *EMG*), other investigations, and radiological tests such as *CT scanning*.

Ewing's sarcoma

A rare malignant bone cancer. Ewing's *sarcoma* arises in a large bone,

E

TYPES OF PHYSICAL EXAMINATION

Examination may include looking for skin changes and feeling organs for size, consistency, and shape. Assessment is made of muscle strength, coordination, joint mobility, and skin sensation. The state of the eyes, ears, mouth, throat, and teeth is checked.

Percussion
The chest is tapped and the vibration felt and heard. A loss of resonance suggests a lung disorder.

Auscultation
The physician uses a stethoscope to listen to lung and heart sounds. Abnormal sounds suggest disease.

Tendon reflexes
One test of the nervous system is to tap a stretched tendon. If the reflex is normal, the muscle should contract.

most commonly the femur (thighbone), tibia (shin), humerus (upperarm bone), or one of the pelvic bones, and spreads to other parts of the body at an early stage. The condition is most common in children between 10 and 15 years of age; it affects twice as many boys as girls and is only rarely seen in black children.

SYMPTOMS

The affected bone is painful and tender and part of it may swell. The bone may also become weakened and fracture easily. Other symptoms include weight loss, fever, and anemia.

DIAGNOSIS

The sarcoma is diagnosed by X rays and a bone *biopsy* (removal of a small piece of bone for analysis). If cancer is found, the complete skeleton is examined by X rays and *radionuclide scanning*, and the lungs by CT *scanning*, to determine if, and how far, the cancer has spread. Spreading by the time of diagnosis is found in 15 to 20 percent of cases.

TREATMENT

Treatment is with *radiation therapy* and *anticancer drugs*. Before the introduction of chemotherapy, death usually occurred within two to three years of diagnosis. Today, the chances of survival have improved considerably; 65 percent of those affected are still alive five years after diagnosis and most of them remain well.

Examination, physical

The part of a medical consultation in which the physician looks, feels, and listens to various parts of the patient's body in order to assess the patient's condition. The physical examination usually follows history-taking, in which the physician listens to the patient's complaints and then asks questions. Physical examination and history-taking together may provide the physician with sufficient information to make a *diagnosis*, or provide clues that will aid the selection of appropriate diagnostic studies.

HOW IT IS DONE

A complete physical examination may be performed if a patient visits a physician for the first time, if a patient complains of generalized symptoms, or if an examination is required for employment or insurance purposes. A more limited examination will be performed if a patient has a disorder or injury in one part of the body.

The main techniques used by a physician during a physical examination are inspection, palpation, percussion, and auscultation.

The physician begins by assessing the patient's general appearance and by looking at any specific problem area, such as a lump, that might be drawn to the physician's attention.

Most physical examinations include palpation (feeling with the hands), by which the physician examines relevant parts of the body for signs such as swelling, tenderness, or enlargement of organs.

In some cases, percussion of the chest over the lungs or of other parts of the body may be performed. Percussion is performed by tapping the patient's body with the fingers and listening to the resonance of the sound produced.

Auscultation (listening with a *stethoscope*) may also be needed. This technique is used mainly to listen to sounds made by the heart and lungs, and to listen to the flow of blood through arteries.

The physician will apply these techniques, sometimes using special equipment, to examine different body systems. For example, he or she may take the pulse or blood pressure, examine the eyes, ears, mouth, throat, and teeth, and assess the strength and coordination of muscles, the mobility of joints, and skin sensation as a reaction to touch and pain.

Excision

Surgical cutting out of diseased tissue from surrounding healthy tissue, such as the removal of a breast lump or gangrenous skin.

Excoriation

Injury to the surface of the skin or of a *mucous membrane* caused by physical abrasion, such as by scratching. The loss of surface cells causes a raw area to develop.

Excretion

The discharge of waste material—carbon dioxide, sweat, urine, and feces—from the body. To maintain health, the body must dispose of the by-products of digestion (such as food residues and an excess of salt or other substances), waste products from the repair of body tissues, medication or its breakdown products, poisonous substances, and water (to maintain the correct fluid volume and to remove solid wastes in solution).

ORGANS OF EXCRETION

The *kidneys* excrete excess nitrogen in the *urine* in the form of urea, along with excess water, salts, some acids, and most drugs.

E

THE EFFECTS OF EXERCISE

There are many changes in different body organs during exercise. Muscles require an increase in blood flow because of their greater energy requirements; the heart and lungs work faster and more efficiently. These changes are controlled by the release of the chemicals epinephrine and norepinephrine from the sympathetic nervous system.

The lungs

The rate and depth of breathing increase to ensure sufficient flow of oxygen from the lungs into the blood. This also helps remove additional carbon dioxide produced by muscle cells during exercise.

The joints

Regular exercise helps maintain the mobility of joints. Increased strength in the muscles and tendons around joints makes them more resistant to injury.

The muscles

There is a rise in the chemical activity within muscle cells. The rate of consumption of oxygen and glucose increases.

Flexed muscles

Relaxed muscles

The heart and circulation

The heart beats faster and more powerfully to increase the flow of blood to the working muscles. Blood vessels in the stomach and under the skin are narrowed to compensate for the increased requirements of the muscles.

ECG printouts

Resting heart rate (above) and during exercise (below).

COMMON TYPES OF EXERCISE

Aerobic	Isometric	Isotonic	Isokinetic
Exercise is aerobic when the body continuously needs to take in additional oxygen to meet the muscles' increased demands. Regular aerobic exercise improves the performance of the cardiovascular and respiratory systems. Jogging, swimming, and cycling are examples of aerobic exercise.	Isometric exercise is exercise without movement, in which one group of muscles exerts pressure against an immovable object or an opposing group of muscles. It is an effective means of increasing muscle strength, but does not exercise the cardiovascular system or help in muscular endurance.	Isotonic exercise is exercise with movement, in which muscle tension is more or less constant and the body works against its own weight or external weights. Isotonic exercise includes weight training and calisthenics (repetitive movements with little or no equipment). It increases muscle strength, size, and endurance.	Isokinetic exercise involves both isotonic and isometric exercise. The muscles move reasonably heavy loads, but are also put through their full range of movement. Isokinetics combines strength training with some aerobic exercise, but requires special equipment.

The *liver* excretes bile, which, as well as containing salts that help emulsify fats in the small intestine, consists of waste products and bile pigments formed from the breakdown of red blood cells. Part of the bile is passed from the body in the *feces*, which it colors brown.

The large *intestine* excretes undigested food, some salts, and some excess water in the form of feces.

The *lungs* discharge carbon dioxide and water vapor into the air.

Sweat glands excrete salt and water onto the skin, thus regulating the body's temperature.

Exenteration

The surgical removal of all organs and soft tissue in a body cavity in the hope of arresting the growth of a cancer. Exenteration is occasionally performed for cancer in the orbit (the bony structure surrounding the eye) or in the pelvis.

Exercise

The performance of any physical activity that improves health or that is used for recreation or the correction of physical injury or deformity (see *Physiotherapy*). Different types of exercise affect the body in one or more of the following ways: some improve flexibility, some improve muscular strength, some improve physical endurance, and some improve the efficiency of the cardiovascular and respiratory systems. The various effects of different types of exercise are described above.

BENEFITS OF EXERCISE

There is an established association between high levels of aerobic exercise and low incidence of *coronary artery disease*. Regular exercise usually leads to a reduction in blood pressure. It also increases the amount of high-density lipoprotein in the blood, which is thought to help protect against *atherosclerosis* (narrowing of arteries by deposits of fatty material) and *myocardial infarction* (heart attack). Exercise has also been shown to be valuable in relieving the symptoms of *peripheral vascular disease* and of some psychological disorders such as *depression*.

Vigorous work with a muscle or a group of muscles, even if it is of short duration, leads to an increase in the size, strength, and possibly the number of the muscle cells, and an increase in the strength of their ligamentous attachments to bones. Improving the strength of muscles in the back and abdomen can help prevent or ease lower back pain. The increased strength is also a potentially useful insurance against damage due to an unexpected strain.

Many elderly people become inactive and lose joint mobility. Regular, gentle, rhythmic movements can help maintain the range of movement of important joints. Coordination and balance deteriorate with age; exercise helps maintain muscle strength and reduce the risk of falls. (See also *Aerobics; Fitness; Fitness testing*.)

Exfoliation

Flaking off, shedding, or peeling from a surface in scales or thin layers, as in *exfoliative dermatitis*.

Exfoliative dermatitis

Inflammation, marked redness, and scaling of the skin over most of the body, also called erythroderma.

Exfoliative dermatitis may be the result of an allergic response to a particular drug or may be caused by the worsening of a skin condition, such as *psoriasis* or *eczema*. Sometimes, exfoliative dermatitis occurs in *lymphoma* and *leukemia*.

There is a widespread rash with severe flaking of the skin. The loss of surface skin, with exposure of its deeper layers, results in increased loss of water and protein from the body surface. Protein loss may cause *edema* (accumulation of fluid in tissues) and muscle wasting. Further complications are *heart failure*, due to the pumping of blood through widened blood vessels, and infection.

The treatment and outlook depend on the cause. About 60 percent of sufferers recover within two to three months; about 30 percent die as a result of complications; and in the remainder the disease takes a chronic form unresponsive to treatment.

Exhibitionism

The habit of deliberately exposing the genitals to strangers. This form of behavior is almost always confined to men. The exhibitionist displays his penis to a female passerby, usually in a secluded spot or from a car or house window with the aim of surprising or frightening the victim.

In 80 percent of cases, a single court appearance puts an end to the exhibitionist's behavior. *Psychotherapy* or *behavior therapy* can sometimes help those who relapse.

Exocrine gland

A gland that secretes substances through a duct onto the inner surface of an organ or onto the outer surface of the body.

Examples include the *salivary glands*, which release saliva into the mouth, the *sweat glands*, which carry sweat to the skin's surface, and the lacrimal glands (see *lacrimal apparatus*), which produce and release tears. The release of exocrine secretions can be triggered by a *hormone* or by a *neurotransmitter*. (See also *Endocrine gland*.)

Exomphalos

A rare birth defect in which a membranous sac which contains part of the intestines protrudes through the umbilicus (navel). In mild cases only one or two loops of intestine protrude, but in severe cases most of the abdominal organs are exposed.

Also called omphalocele, exomphalos is associated with other birth defects, including intestinal malformations. Many babies with the condition are stillborn or die soon after birth. Exomphalos is treated by surgery. Prior to operation, the covering membranes may be painted with a drying, antiseptic solution to thicken them, making subsequent surgery easier.

Exophthalmos

Protrusion of one or both eyeballs caused by a swelling of the soft tissue in the bony orbit (eye socket). The eyeball is pressed forward, exposing an abnormally large amount of the front of the eye, forcing the eyelids apart and causing a staring appearance.

CAUSE

The most common cause of exophthalmos is *thyrotoxicosis* (overactivity of the thyroid gland). Other causes include an *eye tumor*, inflammation, or an *aneurysm* behind the eye; in these cases only one eye is affected.

One-sided exophthalmos
The affected eye (shown above) protrudes markedly compared with the normal eye. More commonly, both eyes are affected.

SYMPTOMS AND SIGNS

Exophthalmos may restrict eye movement and cause *double vision*. In severe cases, the pressure in the orbit may be so high that the blood supply to the optic nerve may be restricted; blindness can result. The lids may be prevented from closing, and vision may become seriously blurred due to drying of the cornea.

TREATMENT AND OUTLOOK

In thyroid exophthalmos, treatment of the thyroid disorder may sometimes relieve the exophthalmos, but often it does not. Early treatment usually returns the vision to normal. Occasionally, surgery to decompress the orbit may be required to relieve pressure on the eyeball and on the optic nerve.

Exostosis

A type of benign *bone tumor* in which there is an outgrowth of bone. Exostosis occurs most commonly at the end of the femur (thighbone) or tibia (shin).

Exostoses account for 90 percent of all bone tumors; they affect twice as many men as women. In about 65 percent of cases the condition is due to hereditary factors; another cause is prolonged pressure on a bone.

SYMPTOMS

In most cases, exostosis produces no symptoms and goes unnoticed. Often it is recognized only after an injury, when it appears as a hard swelling. Occasionally the bony outgrowth presses on a nerve, causing pain or weakness in the affected area (usually when it is beneath a fingernail or toenail).

DIAGNOSIS AND TREATMENT

A preliminary diagnosis based on symptoms and signs can be confirmed by X ray. Treatment, by surgical removal, is usually performed only if the tumor is causing symptoms or is unsightly.

E

Exotoxin

 A poison released by some types of bacteria into the bloodstream, from where it causes widespread effects throughout the body. Exotoxins are among the most poisonous substances known. They are produced by certain types of bacteria, such as *tetanus* bacilli (which enter the body through a wound and produce an exotoxin that affects the nervous system to cause muscle spasms and paralysis) and *diphtheria* bacilli (which initially infect the throat, but release an exotoxin that damages the heart and nervous system).

Infections by tetanus, diphtheria, and some other bacteria that release life-threatening exotoxins can be prevented by a program of immunization with vaccines consisting of detoxified exotoxins. Treatment of such infections usually includes the administration of *antibiotic drugs* and an *antitoxin* to neutralize the exotoxin. (See also *Endotoxin; Enterotoxin.*)

Exotropia

A term for a divergent *squint*. One eye is used for detailed vision and the other is directed outward.

Expectorants

Cough remedies that encourage the coughing up of sputum (phlegm) from the respiratory tract.

Expectoration

The coughing up and spitting out of sputum (phlegm). (See also *Cough.*)

Expiration

See *Breathing.*

Exploratory surgery

Any operation to investigate or examine part of the body to discover the extent of known disease or to establish a diagnosis. For example, exploratory *thoracotomy* is performed on the chest and exploratory *laparotomy* on the abdomen.

Exposure

A term used to describe the effects on the body of being subjected to very low temperatures, or to a combination of low temperatures, wetness, and high winds. The primary danger comes from the lowering of body temperature in these conditions (see *Hypothermia*).

The term is also sometimes used to describe subjection to radiation or to a variety of environmental pollutants.

Expressing milk

A technique used by *breast-feeding* women for removing milk from the breasts. Expressing milk may be necessary when the breasts are overfull (see *Engorgement*). A woman may also want to express milk from her breasts so that the milk can be given to the baby in her absence.

EXPRESSING MILK BY HAND

Wash your hands thoroughly before starting, then follow the method below. Repeat the sequence twice on each breast, alternating between breasts. If the breasts are engorged, bathe them in hot water first to help milk flow.

1 Cup the breast in both hands, thumbs on top and fingers underneath. Squeeze the outer part of the breast firmly. Repeat 10 times, moving around the breast.

2 Move hands closer to the nipple area and repeat the squeezing movement 10 more times.

3 Hold the breast in one hand. With the thumb and forefinger of the other hand, squeeze the edge of the areola in and up so that milk squirts out. Move your hand around the areola, squeezing gently and rhythmically for about five minutes.

Most women find it easier to express milk by hand, but a *breast pump* can be used. Milk should be expressed into a sterilized container and sealed. It will keep for up to 48 hours in a refrigerator. When properly prepared, it can be stored in a freezer for up to six months.

Exstrophy of the bladder

A rare birth defect in which the bladder is turned inside out and is open to the outside of the body through a space in the lower abdominal wall.

Usually, there are also other defects, such as *epispadias* (emergence of the urethra through a hole in the shaft of the penis) in males, and failure of the pubic bones to join at the front.

Untreated, an affected child constantly leaks urine. Surgical treatment consists of reconstructing the bladder, if it is big enough, and closing the abdominal wall. If the bladder is very small, it is removed and the urine diverted elsewhere in the abdomen (see *Urinary diversion*).

Extra billing

The practice of a physician billing the patient for the difference between the provincial medical plan fee rate for a procedure and the physician's charge for that procedure.

Extraction, dental

The removal of one or more teeth by a dentist.

WHY IT IS DONE

Extraction may be performed when a tooth is severely decayed, when an abscess has formed, or when a tooth is too badly broken to be repaired by crowning or root canal treatment. Teeth may also be removed if they are causing crowding or malocclusion (incorrect bite), if they are loose because of advanced gum disease, or if they are preventing another tooth from erupting.

HOW IT IS DONE

For most extractions, local anesthesia is used. General anesthesia may be used to extract badly impacted wisdom teeth, to extract several teeth at once, or for extremely anxious or mentally handicapped patients or young children.

Most teeth are extracted with dental forceps, which are designed to grasp the root of the tooth. When gentle but firm pressure is applied, the blades cut through the periodontal ligaments (the tough fibrous membranes supporting the tooth in its socket), the socket is gradually expanded, and the tooth is removed. Occasionally the root of the tooth fractures during this procedure, especially if the bone is dense (as in older people) and may need to be removed separately.

If the tooth is especially difficult to remove—for example, if it is impacted, the crown is missing, or the roots are very curved—it may be necessary to cut a small flap into the gum and remove a small amount of nearby bone. The tooth is then extracted and the gum is sutured.

COMPLICATIONS

Most extractions take place without complications. Occasionally, if a blood clot fails to form in the empty tooth socket, or if the blood clot is dislodged, *dry socket* (infection in the tooth socket) develops. Dislodging a clot can also cause renewed bleeding; this can be eased by placing a tightly folded handkerchief or a gauze pad on the wound and biting on it gently for about 30 minutes. If bleeding continues, suturing of the tissue around the socket may be necessary.

Extradural hemorrhage

Bleeding into the space between the inner surface of the skull and the external surface of the dura mater, the outer layer of the *meninges* (protective covering of the brain).

CAUSES AND SYMPTOMS

An extradural hemorrhage usually results from a blow to the side of the head that fractures the skull and ruptures an artery running over the surface of the dura mater. The person may momentarily lose consciousness and then apparently recover.

A hematoma (collection of clotted blood) forms and enlarges, increasing pressure within the skull and causing symptoms a few hours or even several days after the injury. The affected person develops a headache that gradually increases in severity; other symptoms include drowsiness, vomiting, seizures, and paralysis on one side of the body. He or she eventually lapses into a coma and, without treatment, may die.

DIAGNOSIS AND TREATMENT

CT scanning confirms the diagnosis. Surgical treatment consists of drilling burr holes in the skull (see *Craniotomy*), draining the blood clot, and clipping the ruptured blood vessel. If the bleeding is diagnosed early (before serious symptoms develop), the outlook is excellent; hence the importance of seeking medical advice and investigation following even a moderate blow to the head (see *Head injury*).

Extrapyramidal system

A network of nerve pathways that links nerve nuclei in the surface of the *cerebrum* (the main mass of the brain), the *basal ganglia* deep within the brain, and parts of the *brain stem*. The system influences and modifies electrical impulses that are sent from the brain to initiate movements in the skeletal muscles.

Damage or degeneration of components in the extrapyramidal system can cause a disturbance in the execution of voluntary (willed) movements and in muscle tone, and can also cause the appearance of involuntary (unwilled) tremors, jerks, or writhing movements. Such disturbances are seen in *Huntington's chorea*, *Parkinson's disease*, some types of *cerebral palsy*, and can also occur as a side effect of taking *phenothiazine drugs*.

Extrovert

A person whose interests are constantly directed outward, to other people and the environment. Extroverts are active, energetic, sociable, easy to talk to, and have many outside interests and concerns. (See also *Personality*.)

Exudation

The discharge of fluid from blood vessels into a tissue or onto the tissue's surface. An exuded fluid (called an exudate) contains cells and a large amount of protein. Most exudates are produced as a result of *inflammation*. When tissue is inflamed, its small blood vessels become wider and the tiny pores in the vessel walls become enlarged, which allows fluid and cells (mainly white blood cells) to escape.

Eye

The organ of sight. The eye consists of structures that focus an image onto the *retina* at the back of the eye and nerve cells that convert this image into electrical impulses that are carried by the *optic nerve* for interpretation by a specialized region of the brain.

The two eyes work in conjunction under the control of the brain, aligning themselves on an object so that a clear image is formed on each retina. If necessary, the eyes sharpen images by altering focus in an automatic process known as *accommodation*.

The pattern of light falling on the retina stimulates a complex flow of impulses along the optic nerves to the brain. The two optic nerves pass into the skull, meet, partially cross over, and run back, at first on the underside of the brain, and then through its substance to the visual cortex—the area of the back surface of the brain concerned with *vision*.

STRUCTURE

EYEBALL The eyeballs lie in pads of fat within the orbits, bony eye sockets that provide protection from injury. Each eyeball is moved by six delicate muscles, the action of these muscles for both eyes being coordinated by a nerve network in the brain stem.

The eyeball has a tough outer coat, the *sclera* (white of the eye). The front, circular part of the outer coat, the *cornea*, is transparent and protrudes slightly. The cornea serves as the main "lens" of the eye and performs most of the focusing. Behind the cornea is a shallow chamber full of aqueous humor (watery fluid), at the back of which is the *iris* (colored part) with its *pupil* (central hole) which appears black. Tiny muscles alter the size of the pupil with changes in light intensity to control the amount of light entering the eye.

Immediately behind the iris, and in contact with it, is the crystalline *lens*, suspended by delicate fibers from a circular muscle ring called the ciliary body. Contraction of the ciliary body alters the shape of the lens; this provides the eye with some focusing power additional to that provided by the cornea. Behind the lens is the main cavity of the eyeball, filled with a clear gel (the vitreous humor).

On the inside of the back of the eye is the retina, a complex structure of nerve tissue on which the image formed by the cornea and the crystalline lens falls. The retina requires a constant supply of oxygen and glucose. To meet this need, a thin network of blood vessels, the choroid plexus, lies immediately under it. The *choroid* is continuous at the front with the ciliary body and the iris; these three parts constitute the uveal tract.

CONJUNCTIVA The eyeball is sealed off from the outside by a flexible membrane called the *conjunctiva*, which is firmly secured around the margin of the cornea but lies freely on the sclera over the front third of the globe. It is attached to the skin at the corners of the eye and forms the inner lining of the lids, with a deep cul-de-sac above and below. This arrangement provides a permanent seal while allowing free mobility of the eyeball.

The conjunctiva contains many tiny tear-secreting and mucus-producing glands. They, along with an oily secretion from the meibomian glands in the eyelids, provide the important, three-layer tear film that must constantly cover the cornea and conjunctiva.

EYELIDS Each lid contains about 30 meibomian glands, with their openings along the lid margin just behind the roots of the lashes. The glands secrete an oil that prevents adhesion of the lid margins during sleep and forms the outer layer of the tear film—a layer that retards evaporation and helps maintain the continuity of the tear film. The blink reflex is protective and helps to spread the tear film evenly over the cornea. This is essential for clear vision. Should the tear film dry out, *corneal abrasion* is more likely.

Just under the skin of the lid is a flat but powerful muscle. Screwing up of the eye in response to danger contracts this muscle, pushing the globe back into the orbit and covering the eye with a bunched-up mass of tissue.

Eye, artificial

A prosthesis to replace an eye that has been removed. Artificial eyes, which were first seen in the 17th century, are worn for cosmetic and psychological reasons.

Often called a "glass eye," the ocular prosthesis is usually a thin, curved, hollow plastic shell. The artificial iris behind the transparent artificial cornea may be produced by hand-painting or using a photograph.

The prosthesis fits neatly behind the eyelids into the cavity from which the natural eye has been removed. Some movement of the artificial eye is achieved by attaching the eye-moving muscles to the remaining conjunctival membrane. In some cases, the eye-moving muscles may be attached to a plastic implant in the eye socket, which allows greater movement of the prosthesis.

Eye drops

Medication in solution used to treat eye disorders or to aid in diagnosis. Common examples of drugs given in this form are *antibiotic drugs, corticosteroid drugs, antihistamine drugs*, drugs to control *glaucoma* (raised pressure in the eye), and drugs used to dilate or constrict the pupil.

To use eye drops, first pull the lower lid away from the eye by using a fingertip to draw down the skin below the eye, and then allow drops to fall behind the lid. To reduce the risk of contamination, avoid touching the skin or eye with the dropper.

Eye, examination of

An inspection of the external and internal structure of the eyes either as part of a standard *vision test* or to make a diagnosis when some disorder is suspected.

ANATOMY OF THE EYE

The eye is a complex organ that focuses light rays to form an image on the retina, which then converts this image into a pattern of nerve impulses that are transmitted to the brain. The cornea and lens focus the light, the pupil controls the amount of light entering the eye, the ciliary body alters the shape of the lens to adjust the focus, and the retina contains millions of nerve cells that respond to light.

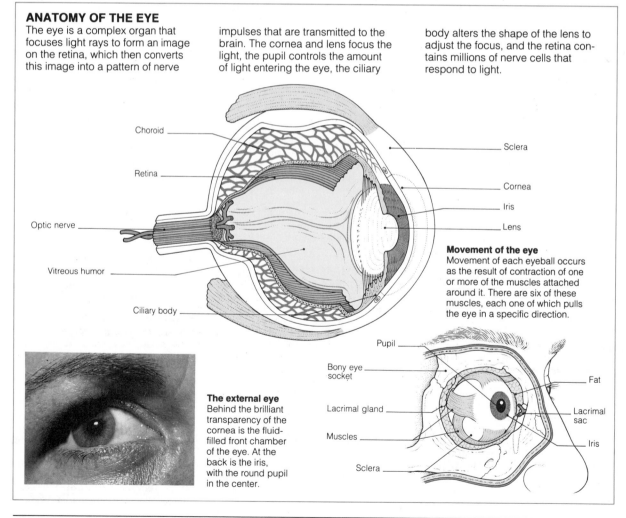

Choroid

Retina

Optic nerve

Vitreous humor

Ciliary body

Sclera

Cornea

Iris

Lens

Movement of the eye
Movement of each eyeball occurs as the result of contraction of one or more of the muscles attached around it. There are six of these muscles, each one of which pulls the eye in a specific direction.

Pupil

Bony eye socket

Lacrimal gland

Muscles

Sclera

Fat

Lacrimal sac

Iris

The external eye
Behind the brilliant transparency of the cornea is the fluid-filled front chamber of the eye. At the back is the iris, with the round pupil in the center.

CONDUCTING AN EYE EXAMINATION

During an eye examination, the ophthalmologist checks external appearance, eye movement, visual acuity, visual field, and color vision. The eyes are checked for the presence of a squint, abrasions, and ulcers. Applanation tonometry and a refraction test are also done.

View of retina through ophthalmoscope
The retina (inner back surface of the eye) is examined to assess conditions such as hypertensive *retinopathy*, as seen here.

Applanation tonometry
Measurement of the pressure within the eye is a routine test for glaucoma.

Snellen's chart
The chart is used to check visual acuity of each eye; the patient's ability to read letters of different sizes from the same distance is assessed.

WHY IT IS DONE

Eye examinations are performed to determine the cause of visual disturbance or other symptoms relating to the eye, and to assess whether or not glasses (or contact lenses) are necessary. Some serious eye disorders, such as *glaucoma*, are symptomless in the early stages and can be detected only by an eye examination.

HOW IT IS DONE

The examination begins with an inspection of the external appearance of the eyes, the lids, and the surrounding skin. A check of eye movements is usually performed. The examiner looks for *squint* and may perform a cover test, which will show if a person has a squint because a squinting eye will move to look directly at a designated object when the other eye is covered. A check of the *visual acuity* (sharpness of vision) in each eye using a *Snellen chart* (the standard eye testing wall chart) follows. Refraction testing (using lenses of different strengths) may be done to determine what glasses or contact lenses may be needed.

A test of the *visual fields* (extent of the peripheral vision) may also be performed, especially in suspected glaucoma or neurological conditions. *Color vision* may also be checked because loss of color perception is an early indication of certain disorders of the retina or optic nerve.

To check for abrasions or ulcers, the conjunctiva and cornea may be stained with *fluorescein* (an orange dye). After staining, conjunctival abrasions appear yellow; corneal abrasions or ulcers show as green areas under white light or fluoresce brilliantly under ultraviolet light.

Applanation *tonometry* (measurement of the pressure within the eye) is an essential test for glaucoma. It is done using a tonometer attached to a slit-lamp microscope.

EQUIPMENT

The *ophthalmoscope* is a an instrument used to examine the inside of the eye, especially the retina.

The slit lamp microscope, with its brilliant illumination and lens magnification, allows meticulous examination of the conjunctiva, cornea, front chamber of the eye, iris, and crystalline lens.

By means of special corneal contact lenses, the magnified view through the slit lamp microscope may be extended to include the vitreous gel behind the lens and the retina. These contact lenses incorporate mirrors to allow examination of structures at the base of the iris and the front edge of the retina. For a full view of the crystalline lens and the structures behind it, the pupil must be widely dilated with drops, such as tropicamide or cyclopentolate.

Eye, foreign body in

Any material on the surface of the eye or under the eyelid, or an object that penetrates the eyeball. Foreign bodies in the eye are very common; most are easily removed at home with a clean cloth and cause no damage.

CAUSES

Particles of dust are the most common type of foreign body in the eye. Occasionally, a fragment of metal, plastic, or wood may be deflected into the eye—for example, when a person is doing a job in the home or on a car. Rarely, an object traveling at high speed actually penetrates the eyeball—for example, a piece of metal in an industrial accident.

SYMPTOMS

A foreign body irritates the eye, causing pain, redness, increased tear production, and usually blepharospasm (uncontrollable closure and squeezing of the eyelid). These symptoms may diminish even if the foreign body remains. Occasionally, there are no symptoms, especially if the eye has been penetrated.

COMPLICATIONS

Some foreign bodies left within the eyeball may change chemically and release damaging ingredients into the substance of the eye, causing blindness. Other foreign bodies may remain whole but may cause infection that leads to blindness. Sympathetic *ophthalmia* is a rare condition that may threaten sight in the uninjured eye.

TREATMENT

Foreign bodies on or in the conjunctiva (the transparent membrane covering the white of the eye and the inside of the eyelids) may be removed at home (see *First aid* box, p. 428).

If a foreign body lies on the cornea (the transparent front part of the eyeball) or may have penetrated the eye, a physician should be consulted. He or she will examine the eye and eyelids and may insert *fluorescein* (an orange stain) into the eye to show up *corneal abrasions* or sites of penetration. If a penetrating injury is suspected, imaging techniques, such as *ultrasound scanning* or an *X ray*, may be performed.

A physician may anesthetize the surface of the eye with eye drops containing a local anesthetic, and then use a sharp spatula to remove a

E

FIRST AID: FOREIGN BODY IN THE EYE

WARNING
Never attempt to remove a particle embedded in the eyeball. Do not remove a foreign body if it is resting on the cornea.

LOWER LID

1 Wash your hands. Ask the victim to look up while you separate the lids and examine the eye.

2 First try floating an object out with water; then try lifting it out with the moistened corner of a clean cloth or folded paper.

UPPER LID

1 Grasp the lashes and carefully draw the upper lid outward and downward. If this does not dislodge the object, try floating it off by getting the victim to blink under water or follow 2 below.

2 Have the victim look down while you place a matchstick across the upper lid and fold the lid up over it. Then exchange the matchstick for a clean cloth and pick off the object.

IRRIGATION OF THE EYE

Flush continuously with running water—some corrosives penetrate deeply and take longer to wash out.

rupture of the *sclera* (white of the eye), with collapse of the eyeball and possible blindness. Lesser injuries may lead to a vitreous hemorrhage (bleeding into the space behind the lens), *hyphema* (bleeding into the front chamber of the eye), *retinal detachment*, or injury to the trabeculum (the channel through which aqueous humor drains from the eye). Hyphema affects vision until the blood is reabsorbed. Injury to the trabeculum can lead to *glaucoma*.

Injuries to the center of the cornea invariably impair vision by causing scarring. Damage to the crystalline lens may cause a *cataract* to form, with resultant loss of vision in that eye. Some injuries also damage the *retina* and the *sclera* at the back of the eye.

Eyelashes, disorders of

The eyelashes are arranged in two rows at the front edge of each lid and normally curve outward. Growth in an abnormal direction may be due to injury to the lid or, more commonly, to infection. Occasionally, lashes grow in an abnormal direction for no obvious reason. With age, the lashes become finer and fewer.

Severe *blepharitis* (inflammation of the lid margins) may cause the margins to be so damaged that lash roots are destroyed. *Trachoma*, an infection in which the lid is distorted by scarring, may lead to trichiasis, in which the lashes turn inward toward the eyeball, rub against the cornea, and cause *corneal abrasion*.

Eye, lazy

A popular term for *amblyopia*, in which normal vision has failed to develop in an otherwise healthy eye. The term is also sometimes used to refer to a convergent *squint*.

Eyelid

A fold of tissue at the upper or lower edge of an *orbit* (eye socket). The eyelids provide protection for the eye.

The eyelids are held in position by ligaments attached to the socket's bony edges. They consist of thin plates of fibrous tissue (called the tarsal plates) covered by muscle and a very thin layer of skin. The inner layer is covered by an extension of the *conjunctiva* (the transparent membrane that covers the white of the eye). Along the edge of each eyelid are two rows of eyelashes. Immediately behind are the openings of the ducts leading from the meibomian glands, which secrete the oily part of the tear film from within the tarsal plates.

foreign body from the cornea. Metallic objects that have penetrated the eye can sometimes be extracted using a powerful magnet. The eye may be covered with a patch and *antibiotic drugs* in the form of eye drops or ointment may be prescribed.

Eye injuries

Serious eye injuries may be caused either by penetration of the eye or by a blow to the eye. Often, however, the eye escapes serious injury because it is well protected by surrounding bone and by the rapid lid-squeeze reflex.

Penetrating injuries are most commonly caused by relatively small objects traveling at high speeds, such as gun pellets, small stones thrown up by rotary lawnmowers, and objects from high-speed machinery used for drilling, sawing, hammering, or grinding. Penetrating injuries can also occur from wind-shield glass in car accidents. Foreign bodies within the eye can cause serious problems (see *Eye, foreign body in*).

Blunt trauma to the eyeball, such as a blow from a stick, may cause tearing of the *iris* (colored part of the eye) or

DISORDERS OF THE EYE

Many eye disorders are minor, but some lead to serious complications unless treated. (See also *Cornea* disorders box; *Retina* disorders box.)

CONGENITAL DEFECTS

Squint (malalignment of the eyes) is sometimes congenital (present at birth). *Cataracts* (opacity of the lens of the eye) can occur in infants, when the cause may be maternal *rubella* infection early in pregnancy. Very rarely, babies are born with microphthalmos (abnormally small eye). Vision in a microphthalmic eye is usually very poor. *Nystagmus* (uncontrollable movement in the eyes) is often congenital.

Retinoblastoma is a malignant tumor of the retina that appears in early life and may occur in one or both eyes. Other congenital disorders affecting the eye include *albinism* (absence of pigment) and abnormalities of development of the cornea and retina.

INFECTION

Conjunctivitis, the most common infection, rarely affects vision. In the late stages of neglected conjunctival infection, such as *trachoma* or severe bacterial conjunctivitis, vision can be impaired.

Corneal infections are more serious and can lead to blurred vision or corneal perforation if not treated early. Endophthalmitis (infection within the eye), which may make it necessary to remove the eye surgically, can occur after a penetrating injury, after severe ulceration, (rarely) after major eye surgery, or from infections elsewhere in the body.

IMPAIRED BLOOD SUPPLY

Narrowing, blockage, inflammation, or other abnormalities of the blood vessels of the retina may cause partial or total loss of vision.

TUMORS

Malignant melanoma of the choroid (the layer of tissue between the retina and the sclera, which is the fibrous outer wall of the eyeball) is the most common primary malignant eye tumor. It can be found without symptoms during routine examinations or can cause a decrease in vision.

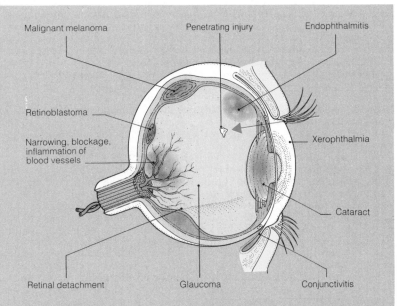

Malignant melanoma — Penetrating injury — Endophthalmitis — Retinoblastoma — Narrowing, blockage, inflammation of blood vessels — Xerophthalmia — Cataract — Retinal detachment — Glaucoma — Conjunctivitis

NUTRITIONAL DISORDERS

Various vitamin deficiencies (particularly vitamin A deficiency) can affect the eye. This may lead to *xerophthalmia* (dryness of the cornea and conjunctiva), night blindness, or, ultimately, *keratomalacia* (corneal softening and destruction).

AUTOIMMUNE DISORDERS

Uveitis (inflammation of the uveal tissues—iris, choroid, and/or ciliary body), when not caused by an infectious agent, may have an autoimmune basis (when the defense mechanisms of the body attack its own tissues). It is common in people with *ankylosing spondylitis* and *sarcoidosis*.

DEGENERATION

Macular degeneration of the retina is common in the elderly. It causes loss of fine, detailed vision, although peripheral vision remains.

Cataract is also common in the elderly; the exact cause is unknown.

OTHER DISORDERS

Glaucoma, a condition in which the pressure in the fluid maintaining the normal shape of the eye is raised, may take various forms. If untreated, glaucoma can lead to permanent loss of vision.

In *retinal detachment*, the retina lifts away from the underlying (choroidal) layer of the eye.

Ametropia is a general term that means the eye has a refractive error (an error in focusing), such as *myopia* (nearsightedness), *hypermetropia* (farsightedness), or *astigmatism*. None of these is a disease in the ordinary sense of the word; they are caused simply by variations of shape and focusing ability of the eye. *Presbyopia* is the (normal) progressive loss of accommodation (ability to focus at near range) with age. *Amblyopia* (poor vision in one eye without any obvious structural abnormality) is often due to squint.

INVESTIGATION

Because of the transparency of its structures, the eye is particularly accessible for examination, and many of the diseases affecting it can be viewed directly by use of the *ophthalmoscope* and *slit lamp*. Photography of the retina and *fluorescein* angiography are also used. (See also *Eye, examination of.*)

E

The eyelids act as protective shutters, closing practically instantaneously as a reflex action if anything approaches the eye. The eyelids also act as wipers to smear the tear film across the *cornea* (the transparent front part of the eyeball).

DISORDERS

Disorders include a *chalazion* (a swelling of a meibomian gland), *blepharitis* (inflammation of the edge of the eyelid), and a *stye* (an abscess at the root of one of the eyelashes).

The shape and position of the eyelids are abnormal in a number of disorders, including *entropion* (the eyelid margin turning inward), *ectropion* (the eyelid margin turning outward), *ptosis* (a drooping eyelid covering all or part of the eye), and baggy eyelids due to dermatochalasis (excess skin on the lid) or blepharochalasis (excess fat under the skin of the lid).

Myokymia (twitching of the eyelid) is a common phenomenon usually due to fatigue. *Blepharospasm* (tight contraction of the eyelid) is usually caused by a foreign body in the eye.

The skin of the eyelid is a common site for a *basal cell carcinoma*.

Eyelid, drooping
See *Ptosis*.

Eyelid surgery
See *Blepharoplasty*.

Eye, painful red
A very common combination of eye symptoms that may be due to any of several different eye disorders. The presence of pain and redness in one or both eyes requires examination and treatment by a physician.

Uveitis (inflammation of all or a part of the uvea) is a common cause. The dull, aching pain may be due to swelling within the front of the eye and spasm in muscles around the iris. The redness is caused by widening of blood vessels around the iris.

Another serious cause of pain and redness in one eye is acute closed-angle *glaucoma* (sudden increase in pressure within the eyeball). The pain is severe and may be accompanied by nausea, vomiting, blurred vision, and seeing haloes. There is redness of the white of the eye

Other important causes of painful red eye include *keratitis* (inflammation of the outer protective layer of the eye), usually as a result of a *corneal ulcer*, or a foreign body on the surface of the eye or under one of the eyelids (see *Eye, foreign body in*).

The most common cause of redness and severe irritation (although not strictly pain) affecting the eye is *conjunctivitis*. The redness is due to dilation (widening) of blood vessels in the conjunctiva. The irritation is similar to that caused by grit in the eye. Conjunctivitis can be due to viral or bacterial infections, irritants (such as chemicals), or allergies. Viral conjunctivitis usually eventually affects both eyes and is mildly infectious.

Eyestrain
A term often used to describe aching or discomfort in or around the eye. Eyestrain is not a medical term; the eyes cannot be damaged by being used, by wearing spectacles of the wrong strength, or by not wearing spectacles when they should be worn.

The vague aches that are commonly called eyestrain are usually a form of headache stemming from fatigue, tiredness of muscles around the eye, *sinusitis*, or mild *blepharitis* (inflammation of the eyelid margins) and *conjunctivitis*.

Eye teeth
A common name for canine *teeth*.

Eye tumors
Tumors of the eye are rare. When eye tumors do occur, they are usually malignant and painless.

TYPES AND TREATMENT

RETINOBLASTOMA This is a *congenital* malignant tumor of the retina that occurs in one or both eyes. If the central vision in one eye is affected, the child may have a squint. If the tumor is not discovered in the early stages, it may be seen as a white or yellowish mass in one pupil. Retinoblastoma may sometimes be treated by *radiation therapy*, *laser treatment*, or *cryosurgery* (freezing), but the eye may require removal to prevent spread of the tumor.

MALIGNANT MELANOMA This is a cancer of the choroid layer, under the retina. It usually affects middle-aged and elderly people and is the most common malignant eye tumor. There are no symptoms in the early stages, but the tumor eventually causes detachment·of the retina and distortion of vision. Small malignant melanomas can be destroyed by laser treatment, but removal of the eye is often advised to avoid spread of the tumor.

SECONDARY EYE TUMORS These occur when cancer in another part of the body spreads to the eye. If the secondary tumor grows behind the eyeball, it

Malignant melanoma of the eye
This shows a well-developed tumor that will cause gradual loss of vision. The amount of sight loss is often surprisingly great for the size of the growth.

may cause bulging of the eye. The effect on vision varies, depending on the location and growth rate. Secondary tumors may sometimes be controlled by radiation therapy; the primary tumor will need to be dealt with separately.

BASAL CELL CARCINOMA This is the most common tumor of the eyelid and is believed to be caused by excessive exposure to sunlight. The tumor usually has a small crusty central crater and a hard rolled edge. Although tumors of this type may grow large, they very rarely spread to other parts of the body. In the early stages, a basal cell carcinoma of the eyelid may be treated by surgery, radiation therapy, or cryosurgery. Extensive plastic surgery or removal of the eye may be necessary if the tumor becomes large.

Face-lift

A cosmetic operation to smooth out wrinkles and lift sagging skin on an aging face to make it look younger. A face-lift is usually performed as an outpatient procedure under a local anesthetic. The two sides of the face are treated during the same operation.

OUTLOOK

Some bruising of the face is common, but there is usually no pain. The stitches are removed three to five days after the operation. In most cases the scars, which fade within a year, are hidden by natural crease lines or by the hair. The effect of a face-lift usually lasts about five years.

In a few cases, satisfactory healing does not occur because of the accumulation of blood under the skin or because of infection that leads to severe scarring.

Facial nerve

The seventh *cranial nerve*. The facial nerve arises from the pons and medulla oblongata (parts of the *brain stem*) and sends branches to the face, neck, salivary glands, and outer ear.

LOCATION OF THE FACIAL NERVE
Arising from the brain stem, the facial nerve has branches that connect to the outer ear, tongue, salivary glands, and muscles of the neck and face.

Brain
Facial nerve
Salivary glands

FACE-LIFT

A face-lift is really a skin-lift operation. Its effects are not always permanent. There is some discomfort after a face-lift and the cosmetic effects are not immediately apparent. Care should be taken in choosing a highly reputable surgeon.

Skin removed

Line of incision

Before and after treatment
The results of most face-lifts are excellent. However, it should be realized that the outcome may not be exactly as expected, and there is always some risk associated with any operation.

How it is done
An incision is made where shown. The skin is undercut as far as the crease running from the nose to the corner of the mouth. It is then pulled upward and backward, and its margins are sewn near the hairline.

The facial nerve performs both motor and sensory functions. It controls the muscles of the neck and of facial expression (including muscles in the forehead); it also stimulates secretion by the submandibular and sublingual salivary glands. In addition, the facial nerve conveys taste sensations from the front two thirds of the tongue and carries sensations from the outer ear.

Damage to the facial nerve causes weakness of the facial muscles (see *Facial palsy*) and, in some cases, loss of taste. Such damage is most commonly due to a viral infection. It may also be a feature of a *stroke*; more rarely, damage to the facial nerve may occur as a result of surgery (typically for a tumor) on the parotid gland (one of the salivary glands) or on the ear.

Facial pain

Pain in the face may be due to a variety of causes or may occur for no known reason. In some cases, the cause of pain affects the face directly. In others, a disorder elsewhere in the body results in *referred pain* in the face.

CAUSES

Injury to the face, such as by blows or cuts, is a common cause of facial pain.

Facial pain is also commonly due to infection. *Sinusitis* (inflammation of the air spaces in the facial bones) can cause pain around the eyes and in the cheek bones. The onset of *mumps* can cause pain in the cheeks before any swelling appears in front of and/or below the ears. Pain from a *boil* in the nose or ear may also be felt in the face.

Problems relating to the teeth and jaws are another common cause of facial pain. Pain may be due to dental caries (see *Caries, dental*) or to a tooth abscess (see *Abscess, dental*). In a baby, *teething* can be a painful process. In an adult, facial pain may be due to impacted wisdom teeth (see *Impaction, dental*) or possibly partial dislocation of the jaw (see *Jaw, dislocated*).

Damage to a nerve that supplies the face can result in severe pain. Examples include the knifelike pain that precedes the one-sided rash in *herpes zoster* (shingles), and the intermittent shooting pain of *trigeminal neuralgia* (tic douloureux), which usually affects only one side of the face and is often brought on by touching the face or chewing.

The referral of pain to the face occurs in several disorders. In *angina pectoris* (pain in the chest due to lack of oxygen to the heart), pain may be felt in the jaw. With *migraine* headaches, pain may occur on one side of the face. When facial pain occurs for no reason, it may be a symptom of *depression*.

TREATMENT

Analgesic drugs (painkillers) can provide temporary relief. If facial pain is severe or persistent, however, a physician or dentist should be consulted.

F

Facial palsy

Weakness of the facial muscles due to inflammation of or damage to the *facial nerve*. The condition is usually temporary and affects only one side of the face.

CAUSES

Facial palsy is most commonly due to Bell's palsy (named after the Scots surgeon Sir Charles Bell), which occurs for no known reason.

Less commonly, facial palsy is associated with *herpes zoster* (shingles) affecting the ear and facial nerve. Facial palsy may also result from accidental or surgical damage to the facial nerve, or from compression of the nerve by a tumor (e.g., by an *acoustic neuroma* affecting the auditory nerve).

SYMPTOMS

Facial palsy usually comes on suddenly. The eyelid and corner of the mouth droop on one side of the face and there may be pain in the ear on that side. It may be impossible to wrinkle the brow or to close the eye, and smiling is distorted. Depending on which branches of the nerve are affected, taste may be impaired or sounds may seem unnaturally loud.

TREATMENT

Facial palsy often clears up without treatment. Taking *analgesic drugs* may help relieve pain, and exercising the facial muscles may facilitate recovery. In some cases, it may be necessary to tape the eyelid shut at bedtime to avoid *corneal abrasion*.

Bell's palsy is sometimes treated with *corticosteroid drugs* or *ACTH* to reduce inflammation of the facial nerve. Electrostimulation of the nerve is of unproved value. Surgical decompression of the facial nerve is of dubious value in persistent cases of Bell's palsy, but re-routing or grafting of nerve tissue may help people with palsies due to injury or tumor.

Facial spasm

An uncommon disorder in which there is frequent twitching of facial muscles supplied by the *facial nerve*. (This condition is often called a tic, but, in fact, tic is a general term that can refer to spasmodic twitching in any part of the body.) The disorder, which affects mainly middle-aged women, is of unknown cause.

Facies

A medical term for the appearance of the face, as in *adenoid* facies: the dull, open-mouthed expression seen in many children whose nasal passages are blocked due to enlarged adenoids.

Factitious disorders

A group of disorders in which a patient's symptoms mimic those of a true illness but which have in fact been invented by, and are under the control of, the patient. There is no apparent cause other than a wish to receive attention.

The most common type of factitious disorder is *Munchausen's syndrome*, which is characterized by real physical symptoms. In a second form, called *Ganser's syndrome*, there are psychological symptoms.

These disorders differ from *malingering*, in which the person claims to be ill for a particular purpose, such as obtaining time off work or claiming compensation.

Factor VIII

One of the blood proteins (coagulation factors) that take part in the "coagulation cascade"—an important process in *blood clotting*. Some people with the inherited condition *hemophilia* have a reduced level of factor VIII in their blood and, consequently, have a tendency to abnormal bleeding and to prolonged bleeding when injured.

Freeze-dried concentrates of factor VIII are given to hemophiliacs by regular intravenous injection, which reduces the bleeding tendency and improves the quality of life. Some hemophiliacs administer the treatment themselves at home.

Fahrenheit scale

A temperature scale in which the melting point of ice is 32° and the boiling point of water is 212°. On this scale, normal body temperature is 98.6°F (37°C). The scale is named after the German physicist Gabriel Fahrenheit. (See also *Celsius scale*.)

Failure to thrive

Failure of expected growth in an infant or toddler, usually assessed by comparing the rate at which a baby gains weight with a standardized growth chart.

Undernourishment may be due to some problem at home, e.g., an unsatisfactory relationship between parent and child. In some cases, the child is actually neglected. Deprived children often have delayed emotional and intellectual development as well as failure to grow.

If a baby fails to gain weight despite receiving an adequate diet and having a stable family background, other conditions may be responsible. Failure to thrive can suggest a serious physical disorder, such as congenital *heart disease*, *kidney failure*, or *malabsorption*.

A baby who fails to thrive is often observed (along with the parent) for a week or two to see how the parent feeds and handles the baby. The baby's diet and weight are carefully monitored. If there are social problems, support for the family can be initiated. (See also *Short stature*.)

Fainting

Temporary loss of consciousness due to insufficient oxygen reaching the brain. The medical term for fainting is syncope.

FIRST AID: FAINTING

1 Anyone who feels faint should sit down and lean forward, head between the knees.

2 If a fainting victim is unconscious and breathing normally, lay the person down and raise his or her legs above chest level.

CAUSES

Fainting often occurs as result of a vasovagal attack, in which overstimulation of the *vagus nerve* causes slowing of the heartbeat and a fall in blood pressure, so reducing the flow of blood to the brain. This type of fainting is usually preceded by sweating, nausea, dizziness, ringing in the ears, dimmed vision, and weakness. Vasovagal attacks are commonly caused by pain, stress, shock, fear, or by being in a stuffy atmosphere that has little oxygen. Other causes include prolonged coughing, straining to defecate or urinate, or blowing an instrument, particularly the trumpet. Fainting is often attributed to a vasovagal attack in cases where no other cause can be determined.

Fainting may also result from postural *hypotension*, in which pooling of blood in the veins of the legs reduces the amount available for the heart to pump to the brain, with a resultant drop in blood pressure. This may occur when a person stands still for a long time, or suddenly stands up. Postural hypotension is common in the elderly, in sufferers from *diabetes mellitus*, and in people taking *antihypertensive drugs* or *vasodilator drugs*.

In some people, episodes of fainting may be associated with temporary difficulty in speaking or weakness in the limbs; this may indicate a disorder called *vertebrobasilar insufficiency*, in which there is an obstruction to the blood flow in vessels that pass through the neck to the brain. This is one form of *transient ischemic attack*.

Fainting may be a symptom of *Stokes-Adams syndrome*, in which blood flow to the brain is temporarily inadequate due to cardiac *arrhythmia* (irregularity of the heartbeat), usually associated with a form of *heart block* (interruption of electrical impulses in the heart).

PREVENTION

A person who experiences warning signs of a faint can sometimes avoid fainting by putting his or her head between the knees or by lying flat on his or her back with the legs raised.

TREATMENT

Recovery from fainting takes place when normal blood flow to the brain is restored. This usually happens within a couple of minutes because falling to the ground places the head at the same level as the heart. To ensure another attack does not occur, the person should remain lying down for 10 to 15 minutes after regaining consciousness.

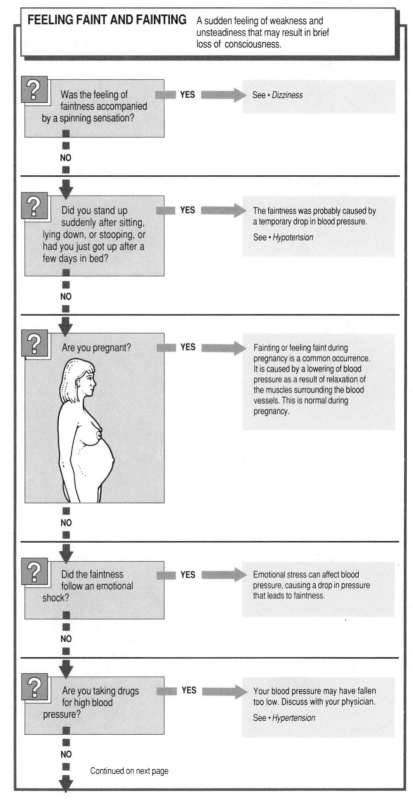

FEELING FAINT AND FAINTING   A sudden feeling of weakness and unsteadiness that may result in brief loss of consciousness.

Was the feeling of faintness accompanied by a spinning sensation? **YES** → See • *Dizziness*

NO

Did you stand up suddenly after sitting, lying down, or stooping, or had you just got up after a few days in bed? **YES** → The faintness was probably caused by a temporary drop in blood pressure.
See • *Hypotension*

NO

Are you pregnant? **YES** → Fainting or feeling faint during pregnancy is a common occurrence. It is caused by a lowering of blood pressure as a result of relaxation of the muscles surrounding the blood vessels. This is normal during pregnancy.

NO

Did the faintness follow an emotional shock? **YES** → Emotional stress can affect blood pressure, causing a drop in pressure that leads to faintness.

NO

Are you taking drugs for high blood pressure? **YES** → Your blood pressure may have fallen too low. Discuss with your physician.
See • *Hypertension*

NO

Continued on next page

F

433

F

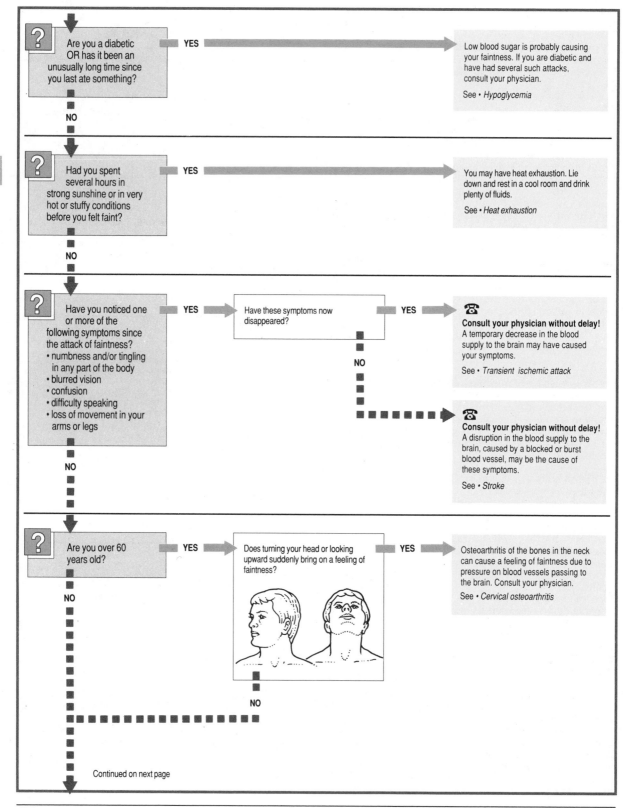

Are you a diabetic OR has it been an unusually long time since you last ate something?

YES → Low blood sugar is probably causing your faintness. If you are diabetic and have had several such attacks, consult your physician.

See • *Hypoglycemia*

NO ↓

Had you spent several hours in strong sunshine or in very hot or stuffy conditions before you felt faint?

YES → You may have heat exhaustion. Lie down and rest in a cool room and drink plenty of fluids.

See • *Heat exhaustion*

NO ↓

Have you noticed one or more of the following symptoms since the attack of faintness?
• numbness and/or tingling in any part of the body
• blurred vision
• confusion
• difficulty speaking
• loss of movement in your arms or legs

YES → Have these symptoms now disappeared?

YES → ☎ **Consult your physician without delay!** A temporary decrease in the blood supply to the brain may have caused your symptoms.

See • *Transient ischemic attack*

NO →

☎ **Consult your physician without delay!** A disruption in the blood supply to the brain, caused by a blocked or burst blood vessel, may be the cause of these symptoms.

See • *Stroke*

NO ↓

Are you over 60 years old?

YES → Does turning your head or looking upward suddenly bring on a feeling of faintness?

YES → Osteoarthritis of the bones in the neck can cause a feeling of faintness due to pressure on blood vessels passing to the brain. Consult your physician.

See • *Cervical osteoarthritis*

NO ↓

NO ↓

Continued on next page

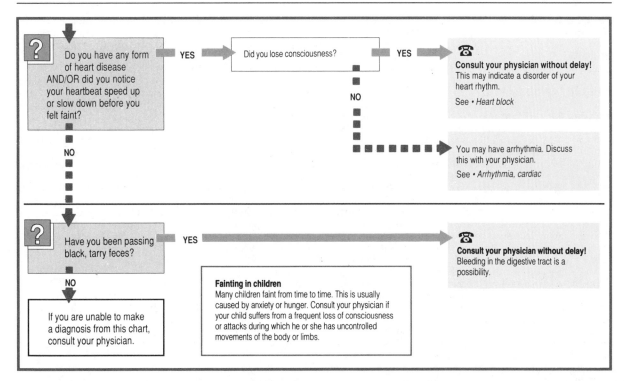

? Do you have any form of heart disease AND/OR did you notice your heartbeat speed up or slow down before you felt faint?

YES → Did you lose consciousness? **YES** →

☎ **Consult your physician without delay!** This may indicate a disorder of your heart rhythm.

See • *Heart block*

NO

You may have arrhythmia. Discuss this with your physician.

See • *Arrhythmia, cardiac*

NO

? Have you been passing black, tarry feces?

YES →

☎ **Consult your physician without delay!** Bleeding in the digestive tract is a possibility.

NO

If you are unable to make a diagnosis from this chart, consult your physician.

Fainting in children
Many children faint from time to time. This is usually caused by anxiety or hunger. Consult your physician if your child suffers from a frequent loss of consciousness or attacks during which he or she has uncontrolled movements of the body or limbs.

F

If a person fails to regain consciousness within a minute or two of fainting, medical help should be obtained promptly and appropriate first aid given (see *Unconsciousness*) until help arrives. Repeated attacks require investigation by a physician.

Faith healing

The supposed ability of certain people to cure disease by their possession of a healing force inexplicable to science. The healer usually transmits this supposed force to the sufferer by direct contact, placing his or her hands on the body ("the laying on of hands"). Often the healer and patient have a deep religious faith and believe the force to be divine. In other cases, no religious faith is involved—only a firm belief in the powers of the healer.

Cures by faith healing have on occasion been demonstrated to the satisfaction of medical observers. However, people who turn to faith healing rather than to orthodox medicine may deprive themselves of the possibility of receiving effective treatment for their condition.

Fallen arches

A cause of *flatfeet*, which can develop as a result of weakness of the muscles that support the arches of the foot. Exercises and arch supports may help.

Fallopian tube

The tube that extends from the *uterus* to the *ovary*. The fallopian tube transports eggs and sperm and is where *fertilization* takes place.

STRUCTURE
The funnel-shaped tube is about 7.5 cm long. The narrow end opens into the uterus and the free, expanded end, divided into fimbriae (fingerlike projections), lies close to the ovary. Its muscular wall is lined by cells with cilia (hairlike projections).

FUNCTION
The fimbriae sweep up the egg after it is expelled from the ovary. The beating cilia and waves of muscular contractions propel the egg toward the uterus. After intercourse, sperm swim up the fallopian tube from the uterus. The lining of the tube and its secretions sustain the egg and sperm, encouraging fertilization, and nourish the egg until it reaches the uterus.

DISORDERS
Salpingitis is inflammation of the fallopian tube, usually following bacterial infection. It accounts for almost 15 percent of cases of *infertility*.

Ectopic pregnancy (development of an embryo outside the uterus) most commonly occurs in the fallopian tube. A delay in the passage of the fertilized egg along the tube results in implantation within the tube wall, which is too thin to sustain growth. As the pregnancy progresses, the fallopian tube may rupture and cause internal bleeding.

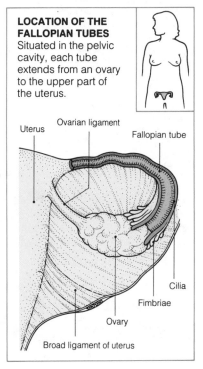

LOCATION OF THE FALLOPIAN TUBES
Situated in the pelvic cavity, each tube extends from an ovary to the upper part of the uterus.

Uterus
Ovarian ligament
Fallopian tube
Cilia
Fimbriae
Ovary
Broad ligament of uterus

Fallot's tetralogy
See *Tetralogy of Fallot.*

Fallout
See *Radiation hazards.*

Falls in the elderly
Falls are frequent in the elderly, and are by far the leading cause of accidental injury and death in those aged 65 and over. Although most falls are not fatal, they are a major source of disability in this group; about 2.5 percent of Canada's elderly population is hospitalized each year as the result of a fall.

CAUSES
Reflex actions in the elderly are much slower than in younger people, and an elderly person who trips or stumbles is often too slow to prevent a fall.

An elderly person may fall either as a result of an accident, commonly caused by a hazard in the home (see illustrated box), or as a result of a medical problem. Medical causes include poor sight, *walking* disorders, cardiac *arrhythmias* (heartbeat irregularities), *hypotension* (reduced blood pressure), *dizziness* for various reasons, *Parkinson's disease*, and the action of various drugs, including *alcohol*, *sleeping drugs*, and *tranquilizer drugs*. Falls

sometimes herald the onset of a serious illness, such as *pneumonia*, or *myocardial infarction* (heart attack).

COMPLICATIONS
Fractures of the hip are a serious complication of falls in the elderly, especially in women. Not only do women have more falls, they are also more likely to suffer from fractures because their bone strength is reduced as a result of the calcium loss that ordinarily follows the menopause (see *Osteoporosis*).

Falls may sometimes have serious indirect consequences in elderly people. The outlook is particularly grave for those who fall and lie on the floor for more than an hour, particularly if it is cold. This may lead to *hypothermia* (low body temperature) or pneumonia.

A serious fall or fear of such a fall, and the helplessness and dependence it could bring, can have adverse psychological effects on an elderly person, sometimes causing a previously active person to become demoralized and housebound.

ACTION AFTER A FALL
Immediate medical help should be obtained if a person is found unconscious, is in severe pain, is bleeding profusely, is burned, has suspected

broken bones, or is showing signs of *shock*. Appropriate first-aid measures should be carried out while awaiting medical help.

PREVENTION
Several simple measures can be taken to guard against falls: ensure that handles in bathrooms and on stairs are secure, good lighting is available, suitable footwear is worn, floor coverings and wiring are safe, and that there is minimal clutter on the floor. Elderly people who live alone can arrange for an alarm system to be installed or for a regular visit by a neighbor. It may also be worthwhile to teach the elderly person a number of techniques for getting up from the floor after a fall.

False teeth
See *Denture.*

Familial
A term applied to a characteristic or disorder that runs in families (that is, it occurs in more members of a particular family than would be expected from the occurrence in the population as a whole). An example of a familial characteristic is male-pattern baldness (see *Alopecia*); an example of a familial disorder is *hyperlipidemia* (abnormally high levels of fat in the blood).

PREVENTING FALLS
Half of all falls are accidental, caused by hazards in the home such as poor lighting, worn carpets, rickety handrails, trailing cords, loose rugs and mats, ill-fitting shoes, and inaccessible cupboards. Snow and ice on paths outside are also a major hazard. The illustration shows some of the main hazards in a typical living room, and ways to remedy them.

Worn areas of carpet
Make safe by tacking down loose edges.

Trailing cords
Secure to a wall or molding.

Loose rugs and mats
All should have nonslip backing; they should never be used to cover a slippery floor.

Uncovered floor areas
Do not polish to a slippery finish. Carpet edges should be firmly fixed to the floor.

Furniture with protruding legs
Do not place in frequently used areas of a room.

Shoes and other clutter
Floors should be free of all clutter.

Familial Mediterranean fever

An inherited condition that affects certain Sephardic Jewish, Armenian, and Arab families. Its cause is unknown. Symptoms usually begin between the ages of 5 and 15 years. The main symptoms are recurrent episodes of fever, abdominal pain, arthritis, and chest pain. Red skin swellings sometimes occur, and affected people may also suffer psychiatric problems.

Attacks usually last from 24 to 48 hours, but may last longer. Between attacks there are usually no symptoms. There is no specific treatment, but known sufferers are able to reduce the incidence of attacks by taking *colchicine*, a drug usually used to treat gout. Death may eventually occur from *amyloidosis*, which is a complication of the condition.

Family medicine

Family medicine refers to the professional services provided by family physicians, who offer continuous and comprehensive care to people of all ages in the office, the patient's home, in clinics, and in hospitals. Such care includes consideration of the health needs of the family as a unit, work with community groups, provision of preventive services, and referral to specialists when indicated.

To obtain certification by the College of Family Physicians of Canada, medical school graduates must undergo two further years of training (see *Resident physician*), or qualify by meeting specified standards of practice and passing a special examination set by the college.

About 50 percent of practicing physicians in Canada are family physicians or general practitioners. Most people seeking medical or surgical treatment make their first contact with the health care system through family or general practitioners.

Family planning

The deliberate limitation or spacing of births. In most developed countries, strategies for family planning include the different methods of *contraception*, and elective abortion (see *Abortion, induced*).

Decisions concerning family planning are usually made on an individual basis, taking social and economic factors into account, but some governments have used financial incentives or penalties in an attempt to influence individual decisions. Most nations have discouraged large families. (See also *Birth control*.)

Family therapy

Treatment of the family as a whole rather than treatment of one or more family members on an individual basis. Family therapy is based on the belief that a troubled person should not be seen in isolation from the family unit. For example, some therapists believe that the conditions of disturbed children may merely reflect parental conflicts. This approach has become popular in recent years for dealing with the problems of children and adolescents.

Usually the therapist arranges regular meetings with the family to find out what feelings lie behind the way parents and children deal with each other. Through discussion and confrontation, these feelings can gradually be changed, leading to greater harmony and understanding.

Famotidine

A recently released *ulcer-healing drug* related to the *antihistamine drugs*. Famotidine reduces the secretion of acid in the stomach and, by doing so, promotes healing of *peptic ulcers* and reduces *esophagitis* (inflammation of the esophagus).

Fanconi's anemia

A rare type of aplastic *anemia*, characterized by severely reduced production of all types of blood cells by the bone marrow.

Fanconi's syndrome

A rare kidney disorder, occurring mainly in childhood, in which various important nutrients and chemicals, such as amino acids, phosphate, calcium, and potassium, are lost in the urine; this leads to failure to thrive, stunting of growth, and bone disorders such as *rickets*.

Fanconi's syndrome has a wide variety of possible causes, including a number of rare inherited abnormalities of body chemistry; it may also occur as a side effect of some drugs, such as out-of-date *tetracycline*. In some cases there is no obvious immediate cause.

The child may resume normal growth if an underlying chemical abnormality can be corrected. Alternatively, he or she may benefit from a *kidney transplant*. In some cases, neither of these measures is possible or beneficial and kidney function progressively worsens, leading to death in childhood or early adolescence. Fanconi's syndrome in adults has a much brighter outlook.

Fantasy

The process of imagining events or objects that are not actually occurring or present. The term also refers to the mental image itself. Fantasy can give the illusion that wishes have been met. In this sense, it provides satisfaction and can be a means of helping people to cope when reality becomes too unpleasant. Fantasy can also stimulate creative ideas and activities by presenting mental images in new combinations.

Psychoanalysts believe that some fantasies are unconscious and represent certain primitive instincts; these fantasies are always presented to the conscious mind in symbols. For example, the fantasy of returning to the womb might be represented by the image of a cave.

Farmer's lung

 An occupational disease affecting the lungs of farm workers. Farmer's lung is a type of allergic *alveolitis*, in which affected people develop *hypersensitivity* (an excessive allergic reaction) to certain molds or fungi that grow on hay, grain, or straw. The causative organisms thrive in warm, damp conditions, and outbreaks are most common in areas of high rainfall.

SYMPTOMS
Typical symptoms develop about six hours after exposure to dust containing fungal spores. The symptoms may include shortness of breath and flu-like symptoms of fever, headache, and muscle aches. In single acute attacks, the symptoms persist for about a day. Repeated exposure to the molds or fungi that provoked the attack may lead to a chronic form of the disease, causing permanent scarring of lung tissues.

DIAGNOSIS AND TREATMENT
The physician takes a full occupational history and listens through a stethoscope for abnormal sounds in the chest. A *chest X ray* may show abnormalities; *pulmonary function tests* show that the efficiency of the lungs is reduced. Blood tests for specific *antibodies* indicate exposure to the fungus.

The sufferer should avoid further exposure to moldy hay or grain; if symptoms persist, *corticosteroid drugs* may be prescribed. Complete recovery can be expected if the disease is diagnosed before permanent lung damage has occurred.

PREVENTION
Farmers can reduce their own and their workers' chances of developing

the condition by reducing the water content of hay and grain before storage and by ensuring that storage conditions are cool and dry (to discourage growth of fungi). Well ventilated work areas help prevent a buildup of fungal spores in the air; wearing protective masks when handling hay, straw, or grain may also help.

Farsightedness

See *Hyperopia*.

Fascia

Fibrous *connective tissue* that surrounds many structures in the body. One layer of the tissue, known as the superficial fascia, envelops the entire body just beneath the skin. Another layer, the deep fascia, encloses muscles, forming a sheath for individual muscles and separating them into groups. The deep fascia also holds in place soft organs, such as the kidneys. Thick fascia in the palm of the hand and sole of the foot have a cushioning, protective function.

Fasciculation

Spontaneous, irregular, and usually continual contractions of a muscle apparently at rest. Unlike the contractions of *fibrillation*, fasciculation is visible under the skin and is described as fine or coarse.

A minor degree of fasciculation is quite common and by and large is no cause for concern. However, persistent fasciculation with weakness in the affected muscle indicates damage to (or possibly disease of) nerve cells in the spine that control the muscle or nerve fibers that connect the spinal nerves to the muscle; *motoneuron disease* is one such disorder.

Fasciitis

Inflammation of a layer of *fascia* (fibrous connective tissue), causing pain and tenderness. Fasciitis is usually the result of straining or injuring the fascia surrounding a muscle; it most commonly affects the sole of the patient's foot (a condition often called plantar fasciitis). Fasciitis may occur in people who suffer from *ankylosing spondylitis* (a rheumatic disorder of the spine) or *Reiter's syndrome* (inflammation of the urethra, conjunctivitis and arthritis).

Treatment consists of resting the affected area and protecting it from pressure (e.g., by wearing cushioned pads in the shoes if the foot is affected). In some cases, injections of *corticosteroid drugs* are given.

Fasciotomy

An operation to relieve pressure on muscles by making an incision in the fascia (fibrous connective tissue) that surrounds them.

WHY IT IS DONE

Fasciotomy is usually performed to treat *compartment syndrome*, a painful condition in which constriction of a group of muscles causes obstruction of blood flow. The condition can result in damage to, or even the death of, affected muscles. Fasciotomy gives the muscles space in which to expand.

The operation is also sometimes performed as a surgical emergency after an injury has caused muscle swelling or bleeding within a muscle compartment.

HOW IT IS DONE

Fasciotomy is performed under a general anesthetic. An incision is made in the skin over the affected muscle group and then in the underlying fascia to allow the muscles to bulge through. Nonemergency fasciotomy usually requires only a small incision; in an emergency procedure, a much larger incision may be needed. Once the muscles have expanded through the opening, the wound is sewn up. In some cases, the muscles bulge out so much that a *skin graft* is required to repair the incision.

Fasting

Abstaining from all food and drinking only water. In temperate conditions and at moderate levels of physical activity, a person can survive on water alone for more than two months; without food or drink, death usually occurs within about 10 days (survival times are shorter in hot or cold conditions and if activity levels are high).

EFFECTS ON THE BODY

Without food, the energy needed to maintain essential body processes is supplied by substances stored in the body tissues.

About six hours after the last meal, the body starts to use glycogen (a carbohydrate stored in the liver and muscles). This continues for about 24 hours, after which the body adapts to obtaining energy from stored fat and from protein obtained from the breakdown of muscles.

After a few days, most energy is obtained from fat, although some continues to come from muscle breakdown. If fasting continues, the body's *metabolism* slows to conserve energy. As a result of this slowdown, the fat and protein from muscles are consumed more slowly.

In the initial stages of fasting, weight loss is rapid. Later it slows, not only because metabolism slows down, but also because the body starts to conserve its salt supply, which causes water retention. Water that would normally be excreted in the urine is absorbed by the tissues. The accumulated fluid causes edema (swelling), mainly affecting the legs and abdomen.

In prolonged fasting, the ability to digest food may be impaired or lost entirely because the stomach gradually stops secreting digestive juices. If this occurs, medical supervision may be necessary when eating resumes. Prolonged fasting also halts the production of sex hormones, causing *amenorrhea* (absence of periods) in women. The body's ability to fight infection deteriorates, and either this or degeneration of the heart muscle may lead to death.

FASTING TO REDUCE WEIGHT

Omitting a main meal each day for a limited period, or occasionally not eating anything for up to 24 hours, may be an effective means of losing weight. However, nobody should go without food for more than 24 hours without consulting a physician. (See also *Weight reduction*.)

Fatigue

See *Tiredness*.

Fats and oils

Nutrients that provide the body with its most concentrated form of *energy*; 1 g of fat provides 9 calories whereas 1 g of carbohydrate produces only 4 calories.

Fats, also called lipids, are compounds containing chains of carbon and hydrogen with very little oxygen. Chemically, fats consist mostly of *fatty acids* combined with *glycerol*. They are divided into two main groups, saturated and unsaturated, depending on the proportion of hydrogen atoms. If the fatty acids contain the maximum quantity possible of hydrogen, they are said to be saturated. If there are some sites on the carbon chain unoccupied by hydrogen, they are unsaturated; when many sites are vacant, they are polyunsaturated. Monounsaturated fats are unsaturated fats with one double bond. Animal fats, such as those found in meat and dairy products, are largely saturated, while vegetable fats tend to be unsaturated to varying degrees.

Fats and oils differ in their consistency: fats are usually solid at room temperature but liquefy when heated; oils are usually liquid at ordinary room temperature.

TYPES

Some dietary fats are sources of the fat-soluble vitamins A, D, E, and K and of essential fatty acids. They are mainly triglycerides (combinations of glycerol and three fatty acids) but also comprise other types of fats. Sources in the diet include not only the visible fats (such as butter, margarine, and vegetable oils) but also the so-called invisible fats found in meat, fish, poultry, and dairy products. The oils of certain cold-water ocean fish may protect against *coronary artery disease*.

Structural fats include triglycerides, phospholipids, and sterols. Triglycerides are the main form of fat found in stores of body fat (adipose tissue). These stores act as an energy reserve as well as providing insulation and a protective layer for delicate organs. Phospholipids are structural fats found in cell membranes. Sterols, such as *cholesterol*, are found in animal and plant tissues; they have a variety of functions, often being converted by chemical actions into hormones or vitamins. Phospholipids and sterols are made in the body from the diet and are not essential in the diet.

FAT METABOLISM

Dietary fats are first emulsified by the action of bile salts and then broken down into fatty acids and glycerol by lipase, a pancreatic enzyme. They are absorbed via the lymphatic system before entering the bloodstream.

The lipids are carried in the blood bound to a protein, when they become known as lipoproteins. There are actually four classes of lipoprotein—chylomicrons, very low-density lipoproteins (VLDLs), high-density lipoproteins (HDLs), and low-density lipoproteins (LDLs). LDLs and VLDLs contain large amounts of cholesterol, which they carry through the bloodstream and deposit in cells. The HDLs pick up cholesterol and carry it back to the liver for processing and excretion. (See also *Nutrition*.)

Fatty acids

Organic acids, containing carbon, hydrogen, and oxygen, that are constituents of *fats and oils*. There are more than 40 different fatty acids found in nature, distinguished by their constituent number of carbon and hydrogen atoms.

Certain fatty acids cannot be synthesized by the body and must be provided by the diet. These fatty acids are linoleic, linolenic, and arachidonic acids, sometimes referred to collectively as the essential fatty acids and at one time called vitamin F. Strictly speaking, only linoleic acid is essential, since the body can make the other two from linoleic acid obtained from food. (See also *Nutrition*.)

Favism

A disorder characterized by an extreme sensitivity to the broad bean VICIA FABA (fava). If an affected person eats these beans, a chemical in the bean causes rapid destruction of his or her red blood cells, leading to a severe type of anemia (see *Anemia, hemolytic*). Favism is uncommon except in some areas of the Mediterranean, especially lowland Greece, where up to 10 percent of the population is affected. Favism is an inherited condition caused by a sex-linked *genetic disorder*. Affected people have a defect in a chemical pathway within their red blood cells that helps to protect the cells from injury. This defect is called *G6PD deficiency* (glucose-6-phosphate dehydrogenase deficiency).

Children in any family with a history of favism should be screened for the condition at an early age. If the disorder is found, they must avoid broad beans and certain drugs (including some *antimalarial drugs* and *antibiotic drugs*) that can have a similar destructive effect on their red blood cells. A list of drugs to avoid can be obtained from a physician when the disorder is diagnosed. With these precautions, affected people are able to remain in good health.

Febrile

Feverish or related to *fever*, as in febrile *convulsions* which occur mainly in young children who have high temperatures.

Fecal impaction

A condition in which a large mass of hard *feces* cannot be evacuated from the rectum. It is usually associated with long-standing *constipation* and dehydrated feces. Fecal impaction is most common in very young children and in the elderly, especially those who are bedridden.

The main symptoms are an intense desire to pass a bowel movement, pain in the rectum, anus, and center of the abdomen and, in some cases, watery feces (which may be mistaken for diarrhea) that are passed around the impacted mass.

To diagnose the condition, the physician inserts a gloved finger into the rectum. Treatment is with *enemas* or, if these are ineffective, by manual removal of the fecal mass.

Fecalith

A small, hard, almost stonelike piece of impacted feces which occasionally forms in a *diverticulum* (a pouch or sac, usually in the large intestine). A fecalith is harmless unless it blocks the entrance to the appendix, causing *appendicitis*, or a diverticulum, causing *diverticulitis*.

Feces

Waste material from the digestive tract that is expelled through the anus. Solidified in the large intestine, feces consist of indigestible food residue (roughage, or dietary *fiber*), dead bacteria (which may account for as much as half the weight of the feces), dead cells shed from the intestinal lining, secretions from the intestine (such as mucus), bile from the liver (which colors the feces brown), and water.

Examination of the feces—for color, odor, consistency, or the presence of blood, pus, fat, parasites, or unusual microorganisms—is important in the diagnosis of digestive tract disorders. (See also *Feces, abnormal*.)

Feces, abnormal

Feces that differ from normal in color, odor, consistency, or content. The changes may be the result of a harmless condition, but in some cases are due to a disorder of the *digestive system* or to a disorder of a related organ, such as the *liver*.

Diarrhea (frequent passage of liquid or very loose feces) may be due simply to anxiety or may be caused by an intestinal infection (see *Gastroenteritis*); by an intestinal disorder such as *ulcerative colitis* or *Crohn's disease*; or by *irritable bowel syndrome*. Loose stools may also indicate *malabsorption*.

Constipation (infrequent passage of very hard feces) is usually harmless but may be a symptom of a disorder of the large intestine.

Pale feces may be due to diarrhea, to a lack of bile in the intestine as a result of *bile duct obstruction*, or to a disease that causes malabsorption (such as *celiac disease*). In malabsorption, the paleness of the feces is due to the high fat content. Such feces may be oily, frothy, foul-smelling, and difficult to flush away.

Dark feces may simply be the result of unusually large amounts of iron or red wine in the diet. However, if feces are black, there may be bleeding in the stomach, duodenum, small intestine, or cecum.

Slimy feces, which contain excessive mucus, may occur for no significant reason, but are sometimes associated with constipation or irritable bowel syndrome. *Enteritis*, *dysentery*, or a tumor (see *Intestine, tumors of*) may also cause slimy feces.

Blood in the feces differs in appearance according to the site of bleeding. Blood that originates in the stomach or duodenum is usually passed in the form of black, tarry feces. Blood due to a disease of the colon, such as ulcerative colitis or a tumor, is red and is usually passed at the same time as the feces. Blood originating in the rectum or anus, which may be due to tumors or to *hemorrhoids* (piles), is usually bright red; the blood often streaks the feces but may be visible only on toilet paper or may drip into the toilet bowl.

INVESTIGATION

Severe or persistent abnormality of the feces should be reported to a physician. The physician may ask for a sample of feces, may perform a *rectal examination*, or may arrange for other tests depending on the suspected diagnosis. (See also *Rectal bleeding*.)

Feces, blood in the

See *Feces, abnormal*; *Rectal bleeding*.

Feeding, artificial

Administration of nutrients other than by mouth, usually through a tube inserted into the stomach or small intestine. Occasionally, a tube is inserted directly into the stomach or jejunum (upper part of the small intestine) by surgical means. This is called enteral nutrition. If the gastrointestinal tract is not functioning, food must be introduced into the bloodstream by *intravenous infusion*. This technique is known as total parenteral nutrition.

WHY IT IS DONE

Tube feeding may be necessary for people who have gastrointestinal disorders (such as those resulting in *malabsorption*) or disorders affecting the nervous system or kidneys. Premature babies often require tube feeding if their sucking reflexes are undeveloped, as do burn or fever patients because of their increased nutritional requirements.

Intravenous feeding is usually necessary when large areas of the absorbing surface of the small intestine have been damaged by disease or have been surgically removed.

HOW IT IS DONE

TUBE FEEDING Suitable food mixtures or preparations of predetermined levels of nutrients are administered via a narrow plastic tube. The tube is passed through the patient's nose (guided via the nasopharynx to the esophagus) and into either the stomach or the duodenum.

If tube feeding is the sole means of nutrition, it must provide all of the essential nutrients (and adequate fluids) to meet the person's daily needs, which can vary markedly.

There are two alternative methods of tube feeding—continuous drip feeding and bolus feeding. Continuous drip feeding is generally preferred because it is tolerated better by patients. Bolus feeding allows rapid administration of a set amount of nutrients at intermittent periods throughout the day. In both methods the rate of flow can be controlled by a pump.

The tube is usually left in place for adults and older children, but for infants and young children it may be removed and later reinserted for each feeding.

INTRAVENOUS FEEDING This method is generally used only when tube feeding is impractical or ineffective; its main drawback is the risk of introducing infection directly into the bloodstream or of blocking a blood vessel. In some cases, there may be problems affecting the liver or gallbladder.

Nutrient preparations are given into an arm vein or directly into a large central vein near the heart via a *catheter* (thin, flexible tube) inserted under local anesthetic and strict *aseptic technique*. Intravenous feeding is sometimes used to supplement feeding by mouth, but can if necessary provide all the nutrients needed to meet a patient's requirements.

Feeding, infant

A baby grows more rapidly in its first year than at any future time in its life. A good diet is essential for healthy growth and development.

BREAST- OR BOTTLE-FEEDING

NUTRITIONAL REQUIREMENTS During the first four to six months, most babies' nutritional requirements are met by milk alone, whether by *breast-feeding* or *bottle-feeding*. Both human milk and artificial milk (cow's milk modified to resemble human milk) contain carbohydrate, protein, fat, vitamins, and minerals in similar proportions (see *Milk* for components), but human milk is the food of choice because it

provides these nutrients in the perfect blend as well as containing *antibodies* and white blood cells that protect the baby against infections.

After the baby is 6 weeks old, supplementary *vitamin D* should be given to breast-fed babies; multivitamin drops containing vitamins A and C in addition to vitamin D are usually given. Most bottle-fed babies do not need extra vitamins because modified dried cow's milk preparations are supplemented with vitamins. Additional vitamins should, however, be given to bottle-fed babies who are at risk of *rickets* (e.g., Asian babies in northern climates).

At 6 months a baby can be safely taken off artificial milk and fed with unchanged cow's milk. Supplementary vitamins should then be given until the baby is established on a mixed diet.

If a baby seems unable to tolerate milk of any kind (see *Food allergy*; *Food intolerance*), a physician should be consulted; he or she may recommend a preparation based on soybeans, vegetable oils, glucose, sucrose, corn syrup, modified meat protein, and other substances. Babies should not be fed skimmed milk, or semiskimmed milk, which has relatively too much protein and minerals and insufficient calories compared with whole milk.

EMOTIONAL REQUIREMENTS For healthy emotional development, a baby requires warmth, security, and contentment; the act of feeding plays an important part in meeting these needs. Breast-feeding is again preferable in this respect because it establishes an intimate bond between mother and child, but bottle-feeding is a perfectly satisfactory alternative if the baby is cuddled and talked to while he or she is fed.

INTRODUCING SOLIDS

Solid foods, initially in the form of purees and cereals, should be introduced into an infant's diet at some time between the ages of 3 and 6 months, depending on the baby's birth weight and rate of growth. By 6 months the baby should be eating some true solids, such as chopped up meat and vegetables. The accompanying chart (facing page) gives the optimum times for the introduction of solids, but a baby's general contentment also provides some guide. A rapidly growing baby who is unable to drink enough milk to satisfy his or her hunger should be given the more concentrated calories of solid food.

Many parents prefer to give their infants home-prepared purees rather than prepared foods. In this case, there are important things to remember: salt and other additives should not be used, since too much salt and other minerals can dangerously overburden a baby's kidneys. Sugar, too, should be kept to a minimum in the diet; a baby easily learns to have a "sweet tooth," which will lead to future dental decay; for the same reason, babies should not be given bottles of sweetened drinks.

A baby can live healthily on a vegetarian diet (one that contains no meat or fish) provided eggs are included, but a baby fed on a vegan diet (one that also excludes dairy produce and eggs as well as all other animal products) is at risk of severe malnutrition. A vegan diet makes it very hard to obtain enough calories, calcium, essential fatty acids, vitamins (especially the fat-soluble vitamins A,D,E, and K, and vitamin B_{12}), and protein. Overall, it is a very bad diet for infants and growing children whose nutrient requirements are relatively much greater than adults'.

FEEDING PROBLEMS

Any difficulties associated with milk usually appear within the first month.

Some babies have an intolerance to certain foods; reactions can include vomiting, diarrhea, or allergic rashes. For this reason, solids should be introduced one by one so that any that cause problems can be identified.

Prolonged crying after feeds may mean that the baby needs help bringing up wind, that artificial milk is not being digested properly, or that the baby has colic (see *Colic, infantile*). (See also *Nutritional disorders*.)

Femoral epiphysis, slipped

Displacement of the upper *epiphysis* (growing end) of the *femur* (thighbone). Such displacement is rare, usually affects those between the ages of 11 and 13, and occurs more often in boys, in obese children with delayed sexual and physical development, and in children who grow rapidly.

While the bone is still growing, the epiphysis is separated from the shaft of the bone by a plate of cartilage. This constitutes a zone of relative weakness in the bone, so that a fall or other injury, even a minor one, can cause the epiphysis to slip out of position. A limp develops and the child feels pain in the knee rather than in the hip. The leg tends to turn outward and hip movements are restricted.

APPROXIMATE AGES FOR INTRODUCING SOLIDS

4 months	At second breast- or bottle-feeding offer one or two teaspoons of	vegetable or fruit puree or cereal.
4½ months	At second breast- or bottle-feeding offer two teaspoons of cereal. At third breast- or bottle-feeding offer	two teaspoons of vegetable or fruit puree.
5 to 6 months	*Early morning* Breast- or bottle-feeding. *Breakfast* Two teaspoons of cereal and mashed hard-boiled egg yolk, followed by breast- or bottle-feeding. *Lunch* One teaspoon of meat or fish puree with three teaspoons of	strained vegetables. Offer water or well-diluted fruit juice instead of milk. *Mid-afternoon* Mashed banana or other soft fruit followed by usual milk feeding. *Dinner* Breast- or bottle-feeding if the baby is still hungry.
6 to 7 months	*Early morning* Breast- or bottle-feeding. *Breakfast* Two teaspoons of cereal with well-cooked scrambled egg. Offer cow's milk from a cup. *Lunch* Offer minced or mashed	food instead of pureed. Give meat or fish with some vegetables, then offer yogurt and fruit. Give a drink of water or well-diluted fruit juice. *Late afternoon/dinner* Meat or cheese sandwich. A drink of cow's milk.
7 to 8 months	*Early morning* Offer a drink of water or well-diluted fruit juice instead of milk. *Breakfast* Cereal and hard-boiled egg with whole-grain bread and butter. A drink of cow's milk.	*Lunch* Cheese, fish, or minced meat with mashed vegetables. Pudding or fresh fruit. A drink of water or well-diluted fruit juice. *Late afternoon/dinner* Meat or cheese sandwich. A drink of cow's milk.
9 to 12 months	*Early morning* A drink of water or well-diluted fruit juice. *Breakfast* Cereal, then well-cooked egg or fish with whole-grain toast and butter. A drink of cow's milk.	*Lunch* Chopped meat or fish, or cheese, with vegetables. Pudding or fresh fruit. A drink of water or well-diluted fruit juice. *Late afternoon/dinner* Meat or cheese sandwiches. A drink of cow's milk.

TREATMENT

An operation is performed under general anesthesia to manipulate the displaced parts of bone back into position and fix them together with metal pins. To prevent possible damage to the other thigh, it, too, may be strengthened with pins during the same operation.

OUTLOOK

Surgery usually provides an effective repair and prevents further accidents of the same type. However, after the injury, the hip tends to be more susceptible than normal to *osteoarthritis*. In rare cases, the hip becomes stiff and painful.

Femoral nerve

One of the main nerves of the leg. The femoral nerve is made up of fibers from nerves in the second, third, and fourth segments of the lumbar spinal cord. The nerves emerge from the lower back region of the spine and run down into the thigh, where they branch to supply the skin and muscles of the front of the thigh. The nerve branches that supply the skin convey sensation; the branches that supply the muscles stimulate contraction of the *quadriceps muscle* of the thigh, causing the knee to straighten.

Damage to the femoral nerve (which impairs the ability of the knee to straighten) is usually caused by a slipped disk in the lumbar region of the spine (see *Disk prolapse*). Damage may also occur as the result of a backward dislocation of the hip or, rarely, as a result of a *neuropathy*.

Femur

The medical name for the thighbone, the longest bone in the body. The lower end hinges with the tibia (shin) to form the knee joint. The upper end is rounded into a ball (head of the femur) that fits into a socket in the pelvis to form the hip joint. The head of the femur is joined to the bone shaft by a narrow piece of bone called the neck of the femur. The neck of the femur is a point of structural weakness and a common fracture site (see *Femur, fracture of*).

The femur can be felt through the skin at two sites. At the lower end, the bone is enlarged to form two lumps (the condyles) that distribute the weight-bearing load on the knee joint. On the outer side of the upper end of the femur is a protuberance called the greater trochanter.

The shaft of the femur is surrounded by powerful muscles whose principal functions are to move the hip and knee joints. The shaft is also well supplied with blood vessels; because of this, a fracture can result in considerable blood loss.

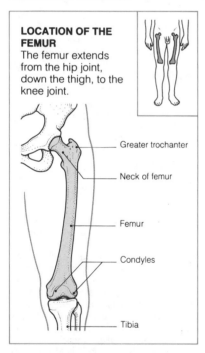

LOCATION OF THE FEMUR

The femur extends from the hip joint, down the thigh, to the knee joint.

Greater trochanter

Neck of femur

Femur

Condyles

Tibia

Femur, fracture of

The symptoms, treatment, and possible complications of a fracture of the femur (thighbone) depend on whether the bone has broken across its neck (the short section between the top of the shaft and the hip joint) or across the shaft.

FRACTURE OF NECK OF FEMUR
This type of fracture, often called a broken hip, is very common in elderly people, especially in women suffering from *osteoporosis* (thinning of the bone) and is usually associated with a fall. The incidence of this type of fracture doubles approximately every seven years after the age of 65, so that by the age of 90 one woman in four has suffered this type of fracture.

In a fracture of the neck of the femur, the broken bone ends are often considerably displaced; in such cases there is usually severe pain in the hip and groin (made worse by movement) and the leg cannot bear any weight. Occasionally, the broken ends of bone become impacted (wedged together). In this case there is less pain and walking is often still possible, which may delay reporting of the injury and detection of the fracture.

DIAGNOSIS AND TREATMENT Diagnosis of a suspected fracture is confirmed by X ray. If the bone ends are displaced, an operation under general anesthesia is necessary, either to realign the bone ends (a procedure called reduction) and to fasten them together with metal screws, plates, or nails, or to replace the entire head and neck of the femur with a metal or plastic substitute (see *Hip replacement*). Both procedures produce a stable repair, and hip and knee movement can be resumed immediately.

If the bone ends are impacted, the person is kept in bed for a few weeks to prevent any jarring movement that might dislodge the bones. The fracture heals naturally without surgery, but supervised exercise is necessary to maintain hip and knee mobility. X rays are taken periodically to determine how well the fracture is healing.

With either type of repair, walking is started with the aid of crutches, progresses to walking with a walking frame, walking with a stick, and, finally, without aid.

COMPLICATIONS These depend on the site of the fracture. A break at the union of the neck and shaft may result in hip deformity (see *Coxa vara*). A fracture across the neck itself may damage the blood supply to the head of the femur, causing the head to crumble (a condition called avascular necrosis). As a result, the bone ends may fail to fuse, or *osteoarthritis* may develop in the joint. In either case, more surgery (usually hip replacement) is required. Osteoarthritis may also develop even if avascular necrosis does not occur.

FRACTURE OF SHAFT OF FEMUR
This type of fracture usually occurs when the femur is subjected to extreme force, such as in a road traffic accident. In most cases, the bone ends are considerably displaced, causing severe pain, tenderness, and swelling.

DIAGNOSIS AND TREATMENT Diagnosis of this injury is confirmed by X ray. With a fractured femoral shaft there is often substantial blood loss from the bone. In most cases, the fracture is repaired by an operation (under general anesthesia) in which the two ends of the bone are realigned and fastened together with a long metal pin. However, sometimes the bone ends can be realigned by manipulation, and surgery is not necessary. After realignment of the bones, the leg is supported with a *splint* and put in *traction* to hold the bone together correctly while it heals.

Following both types of treatment, supervised exercise and massage of the knee, ankle, and foot is started to prevent the joints from becoming stiff. The progress of healing is checked regularly by X rays; when it is complete, weight bearing and walking is started gradually.

COMPLICATIONS These include failure of the bone ends to unite or successful fusion of the broken ends at the wrong angle, infection of the bone, or damage to a nerve or artery. All of these complications usually require more surgery. A fracture of the lower end of the shaft can result in permanent stiffness of the knee.

Fenoprofen

A *nonsteroidal anti-inflammatory drug* (NSAID). Fenoprofen is used to relieve pain and stiffness caused, for example, by *rheumatoid arthritis*, *osteoarthritis*, and *gout*. Fenoprofen is also used in the treatment of muscle and ligament sprains; it reduces pain and helps speed recovery. In common with all NSAIDs, fenoprofen may have side effects, especially irritation of the stomach and an increased risk of peptic ulcer.

Ferrous sulfate

Iron sulfate (see *Iron*).

Fertility

The ability to produce children without undue difficulty.

MALE FERTILITY
A man's fertility depends on the production of normal quantities of healthy *sperm* in the testes, and on the ability to achieve *erection* and to ejaculate *semen* into the vagina during *sexual intercourse*.

The *testes*—under the influence of *gonadotropin hormones* from the pituitary gland—produce hundreds of millions of sperm. The large output is necessary for normal fertility because only about one in 80,000 sperm ejaculated into the vagina reaches a fallopian tube (see *Fertilization*).

Normal fertility also requires a large proportion of the sperm to be healthy. After ejaculation, the sperm must be able to pass through the hostile environment of acid secretions in the vagina, to penetrate a barrier of mucus around the cervix, and to swim into the fallopian tubes.

Men become fertile at puberty and usually remain so (although to a lesser degree) well into old age.

FEMALE FERTILITY

The ability of a woman to conceive depends on normal *ovulation* (the monthly production of a healthy *ovum* by one of the *ovaries*) and the ovum's unimpeded passage down a fallopian tube toward the uterus; on thinning of the mucus surrounding the mouth of the cervix to enable sperm to penetrate more easily; and on changes in the lining of the uterus that prepare it for the implantation of a fertilized ovum. These processes are in turn dependent on normal production of gonadotropins by the pituitary gland, and on production of the sex hormones *estrogen* and *progesterone* by the ovaries.

Women become fertile at puberty and remain so until the *menopause*. (See also *Fertility drugs; Infertility*.)

Fertility drugs

A diverse group of hormonal or hormone-related drugs used in certain circumstances to treat some cases of female and male *infertility*.

In women, fertility drugs may be prescribed when abnormal hormone production by the pituitary gland or ovaries disrupts *ovulation* or causes mucus around the cervix to become so thick that sperm cannot penetrate it.

In men, fertility drugs are less effective, but may be used when abnormal hormone production by the pituitary gland or the testes interferes with normal sperm production. (See also *Clomiphene; Gonadotropin hormones; Infertility; Testosterone*.)

Fertilization

The union of a *sperm* and an *ovum* (egg). In natural fertilization (see illustrated box overleaf), the sperm and ovum unite after *sexual intercourse*. Fertilization may also occur as a result of semen being artificially introduced into the cervix (see *Artificial insemination*), or may take place in the laboratory (see *In vitro fertilization*).

Fetal alcohol syndrome

A combination of *congenital* defects resulting from high *alcohol* consumption by the mother during *pregnancy*.

Even small amounts of alcohol may be harmful in pregnancy, because (like *tobacco-smoking*) alcohol seems to affect fetal growth. The risks of *miscarriage* and *birth defects* may also be increased. Fetal alcohol syndrome, however, is a rare condition, which occurs only if there is persistent alcohol consumption during pregnancy. It has been reported in approximately one third of infants born to mothers with chronic *alcohol dependence* who go on drinking throughout pregnancy.

Fetal alcohol syndrome may occur in babies of women who consistently drink the equivalent of as little as 30 ml of pure alcohol (the equivalent of two mixed drinks or two to three bottles of beer or glasses of wine) per day. Today, the accepted medical advice is that women should abstain completely from alcohol during early pregnancy.

The affected baby has diminished growth, delayed mental development, a small head, a small brain, and small eyes with short eye slits. He or she may have a cleft palate, a small jaw, heart defects, and joint abnormalities. The baby, who is suffering from alcohol withdrawal, sucks poorly, sleeps badly, and is irritable.

Almost one fifth of affected babies die during the first few weeks of life; many who survive are physically and mentally retarded to some degree. (See also *Alcohol dependence*.)

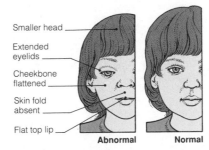

Smaller head
Extended eyelids
Cheekbone flattened
Skin fold absent
Flat top lip

Abnormal   **Normal**

Fetal alcohol syndrome
The left side of the child's face shows some typical features of severe fetal alcohol syndrome. The head is smaller (microcephaly), the cheekbone flattened, and the upper lip small and flat, the eyelids extend further over the eye, and the philtrum (the fold between the nose and lip) is absent.

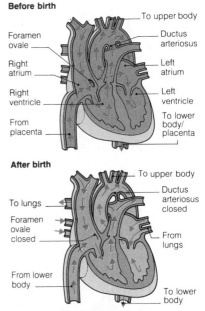

Before birth

Foramen ovale
Right atrium
Right ventricle
From placenta

To upper body
Ductus arteriosus
Left atrium
Left ventricle
To lower body/placenta

After birth

To lungs
Foramen ovale closed
From lower body

To upper body
Ductus arteriosus closed
From lungs
To lower body

Fetal heart circulation
In the fetus, blood passes from the right atrium of the heart to the left atrium through the foramen ovale. Another channel, the ductus arteriosus, allows blood to pass from the pulmonary artery to the aorta. Both channels close after birth.

Fetal circulation

Blood circulation in the fetus is different from the normal circulation after birth (see *Circulatory system*). The fetus neither breathes nor eats, so oxygen and nutrients are obtained—via the *placenta* and *umbilical cord*—from the mother's blood. The other fundamental difference in circulation is that blood bypasses the lungs in the fetus.

Oxygen and nutrients enter the fetal blood in the placenta, an organ embedded in the inner lining and wall of the uterus and connected to the fetus by the umbilical cord. The oxygenated blood flows to the fetus along a vein in the umbilical cord, then enters the right atrium (right upper chamber) of the heart, after which, instead of flowing to the lungs, it bypasses them. It does this by flowing into the left atrium through a hole called the foramen ovale.

The blood then passes to the left ventricle (left lower chamber), from where it is pumped to the upper parts of the body to provide the tissues with oxygen. It then returns to the heart, flowing into the right atrium and from there into the right ventricle. (After birth, blood pumped from this ventricle passes via the pulmonary artery to

F

F

THE PROCESS OF FERTILIZATION

Fertilization occurs when the head of a sperm penetrates a mature ovum in a fallopian tube. After penetration, the nuclei (which contain the genetic material) of the sperm and ovum fuse, and the body and tail of the sperm drop off. The newly fertilized ovum, called a zygote, then forms an outer layer that is impenetrable to other sperm. The zygote undergoes repeated cell divisions as it passes down the fallopian tube, so that, by the time it reaches the uterus, it has grown into a solid ball of cells called a morula. It then develops an inner cavity with a small cluster of cells to one side; this is called a blastocyst.

FERTILE PERIOD

Ovulation occurs about halfway through the menstrual cycle (14 to 16 days before the start of a period), after which the released ovum is available for fertilization for about two days. Sperm can also live for approximately two days, so the peak fertile period is about four days.

Peak and possible fertile periods

Although the peak fertile period is about four days, the possible fertile period may last seven to 12 days, due to variations in how long the ovum and sperm can survive and the timing of ovulation. The illustration shows the peak and maximum possible fertile periods in a 28-day cycle.

Sperm and ovum
A single sperm penetrates the ovum, thereby fertilizing it. To achieve this, the sperm releases enzymes that dissolve a path through the ovum's outer layers.

Morula
The fertilized ovum (zygote) divides repeatedly to form a ball of cells (morula).

Blastocyst
The morula develops a cavity, thereby becoming a blastocyst.

Fallopian tube

Fimbriae

Ovary

Ovarian follicle
A mature ovum is released from the follicle into the fallopian tube

Ovarian follicle

Uterus

Blastocyst

Uterine wall

Blastocyst
The blastocyst embeds in the uterine wall (implantation), where it develops into an embryo and also forms the placenta.

JOURNEY OF THE SPERM

When semen is ejaculated into the vagina, as many as 500 million sperm are released, most of which are capable of fertilizing an ovum. But, as they travel upward (propelled by their whiplike tails), more than half are killed by acidic vaginal secretions; many more die during the journey up through the cervix and uterus and into the fallopian tubes. The journey can take from one to five hours, and, in the end, only a few thousand sperm have survived.

Fallopian tube

Sperm

Ovum

Ovary

Uterus

Cervix

Vagina

Penis

Life span of sperm
A sperm can live in a fallopian tube for up to 48 hours, during which time it is capable of fertilizing an ovum.

the lungs for reoxygenation and elimination of carbon dioxide and other wastes.) However, in the fetus, the blood is only partly deoxygenated at this stage and has more tissues to supply with oxygen. Bypassing the lungs again, it flows from the pulmonary artery into the aorta; it does this through a channel called the ductus arteriosus which, like the foramen ovale, closes after birth.

The aorta carries the blood to the lower parts of the body, from where, completely deoxygenated, it is carried by two arteries in the umbilical cord to the placenta. There, carbon dioxide and other waste products are carried away by the mother's blood.

In rare cases, the foramen ovale or ductus arteriosus fails to close after birth, causing a congenital heart disorder (see *Heart disease, congenital*).

Fetal distress

Physical stress experienced by a fetus during labor as a result of not receiving enough oxygen. The most stressful period of labor for a baby is during a contraction, when the uterus tightens and thus reduces the baby's supply of oxygen from the placenta. If, in addition, there are problems with the labor, such as the mother's losing blood or having a pelvis too small for the size of the baby's head, the amount of oxygen reaching the baby may be inadequate.

MONITORING

Fetal distress causes the baby's heart rate to slow, which shows as a dip on a cardiotocograph (see *Fetal heart monitoring*). Alternatively, a distressed baby may show no variability in heart rate. This is in contrast to a healthy baby, whose heart rate varies within a normal range of from 120 to 160 beats per minute. The obstetrician keeps a close watch on the heart rate and, if necessary, may obtain a blood sample from the baby's scalp for analysis. *Acidosis* (high acidity) indicates that the baby is not getting enough oxygen. The amniotic fluid around the baby is examined for signs of *meconium* because passing of these fetal feces can be an indication of fetal distress.

DELIVERY

Fetal distress sometimes occurs as a temporary episode, but if acidosis is severe, the distressed fetus may need to be delivered promptly—by *cesarean section* if oxygen shortage occurs during the first stage of labor, and by *forceps delivery* or *vacuum extraction* during the second stage. (See also *Childbirth*.)

Fetal heart monitoring

Use of an instrument to record and/or listen to an unborn baby's heartbeat during pregnancy and labor. Some form of monitoring of fetal well-being is performed during labor in all hospitals.

WHY IT IS DONE

In pregnancy, monitoring is carried out at intervals if tests indicate that the placenta is not functioning normally or if the baby's growth has been slow. Uterine contractions or other stimuli, such as reflex kicking, increase the heart rate in a healthy fetus; the obstetrician can detect this using a fetal heart monitor.

During labor, monitoring can detect *fetal distress*, caused by the baby's not receiving enough oxygen. A fetus deprived of oxygen usually has an abnormal heart rate. Fetal monitoring can detect this abnormality and allows the obstetrician to take appropriate action, which may include emergency delivery procedures.

HOW IT IS DONE

In the simplest form of fetal heart monitoring, the obstetrician uses a special fetal stethoscope to listen to the baby's heartbeat.

In a more sophisticated version, known as cardiotocography, an electronic fetal heart rate monitor is used to make a continuous paper or sound recording of the heartbeat together with a recording of uterine contractions. The heartbeat is picked up either externally by an *ultrasound* transmitter strapped to the mother's abdomen or, as an alternative during labor, internally by an electrode attached to the baby's head and linked to the recording device by a wire inserted through the mother's vagina. The fetal heartbeat is amplified and heard as a beeping noise or printed as a paper trace.

Meantime, the mother's uterine contractions are measured and recorded either by an external pressure gauge strapped to the mother's abdomen or by an internal plastic tube that is inserted through the vagina into the amniotic fluid.

ADVANTAGES AND DISADVANTAGES

Electronic fetal monitoring has the advantage of giving the physician a minute-by-minute assessment of the baby's condition. Many obstetricians are convinced that babies are less likely to become hypoxic (deprived of oxygen) during labor with continuous monitoring and that monitoring therefore results in the bringing to birth of healthier babies.

However, routine electronic fetal monitoring has been controversial for a number of reasons. Critics have claimed that it limits maternal mobility during labor and that it leads to overdiagnosis of fetal distress and therefore to unnecessary cesarean sections. Critics also claim that external monitoring unnecessarily exposes healthy babies to ultrasound and that internal monitoring may increase the risk of infection during labor without resulting in improvement in the outcome of low-risk pregnancies.

Fetishism

Reliance on special objects in order to achieve sexual arousal. Fetishism is thought to be rare and restricted to men; because of the nature of the practice, there are no reliable statistics.

The objects need not have an obvious sexual meaning; they include shoes, gloves, rubber or leather garments, and parts of the body such as the feet or ears. It seems that once a particular fetish has led to successful orgasm, it becomes increasingly difficult to obtain sexual satisfaction without it. Nevertheless, many fetishists are able to have a stable sexual relationship, provided their partners join in the practice.

CAUSES

Fetishism usually has no obvious cause, although it may, rarely, result from certain forms of brain damage. According to psychoanalysts, the origin may be a childhood *fixation* of sexual interest upon some aspect of the mother's body or appearance.

TREATMENT

As long as fetishism does not impair sexual or social life, there is no reason for any form of medical interference. Treatment is needed only if the behavior is causing distress or if there are persistent criminal acts, such as stealing underwear.

Fetoscopy

A procedure for directly observing a fetus inside the uterus by means of a fetoscope, a type of *endoscope* (viewing instrument). The fetoscope can also be used to take samples of fetal blood and tissue for analysis and to permit treatment of some fetal disorders.

WHY IT IS DONE

Fetoscopy is used to diagnose various *congenital* abnormalities and *genetic disorders* before the baby is born. Because the technique carries some risks, it is performed only if there is a greater-than-normal chance that the baby will have some abnormality (for

F

F

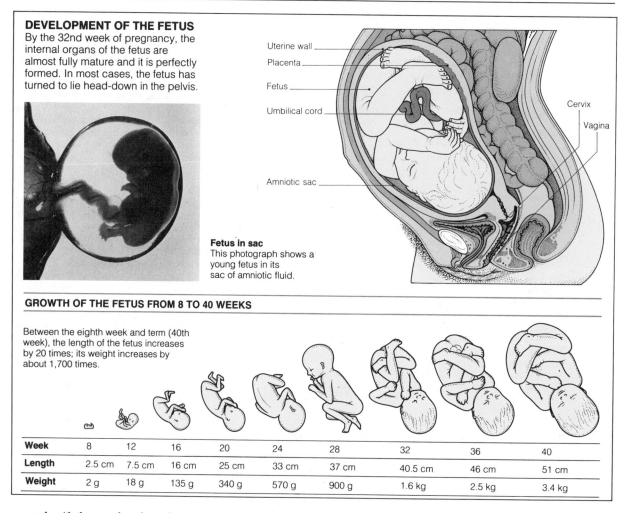

DEVELOPMENT OF THE FETUS

By the 32nd week of pregnancy, the internal organs of the fetus are almost fully mature and it is perfectly formed. In most cases, the fetus has turned to lie head-down in the pelvis.

Uterine wall
Placenta
Fetus
Umbilical cord
Amniotic sac
Cervix
Vagina

Fetus in sac
This photograph shows a young fetus in its sac of amniotic fluid.

GROWTH OF THE FETUS FROM 8 TO 40 WEEKS

Between the eighth week and term (40th week), the length of the fetus increases by 20 times; its weight increases by about 1,700 times.

Week	8	12	16	20	24	28	32	36	40
Length	2.5 cm	7.5 cm	16 cm	25 cm	33 cm	37 cm	40.5 cm	46 cm	51 cm
Weight	2 g	18 g	135 g	340 g	570 g	900 g	1.6 kg	2.5 kg	3.4 kg

example, if the mother has already had an abnormal baby or if there is an established family history of genetic disorders).

Fetoscopy allows a close-up look at the developing fetus, particularly the face, limbs, genitals, and spine, and can detect abnormalities, such as spinal column defects, facial defects, and limb defects. By attaching additional instruments, the fetoscope can also be used for the surgical correction of some defects, such as certain urinary system disorders. (See also *Amniocentesis; Chorionic villus sampling*.)

Fetus

The unborn child from the end of the eighth week after conception until birth. For the first eight weeks, the unborn child is called an *embryo*.

The fetus develops in the mother's *uterus* in a sac filled with *amniotic fluid*, which cushions it against injury. The oxygen and nutrients the fetus needs are supplied through the *placenta*, an organ embedded in the inner wall of the uterus and attached to the fetus by the umbilical cord.

Fever

Known medically as pyrexia, a fever is defined as a body temperature above 37°C, measured in the mouth, or 37.7 °C, measured in the rectum.

A fever may be accompanied by other symptoms, such as shivering, headache, sweating, thirst, a flushed face, hot skin, and faster than normal breathing. In some cases there may be rigors (attacks of severe shivering followed by drenching sweats and a sudden fall in body temperature). *Confusion* or *delirium* sometimes occurs with fever, especially in the elderly; a very high fever may also cause seizures (see *Convulsion, febrile*) or *coma*, especially in children.

CAUSES

Most fevers are caused by bacterial or viral infections, such as *typhoid fever, tonsillitis, influenza,* or *measles*. In these cases, proteins called pyrogens are released when the white blood cells of the body's defense system fight the microorganisms responsible for the illness. These pyrogens act on the temperature-controlling center in the brain, causing it to raise body temperature in an attempt to destroy the invading microorganisms.

Fever may also occur in noninfectious conditions, such as *dehydration, thyrotoxicosis* (a condition that results from overactivity of the thyroid gland), *myocardial infarction* (heart attack), and *lymphoma* (a tumor of the lymphatic system). The function of fever is not understood in such cases. (See also *Fever* symptom chart.)

TREATMENT

A physician should be consulted if a

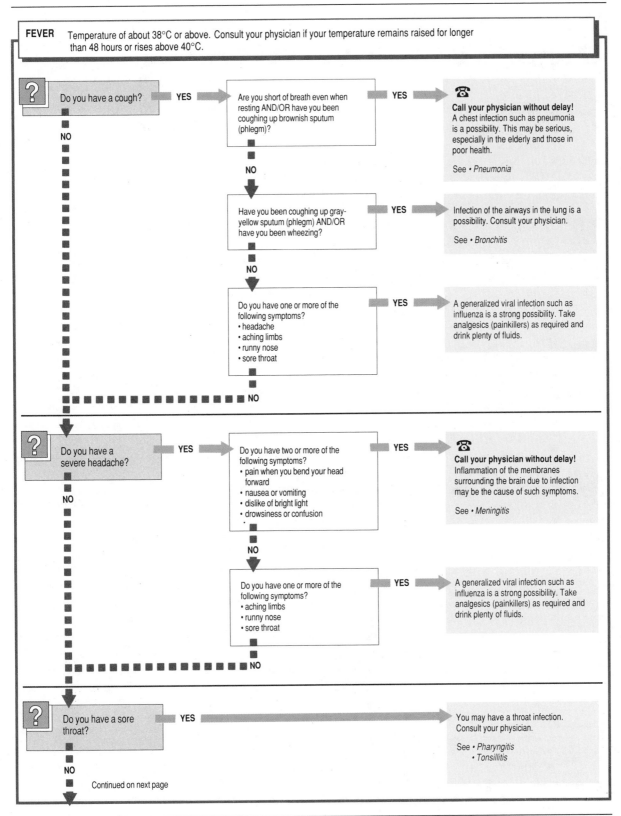

FEVER Temperature of about 38°C or above. Consult your physician if your temperature remains raised for longer than 48 hours or rises above 40°C.

? Do you have a cough? → **YES** →

Are you short of breath even when resting AND/OR have you been coughing up brownish sputum (phlegm)? → **YES** →

☎ **Call your physician without delay!** A chest infection such as pneumonia is a possibility. This may be serious, especially in the elderly and those in poor health.

See • *Pneumonia*

NO ↓

Have you been coughing up gray-yellow sputum (phlegm) AND/OR have you been wheezing? → **YES** →

Infection of the airways in the lung is a possibility. Consult your physician.

See • *Bronchitis*

NO ↓

Do you have one or more of the following symptoms?
• headache
• aching limbs
• runny nose
• sore throat
→ **YES** →

A generalized viral infection such as influenza is a strong possibility. Take analgesics (painkillers) as required and drink plenty of fluids.

NO

? Do you have a severe headache? → **YES** →

Do you have two or more of the following symptoms?
• pain when you bend your head forward
• nausea or vomiting
• dislike of bright light
• drowsiness or confusion
→ **YES** →

☎ **Call your physician without delay!** Inflammation of the membranes surrounding the brain due to infection may be the cause of such symptoms.

See • *Meningitis*

NO ↓

Do you have one or more of the following symptoms?
• aching limbs
• runny nose
• sore throat
→ **YES** →

A generalized viral infection such as influenza is a strong possibility. Take analgesics (painkillers) as required and drink plenty of fluids.

NO

? Do you have a sore throat? → **YES** →

You may have a throat infection. Consult your physician.

See • *Pharyngitis*
    • *Tonsillitis*

NO

Continued on next page

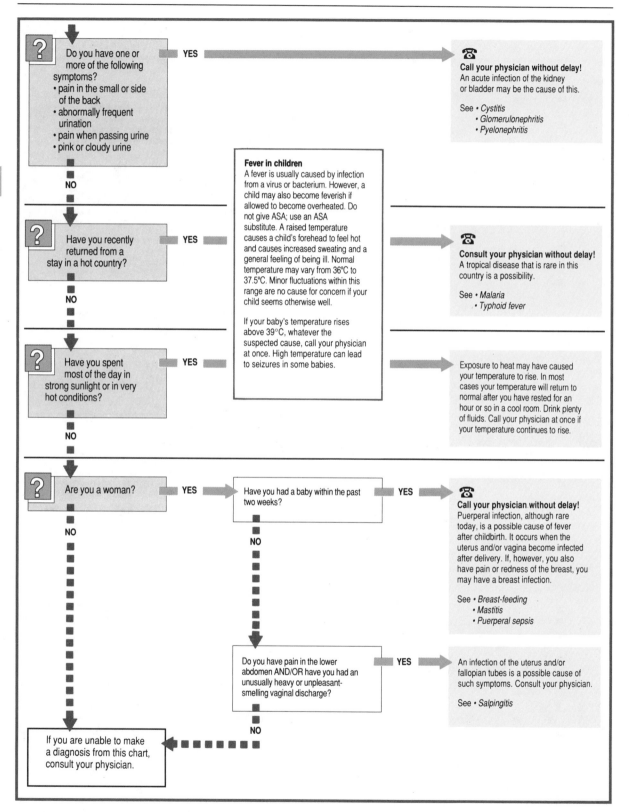

Do you have one or more of the following symptoms?
- pain in the small or side of the back
- abnormally frequent urination
- pain when passing urine
- pink or cloudy urine

YES → ☎ **Call your physician without delay!** An acute infection of the kidney or bladder may be the cause of this.

See • *Cystitis*
• *Glomerulonephritis*
• *Pyelonephritis*

NO

Have you recently returned from a stay in a hot country?

YES → ☎ **Consult your physician without delay!** A tropical disease that is rare in this country is a possibility.

See • *Malaria*
• *Typhoid fever*

NO

Fever in children
A fever is usually caused by infection from a virus or bacterium. However, a child may also become feverish if allowed to become overheated. Do not give ASA; use an ASA substitute. A raised temperature causes a child's forehead to feel hot and causes increased sweating and a general feeling of being ill. Normal temperature may vary from 36°C to 37.5°C. Minor fluctuations within this range are no cause for concern if your child seems otherwise well.

If your baby's temperature rises above 39°C, whatever the suspected cause, call your physician at once. High temperature can lead to seizures in some babies.

Have you spent most of the day in strong sunlight or in very hot conditions?

YES → Exposure to heat may have caused your temperature to rise. In most cases your temperature will return to normal after you have rested for an hour or so in a cool room. Drink plenty of fluids. Call your physician at once if your temperature continues to rise.

NO

Are you a woman?

YES → **Have you had a baby within the past two weeks?**

YES → ☎ **Call your physician without delay!** Puerperal infection, although rare today, is a possible cause of fever after childbirth. It occurs when the uterus and/or vagina become infected after delivery. If, however, you also have pain or redness of the breast, you may have a breast infection.

See • *Breast-feeding*
• *Mastitis*
• *Puerperal sepsis*

NO

Do you have pain in the lower abdomen AND/OR have you had an unusually heavy or unpleasant-smelling vaginal discharge?

YES → An infection of the uterus and/or fallopian tubes is a possible cause of such symptoms. Consult your physician.

See • *Salpingitis*

NO

NO

If you are unable to make a diagnosis from this chart, consult your physician.

fever lasts more than three days or if there are worrying accompanying symptoms, such as severe headache with stiff neck, abdominal pain, or pain when passing urine. Prompt medical advice is also necessary if fever occurs in a baby less than 6 months old, in a child with a history of febrile convulsions, or in an elderly person. Antipyretic (fever-reducing) drugs, such as *ASA* (adults only) and *acetaminophen*, may be given to treat fevers due to infections; such drugs also help relieve any aches and pains accompanying the fever. Otherwise, treatment is directed toward the underlying cause (for example, giving *antibiotic drugs* for a bacterial infection).

Febrile convulsions can often be prevented by cooling the entire body, either in a lukewarm bath or by sponging with lukewarm water, as soon as the fever starts.

Fever of unknown origin
Persistent fever for which no cause is readily apparent despite extensive medical investigations. The cause is usually an illness that is difficult to diagnose or a common disease that presents itself in an unusual way.

Common causes include various viral infections; *tuberculosis*; cancer, particularly *lymphoma* (cancer of the lymphoid tissue); and *collagen diseases*, such as systemic *lupus erythematosus*, *temporal arteritis*, and, in children, Still's disease (see *Rheumatoid arthritis, juvenile*). Another possible cause is a *drug* reaction.

Fiber, dietary
Indigestible plant material in food. Dietary fiber includes certain types of polysaccharides, cellulose, hemicelluloses, gums, and pectins (see *Carbohydrates*) and also lignin.
STRUCTURE
Cellulose, hemicelluloses, and lignin form the main structural components of plant cell walls. Pectins and gums are viscous (sticky) substances in plant sap. Together, these five substances provide the plant with a structure that is stable and partly rigid. Humans do not possess the necessary enzymes to digest these substances, which pass through the digestive system virtually unchanged and cannot be used as a source of energy. Some substances in dietary fiber are fermented by bacteria in the large intestine to produce acids and gas.
FUNCTION
Some components of dietary fiber have the capacity to hold water and

GOOD SOURCES OF FIBER

Recommended daily intake 25 to 30 grams

	Grams
Whole-grain flour	9.6
Dried apricots	24
Peanuts	8.1
Celery	4.9
Peas	12
Raisins	6.4
Green beans	7.4
Prunes	16.1
Bran	44

Grams: 0 5 10 15 20 25 30 35 40 45

Essential for the efficient working of the digestive system, fiber is usually eaten as fruit or grains. Among the best sources are bran, apricots, prunes, and whole-grain bread. Eating sufficient fiber in food can reduce constipation.

thus add bulk to the feces, which then pass through the intestines more easily, aiding normal bowel function. For this reason, dietary fiber can be effective in treating *constipation* and disorders such as *diverticular disease*. Dietary fiber may also be useful in the treatment of *irritable bowel syndrome*.

The easiest way to increase the amount of fiber in the diet is to increase the intake of unrefined carbohydrate foods such as wholegrain bread, cereals, and grains, root vegetables, and fruits. (See also *Nutrition*.)

Fiberoptics
The transmission of images through bundles of thin, flexible, glass or plastic threads that propagate light by total internal reflection. This means that all the light from a powerful external source travels the full length of the fiber without losing its intensity.

Fiberoptics has led to the development of *endoscopes*, instruments that enable structures deep within the body to be viewed directly. One bundle of fibers carries light to the penetrative end of the instrument and a parallel bundle transmits the image of what is illuminated to the viewer's eye or to a still or video camera. The flexibility of the fibers allows them to be passed through the loops of the large intestine or down through the curve of the stomach and into the duodenum without distorting the image. (See also *Endoscopy*.)

Fibrillation
Localized, spontaneous, rapid contractions of individual muscle fibers. Unlike *fasciculation* (a similar muscular

"quivering"), fibrillation cannot be seen under the skin. In skeletal muscles, fibrillation is detected by an *EMG* (electromyogram). In heart muscle it is detected by an *ECG* (electrocardiogram).

Fibrillation usually occurs after a nerve supplying a muscle is destroyed, which causes the affected muscle to become weak and waste away. Fibrillation of the heart muscle is caused by disruption of the spread of nerve impulses through the muscle wall of a heart chamber. As a result, the chamber no longer contracts as a single unit; instead, it produces a rapid, irregular rhythm (see *Atrial fibrillation*; *Ventricular fibrillation*).

Fibrinolysis
The breakdown or dissolution of fibrin, the principal component of any blood clot. Fibrin is a stringy protein that is formed in blood from a precursor substance, fibrinogen, as the end product of coagulation. Along with platelets and red blood cells, fibrin forms the final clot that plugs and seals a damaged blood vessel wall (see *Blood clotting*).

In addition to the coagulation system, blood contains a fibrinolytic system, the end product of which is an enzyme called plasmin, formed from a precursor called plasminogen. Plasmin acts directly to break up fibrin filaments with the effect thus of dissolving clots.

The fibrinolytic system is activated in parallel with the coagulation system when a blood vessel is damaged. It helps restrain clot formation in blood vessels (thus helping to prevent clots from blocking blood vessels) and eventually dissolves a clot once a broken blood vessel wall has healed. *Thrombosis* (abnormal clot formation) occurs only if there is a disturbance in the balance between mechanisms that promote clot formation, such as sluggish blood flow, and those, such as fibrinolysis, that restrain clot formation or dissolve blood clots.

Fibrinolytic drugs
Drugs used to dissolve blood clots. (See *Thrombolytic drugs*.)

Fibroadenoma
A benign, fibrous tumor found commonly in the breast. Fibroadenomas of the breast are painless, firm, round lumps, usually 1 to 5 cm in diameter, and movable. Fibroadenomas occur most often in women under 30 and are more common in black women. Multiple tumors may develop in one or both breasts.

Removal is performed under either a local or a general anesthetic. After removal, lumps believed to be fibroadenomas are examined by a pathologist to rule out the small chance of *breast cancer*.

Fibroadenosis
Overgrowth of glandular and fibrous tissue in the breasts, causing pain, tenderness, swelling, and cysts or other lumps in the breast. This common disorder is also known as benign mammary dysplasia, chronic mastitis, fibrocystic disease of the breast, cystic mastitis, or benign breast disease. The development of fibroadenosis may be related to fluctuating levels of female sex hormones; it is most common in women between the ages of 30 and 50.

SYMPTOMS
Fibroadenosis usually causes one or both breasts to become lumpy and tender. There may be either diffuse lumpiness of the breasts or a single breast lump, usually affecting the upper, outer part of the breast. There may also be a feeling of heaviness in an affected breast and occasionally a discharge from the nipple. The symptoms are worse during the second half of the menstrual cycle.

DIAGNOSIS AND TREATMENT
Mammography or a *biopsy* (removal of a sample of tissue for microscopic analysis) may be performed to rule out the possibility of *breast cancer*.

No specific treatment is generally required, but *diuretic drugs* may help relieve symptoms. If symptoms are severe, *progestogen drugs*, *danazol*, or *bromocriptine* may be prescribed. Any cysts in the breasts may be aspirated (drained using a needle and syringe).

Women with fibroadenosis should examine their breasts carefully each month (see *Breast self-examination*) so that any changes can be reported promptly to a physician.

Fibrocystic disease
A term that is used to refer either to the inherited disorder *cystic fibrosis*, characterized by the secretion of abnormal mucus by various glands and by recurrent respiratory infection, or to the presence of single or multiple benign tumors or cysts in the breast (see *Fibroadenosis*).

Fibroid
A benign tumor of the *uterus*. Fibroids consist of smooth muscle bundles and *connective tissue* that grow slowly within the uterine wall. As a fibroid enlarges, it may grow within the muscle so that the uterine cavity is distorted, or it may protrude from the uterine wall into the uterine cavity but remain attached by a stalk. Fibroids may be as small as a pea or as large as a grapefruit, and there may be one or more of them.

INCIDENCE AND CAUSE
Fibroids are among the most common tumors, occurring in about 20 percent of women over 30. They appear most often in women aged 35 to 45 and seldom before the age of 20.

The cause of fibroids is still unknown, but it is generally thought to be related to an abnormal response to *estrogen hormones*. Oral contraceptives containing estrogen can cause fibroids to enlarge, as can *pregnancy*. Decreased estrogen production such as occurs after the *menopause* usually causes them to shrink.

SYMPTOMS
In many cases there are no symptoms, especially if a fibroid is small. If a fibroid grows and erodes the lining of the uterine cavity, it may cause heavy or prolonged menstrual periods; severe bleeding can lead to iron-deficiency *anemia*. Large fibroids may exert pressure on the bladder, causing discomfort or frequent passing of urine, or on the bowel, causing backache or constipation. Occasionally, a fibroid attached to the uterine wall becomes twisted and causes a sudden pain in the lower abdomen. Fibroids that distort the uterine cavity may be responsible for recurrent miscarriage or infertility.

Symptomless fibroids are often discovered during a routine pelvic examination. When fibroids are thought to be the cause of menstrual disturbances or responsible for other symptoms, *ultrasound scanning* can confirm the diagnosis.

TREATMENT
Small, symptomless fibroids usually require no treatment, but regular examinations may be necessary to determine whether they are growing. Surgery is required for fibroids that cause serious symptoms or complications. A *hysterectomy* (removal of the uterus) is sometimes considered if there are large numbers of fibroids. Myomectomy (shelling out the fibroid from its capsule) saves the uterus and is another alternative.

Uterus

Fibroids

Uterine wall

Location of fibroids

Fibroma
A benign tumor of the cells that make up *connective tissue* (material that surrounds body structures and holds them together). For example, a neurofibroma is a tumor of the cells that surround nerve fibers (see *Neurofibromatosis*). An ovarian fibroma is a tumor of the cells that surround the follicles from which ova (eggs) develop. Treatment is not required unless the tumor is causing symptoms.

Fibrosarcoma
A rare, malignant (cancerous) tumor of the cells that make up *connective tissue* (material that surrounds body structures and holds them together). A fibrosarcoma may develop from a *fibroma* (a benign tumor of connective tissue) or it may be malignant from the start.

A fibrosarcoma most often develops in tissues around the muscles in a limb but can also affect a bone or the cells around nerve fibers. The tumor can spread to damage nearby structures.

A fibrosarcoma causes a localized swelling, which may not be noticed at first, depending on its site and how deep it is. Occasionally, widened veins appear on the skin over the growth; the fibrosarcoma may feel warm or may pulsate.

Treatment is by surgical removal or *radiation therapy*; this may be only temporarily successful if cells from the tumor have spread via the bloodstream to start growths elsewhere in the body.

Fibrosis

An overgrowth of scar tissue or *connective tissue* (material that surrounds body structures and holds them together).

Fibrous tissue may be formed as an exaggerated healing response to injury, infection, or inflammation. It can also result from a lack of oxygen in a tissue, usually due to inadequate blood flow through it—for example, in heart muscle damaged by a *myocardial infarction* (heart attack).

In fibrosis, specialized structures (such as kidney cells or muscle cells) are replaced by fibrous tissue, which causes impaired function of the organ concerned. An overgrowth of fibrous tissue can compress hollow structures, as occurs in *retroperitoneal fibrosis*, in which the ureters (tubes draining urine from the kidneys into the bladder) become blocked. Fibrous tissue formed within a muscle after a tear shortens the muscle and disrupts the normal contraction of fibers. This increases the likelihood of further tears unless the muscle is stretched and exercised.

Fibrositis

Pain and stiffness in the muscles around joints and sometimes in the back. Fibrositis is not a medical term, and some physicians refuse to recognize the condition because investigation usually fails to reveal any detectable reason for the symptoms.

Tension and bad posture may cause the condition, which seems to occur more often in anxious people and in those who spend time sitting in a cramped position. Sometimes, an attack occurs after an infection or new exercise. Fibrositis is most common in middle-aged and elderly people.

SYMPTOMS

Pain and stiffness may be felt in the neck, shoulders, chest, buttocks, knees, and back. There is usually no restriction of movement. Tender areas can sometimes be felt in the affected muscles. In some cases, the attacks (which are generally worse in cold, damp weather) are accompanied by exhaustion and disturbed sleep.

TREATMENT

Analgesic drugs (painkillers), hot baths, massage, and relaxation exercises usually relieve the pain and stiffness. A series of exercises designed to improve posture, starting with a gradual program to tone the muscles, may help prevent attacks. (See also *Back pain*.)

Fibula

The outer and thinner of the two long bones of the lower leg. The fibula is much narrower than the other lower-leg bone, the *tibia* (shin), to which it runs parallel and to which it is attached at both ends by ligaments. The top end of the fibula does not reach the knee, but the lower end extends below the tibia and forms part of the *ankle*.

The main function of the fibula is to provide an attachment for muscles. It provides little supportive strength to the lower leg, which is why pieces of bone can safely be taken from it for grafting elsewhere in the body.

FRACTURE

The fibula is one of the most commonly broken bones. Fracture of the fibula just above the ankle may occur with a severe ankle sprain as a result of a violent twisting movement. *Pott's fracture* is fracture of the fibula just above the ankle combined with dislocation of the ankle and sometimes with fracture of the tibia.

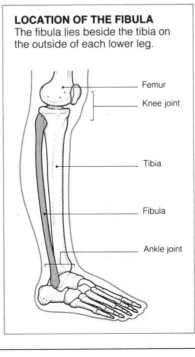

LOCATION OF THE FIBULA
The fibula lies beside the tibia on the outside of each lower leg.

Femur

Knee joint

Tibia

Fibula

Ankle joint

A suspected fracture of the fibula is X-rayed to confirm the diagnosis. In some cases the lower leg is immobilized in a plaster *cast* to allow the bone to heal. If the fracture occurs in the middle portion of the fibula, immobilization may not be needed. If the fracture is severe (especially if it is accompanied by dislocation of the ankle), surgery may be necessary to fasten the broken pieces of bone with metal pins.

A fractured fibula may take up to six weeks to heal, depending on the severity of the fracture and the age of the patient.

Fifth disease

An infectious disease of childhood that causes a widespread rash. It is also known as "slapped cheek" disease or as erythema infectiosum. Fifth disease is the least well known of the five common childhood infections.

Fifth disease affects children between the ages of 2 and 14 and usually occurs in small outbreaks in the spring. It is caused by a virus known as parvovirus. The incubation period is four to 14 days.

SYMPTOMS AND TREATMENT

The rash starts on the cheeks as separate, rose-red, raised spots, which subsequently converge. Within a few days the rash spreads in a lacy pattern over limbs but only sparsely on the trunk. It is often accompanied by mild fever. The rash usually clears after about 10 days but may recur over several weeks. Adults, who contract the disease only rarely, may have joint pain and swelling.

The only treatment required is bed rest, plenty of clear fluids, and *acetaminophen* to reduce any fever.

Fight or flight response

The physical response when the sympathetic division of the *autonomic nervous system* is aroused. The fight or flight response is both primitive and universal, is common to all animals, including man, and is a reaction to sensing a threat of any kind. The physiological changes occur in response to fear and also in *anxiety disorders*. *Epinephrine, norepinephrine,* and other hormones are released from the adrenal glands and the nervous system, leading to a raised heart rate, dilation of the pupils, the hair standing on end, and increased flow of blood to the muscles. All these responses make the body more efficient in either fighting or fleeing the apparent danger.

Filariasis

A group of tropical diseases caused by various parasitic worms or their larvae, which are transmitted to man by insect bites. Adult females, which vary in length from 2 to 50 cm, produce thousands of microfilariae (larvae) which are carried throughout the body in the bloodstream. Blood-sucking insects (primarily certain species of mosquito and fly) ingest the microfilariae in blood from infected people and transmit them by biting others.

Filariasis is prevalent in tropical Africa, Indonesia, the South Pacific, coastal Asia, southern Arabia, southern Mexico, and Guatemala.

TYPES AND SYMPTOMS
Some species of worm live in the lymphatic vessels. Swollen lymph nodes and recurring attacks of fever are early symptoms. Inflammation of lymph vessels results in localized *edema* (an accumulation of fluid in the tissues, causing swelling). Following repeated infections, the affected area—commonly a limb or the scrotum—becomes enormously enlarged and the skin becomes thick, coarse, and fissured, leading to a condition known as *elephantiasis*.

The larvae of another type of worm invade the eye, causing blindness (see *Onchocerciasis*). A third type, which may sometimes be seen and felt moving just beneath the skin, causes *loiasis*, characterized by irritating and sometimes painful areas of edema called Calabar swellings.

DIAGNOSIS AND TREATMENT
The diagnosis of filariasis is confirmed by microscopic examination of blood for the presence of microfilariae.

A three-week course of the *anthelmintic drug* diethylcarbamazine most often cures the infection, but may cause a reaction marked by fever, sickness, and muscle and joint pains.

PREVENTION
Where resources are available, filariasis can be controlled by the administration of diethylcarbamazine preventively and by the use of insecticides, repellents, nets, and protective clothing to help avoid insect bites. (See also *Insects and disease; Roundworms*.)

Filling, dental

The process of replacing a chipped or decayed area of tooth with an inactive material. The term is also used to describe the restorative (filling) material itself. Amalgam, a hard-wearing mixture of silver, mercury, and other metals, is generally used for back teeth, where the filling will not show. Tooth-colored plastic material, porcelain, or acrylic is more likely to be used for front teeth. Other substances, such as gold, are also sometimes used.

WHY IT IS DONE
When enamel is damaged, bacteria can invade the dentin beneath and eventually attack the pulp (blood vessels and nerves), causing the tooth to die. It is therefore preferable to repair teeth at as early a stage as possible—ideally when only the enamel is affected. Filling also restores a tooth to its original shape, which is important not only for appearance but for maintaining a correct bite.

HOW IT IS DONE
If the filling required is large or in a sensitive area, the dentist will numb the surrounding gum with a local anesthetic. Any soft, decayed material is scooped out with sharp instruments. A high-speed drill is used to remove harder material and to shape a hole that will hold the filling securely. While the dentist works, a suction tube placed in the patient's mouth draws away saliva; the cavity is kept as dry as possible with occasional bursts of compressed air.

If the pulp is almost exposed, the bottom of the cavity is lined with a sedative paste to protect the sensitive pulp from pressure and temperature changes. If one or more of the walls of the tooth is missing because of extensive decay, a matrix (steel band) may be placed around the tooth to support the filling. The dentist then mixes the amalgam (or other filling material), which at first has a gummy consistency, and packs it into the cavity, contouring the surface so that it is smooth. The filling sets sufficiently to allow the matrix to be removed after a few minutes. The amalgam hardens completely over the next 24 hours.

If a front tooth is chipped, the dentist may use a *bonding* technique in which the surface of the tooth is etched with a mild acid solution and plastic or porcelain material is then attached to the roughened surface, shaped, polished, and finished.

OUTLOOK
Amalgam fillings have a limited life and may need to be replaced after about 10 years. Occasionally, a filling needs to be replaced earlier—for example, if decay has continued to spread underneath the filling, either because of leakage at the filling margins or due to recurrent decay. Occasionally, fillings are dislodged, usually by chewing on sticky candy, or they fracture as a result of biting something hard.

Film badge

A device that enables hospital staff members to monitor their exposure to *radiation*. Film badges are worn by those who perform X-ray procedures and radiation therapy.

The badge consists of a piece of photographic film in a holder that is worn

THE CYCLE OF FILARIASIS
Filariasis is caused by parasitic worms and/or their larvae. There are several stages in the development of this infection as it spreads through the body.

Larvae enter the body through the bite of a blood-sucking insect

Larvae spread throughout the body via the bloodstream and lymphatic vessels

In the lymphatics, larvae develop into adult worms, which produce more larvae

The new larvae enter the blood and are ingested by a blood-sucking insect on the clothing. The film has a fast (sensitive) emulsion on one side and a slow emulsion on the other. Small doses of radiation blacken only the fast emulsion; higher doses start to blacken the slow emulsion and make the fast emulsion opaque.

Finger

One of the digits of the *hand*. Each finger has three phalanges (finger bones), except for the thumb, which has two. The phalanges join at hinge joints moved by muscle tendons that flex (bend) or extend (straighten) the finger. The tendons are covered by synovial sheaths that contain fluid, to enable the muscles to work without friction. A small artery, vein, and nerve run down each side of the finger. The entire structure is enclosed in skin with a *nail* at the tip.

DISORDERS

Congenital disorders include *polydactyly* (extra fingers), *syndactyly* (fused fingers), or missing fingers. Sometimes the skin membrane between the fingers is very long and deep, giving an appearance of *webbing*.

Injuries to the finger are common, particularly *lacerations*, *fractures*, and tendon ruptures. *Baseball finger* occurs when the extensor tendon that runs along the back of the finger is pulled from its attachment following a blow to the fingertip.

Inflammation due to *rheumatoid arthritis* or *osteoarthritis* may affect the finger joints, causing stiffness, pain, swelling, and deformity. The flexor tendons, which run along the front of the fingers, may become inflamed and stuck in the tendon sheath, causing *trigger finger*.

Infections may occur in the finger pulp at the tip; *paronychia* (infection of the tissue around the nail) sometimes follows a minor cut.

Altered control of the muscles in the walls of the vessels and impaired blood supply to the hands and fingers may cause *Raynaud's disease*. Dactylitis is a spindle-shaped swelling of the fingers, which occurs in *sickle cell anemia* and is an uncommon feature of tuberculosis and syphilis.

Clubbing of the fingers may occur as a sign of chronic lung disease, lung cancer, and some forms of congenital heart disease, especially in untreated *tetralogy of Fallot*.

Tumors of the finger are rare but may occur nonetheless in *chondromatosis*, a condition characterized by multiple benign cartilage tumors. (See also *Hand*, *Nail*.)

STRUCTURE OF A FINGER

The phalanges (bones) are joined at hinge joints and are moved by tendons.

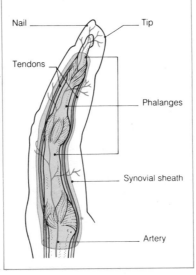

Nail — Tip
Tendons —
Phalanges
Synovial sheath
Artery

Finger joint replacement

A surgical procedure in which artificial joints made of metal, plastic, or silicone rubber are used to replace finger joints destroyed by disease.

WHY IT IS DONE

The main use of the operation is to relieve pain and to restore some degree of movement to hands that have been crippled by *rheumatoid arthritis*, which destroys the cartilage, bone, and lining of joints, leaving them weak and unstable.

Less commonly, surgery is performed to relieve pain and to improve mobility in joints in which *osteoarthritis* has destroyed the cartilage and created new bone.

HOW IT IS DONE

The operation is performed under local or general anesthetic. Several finger joints are usually treated simultaneously.

An incision is made to expose the joint; the ends of the two diseased bones in the joint are cut away, along with diseased cartilage. An artificial joint is then inserted into the bone ends. The tissue covering the joint and the overlying skin are sewn up and the finger is immobilized in a splint until the wound has healed.

RECOVERY PERIOD

The hand is bandaged and raised in a sling to prevent swelling. The stitches are removed after about 10 days, after which the patient is encouraged to

move the fingers and return to normal activities. Exercises for the fingers may be required later to maintain finger function.

RESULTS

The procedure is usually successful in relieving pain and enabling the patient to use his or her hands again. However, it can rarely restore normal movement to the hand because joint diseases affect not only bones and cartilage in the joints, but also surrounding tissue that contributes to the flexibility of joints.

Fingerprint

An impression left on a surface by the pattern of fine curved ridges on the skin of the fingertips. The ridges occur in four main patterns—loops, arches, whorls, and compounds (combinations of the other three). It is on these ridges that fingerprint classification is based.

In law, fingerprints are accepted as a means of identification, since no two people—not even identical twins—have the same fingerprints. (See also *Genetic fingerprinting*.)

First aid

The treatment of any injury or sudden illness given before professional medical care can be provided.

MINOR INJURIES

Most first aid consists of treating minor injuries, such as small *wounds*, *sprains*, foreign bodies in the eye (see *Eye, foreign body in*), minor *burns*, and *fractures*. Coping with these injuries requires proficiency in applying *bandages*, *dressings*, and *splints*.

EMERGENCY FIRST AID

The aims of first aid treatment in an emergency are to preserve life, to prevent the condition from worsening, to protect the individual from further harm, to aid recovery, to provide reassurance to victim and family, and to make the ill or injured person as comfortable as possible.

The role of the person giving first aid is to assess the situation, to give immediate and appropriate treatment, and to arrange for the ill or injured person to be seen by a physician or taken to hospital without delay. Additionally, the person administering first aid should find out as much as possible about the events surrounding the accident or injury from the victim or from bystanders.

If the victim is unconscious or losing consciousness, the person giving first aid must first ensure that the airway is clear, that breathing is satisfactory (by

F

F

FIRST AID: FIRST AID KIT

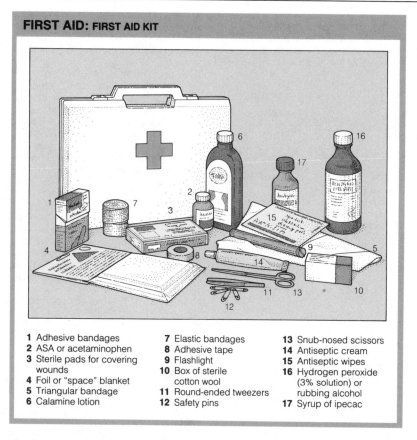

1 Adhesive bandages	**7** Elastic bandages	**13** Snub-nosed scissors
2 ASA or acetaminophen	**8** Adhesive tape	**14** Antiseptic cream
3 Sterile pads for covering	**9** Flashlight	**15** Antiseptic wipes
wounds	**10** Box of sterile	**16** Hydrogen peroxide
4 Foil or "space" blanket	cotton wool	(3% solution) or
5 Triangular bandage	**11** Round-ended tweezers	rubbing alcohol
6 Calamine lotion	**12** Safety pins	**17** Syrup of ipecac

checking breathing rate), and that the circulation is good (by checking pulse and skin color). Airway, breathing, and circulation are easily remembered by the letters ABC.

The *recovery position* helps maintain an open airway in an unconscious person who is breathing. *Artificial respiration* is necessary if a patient is not breathing. *Cardiopulmonary resuscitation* is essential if the person is not breathing and has no heartbeat. Any significant *bleeding* must be controlled by the rescuer applying pressure at the appropriate *pressure point*.

No severely injured or ill person should be moved without trained help unless life is in immediate danger. This especially applies to anyone with a suspected *spinal injury*. The person should be kept warm, and any tight clothing should be loosened.

If many people are injured, the person giving first aid must establish an order of priority for their care. Highest priority is for those who have no pulse, are breathing with difficulty or not at all, are unconscious, or bleeding severely. Such people may die unless immediate treatment is given.

First aid training is provided by various organizations, which award certificates to all those who have attended courses and thereafter passed an examination. (See also *Childbirth* emergency box; *Choking*; *Drowning*; *Frostbite*; *Heatstroke*; *Hypothermia*; *Poisoning*. First aid treatment for other specific conditions appears under the appropriate heading—for example, *Epilepsy*; *Nosebleed*.)

Fistula

An abnormal passage from an internal organ to the body surface or between two organs.

Fistulas may be congenital (present from birth) or may be acquired as a result of tissue damage. Congenital types include *tracheoesophageal fistulas*, branchial fistulas (see *Branchial disorders*), and thyroglossal fistulas (see *Thyroglossal disorders*). Acquired fistulas may result from injury, infection, or cancer. Some types of *arteriovenous fistula* (between an artery and a vein) are constructed artificially to provide ready access to the blood circulation, which may be necessary in people who are having *dialysis*.

Fistulas of the urinary tract, which open from the urethra or bladder to the perineum (the area between the anus and the genitals), may be a complication of radiation therapy to the pelvis or a complication of damage caused by a difficult childbirth. Such fistulas may cause urinary *incontinence* or *urinary tract infection*.

Fistulas between the intestine and the skin may occur in *Crohn's disease* and may also occur as complications of abdominal surgery. The intestinal contents may escape through an opening to the skin or through a surgical wound.

Some types of fistula close spontaneously, but most need to be cut out and repaired surgically.

Fitness

Having the capacity for physical work so that normal daily activities can be performed without exhaustion. Fitness depends on strength (the ability to exert force for pushing, pulling, lifting, and other bodily functions), flexibility (the ability to bend, stretch, and twist through a full range of movements), and endurance (the ability to maintain a certain amount of effort for a certain period of time).

HOW FITNESS IS ACHIEVED
Because cardiovascular fitness is the precondition for all other forms of fitness, aerobic exercise, which increases the efficiency of the body's use of oxygen, is the basis for any fitness program. Exercises to develop flexibility and strength should be combined with aerobic exercise for a total fitness program. Although fitness training has cumulative effects that build up over many months (provided that there is a sustained increase in activity levels), the effects are specific to the muscles used and the ways in which they are used. A variety of activities is necessary to achieve a general training effect.

BENEFITS OF FITNESS
A person who is fit has a better chance of avoiding *coronary artery disease* and preventing the effects of age and chronic disease. When the body is fit, the maximum work capacity is increased, endurance is increased, and a particular task utilizes a smaller proportion of the work capacity.

The strength, endurance, and efficiency of the heart are also increased by exercise. A fit heart pumps 25 percent more blood per minute when at rest and over 50 percent more blood per minute during physical exertion than an unfit heart. A fit person's heart normally beats 60 to 70 times a minute; an unfit person's heart beats 80 to 100 times per minute. The heart of a fit person is more efficient than that of an unfit person and is therefore less subject to strain. (See also *Aerobics*; *Exercise*.)

Fitness testing

A series of exercises designed to determine an individual's level of *fitness*, primarily cardiovascular fitness and muscle performance.

WHY IT IS DONE

Fitness testing is usually performed to determine a person's level of fitness before starting an exercise program. It also determines whether or not a person will be at risk when starting to exercise, particularly following a *myocardial infarction* (heart attack). Fitness testing is also done periodically to assess and monitor progress during an exercise program.

HOW IT IS DONE

The tests are usually carried out by a physician in his or her office or in the outpatient department of a hospital. A physical examination is usually performed, including measurements of height, weight, and body fat. Blood and urine tests may be carried out, including an analysis of blood *cholesterol* and high-density and low-density lipoprotein content, since high cholesterol levels are related to *atherosclerosis* (narrowing of the arteries).

One test involves measuring the performance of the heart during physical work. The heart's efficiency at pumping blood is measured using the pulse rate (number of heartbeats) per minute. The more efficient the heart, the slower it works during exercise and the quicker it returns to normal afterward. The pulse is taken at rest, and then the heart performance is measured during exercise at one or more intensities. This exercise may include step climbing, riding a stationary bicycle, or walking or running on a treadmill. After a specific period, the exercise is stopped and the pulse is taken to determine how hard the heart is working at its maximum level. The pulse is usually taken again after a minute to determine how long it takes for the heartbeat to return to normal. The blood pressure response to exercise also gives useful information to the physician and patient.

Another type of exercise test involves measuring a person's overall performance in a standard exercise. This is most suitable for monitoring progress through an exercise program and for setting goals. The test may be based either on measuring the distance covered in a fixed time or the time needed to cover a fixed distance. (See also *Aerobics*; *Exercise*.)

Fixation

A term used by Sigmund Freud to describe the attachment of a person's libido (sexual drive or interest) to real or imagined events during early childhood. Freud suggested that young children go through various stages related to certain parts of the body. These stages were called the oral, anal, and phallic stages because putting things in the mouth, concern about feces, and playing with the penis or clitoris were prominent behaviors during the different stages. In modern *psychoanalytic theory*, childhood stages are viewed within the context of the child's early relationships, starting with the mother.

EFFECTS

Fixations are unconscious and exist to some extent in all human beings; experiences from childhood are seen as permanently affecting the adult's thoughts and feelings. However, when the fixations are very powerful, resulting from especially traumatic relationships or series of events or experiences, they lead to the sort of behavior that would be expected from an immature child. Regression (going back) to one of these early stages is thus regarded by some analysts as the underlying cause of certain emotional disorders.

Flail chest

A type of chest injury, usually resulting from a road traffic accident or from violence. In flail chest, multiple rib fractures, usually at the front and side of the chest, produce an isolated portion of the chest wall. This portion moves in when the victim breathes in and moves out when he or she breathes out; this motion is opposite to the normal direction.

The injury may severely impair the efficiency of breathing and result in collapse due to *respiratory failure* and *shock*. It makes breathing and coughing very painful, which can increase the likelihood of chest infection and collapse of the lung (see *Atelectasis*).

TREATMENT

Emergency treatment consists of turning the person onto the affected side or supporting the flail segment by firm strapping. In the most severe cases, the patient may need immediate admission to an intensive care unit, where artificial *ventilation* can be maintained. This treatment is continued for about 10 days until the ribs are sufficiently healed.

Flatfeet

A condition, usually affecting both feet, in which the arch is absent and the sole rests flat on the ground. The medical term for this condition is the Latin equivalent: *pes planus*.

CAUSES

Almost everyone is born with flatfeet. The arches form gradually as supportive ligaments and muscles in the soles of the feet develop, and are not usually fully formed until about the age of 6.

In some people, however, the ligaments and muscles are weak for unknown reasons and the feet remain flat. Less commonly, the arches do not form because of a hereditary defect in the structure of the small bones of the foot.

Flatfeet can also be acquired in adult life because of fallen arches, sometimes as the result of a rapid increase in weight. Flatfeet may also be caused by a weakening of the muscles and ligaments that support the arch, which sometimes occurs in a neurological or muscular disease such as *poliomyelitis*.

SYMPTOMS AND TREATMENT

Most flatfeet—due to ligaments and muscles that have never developed fully—are usually painless and require no treatment. When the condition is caused by a defect in the foot bones or develops in adult life, the feet may ache when walking or standing. A few affected children require an operation to correct the bones in the feet. In adults, treatment consists of wearing arch supports and performing exercises to strengthen the weakened ligaments and muscles.

Flatulence

Abdominal discomfort or fullness, relieved by belching or passage of wind through the anus. Flatulence is a feature of many gastrointestinal conditions, in particular *dyspepsia*, *irritable bowel syndrome*, and disease of the *gallbladder*.

When a person is in an upright position, most swallowed air passes back up the esophagus to be expelled through the mouth. When a person is in a prone position, the air may pass through the intestine and anus instead. Gas formed in the intestine is passed only through the anus.

F

Flatus

Gas passed through the anus, sometimes called "wind." Gas is formed in the large intestine as a result of the action of bacteria on carbohydrates and amino acids in digested food; the gas consists of hydrogen, carbon dioxide, and methane. Air may be swallowed while eating and enter the stomach or intestine. Excessive swallowing of air, known as aerophagia, may occur during rapid eating or at times of stress.

Large amounts of gas may cause considerable abdominal discomfort, which may be relieved by the passage of wind through the anus or by defecation. Normal amounts of gas may cause abdominal discomfort in people whose intestines are abnormally sensitive. (See also *Flatulence*.)

Flatworm

 Any species of worm that has a flattened shape—as opposed to a *roundworm* or nematode, which has a cylindrical shape. Flatworms are also sometimes called platyhelminths.

Two types of flatworm are parasites of humans—cestodes (tapeworms) and trematodes (flukes and schistosomes). (See also *Liver fluke*; *Schistosomiasis*; *Tapeworm infestation*.)

Flavoxate

An *antispasmodic* drug that also relieves pain. Flavoxate is used primarily to ease the discomfort of urinary tract infections or of frequent urination. Side effects may include blurred vision and dry mouth.

Flea bites

See *Insect bites*.

Flies

See *Insects and disease*.

Floaters

Fragments perceived to be floating in the field of vision. Floaters move rapidly with eye movement but drift slightly when the eyes are still. They do not usually affect vision.

Most floaters are shadows cast on the retina by microscopic structures in the vitreous humor, a jellylike substance that lies behind the lens. In older people, the vitreous humor tends to shrink slightly and detach from the retina, often causing conspicuous floaters, which usually decrease with time.

The sudden appearance of a cloud of dark floaters, especially if accompa-nied by bright light flashes, suggests *retinal tear* or *retinal detachment*. A large red floater that obscures vision is usually due to a *vitreous hemorrhage*.

Flooding

A technique used in *behavior therapy* for treating *phobias*.

Floppy infant syndrome

A condition in which a baby's muscles lack normal tension or tone. Careful medical investigation is required. (See *Hypotonia in infants*.)

Floppy valve syndrome

See *Mitral valve prolapse*.

Floss, dental

Soft nylon or silk thread, waxed or unwaxed, used to remove dental *plaque* and food particles from between the teeth and around the gum.

Flow cytometry

A test that reveals the arrangement and amount of *DNA* (genetic material) within cells as a means of diagnosing malignancy. The pattern of DNA in cancer cells is different from that of normal cells. The test is helpful in distinguishing benign from malignant cells, and also in monitoring the effects of *anticancer drug* treatment. (See also *Cytology*.)

Flu

See *Influenza*.

Flucloxacillin

A *penicillin drug*. Flucloxacillin is usually prescribed to treat *staphylococcal infections*, such as wound and skin infections and certain types of pneumonia.

Fluctuant

A term used medically to describe the movement within a swelling when the swelling is palpated (examined by touch). Such a movement is a sign that the swelling contains liquid (such as pus in an abscess).

Fluke

 A type of flattened worm, also called a trematode, which may infest humans or animals. The two main diseases caused by flukes are *liver fluke* infestation, which occurs worldwide, and *schistosomiasis*, a common and debilitating tropical disease.

Fluocinolone

A topical *corticosteroid* that comes in the form of an ointment, cream, or solution. Fluocinolone can be applied to the skin to relieve the itching, swelling and discomfort of skin inflammation or allergy.

Fluorescein

A harmless orange dye used in *ophthalmology* as an aid to the diagnosis of certain types of *eye* disorders.

Fluorescein drops can be applied to the eye to check for the presence of conjunctival abrasions, which show up yellow when stained, or of *corneal abrasions* or *corneal ulcers*, which look green under white light or fluoresce brilliantly under ultraviolet light.

The dye is also used in a technique known as fluorescein angiography, which shows details of the blood circulation in the *retina* and *choroid* (the innermost layers of the eye). For this technique, a sterile solution of fluorescein is injected into a vein, and then photographs of the retina, using

---

HOW TO USE DENTAL FLOSS

Floss should be used as an adjunct to toothbrushing to remove plaque and food particles from gaps between teeth and around gums. Care should be taken to avoid damaging the gum margins.

1 Break off a generous length of floss (about 50 cm) and wrap the ends around one finger of each hand. Do not use the same length of floss twice.

2 Holding the floss taut, guide it gently into the gap between the teeth until it reaches the gum line. Then rub the sides of each tooth with the floss using an up-and-down motion.

blue light and a green filter on the camera, are taken while the fluorescein is passing through the blood vessels in the eye.

Fluoridation

The addition of *fluoride* to the water supply as a means of reducing the incidence of dental *caries* (tooth decay). Some areas have naturally high levels of fluoride in the drinking water; in other areas, fluoride may be added to bring the concentration up to a recommended level of 1 part per million. In Canada, 37 percent of the population drinks naturally or artificially fluoridated water, although the municipal water systems of Montreal and Vancouver are not fluoridated. Although considerable political controversy has surrounded fluoridation programs, there is no firm evidence that fluoridation at the recommended level has any harmful effects.

Fluoride

A mineral compound that is useful in helping prevent dental *caries* (tooth decay). Fluoride is thought to work by strengthening the mineral composition of the tooth enamel (see *Teeth*), making it more resistant to acid attacks. Fluoride may also reduce the acid-producing ability of microorganisms in dental *plaque*.

Fluoride that is ingested during the formation of teeth produces a lifelong beneficial effect because it is incorporated into the developing tooth substance. Children who from birth drink water fluoridated at a recommended level of 1 part per million have on average 50 percent fewer cavities in their primary teeth and 44 percent fewer cavities in their permanent teeth. If the local water supply does not provide the recommended level of fluoride, children may be given drops or tablets.

Fluoride is also beneficial to both children and adults when applied directly to the teeth. The dentist may treat children's teeth by painting on a fluoride solution or by holding a fitted tray filled with fluoride gel against the teeth for a few minutes. Fluoride mouthwashes and toothpastes are available for use at home.

Ingestion of excess fluoride during tooth formation may lead to *fluorosis*, mottling of the tooth enamel, sometimes with brown discoloration.

Fluorosis

Mottling of the tooth enamel caused by ingestion of excess *fluoride* as the teeth are formed. In the most severe cases, mottling is so great that the enamel develops unsightly brown stains. Severe cases usually occur only in areas where the level of fluoride in water for one reason or another is many times greater than the recommended level of 1 part per million. Fluorosis can occur in other areas if excessive additional fluoride is consumed—for instance, because of the unsupervised use of fluoride tablets.

Mild white mottling of the teeth may occur in a small percentage of children ingesting water at the recommended level, but this form of fluorosis does not usually impair appearance.

Fluorouracil

An anticancer drug that inhibits the growth of tumor cells. Fluorouracil is given in conjunction with other drugs to treat cancers of the colon, rectum, breast, and liver. It can also be used as a cream to treat *basal cell* cancers of the skin. Like other cancer drugs, it affects the growth of normal cells as well, and can cause gastrointestinal symptoms, anemia, and increased susceptibility to infections.

Fluphenazine

A potent long-acting *phenothiazine* drug used to suppress abnormal aggressive behavior and anxiety. It may cause drowsiness and tremors.

Flurazepam

A *benzodiazepine drug* used in the treatment of *insomnia*.

Flush

Reddening of the face and sometimes of the neck, caused by dilation of the blood vessels close to the surface of the skin. Flushing may occur during *fever*.

Foam, contraceptive

See *Spermicides*.

Folic acid

A *vitamin* essential for the production of red *blood cells* by the *bone marrow*. Folic acid is contained in a variety of foods, particularly liver and raw vegetables; adequate amounts are usually included in a normal diet.

During pregnancy, folic acid plays an important part in fetal growth—in the development of the nervous system and in the formation of blood cells. During the last three months of pregnancy, folic acid tablets may be necessary to supplement the diet.

Folic acid deficiency is a cause of megaloblastic *anemia*, which causes symptoms such as fatigue, depression, and pallor. Deficiency can occur during any serious illness or can result from a poor diet, especially in people who drink large amounts of alcohol.

Folie à deux

A French term used to describe the unusual occurrence of two people's sharing the same psychotic illness (see *Psychosis*). Commonly the two are closely related (e.g., a married couple or a brother and sister) and share one or more paranoid *delusions*. If the sufferers are separated, one of them almost always quickly loses the symptoms, which have been imposed or communicated by the dominant, and genuinely psychotic partner.

Folk medicine

Any form of medical treatment based on popular tradition. Examples include the charming of warts, the use of copper bracelets for the treatment of rheumatism, and the piercing of ears to improve the eyesight. What these remedies have in common is their support by local conviction and their lack of a professional practitioner. By contrast, the diagnostic and healing techniques used by a witch doctor are known as traditional medicine; those used by a chiropractor or a homeopathist are known as *alternative medicine*.

Follicle

A small cavity in the body. One example is a *hair* follicle, a pit on the surface of the skin from which a hair grows. Another is an ovarian follicle, one of the many fluid-filled cavities in the female *ovary* in which an ovum (egg) develops.

Follicle-stimulating hormone

A *gonadotropin hormone*, also known as FSH, produced and secreted by the pituitary gland.

Folliculitis

Inflammation of one or more hair follicles as a result of a *staphylococcal infection*. Folliculitis may occur almost anywhere on the skin. It is commonly found on the neck, thighs, buttocks, or armpits, causing a *boil*, or it may affect the bearded area of the face, leading to the development of pustules (see *Sycosis vulgaris*).

Treatment is with *antibiotic drugs*. The infection often spreads to other members of the family. To prevent this or to control an outbreak that has already occurred, each person should wash frequently and use a separate facecloth and towel; clothes worn next to the skin should be washed daily in boiling water.

Fomites

Inanimate objects, such as clothing, books, bed linen, or a telephone receiver, which are not harmful in themselves, but which may be capable of harboring bacteria, viruses, parasites, or other harmful organisms and thus may convey an infection from one person to another. Fomites mainly transmit respiratory infections, such as influenza.

Fontanelle

One of the membrane-covered spaces between the bones of a baby's skull. At birth, the skull bones are not yet fully fused and two soft areas between the skull bones can be felt on the scalp. These soft areas are the anterior (front) fontanelle, which is diamond-shaped, about 2.5 cm across, and usually closes up by the age of 18 months, and the posterior (rear) fontanelle, which is triangular, about 6 mm across, and closes within about 2 months of birth.

DISORDERS

It is normal for the fontanelles to bulge and become tense when a baby cries. However, persistent tension at other times may indicate an abnormality, particularly *hydrocephalus* (an accumulation of fluid within the baby's skull). A sunken fontanelle may be a sign of *dehydration*. If a fontanelle is abnormally large or takes a long time to close, the cause may be a brain abnormality or a disorder, such as *rickets*, affecting the skull bones. Early closure of the fontanelles results in deformity called *craniosynostosis*.

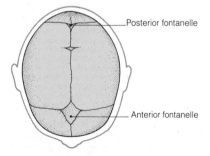

Location of the fontanelles
There are two soft areas on the baby's skull—the anterior fontanelle is diamond-shaped, the posterior fontanelle is triangular.

Occasionally, a third fontanelle is present between the other two; this occurs in *Down's syndrome*. Some babies have extra bones in the anterior fontanelle; this is not abnormal. The extra bones fuse into the skull when the gap closes.

Food additives

Food additives are chemical substances added to food for a specific reason, such as to modify the texture or improve the appearance of the food. Contrary to popular belief, not all food additives are artificial; for example, lecithin, extracted from soybeans, is added to whole milk powder to help it dissolve in water.

Only additives that are listed in the Canadian Food and Drug Regulations are permitted in food processing or for sale. Some 300 substances are classified as food additives, but other substances commonly mixed with foodstuffs, such as starch, salt, and sugar, are classed as nutritive ingredients. Other ingredients of food not defined as additives are listed in the food and drug regulations. These include vitamins, amino acids, spices,

flavorings, and veterinary drugs. Additives are classified in 15 groups according to their function. The table gives examples of some of the agents in some of these classes and shows how they are used.

Preservatives, such as sodium nitrate, are added to food to control the growth of bacteria, molds, and yeasts, especially those that might contaminate the food after it has left the manufacturer. Other additives, such as antioxidants, improve the keeping quality of the food by preventing undesirable changes (such as by stopping rancidity in foods containing fat).

Additives that improve texture include emulsifiers, stabilizers, thickeners, and gelling agents. They alter the consistency of food and how it feels in the mouth.

Appearance and taste are often improved by the use of colorings, flavorings, sweeteners, and flavor enhancers. Colors and flavors are used mainly to compensate for losses during processing, to strengthen existing colors or flavors, and to ensure standardization in products.

SOME FOOD ADDITIVES AND THEIR USES

Type	Possible use in	Reasons for use
Antioxidants L-ascorbic acid Synthetic alpha-tocopherol Lecithins	Fruit drinks Cereal-based baby foods Low-fat spreads	Improve keeping quality by preventing undesirable chemical reactions
Coloring agents Tartrazine (yellow/orange) Carotenes (orange) Caramel	Soft drinks Cheese Soft drinks	Restore color lost in processing, ensure uniform color
Emulsifiers and stabilizers Agar (extracted from seaweed) Guar gum (from cluster beans) Pectin (occurs naturally in fruits and plants)	Ice creams Packet soups Jams, preserves	Improve texture, consistency, alter "mouth feel"
Preservatives Benzoic acid/benzoates Sulfur dioxide/sulfites Nitrites/nitrates	Fruit products Meat products Cooked and cured meats	Improve keeping quality by inhibiting growth of microorganisms
Enzymes Rennet Papain Lactase	Cheese Meat tenderizer Milk products for special diets for lactose intolerance	Render food more easily digestible

Food additives
Canadian law specifies that prepackaged foods must list all ingredients including additives on the package label. Additives are not permitted in certain prepackaged products including milk, meat, and fresh eggs.

Color may not be added to meat to make it look redder or fresher. *Artificial sweeteners*, such as aspartame, are used in place of sugar, especially in products designed for diabetics or slimmers.

RISKS

Food additives are carefully monitored and regulated; there is no evidence that any additives in general use can harm the population as a whole. However, even though an additive may be harmless to most people, it may produce an allergic reaction in others. The best known flavor enhancer, *monosodium glutamate* (MSG), may cause *Chinese restaurant syndrome*. (MSG is not considered an additive in Canada.) Tartrazine, a widely used yellow food coloring, produces an allergic reaction in a very small number of people.

Additives are sometimes blamed for causing *hyperactivity* in children, but most physicians believe that the majority of hyperactive children are not allergic to food additives.

Food allergy

An inappropriate or exaggerated reaction of the *immune system* to a food. Sensitivity to cow's milk protein is a fairly common food allergy in young children. Other foods most commonly implicated in food allergy include wheat, fish, shellfish, and eggs. Allergy to food is much more common than allergy to food additives.

Food allergy is more common in people who suffer from other forms of *allergy* or *hypersensitivity*, such as *asthma*, allergic *rhinitis* (hay fever), and *eczema*.

Immediate reactions, occurring within an hour or sometimes minutes of eating the trigger food, include lip swelling, tingling in the mouth or throat, vomiting, abdominal distention, abnormally loud bowel sounds, and diarrhea.

The only effective treatment of food allergy is to avoid the offending food. (See also *Food intolerance*.)

Food-borne infection

Any infectious illness caused by eating food contaminated with viruses, bacteria, worms, or other organisms.

CAUSES

There are two main mechanisms by which food can become infected.

First, many animals that are kept or caught for food may harbor disease organisms in their tissues or internal organs. If meat or milk from such an animal is eaten without being thor-oughly cooked or pasteurized, the organisms may cause illness in their human host. In Canada, the only common infection of this type is *food poisoning* from improperly cooked meat, poultry, fish, shellfish, or eggs.

Second, food may be contaminated with disease organisms spread from an infected person or animal—usually by flies moving from feces to food.

PREVENTION

In developed countries, food-borne infections are controlled or prevented by adequate sanitation and sewage treatment; by multiple laws and regulations that govern animal husbandry, the production of food in farms and factories, and its subsequent storage and distribution; and by generally high standards of personal hygiene in handling and eating food.

In some less affluent parts of the world, many of these controls do not exist and the chances of a food-borne infection are thus much higher. When visiting such countries, it is wise to avoid certain foods, particularly salads, any meat or fish that looks suspect or not thoroughly cooked, shellfish, milk, butter, cream, and ice cream. Raw fruits and vegetables are generally safe once the exterior peel or skin has been removed.

Immunization is available against certain food-borne and water-borne infections, such as *typhoid fever* and *cholera*, but immunization usually provides only partial protection and is no substitute for good food hygiene. (See also *Water-borne infection*.)

Food fad

A like or dislike of a particular food or foods that is carried to extremes. A food fad may lead to an undue reliance on, or avoidance of, a particular foodstuff.

Fads are especially common in toddlers and adolescents and in those under stress. For most people, food fads are not serious since they are either short-lived or restricted to a limited number of foods. However, when food fadism or food aversion has an obsessional quality about it, or is persistent, it may be indicative of a more serious eating disorder. (See also *Anorexia nervosa*; *Bulimia*.)

Food intolerance

An adverse reaction to a food or food ingredient that occurs each time the substance is eaten, that is not due to a psychological cause or to *food poisoning*, and that does not affect the *immune system*.

CAUSES

Food intolerance is mainly of unknown cause, but is sometimes due to various unknown irritants, *toxins*, or *food additives*. The condition may be associated with an adverse reaction to foods such as green peppers, fried foods, or onions. Food intolerance can be caused by an inborn or acquired biochemical defect, such as *lactase deficiency* (an inability to digest milk sugar).

Food poisoning

A term used for any illness of sudden onset, usually with stomach pain, vomiting, and diarrhea, suspected of being caused by eating contaminated food. Most cases are the result of contamination of food by bacteria or viruses.

Food poisoning is usually suspected when, for example, several members of a household (or customers at a restaurant) become ill after eating the same food.

TYPES AND CAUSES

Food poisoning can be classified, according to cause, into infective and noninfective types. Some foods can cause poisoning of either type. For example, shellfish such as mussels, clams, and oysters can become contaminated by bacteria or viruses, by toxins acquired from poisonous plankton (tiny marine animals and plants), or by chemical pollutants in the water.

INFECTIVE CAUSES In Canada, food-borne illness is on the increase despite educational programs and legislation to improve standards of food preparation. Some of this increase is due to better reporting of outbreaks and isolated cases. It is estimated that there are more than 2 million cases of food poisoning each year in Canada: most of these are mild, but about 6,000 cases are investigated annually by health officials. *SALMONELLA* bacteria are the most common causes of food poisoning. Certain strains of *ESCHERICHIA COLI* (see *Water-borne infections*) cause a severe and potentially fatal inflammation of the colon called hemorrhagic colitis. *CAMPYLOBACTER BACILLI* are another cause of food poisoning, as is *LISTERIA* (see *Listeriosis*), which is harder to detect and generally produces a milder infection. Most of these bacteria are able to multiply rapidly in the intestine, and cause inflammation by releasing an *enterotoxin*.

Some farm animals, especially poultry, commonly harbor bacteria re-

F

INFECTED ANIMAL PRODUCTS

Some animals harbor disease organisms (e.g., bacteria, worms, and parasites) in their tissues and these may cause infection if meat or dairy products are consumed raw or improperly cooked. Beef, pork, and fish tapeworm infestations, salmonella poisoning, and (rarely) brucellosis can be transmitted in this way.

1 Cows, pigs, poultry, eggs, fish, and shellfish are sources of bacterial, viral, or worm infection or infestation.

2 Adequate milk pasteurization and inspection of meat and fish before sale prevent most infections and infestations of this type.

3 Thorough preparation and cooking of meats, fish, shellfish, poultry, and eggs further reduces the risk of infection.

FOOD CONTAMINATION

Intestinal infections may be spread from person to person if organisms in feces contaminate food, directly or indirectly. This can occur if vegetable crops are sprayed with sewage, flies settle on feces and then on food, or if food is handled by a person who has not washed his or her hands.

Contaminating organism
The photograph (left), taken through an electron microscope, shows a typical *SALMONELLA* bacterium. The organism uses its many flagellae (whiplike structures) to move. *SALMONELLA* is a common contaminant of poultry, eggs, and egg products and may cause severe food poisoning.

sponsible for food poisoning. If frozen poultry is not completely thawed before being cooked, or is not cooked sufficiently thoroughly, it is liable to cause poisoning. Eggs laid by affected poultry may also contain disease-causing bacteria. Unless eggs are known to be disease-free, they should be well cooked before eating, especially if they are to be eaten by babies, the sick, or the elderly.

Bacteria may also be transferred to food from the excrement of infected animals or people, either by flies or by the handling of food by an infected person—especially if the hands have not been washed after using the toilet. If contaminated food is left for any time in warm conditions, a large colony of bacteria may develop without obvious food spoilage.

Some types of bacteria cause the formation of toxins which may be difficult to destroy even with thorough cooking. Toxin-forming strains of *STA-PHYLOCOCCUS*, for example, may spread to food from a septic abscess on a food-handler's skin. The organism *CLOSTRIDIUM PERFRINGENS* is resistant to heat and may survive in precooked foods, such as stews and pies, which are not correctly stored.

A few cases of *botulism*, a potentially fatal form of food poisoning, are reported in Canada each year. Outbreaks are attributed to improper storage of foods prepared in restaurants, or to eating fermented marine animal products (muktuk), which may occur in Inuit communities.

Some viruses can also cause food poisoning. Like bacteria, they can be transferred from water contaminated with human excrement to partially cooked or raw food. Parasites can also cause food poisoning; the commonest form in Canada is *trichinosis*, usually acquired from eating bear meat.

NONINFECTIVE CAUSES Paralytic shellfish poisoning can result from a toxin in shellfish harvested at certain times of the year on the West Coast or in the Bay of Fundy. Shellfish absorb the toxins from small marine organisms called dinoflagellates, which produce a reddish discoloration of the water called "blooms." Levels of the toxin in the shellfish are carefully monitored, and when they exceed acceptable limits, they cannot be used for human consumption. A different toxin absorbed by mussels has also been responsible for an outbreak of food poisoning. Certain mushrooms and toadstools (see *Mushroom poisoning*) also contain dangerous toxins. Purely chemical poisoning can result from eating food contaminated with high levels of insecticide, food stored in a container that formerly contained chemicals, or acidic food such as fruit juices or tomatoes stored too long in a can coated with tin, zinc, or other heavy metal.

SYMPTOMS

The onset of symptoms varies according to the cause of poisoning. Symptoms usually develop within 30 minutes in cases of chemical poisoning, between one and 12 hours in cases of bacterial toxins, and between 12 and 48 hours with most bacterial and viral infections.

Symptoms vary considerably according to how badly the food responsible for the poisoning was contaminated, but usually include nausea, vomiting, diarrhea, stomach pain, and, in severe cases, *shock* and collapse.

The symptoms of botulism are markedly different, affecting the nervous system and causing difficulty in speaking, visual disturbances, muscle paralysis, and vomiting.

DIAGNOSIS

The diagnosis of bacterial food poisoning can sometimes be confirmed from a culture of a sample of the person's vomit or feces. Chemical food poisoning can often be diagnosed from a description of what the person has eaten, and from analysis of a sample of the suspect food, if available.

TREATMENT

Mild cases can be treated at home. The affected person should eat no solid food but should drink plenty of fluids, which should include some salt and sugar to replace what is being lost (see *Rehydration therapy*).

If vomiting and diarrhea are severe, or if an affected person collapses, medical assistance should be sought. If possible, samples of food left from a recent meal should be kept; they may help pinpoint the cause.

Hospital treatment may be necessary in severe cases. If poisoning by a chemical or bacterial toxin is suspected, gastric *lavage* (washing out the stomach) may be carried out. Otherwise, treatment usually concentrates on preventing or treating dehydration; fluids and electrolytes (salts) are given by mouth or intravenously.

Except for botulism and some cases of mushroom poisoning, most food poisoning is not serious. Recovery generally occurs within three days.

PREVENTION

Some simple measures can virtually eliminate the chances of food poisoning. Hands should always be washed before handling food, and fresh vegetables and fruit rinsed in clean water. Cutting boards and implements used on raw meat should also be rinsed before they are used for other food. Frozen poultry should always be completely thawed before cooking and then should be well cooked. Because raw meat and poultry carry disease-causing organisms, it is important to wash the hands immediately after handling these foods and before proceeding with further food preparation. Such organisms are destroyed by proper cooking.

Ask for advice on the preparation of any food that is unfamiliar to you. Suspect items—such as mussels that do not open when boiled, bulging tin cans, or any food that smells or looks obviously spoiled—should be rejected. People who preserve food at home should take care to sterilize food thoroughly by heating it in a pressure cooker at 120°C for 30 minutes. (See also *Cholera; Dysentery; Typhoid fever*.)

Foot

The foot has two vital functions—to support the weight of the body in standing or walking and to act as a lever to propel the body forward.

ANATOMY OF THE FOOT

An adult has 26 bones in each foot—one eighth of the total number in the entire skeleton. The calcaneus is attached to the talus. In front are the navicular, cuboid, and cuneiform bones, which are attached to the metatarsals. Phalanges form the toes.

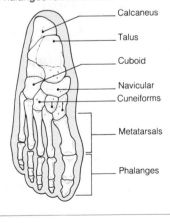

- Calcaneus
- Talus
- Cuboid
- Navicular
- Cuneiforms
- Metatarsals
- Phalanges

STRUCTURE

The largest bone of the foot is the *calcaneus* (heel bone); it is jointed with the talus, the second largest bone. In front of the talus and calcaneus is a series of smaller bones—the navicular, cuboid, and cuneiform. These in turn are jointed with five long bones called the metatarsals. The phalanges are the bones of the toes; the big toe has two phalanges, all the other toes have three.

Tendons passing around the ankle connect the muscles that act on the various bones of the foot and toes. The main blood vessels and nerves pass in front of and behind the inside of the ankle joint to supply the foot. The undersurface of the normal foot forms a natural arch which is supported by ligaments and muscles. Fascia (fibrous tissue) and fat form the sole of the foot, which is covered by a layer of tough skin.

DISORDERS

Injuries to the foot commonly result in *fracture* of the metatarsals and phalanges. The calcaneus may fracture following a fall from a height onto a hard surface.

Deformities of the foot are fairly common and include *talipes* (clubfoot), *flatfeet*, and *clawfoot*. Another common deformity is a *bunion*, which is a thickened *bursa* (fluid-filled pad) overlying the joint at the base of the big toe.

A number of disorders can affect the skin of the foot. *Corns*, a common complaint, are small areas of thickened skin which are usually caused by tight-fitting shoes. *Plantar warts* (verrucae) are warts that develop on the skin on the sole. *Athlete's foot*, a fungal infection, mainly affects the skin between the toes, causing it to become itchy, sore, and cracked.

Gout, a fairly common type of arthritis, often affects the joint at the base of the big toe or one of the joints in the foot. Ingrowing of the toenail (see *Toenail, ingrown*) commonly affects the nail of the big toe, causing inflammation of the surrounding tissues and *paronychia* (infection of these tissues). *Footdrop* (inability to raise the foot properly) may be due to damage to the muscles in the leg that perform this movement or to the nerves that supply these muscles.

Footdrop

A condition in which the foot cannot be raised properly. It hangs limp from the ankle joint, causing it to catch on the ground when walking.

COMMON FOREIGN BODIES IN CHILDREN

Children constantly experiment with objects in the environment. They frequently place small objects into their mouths, noses, or ears. As a result, a swallowed or stuck foreign body is a common occurrence. It is wise to keep all small objects well out of reach of children.

Ear and nose
Attempting to remove a foreign body from the ear can be dangerous because of the risk of pushing the object further in. The physician uses a syringe, suction, or forceps. A foreign body in the nose may be taken out with forceps by the physician; an older child may be able to blow it out while the other nostril is blocked.

Lungs
Inhaled objects such as peanuts or teeth may become lodged in the bronchi and cause obstruction of air flow, resulting in pneumonia or lung collapse. Symptoms may include choking, coughing, and breathing difficulty. If the child is choking, call an ambulance or take him or her to hospital immediately.

X ray of foreign body
This X ray shows that the child has swallowed a closed hair barrette.

Stomach
Foreign bodies commonly found in the stomach include coins, batteries, marbles, and buttons. Most small, smooth objects pass safely out of the body in feces, but an object that has failed to pass through the body after seven to 10 days, or sharp objects or batteries, usually require removal by endoscopy or surgery.

CAUSES

Neuritis (inflammation of a nerve) affecting the nerves that supply muscles that move the foot is a common cause of footdrop; it may be due to *diabetes mellitus, multiple sclerosis,* or to a *neuropathy.* Weakness in the foot muscles can also result from pressure on a nerve root as it leaves the spinal cord, due perhaps to a *disk prolapse* (slipped disk) or, rarely, to a tumor.

TREATMENT

Treatment is of the underlying cause, but in many people the weakness persists. A footdrop splint (see *Caliper splint*) can be worn to keep the foot fixed in place when walking.

Foramen

A natural hole or passage in a bone or other body structure, usually to allow the passage of nerves or blood vessels. The foramen magnum is the large opening in the base of the skull through which the spinal cord passes.

Forceps

A tweezerlike instrument used for handling tissues or equipment during surgical procedures. Various types of forceps are designed for specific purposes. For example, forceps used for dressings have scissor handles for easy manipulation, and tissue forceps have fine teeth at the tip of each blade so that tissues can be handled delicately during operations. (See also *Forceps delivery; Forceps, obstetric.*)

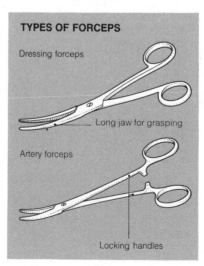

TYPES OF FORCEPS

Dressing forceps

Long jaw for grasping

Artery forceps

Locking handles

Forceps delivery

The use of forceps (see *Forceps, obstetric*) by an obstetrician to ease out the baby's head during a difficult birth (see *Childbirth*). *Vacuum extraction,* a procedure introduced in the 1950s, may be used as an alternative when the birth is prolonged.

WHY IT IS DONE

Forceps delivery is used if the mother is overtired or unable to push out her baby unaided, or if the baby is showing signs of *fetal distress.* (If fetal or maternal distress occurs before the second stage of labor begins, a *cesarean section* rather than forceps delivery is necessary.)

Forceps are used to control the head in *breech delivery* (in which the baby's buttocks are delivered before the head) to prevent a too-rapid delivery. Forceps are also used if the baby's head is stuck in the middle of the mother's pelvis and needs to be rotated to make delivery possible. This type of delivery, called a mid-forceps delivery, requires extreme skill on the part of the obstetrician; a *cesarean section* is sometimes performed instead.

OBSTETRIC FORCEPS

The two wide, blunt blades are designed to fit around the baby's head. The handles lock together so that the blades are held apart.

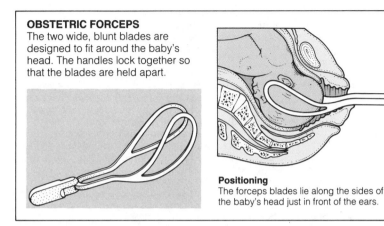

Positioning
The forceps blades lie along the sides of the baby's head just in front of the ears.

HOW IT IS DONE

The mother is given an *analgesic drug* (painkiller) and either local or *epidural anesthesia*. She then lies on her back, with her legs raised in stirrups, and her bladder may be emptied with a *catheter*. The obstetrician then examines the mother. Forceps can be applied only if the cervix (neck of the uterus) is fully dilated and the baby's head is engaged in the pelvis. An *episiotomy* (making of a cut in the perineum) is usually performed before a forceps delivery.

The forceps blades are placed on either side of the baby's head, just in front of the ears. If the baby's chin points downward, gentle traction is applied to the forceps and the baby is delivered. If the chin is pointing sideways or upward, rotation of the head is usually necessary before traction can be applied; in such cases, rotation forceps are used.

RECOVERY PERIOD

After a forceps delivery, care is similar to that following a spontaneous (unassisted) vaginal delivery. Sometimes there is greater bruising of the perineum, but this usually heals rapidly and can be eased by the application of ice packs. After a forceps delivery, the baby may have forceps marks on the face but these disappear after a few days. The length of stay in hospital for both mother and child is usually the same as after a spontaneous vaginal delivery.

Forceps, obstetric

Surgical instruments used in *forceps delivery* to deliver the head of a baby in a difficult labor.

Obstetric forceps consist of two blades that cup the baby's head. Each blade is joined to a separate handle and the two handles are fitted together; when assembled, the blades are separated by a fixed distance (see illustrated box).

Foreign body

An object that is present in an organ, opening, or passage of the body but that should not be there. A foreign body may enter the body accidentally (by inhalation or swallowing, for example) or it may be deliberately introduced. Common sites include the airways (see *Choking*), ear (see *Ear, foreign body in*), eye (see *Eye, foreign body in*), rectum, urethra, and vagina. Splinters or other objects that enter via the skin and become embedded in body tissues are also classed as foreign bodies. (See also illustrated box.)

Forensic medicine

The branch of medicine concerned with the law, especially criminal law. The forensic pathologist is a physician who specializes in the examination of bodies when circumstances suggest death was unnatural (i.e., suicide, homicide, or an accident). The examination usually includes an assessment of the time of death (from data such as the temperature of the corpse and its state of decomposition), deduction of the likely nature of any weapon used (from study of the injuries), and matching of blood, hair, and skin from the victim with those on any weapons, on the clothing of suspects, or on parts of a vehicle.

Forensic pathologists may also be asked to examine victims of alleged sexual assault or child abuse. They also consult in cases of poisoning and possible drug deaths.

Forensic scientists use laboratory methods to study body fluids (such as blood, semen, and saliva) found on or near the victim and compare the fluids with those from suspects. They are also trained in ballistics and the identification of fibers from clothing.

In addition, scientists may advise on *blood groups* and *genetic fingerprinting* in criminal investigations and in cases of disputed paternity.

Foreskin

The popular name for the prepuce, the loose fold of skin that covers the glans of the *penis* when it is flaccid and which retracts during erection.

At birth, the foreskin is attached to the glans and slowly separates over the first 3 to 4 years of life. No attempt should be made to retract the foreskin in a young boy. If tightness persists after the age of 5, there is no need to consult a physician unless the child is unable to pass urine normally or suffers from recurrent infection (because the glans cannot be cleaned adequately).

In some societies, the foreskin is routinely removed from newborn boys, an operation called *circumcision*, usually for religious or hygienic reasons. Circumcision may be performed at any age as a treatment for disorders of the foreskin.

DISORDERS

In *phimosis*, the foreskin remains persistently tight after the age of 5, causing difficulty in passing urine and ballooning of the foreskin. There may be recurrent *balanitis* (infection and inflammation of the glans and foreskin). Erection is often painful, which is why the condition is frequently discovered only at puberty.

In the related disorder *paraphimosis*, the foreskin becomes stuck in the retracted position, causing painful swelling of the glans.

Forgetfulness

Inability to remember. (See *Memory*.)

Formaldehyde

A colorless, pungent, irritant gas. In medicine, a solution of formaldehyde and a small amount of alcohol in water—a preparation known as formalin—is used to preserve tissue specimens or to harden them (a procedure called fixation) before they are stained and examined. Formalin is also used as a *disinfectant*. In a few people, formaldehyde causes an allergic reaction affecting the skin or lungs.

Formication

An unpleasant sensation, as if ants were crawling over the skin. Formication may occur following abuse of certain drugs, such as alcohol, cocaine, or morphine. Scratching of the skin may cause a rash and occasionally lead to an incorrect diagnosis of a skin disease.

Formula, chemical

A way of expressing the constituents of a chemical in symbols and numbers. Every known chemical substance has a formula. Water, for example, has the formula H_2O, indicating that it is composed of molecules of two hydrogen atoms (H_2) and one oxygen atom (O).

Fracture

A break in a bone, most commonly caused by a fall. A bone is usually broken directly across its width, but can also be fractured lengthwise, obliquely, or spirally.

TYPES OF FRACTURE

Fractures are divided into two main types: closed (or simple) and open (or compound). In a closed fracture the broken bone ends remain beneath the skin and little or no surrounding tissue is damaged; in an open fracture one or both bone ends project through the skin. Fractures may also be classified according to the shape or pattern of the break (see box).

If the two bone ends have moved apart, the fracture is termed displaced; in an undisplaced fracture the ends remain in alignment and there is simply a crack in the bone.

CAUSES AND INCIDENCE

Most fractures are caused by a sudden injury that exerts more force on the bone than it can withstand. The force may be direct, as when a finger is hit by a hammer, or indirect, as when twisting the foot exerts severe stress on the *tibia* (shin).

Some diseases, such as *osteoporosis* and certain forms of cancer, weaken bone so much that it takes only a minor injury—or none at all—for the bone to break. This type of fracture is termed pathological.

Common sites of fracture include the hand, the wrist (see *Colles' fracture*), the *ankle joint*, the *clavicle* (collarbone), and the neck of the femur or hip (see *Femur, fracture of*), usually as a result of a fall.

Elderly people are the most prone to fractures because they fall more, accidents that generally occur in their own homes, and because their bones are fragile.

SYMPTOMS AND SIGNS

There is usually swelling and tenderness at the site of the fracture and, in some cases, deformity or projecting bone ends. The pain is often severe and is usually made worse by any movement of the area.

FIRST AID TREATMENT

Anyone suffering a suspected or known fracture should be taken to hospital; if the injured person cannot walk, medical help should be summoned. Do not try to force back a displaced bone yourself.

Treat severe bleeding (see *Bleeding, treatment of*), covering any open wounds with a clean dressing. Move the patient as little as possible. *Splinting* is usually necessary, especially if the injured person needs to be moved or if there is a long delay before help arrives. If an injured arm can be bent comfortably across the chest, splint it first and then apply a *sling*. If *spinal injury* is suspected, do not move the person at all unless his or her life is in immediate danger.

Do not give the injured person any food or liquid in case an operation requiring a general anesthetic has to be performed later.

PROFESSIONAL TREATMENT

X rays are taken to confirm the diagnosis and to provide a clear picture of the type of fracture and the degree of any displacement or malalignment.

Bone begins to heal immediately after it has broken. The first aim of treatment is therefore to ensure that the bone ends abut each other and are in alignment so that the bone will retain its previous shape after the fracture heals.

Bone ends that have been displaced by the fracture are maneuvered back into position—a procedure known as reduction. The bone may be manipulated through the skin (closed reduction) while the patient is under a local or general anesthetic. Alternatively, the bone may be repositioned through an incision under general anesthesia (open reduction).

Once the fracture has been reduced, the bone is immobilized to allow the broken pieces to reunite firmly while the healing process takes place.

In some cases the ends of the fractured bone may be fixed together by metal pins inserted through the skin and into the bone and kept in position by attachment to an external frame (external fixation); once the fracture has healed, the pins and frame are removed. In other cases an operation is done to open up the injury site and fasten together the bone pieces with metal screws, nails, plates, rods, or wires (internal fixation).

RECOVERY PERIOD

The time taken for fractures to heal varies considerably and depends on many factors. Fractures mend much more easily in children than in adults, and in babies they can heal in as little as two weeks. In an adult a weight-bearing bone, such as the tibia, may take up to six months to knit together completely; bones that do not bear weight, such as the *radius* (one of the lower-arm bones) and clavicle (collarbone), generally take no longer than eight weeks.

COMPLICATIONS

Most fractures heal without problem. Healing is sometimes delayed because the blood supply to the affected bone is inadequate (as a result of damaged vessels) or because the bone ends are not close enough together. If the fracture fails to unite, internal fixation or a *bone graft* may be required.

Occasionally, bone ends reunite at the wrong angle. If this causes deformity, an operation may be necessary to break the bone again, set it correctly, and fix it with nails. *Osteomyelitis* is a possible complication of open fractures and may be difficult to cure.

REHABILITATION

Physiotherapy plays an important part in rehabilitation after a fracture because complete immobility of a bone for a prolonged period can result in loss of muscle bulk, stiffness in nearby joints, and *edema* (accumulation of fluid), with a risk of permanent disability. The patient is encouraged to begin gradually using the affected part as soon as is safely possible, and is given exercises that will restore flexibility to the joints and strength to the muscles. (See also *Monteggia's fracture*; *Pelvis*; *Pott's fracture*; *Rib, fracture of*; *Skull, fracture of*.)

Fracture, dental

A break in a *tooth*. Tooth fractures are most commonly caused by falling onto a hard surface or by being hit in the mouth by a hard object, as may occur when playing sports. Front teeth that project more than normal are especially vulnerable to accidental fracture. Fractures may involve the crown or the root of the tooth, or both. In most cases, only the enamel (the hard, brittle covering of the crown) is fractured.

Fractures of the enamel or of the enamel and dentin can usually be repaired by dental *bonding*; in some cases, a replacement crown may be fitted (see *Crown, dental*). If the pulp of a tooth is damaged, *pulpotomy* may be

FRACTURES: TYPES AND TREATMENT

There are two main types of fractures: simple (closed) and compound (open). Within these two categories are several other types, three of which are illustrated here.

Compound fracture
A sharp piece of bone punctures the skin and is therefore exposed to organisms. There is a high risk of infection.

Transverse fracture
This may result from a sharp, direct blow or be a stress fracture caused, for example, by prolonged running.

Greenstick fracture
This type usually occurs in children. Sudden force causes only the outer side of the bent bone to break.

Comminuted fracture
The bone shatters into more than two pieces. This fracture is usually caused by severe force, such as in a car accident.

Simple fracture
The broken bone does not break the skin. Because organisms do not come into contact with the fracture, infection is rare.

F

REPAIR OF FRACTURES

There are various ways of repairing fractures depending on the particular bone, the severity of the fracture, and the age of the patient.

Internal fixation
The photograph (left) shows immobilization of an unstable ankle fracture by the insertion of metal screws across the bone ends.

External fixation
Immobilization may be achieved by means of a plaster cast (above) or, in cases such as an unstable fracture of the tibia (left and above left), through the use of metal pins inserted into the bone on either side of the break and locked into position on an external metal frame.

THE BONE HEALING PROCESS

After a fracture, the bone starts to heal immediately. Any displacement of the bone ends must therefore be corrected without delay to minimize deformity.

1 A blood clot forms between the bone ends, sealing off the ends of the damaged vessels.

2 Macrophages invade the fracture site to remove wound debris. Fibroblasts then create a mesh to form a base for new tissue.

3 New bone (callus) is laid down between the bone ends and over the fracture line.

4 Remodeling takes place, with more dense, stronger bone laid down. New blood vessels have formed.

5 Over a period of weeks, the bone returns to its former shape.

F

performed. Fractures of the root of a tooth may be treated by splinting (see *Splinting, dental*), by *root-canal treatment*, by the fitting of a replacement crown over the root, or by removing the tooth (see *Extraction, dental*).

Fragile X syndrome

An inherited defect of the X *chromosome* that causes mental retardation. Fragile X syndrome is the most common cause of mental retardation after *Down's syndrome*.

The disorder occurs within families according to an X-linked recessive pattern of inheritance (see *Genetic disorders*). Although males are mainly affected, women are able to carry the genetic defect responsible for the disorder and pass it on to some of their sons, who are affected, and some of their daughters, who in turn become carriers of the defect.

Approximately one in 1,500 men is affected by the condition; one in 1,000 women is a carrier. In addition to being mentally retarded, affected males are generally tall, physically strong, have a prominent nose and jaw, increased ear length, large testes, and are prone to epileptic seizures. About one third of female carriers show some intellectual impairment.

There is no treatment for the condition. If a woman has a history of the syndrome in her family, it is useful to seek *genetic counseling* regarding the risk of a child's being affected.

Freckle

A tiny patch of pigmented skin, often round or oval in shape. Freckles occur on sun-exposed areas of skin and tend to become more numerous as a result of continued exposure. The tendency to freckling is inherited and occurs most in fair and red-haired people.

Freckles are harmless, but people with highly freckled complexions should avoid excess sunlight and should use *sunscreens*.

Free-floating anxiety

Vague apprehension and tension associated with *generalized anxiety disorder*.

Frequency

See *Urination, frequent*.

Freudian slip

A slip of the tongue or a minor error in action that could be what the person really wanted to say or do. The term, also called a parapraxia, is derived from Sigmund Freud's book "The Psychopathology of Everyday Life."

As the error tends to be laughed off, Freud saw the process as a compromise between the fulfillment of an unconscious wish and the conscious effort to repress it.

Freudian theory

A discipline developed by Sigmund Freud (1856-1939), a Viennese neurologist. The theory developed out of his treatment of neurotic patients using hypnosis and later the interpretation of dreams. This formed the basis of his technique of *psychoanalysis*. Freud believed that feelings, thoughts, and behavior were controlled by unconscious wishes and conflicts and that problems occurred when these desires were not fulfilled or the conflicts remained unresolved.

According to Freud, the conflicts originated in childhood and persisted into adulthood. The essence of his theory concerns early psychological development, particularly sexual development. Freud defined a number of stages—oral, anal, and genital (representing the areas of the body on which an infant's attention becomes fixed at different ages)—and three components of personality—the *id*, *ego*, and *superego* (based respectively on pleasure, reality, and moral and social constraints). The classic Freudian model sees all behavior as having its roots in unconscious instincts, but ultimately being determined by the interplay between the id, ego, and superego. (See also *Psychoanalytic theory; Psychotherapy*.)

Friar's balsam

A name for tincture of benzoin. Friar's balsam is used as an *inhalation* for the relief of nasal congestion, acute rhinitis, sinusitis, and to loosen coughs. It is available over-the-counter.

Friedreich's ataxia

A very rare inherited disease in which degeneration of nerve fibers in the spinal cord causes *ataxia* (loss of coordinated movement and balance). The disease is the result of a genetic defect, usually of the autosomal recessive type (see *Genetic disorders*). It affects about two people per 100,000.

SYMPTOMS

Symptoms first appear in late childhood or adolescence. The main symptoms are unsteadiness when walking, clumsy hand movements, slurred speech, and rapid, involuntary eye movements. In many cases there are also abnormalities of bone structure and alignment.

TREATMENT AND OUTLOOK

There is as yet no cure for the disease. Once symptoms have developed, the disease becomes progressively more severe, and, within 10 years of onset, more than half the sufferers are confined to wheelchairs. If *cardiomyopathy* (heart muscle disease) develops, it may contribute to an early death. People who have blood relatives with Friedreich's ataxia may benefit from *genetic counseling* before deciding whether to have children.

Frigidity

Lack of desire for or inability to become aroused during sexual intercourse (see *Sexual desire, inhibited*). The term has been used almost exclusively with reference to women and is now being discouraged because of its negative connotations—blaming a woman for something that may exist only in the mind of her partner. (See also *Orgasm, lack of*.)

Frostbite

Damage to tissues caused by extremely cold temperatures. Frostbite can affect any part of the body that is not properly covered against the elements, but the nose, ears, fingers, and toes are most susceptible to this condition. The lower the temperature, the shorter the time required to cause damage; wind and blizzard conditions also harm more quickly.

The first symptoms are a pins and needles sensation, followed by complete numbness. The skin appears white, cold, and hard, and then becomes red and swollen. If only the skin and immediately underlying tissues are damaged, recovery may be complete. If blood vessels are affected, *gangrene* (tissue death) can follow. After the tissue has thawed, blisters form and some areas of skin eventually become black, indicating that the tissue is dead. In such cases, the damage is permanent and amputation of the affected part may be necessary.

TREATMENT

Frostbite must be treated promptly but thawing should be undertaken only when there is no risk of further freezing. The person should be sheltered from the cold and the affected parts warmed as quickly as possible by immersing them in water at 40°C— hot but not uncomfortable to the rescuer's elbow. Movement of the affected parts should be avoided; massage is not helpful. (See also *First aid* box on facing page.)

FIRST AID: FROSTBITE

DO NOT
- rub the affected parts
- attempt to burst blisters
- warm the affected area with direct heat
- allow the victim to walk on a frostbitten foot

WARNING
Frostbite is often accompanied by hypothermia, which must be treated first. Proper medical attention should be sought promptly, but first aid should be given immediately.

1 Shelter the victim from the cold and remove clothing from the affected part. Remove anything that constricts, such as rings or a watch.

2 Rewarm the affected area by covering it with warm hands or clothing. Frostbitten hands can be warmed in the victim's armpits; feet can be warmed in the rescuer's armpits.

3 If warm water (no hotter than 40°C) is available, immerse the affected part. The area should then be covered with a sterile dressing.

Frottage

The act of rubbing against another person to achieve sexual arousal. Also called frotteurism, it is usually carried out in a densely packed crowd or on crowded buses or subway cars, where a man rubs his (clothed) genitals against a woman's buttocks or thigh. Such men commonly indulge in other sexual *deviations*, may have an abnormal interest in buttocks or perhaps various articles of clothing (see *Fetishism*), and are unable to form successful sexual relationships.

Frozen section

A method of preparing a *biopsy* specimen (tissue removed for microscopic examination) that provides a rapid indication of whether or not the tissue is malignant. Frozen section does not yield sufficient detail for routine use and cannot replace the more lengthy conventional preparation of biopsy specimens. It was formerly used to provide information while a patient was undergoing surgery, but has now been largely superseded by other techniques, such as aspiration biopsy, which can be performed before the operation.

WHY IT IS DONE

Frozen section is primarily used to determine whether *breast lumps* are benign or malignant. It can also be used to check whether thyroid or intestinal tumors are malignant, and to diagnose *lymphomas*.

HOW IT IS DONE

Frozen section is performed during a surgical procedure and provides information that will allow the surgeon to decide whether or not further tissue should be removed before the operation is completed.

The surgeon removes a sample of tissue and sends it to the pathology laboratory for analysis. The sample is quickly frozen in liquid nitrogen, cut into very thin sections, placed on a glass slide, and stained so that the cells can be examined under the microscope. The entire process takes about 20 minutes. Information about the sample is then conveyed to the operating room and the surgeon decides what action is needed.

Frozen shoulder

Stiffness and pain in the *shoulder*, making normal movement of the joint impossible. In severe cases, the shoul-der may be completely rigid and pain may be intense.

Frozen shoulder is caused by inflammation and thickening of the lining of the capsule in which the joint is contained. The problem usually develops for no known reason, but in some cases it follows a minor injury to the shoulder, a *stroke*, chronic *bronchitis*, or *angina pectoris*.

The condition mainly affects middle-aged people, and there is a higher-than-average incidence among people with *diabetes mellitus*.

TREATMENT

Moderate symptoms can be eased by exercise and by taking *analgesic drugs* (painkillers) and *nonsteroidal anti-inflammatory drugs*, and by applying *ice packs* to the shoulder or using a heat lamp. In severe cases, injections of *corticosteroid drugs* into the joint may be required to relieve pain. Manipulation of the joint under a general anesthetic can also restore mobility, but carries the risk of initially increasing pain in the joint. Whatever the severity and treatment, recovery from this condition is usually slow.

Frusemide

See *Furosemide*.

Frustration

A deep feeling of discontent and tension because of unresolved problems, unfulfilled needs, or because the path to a goal is blocked.

In a person who is mentally healthy, frustration can be dealt with in a socially acceptable way. In less well-adapted people, however, such discontent and tension may lead to *regression* (childlike behavior), *aggression*, or *depression*.

FSH

Abbreviation for *follicle-stimulating hormone*, a *gonadotropin hormone* (one that stimulates the gonads—the ovaries and testes) produced by the anterior part of the pituitary gland.

Fugue

An episode of altered consciousness in which a person apparently purposefully wanders away from home or work and, in some cases, adopts a new identity. When the fugue ends, the affected person has no recollection of what has occurred.

Fugues may last for hours or days. During a short fugue, the sufferer may be confused and agitated. During a longer fugue, behavior may appear normal but there may be accompany-

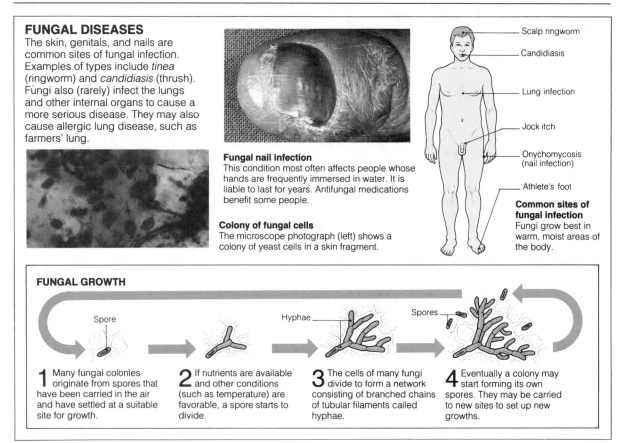

FUNGAL DISEASES

The skin, genitals, and nails are common sites of fungal infection. Examples of types include *tinea* (ringworm) and *candidiasis* (thrush). Fungi also (rarely) infect the lungs and other internal organs to cause a more serious disease. They may also cause allergic lung disease, such as farmers' lung.

Fungal nail infection
This condition most often affects people whose hands are frequently immersed in water. It is liable to last for years. Antifungal medications benefit some people.

Colony of fungal cells
The microscope photograph (left) shows a colony of yeast cells in a skin fragment.

Scalp ringworm
Candidiasis
Lung infection
Jock itch
Onychomycosis (nail infection)
Athlete's foot

Common sites of fungal infection
Fungi grow best in warm, moist areas of the body.

FUNGAL GROWTH

Spore — Hyphae — Spores

1 Many fungal colonies originate from spores that have been carried in the air and have settled at a suitable site for growth.

2 If nutrients are available and other conditions (such as temperature) are favorable, a spore starts to divide.

3 The cells of many fungi divide to form a network consisting of branched chains of tubular filaments called hyphae.

4 Eventually a colony may start forming its own spores. They may be carried to new sites to set up new growths.

---

ing symptoms, such as hallucinations, feeling unreal, or an unstable mood.

Fugues are uncommon. Causes include *dissociative disorders, temporal lobe epilepsy, depression, head injury,* and *dementia.* (See also *Amnesia.*)

Fulminant

A medical term used to describe a disorder that develops and progresses suddenly and with great severity. The term is usually applied to an infection that has spread rapidly through the bloodstream to affect several organs and cause a high fever.

The term may also be applied to types of arthritis in which many joints are painful and stiff and deformities appear soon after the onset of symptoms, or to a cancer that has spread rapidly to cause dramatic weight loss and debility.

Fumes

See *Pollution.*

Functional disorders

This term is generally used to describe illnesses in which there is no evidence of organic disturbance even though the patient's physical performance is impaired.

Fungal infections

Diseases of the skin or other organs caused by the multiplication and spread of *fungi.* Fungal infections, also known as *mycoses,* range from the mild and unnoticed to the severe and sometimes fatal.

In addition to infections, fungi can also cause a number of allergic disorders, such as *asthma* and allergic *alveolitis.*

CAUSES
Some fungi are harmlessly present all the time in areas of the body such as the mouth, skin, intestines, and vagina, but are prevented from multiplying through competition from bacteria. Other fungi are dealt with by the body's *immune system* (defenses against infection).

Fungal infections are more common and serious in people who are taking long-term *antibiotic drugs* (which destroy the bacterial competition) and in those who are taking *corticosteroid* *drugs* or taking *immunosuppressant drugs* (used to suppress the immune system). Fungal infections more commonly affect people with an immune deficiency disorder, such as *AIDS.* Such infections are described as opportunistic infections because they take advantage of the victim's lowered defenses. *Aspergillosis, candidiasis, cryptococcosis* and *nocardiosis* are typical opportunistic infections. Some fungal infections are also more common in people with *bronchiectasis, diabetes mellitus, emphysema, tuberculosis,* and *Hodgkin's disease.*

Fungi that cause skin infections thrive in warm, moist conditions, such as may occur between the toes especially in the summer months, and in the genital area year-round.

TYPES
Fungal infections can be broadly classified into superficial infections (those that affect the skin, hair, nails, genital organs, and the inside of the mouth, producing diseases such as athlete's foot and ringworm); subcutaneous infections (those beneath the skin); and "deep" infections (those affecting

tissues of major internal organs, such as the lungs or, more rarely, the liver, bones, lymph nodes, brain, heart, or urinary tract).

SUPERFICIAL INFECTIONS The main superficial fungal infections are *candidiasis* (thrush) and *tinea* (including ringworm and athlete's foot), both of which are very common. Candidiasis is caused by the yeast CANDIDA ALBICANS and usually affects the genitals or inside of the mouth. Tinea affects external areas of the body.

SUBCUTANEOUS INFECTIONS These are rare. The one most commonly seen is called *sporotrichosis* and may follow contamination of a scratch. Most other conditions of this type occur mainly in tropical countries, the most important being *mycetoma* (sometimes called Madura foot).

DEEP INFECTIONS These are rare or uncommon (although becoming more common), but can be a serious threat to people who have an immune deficiency disorder or who are taking immunosuppressant drugs. Fungal infections of this sort include *aspergillosis*, *histoplasmosis*, *cryptococcosis*, and *blastomycosis*, all caused by different fungi. The fungal spores enter the body by inhalation into the lungs. Candidiasis can also spread from its usual sites to infect the esophagus, urinary tract, and numerous other internal sites.

Fungi

Simple parasitic life-forms including molds, mildews, yeasts, mushrooms, and toadstools. There are more than 100,000 different species of fungi with widely different characteristics worldwide. Of these, most are either harmless or positively beneficial to human health, including various yeasts used in baking and brewing, some molds that are the source of certain antibiotic drugs, and various edible mushrooms and truffles that are considered gastronomic delicacies in many parts of the world. Of the edible varieties, only a few—the mushroom being the most notable—have been successfully cultivated. This usually occurs in caves or special buildings where growth can take place in the dark under controlled temperature and humidity.

There are, however, also a number of fungi that can cause sometimes fatal disease and illness in humans. There is evidence, too, that the toxic effects of particular fungi can vary among people, so what may be consumed without harm by one may be fatal to another. For example, some Siberian tribes use as an intoxicant a species of mushroom that is ordinarily poisonous to humans.

Fungi are particularly abundant in the tropics, but certain species also appear during the short summers in the Arctic. Numerous fungi are found in water, both fresh and saltwater. The study of fungi and fungal diseases is known as mycology.

Except for the absence of chlorophyll, fungi and algae are similar structurally. Some fungi, notably the yeasts, occur as colonies of individual cells. In others, the cells divide to form chains of tubular filaments called hyphae, which are organized into a complex network called a mycelium. By and large, mycelia are colorless although they may contain pigments of every color.

With some soil-living fungi, parts of the mycelium form into large fruiting bodies, seen as mushrooms, puff balls, or toadstools. Many fungi form minute bodies called spores, which are like seeds. These spores can be carried in the air and, if they settle in a suitable location with nutrients available, they divide to form a new mycelium; the molds that eventually form on exposed food are a type of mycelium. Fungal spores are ever present in the air and soil.

FUNGI AND DISEASE

Fungi can cause illness and disease in a variety of ways.

First, the fruiting bodies of some soil-living fungi contain toxins that can produce direct poisoning if eaten (see *Mushroom poisoning*).

Second, certain fungi that infect food crops produce dangerous toxins that can cause a type of food poisoning if contaminated food is eaten. The best known of these are a fungus that infects rye and other cereals and produces a toxin called *ergot*, and another that grows on peanuts and produces the poison *aflatoxin*. Ergot poisoning is rare today, but chronic aflatoxin poisoning from eating moldy peanuts is a suspected cause of liver cancer in some regions of Africa.

Third, the inhaled spores of some fungi can cause a persistent allergic reaction in the lungs, known as allergic *alveolitis*. Farmers' lung, caused by spores from moldy hay, is an example of such a reaction. Fungal spores are also sometimes responsible for other allergic disorders such as *asthma* and allergic *rhinitis* (hay fever).

Fourth, some fungi are able to invade and form colonies within the lungs, in the skin, beneath the skin, or sometimes in various tissues throughout the body, leading to conditions ranging from mild skin irritation to severe, even fatal illness.

The outstanding characteristic of a systemic fungal infection is its chronic course. It develops slowly and symptoms—fevers, chills, night sweats, anorexia, weight loss, general malaise, and depression—are rarely acute. Years may elapse before the patient seeks medical attention for the condition. Caught early, fungal diseases have an excellent prognosis. Surgery and chemotherapy may be part of the treatment prescribed.

Diagnosis may be difficult because symptoms of fungal disease resemble those of other diseases such as cancer and tuberculosis. In fact some researchers claim that many people once treated for tuberculosis may not have had that disease at all but rather were suffering from fungal lung infections. (See *Fungal infections*.)

Fungicidal

A term describing an ability to kill *fungi*. (See *Antifungal drugs*.)

Funny bone

Popular term for the small area at the back of the *elbow* where the ulnar nerve passes over a prominence of the humerus (upper arm bone). A blow to the nerve causes acute pain, numbness, and a tingling sensation in the forearm and hand.

Furosemide

A loop diuretic used to reduce *edema* due to kidney, heart, or liver disease. Furosemide increases the loss of potassium through the kidneys, and should be used in conjunction with potassium supplements or a *potassium-sparing* diuretic.

Furuncle

Another name for a *boil*.

G6PD deficiency

An inherited disorder that affects the chemistry of red blood cells, making them prone to damage by infectious illness or certain drugs or foods.

CAUSES AND INCIDENCE

G6PD deficiency is caused by the production within red blood cells of abnormal molecules of an enzyme (a type of protein) called glucose-6-phosphate dehydrogenase. Because the molecules of this substance are defective, they cannot carry out their normal function, which is to help in a chemical process that protects the cells from damage.

The disorder is the result of an abnormality in the affected person's genetic material and is inherited in an X-linked recessive pattern (see *Genetic disorders*). This means that most of those affected are male, but women may carry the defective gene in a hidden form and pass it on to some of their sons. The disorder is very rare in people of northern European stock but affects as many as 15 percent of southern Europeans and black males.

The drugs that can precipitate hemolysis (red cell destruction) in affected people are listed in the accompanying table. In one form of G6PD deficiency, known as *favism*, affected people are extremely sensitive to a chemical in broad beans, which they must avoid eating.

SYMPTOMS

A few days after taking a precipitating drug or food, or during the course of an infectious illness, a person with G6PD deficiency develops symptoms of hemolytic *anemia* (such as jaundice, fatigue, headaches, shortness of breath on exertion, and sometimes darkening of the urine due to the destruction of red blood cells).

DIAGNOSIS AND TREATMENT

The presence of G6PD deficiency can be established by a blood test. The deficiency cannot be treated but any episode of hemolytic anemia caused by a drug can be halted by stopping use of the drug. Full recovery then takes place within a few days.

Anyone with a history of G6PD deficiency in the family should ask for a screening test before taking any of the incriminated drugs. If the test result is positive, these drugs should be avoided. Anyone known to have the condition should also seek prompt treatment for any infectious illness to prevent a hemolytic crisis.

GABA

Common abbreviation for gamma-aminobutyric acid, a *neurotransmitter* (chemical released from nerve endings that conveys messages within the nervous system). GABA controls the flow of nerve impulses by blocking the release of other neurotransmitters (e.g., *norepinephrine* and *dopamine*) that stimulate nerve activity. The activity of GABA is increased by *benzodiazepine drugs* and by *anticonvulsant drugs*.

It has been suggested that people with *Huntington's chorea* (a hereditary disease characterized by mental retardation and involuntary movements) have insufficient GABA-producing nerve cells in the brain centers that coordinate movement.

Gait

The style or manner of *walking*. Some neuromuscular disorders are evaluated on the basis of altered gait.

Galactorrhea

Spontaneous, persistent production of milk by a woman who is not pregnant or lactating (producing milk after childbirth), or, very rarely, production of milk by a man.

CAUSES

Lactation is initiated by a rise in the level of *prolactin* (a hormone produced by the pituitary gland). Galactorrhea is caused by an excessive amount of prolactin being secreted as a result of a *pituitary tumor* or as a result of other endocrine diseases, such as *hypothyroidism*. Certain *antipsychotic drugs* (such as chlorpromazine) and some

brain diseases (for example, *meningitis*) may be associated with increased prolactin production. However, in about 50 percent of cases, no cause can be found.

SYMPTOMS AND SIGNS

The breast secretion is obviously milk-like. If it is of any other color or blood-stained, another cause (such as a breast tumor) should be suspected. Excessive levels of prolactin may also adversely affect the ovaries, causing *amenorrhea* (absence of menstrual periods) or *infertility*. If the underlying cause is a pituitary tumor, the symptoms may include headache and visual disturbances.

TREATMENT

Surgery or *radiation therapy* may be required if there is a pituitary tumor, but the symptoms are often controlled and the size of the tumor decreased by treatment with *bromocriptine*.

In addition to treating the underlying cause, hormone or drug therapy may be used to suppress prolactin and thus prevent milk production. Bromocriptine, which suppresses prolactin production, can successfully treat galactorrhea when the cause is unknown, and in most instances may also allow the subsequent return of periods and fertility.

Galactosemia

An extremely rare inability of the body's biochemical system to change galactose (a sugar derived from the milk sugar lactose) into glucose because of the absence of an enzyme in the liver. Galactosemia is caused by an autosomal recessive genetic defect (see *Genetic disorders*).

SYMPTOMS

Galactosemia causes no symptoms at birth, but jaundice, diarrhea, and vomiting soon develop and the baby fails to gain weight. If untreated, the condition results in liver disease, *cataract* (opacity in the lens of the eye), and *mental retardation*.

DRUGS TO BE AVOIDED BY PEOPLE WITH G6PD DEFICIENCY

Class	Drugs to avoid
Antimalarial drugs	Primaquine, chloroquine, quinine*, dapsone
Antibacterial and antibiotic drugs	Nitrofurantoin, sulfonamides (such as co-trimoxazole and sulfacetamide), chloramphenicol*, nalidixic acid
Analgesics (painkillers)	ASA
Miscellaneous	Vitamin K (water-soluble form), probenecid, quinidine*

*These drugs do not usually cause problems in the type of G6PD deficiency that affects black people.

DIAGNOSIS AND TREATMENT

The diagnosis is confirmed by urine and blood tests. Feeding with a special lactose-free milk leads to dramatic improvement; normal milk must be avoided throughout life.

Gallbladder

A small, pear-shaped sac situated underneath the liver, to which it is attached by fibrous tissue. *Bile* produced by the liver passes to the gallbladder by means of a small tube, the cystic duct. This duct branches off from the bile duct, which carries bile from the liver to the duodenum.

Within the gallbladder, bile is stored and concentrated (by absorption of its water content through the gallbladder walls). When food passes from the stomach to the duodenum, secretin and cholecystokinin (gastrointestinal hormones) cause the gallbladder to contract and expel bile into the duodenum, where the bile emulsifies fats contained in the food. (See also *Biliary system*.)

Gallbladder cancer

A rare cancer of unknown cause, occurring mainly in old age. It usually occurs in gallbladders with *gallstones*, but affects only a minute number of gallstone sufferers. There are about 600 new cases of this cancer in Canada each year.

The cancer may cause *jaundice* and tenderness in the upper right abdomen but is sometimes symptomless. It is diagnosed by *ultrasound scanning*; occasionally, the cancer is discovered during surgery on the gallbladder.

Cancer of the gallbladder is treated by removal of as much of the tumor as possible. The cancer has often invaded the liver by the time it is detected, making the outlook poor.

Gallium

A metallic element whose radioactive form is used in *radionuclide scanning* (a technique for obtaining images of internal organs). Gallium is injected into the bloodstream and, about 72 hours later, scanning is performed.

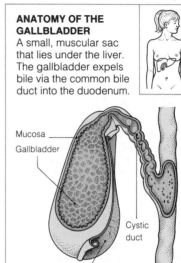

ANATOMY OF THE GALLBLADDER

A small, muscular sac that lies under the liver. The gallbladder expels bile via the common bile duct into the duodenum.

Mucosa

Gallbladder

Cystic duct

Serous coat

Common bile duct

G

DISORDERS OF THE GALLBLADDER

The gallbladder rarely causes problems in childhood or early adulthood but, from middle age onward, the increasing occurrence of gallstones can sometimes give rise to symptoms.

Because the digestive system can function normally without a gallbladder, its removal has little known long-term effect.

CONGENITAL AND GENETIC DEFECTS

Abnormalities present from birth may include no gallbladder, an oversized gallbladder, or two gallbladders; these defects rarely cause problems.

METABOLIC DISORDERS

The principal disorder of the gallbladder, with which most other problems are associated, is the formation of *gallstones*. Gallstones are common, but only about 20 percent of people with gallstones have symptoms or complications. Attempts by the gallbladder to expel the stone or stones can cause severe *biliary colic* (abdominal pain). There are three main types of gallstones: cholesterol gallstones, pigment gallstones, and mixed gallstones. The great majority are cholesterol or mixed gallstones, and women are affected four times as often as men. Every year thousands of people

develop gallstones. Many people carry "silent" gallstones, which produce no symptoms.

INFECTION AND INFLAMMATION

If a gallstone becomes stuck in the outlet from the gallbladder, the trapped bile may irritate and inflame the gallbladder walls and the bile itself may become infected. This is called acute *cholecystitis*. The first symptom may be biliary colic, which is followed by fever and abdominal tenderness.

Repeated attacks of biliary colic and acute cholecystitis can lead to chronic cholecystitis, in which the gallbladder becomes shrunken and thick-walled and ceases to function. Rarely, the gallbladder may become inflamed without the presence of gallstones —a condition that is called acalculous cholecystitis.

Occasionally, cholecystitis proceeds to a condition in which the gallbladder fills with pus, called *empyema* of the gallbladder. This can cause a high fever and severe abdominal pain.

TUMORS

Gallbladders harboring *gallbladder cancer* usually contain gallstones. However, this cancer is extremely uncommon compared to the high prevalence of gallstones.

OTHER DISORDERS

In rare cases where a gallbladder is empty when a stone obstructs its outlet, it may fill with mucus secreted by the gallbladder walls, resulting in a distended, mucus-filled gallbladder known as a *mucocele*.

INVESTIGATION

Gallbladder problems are investigated by physical examination and techniques such as *ultrasound scanning*, *radionuclide scanning*, or *cholecystography* (X rays of the gallbladder after it has been filled with radiopaque substance). Blood tests may also be carried out.

Gallium tends to accumulate in tumors and pus; its main uses in scanning are to detect malignant diseases, such as *Hodgkin's disease*, and abscesses or areas of *osteomyelitis*.

Gallstones

Round or oval, smooth or faceted lumps of solid matter found in the *gallbladder* (the sac under the liver where bile is stored and concentrated). Gallstones are sometimes found in the bile ducts (which connect the gallbladder and liver to the duodenum). In these cases, the symptoms can be severe. There may be one to 10 or more stones, ranging in size from about 1 to 25 mm across. Gallstones composed principally of *cholesterol* are the most common type, but some contain a high content of bile pigments and other substances, such as calcium compounds.

CAUSES AND INCIDENCE
Gallstones develop when an upset occurs in the chemical composition of bile. This most commonly occurs when the liver either puts too much cholesterol into the bile (which occurs in obesity) or fails to put in enough of the detergent substances that normally keep cholesterol in solution.

Excess cholesterol in the bile may lead to the formation of solid cholesterol fragments, which may build up to form stones. In some cases, this process may be triggered by bacteria within the gallbladder. Fasting for long periods may help gallstones to develop by causing bile to stagnate in the gallbladder.

Gallstones are rare in childhood and become progressively more common with age. Two to three times more women than men are affected by gallstones; autopsies show that 20 percent of all women have gallstones when they die.

Risk groups include overweight people and women who have had many children. Use of oral contraceptives may cause gallstones to form earlier than they would otherwise.

PREVENTION
People should avoid becoming overweight and should limit their consumption of sugar and fat. Some experts believe a high intake of fiber helps prevent gallstones and that drinking one alcoholic drink a day has a protective effect.

SYMPTOMS
Only about 20 percent of gallstones cause symptoms or complications. Symptoms commonly begin only when a gallstone gets stuck in the duct leading from the gallbladder. This causes *biliary colic* (intense pain in the upper right side of the abdomen or between the shoulder blades) and may make the sufferer feel sick and possibly vomit. Indigestion made worse by fatty foods often seems to be associated with gallstones. Flatulence is common. Other possible complications include *cholecystitis* (inflammation of the gallbladder) and *bile duct obstruction* leading to jaundice.

DIAGNOSIS AND TREATMENT
Ultrasound scanning can detect 95 percent of gallstones and is therefore the first test to be performed. An older and slightly less sensitive method is X-ray oral *cholecystography*, which utilizes an iodine-containing dye taken by mouth. Blood tests may also be performed. If the physician suspects that the gallstones may have escaped into the bile ducts, *cholangiography* may be carried out.

Stones that do not cause symptoms can safely be left alone, as they are unlikely to cause trouble. When symptoms are severe, *cholecystectomy* (surgical removal of the gallbladder) is carried out; this cures the problem in 95 percent of cases.

In some cases, drug treatment may be used, especially if the stones are small and do not contain calcium. Drug treatment with *chenodeoxycholic acid* or *ursodeoxycholic acid* can dissolve stones over a period of several months. X rays or ultrasound scans of the gallbladder are performed to check progress. However, stones recur after drug treatment is stopped in about 50 percent of cases, and ultrasound scans are therefore carried out to monitor patients for the following few years.

OUTLOOK
New treatments are being developed. Extracorporeal shock-wave *lithotripsy* uses shock waves to shatter the stones. In another technique a tube is inserted into the gallbladder and a strong solution that dissolves cholesterol is flushed through. The safety and long-term value of these treatments is still being investigated.

Gambling, pathological
Chronic inability to resist impulses to gamble, resulting in personal or social problems. Most gamblers can stop at a given point; pathological or "compulsive" gamblers seem unable to control the amount they spend and are unable to stop even when they continue to lose. The urge to gamble is so great that tension can be relieved only by more gambling. Family problems, bankruptcy, and crime may be the consequences.

Gamma globulin
A substance prepared from human blood that contains *antibodies* against most common infections. (See *Immunoglobulin injection*.)

Ganglion
A cystic swelling associated with the sheath of a *tendon*. It is a common condition and usually occurs on the wrist, although a finger or foot may sometimes be affected. The cyst, which contains thick fluid derived from the synovial fluid that lubricates tendons and joints, can vary from the size of a small pea to, rarely, the size of a golf ball.

A ganglion may disappear spontaneously; if it does not, treatment is usually necessary only if the cyst is painful or unsightly. The fluid may be sucked out with a needle and syringe, but ganglions treated in this way commonly recur. The best treatment is surgical removal, after which ganglions rarely recur.

Gangrene
Death of tissue, usually as a result of loss of blood supply. It may affect a small area of skin, a finger, or a substantial portion of a limb.

SYMPTOMS
Pain is felt in the dying tissues, but once they are dead they become numb. The affected skin and underlying tissue turn black. Bacterial infection may develop, causing the gangrene to spread and give off an unpleasant smell. There may be redness, swelling, and oozing pus around the blackened area.

There are two types of gangrene (dry and wet). In dry gangrene there is usually no bacterial infection; the deprived area dies because its blood

Gangrene of the foot
This photograph shows a foot with an extensive area of dead tissue, with blackening of the overlying skin.

supply is blocked. This type of gangrene does not spread to other tissues. It may be caused by *arteriosclerosis, diabetes mellitus, thrombosis,* an *embolism,* or *frostbite.* Wet gangrene develops when dry gangrene or a wound becomes infected by bacteria. A particularly virulent type—known as gas gangrene—is caused by a dangerous strain of bacteria that destroys muscles and produces a foul-smelling gas. Gas gangrene has caused millions of deaths in war.

TREATMENT
Treatment of dry gangrene consists of improving circulation to the affected body part before it is too late. If the tissue becomes infected, the patient is given *antibiotic drugs* to prevent wet gangrene from setting in.

If wet gangrene is diagnosed, *amputation* of the affected part is unavoidable. Usually, some of the adjacent living tissue must be removed as well.

Ganser's syndrome
A rare, *factitious disorder* in which a person seeks, consciously or unconsciously, to mislead others regarding his or her mental state.

Ganser's syndrome occurs most often in prisoners. A characteristic of the disorder is the giving of "approximate answers." If presented with a 2 × 2 equation, for example, a Ganser's syndrome victim may say it equals 5. The choice of an answer near the correct one suggests that the person knows the real response. The sufferer also displays symptoms that simulate *psychosis,* such as episodes of intense agitation or stupor.

Gardnerella vaginalis
A bacterium commonly found in the vaginal discharge of women with nonspecific *vaginitis.*

Gargle
A liquid preparation to wash and freshen the mouth and throat, usually not meant to be swallowed. Gargles may contain mouth fresheners, flavorings, *antiseptics,* or local anesthetics. Those containing antiseptics and local anesthetics relieve the irritation associated with sore throats, but do not cure the underlying cause. The home remedy of gargling with salt water is usually equally effective.

Gas
A common name for air or products of intestinal fermentation in the gastrointestinal tract. Gas may be expelled through the mouth (see *Belching*) or passed through the anus (see *Flatus*).

During feeding babies often swallow air, which may accumulate in the stomach and cause discomfort unless they are "burped" by gently patting the back. Air is often swallowed during *hyperventilation.*

Gas-and-air
A mixture of *nitrous oxide* and *oxygen,* used chiefly as an *analgesic drug* (painkiller) during *childbirth.* It is usually available in premixed cylinders and may be self-administered, through a gas mask, as required.

Gastrectomy
Removal of the whole stomach (total gastrectomy) or, more commonly, a part of the stomach (partial gastrectomy). Gastrectomy is a major operation requiring hospitalization and extensive postoperative care.

WHY IT IS DONE
Total gastrectomy is a rare operation used to treat some *stomach cancers.* Partial gastrectomy is fairly common. It is usually performed to deal with *peptic ulcers* (ulcers of the stomach or duodenum), especially ulcers that have failed to heal after changes in diet or drug treatment, ulcers that bleed very badly or perforate (make a hole in) the stomach or duodenal wall.

In the treatment of duodenal ulcers, partial gastrectomy may be combined with *vagotomy* (cutting of the nerves to the acid-secreting part of the stomach) to prevent more ulcers. Partial gastrectomy is sometimes performed to treat cancers located near the stomach's outlet.

HOW IT IS DONE
A general anesthetic is given and the stomach emptied by means of a *naso-*

G

TYPES OF GASTRECTOMY
There are several different types of gastrectomy operations. In total gastrectomy, the whole stomach is removed; in partial gastrectomy, between one half and two thirds of the stomach is removed. There are two common types of partial gastrectomy operation—the Billroth I and the Billroth II.

Esophagus
Duodenum
Stomach
Jejunum

Total gastrectomy
The whole stomach is removed and the esophagus is joined directly to the jejunum (the middle section of the small intestine).

Billroth I gastrectomy
The remaining part of the stomach is joined to the duodenum (the first part of the small intestine).

Billroth II gastrectomy
The surgeon performs a *gastroenterostomy* (a procedure in which the stomach is joined to the jejunum) and seals the end of the duodenum to form a blind loop.

gastric tube (a tube passed through the nose down the esophagus into the stomach). Different gastrectomy procedures are shown in the illustrated box on page 473.

RECOVERY PERIOD

After the operation, the nasogastric tube is left in position to allow digestive secretions to drain. When the volume of these secretions diminishes and normal *peristalsis* (the rhythmic contractions that force food through the digestive system) returns, the patient is given small amounts of water. If these do not cause abdominal pain or nausea, the nasogastric tube is removed. The intake of fluids is gradually increased and, within a few days, a light diet can be started.

COMPLICATIONS

Only about 10 percent of patients suffer complications requiring further treatment after partial gastrectomy. There is a higher risk of complications after total gastrectomy.

Because removal of the stomach disturbs normal digestion, postgastrectomy syndromes (side effects after gastric surgery) develop in some patients. The most troublesome are fullness and discomfort after meals; formation of an ulcer at the new junction between stomach and small intestine; regurgitation of bile, which may lead to *gastritis* (inflammation of the stomach), *esophagitis* (inflammation of the esophagus), and vomiting of bile; diarrhea; and *dumping syndrome* (sweating, nausea, dizziness, and weakness felt soon after eating a meal because food leaves the stomach too quickly). These side effects usually disappear in time, but diet and drug treatment or another operation may be necessary.

Other complications include *malabsorption* (a reduced ability to absorb food, minerals, and vitamins), which may lead to *anemia* or *osteoporosis* (thinned bones). After total gastrectomy, patients cannot absorb vitamin B_{12} and are therefore given monthly injections for the rest of their lives.

Gastric erosion

A break in the surface layer (mucosa) of the membrane lining the stomach. If a break extends deeper than this layer, it is called a gastric ulcer (see *Peptic ulcer*). Gastric erosion occurs in some cases of *gastritis* (inflammation of the stomach lining).

CAUSES AND SYMPTOMS

The causes of gastric erosions are not clear, but many cases are the result of the ingestion of *alcohol*, *iron* tablets,

ASA, or other *nonsteroidal anti-inflammatory drugs* (NSAIDs), such as phenylbutazone or indomethacin. The stress of serious illness, such as *septicemia* or *kidney failure*, or of *burns* may bring on a gastric erosion. Often there are no symptoms, although erosions may bleed, resulting in *vomiting blood* or *melena* (black feces containing blood). Slight but persistent blood loss may eventually cause *anemia*.

DIAGNOSIS AND TREATMENT

Gastric erosions are diagnosed by *gastroscopy* (examination of the stomach by means of a flexible viewing instrument), which reveals small bleeding points in the stomach lining.

Gastric erosions usually heal completely in a few days when treated with *antacid drugs* and with *ulcer-healing drugs*, such as cimetidine, ranitidine, or famotidine.

Gastric ulcer

A raw area in the wall of the stomach caused by a breach of its inner surface lining. (See *Peptic ulcer*.)

Gastritis

Inflammation of the mucous membrane that lines the stomach. The illness may be acute, occurring as a sudden attack, or chronic, developing gradually over a long period.

CAUSES

Acute gastritis may be caused by irritation of the stomach lining by a drug, most commonly *ASA*; by *alcohol*; by infection of the stomach by a bacterium of the *CAMPYLOBACTER* genus; or by extreme physical stress such as *head injury*, severe *burns*, or the development of *liver failure*.

Chronic gastritis may be caused by prolonged irritation of the stomach by alcohol, *tobacco-smoking*, or *bile*; by an *autoimmune disorder* that damages the stomach lining (see *Anemia, megaloblastic*); or by degeneration of the stomach lining with age.

SYMPTOMS

Gastritis produces similar symptoms to a gastric ulcer, with which it may be confused. Symptoms include discomfort in the upper abdomen (often aggravated by eating), nausea, and vomiting. In acute gastritis, the feces may be blackened by blood lost from the stomach; in chronic gastritis, slow blood loss may cause anemia (see *Anemia, iron-deficiency*), resulting in symptoms such as pallor, tiredness, and breathlessness.

DIAGNOSIS AND TREATMENT

The diagnosis is made using *gastroscopy* (direct examination of the stom-

ach lining through a flexible viewing instrument called a gastroscope). A stomach *biopsy* (removal of a sample of tissue for analysis) may be performed at the same time, using an attachment at the end of the gastroscope. Microscopic examination of the sample indicates the type of inflammation. The correlation between the microscopic findings and the symptoms is not always clear.

A person with gastritis should take *acetaminophen*, not *ASA*, for pain relief, should avoid alcohol, and should not smoke. *Ulcer-healing drugs*, especially *bismuth* preparations, may help heal the inflamed stomach lining.

Gastroenteritis

Inflammation of the stomach and intestines, often causing sudden and sometimes violent upsets. The illness does not usually last for more than two or three days and the sufferer tends to recover without any specific treatment other than replacement of lost fluid and salt. *Dysentery, typhoid fever, cholera, food poisoning,* and *travelers' diarrhea*—as well as many milder stomach upsets—are all forms of gastroenteritis.

CAUSES AND INCIDENCE

Gastroenteritis is an extremely common cause of mild illness in developed countries and a major cause of death in some developing ones, especially among infants.

The illness may be caused by any of a variety of bacteria, bacterial toxins, viruses, and other small organisms that have contaminated food or water supplies. There are also a number of noninfectious causes of gastroenteritis—for example, *food intolerance*, very spicy foods, certain irritant drugs and poisons, and excessive intake of *alcohol*. In many people, *antibiotic drugs* cause symptoms similar to those of gastroenteritis because the drugs can upset the balance of bacteria that occur naturally in the intestines.

SYMPTOMS

The onset and severity of symptoms depends on the type and concentrations of the microorganisms, food, or toxic substance causing the illness. Appetite loss, nausea, vomiting, cramps, and diarrhea are the symptoms; these may come on gradually, but more often appear suddenly. The combination of symptoms may be so mild that they cause little disruption to daily routine, or the attack may be so severe that *dehydration, shock,* and collapse occur. Severe symptoms are most likely in babies and the elderly.

DIAGNOSIS

In mild attacks, no detailed inquiries or investigations are usually made, but in more serious cases the physician may try to find out if other people have been affected and may ask about food that has been eaten and any recent travel abroad.

TREATMENT AND OUTLOOK

Mild cases are treated at home. The affected person should rest, preferably in bed, and take plenty of fluids in frequent small amounts. If much fluid is being lost by vomiting and diarrhea, *rehydration therapy* to replace lost fluids is necessary. Ready-prepared salt and glucose rehydration mixtures can be obtained from pharmacists. If commercial preparations are not available, the patient may be given a solution of one teaspoon of salt and eight teaspoons of sugar in a litre of water. Avoid solid food until symptoms subside.

If the illness is severe, hospital treatment may be necessary. Fluids may be given by *intravenous infusion* to replace the vital body salts lost by vomiting and diarrhea. After the acute phase, water and then other clear fluids are given by mouth; if these fluids do not cause further upset, a bland diet is introduced. Treatment with *antibiotic drugs* is reserved for specific bacterial infections such as typhoid fever.

In most cases the illness subsides gradually without any special measures; recovery is usually complete with no complications.

PREVENTION

Care taken in food preparation and hygiene can substantially reduce the chances of gastroenteritis (see *Foodborne infection*; *Food poisoning*). Some protection against typhoid fever and cholera can be acquired by vaccination before traveling to countries where these diseases occur. Avoidance of substances known to cause upset will minimize noninfectious attacks.

Those caring for a person with the symptoms of gastroenteritis should be scrupulous about personal hygiene to prevent the illness from spreading.

Gastroenterology

The study of the *digestive system* and the diseases and disorders affecting it. The major organs involved include the mouth, esophagus, stomach, duodenum, small intestine, colon, and rectum. Diseases of the liver, gallbladder, and pancreas are also included in this specialty.

A specialist in this branch of medicine is called a gastroenterologist.

The work of the gastroenterologist has been revolutionized in recent years by the development of *fiberoptic endoscopes*. Much of the gastrointestinal tract can now be visualized directly by these instruments and samples can be taken for laboratory examination.

The gastroenterologist, whenever possible, treats patients by advising on diet and lifestyle and/or by prescribing medication; if necessary, the gastroenterologist refers patients for surgical treatment.

Gastrointestinal hormones

A group of hormones released from specialized endocrine cells in the stomach, pancreas, and intestine that controls various functions of the digestive organs. Gastrin, secretin, and cholecystokinin are probably the best documented of these hormones. (See illustrated box.)

Other gastrointestinal hormones released by the intestine include motilin, neurotensin, and enteroglucagon; their precise functions are still being studied.

DISORDERS

Disorders produced by gastrointestinal hormones are relatively rare. The most notable example is a tumor of gastrin-secreting cells in the pancreas or the wall of the intestine, a condition called *Zollinger-Ellison syndrome*.

Gastrointestinal tract

The part of the *digestive system* that consists of the *mouth, esophagus, stomach*, and *intestine*; it excludes the liver, gallbladder, and pancreas.

Gastrojejunostomy

A surgically created connection between the stomach and the jejunum (the middle two thirds of the small intestine). Gastrojejunostomy is occasionally combined with partial *gastrectomy* (removal of the lower part of the stomach).

WHY IT IS DONE

The operation was formerly performed as part of the treatment of a duodenal ulcer (see *Peptic ulcer*) but is now rare. The purpose of gastrojejunostomy is to allow food to pass directly from the stomach to the small intestine, thereby avoiding faulty emptying arising as a complication of *vagotomy*, or permitting a bypass around a duodenum that is scarred and obstructed.

HOW IT IS DONE

The patient is given a general anesthetic and the stomach is emptied by means of a *nasogastric tube* (a tube passed through the nose down the esophagus into the stomach). If the gastrojejunostomy is to be combined with partial gastrectomy, some of the lower part of the stomach is removed.

G

HORMONES IN THE DIGESTIVE TRACT

Hormones released from endocrine cells in the stomach, pancreas, and intestine aid digestion by stimulating the release of bile from the gallbladder and enzymes from the pancreas into the duodenum.

Cholecystokinin
Released by the duodenum in response to fats and acid, cholecystokinin causes the gallbladder to squeeze bile into the duodenum and stimulates the production of pancreatic enzymes, which pass into the duodenum through the pancreatic duct.

Secretin
Secreted by the lining of the duodenum in response to acid entering from the stomach, secretin acts on the pancreas to increase the output of bicarbonate, which neutralizes acid from the stomach. It also increases the release of enzymes from the pancreas.

Gastrin
Secreted mainly by cells in the stomach in response to eating food (especially protein), gastrin causes the stomach to produce more acid and stimulates contraction of muscle in the wall of part of the stomach, ileum, and colon. This contraction propels food through the digestive tract.

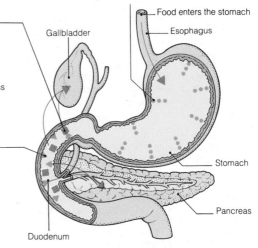

Food enters the stomach
Esophagus
Gallbladder
Stomach
Pancreas
Duodenum

The surgeon then pulls up the first part of the jejunum and stitches it to the lower part or remnant of the stomach; a new opening is made through which food will pass to the small intestine. The nasogastric tube is left in position for a few days after the operation to allow digestive secretions to drain. The intake of fluids is gradually increased after the operation and, after a few days, a light diet can be started.

Gastroscopy

Examination of the lining of the esophagus, stomach, and duodenum (first part of the small intestine) by means of an *endoscope* (long, flexible viewing instrument), called a gastroscope or esophagogastroduodenoscope, inserted through the mouth.

WHY IT IS DONE

Gastroscopy is used to investigate symptoms, such as severe pain in the upper abdomen or bleeding from the upper gastrointestinal tract, and to look for disorders of the esophagus, stomach, and duodenum. The procedure may also be used to assess how these disorders are responding to treatment. Gastroscopy is used to identify the source of bleeding and sometimes to treat bleeding sites in the esophagus, the stomach, and the duodenum.

Special attachments at the end of the instrument enable the physician to remove *biopsy* samples (small amounts of tissue for microscopic examination).

Various other procedures may be carried out using a gastroscope, such as injecting *esophageal varices* (abnormally enlarged veins in the esophagus) or *esophageal dilatation* (stretching) of an *esophageal stricture*. The gastroscope is also used to facilitate passage of a gastric feeding tube through the skin (see *Gastrostomy*).

HOW IT IS DONE

The procedure is performed when the stomach is empty; patients are therefore asked to fast for at least six hours beforehand. In most cases, a *sedative drug* is given to relax the patient and a local anesthetic may be sprayed onto the back of the throat. A general anesthetic may be used if a patient appears particularly anxious or if elaborate investigations or treatments are required.

A diagnostic examination usually lasts for between five and 20 minutes. Some discomfort may be felt as the tube passes down the throat; there may be a sore throat afterward.

Complications from gastroscopy are rare. Most are caused by inhalation of vomit or adverse reactions to sedative drugs.

Gastrostomy

A surgically produced opening in the stomach, usually connecting the stomach to the outside so that a feeding tube can be placed in the stomach or passed into the small intestine.

Gastrostomy may be performed on people who are starving from cancer of the esophagus (see *Esophagus, cancer of*) or who are unable to chew and swallow due to a *stroke* or other neurological disease. (See also *Feeding, artificial*.)

Gauze

An absorbent, open-weave fabric, usually made of cotton. For medical purposes it is usually sterilized and sealed in a package.

Gauze is often used as a *dressing* for wounds. It can be applied dry or can be immersed in an *antiseptic* fluid or cream; a bandage or adhesive tape is used to hold it in place. The gauze absorbs blood and other fluids oozing from the wound. Gauze is usually not used to dress skin ulcers because it tends to stick to moist surfaces and, when removed, dislodge new tissue.

Surgeons sometimes insert pieces of gauze into wounds during surgery to soak up blood and keep the operation site clear.

Gavage

The process of feeding liquids through a *nasogastric tube* (one passed into the stomach through the nose). (See *Feeding, artificial*.)

Gavage also refers to hyperalimentation (treatment of a patient by excessive feeding beyond the requirements of appetite).

Gay bowel syndrome

A combination of conditions affecting the anus, rectum, and colon that occurs mainly, but not exclusively, in male homosexuals.

The conditions in gay bowel syndrome result from various types of sexual activity, such as penile-anal contact, oral-anal contact, and fisting (insertion of the fist into the rectum). Gay bowel syndrome includes noninfectious disorders, such as *hemorrhoids*, *polyps*, foreign bodies in the rectum, and injury to the anus and rectum. *Proctitis* (inflammation of the rectum) is common and there may

also be *anal fistulas*, rectal abscesses, and rectal ulcers. Infections occurring in gay bowel syndrome include anal warts (see *Warts, genital*), amebiasis, viral *hepatitis*, *gonorrhea*, *syphilis*, *shigellosis*, and *lymphogranuloma venereum*.

Gemfibrozil

A drug that lowers the levels of fats (*lipids*) in order to reduce the risk of atherosclerosis, which leads to coronary heart disease and stroke. It is usually given to people with *hyperlipidemia* only after a low-fat diet has failed to reduce blood fat levels significantly. Gemfibrozil may cause nausea and diarrhea, and is contraindicated in people with kidney or liver disease.

Gender identity

The inner feeling of maleness or femaleness. Gender identity is not necessarily the same as biological sex. Gender identity is fixed within the first two to three years of life and is reinforced during puberty; once established, it usually cannot be changed. Gender role is the public declaration of gender identity—that is, the image people present outwardly that confirms their inner feelings about their gender.

Gender identity problems occur when a person has persistent feelings of discomfort about his or her sexual identity. *Transsexualism* is the most common example of this problem.

Gene

A unit of the material of heredity. In physical terms, a gene consists of a short section of the substance *DNA* (deoxyribonucleic acid) contained within the nucleus of a cell. In functional terms, a particular gene has a specific influence on the workings of a cell; the activities of the same gene in many different cells specify a particular physical or biochemical feature of the whole body (e.g., hair color or a chemical step in the digestion of food).

Every human cell holds, within its nucleus, more than 50,000 different genes. Through the sum of their effects, genes influence and direct the development and functioning of all organs and systems within the entire body. In short, they provide an instruction manual or program for growth, survival, reproduction, and possibly also for aging and death.

Each of a person's cells (with the exception of egg and sperm cells) contains an identical set of genes. This is because all the cells are derived, by a process of division, from a single fertilized egg, and with each division the genes are copied to each offspring cell. Within any cell, however, some genes are active and others are idle, according to the specialized nature of the cell.

If the genes from any two people (other than identical twins) are compared, they always show a number of differences. These differences account for all or much of the variation among people in such aspects as gender, height, skin, hair and eye color, and body shape, and in susceptibility to certain diseases and disorders (see *Genetic disorders; Inheritance*). Genes also influence intelligence, personality, physical and mental talents, and behavior, although the extent of their contribution here is less clear-cut because environment and learning also play an important role.

GENE STRUCTURE AND FUNCTION

The physical material of inheritance, DNA, is an extremely long, chainlike structure. Together with some protein, it makes up the 23 pairs of *chromosomes* in the nuclei of all cells. A gene corresponds to a small section of DNA within a chromosome.

All genes fulfil their function, or exert an influence in cells or in the body at large, by directing the manufacture of particular proteins. (See illustrated box overleaf.)

Although many proteins have a particular structural or catalytic role in the body, others are synthesized solely for the purpose of influencing the activity of other genes, which they are able to switch "on" or "off." These genes responsible for making these proteins are termed "control" genes. The whole process of development and growth can be thought of as being programmed by the sequential switching "on" or "off" of particular genes; this control program is exceedingly complex.

The activities of control genes help differentiate, for example, between nerve and liver cells, where quite different sets of genes are active or idle. If the control genes are disrupted, cells may lose their specialist abilities and begin to multiply out of control; this is the probable mechanism by which cancers and other tumors are started (see *Carcinogenesis; Oncogenes*).

MUTANT GENES

Whenever a cell divides, copies of all of its genetic material are made for the two daughter cells by the process of DNA replication (see *Nucleic acids*) and chromosomal division (see *Meiosis; Mitosis*). However, the copying process is not perfect, and very occasionally a fault occurs, leading to a *mutation* (change) in the nucleic acid sequence; this, in turn, alters the structure of the DNA in one of the daughter cells—and thus leads to a

change in one of its genes. This mutant gene is then passed on each time the cell subsequently divides. If a gene mutation occurs during the formation of an egg or sperm cell that later takes part in fertilization, the person who develops from the fertilized egg will have the mutant gene present in each of his or her cells.

Carrying a mutant gene can have various effects. In some cases, it affects the structure of the protein whose manufacture is directed by the gene. Depending on the importance of the protein and the change in its structure, this usually has a disadvantageous effect, ranging from mild to lethal. Moreover, the mutant gene may be passed on to some of the person's own children. Diseases or disorders that result from such mutant genes are termed *genetic disorders*. Very rarely, genetic mutations occur that have a positively beneficial effect.

ALLELES, DOMINANCE, AND RECESSIVENESS

The consequences of inheriting a mutant gene are influenced by further factors. For every protein in the body, there are normally two genes capable of directing the manufacture of that protein—one inherited from the mother and one from the father. These may or may not be identical. The two genes are carried at the same location on each of a pair of chromosomes. If one of the genes mutates, leading to production of an altered

G

WHERE DO YOUR GENES COME FROM?

A person's genes are inherited from his or her parents. Half come from the mother and half from the father via the egg and sperm cells. Each parent provides a different selection, or "mix," of his or her genes to each child; this accounts for the marked differences in appearance, health, and personality among most brothers and sisters. Everyone holds a copy of his or her genes within each body cell.

Gene transmission

In this diagram, only eight genes are shown—in reality, each cell in the body contains about 50,000 genes. Half of them come from the mother and half from the father—thus a quarter of the genes originate from each of the four grandparents.

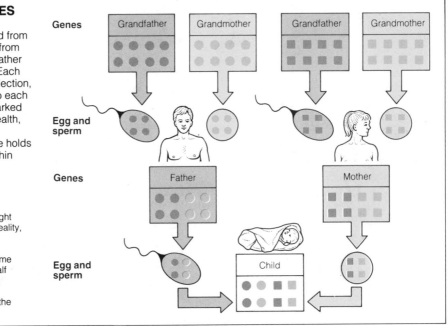

G

WHAT GENES ARE AND WHAT THEY DO

Genes are units of hereditary material contained in a person's cells. They hold information for all aspects of bodily growth and development, exerting their effects by directing the manufacture of proteins. All of a person's genes come from his or her parents. The physical differences between people, such as in eye, hair, and skin color, arise from slight differences in gene structure.

DNA PRINTOUT

Through painstaking laboratory research, the exact structure of many genes is now known.

```
TTC-GAG-CAT-CTG-GGG-ATG-
TCA-TGT-CCT-TCA-TCG-TTT-
TGA-TTA-CCG-ACC-CCA-TCG-
TAT-GAC-ACG-CAA-GTT-CCG-
CGG-TCA-CGC-ACG-TCA-TGT-
GGG-GAC-TCG-TAA-TCA-CGT-
CAA-GCG-AGT-TTA-AAT-AGA-
CGA-CGC-AGC-TTT-GAA-TTC-
TAT-AAC-TAC-TAA-CTG-TTA-
TTG-TTA-TGT-GAT-GGG-TTA-
ATG-AGC-GGA-GTG-CAT-TAT-
```

This printout shows a small part of the DNA base sequence in the gene that codes for the protein trypsin, a digestive enzyme.

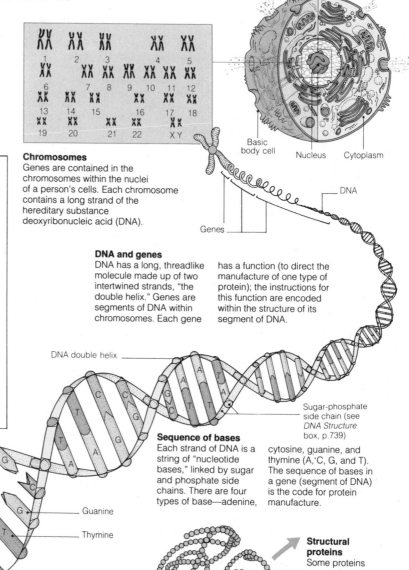

Chromosomes
Genes are contained in the chromosomes within the nuclei of a person's cells. Each chromosome contains a long strand of the hereditary substance deoxyribonucleic acid (DNA).

Basic body cell

Nucleus

Cytoplasm

Genes

DNA

DNA and genes
DNA has a long, threadlike molecule made up of two intertwined strands, "the double helix." Genes are segments of DNA within chromosomes. Each gene has a function (to direct the manufacture of one type of protein); the instructions for this function are encoded within the structure of its segment of DNA.

DNA double helix

Sugar-phosphate side chain (see *DNA Structure* box, p.739)

Sequence of bases
Each strand of DNA is a string of "nucleotide bases," linked by sugar and phosphate side chains. There are four types of base—adenine, cytosine, guanine, and thymine (A, C, G, and T). The sequence of bases in a gene (segment of DNA) is the code for protein manufacture.

Guanine

Thymine

Adenine

Cytosine

Decoding apparatus
To decode a gene, a negative copy of it is made, using the gene as a template; this copy (called messenger RNA) then passes to the cytoplasm of the cell for decoding (see *Protein synthesis*).

Protein molecule

Protein molecule
The information in a gene is decoded to make a protein molecule, which is folded and consists of a string of amino acids.

Structural proteins
Some proteins are used as structural components of cells, tissues, and organs.

Enzymes
Other proteins are enzymes, which promote important chemical processes vital to bodily growth and functioning.

protein, it can often be "masked" by the presence of a normal gene on the other chromosome of the pair.

In fact, the gene at any particular location on a chromosome can exist in any of various forms, called alleles, consisting usually of a normal form and one or more mutant forms, which cause the production of altered proteins. If the effects of a particular allele mask or override those of the allele at the same location on its partner chromosome, it is said to be dominant. The masked allele is recessive.

Dominant genetic traits, such as brown eyes and blood group A, are those in which the allele producing the trait needs to be present only in a single dose for it to have an outwardly apparent effect. Recessive traits, such as blue eyes and blood group O, are those in which an allele for the trait must usually be present in a double dose for it to have an outward effect.

The patterns by which various traits and disorders are passed on from parents to children, including the further complication of sex-linked and multifactorial inheritance and disorders, are discussed under *Inheritance* and *Genetic disorders*. Medical advice on genetic matters—for example, to parents on the chances of an intended child being affected by a particular genetic disorder—is the province of *genetic counseling*.

Generalized anxiety disorder

A neurotic illness in which the main symptoms are chronic and persistent apprehension and tension about nothing in particular ("free-floating anxiety"). There may also be physical reactions such as trembling, sweating, lightheadedness, and irritability.

Symptoms may be so severe that they interfere with everyday living and require medical attention. Psychological treatments (such as *psychotherapy*) or drugs may be helpful, although *sedative drugs* and *tranquilizer drugs* are kept to a minimum because dependence can result. (See also *Anxiety; Anxiety disorders*.)

General paralysis of the insane

The late stage of mental and physical deterioration that occurs in untreated or unsuccessfully treated *syphilis*.

General practice

A term for the medical practice of a non-specialized physician who is often the patient's first point of contact with the medical care system, and who may offer continuous and comprehensive medical care. The term is gradually being replaced by *family physician*. At present, a physician may practice under either designation.

Generic drug

The common term "generic drug" is not strictly correct. Any drug licensed for public use has three kinds of names: a chemical name, a generic (nonproprietary) name, and at least one brand (proprietary) name.

In Canada, the generic name is chosen by drug experts and approved by Health and Welfare Canada (HWC). The generic name will apply to a single, therapeutically active drug recognized or recommended for public use by government agencies such as HWC's Health Protection Branch, and organizations such as the World Health Organization and the British Pharmacopoeia Commission. A generically named drug may also be marketed under one or more brand names. For example, diazepam is the generic (nonproprietary) name for a drug sold under the brand (proprietary) names Apo-Diazepam, Nova-Dipam and Valium.

"Generic prescribing" is a more useful term than "generic drug." Generic prescribing occurs in two situations. A physician may write a prescription using a generic rather than a brand name or, because of certain regulations, the pharmacist may be required to fill the prescription with the cheapest form of the drug—unless the physician specifically forbids it. A drug sold under a generic name usually costs less than one sold under a brand name.

Genetic code

The inherited instructions, contained in chemical form within the nuclei of cells, that specify the activities of cells and thus the development and functioning of the whole body. The term "genetic code" is also used more widely to include the system by which the instructions are copied from a cell to its offspring, the chemical basis by which the instructions are encoded, and the "key" by which the coded instructions are translated.

The basis of the genetic code is contained within molecules of the long, chain-like substance deoxyribonucleic acid (DNA). DNA, along with some protein, makes up the *chromosomes* present in the nuclei of cells. A particular *gene*, or unit of inheritance, corresponds to a section of DNA within a chromosome. Each gene contains the coded instructions for a cell to manufacture a particular protein, which may be an *enzyme* with a vital role in the cell's activities or may have some other function or structural use in the body. Most biochemical activity in the body stems from the manufacture of proteins under the guidance of genetic coding.

Little was known about how bits of DNA could specify the manufacture of proteins until the chemical structure of DNA was worked out in 1953. It was found that DNA consists of two long intertwined strands (the "double helix"), each consisting of a sequence of simple chemicals called nucleotide bases. Four different types of base—adenine, cytosine, guanine, and thymine, ordinarily abbreviated to the letters A, C, G, and T—occur in DNA. The sequence of these bases along particular sections of one of the strands provides the instructions for protein manufacture.

The bases A, C, G, and T can be thought of as the letters of the code. Their sequence along a section of DNA (for example, CGGATCCTAGTTGATCATGAC) would be completely meaningless without the key to the code, employed by the cell's decoding apparatus. This decoder reads the bases three at a time, and each triplet of bases codes for a particular amino acid, the chemical unit from which proteins are made. For example, the base sequence ACG in a section of DNA codes for the amino acid cysteine and the sequence TGA codes for threonine. As triplets of nucleotide bases are read in turn, the corresponding amino acids are brought together and linked, and, as a complete sequence of bases is read, a chain of amino acids (a polypeptide chain) is formed. This may be a protein molecule itself or may form part of a larger protein structure. Certain base triplets, found at the end of gene sequences, code for termination of *protein synthesis*.

A complication of the system is that the decoding apparatus does not read directly from DNA but from an intermediary substance, messenger *RNA* (ribonucleic acid). The DNA acts as a template for RNA manufacture which in turn provides the coded instructions necessary for protein synthesis.

See *Nucleic acids* for a description of the process by which DNA is copied and passed on from each cell to its offspring (and via egg and sperm cells to a new individual).

G

Genetic counseling

Guidance given (usually by a physician with experience in genetics) to a person or persons who are considering having a child but are concerned because there is a blood relative (perhaps a previous child) with an inherited disorder, or because they are at risk for some other reason of bearing a child with such a disorder.

In most cases, genetic counseling entails predicting the chances of recurrence of a condition that has already affected one or more members of a family. Such counseling depends on a correct diagnosis of the disorder. The counselor can then explain why the disorder occurred and how it is inherited.

Genetic counseling also includes discussing the outlook for an affected child, advising couples about contraception if they decide not to have children or not to have any more children, and discussing the alternative routes to parenthood.

WHO IS COUNSELED?

Counseling is important for parents of a child with a *genetic disorder*, such as cystic fibrosis or hemophilia, or a *chromosomal abnormality*, such as Down's syndrome or Turner's syndrome. It may be useful if a child is born with *birth defects*, such as a cleft lip or congenital heart disease, and may be helpful in many other conditions, such as epilepsy, mental retardation, or abnormal sexual development. Counseling may be useful for prospective parents if there is a history of any of these conditions in a blood relative, or if a woman has had several *miscarriages* or *stillbirths*.

Genetic counseling may also be advisable in cases of first-cousin marriages and advanced maternal age.

HOW IT IS DONE

Genetic counseling may be provided by a clinical geneticist, by a pediatrician, or by the family physician.

The counselor makes a pedigree (family tree) of the family. This includes details of any diseases in the family, any blood relationship between partners, or any history of miscarriages. Information from death certificates or postmortem reports of relatives may also be needed.

When a couple have already had an abnormal child, the counselor will ask if there was any exposure to radiation or drugs during pregnancy, or if there was any injury to the child at birth, as these can cause abnormalities in otherwise healthy families. The counselor examines the affected child and his or her parents and arranges for any necessary tests, such as *chromosome analysis*. Certain conditions, such as Down's syndrome, sometimes result from abnormalities in the parents' chromosomes.

For many genetic disorders, it is now possible to establish with some certainty whether or not the parents of an affected child are "carriers" of a defective gene, which can significantly affect the chances of recurrence. Although the actual genes are not identified, DNA markers (fragments of genetic material known to be close to the defective gene on a chromosome) have been identified, and these can be looked for on the parents' chromosomes by advanced laboratory techniques (see *Genetic probe*), which are becoming more readily available.

Virtually every case investigated by a genetic counselor is unique. Several factors may influence the chances of a disorder recurring, and, in some cases, complex mathematical calculations must be carried out to estimate the risk for a couple.

WHAT IT CAN OFFER

When a couple have had an abnormal child, an important aspect of counseling is the explanation of how it occurred and how the child will progress, including the chances of the child having children and whether they, too, will be affected.

Otherwise, advice consists mainly of an estimate of the risk of occurrence or recurrence of the disorder in question. The couple's decision to have children or to have more children of their own depends partly on how they view the risk estimate; and also on other factors, such as the severity of the disorder, the burden an affected child would place on the family, and the availability of alternative routes to parenthood.

The decision on the best course of action is left to the parents after they have had detailed discussions with the counselor and feel satisfied that they understand the condition in question and its implications.

When there is a significant risk of producing an abnormal child, the parents may choose to try for a healthy child (allowing the pregnancy to continue to term only if no abnormality is found during prenatal testing). In certain conditions, such as spina bifida, Down's syndrome, hemophilia, muscular dystrophy, and cystic fibrosis, prenatal diagnosis by *amniocentesis* or *chorionic villus sampling* can reveal (with reasonable accuracy) an abnormality early in pregnancy. In such cases, an induced abortion may be chosen if an abnormality is found.

If a couple decide against having children, options for parenthood include adoption and *artificial insemination* by donor (the mother's egg is fertilized by a donor sperm). The latter is worth considering if both parents are carriers of a rare inherited condition or if the father has a dominant genetic disorder.

Test-tube fertilization of a donor egg by the father's sperm, in cases where the mother carries an abnormal gene, is not yet widely available.

Genetic disorders

Any disorder caused, wholly or partly, by a fault or faults in the inherited, genetic material in a person's cells—that is, in the *genes*, which are formed from *DNA* (deoxyribonucleic acid) and make up the *chromosomes* in the cells. A large number of diseases have a genetic cause.

Many genetic disorders are apparent at birth and are thus also *congenital*. However, the terms genetic and congenital are not synonymous; many genetic defects do not become apparent until many years after birth, and many congenital abnormalities are not genetic in origin.

Many people with a genetic disorder have one or more relatives affected by the same disorder—that is, the disorder is also *familial*. However, there are also occasions when a child is born unexpectedly with a genetic disorder (that is, with no previous family history). There are a number of mechanisms by which this can occur.

CAUSES AND TYPES

The reason abnormal genetic material can lead to disorders or disease is that genes control the manufacture in cells of *enzymes* and other proteins that play roles of varying importance in cells and in the body as a whole. If the genetic material is defective, abnormal proteins (or abnormal amounts of proteins) may be produced, causing disturbances in body chemistry that lead to disease.

For a person to exhibit a genetic disorder, the abnormality in the genetic material must usually be present in each of his or her cells, which means that it must also have been present in either the egg or the sperm cell (or both) from which the individual was derived. There are two ways in which this can happen. The first is that one or both parents carried a defect in their own genetic material; the second is

UNIFACTORIAL GENETIC DISORDERS

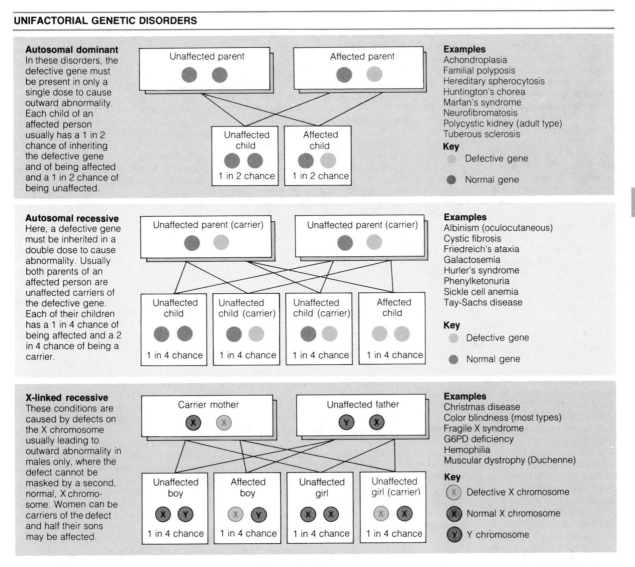

Autosomal dominant
In these disorders, the defective gene must be present in only a single dose to cause outward abnormality. Each child of an affected person usually has a 1 in 2 chance of inheriting the defective gene and of being affected and a 1 in 2 chance of being unaffected.

Unaffected parent | Affected parent

Unaffected child — 1 in 2 chance
Affected child — 1 in 2 chance

Examples
Achondroplasia
Familial polyposis
Hereditary spherocytosis
Huntington's chorea
Marfan's syndrome
Neurofibromatosis
Polycystic kidney (adult type)
Tuberous sclerosis

Key
Defective gene
Normal gene

Autosomal recessive
Here, a defective gene must be inherited in a double dose to cause abnormality. Usually both parents of an affected person are unaffected carriers of the defective gene. Each of their children has a 1 in 4 chance of being affected and a 2 in 4 chance of being a carrier.

Unaffected parent (carrier) | Unaffected parent (carrier)

Unaffected child — 1 in 4 chance
Unaffected child (carrier) — 1 in 4 chance
Unaffected child (carrier) — 1 in 4 chance
Affected child — 1 in 4 chance

Examples
Albinism (oculocutaneous)
Cystic fibrosis
Friedreich's ataxia
Galactosemia
Hurler's syndrome
Phenylketonuria
Sickle cell anemia
Tay-Sachs disease

Key
Defective gene
Normal gene

X-linked recessive
These conditions are caused by defects on the X chromosome usually leading to outward abnormality in males only, where the defect cannot be masked by a second, normal, X chromosome. Women can be carriers of the defect and half their sons may be affected.

Carrier mother | Unaffected father

Unaffected boy — 1 in 4 chance
Affected boy — 1 in 4 chance
Unaffected girl — 1 in 4 chance
Unaffected girl (carrier) — 1 in 4 chance

Examples
Christmas disease
Color blindness (most types)
Fragile X syndrome
G6PD deficiency
Hemophilia
Muscular dystrophy (Duchenne)

Key
X — Defective X chromosome
X — Normal X chromosome
Y — Y chromosome

---

that a *mutation* (a change in the genetic material) occurred during the formation of the egg or sperm cell. Mutations are one of the mechanisms by which a child affected by a genetic disorder can be born into a family that has never had a known history of genetic disorders. With some of the more common genetic disorders, such as Duchenne *muscular dystrophy*, about one third of cases are due to new mutations.

Genetic disorders fall into three broad classes: *chromosomal abnormalities*, unifactorial defects, and multifactorial defects. In the first, a child is born with an abnormal number of whole chromosomes, or extra or missing bits of chromosomes, in the cells.

Since chromosomes contain many genes, this can lead to multiple disturbances and disorders.

Unifactorial disorders are caused by a single defective gene or pair of genes; these disorders are distributed among the members of an affected family according to relatively simple laws of inheritance. Multifactorial disorders are caused by the additive effects of several genes, along with environmental factors; the pattern of inheritance is less straightforward.

UNIFACTORIAL DISORDERS
These disorders are rare, but there are many of them, and in total they cause a considerable amount of disability.

All unifactorial genetic disorders are the result of defects in a gene, or in

a pair of genes, controlling the production of a particular protein. They can be divided into two groups—called sex-linked and autosomal disorders—according to whether the affected gene or genes are located on the sex chromosomes (nearly always the X chromosome) or on any of the other 22 pairs of chromosomes, which are known as autosomes (see *Chromosomes*).

Autosomal disorders generally affect both sexes equally and are further divided into two groups, called autosomal dominant and autosomal recessive, according to whether the defective gene needs to be present in a single or double dose to cause an outward abnormality.

Sex-linked disorders show a bias in their incidence among the sexes. Most are of one type—X-linked recessive disorders—and primarily affect males. Some examples of the three varieties of unifactorial disorder are shown in the table on the previous page.

AUTOSOMAL DOMINANT DISORDERS With these disorders, a person needs to carry the defective gene in only a single dose for it to have an outwardly apparent effect. Such individuals are termed *heterozygotes* with respect to the gene, which means they carry one normal copy and one defective copy of the gene. Because the defective gene is dominant—that is, it overrides the normal gene—its presence usually leads to an outward abnormality (but not always a severe one).

Some affected people have inherited the defective gene from one of their parents. In other cases, there is no family history of the condition and the defect has usually arisen as a result of a mutation.

If an affected individual has children, each one has a 50 percent chance of inheriting the defective gene and of being affected. Often these disorders appear in each of several generations, finally disappearing only when the affected individuals in a generation have no affected children or no children at all.

AUTOSOMAL RECESSIVE DISORDERS People who manifest these disorders have always acquired the particular gene defect in a double dose—they are said to be *homozygotes* with respect to the defective gene. In most cases, both parents of an affected person are heterozygotes—they carry the defective gene in a single dose along with a normal gene. But, because the defective gene is recessive and "masked" by the normal gene, the parents display no outward abnormality.

With all autosomal recessive defects, the number of such carriers in the population always outnumbers those who are actually affected. For example, with *cystic fibrosis* (the most common disorder of this type), one in 22 of the population is a carrier of the defective gene, but only one person in 2,000 is born with the condition. The majority of carriers are unaware of the fact and have no family history of the condition—the defective gene has been passed on to them silently over many generations. When two carriers have children and one is born with an autosomal recessive condition, the manifestation of the defect thus usually comes as a complete surprise.

Because both parents are carriers, any subsequent child will have a one in four chance of also being affected.

X-LINKED RECESSIVE DISORDERS In these conditions, the defective gene is on the X chromosome. Women have two X chromosomes in their cells; men have only one, which they inherit from their mothers and pass on to their daughters.

When a woman inherits the defective gene in a single dose, its effect is masked by the normal gene on her other X chromosome because it is recessive and she displays no outward abnormality. She is a heterozygote carrier of the defective gene. However, when a male inherits the defective gene, there is no normal gene on a second X chromosome to mask it, and he will thus display the abnormality.

The familial pattern of these disorders is as follows. Affected males far outnumber affected females and in all cases have inherited the genetic defect from their mother (who is a carrier). They pass the defective gene to none of their sons but to all of their daughters, who become carriers in turn. Carrier females transmit the defective gene on average to half their sons, who are affected, and to half their daughters, who become carriers in turn. This type of disorder cannot be passed on by an unaffected male. Thus, the pattern is for some of the males in an affected family to have the disorder, while the females in the family are either known or possible carriers.

MULTIFACTORIAL DISORDERS
A large number of disorders fall into this category—including *asthma*, insulin-dependent *diabetes mellitus*, *schizophrenia*, and a number of conditions present at birth, such as *talipes* (clubfoot) and *cleft lip and palate*.

In each case, susceptibility to the disorder is thought to be determined by a number of different genes which, along with environmental influences, have an additive effect. The degree to which susceptibility to each of these various disorders is determined by genes has been estimated and is termed *heritability*.

AFFECTED FAMILIES
The underlying cause of genetic disorders (defects in genes) cannot be treated. However, there are a number of methods by which the chances of a child being born with a genetically based disorder can be reduced.

If a couple is considering having children and if either of them or any of

their parents or close blood relatives has a genetically based disorder, they would be wise to obtain *genetic counseling*. This is especially important if the couple have had a child with a genetically based condition.

Once a pregnancy is established, study of the genetic material in fetal cells obtained by techniques such as *chorionic villus sampling* and *amniocentesis* can establish whether or not certain genetic disorders are present. In cases where a serious disorder is found, a termination of the pregnancy may be considered.

Genetic engineering
A branch of *genetics* concerned, in its broadest sense, with the alteration of the inherited, genetic material carried by a living organism, in order to produce some desired change in the characteristics of the organism.

In practice, the main application of genetic engineering to date has been to mass-produce a variety of substances—all proteins of various sorts—that have uses in medical treatment and diagnosis. The function of any *gene* is to control the production of a particular protein in a living cell. If the gene responsible for synthesizing a useful protein can be identified, and if such a gene can be inserted into another cell that can be made to reproduce rapidly, then a colony of cells containing the gene can be grown. The colony will then produce the protein in large amounts.

WHY IT IS DONE
Genetic engineering has been used for producing some human hormones (notably *insulin* and *growth hormone*), some proteins for use in *vaccines* (e.g., against hepatitis), and *interferon*, a substance with potential for treating viral infections. Many other medically useful substances are also genetically engineered, including *factor VIII* (a blood protein used in the treatment of hemophilia) and *tissue plasminogen activator* (TPA), a substance that dissolves blood clots.

HOW IT IS DONE
The main technique for mass-producing useful proteins by genetic engineering is called recombinant *DNA technology*. DNA (deoxyribonucleic acid) is the genetic material in cells that controls the manufacture of different proteins.

The first step is to identify a specific gene within the DNA of a cell that controls the manufacture of a particularly useful protein. This involves a number of highly sophisticated laboratory techniques. The next step is either to extract the gene from the cell or, if the exact chemical structure of the gene can be worked out, to synthesize it.

The final step is to introduce the gene into the DNA of a suitable recipient cell. *Enzymes* can be used to split the recipient cell's DNA at a certain site and so produce a gap into which the gene can be spliced (hence the term recombinant DNA).

The types of cells or organisms suitable for such genetic alteration are those that can subsequently be made to reproduce rapidly and indefinitely. The most popular organisms to date have been the common intestinal bacterium *ESCHERICHIA COLI* and various yeasts, but cells of other organisms, including human cancer cells, have also been used with success.

OUTLOOK
In view of the ease with which some of the bacteria and other organisms used for genetic engineering can reproduce, and the possibility of accidentally creating and liberating highly dangerous microorganisms, doubts have frequently been expressed about the dangers of "tampering with nature" in this way. These dangers are real but are well recognized by researchers in the field, who have produced stringent codes of practice and regulations to ensure safety.

In the future, it may be possible to extend genetic engineering to the manipulation of human genetic material to treat *genetic disorders*.

Genetic fingerprinting
A technique, also known as DNA fingerprinting, which is able to reveal relationships between individuals. Genetic fingerprinting, which was first used in 1984, can be used to prove paternity (see *Paternity testing*) or to identify a criminal suspect by comparing *DNA* samples.

DNA is the genetic material contained in all living cells and can be extracted from blood, semen, and other body tissues. A pattern of chemical signals within the DNA molecule is unique to each person (except for identical twins) and this unique pattern can be used to provide the genetic "fingerprint."

HOW IT IS DONE
A sample, usually a blood sample, is taken from the suspected person and DNA is extracted from it. The DNA is cut into fragments by an *enzyme* and the fragments are separated into bands in an agar gel by a process called electrophoresis. The band pattern is transferred to a nylon membrane, after which a radioactive DNA "probe" is added; the probe binds to specific sequences of DNA on the membrane. X-ray film is placed next to the membrane to detect the radioactive pattern. The film is developed and the unique pattern of bands, known as the genetic fingerprint, becomes visible.

USES
The genetic fingerprint in one sample can be compared with the genetic fingerprint in samples taken from another individual or in forensic samples. In this way, genetic fingerprinting can be used to resolve cases of disputed paternity or maternity, showing with certainty whether an individual is or is not the parent of a particular child. Such information may be needed, for example, to resolve civil paternity disputes or to provide further evidence in immigration disputes.

Genetic fingerprinting has important applications in forensic science. Forensic samples may be analyzed to identify or eliminate suspects. For example, a blood sample at the scene of a crime or a semen sample in a rape case can be analyzed and its genetic fingerprint compared with that of a suspect's sample.

Genetic probe
A specific fragment of *DNA* (deoxyribonucleic acid) used in laboratory tests to determine whether particular gene defects or genetic "markers" are present in a person's or a fetus's genetic material (i.e., the DNA contained in the *chromosomes* of all cells).

Genetic probes have their main use in prenatal diagnosis of *genetic disorders*, and in investigating whether individuals with a family history of a genetic disorder carry the defective gene themselves. This is appropriate for dominant genes that cause disease in adult life, and for recessive genes that do not cause disease in healthy gene carriers but may be passed on by them to their children who would develop the disease.

Some genetic probes detect the abnormal gene directly, and this type of probe can be used to diagnose genetic disorders. However, many defective genes cannot be identified directly, and gene probes have to be used to demonstrate genetic markers, which are themselves harmless, but may be inherited along with a particular defective gene. The inheritance of the defective gene can be predicted by tracking the genetic markers through an individual family.

One of the main laboratory techniques using genetic probes involves isolating DNA from the chromosomes of cells from the person or fetus being tested. This DNA is split up using *enzymes* in a test tube, and the fragments are fixed onto a filter. A radioactively labeled sequence of DNA (the probe) is added, and this will bind to the gene or marker sequence in the DNA of the individual being tested. This binding can then be visualized as a variety of patterns on an X-ray film.

Genetics
The study of *inheritance*—that is, how the characteristics of living organisms are passed from one generation to another, the chemical basis by which such characteristics are determined, and the causes of the similarities and differences among individuals of one species or between different species. More particularly, genetics includes the study of *DNA* (deoxyribonucleic acid), the substance in cells that determines the characteristics of an organism, and of *genes*, which are units of inheritance corresponding to specific bits of DNA.

Particular branches of human genetics include population genetics, which studies the relative frequency of various genes in different human races; molecular genetics, which is concerned with the structure, function, and copying of DNA from one cell to another, and also how *mutations* (changes) occur in DNA; and medical or clinical genetics, which is concerned with the study and prevention of *genetic disorders*.

Genital herpes
See *Herpes, genital.*

Genitalia
The reproductive organs, especially the external (visible) ones. The male genitalia include the *penis*, *testes* (within the *scrotum*), *prostate gland*, seminal vesicles, and associated ducts, such as the *epididymis* and *vas deferens*. The female genitalia include the *ovaries*, *fallopian tubes*, *uterus*, *vagina*, *clitoris*, *vulva*, and *Bartholin's glands*.

Genitalia, ambiguous
A group of conditions, also known as intersex, in which the external sex organs are not clearly male or female,

or in which the external sex organs resemble those of people with the opposite chromosomal sex.

A person with ambiguous genitalia may have true *hermaphroditism*, possessing both testicular and ovarian tissue, or *pseudohermaphroditism*, possessing only testicular or ovarian tissue. These disorders of sexual differentiation may result from abnormality of the sex chromosomes, abnormality of the testes or ovaries, or a hormonal disorder (see *Sex determination*).

Genital ulceration

An eroded area of skin on the *genitalia*. In men, the ulcer may be on the skin of the penis or scrotum; in women, it may be on the vulva or within the vagina.

CAUSES

The most common cause of genital ulceration is a *sexually transmitted disease*. The early stages of syphilis are characterized by a hard chancre, a painless ulcer at the site where the bacteria penetrated the skin. This may be followed by the development of shallow, elongated ulcers after the chancre has healed. The HERPES SIMPLEX virus may cause painful, fluid-filled blisters to develop on the genitalia; infection of the blisters by bacteria can cause ulceration (see *Herpes, genital*). *Chancroid* is a common tropical bacterial infection that causes painful genital ulcers. *Granuloma inguinale*, also common in the tropics, is a bacterial infection that causes painless genital ulcers. *Lymphogranuloma venereum* is a chlamydial infection resulting in blisters that occasionally ulcerate.

Genital ulceration may also develop as a result of injury or damage, which may occur during sexual intercourse.

Genital ulceration is sometimes a side effect of drugs. It can be caused by solutions applied to genital warts in high concentrations. It can also be a reaction to a drug taken by mouth; *sulfonamide drugs*, for example, can cause mouth and genital ulcers (see *Stevens-Johnson syndrome*).

Behçet's syndrome is a rare condition that causes tender, recurrent ulcers in the mouth and on the genitals. Cancer of the penis or vulva may cause a painless ulcer with raised edges that turn outward.

DIAGNOSIS

The diagnosis of the underlying cause of genital ulceration is made from the appearance of the ulcer and from any other signs, such as enlarged lymph nodes or a skin rash. Swabs from the ulcer are taken and the material is examined and cultured to look for a specific bacterium or virus. Blood tests to detect *antibodies* to a specific type of infection may be performed.

Genital warts

See *Warts, genital*.

Genitourinary medicine

The branch of medicine concerned with *sexually transmitted diseases* and their effects on the *reproductive system*, *urinary tract*, and other parts of the body. There is some overlap between this specialty and *urology* (which deals with reproductive system disorders in men) and *gynecology* (which is concerned with reproductive system disorders in women).

Gentamicin

An *antibiotic drug* given by injection to treat serious infections, or in the form of drops or ointment to treat eye or ear infections.

Gentamicin cannot be given by mouth because it is inactivated by the digestive process. It is given by injection, often in combination with other antibiotic drugs, to treat serious infections, such as *meningitis*, *septicemia* (blood poisoning), and *endocarditis* (inflammation of the heart lining). Because gentamicin can damage the kidneys or inner ear, blood tests may be performed during treatment to determine gentamicin levels in the blood and so allow careful monitoring of the dose.

Gentian violet

A purple dye used mainly by microbiologists to make bacteria visible under the microscope. Gentian violet also has antiseptic properties and was formerly used to treat burns, boils, carbuncles, fungal infections, and mouth ulcers.

Genu valgum

The medical term for *knock-knee*.

Genu varum

The medical term for *bowleg*.

Geriatric medicine

The medical specialty concerned with care of the elderly. Many diseases and disorders that affect the elderly may occur in patients of all ages, but older people tend to respond differently to sickness and treatment. For example, *aging* is associated with a progressive decline in the functioning of major organs—the heart, lungs, kidneys, liver, and brain. Consequently, an infection in one of these organs or elsewhere in the body that would cause only minor illness in a young adult might be life-threatening in an older person. Any illness in an elderly person may cause a temporary but marked slowing of thought processes, and may lead to *confusion* and other features that may be mistaken for *dementia*. This is due to the added stress placed on the brain during the illness. Furthermore, many drugs are eliminated from the body by the liver or kidneys and, if these organs are affected by aging, drug dosages may require modification to avoid dangerous side effects.

A geriatrician is a physician with special training in care of the elderly sick. He or she takes particular care not to give excessive doses of drugs and also tries to avoid moving patients away from familiar surroundings unless hospital admission is essential. The geriatrician is also involved in preparing patients to cope with everyday tasks after they leave hospital, and will make contact with social services and voluntary agencies. (See also *Elderly, care of; Rehabilitation*.)

Germ

 The popular term for any microorganism that causes disease. Examples include *viruses* and *bacteria*. In medicine, the word germ is used in a different sense to describe simple, undifferentiated cells that are capable of developing into specialized tissues, such as the cells of the early embryo.

German measles

Another name for *rubella*.

Germ cell tumor

A growth comprised of immature sperm cells in the male testis or of immature ova (eggs) in the female ovary. A seminoma is one type of germ cell tumor (see *Testis, cancer of*).

Gerontology

The study of *aging* in all its aspects (developmental, biological, medical, sociological, and psychological). The specialty that treats the medical problems of the elderly is called *geriatric medicine* or geriatrics.

Gestalt theory

A school of psychology based on the idea that a sense of wholeness is more important than the individual bits and pieces of perception and behavior. It was founded in Germany early this century by a group that adopted the name gestalt, meaning "form," "pattern," or "configuration". In a broad sense, gestalt refers to any idea based on the notion that the whole is more than the sum of its parts.

In studying emotional states and social issues, Gestalt theory emphasizes viewing things as a whole rather than breaking them down into collections of stimuli and responses. Gestalt therapy became popular as a means of coping with personal problems and is still practiced today by some therapists; this type of therapy aims to increase self-awareness by looking at all aspects of an individual within his or her environment.

Gestation

The period from *conception* to birth, during which the developing infant is carried in the uterus.

Gestation normally lasts around 270 days, about nine months. Because of the difficulty in determining the precise date of conception, physicians time pregnancies from the first day of the last normal menstrual period, giving a gestation period of 284 days. (See also *Childbirth*; *Embryo*; *Fetus*; *Pregnancy*.)

Giardiasis

 An infection of the small intestine, caused by the protozoan (single-celled) parasite GIARDIA LAMBLIA. Giardiasis is most common in tropical areas and in people who have visited the tropics. Recently it has become more common in developed countries, mainly affecting homosexual men, people living in institutions, and preschool children in nurseries. Giardiasis is spread by contaminated food or water or by direct contact with an infected person.

SYMPTOMS
About two thirds of those infected have no symptoms. When symptoms do occur they begin one to three days after the parasite has entered the body. The person has violent attacks of diarrhea accompanied by flatus (wind); the feces are foul-smelling, may be greasy, and tend to float in the toilet bowl. Abdominal discomfort, cramps, and swelling, loss of appetite, and nausea may also occur. In some cases, the infection becomes chronic.

DIAGNOSIS AND TREATMENT
The infection is diagnosed from microscopic examination of a sample

of feces for the presence of the parasites. If there is any doubt, a *jejunal biopsy* (removal of a small sample of tissue for microscopic analysis) may be carried out. Acute giardiasis usually clears up without treatment. However, drug treatment with *metronidazole* quickly relieves symptoms.

PREVENTION
Infection can be prevented by thorough hand washing before handling food and by avoiding food or water that could possibly be contaminated.

Giddiness

See *Dizziness*.

Gigantism

Excessive growth (especially height) resulting from overproduction, during childhood or adolescence, of growth hormone by a tumor of the *pituitary gland*. Untreated, the tumor may eventually destroy the pituitary gland and cause death during early adult life. If the tumor develops after growth has stopped, the result is *acromegaly* rather than gigantism.

Oversecretion of growth hormone from early life can result in an individual attaining an immense height. The tallest documented giant in medical history, Robert Wadlow, reached a height of 2.72 m before he died, aged 22. Such instances are rare, however. By far the most common reason for a child being tall is that his or her parents are tall. Other rare causes of excessive height in childhood are *Marfan's syndrome* and *thyrotoxicosis*.

DIAGNOSIS AND TREATMENT
The diagnosis of gigantism is made when *brain imaging* and blood tests confirm the presence of a pituitary tumor and excessive amounts of growth hormone. The condition may be treated with *bromocriptine*, a drug that blocks the release of growth hormone, or by surgery or *radiation therapy* to remove or destroy the tumor.

Gilbert's disease

An inherited disorder that affects the way in which *bilirubin* is processed by the *liver*.

Gilbert's disease is common, affecting about two per cent of the population. Usually there are no symptoms, but mild jaundice, sometimes with malaise, anorexia, and abdominal pain, may be brought on by an illness. Sufferers are otherwise healthy. No treatment is necessary.

Gilles de la Tourette's syndrome

A rare disorder of movement, named after the French neurologist who first described it in 1885, now commonly termed Tourette syndrome. It starts in childhood with repetitive grimaces and tics, usually of the head and neck, sometimes of the arms, legs, and trunk. Involuntary barks, grunts, or other noises may appear as the disease progresses. In about half the cases, the sufferer has episodes of coprolalia (using foul language).

The syndrome is more common in males, and is probably underdiag-

G

HOW GIARDIASIS IS SPREAD

Giardiasis is spread by contaminated water or food, or by personal contact. This parasitic infection is most common in the tropics, but recently it has become a more frequent occurrence in developed countries, especially among groups of preschool children.

The parasites are acquired from drinking untreated water or food that has been contaminated by sewage or through hand-to-hand or sexual contact with an infected person.

The parasites enter and multiply within the intestines, where they adhere to the intestinal walls.

Symptoms occur 1 to 3 days after infection and include diarrhea and stomach cramps.

The parasites are in the feces and in areas of poor sanitation may contaminate water and food.

nosed because of its strange symptoms. It is usually of lifelong duration but *antipsychotic drugs*, such as *haloperidol*, can provide effective relief in some cases.

Gingiva

The Latin name for the *gums* surrounding the base of the teeth.

Gingivectomy

Surgical removal of part of the gum margin. Gingivectomy may be used to treat severe cases of gingival *hyperplasia* (thickening of the gums), a condition usually caused by the anticonvulsant drug *phenytoin*. Gingivectomy is also used to remove pockets of infected gum formed during the advanced stages of *periodontitis* (gum disease).

Gingivectomy is performed by a dentist using local anesthetic. After surgery, the newly exposed area around the base of the teeth may initially be sensitive; the exposure also makes the teeth appear to be longer. There are no complications as long as scrupulous *oral hygiene* is maintained after surgery.

Gingivitis

Inflammation of the gingiva (gums), often due to infection. Gingivitis is a reversible stage of gum disease.

CAUSES

Gingivitis is usually caused by the buildup of dental *plaque* (a sticky deposit of bacteria, mucus, food particles, and other irritants) around the base of the teeth. It is thought that toxins produced by bacteria within the plaque irritate the gums, causing the gums to become infected, tender, and swollen. Gingivitis can result from injury to the gums, usually from rough toothbrushing or flossing.

INCIDENCE

Mild gingivitis is very common in young adults. Pregnant women and people with *diabetes mellitus* are susceptible because of changes in their hormone levels.

SYMPTOMS

Healthy gums are pink or brown and firm; in people with gingivitis, they become red-purple, soft, shiny, and swollen. The gums bleed easily, especially during toothbrushing, and are often tender.

PREVENTION AND TREATMENT

Good *oral hygiene* is the main means of preventing and treating gingivitis. Teeth should be thoroughly brushed with a *fluoride* toothpaste at least once a day and preferably after all meals;

dental floss should be used at least once a day. A dentist should be consulted at least once a year so that dental plaque and *calculus* (mineralized plaque) can be removed (see *Scaling, dental*). The dentist may recommend a mouthwash for use at home.

COMPLICATIONS

Untreated gingivitis may damage gum tissue around the base of the teeth, leading to the formation of pockets in which plaque and calculus can collect. Bacteria within the plaque may cause inflammation to spread, eventually leading to chronic *periodontitis*, an advanced stage of gum disease in which the supporting tissues of the teeth and the surrounding bone become eroded, loosening the teeth.

Acute ulcerative gingivitis may develop due to invasion of tissue by *anaerobic* bacteria in people with chronic gingivitis, especially those with lowered resistance to infection (see *Gingivitis, acute ulcerative*).

Gingivitis, acute ulcerative

Painful bacterial infection and ulceration of the gums, also known as acute necrotizing ulcerative gingivitis, trench mouth, Vincent's stomatitis, or Vincent's disease.

CAUSES AND INCIDENCE

The condition is caused by abnormal growth of microorganisms which usually exist harmlessly in small numbers in gum crevices. Predisposing factors include poor *oral hygiene*, smoking, throat infections, and emotional stress. In many cases acute ulcerative gingivitis is preceded by *gingivitis* or by *periodontitis*. The condition is relatively rare, primarily affecting young adults aged 15 to 35.

SYMPTOMS

The symptoms appear over the course of a day or two. The gums become sore and inflamed and bleed at the slightest pressure. Craterlike ulcers, which bleed spontaneously, develop on the gum tips between teeth, and there is a foul taste in the mouth, bad breath, and sometimes swollen lymph nodes. As the disease advances, ulcers spread along the gum margins and into deeper tissues. Occasionally, the infection spreads to the lips and the lining of the cheeks, resulting in destruction of tissues (see *Noma*).

TREATMENT

The dentist usually prescribes a mouthwash containing hydrogen peroxide to relieve pain and inflammation. After a few days, when the gums are less tender, scaling (see *Scaling, dental*) is performed to remove

Example of gingivitis
The gums around the bases of the upper teeth are puffy, shiny, and tender. They overhang the teeth margins. Affected gums often bleed when brushed.

dental *plaque* and *calculus* from the teeth. In severe cases, the antibacterial drug *metronidazole* may be prescribed to control infection.

Regular follow-up visits to the dentist may be necessary. Counseling may focus on maintaining oral hygiene, giving up smoking, or learning to cope with stress.

Gland

A group of specialized cells that manufacture and release chemical substances, such as *hormones* and *enzymes*, for use in the body.

There are two main types of glands: endocrine and exocrine. *Endocrine glands* do not have ducts and thus release their secretions directly into the bloodstream; examples include the pituitary, thyroid, and adrenal glands. *Exocrine glands* have ducts and release their secretions either onto the surface of the skin or into a hollow structure such as the mouth or digestive tract; examples include the sebaceous glands, which secrete sebum onto the skin, and the salivary glands. The pancreas releases endocrine secretions (insulin) and exocrine secretions (cholecystokinin).

Lymph nodes (collections of cells in the *lymphatic system*) are sometimes referred to as glands. Strictly speaking, this is an incorrect usage of gland because lymph nodes do not secrete chemical substances. However, they do release white blood cells, which play an important role in fighting infections and in allergic reactions.

Glanders

An infection of horses caused by the bacterium *PSEUDOMONAS MALLEI*, which is only very rarely transmitted to humans.

Initial symptoms include mild fever, headache, general aches and pains, and possibly some generalized swelling of the lymph nodes. Ulcers or abscesses may develop where bacteria entered through the skin; if entry of bacteria was through the lungs, *pneumonia* may develop. In severe cases, *septicemia* (blood poisoning) may then follow. Treatment is with *antibiotic drugs*.

Glands, swollen

Enlargement of the *lymph nodes* (glands) as a result of inflammation and/or proliferation of white blood cells within them. The medical term for this common condition is lymphadenopathy.

CAUSES

Swollen glands are a very common symptom and are usually caused by a minor infection. Children are especially prone to swollen glands as a result of infections, partly because the lymphatic system plays a more important part in combating infections in childhood than in adult life. Swollen glands may also be caused by an allergic reaction (see *Allergy*).

Rarer causes of swollen glands include *Hodgkin's disease* and other forms of *lymphoma* (lymph gland tumor), *leukemia* (cancer of the white blood cells), or a *metastasis* (secondary cancer that has spread from elsewhere in the body).

When the underlying cause affects only a limited area, swollen glands also tend to be localized; for example,

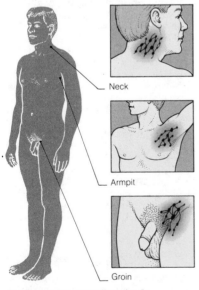

Common sites of swollen glands
The three most common sites where swollen glands can be felt are in the neck, armpit, and groin.

a throat infection may result in swelling only of the lymph glands situated in the neck.

Swollen glands near the surface of the skin—in the groin or neck, for example—are usually felt as tender, slightly warm lumps. However, swelling of deeper glands, such as those in the lungs or abdomen, is almost invariably unnoticeable.

INVESTIGATION AND TREATMENT

In many cases, the cause of swollen glands is obvious from the presence of a localized infection or something such as a bee sting that has caused an allergic reaction. In other cases, the accompanying symptoms usually indicate the cause; for example, swollen glands with a sore throat, fever, and tiredness suggest infectious *mononucleosis* (glandular fever).

If swollen glands persist or there is no obvious cause, tests may be necessary. These may include a blood count, chest X rays to look for swollen glands in the lungs, or a *biopsy* (removal of tissue for microscopic analysis) of an affected lymph node. Treatment depends on the underlying cause. *Antibiotic drugs* may be given for an infection, *antihistamine drugs* for an allergy, and *radiation therapy* and/or *anticancer drugs* for a tumor.

Glandular fever

See *Mononucleosis, infectious*.

Glasses

Simple optical devices used to correct focusing errors in the eyes so that clear vision is achieved. The lenses are made of glass or plastic and the shape and thickness are chosen during an eye test (see *Vision tests*).

TYPES OF LENSES

Lenses may be convex (outwardly curved), concave (inwardly curved), or cylindrical (see illustrated box overleaf). Most are single-vision lenses, but bifocal or trifocal lenses, with smaller areas differing in power from the main lens, are common. Varifocal lenses, with power increasing gradually from the center to one edge, are becoming popular. Lenses may have a permanent tint or may incorporate chemicals that produce darkening on exposure to light.

Glass eye

See *Eye, artificial*.

Glaucoma

A condition in which the pressure of the fluid in the *eye* is so high that it causes damage. A minimal pressure is

required to maintain the shape of the eyeball, but excessive pressure may result in the compression and obstruction of the small blood vessels that nourish the fibers of the *optic nerve*. The result is nerve fiber destruction and gradual loss of vision.

TYPES AND CAUSES

The most common form is chronic simple (open-angle) glaucoma, which rarely occurs before the age of 40 and often causes no symptoms until blindness is advanced. It is due to a gradual blockage of the outflow of aqueous humor (fluid in the front compartment of the eye) over a period of years, causing a slow rise in pressure. This type tends to run in families.

In acute (closed-angle) glaucoma, there is a sudden obstruction to the outflow of aqueous humor from the eye and the pressure rises suddenly. Subacute glaucoma causes similar but transient bouts of acute glaucoma.

Congenital glaucoma is due to a structural abnormality in the drainage angles of the eyes.

Glaucoma can also be caused by injury to the eye, or by a serious eye disease such as *uveitis, lens dislocation,* or adhesions (abnormal bands of tissue) between the iris and the cornea.

PREVALENCE

The prevalence of simple glaucoma requiring treatment because of a visual field defect rises with age, increasing from 0.5 percent at 40 years of age to 7 percent at 80 years. In Canada, glaucoma accounts for about 10 percent of functional blindness in people aged 70 and over.

SYMPTOMS AND SIGNS

Chronic simple glaucoma often causes no symptoms because the gradual loss of peripheral vision is not apparent to the affected person. Only late in the disease, when there is severe, irreversible damage, may the person be aware of some visual loss.

The symptoms of acute glaucoma include a dull, severe, aching pain in and above the eye, some fogginess of vision, and (in subacute bouts) the perception of halos (rainbow rings around lights) at night. Nausea and vomiting may occur and the eye may become red and have a partly dilated pupil and a hazy cornea.

DIAGNOSIS

Chronic simple glaucoma often causes no symptoms and is usually detected only by routine eye examinations. Applanation *tonometry* (measuring the pressure in the eye) is an essential check for glaucoma, especially if there is a family history of the disorder. Use

G

G

WHY GLASSES ARE USED

For *hyperopia* (farsightedness), convex (or plus) lenses are needed. Sufferers of *presbyopia* also need plus (magnifying) lenses. *Myopia* (nearsightedness) requires concave (or minus) lenses.

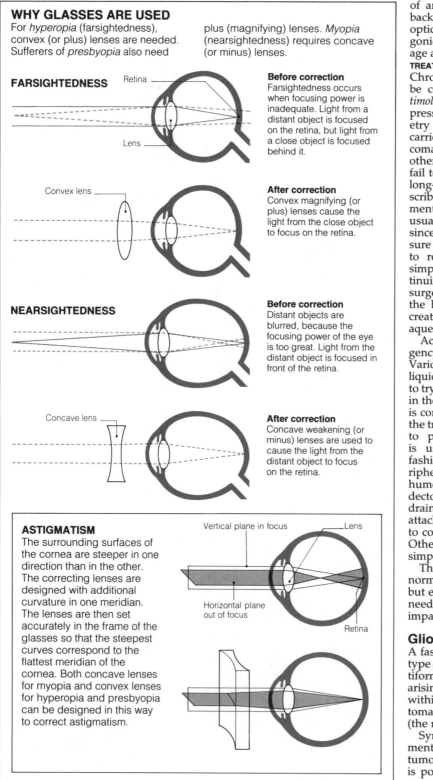

FARSIGHTEDNESS

Retina

Lens

Before correction
Farsightedness occurs when focusing power is inadequate. Light from a distant object is focused on the retina, but light from a close object is focused behind it.

Convex lens

After correction
Convex magnifying (or plus) lenses cause the light from the close object to focus on the retina.

NEARSIGHTEDNESS

Before correction
Distant objects are blurred, because the focusing power of the eye is too great. Light from the distant object is focused in front of the retina.

Concave lens

After correction
Concave weakening (or minus) lenses are used to cause the light from the distant object to focus on the retina.

ASTIGMATISM

The surrounding surfaces of the cornea are steeper in one direction than in the other. The correcting lenses are designed with additional curvature in one meridian. The lenses are then set accurately in the frame of the glasses so that the steepest curves correspond to the flattest meridian of the cornea. Both concave lenses for myopia and convex lenses for hyperopia and presbyopia can be designed in this way to correct astigmatism.

Vertical plane in focus

Lens

Horizontal plane out of focus

Retina

---

of an *ophthalmoscope* to examine the back of the eye may show an abnormal optic nerve. Visual field testing and gonioscopy (examination of the drainage angle) can also be important.

TREATMENT

Chronic simple glaucoma can usually be controlled with eye drops (e.g., *timolol* twice daily), which reduce the pressure in the eye. Repeated tonometry and visual field testing may be carried out to ensure that the glaucoma is being controlled; if necessary, other eye drops will be given. If drops fail to control the pressure, tablets or long-acting capsules may also be prescribed. The medicines for treatment of chronic simple glaucoma usually need to be continued for life since, if they are stopped, the pressure generally rises. If medicines fail to reduce the pressure in chronic simple glaucoma, and if there is a continuing loss of visual field or vision, surgery may be necessary to open up the blocked drainage channel or to create an artificial channel for the aqueous humor.

Acute glaucoma is a medical emergency calling for urgent treatment. Various treatments (eye drops, pills, liquids, intravenous fluids) are given to try to reduce the very high pressure in the eye. Usually, after the pressure is controlled, surgery is necessary for the treatment of acute glaucoma to try to prevent a further attack. This is usually a peripheral *iridectomy*, fashioning a small opening at the periphery of the iris so that aqueous humor can drain more easily. The iridectomy is often curative but, if the drainage angle was damaged by the attack, drug treatment may be needed to control the pressure after surgery. Other types of surgery, as for chronic simple glaucoma, may be necessary.

The pressure rise of glaucoma can normally be prevented by treatment, but early diagnosis and treatment are needed in order to prevent any impairment of vision.

Glioblastoma multiforme

A fast-growing and highly malignant type of *brain tumor*. Glioblastoma multiforme is a type of *glioma*, a tumor arising from glial (supporting) cells within the brain. Most glioblastomas develop within the cerebrum (the main mass of the brain).

Symptoms, diagnosis, and treatment are as for other types of brain tumor. Despite treatment, the outlook is poor, with few patients surviving more than two years.

Acute closed-angle glaucoma
This type of glaucoma is caused by an unduly narrow angle between the iris and the back of the peripheral cornea. Dilation of the pupil may therefore lead to a sudden complete blockage of the outflow, causing a rapid increase in pressure in the eyeball.

Ciliary body
Blocked drainage channel
Cornea
Iris
Aqueous humor
Lens

Glioma

A type of *brain tumor* arising from the supporting glial cells within the brain.

Gliomas make up about 60 percent of all primary brain tumors (originating from the brain rather than spread from elsewhere). There are about 1,800 new cases of primary brain tumors (glioblastomas and glioblastomas multiforme combined) in Canada each year.

Types of glioma include *astrocytoma*, *glioblastoma multiforme* (a highly malignant variety of astrocytoma), *ependymoma* and *medulloblastoma* (more common in children), and *oligodendroglioma*. Symptoms, diagnosis, and treatment are as for other types of brain tumor.

Globulin

Any of a group of proteins characterized by being insoluble in water but soluble in dilute salt solutions; *antibodies* (also known as *immunoglobulins*) are an example.

TYPES
Globulins in plasma can be divided into three main groups, known as alpha-, beta-, and gamma globulins.

Alpha-globulins include alpha$_1$-antitrypsin and haptoglobin. The former is an *enzyme* produced by the

lungs and liver; deficiency is associated with *hepatitis* in children and *emphysema* (a lung disorder) in young adults. Haptoglobin is found in the blood plasma, where it binds together *hemoglobin* (the oxygen-carrying protein in red blood cells) and prevents it from being excreted in the urine by the kidneys. Various other alpha-globulins are produced as a result of inflammation, tissue damage, *autoimmune disorders* (in which the immune system attacks the body's own tissues), or certain cancers.

Beta-globulins consist mainly of low-density lipoproteins (LDLs), substances involved in the transport of fats in the blood circulation, and transferrin, which carries iron in the blood. The amount of beta-globulins is increased in certain types of *hyperlipidemia* (a condition in which abnormally high levels of fats are present in the blood).

All of the gamma globulins are antibodies, which are proteins produced by the immune system in response to infection, as part of an allergic reaction, and after an organ transplant. Gamma globulins may also be produced in any disorder that causes persistent inflammation of an organ, such as *rheumatoid arthritis* or *cirrhosis* of the liver. Certain conditions, such as *multiple myeloma*, result in the production of large amounts of a specific gamma globulin.

Globus hystericus

A condition, also called globus pharyngis, in which there is an uncomfortable feeling of a "lump in the throat." This lump is felt to interfere with swallowing and breathing, sometimes so much so that the sufferer is convinced that he or she cannot breathe. Respiration comes in sighs or gasps, anxiety increases, and *hyperventilation* (rapid breathing) and symptoms of a *panic attack* often

Cross section of a brain
This photograph (taken from an autopsy specimen) shows a large area of brain infiltrated by a glioma (dark color).

ensue. Some patients insist that their Adam's apple has become larger or displaced in some way.

In most cases there is no physical basis for these attacks, which occur most commonly in people who are feeling anxious or depressed. The condition is not life-threatening. Breathing in and out of a small paper bag fitted tightly around the nose and mouth will alleviate the symptoms brought on by hyperventilation.

Unless a physical cause is found, treatment is by reassurance, breath-control training, and, in some instances, psychological treatments (e.g., *psychotherapy*). Use of *antianxiety drugs* or *antidepressant drugs* to treat the condition is rarely helpful.

Glomerulonephritis

Inflammation of the glomeruli (filtering units of the *kidney*). Both kidneys are affected, although not all the glomeruli are affected simultaneously. Damage to the glomeruli hampers the removal of waste products, salt, and water from the bloodstream, which may cause serious complications.

CAUSES AND INCIDENCE
The incidence of glomerulonephritis differs markedly around the world, mainly because some common tropical diseases (such as *malaria* and *schistosomiasis*) are important causes. Although these diseases are rarely responsible for glomerulonephritis in developed countries, glomerulonephritis is still the most common cause of chronic *kidney failure* in North America and Europe.

Some types of the disease are caused by the patient's *immune system* making *antibodies* to eliminate microorganisms—usually bacteria responsible for an infection, such as a *streptococcal infection* of the throat. These antibodies combine with bacterial *antigens* to form particles called immune complexes, which circulate in the bloodstream and become trapped in the glomeruli; this triggers an inflammatory process that may damage the glomeruli and prevent them from working normally. Glomerulonephritis also occurs in some *autoimmune disorders*, such as systemic *lupus erythematosus* (a chronic disease of connective tissues).

SYMPTOMS
Mild forms of glomerulonephritis may produce no symptoms and the disease may be discovered only when a urine sample is tested for some other reason. In some cases, glomerulonephritis comes to light only when

G

489

G

kidney failure has reached an advanced stage and causes symptoms due to the accumulation of waste products and fluid that are usually eliminated in the urine.

Some sufferers experience a dull ache over the kidneys. The urine may become bloodstained because damaged glomeruli can allow red blood cells into the urine. Proteinuria (loss of protein into the urine) may cause *edema* (accumulation of fluid in body tissues), causing swelling of parts of the body (see illustrated box). Such swelling may cause mild puffiness around the eyes.

The combination of proteinuria, low albumin (protein) in the blood, and edema, is called *nephrotic syndrome*. *Hypertension* (high blood pressure) may develop in these circumstances and is a possibly serious complication of glomerulonephritis.

In some cases, glomerulonephritis is severe and sudden, so that kidney failure develops over a few days; sufferers often notice that they are passing very small quantities of urine.

DIAGNOSIS

There are many types of glomerulonephritis and the same cause may produce different types in different individuals. Diagnosis involves *urinalysis* (microscopic and chemical analysis of urine) and *kidney biopsy* (removal of a small amount of kidney tissue for microscopic analysis). *Kidney-function tests* may also be performed to measure how well the kidneys are removing waste products and how much protein is being lost in the urine.

TREATMENT

Treatment usually involves admission to hospital and depends on the type and severity of the disease.

Children with nephrotic syndrome usually respond to treatment with *corticosteroid drugs*, such as *prednisolone*. Glomerulonephritis following a streptococcal infection usually clears up after the infection is successfully treated with *antibiotic drugs*.

In general, adults respond less well to treatment but eventual kidney failure may sometimes be prevented or delayed. Drugs may be prescribed to control hypertension and a special diet may be given to reduce the kidneys' load. A few patients with severe glomerulonephritis respond to treatment with *immunosuppressant drugs* (which dampen the body's natural defense system) or *plasmapheresis* (which rids the bloodstream of immune complexes and substances that damage the glomeruli).

Glomerulosclerosis

Scarring that occurs as a result of damage within the glomeruli (filtering units of the *kidney*).

Mild glomerulosclerosis occurs normally with age; a 10 percent decrease in kidney function is common each decade after a person reaches the age of 30. However, even a 75 percent reduction is compatible with a normal life.

Glomerulosclerosis may occur in some severe types of *glomerulonephritis* that are difficult to treat and in which damage progresses to destroy the kidneys. Typically, patients suffering from this condition develop severe *proteinuria* (the presence of protein in the urine) and severe *edema* (accumulation of fluid in body tissues), resulting in swelling of parts of the body.

Glomerulosclerosis is also found in some people with *diabetes mellitus*. It is seen in reflux nephropathy (kidney damage associated with backflow of infected urine from the bladder) and in some people with *hypertension* (high blood pressure). Intravenous drug abuse may cause glomerulosclerosis. The condition has also been found in some people with *AIDS*.

Glomus tumor

A small, painful, bluish swelling in the skin, usually on a finger or toe near or under the nail, which is tender to touch and more painful if the limb is hot or cold. Glomus tumors result from an overgrowth of glomus bodies, structures with numerous nerve endings that normally control blood flow and temperature in the skin. The tumors are surgically removed.

Glossectomy

Removal of all or part of the *tongue*. Glossectomy may be performed to treat *tongue cancer* although this condition is more commonly treated by *radiation therapy*. If a large part of the tongue is removed, speech is impaired and eating is difficult. A liquid diet is then necessary.

Glossitis

Inflammation of the *tongue*. The tongue feels sore and swollen and looks red and smooth; adjacent parts of the mouth may also be inflamed.

Glossitis occurs in various forms of *anemia* and in *vitamin B* deficiency. Other causes include infection of the mouth (especially by *herpes simplex*), irritation by dentures, and excessive

---

THE EFFECTS OF GLOMERULONEPHRITIS

The glomeruli are damaged as a result of inflammation. Red blood cells and protein leak into the urine.

Protein loss from the circulation causes fluid to accumulate in body tissues, causing edema.

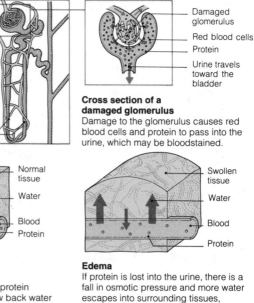

Kidney

Kidney tubule

Damaged glomerulus

Red blood cells

Protein

Urine travels toward the bladder

Cross section of a damaged glomerulus
Damage to the glomerulus causes red blood cells and protein to pass into the urine, which may be bloodstained.

Normal tissue

Water

Blood

Protein

Healthy tissue
Through osmotic pressure, protein molecules in the blood draw back water lost to surrounding tissues.

Swollen tissue

Water

Blood

Protein

Edema
If protein is lost into the urine, there is a fall in osmotic pressure and more water escapes into surrounding tissues, causing swelling.

use of alcohol, tobacco, or spices. A congenital form of glossitis affects the middle portion of the back of the patient's tongue.

Treatment is for the underlying cause. Self-help measures include maintaining good *oral hygiene*, by not smoking, and by avoiding acidic or spicy foods that aggravate the soreness. Regular rinsing of the mouth with a salt solution may help.

Glossolalia
Speaking in an imaginary language that has no actual meaning or syntax. Some Christians regard glossolalia as a sign of possession by the Holy Spirit; scientists tend to view it as a form of *hypnosis* or *hysteria*. (See also *Neologism*.)

Glossopharyngeal nerve
The ninth *cranial nerve*. This nerve performs both sensory and motor functions. It conveys sensations, especially taste, from the back of the tongue, regulates secretion of saliva by the parotid gland, and controls movement of the throat muscles.

Glottis
The part of the *larynx* (voice box) that consists of the vocal cords and the slit-like opening between them.

Glucagon
A hormone produced by the *pancreas* that opposes the action of *insulin*. Glucagon stimulates the breakdown of glycogen (a carbohydrate stored in the liver and muscles) into glucose (sugar). The glucose is then released into the bloodstream, where it is available as a source of energy for cells anywhere in the body. Glucagon thus regulates the level of glucose in the blood; when the level falls, glucagon is released from the pancreas.

USE AS A DRUG
Glucagon is extracted from the pancreas of pigs or cows for use as a drug. It is given by subcutaneous (under the skin) injection in the emergency treatment of people with *diabetes mellitus* who are unconscious as a result of hypoglycemia (low blood sugar). Glucagon produces recovery within 15 to 20 minutes; the patient is then given glucose by mouth to prevent a relapse. Nausea and vomiting are occasional adverse effects.

Glucocorticoids
Hormones produced by the cortex (outer layer) of the *adrenal glands* that affect carbohydrate metabolism by

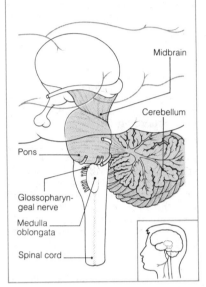

increasing the blood sugar level and the amount of glycogen in the liver. The principal glucocorticoid is *hydrocortisone* (also called cortisol), which also has a *mineralocorticoid* (affecting the body's sodium and potassium balance) effect.

Glucose
A simple sugar (monosaccharide) produced by the digestion of starch and sucrose; also called dextrose. Glucose is a fruit sugar, present in fruits and fruit juices together with fructose. It is the chief source of energy for the body and is carried to all tissues in the blood. The term blood sugar refers to glucose in the bloodstream.

BLOOD SUGAR LEVELS
Despite wide variation in carbohydrate intake (and, therefore, large fluctuations in the amount of glucose in the body), the blood sugar level is normally kept within narrow limits. This is achieved by the actions of several hormones, notably *insulin, glucagon, adrenaline, corticosteroid hormones,* and *growth hormone*. If the blood sugar level is abnormally high (known as *hyperglycemia*), it may cause *glycosuria* (glucose in the urine). An abnormally low blood sugar level is called *hypoglycemia*.

Insulin, released by the pancreas in response to increased blood sugar

levels, lowers the level by stimulating the uptake of glucose by cells. Inside the cells, glucose may be "burned" to produce energy, converted to *glycogen* for storage (mainly in the liver and muscles), or used in the production of triglycerides (fats).

Glucagon is released by the pancreas when the blood sugar level is low. It stimulates the breakdown of stored glycogen to glucose, which is then released into the bloodstream.

Adrenaline and corticosteroid hormones released by the adrenal glands in response to stress have the same basic effect as glucagon—that is, they stimulate the release of glucose to increase the blood sugar level.

Glue ear
Accumulation of fluid in the middle ear cavity, causing impaired hearing. Persistent glue ear is most common in children. It is often accompanied by enlarged *adenoids* and frequently occurs with viral upper respiratory tract infections, such as the common *cold*. Usually both ears are affected. The condition is also known as otitis media with effusion, persistent middle ear effusion, and secretory otitis media.

CAUSES
The mucus-secreting lining of the middle ear cavity sometimes becomes overactive, producing large amounts of sticky fluid. If there is blockage of the *eustachian tube*, the passageway that links the middle ear to the back of the nose, the fluid cannot drain away properly. The fluid subsequently accumulates and eventually interferes with the movement of the delicate bones in the middle ear.

SIGNS
The first, and often the only, sign is some degree of *deafness*. The child may be unaware of this and, unless his or her unresponsiveness is noticed by parents or teachers, the condition may pass undetected.

DIAGNOSIS
Glue ear is sometimes first detected through *hearing tests*, which should be carried out routinely on all children. Once any hearing loss is detected or suspected in a child, a physician uses an *otoscope* (viewing instrument) to examine each eardrum for the characteristic changes in appearance and color that occur in glue ear.

TREATMENT
In mild cases the patient is given nose drops containing *decongestant drugs* to unblock the affected eustachian tube, so that the fluid can drain through it.

G

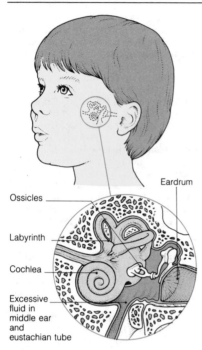

Ossicles

Labyrinth

Cochlea

Excessive fluid in middle ear and eustachian tube

Eardrum

Effects of glue ear
In this condition, sticky fluid in the middle ear prevents free movement of the eardrum and ossicles, causing deafness.

When the condition is severe, a *myringotomy* (a surgical opening in the eardrum to permit drainage of the middle ear cavity) and insertion of a *grommet tube* (to equalize pressure on both sides of the eardrum) may be needed. Removal of the adenoids may also be required (see *Adenoidectomy*).

Glue sniffing
See *Solvent abuse*.

Gluten

 A combination of gliadins and glutenins (types of proteins) formed when certain cereal flours (most notably wheat flour) are mixed with water. Sensitivity to part of the gliadin in gluten causes *celiac disease*.

Gluten enteropathy
See *Celiac disease*.

Gluten intolerance
See *Celiac disease*.

Gluteus maximus
The large, powerful muscle in each of the buttocks which helps give them their rounded shape. The gluteus maximus is responsible for moving the thigh sideways and backward.

Glyburide
An oral *hypoglycemic drug* used to treat non-insulin-dependent *diabetes mellitus*. Glyburide stimulates the pancreas to produce *insulin*, which promotes the uptake of glucose (sugar) into muscle and fat tissue, thereby lowering the level of glucose in the blood.

Glycerine
See *Glycerol*.

Glycerol
A colorless syrupy liquid which has a sweet taste. Glycerol, also known as glycerine, is used in several drug preparations and in the food processing industry.

Glycerol is prepared commercially from *fats and oils*; it is an essential constituent of triglycerides (simple fats). The triglyceride molecule consists of one molecule of glycerol combined with three molecules of fatty acids.

During digestion, glycerol is split from the fatty acids and may recombine with them to form stored fat in the body or be used as a body fuel to provide energy.

In the form of rectal *suppositories*, glycerol relieves *constipation* by softening hard feces. Glycerol is used in moisturizing creams to help prevent dryness and cracking of the skin (for example, it is used to protect the nipples during breast-feeding). Glycerol is also used in eardrops to help soften *earwax* prior to syringing of the ears, and in *cough remedies* to help soothe a dry, irritating cough. Glycerol is sometimes added to foods, such as cakes, to keep them moist.

Glyceryl trinitrate
A *vasodilator drug* used to treat and prevent symptoms of *angina pectoris* (chest pain due to inadequate blood supply to the heart).

Glyceryl trinitrate may cause a headache, flushing, and dizziness. Adverse effects are usually relieved by a reduction in the dose; this can be achieved by putting a tablet under the tongue and then spitting it out when sufficient of the preparation has dissolved to cause the chest pain to cease.

Glycogen
The principal *carbohydrate* storage material in the body. Glycogen is a polysaccharide, consisting of many glucose molecules linked to form long chains, and is found mainly in the liver and in muscles.

Glycogen plays an important role in controlling blood sugar levels. When there is too much sugar (glucose) in the blood, the excess is converted to glycogen. This conversion (controlled by *insulin* and *corticosteroid* hormones) takes place chiefly in the liver and in muscles. When the blood sugar level is low, glycogen is converted back to glucose (a process regulated by the hormones *glucagon* and *adrenaline*) and released into the bloodstream.

Glycosuria
The presence of *glucose* in the urine. Glycosuria results from failure of the *kidneys* to reabsorb glucose back into the bloodstream after the blood has been filtered. Glycosuria by itself does not necessarily indicate that a serious condition is present.

In the normal filtering process in the kidneys, glucose is removed from the bloodstream along with many other normal blood constituents. The filtered fluid passes down the many tubules of the kidneys, where wanted substances are reabsorbed and returned to the bloodstream and unwanted substances are excreted as urine. In most healthy people, glucose is one of the substances that are almost completely reabsorbed.

LOCATION OF THE GLUTEUS MAXIMUS
The top is attached to the sacrum, coccyx, and pelvis. The lower part is attached to the femur (thighbone).

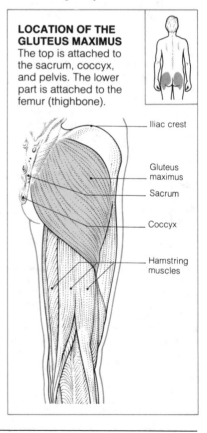

Iliac crest

Gluteus maximus

Sacrum

Coccyx

Hamstring muscles

Glycosuria may be caused by failure of the kidneys to reabsorb all the glucose because of *hyperglycemia* (an abnormally high level of glucose in the blood), as in *diabetes mellitus*.

Alternatively, glycosuria may occur if the kidney tubules have been damaged and are unable to reabsorb even normal amounts of glucose. Damage to the tubules may be a result of rare *metabolic disorders* present from birth or be a consequence of *drug poisoning* or heavy metal poisoning.

Glycosuria also occurs in some healthy people who have kidneys that are unable to reabsorb all the glucose filtered out of the bloodstream. This condition tends to run in families. Glycosuria often occurs during pregnancy as a consequence of hormonal changes; this is usually not serious provided there are no other symptoms and blood glucose is normal.

DIAGNOSIS AND TREATMENT
Glycosuria may be found during a routine examination or if the physician is performing specific tests because diabetes mellitus is suspected. Urine can be tested for glucose by using a chemically impregnated strip that changes color when it comes in contact with glucose. Treatment depends on the underlying cause.

Gnat bites
See *Insect bites*.

Goiter
Enlargement of the *thyroid gland*, visible as a swelling on the neck.
CAUSES
The thyroid gland may enlarge (without any disturbance of its function) at puberty, during pregnancy, or as a result of taking *oral contraceptives*. In many parts of the world the main cause of a goiter is lack of sufficient *iodine* in the diet. The thyroid requires the iodine to produce the hormone thyroxine; a deficiency causes swelling of the thyroid.

A condition known as toxic goiter develops in *Graves' disease* and in other forms of *hyperthyroidism* (overactivity of the thyroid gland) that lead to *thyrotoxicosis*. Typical features of thyrotoxicosis include warm, dry skin, increased appetite, weight loss, tremor, insomnia, and occasional muscle weakness and agitation.

A goiter is also a feature of different types of *thyroiditis* (inflammation of the thyroid gland), including *Hashimoto's thyroiditis* (an autoimmune disorder) and de Quervain's thyroiditis, both of which damage the gland.

Appearance of goiter
The thyroid may become enlarged for various reasons, including dietary deficiency of iodine, inflammation, or an autoimmune disorder affecting the gland.

Other causes of goiter include a tumor or nodule in the gland and, in rare cases, *thyroid cancer*. A goiter can also be caused by drugs given to treat overactivity of the thyroid gland.
SYMPTOMS
A goiter can range in size from a barely noticeable lump to an enormous swelling, depending on the cause. Large swellings may press on the esophagus or trachea, making swallowing or breathing difficult.
DIAGNOSIS AND TREATMENT
Diagnosis is based on the nature of the swelling and any accompanying symptoms. *Thyroid-function tests*, including blood tests and *radionuclide scanning*, may be carried out to determine the activity of the thyroid gland. X rays may be taken to investigate accompanying symptoms.

A goiter that is not caused by disease may eventually disappear or may be so small that it does not require treatment. However, a large or unsightly goiter, or one that is causing difficulty with swallowing or breathing may require total or partial removal (see *Thyroidectomy*).

If iodine deficiency is identified as the cause, the patient will be advised to eat more fish and iodized salt, which are both rich in iodine. When a goiter is the result of disease, treatment will be for the underlying disorder. If a drug is the cause, the goiter usually disappears once the course of treatment is over.

Gold
An *antirheumatic drug* used to treat *rheumatoid arthritis* and, occasionally, arthritis arising as a complication of *psoriasis*. Gold is usually prescribed in severe cases after a *nonsteroidal anti-inflammatory drug* (NSAID) has proved ineffective.
HOW IT WORKS
Gold has an anti-inflammatory action that relieves joint pain and stiffness and may prevent further damage.
POSSIBLE ADVERSE EFFECTS
A common adverse effect of gold is *dermatitis* (inflammation of the skin); if itching occurs, the drug is usually withdrawn. Gold may damage the kidneys, liver, and bone marrow. Blood tests are performed during treatment to check the function of these organs.

Gold may cause loss of appetite, nausea, diarrhea, abdominal pain, and, occasionally, *anaphylactic shock* (a serious allergic reaction that requires emergency treatment).

Golfer's elbow
A condition caused by inflammation of the epicondyle (bony prominence) on the inner side of the *elbow*, at the site of attachment of some forearm muscles. The inflammation causes pain and tenderness at the inner side of the elbow and sometimes in the forearm.

Golfer's elbow is caused by overuse of these muscles, which act to bend the wrist and fingers. Activities that can cause the condition include gripping and twisting (such as using a screwdriver) or playing golf with a faulty grip or swing.
TREATMENT
Treatment consists of resting the elbow, applying ice packs, and taking *analgesic drugs* (painkillers) and/or anti-inflammatory tablets. If the pain is severe or persistent, injection of a *corticosteroid drug* may be helpful.

If the pain is caused by a sport, it is wise to stop playing for a week or two and to seek advice about playing technique.

Gonadotropin hormones
Hormones that stimulate cell activity in the gonads (*ovaries* and *testes*). Gonadotropins are essential for female and male fertility. The two most important gonadotropins are follicle-stimulating hormone (FSH) and luteinizing hormone (LH), which are secreted by the *pituitary gland*. Another gonadotropin, HCG (see *Gonadotropin, human chorionic*), is produced by the placenta.
GONADOTROPIN HORMONE THERAPY
Synthetic HCG is used in the treatment of recurrent *miscarriage* and certain types of female and male

infertility. Menotropin (a gonadotropin extracted from the urine of postmenopausal women) contains both FSH and LH and is used in the treatment of female infertility due to a failure to ovulate.

Gonadotropin, human chorionic

A hormone produced by the *placenta* in early *pregnancy*. Human chorionic gonadotropin (HCG) stimulates the *ovaries* to produce *estrogen* and *progesterone*, hormones needed to maintain a healthy pregnancy.

HCG is excreted in the urine; its measurement forms the basis of most pregnancy tests (a high level confirming pregnancy).

HCG THERAPY

HCG extracted from the urine of pregnant women is given by injection to treat certain types of *infertility*. Along with *clomiphene* tablets, which stimulate gonadotropin release from the pituitary, HCG may induce *ovulation* in women who have not been ovulating. In men, HCG has been used in an attempt to increase sperm production.

HCG is occasionally given to prevent *miscarriage* in women whose production of progesterone is deficient.

HCG is also prescribed for the treatment of cryptorchidism (see *Testis, undescended*) in young boys, although surgical correction is usually required.

Gonads

The sex glands—the *testes* in men and the *ovaries* in women. The testes, situated in the scrotum, produce sperm and secrete the hormone *testosterone*. The ovaries, situated in the abdomen, release usually one ovum (egg) from either the right or the left ovary each month and secrete the hormones *estrogen* and *progesterone*.

The activities of the gonads—both male and female—are regulated by *gonadotropin hormones* released by the pituitary gland.

Gonorrhea

One of the most common *sexually transmitted diseases*, popularly known as "the clap." Gonorrhea occurs throughout the world.

CAUSES AND INCIDENCE

Gonorrhea, caused by the bacterium NEISSERIA GONORRHOEAE, is most often transmitted during sexual intercourse, including oral or anal sex. An infected woman may also transmit the disease to her baby during childbirth.

Gonorrhea is the second most common sexually transmitted disease in Canada, after *nonspecific urethritis*, and is most prevalent among young adults who have had multiple sexual partners.

SYMPTOMS AND SIGNS

Gonorrhea has a short incubation period of two to 10 days. In men, symptoms usually include a urethral discharge and pain on passing urine. About 60 percent of infected women have no symptoms; if symptoms are present, they usually consist of a vaginal discharge or a burning sensation when passing urine.

Infection acquired through anal sex causes gonococcal *proctitis* (inflammation of the rectum and anus). It causes pain and anal discharge in only about 10 percent of infected people. Oral sex with an infected person may lead to gonococcal *pharyngitis*, which may cause sore throat but often causes no symptoms. A baby exposed to infection in the mother's reproductive tract during childbirth may acquire gonococcal *ophthalmia*, a severe inflammation affecting one or both eyes.

COMPLICATIONS

Untreated gonorrhea may spread to other parts of the body. In men, it may cause *prostatitis* (inflammation of the prostate) or *epididymo-orchitis* (inflammation of the epididymides and testes), affecting fertility. In women, untreated gonorrhea affects the fallopian tubes, causing *pelvic inflammatory disease* (PID). Damage to the fallopian tubes causes increased susceptibility to further episodes of PID, increases the risk of an *ectopic pregnancy* occurring in a fallopian tube, and may lead to *infertility*.

Gonococcal bacteria may occasionally spread through the bloodstream to cause gonococcal *arthritis*, with pain and swelling of joints around the body. Multiplication of bacteria in the bloodstream causes *septicemia*, producing generalized symptoms and signs, including fever and malaise. In rare cases, gonococcal septicemia affects the brain or heart and may cause death.

DIAGNOSIS

Many disorders can cause a urethral or vaginal discharge, and laboratory tests are necessary to confirm a diagnosis of gonorrhea. Tests are carried out on a sample of the discharge or on swabs taken from the urethra, cervix, and sometimes the rectum.

TREATMENT

Gonorrhea is treated with an antibiotic, usually a *penicillin drug*, such as procaine penicillin or *ampicillin*. If the infection is caused by penicillin-resistant NEISSERIA GONORRHOEAE or if the infected person is allergic to penicillin, other antibiotics, such as cefotaxime, ciprofloxacin or spectinomycin, may be used. After treatment, tests are performed to ensure that the infection has been cured.

OUTLOOK

Treatment for gonorrhea is effective but does not protect against reinfection. Sexual partners must be told that they might have gonorrhea even if they have no symptoms; many clinics have counselors (known as contact tracers or health advisers) who identify and inform all people who might have been infected by the patient.

Goodpasture's syndrome

A rare condition characterized by *glomerulonephritis* (inflammation of the filtering units of the kidney), coughing up blood, and *anemia*. Goodpasture's syndrome is a serious disease; unless treated early it may lead to life-threatening bleeding into the lungs and progressive *kidney failure*.

Goodpasture's syndrome is an *autoimmune disorder* (one in which the body's *immune system* attacks its own tissues). *Antibodies* are formed that attack the capillaries (tiny blood vessels) in the lungs and kidneys, eventually resulting in inflammation and disruption of the normal functioning of the lungs and kidneys.

The disease usually affects young men, but can develop in women and at any age.

TREATMENT

Mild forms may be treated with *immunosuppressant drugs* (drugs that hamper the normal working of the body's immune system) and *plasmapheresis* (a procedure for removing unwanted antibodies from the blood plasma).

People who suffer from severe and repeated attacks require treatment by *dialysis* (a technique for removing waste products from the blood) and, eventually, a *kidney transplant*.

Good Samaritan laws

The various codes and statutes requiring people to help others who are injured or in danger and protecting those who do are sometimes called Good Samaritan laws. Under such legislation, health professionals are not required to provide care beyond what they are trained and legally licensed to provide. For example, a nurse who arrives at the scene of an accident is not required to perform a physician's function, but only to do what a nurse would normally do. In

Alberta, the Emergency Medical Aid Act relieves anyone of liability who voluntarily comes to the aid of an injured person and acts reasonably in trying to help. In Quebec, the Charter of Human Rights and Freedoms obliges everyone to come to the aid of a person whose life is in peril.

Gout

A metabolic disorder that causes attacks of *arthritis*, usually in a single joint. Gout may be associated with kidney stones (see *Calculus, urinary tract*) which may lead to *kidney failure*.

SYMPTOMS AND SIGNS

An acute attack of gout usually affects a single joint, most commonly the joint at the base of the big toe, but it can affect other joints, including the knee, ankle, wrist, foot, and small joints of the hand.

The affected joint is red, swollen, and extremely tender; the pain reaches a peak level of intensity within 24 to 36 hours. The redness and swelling may spread and be confused with *cellulitis* (inflammation of tissues beneath the skin). The pain is so intense that the sufferer may not be able to stand on an affected foot or even tolerate the pressure of bedclothes on it. Sometimes there is a mild fever.

The first attack usually involves only one joint and lasts a few days. Some people never have another attack, but most have a second attack between six months and two years after the first. After the second attack, more and more joints may be involved, and there may be constant pain due to damage to the joint from chronic inflammation.

TREATMENT

Pain and inflammation in gout can be controlled with large doses of a *nonsteroidal anti-inflammatory drug* (NSAID). *Colchicine* is sometimes prescribed if NSAIDs are not considered suitable. For maximum benefit, treatment should start as soon as an attack begins; patients prone to recurrent attacks should carry their gout medicine with them. As the inflammation subsides, usually within two to three days, the dose is gradually reduced and finally stopped. If an attack of gout is not responding to treatment with an NSAID or colchicine, a *corticosteroid drug* may be injected into the affected joint.

Increased levels of purine (a product of *DNA*) can raise the level of uric acid in the blood. Although a strict low-purine diet is not necessary,

GOUT

Gout is a common joint disease, affecting 10 times more men than women. In men it occurs at any time after puberty; in women it usually occurs only after the menopause. There is often a family history of the

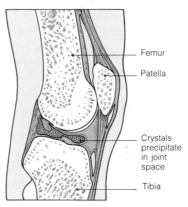

Crystal precipitation
Crystals of uric acid precipitate into the joint space and surrounding tissues of the knee, causing intense inflammation and extreme pain.

Femur
Patella
Crystals precipitate in joint space
Tibia

Appearance of gout
Deposition of uric acid crystals in the joint space has caused inflammation and obvious swelling of the affected right knee.

disorder. Hyperuricemia (excess uric acid in the blood) leads to formation of uric acid crystals in joints; crystals may also be deposited in soft tissues in the ears and around tendons.

DIAGNOSIS
Gout is considered as a diagnosis whenever an attack of arthritis affects a single joint. A blood test is usually performed; a high level of uric acid suggests gout.

Aspiration
Fluid is aspirated (removed through a needle into a syringe) from the swollen knee joint and examined under a microscope.

Microscopic evidence
The presence of uric acid crystals confirms the diagnosis.

people with gout should avoid foods that are high in purine, such as liver and other organ meats, legumes, and poultry. Heavy consumption of alcohol should also be avoided because it may precipitate an acute attack.

Many people never have more than a few attacks of gout, and further treatment is usually unnecessary. If attacks are recurrent, the frequency can be reduced by lowering the urate levels with drugs that either inhibit the formation of uric acid (such as *allopurinol*) or increase the excretion of

uric acid by the kidneys (uricosuric drugs, such as *probenecid* and *sulfinpyrazone*). If the level of uric acid in the blood is very high, drug treatment may be continued for life to prevent *hypertension* or kidney disease.

Grafting

The process of transplanting healthy tissue from one part of the body to another (autografting), from one person to another (allografting or homografting), or from an animal to a person (xenografting).

Grafting is used to repair or replace diseased, damaged, or otherwise defective tissues or organs. Those that are most commonly transplanted (see *Transplant surgery*) include the skin (see *Skin graft*); bone (see *Bone graft*); bone marrow (see *Bone marrow transplant*); the cornea of the eye (see *Corneal graft*); the kidney (see *Kidney transplant*); the heart (see *Heart transplant*); the heart and lungs (see *Heart-lung transplant*); the liver (see *Liver transplant*); the heart valves (see *Heart valve surgery*); and blood vessels and nerves (see *Microsurgery*).

COMPLICATIONS

With autografting, the grafted tissue is usually assimilated at the new site without any trouble and soon grows into the surrounding tissue to provide a good repair.

Problems occur, however, with allografting and xenografting, both of which are usually carried out to replace rather than repair tissue. Xenografting is not performed clinically except for the use of porcine (pig) heart valves. The major disadvantage of allografting is that the recipient's defense system automatically attempts to reject the foreign cells of the donor's tissue and to destroy them in the same way that it would invading microorganisms. The only exceptions are grafts between identical twins (because their tissue matches exactly) and corneal grafting (because the cornea has no blood supply and therefore no white blood cells and antibodies to act as a defense system).

To overcome rejection, as close a match as possible between the tissues of recipient and donor is sought (see *Tissue-typing*). *Immunosuppressant drugs* are given to suppress the body's defense system—although this can cause decreased kidney function. *Cyclosporine*, introduced in the mid-1980s, has been very effective in the control of rejection and *graft-versus-host disease*.

Graft-versus-host disease

A common complication of a *bone marrow transplant*. Graft-versus-host disease is caused by cells called cytotoxic T-*lymphocytes*, present in the transplanted marrow, attacking the transplant recipient's tissues. Lymphocytes form part of the *immune system* and normally play a beneficial role by attacking cells recognized as foreign. However, in transplant procedures, this activity is harmful.

Graft-versus-host (GVH) disease may occur soon after an organ transplant or may appear some months later. The first sign of the disease is usually a skin rash. This may be followed by diarrhea, abdominal pain, jaundice, inflammation of the eyes and mouth, and breathlessness. Most patients recover within a year, but some gradually get weaker and thinner and about one third die.

Graft-versus-host disease can be prevented by giving *immunosuppressant drugs*, such as *cyclosporine*, to all transplant recipients. If the disease develops, it is treated with *corticosteroid drugs* and with other immunosuppressant drugs. It may be possible to prevent GVH in bone marrow transplants by removing cytotoxic T-cells from the donor marrow before the transplant is performed.

Gramicidin

A *topical* antibiotic used for infections of the skin, eyes, and ears. Gramicidin is combined with *nystatin*, another antibiotic, to combat fungal infections, or with *corticosteroids* to reduce inflammation and itching.

Gram's stain

An iodine-based stain widely used in bacteriology to help differentiate between various types of bacteria. It is also known as Gram's iodine.

There are several different methods of Gram staining. Basically, however, the specimen is stained with gentian violet, followed by a solution of Gram's stain, and then treated with a decolorizing agent such as acetone. Finally, the specimen is counterstained with a red dye. Bacteria that retain the dark violet stain are known as gram-positive, whereas those that lose the violet stain after decolorization but take up the counterstain (causing them to appear pink) are gram-negative. Examples of gram-positive bacteria include several species of STREPTOCOCCUS, STAPHYLOCOCCUS, and CLOSTRIDIUM; gram-negative bacteria include VIBRIO CHOLERAE (which causes cholera) and various species of SALMONELLA.

Grand mal

A type of epileptic seizure in which the sufferer, sometimes after warning symptoms, cries out, falls to the ground unconscious, and has generalized jerky muscle contractions. The seizure may last for a few minutes. The person usually remains unconscious for a time and may have no recall of the seizure on awakening. (See also *Epilepsy*.)

Granulation tissue

A mass of red, moist, granular tissue that develops on the surface of an ulcer or open wound during the process of healing. The tissue consists mainly of fibroblasts (which make collagen) and numerous small blood vessels. (See also *Healing*; *Wound*.)

Granuloma

An aggregation of cells, of a type associated with chronic inflammation.

CAUSES AND TYPES

Granulomas usually occur as a reaction to the presence of certain infectious agents or to a foreign body, but may occur in conditions of unknown cause. Certain infections, such as *tuberculosis*, *brucellosis*, *leprosy*, and *syphilis*, although caused by different bacteria, give rise to infective granulomas in many different organs of the body. *Sarcoidosis*, a condition of unknown cause, is also characterized by granulomas in different organs. Granulomas may also occur in parasitic and fungal infections.

A foreign body granuloma can occur as a reaction to inorganic material, such as dust, talcum powder, dirt, or a suture. A pyogenic granuloma is a common benign skin tumor which develops on exposed areas following minor injury and often occurs on the hands of gardeners. The swellings are raised, red, moist, and tender and often disappear gradually without treatment. Pyogenic granulomas can be removed surgically, or by *electrocautery* or *cryosurgery*.

Many other, largely unrelated, conditions are also described as granulomas. For example, a dental granuloma is a swelling arising from poorly fitting false teeth; another type of granuloma is a benign growth on the iris. (See also *Granuloma annulare*; *Granuloma inguinale*; *Granuloma, lethal midline*.)

Granuloma annulare

A harmless skin condition characterized by a circular, raised area of skin, occurring most commonly in children, usually on the knuckles or fingers, and less commonly on the upper part of the feet or on the elbows or ears. The raised area spreads slowly outward to form a ring, 2.5 to 7.5 cm in diameter, with raised edges and a flattened center. Rarely, several of these ringlike patches occur over a wider area. The cause is unknown.

The diagnosis of granuloma annulare is often made simply from its appearance but may be confirmed by means of a skin *biopsy* (removal of a

G

small sample of tissue for microscopic investigation). No treatment is necessary. In most cases, the affected skin heals completely eventually.

Granuloma inguinale

A *sexually transmitted disease* that causes ulceration of the genitals. The infection is caused by bacterialike organisms called Donovan's bodies. Granuloma inguinale is common in certain parts of the tropics, although it is very rare in developed countries.

The first symptoms are painless, raised nodules on the penis or labia or around the anal area. The nodules gradually ulcerate and then form red, raised areas that are usually painless. These areas sometimes contain pus and, if left untreated, may eventually heal with extensive scarring. Diagnosis is based on finding Donovan's bodies in a *biopsy* sample from a sore. The antibiotic drugs *tetracycline* or *gentamicin* are effective treatments.

Granuloma, lethal midline

A rare disorder of unknown cause in which the nose and other facial structures become inflamed and eventually destroyed by progressive damage to the skin and underlying tissues.

Patients with midline granuloma are usually in their 40s or 50s; women are affected more often than men. The first symptoms are usually caused by ulceration within the nose. Tissue destruction may spread to the facial sinuses, the gums, and the orbits (eye sockets).

The most effective treatment is *radiation therapy*, which usually halts the progression of the disease and may improve symptoms for years.

Graves' disease

A disorder characterized by toxic *goiter* (an overactive and enlarged thyroid gland), excessive production of thyroid hormones leading to *thyrotoxicosis*, and sometimes *exophthalmos* (bulging eyeballs). Graves' disease is an *autoimmune disorder* (a disorder in which the *immune system* attacks the body's own tissues).

Gravida

The medical term for a pregnant woman. The term is often combined with a prefix to indicate the total number of pregnancies (including the present one). For example, a primigravida is a woman who is pregnant for the first time, and a secundigravida is a woman who is pregnant for the second time; multigravida is a

general term for a woman who has been pregnant at least once before.

Gray

An SI (International System of Units) unit of radiation dosage (see *Radiation units* box).

Gray matter

Regions of the central nervous system (*brain* and *spinal cord*) consisting principally of closely packed and interconnected nuclei of nerve cells, rather than their filamentous projections or axons, which make up the white matter. In the brain, gray matter is primarily found in the outer layers of the *cerebrum* (the main mass of the brain and the region responsible for advanced mental functions) and in some regions deeper within the brain. Gray matter also makes up the inner core of the spinal cord.

Grief

An intensely unhappy and painful emotion, usually caused by loss of a loved one. (See *Bereavement*.)

Grip

The *hand* is particularly well adapted for gripping, with an opposable thumb (i.e., one that is able to touch each of the fingers), specialized skin on the palm and fingers to provide adhesion, and a complex system of muscles, tendons, joints, and nerves that enables precise movements of the digits.

The hand can perform two basic grips: grasping, which is a strength hold that involves the whole hand, and pinching, which is a precision hold using the thumb and a finger. Both grips are controlled by a combination of long muscles in the forearm and short muscles in the hand itself.

Gripping ability can be reduced by any condition that causes muscular weakness or impairment of sensation in the palms or fingers (e.g., a *stroke* or *nerve injury*) or by disorders that affect the bones or joints of the hand or wrist, such as *arthritis* or a *fracture*.

Grippe

A term of French origin for any illness resembling *influenza*. The term was once used in English-speaking as well as French-speaking countries.

Griseofulvin

A drug given by mouth to treat *tinea* infections (a group of fungal infections) which have not responded to antifungal creams or lotions. Griseo-

fulvin is particularly useful in the treatment of infections affecting the scalp, beard, palms, soles of the feet, and nails. Common side effects are headache, loss of taste, dry mouth, abdominal pain, and *photosensitivity* (increased sensitivity of the skin to sunlight). During long-term treatment, griseofulvin may cause liver or bone marrow damage; blood tests may be carried out to check the function of these organs.

Groin

The hollow between the lower abdomen and top of the thigh. (See also *Groin, lump in the; Groin strain*.)

Groin, lump in the

A swelling in the hollow between the lower abdomen and the top of the thigh. The most common cause of a lump in the groin is enlargement of a lymph node as a result of an infection (see *Glands, swollen*). Another common cause is a *hernia*, in which abdominal contents protrude through a weak area in the abdominal wall.

Other possible causes of a lump in the groin include an *abscess* (a pus-filled sac), a *lipoma* (a painless benign tumor of fat cells), or an undescended testis (see *Testis, undescended*). Rarely, a lump in the groin may be due to a *varicose vein* or to an *aneurysm* (balloonlike swelling of an artery).

The cause of a lump in the groin can usually be ascertained by physical examination by a physician. Treatment depends on the cause.

Groin strain

Pain and tenderness in the groin due to overstretching of a muscle, typically while running or participating in sports. The muscles commonly affected are the adductors (on the inside of the thigh), which help to rotate and flex the thigh and pull it inward, and the rectus femoris (at the front of the thigh), which also flexes the thigh.

Pain and tenderness in the groin that mimics pain due to muscle strain may sometimes be caused by *osteoarthritis* in the hip or lower spine, *osteitis pubis* (inflammation of the pubic bones, situated at the front and base of the spine), or an inguinal *hernia* (a protrusion of abdominal contents through a weak area in the abdominal wall).

Groin strain is difficult to treat and recovery may be slow. When the cause is obviously a simple muscle strain, treatment is by *physiotherapy*.

G

However, if another cause is suspected, or if what was thought to be a muscle strain does not respond to physiotherapy, tests such as X rays may be required. An X ray may show that a muscle has pulled a small piece of bone away from the pelvis; surgery may then be necessary.

Grommet tube

A small tube that may be inserted through the eardrum during a *myringotomy* (a procedure in which an incision is made in the eardrum) in order to treat *glue ear* in children.

The grommet equalizes the pressure on both sides of the eardrum, permitting mucous fluid to drain down the eustachian tube into the back of the throat. Tubes are usually allowed to fall out on their own as the hole in the eardrum closes, which generally occurs between six and 12 months after insertion. Children with grommets should wear special earplugs for swimming.

Group therapy

Any treatment of emotional or psychological problems in which groups of patients meet regularly with a therapist. Interaction among members of the group is thought to be therapeutic and for certain problems is considered to be more effective than the traditional patient-therapist relationship.

A typical therapy group consists of eight to 10 people who meet for an hour or more once or twice a week to discuss their problems. This may be useful for people with personality problems and for sufferers from *alcohol dependence*, *drug dependence*, *anxiety disorders* and eating disorders.

Growing pains

Vague aches and pains that occur in the limbs of children. The pains are usually felt at night and most often affect the calves of children between 6 and 12 years old. The cause of growing pains is unknown.

Growing pains are of no medical significance and require no treatment, although the pains may interfere with the child's sleep and may alarm parents. If pain is severe or associated with other symptoms, such as joint swelling or malaise, a physician should be consulted.

Growth

An abnormal proliferation of cells within a localized area (see *Tumor*); the increase in height and weight as a child develops (see *Growth, childhood*).

Growth, childhood

The period of most rapid growth occurs before birth, during embryonic and fetal development. After birth, although growth is still very rapid in the first few years of life, especially in the first year, the rate of growth steadily decreases. At the onset of *puberty* there is another major period of growth and development which continues until full adult height is reached, usually at about 16 or 17 in girls and 19 to 21 in boys. In general, increase in weight follows the same pattern as increase in height.

Significant variations occur within the typical growth pattern. For example, boys grow faster than girls until the age of about 7 months, after which girls grow more rapidly until about 4 years of age, when the rate of growth becomes the same, and remains so until puberty. In terms of overall height, girls tend to be shorter than boys at all ages until puberty, when they become taller for a few years. But because puberty is later in boys, their final height is greater.

Growth is not simply a process of becoming taller and heavier. The body shape also changes because different areas grow at different rates. At birth, the head is already about three quarters of its adult size; the head grows to almost full size during the first year. Thereafter, it becomes proportionately smaller because the body grows at a much faster rate. The limbs grow faster than the trunk during early childhood but more slowly during puberty.

Different tissues also grow at different rates. For example, lymphatic tissue grows rapidly until just before adolescence, when it begins to shrink. The brain also grows quickly during the early years, but reaches about nine tenths of its adult weight by the age of 5, after which its growth rate decreases markedly.

FACTORS THAT INFLUENCE GROWTH

Growth can be influenced by heredity and by environmental factors, such as nutrition, general health, and emotional welfare. Hormones also play an important role, particularly *growth hormone*, *thyroid hormones*, and, at puberty, the *sex hormones*.

A child with taller-than-average parents also tends to grow to above-average height. However, this may be counteracted by poor health or undernutrition. In infancy, weight is the best indicator of health and nutrition. Thereafter, height is equally important. Regular measurement of height,

CHANGES IN BODY PROPORTIONS BETWEEN BIRTH AND ADOLESCENCE

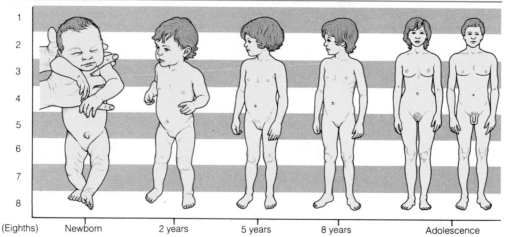

(Eighths) Newborn   2 years   5 years   8 years   Adolescence

If the body is divided into eight equal parts, it can be seen that proportions change radically in relation to the body's overall length. For example, a newborn baby's legs account for only three eighths of his or her height while an adolescent's legs account for one half. A newborn's head accounts for as much as a quarter of his or her height while an adolescent's head accounts for only one eighth.

G

GROWTH CHART: BOYS 1 TO 18 YEARS

Height

Weight

in cm — lbs kg

Age (in years)

Growth in boys

In normal growth, height and weight increase steadily until the onset of puberty. A sudden spurt in growth occurs during puberty (between the ages of 13 and 16). To check your boy's weight range find the age on the bottom line and the weight on the right of the graph. The point where the lines meet will show if the child is heavy, average, or light. To check on height range, follow the age line up to where it intersects with the height scale on the left of the graph.

Key

Height
Tall
Average
Short

Weight
Heavy
Average
Light

GROWTH CHART: GIRLS 1 TO 18 YEARS

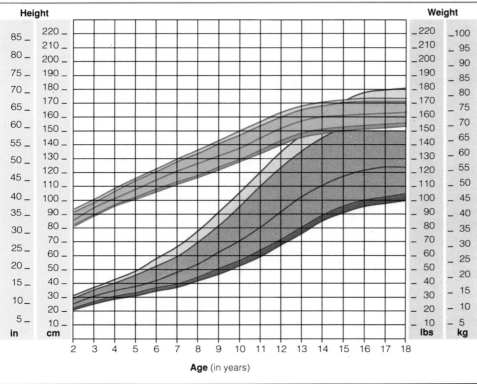

Height

Weight

in cm — lbs kg

Age (in years)

Growth in girls

In normal growth, height and weight increase steadily until the onset of puberty. A sudden spurt in growth occurs during puberty (between the ages of 11 and 14). To check your girl's weight range find the age on the bottom line and the weight on the right of the graph. The point where the lines meet will show if the child is heavy, average, or light. To check on height range, follow the age line up to where it intersects with the height scale on the left of the graph.

Key

Height
Tall
Average
Short

Weight
Heavy
Average
Light

weight, and, in babies, head circumference, provides an invaluable record of a child's growth rate.

A chronic illness, such as *cystic fibrosis*, will retard growth if it is undetected. Even a minor illness can slow growth, although the growth rate usually catches up when the child recovers. In some cases, slow growth may be the only sign that a child is ill, malnourished, emotionally distressed or deprived. However, there is wide individual variation in the growth rate, and *short stature* does not necessarily indicate poor health. Slow growth in a child requires assessment by a pediatrician.

Abnormally rapid growth is rare. Usually, it is a familial trait but it may occasionally indicate an underlying disorder, such as a pituitary gland tumor causing *gigantism*. (See also *Age; Child development*.)

Growth hormone

A substance produced by the *pituitary gland* that stimulates normal body growth and development by altering chemical activity in cells. Growth hormone stimulates the production of protein in muscle cells and the release of energy from the breakdown of fats. Oversecretion of growth hormone may result in *gigantism* or *acromegaly*.

GROWTH HORMONE THERAPY

In the past, growth hormone was extracted from human corpses; it is now prepared synthetically. Growth hormone therapy is used to treat *short stature* when the underlying cause is a pituitary gland disorder. It is also used for children with genetic disorders associated with *short stature*, such as Turner's syndrome. Treatment is usually started in early childhood. Growth hormone is sometimes given with an anabolic *steroid*, which also promotes tissue growth.

POSSIBLE ADVERSE EFFECTS

There is a slight risk that *diabetes mellitus* may develop during treatment. Some people produce *antibodies* to growth hormone, but this does not seem to reduce its effectiveness.

Guaifenesin

An expectorant, guaifenesin is used to increase the production of *phlegm* by the lungs in order to decrease the frequency of coughing spells. Its efficacy in prescribed doses has not been proven. Side effects are rare.

Guanethidine

An *antihypertensive drug* used to treat severe *hypertension* (high blood pres-

sure) that has not responded to other drugs. Adverse effects of guanethidine include dizziness or fainting, diarrhea, and impotence.

Guanethidine is also used in the form of eye drops in combination with *epinephrine* as a treatment for *glaucoma*.

Guar gum

A gum extracted from the cluster bean (*CYAMOPSIS TETRAGONOLABA*). Guar gum is not digested in the body and is therefore classed as dietary fiber. It is used as an aid to controlling the blood sugar level in people with *diabetes mellitus*. Guar gum is sold in some pharmacies and health food stores.

HOW IT WORKS

Guar gum forms a sticky solution in the stomach and slows the movement of nutrients from there into the small intestine. This action slows the rate at which glucose is absorbed from the small intestine into the bloodstream, thus preventing a sudden rise in the blood sugar level after a meal. There is no evidence that guar gum is effective as a slimming aid.

POSSIBLE ADVERSE EFFECTS

Guar gum has an unpleasant taste and may cause flatulence, nausea, and abdominal discomfort.

Guillain-Barré syndrome

A rare form of damage to the peripheral nerves (see *Peripheral nervous system*) that causes weakness of the limbs. The nerves become inflamed, particularly where their roots leave the spine, impairing both movement and sensation. The disease is also known as acute polyneuritis and ascending paralysis.

CAUSES AND INCIDENCE

The cause of the disease is believed to be an allergic reaction to an infection, usually viral; the nerves are inflamed by *antibodies* produced by the reaction. In most cases the disease develops two or three weeks after the onset of an infection, usually an infection of the upper respiratory tract, such as a sore throat or influenza, or a gastrointestinal upset. In 1976, an epidemic occurred in North America following mass vaccination against swine flu.

SYMPTOMS

Weakness, often accompanied by numbness and tingling, usually starts in the legs and spreads to the arms. The weakness becomes progressively worse and may develop into paralysis. The muscles of the face and those controlling speech, swallowing, and breathing may also be affected, causing difficulty with these activities.

DIAGNOSIS

The diagnosis is made from the patient's symptoms and signs, from the results of electrical tests to measure how fast nerve impulses are being conducted, and from a *lumbar puncture*, in which a sample of cerebrospinal fluid is taken from the spinal canal for analysis.

TREATMENT AND OUTLOOK

Patients are treated in hospital, where their condition can be closely monitored. *Intubation* (insertion of a breathing tube down the throat) and mechanical *ventilation* may be necessary to aid breathing. *Plasmapheresis* (in which blood plasma is withdrawn from the patient, treated to remove antibodies, and replaced) may be employed in severe cases.

Most people recover completely without specific treatment, but some are left with permanent weakness in affected areas and/or suffer from further attacks of the disease.

Guilt

A painful feeling that arises from the awareness of having broken a moral or legal code. Guilt is self-inflicted, unlike shame, which depends on how others view the transgression. Some psychoanalysts see guilt as a result of the prohibitions of the *superego* (conscience) instilled by parental authority in early life. Others see guilt as a conditioned response to actions that in the past have led to punishment.

Feeling guilty from time to time is normal. However, feeling very guilty for no reason or experiencing guilt at an imagined crime is one of the main symptoms of psychotic *depression*.

Guinea worm disease

A tropical disease caused by a female parasitic worm more than 1 m long. Infection is the result of drinking water containing the water flea *CYCLOPS*, which harbors larvae of the worm. The larvae pass through the intestinal wall and mature in body tissues. After about a year, the adult female worm, now pregnant, approaches the surface of the skin, and creates an inflamed blister that bursts, exposing the end of the worm.

SYMPTOMS AND TREATMENT

Urticaria (hives), nausea, vomiting, and diarrhea often develop while the blister is forming.

The traditional remedy is to wind the worm gently from the skin onto a small stick. Once the worm is out, the condition usually clears up. *Thiabendazole and niridazole, an investigational drug, are given to reduce inflammation, *antibiotic drugs* are given to control secondary infection, and the patient is immunized against *tetanus*.

Gullet

The common name for the *esophagus*.

Gum

Also called the gingiva, the soft tissue surrounding the *teeth* that protects underlying structures and helps keep the teeth tightly in position in the *jaw*. The gingival margin, a cuff of gum 2 mm thick, fits tightly around the base of the teeth and is anchored within the bony socket by the periodontal ligaments. Normal, healthy gums are pink or brown and are firm. Careful *oral hygiene*, including daily brushing and flossing, is needed to avoid gum disease.

Gingivitis (an early, reversible stage of gum disease, characterized by inflammation of the gums) may occur if dental *plaque* is allowed to collect around the base of the teeth. Bleeding gums are nearly always a symptom of gingivitis; rarely, they are due to *leukemia* or *scurvy* (vitamin C deficiency). Bruised gums are more likely to be caused by a *bleeding disorder*. Gingival *hyperplasia* (fleshy thickening of the gums) occurs most commonly as a side effect of treatment with *phenytoin* (an anticonvulsant drug).

Untreated gingivitis may lead to chronic *periodontitis*, the advanced stage of gum disease, in which infected pockets form between the gums and the teeth.

Gumboil

See *Abscess, dental*.

Gumma

A soft tumor that is characteristic of the late stages of untreated *syphilis* but is now extremely rare.

Gut

A common name for the *intestine*.

Guthrie test

A blood test performed routinely on babies between the eighth and 14th day after birth to check for *phenylketonuria*. This is an inherited disorder in which the *amino acid* phenylalanine accumulates in the blood and tissues, usually leading to severe brain damage unless treated. The Guthrie test measures the amount of phenylalanine in the blood.

HOW IT IS DONE

The baby's heel is pricked with a needle and a few drops of blood are soaked onto a piece of absorbent filter paper. The paper is then placed on a nutrient medium containing bacteria whose growth is activated by phenylalanine. The size of the area of bacterial growth that appears is directly related to the concentration of phenylalanine in the blood.

RESULTS

A concentration of phenylalanine above 20 mg per millilitre indicates that phenylketonuria may be present; other, more accurate tests are performed to confirm the diagnosis.

The Guthrie test may also be used to screen for other disorders of amino acid metabolism, such as tyrosinemia, one of several other disorders in which phenylalanine accumulates in the blood.

Gynecology

The medical specialty concerned with the female *reproductive tract*. Gynecology is involved with the investigation and treatment of menstrual problems (see *Menstruation, disorders of*), *infertility*, *sexual problems*, problems relating to the *menopause*, and other problems affecting the female reproductive tract, such as uterine *fibroids*, *ovarian cysts*, and cervical *polyps*. Gynecologists also give advice about methods of *contraception*. Treatments include drug therapy and surgical procedures, such as *dilatation and curettage* (D and C) and *hysterectomy* (removal of the uterus).

Gynecology covers disorders of early pregnancy, such as recurrent *miscarriage*, although the management of pregnancy falls within the specialty of *obstetrics*. Most specialists in gynecology are also specialists in obstetrics.

Gynecomastia

Enlargement of one or both breasts in the male, almost always due to an excess of the female sex hormone *estrogen* in the blood.

CAUSES

Estrogen, which is responsible for female secondary *sexual characteristics*, is produced in large quantities in women, but is also produced in small amounts in all men (just as all women produce small amounts of male sex hormones). In some males, however, an abnormal amount of estrogen is produced, usually for reasons that are not fully understood, but sometimes because of disease.

Gynecomastia is quite common at *puberty*, taking the form of a slight swelling in one or both breasts, often accompanied by some tenderness. A young boy with gynecomastia is likely to be worried and embarrassed; he should be reassured that his masculinity is not threatened and that the problem will soon pass. Gynecomastia of this mild, temporary kind can also occur at birth.

If the condition develops later—most commonly when a man is over the age of 50—the enlargement may be greater, especially in an already obese man. Such cases are usually not serious, but investigation is necessary to rule out the possibility of an underlying disease. This disease could be *cirrhosis* of the liver, in which the liver is unable to break down estrogen; a tumor of the testis (see *Testis, cancer of*), which can raise the level of estrogen in the blood; or, if only one breast is affected, *breast cancer*.

Adult gynecomastia, which sometimes affects only one breast, can also occur when synthetic hormones and some drugs, such as *digoxin, spironolactone* and *cimetidine*, change the balance of sex hormones in the blood.

DIAGNOSIS AND TREATMENT

A physician may arrange for blood tests. If cancer is suspected, a *biopsy* (removal of the entire lump or a piece of tissue for analysis) will be performed; early treatment is essential if the cause is breast cancer.

The treatment depends on the underlying cause. If a drug is responsible, an alternative drug will be prescribed if possible; otherwise, the gynecomastia must be weighed against the effects of withdrawing the drug treatment, which may in themselves be undesirable.

If there is no underlying disease, the swelling usually subsides without treatment, although it may take a few years. A man who is embarrassed by enlarged breasts may prefer to have cosmetic surgery.

If the swelling is moderate, an operation can be performed that leaves only a small, unnoticeable scar around part of the areola (the dark skin surrounding the nipple). In many cases, this operation can be carried out under a local anesthetic as an outpatient procedure. *Mammoplasty*, an operation more frequently performed on women, is used when breast enlargement is severe. This operation takes longer, requires a general anesthetic, and leaves extensive and obvious scarring.

G

H

Habituation

The effect of becoming accustomed to an experience. In general, the more a person is exposed to a stimulus, the less he or she is aroused by it. Experiments have shown that frightening pictures make the pulse rate rise less the more they are seen. People can also become habituated to certain drugs, and need increasing amounts to receive the same effect (*tolerance*).

Hair

A threadlike structure composed of dead cells containing *keratin* (a fibrous protein that is also the main constituent of the nails and outer skin layer). Hair has little practical function in humans.

The root of each hair is embedded in a tiny pit in the skin called a hair follicle. Each shaft of hair consists of a spongy semihollow core (the medulla), a surrounding layer of long, thin fibers (the cortex) and, on the outside, several layers of overlapping cells (the cuticle). During the growing phase of a hair the root is firmly enclosed by live tissue called a bulb, which supplies the hair with keratin; the bulb is the pale swelling that sometimes can be seen when a hair is pulled out. The upgrowth of dead cells and keratin from the root forms the hair.

TYPES

There are three types of human hair. From the fourth month of gestation, the fetus is covered with downy hair called lanugo, which is shed during the ninth month. After birth and until puberty, vellus hair, which is fine, short, and colorless, covers most of the body. The third type, terminal hair, is thicker, longer, and often pigmented; it grows on the scalp, the eyebrows, and the eyelashes. At puberty, terminal hair replaces vellus in the pubic area and the armpits. In most men and some women the process continues on the face, limbs, and trunk (see *Hirsutism*).

COLOR AND TEXTURE

Hair color is determined by the

THE STRUCTURE OF A HAIR
The hair shaft contains dead cells and keratin (a type of protein). The root is embedded in the skin.

Cuticle
Medulla
Cortex
Hair shaft
Sebaceous gland

Follicle   Root   Bulb   Erector pili muscle

Cross section through hairs
The central medulla, cortex, and outer cuticle can all be clearly differentiated in this microscope photograph.

amount of pigment called *melanin* in the hair shaft. Melanin is produced by cells called melanocytes at the base of the hair follicle. Red melanin is responsible for red and auburn hair, black melanin for all other colors. If cells receive no pigment, the cortex of each hair becomes transparent and the resulting hair appears white.

The degree of curliness of a hair depends on the cross-section shape of its follicle.

DISORDERS

Many hair disorders can be a symptom of a serious underlying disorder.

Brittle hair, which breaks easily and splits at the ends, is usually due to excessive shampooing, combing, or blow-drying. Occasionally, brittle hair can be a sign of severe vitamin or mineral deficiency, or may indicate *hypothyroidism* (underactivity of the thyroid gland). Very dry hair is often the result of excessive use of heated rollers or curling irons, or frequent perming, tinting, or bleaching; it can also be caused by malnutrition.

Ingrown hairs occur primarily in black people or in people with very curly hair. The free-growing end of the hair penetrates the skin near the follicle. Ingrown hairs often cause severe inflammation.

Hairball

A ball of hair in the stomach. Also known as a trichobezoar, it is found in people who nervously pull, suck, or chew their hair. (See *Bezoar*.)

Hairiness, excessive

See *Hirsutism*; *Hypertrichosis*.

Hair removal

Hair is usually removed from different parts of the body for cosmetic reasons. It may also be shaved from around an incision site to allow thorough cleansing before surgical operations.

The method used depends on the part of the body involved and the degree of permanency required.

Shaving removes hair at skin level and is suitable for the legs, for armpit and pubic hair, and for the facial beard in men. Shaving is quick and safe, but the hair soon grows back.

Depilatory creams dissolve the hair just below the skin surface, creating a smoother effect than shaving. However, depilatories may cause irritation and should be used with caution on sensitive areas. Waxing is suitable for the legs and face. The wax is applied to the area and peeled off, pulling out the hair with it. Plucking with tweezers is suitable for small areas. After each of these methods, hair takes several weeks to regrow.

Permanent removal of hair requires *electrolysis*, in which an electric current is used to destroy the growing part of the hair. Electrolysis is very time-consuming and expensive, and is usually used only for small areas.

Hair transplant

A cosmetic operation in which hairy sections of scalp are removed and transplanted to hairless areas to treat *alopecia* (baldness).

HAIR GROWTH

Scalp hair grows about a centimetre per month. There are about 300,000 hairs on the scalp, though there is considerable individual variation. The exact number depends on the number of hair follicles, which is established before birth. Each hair goes through alternating periods of growth and rest. On average, a person sheds 100 to 150 scalp hairs a day.

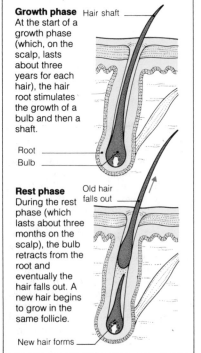

Growth phase
At the start of a growth phase (which, on the scalp, lasts about three years for each hair), the hair root stimulates the growth of a bulb and then a shaft.

Hair shaft

Root
Bulb

Rest phase
During the rest phase (which lasts about three months on the scalp), the bulb retracts from the root and eventually the hair falls out. A new hair begins to grow in the same follicle.

Old hair falls out

New hair forms

HOW IT IS DONE

One or a combination of the following techniques may be employed.

PUNCH GRAFTING This is the most common method of hair transplantation; it is performed using a local anesthetic and is an outpatient procedure. A punch is used to remove small areas of bald scalp, about 6 mm across, which are replaced with areas of hairy scalp. The grafts are taped into position until natural healing takes effect.

STRIP GRAFTING This requires a general anesthetic and is carried out in hospital. Strips of bald skin are cut from the top of the head, and strips of hairy scalp are stitched in their place.

FLAP GRAFTING This is often used to form a new hairline. It is similar to strip grafting, except that flaps of hairy skin are lifted, swiveled, and stitched to replace areas of bald skin.

MALE PATTERN BALDNESS REDUCTION This relatively new technique consists of cutting out areas of bald skin and then stretching surrounding areas of hair-bearing scalp to replace the bald areas.

RESULTS

The success of hair transplantation varies. The hair in punch grafts often falls out after transplantation, leaving unsightly patches for several months until new hair grows. Also, hair does not always grow properly in the areas from which graft skin is taken. Even successful transplants do not last indefinitely; after a time, the transplanted areas also become bald.

Half-life

The time taken for the activity of a substance to reduce to half its original level. The term is usually used to refer to the time taken for the level of *radiation* emitted by a radioactive substance to decay to half its original level. The concept of half-life is useful in *radiation therapy* for assessing how long material will stay radioactive in the body.

Half-life is used in pharmacology to refer to the length of time taken by the body to eliminate half the quantity of a drug in the bloodstream.

Halitosis

The medical term for bad breath. Halitosis is occasionally a sign of illness, but is usually simply a result of smoking, drinking alcohol, eating garlic or onions, or poor oral and dental hygiene. Neither constipation nor indigestion is a cause.

Persistent bad breath not caused by any of these may be a symptom of mouth infection, *sinusitis*, or certain lung disorders, such as *bronchiectasis*.

Hallucination

A perception that occurs when there is no external stimulus (for example, hearing voices or seeing faces when there is no one there). Hallucination differs from an *illusion*, in which a real stimulus is present but has been misinterpreted (thinking that the ticking of a clock is a bomb, for example).

TYPES AND CAUSES

Auditory hallucinations (the hearing of voices) are the most common type. They are a major symptom of *schizophrenia*, but may also be caused by *manic-depressive illness* and certain brain disorders. Visual hallucinations (seeing visions) are most often found in states of *delirium* brought on either by a physical illness (such as *pneumonia*) or by alcohol withdrawal (see *Delirium tremens*). *Hallucinogenic drugs*,

such as mescaline, are another common cause. Hallucinations of smell are often a sign of *temporal lobe epilepsy*, especially when the epilepsy is caused by a tumor. Hallucinations of touch and taste are uncommon and probably occur mainly in people with schizophrenia. There is evidence that people subjected to *sensory deprivation* or to overwhelming physical stress hallucinate temporarily.

Hallucinogenic drug

A drug that causes a *hallucination*. Hallucinogens include certain drugs of abuse, also called psychedelic drugs, such as *LSD*, *marijuana*, *mescaline*, and *psilocybin*. Alcohol may also have an hallucinogenic effect if taken in large amounts; hallucinations also occur during alcohol withdrawal. Certain prescription drugs, including *anticholinergic drugs*, *levodopa*, and *timolol*, may cause takers to have hallucinations in rare instances.

Hallux

The medical name for the big *toe*.

Hallux rigidus

Loss of movement in the large joint at the base of the big toe due to *osteoarthritis*. The condition often follows an injury. The joint is usually tender and swollen, and pain is worse during walking or running.

Hallux rigidus, which may be mistaken for *gout*, is diagnosed if X rays reveal degeneration of the joint. Treatment consists of resting the toe and wearing an insert in the shoe. Surgery is sometimes required.

Hallux valgus

A deformity of the big toe in which the joint at the base projects out from the foot and the top of the toe turns inward. The condition, which is more common in women, is usually associated with wearing narrow, pointed shoes with high heels, but is sometimes caused by an inherited weakness in the joint. A hallux valgus often leads to the formation of a *bunion* (a firm, fluid-filled, sometimes painful swelling over the joint) or to *osteoarthritis* in the joint.

Treatment is required only if the bunion becomes very large or persistently inflamed or if the osteoarthritis causes pain and limits foot movement. In this case, the toe may be straightened by means of *osteotomy* (surgery to remove part of a bone and realign its ends) or *arthrodesis* (surgery to fuse the bones of a joint).

H

H

Haloperidol

An *antipsychotic drug* used in the treatment of mental illnesses such as *schizophrenia* and *mania*.

Haloperidol is also given to control the symptoms of *Gilles de la Tourette's syndrome* (a rare neurological disorder) and may be used, in small doses, to sedate aggressive or hostile people with *dementia*.

POSSIBLE ADVERSE EFFECTS

Adverse effects include drowsiness, lethargy, weight gain, dizziness, and, more seriously, *parkinsonism* (a neurological disorder that causes symptoms such as abnormal involuntary movements and stiffness of the face and limbs).

Halothane

A colorless liquid inhaled as a vapor to induce and help maintain general anesthesia (see *Anesthesia, general*). In rare cases it may cause *arrhythmia* or liver damage.

Hamartoma

A benign, tumorlike mass consisting of an overgrowth of tissues that are normally found in the affected part of the body.

Hamartomas are common in the skin (the most common type is a *hemangioma*, an overgrowth of blood vessels in the skin), but also occur in the lungs, heart, or kidneys.

Hammer toe

A deformity of the *toe* (usually the second toe) in which the main toe joint stays bent. A painful *corn* often develops on this joint because of pressure from the overlying shoe. Hammer toe is caused by an abnormality of the tendons in the toe.

A protective felt pad usually eases pressure on the joint and thus relieves pain. If pain persists, the deformity may require surgical correction.

Appearance of hammer toe
This photograph shows the typical appearance of a hammer toe, in which one of the joints of the second toe is fixed in a bent position.

THE SKELETAL STRUCTURE OF THE HAND AND WRIST

Four of the eight wrist bones (carpals) articulate with the radius and ulna. The rest are connected to the five bones of the palm (metacarpals), each of which articulates with a phalanx.

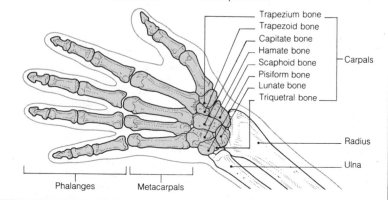

Trapezium bone
Trapezoid bone
Capitate bone
Hamate bone
Scaphoid bone — Carpals
Pisiform bone
Lunate bone
Triquetral bone

Radius

Ulna

Phalanges   Metacarpals

Hamstring muscles

A group of muscles at the back of the thigh. The upper ends of the hamstring muscles are attached by tendons to the pelvis; the lower ends are attached by tendons called hamstrings to the tibia and fibula. The hamstring muscles bend the knee and swing the leg backward from the thigh.

DISORDERS

Tearing of the hamstring muscles is common in sports, particularly in sprinting. The injury happens suddenly and is very painful. Bruising over the area develops several days later. Repeated strenuous exercise may cause a sprain of the muscles, with pain coming on gradually (see *Overuse injury*). Both types of injury can often be prevented by warming-up exercises.

Sciatica (pain down the back of the leg caused by pressure on the sciatic nerve) may be particularly severe in the hamstring muscles.

Painful spasms of the hamstring muscles can also sometimes occur as a protective response to a knee injury; by restricting movement of the damaged knee joint, the muscle spasms limit further injury.

Hand

The hand, which is the most versatile part of the body, allows humans (and other primates) to hold and manipulate objects. This ability is primarily due to the fact that the fingers and thumb can move independently and can form an effective *grip*).

STRUCTURE

The hand is made up of the wrist, palm, and fingers (see above).

Movements of the hand are achieved mainly by tendons that attach the muscles of the forearm to the bones of the hand. These tendons are surrounded by synovial sheaths containing a lubricating fluid that prevents friction. Other movements are controlled by short muscles in the palm of the hand; some of these muscles make up the prominent areas along the sides of the hand from the bases of the thumb and little fingers to the wrist.

Blood is supplied to the hand by two arteries (the radial on the thumb side of the wrist and the ulnar on the little finger side) and is carried away by veins that are prominent on the back of the hand. Sensation and movement are controlled by the radial, ulnar, and median nerves.

DISORDERS

Because they are so frequently used, the hands are susceptible to injury, including cuts, burns, bites, fractures, and, occasionally, tendon injuries. *Dermatitis* is also common, since the hands are exposed to a considerable variety of irritating agents.

The hand may be affected by contracture, a deformity caused by shrinkage of tissues in the palm of the hand (see *Dupuytren's contracture*) or damage to muscles in the forearm (see *Volkmann's contracture*). Degeneration of a synovial sheath on the upper side of the wrist may cause a harmless swelling known as a *ganglion*.

Osteoarthritis commonly attacks the joint at the base of the thumb, rendering it painful and immobile. *Rheumatoid arthritis* may cause deformity by attacking the joints at the base of the fingers and rupturing tendons.

Handedness

Preference for using the right or left hand. Some 90 percent of healthy adults use the right hand for writing; two thirds prefer the right hand for most activities requiring coordination and skill. The rest are either left-handed or ambidextrous (able to use both hands equally well). There is no male-female difference in the proportions preferring each hand.

It is uncertain why all humans are not simply ambidextrous. Up to the age of about 12, it is possible to switch handedness if a person's dominant hemisphere of the brain is damaged.

CAUSES
Inheritance is probably the most important factor in determining handedness. Studies have shown a greater number of nerves going to one side of the brain even in the newborn. A child made to use the right hand despite natural preference, however, may "become" right-handed. In earlier times, left-handed people were considered to be unlucky or evil (the word sinister is derived from the Latin word for left), so children were trained to be right-handed. Even today, so many people are naturally right-handed that the pressure to conform is high, especially in some cultures where the left hand is that used for wiping the anus after defecation. In every country, most tools and gadgets are designed for right-handed use. Some left-handed people may subconsciously resent the change when forced to use the right hand.

Handedness is related to the division of the brain into two hemispheres, each of which controls movement and sensation on the opposite side of the body. In most right-handed people, the speech center is in the left hemisphere, so that a stroke affecting this side of the brain causes aphasia (speech impairment) as well as paralysis and weakness of the right arm and leg. In 70 percent of left-handed people, the speech center is on the right, and left hemisphere damage does not cause aphasia.

EFFECTS OF HANDEDNESS
It is not clear whether handedness is related to special abilities. Left-handed tennis players or bowlers seem to succeed because their shots or balls come from an unusual angle. Although the left brain is related to verbal ability and logical reasoning, and the right to emotional and spatial awareness, there is no evidence that more artists are left-handed or more philosophers right-handed.

Hand-foot-and-mouth disease

A common infectious disease of toddlers, caused by a virus known as a coxsackievirus. Hand-foot-and-mouth disease often occurs in small epidemics in nursery schools, usually in the summer months.

The illness is usually mild and lasts only a few days. Symptoms include blistering of the palms, soles, and inside of the mouth, reluctance to eat, and a slight fever. There is no treatment other than mild analgesic drugs (painkillers) to relieve the discomfort of the blisters. The illness is unrelated to foot-and-mouth disease in cattle.

Handicap

The extent to which a physical or mental disability interferes with normal functioning and causes the person to be disadvantaged.

The management and treatment of a handicap involves assessment of the specific disability, the provision of suitable aids, specific educational help, and, if necessary, longer-term support in an appropriate setting.

Hangnail

A strip of skin torn away from the side or base of a fingernail, exposing a raw, painful area. Hangnails usually occur after frequent immersion in water has dried the skin on the fingers. Biting the nails is another common cause. The raw area may become infected and develop into a paronychia.

A hangnail should be trimmed with scissors and covered until it heals. The condition may be prevented by applying a moisturizing cream.

Hangover

The unpleasant effects sometimes experienced on waking after over-indulgence in alcohol. Characterized by headache, nausea, vertigo, and depression, the severity of a hangover is determined by the amount and type of alcohol consumed. Brandy and red wine have high concentrations of congeners (secondary products of alcohol fermentation), which may produce bad hangovers.

Alcohol increases urine production and some of the symptoms of a hangover are due to mild dehydration; drinking a large quantity of water before going to sleep may help. Recovery from a hangover is usually just a matter of time, but people suffering from alcohol dependence may experience more severe and persistent hangovers or they may suffer from withdrawal symptoms.

Hansen's disease

A chronic bacterial infection, also known as leprosy, that damages nerves, mainly in the limbs and facial area, and may also lead to skin damage. Untreated Hansen's disease can have severe complications, which include blindness and disfigurement. Contrary to popular belief, Hansen's disease is not highly contagious.

CAUSES
Hansen's disease is caused by a bacterium, MYCOBACTERIUM LEPRAE, spread in droplets of nasal mucus. A person is infectious to others only during the first stages of the disease. Only people living in prolonged close contact with an infected person are at risk of infection. This, along with the fact that only 3 percent of the population are susceptible to Hansen's disease at all, means that there is no justification for the practice (still prevalent in some countries) of isolating people with the disease.

INCIDENCE
Worldwide, there are about 20 million sufferers from Hansen's disease, mostly in Asia, Central and South America, and Africa. Probably fewer than 20 percent of these have access to treatment. An average of 26 new cases is reported in Canada each year. Almost all of these are in Canadian residents born abroad in areas where leprosy is endemic; there has been no transmission of leprosy within Canada in recent decades.

SYMPTOMS AND SIGNS
Hansen's disease has a very long incubation period—about three to five years. Most of the destructive effects on nervous tissue are caused not by bacterial growth but by a reaction of the body's immune system to the organisms as they die.

There are two main types of Hansen's disease: the lepromatous type, in which the damage is widespread, progressive, and severe; and the tuberculoid type, which is milder.

Initially, damage is confined to peripheral nerves, which supply the skin and muscles. Skin areas supplied by affected nerves become lighter or darker and sensation and sweating in these areas are reduced.

As the disease progresses, the peripheral nerves swell and become tender. Hands, feet, and facial skin eventually become numb and muscles become paralyzed.

Complications include loss of all sensation in the hands and feet, so that accidental burns or injuries are not noticed, leading to extensive scarring or even to loss of fingers or toes. Muscle paralysis can lead to further deformity. Damage to the facial nerve means that the eyelids cannot be closed; the cornea dries and ulcerates, leading to blindness. Alternatively, direct invasion by bacteria may lead to inflammation of the eyeball, again leading to blindness. The disability caused by the combined effects of blindness and loss of touch sensation is extremely severe.

Cartilage and bone in the nose are often eroded, and bones elsewhere in the body may be destroyed.

The testes may atrophy (waste), leading to sterility.

DIAGNOSIS
Early diagnosis of the disease is essential to prevent permanent disfigurement and disability. A provisional diagnosis is made from a physical examination of the patient; the presence of the bacteria is confirmed by a skin *biopsy* (removal of a sample of tissue for analysis).

TREATMENT
Drug treatment may be with a combination of dapsone, rifampin, and clofazimine, which kills most of the causative bacteria within a few days. Any damage that has already occurred, however, is irreversible. Patients cease to be infectious soon after treatment starts. To prevent a relapse, use of the drug needs to be continued for at least two years after the bacteria have disappeared.

Prevention of damage to the feet and other insensitive areas—through the use of proper footwear and health education—is very important. *Plastic surgery* may be helpful for people with facial deformities. Nerve and tendon transplants may improve the function of damaged limbs.

OUTLOOK
With so many sufferers in poor countries, the battle against Hansen's disease has only just begun. Experimental vaccines against Hansen's disease are under trial.

Hardening of the arteries
The popular term for *arteriosclerosis*, the most common form of which is *atherosclerosis*.

Harelip
A common term for the *birth defect* in which there is a split in the upper lip due to failure of the two sides to fuse during fetal development. Also called cleft lip, it is often associated with a similar failure of the two halves of the palate to join. (See *Cleft lip and palate*.)

Hashimoto's thyroiditis
An *autoimmune disorder* in which the body's immune system develops *antibodies* against its own thyroid gland cells. As a result, the thyroid gland becomes unable to produce enough *thyroid hormones*, a condition called *hypothyroidism*.

The principal symptoms are tiredness, muscle weakness, and weight gain. A goiter (enlargement of the thyroid gland) develops.

The diagnosis is confirmed by blood tests to measure the level of thyroid hormones and to detect the presence of thyroid antibodies. Treatment consists of thyroid hormone replacement therapy, which is continued for life. If a goiter persists despite drug treatment, surgery may be necessary.

Hashish
Another name for *marijuana*.

Hay fever
The popular name for a seasonal form of allergic rhinitis. (See *Rhinitis, allergic*.)

Headache
One of the most common types of pain. A headache is only very occasionally a symptom of a serious underlying disorder. The pain of a headache does not come from the brain, which contains no sensory nerves, but arises from the *meninges* (the membranes around the brain) and from the scalp and its blood vessels and muscles. The pain is produced by tension in, or stretching of, these structures.

The pain may be felt all over the head or may occur in only one part—for example, in the back of the neck, the forehead, or one side of the head. Sometimes the pain moves to another part of the head during the course of the headache. The pain of headache may be superficial or deep, throbbing or sharp, and there may also be accompanying or preliminary symptoms, such as nausea, vomiting, and visual or sensory disturbances.

Many headaches are simply the body's response to some adverse stimulus, such as hunger or a change in the weather. These headaches usually clear up in a few hours and leave no aftereffects.

Tension headaches, caused by tightening in the muscles of the face, neck, and scalp as a result of stress or poor posture, are also common. They may last for days or weeks and can cause varying degrees of discomfort.

Some types of headache are especially painful and persistent but nevertheless are not an indication of a progressive underlying disorder. *Migraine* is a severe, incapacitating headache preceded or accompanied by visual and/or stomach disturbances. Cluster headaches cause intense pain behind one eye and may wake the sufferer nightly for periods of weeks or months.

CAUSES
Common causes of headache include *hangover*, irregular meals, prolonged travel, poor posture, a noisy or stuffy work environment, excitement, and excessive sleep. Recent research has shown that certain foods (such as cheese, chocolate, and red wine) trigger migraine attacks in susceptible people. *Food additives* may also cause headache. Other causes include *sinusitis*, *toothache*, *head injury*, and *cervical osteoarthritis*. Among the rare causes of headache are *brain tumor*, *hypertension* (high blood pressure), *temporal arteritis* (inflammation of arteries in the face, neck, and scalp), *aneurysm* (ballooning of a blood vessel, in this case in the brain), and increased pressure within the skull.

INVESTIGATION
If headaches are persistent, without obvious cause, and do not respond to self-help treatment, medical advice should be sought. The physician will ask about the nature and site of the pain and at what intervals the headaches occur. A careful general physical and neurological examination will be performed. *CT scanning* or *MRI* (magnetic resonance imaging) may be carried out if a neurological cause for the headaches is suspected.

TREATMENT
Prevention is more important than treatment; many of the known causes can easily be avoided, particularly if the sufferer knows what triggers the headaches. Once a headache has started (provided it is not a migraine or cluster headache), one or more of the following measures should ease the pain: relaxing in a hot bath; lying down; avoidance of aggravating factors (such as excessive noise or a stuffy room); stretching and massaging the muscles in the shoulders, neck, face, and scalp; taking a mild *analgesic drug* (painkiller); and sleeping.

Head-banging
Persistent, rhythmic banging of the head, usually against a wall or hard object. Head-banging occurs in mentally retarded people, particularly

HEADACHE
Pain in the head that may be anything from mild to severe and incapacitating.

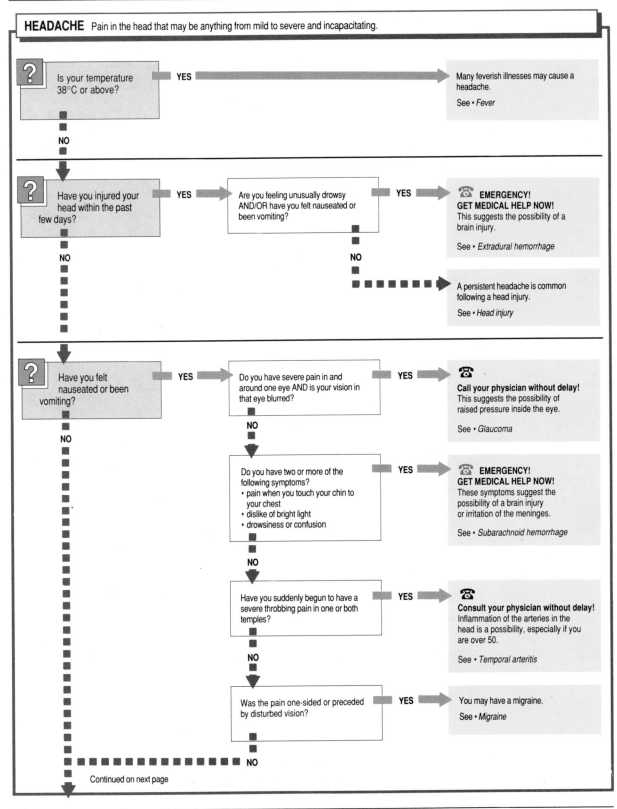

Is your temperature 38°C or above?
→ YES → Many feverish illnesses may cause a headache.
See • *Fever*

NO ↓

Have you injured your head within the past few days?
→ YES → **Are you feeling unusually drowsy AND/OR have you felt nauseated or been vomiting?**
→ YES → ☎ **EMERGENCY! GET MEDICAL HELP NOW!** This suggests the possibility of a brain injury.
See • *Extradural hemorrhage*

NO ┈→ A persistent headache is common following a head injury.
See • *Head injury*

NO ↓

Have you felt nauseated or been vomiting?
→ YES → **Do you have severe pain in and around one eye AND is your vision in that eye blurred?**
→ YES → ☎ **Call your physician without delay!** This suggests the possibility of raised pressure inside the eye.
See • *Glaucoma*

NO ↓

Do you have two or more of the following symptoms?
• pain when you touch your chin to your chest
• dislike of bright light
• drowsiness or confusion
→ YES → ☎ **EMERGENCY! GET MEDICAL HELP NOW!** These symptoms suggest the possibility of a brain injury or irritation of the meninges.
See • *Subarachnoid hemorrhage*

NO ↓

Have you suddenly begun to have a severe throbbing pain in one or both temples?
→ YES → ☎ **Consult your physician without delay!** Inflammation of the arteries in the head is a possibility, especially if you are over 50.
See • *Temporal arteritis*

NO ↓

Was the pain one-sided or preceded by disturbed vision?
→ YES → You may have a migraine.
See • *Migraine*

NO ┈→

NO ↓

Continued on next page

H

H

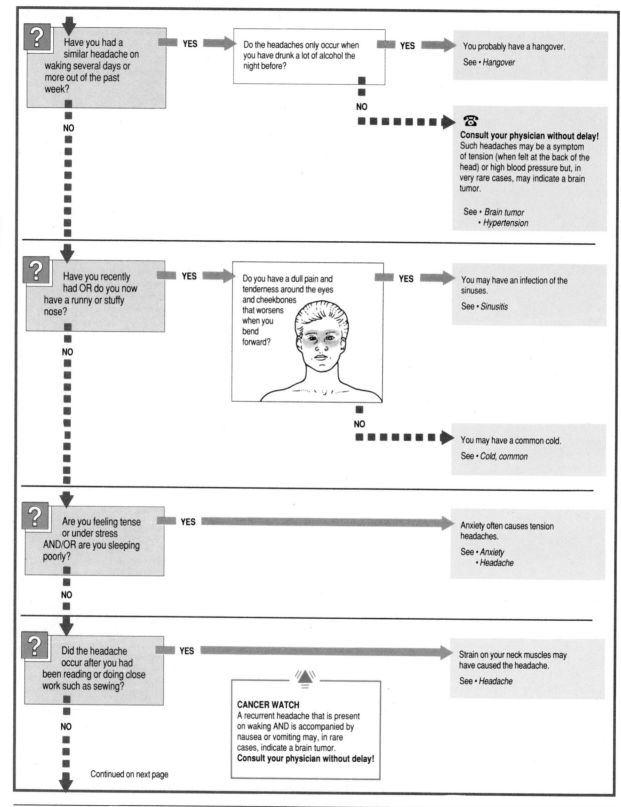

Have you had a similar headache on waking several days or more out of the past week?

YES → **Do the headaches only occur when you have drunk a lot of alcohol the night before?**

YES → You probably have a hangover.

See • *Hangover*

NO → ☎

Consult your physician without delay! Such headaches may be a symptom of tension (when felt at the back of the head) or high blood pressure but, in very rare cases, may indicate a brain tumor.

See • *Brain tumor*
  • *Hypertension*

NO

Have you recently had OR do you now have a runny or stuffy nose?

YES → **Do you have a dull pain and tenderness around the eyes and cheekbones that worsens when you bend forward?**

YES → You may have an infection of the sinuses.

See • *Sinusitis*

NO → You may have a common cold.

See • *Cold, common*

NO

Are you feeling tense or under stress AND/OR are you sleeping poorly?

YES → Anxiety often causes tension headaches.

See • *Anxiety*
  • *Headache*

NO

Did the headache occur after you had been reading or doing close work such as sewing?

YES → Strain on your neck muscles may have caused the headache.

See • *Headache*

CANCER WATCH
A recurrent headache that is present on waking AND is accompanied by nausea or vomiting may, in rare cases, indicate a brain tumor.
Consult your physician without delay!

NO

Continued on next page

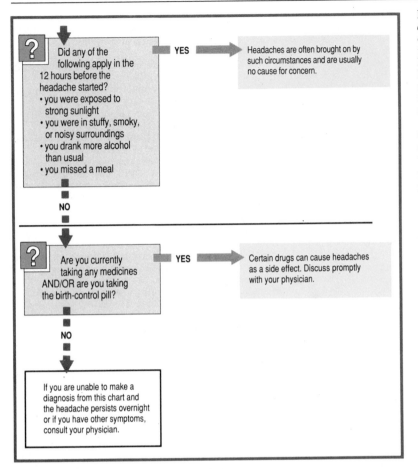

Did any of the following apply in the 12 hours before the headache started?
• you were exposed to strong sunlight
• you were in stuffy, smoky, or noisy surroundings
• you drank more alcohol than usual
• you missed a meal

YES → Headaches are often brought on by such circumstances and are usually no cause for concern.

NO

Are you currently taking any medicines AND/OR are you taking the birth-control pill?

YES → Certain drugs can cause headaches as a side effect. Discuss promptly with your physician.

NO

If you are unable to make a diagnosis from this chart and the headache persists overnight or if you have other symptoms, consult your physician.

children and adolescents in institutions that provide little or no stimulation. Head-banging is a form of self-stimulation and is also an attention-seeking device. It may lead to serious injury. Protective headgear and *behavior therapy* may help.

Head-banging also occurs in some normal toddlers, often when they are frustrated or angry, or as a comfort when going to sleep. It may sometimes occur during sleep.

Most children grow out of head-banging. In the majority of cases, the problem is best ignored, but if head-banging is severe or persistent a physician should be consulted.

Head injury

Injury to the head may occur as a result of traffic accidents, sports injuries, falls, assault, accidents at work and at home, or bullet wounds. Most people have a minor head injury at least once in their lives. One percent of all deaths are caused by head injury, half as a result of traffic accidents.

A head injury can damage the scalp, skull, or brain. Minor injuries cause no damage to the underlying brain. Even when there is a *skull fracture*, or the scalp is split, the brain may not be damaged. However, a blow may severely shake the brain, sometimes causing *brain damage*, even when there are no external signs of injury.

A blow often bruises the brain tissue, causing death of some of the brain cells in the injured area. When an object actually penetrates the skull, foreign material and dirt may be implanted into the brain and lead to infection. A blow or a penetrating injury may tear blood vessels and cause *brain hemorrhage*. Head injury may cause swelling of the brain; this is particularly evident after bullet wounds because their high velocity causes extensive damage. If the skull is fractured, bone may be driven into the underlying brain.

SYMPTOMS AND SIGNS

If the head injury is mild, there may be no symptoms other than a slight headache. In some cases there is *concussion*, which may cause confusion, dizziness, and blurred vision (sometimes persisting for several days). More severe head injuries, particularly blows to the head, may result in unconsciousness that lasts longer than a few minutes, or *coma*, which may be fatal.

Postconcussive *amnesia* (loss of memory of events that occurred after an accident) may occur, especially if the skull has been fractured. This amnesia usually lasts more than an hour after consciousness is regained. There may also be preconcussive amnesia (loss of memory of events that occurred before the accident). The more serious the injury to the brain, the longer unconsciousness and amnesia are likely to last.

After a severe brain injury, a person may suffer some muscular weakness or paralysis and loss of sensation.

Symptoms such as persistent vomiting, pupils of unequal size, double vision, or a deteriorating level of consciousness suggest progressive brain damage.

INVESTIGATION

Any person suffering loss of consciousness, however brief, should be seen by a physician. The person may be hospitalized for observation; *skull X rays* are performed to identify any fracture. If a brain hemorrhage is suspected, *CT scanning* may be carried out.

TREATMENT

Cuts to the scalp may require stitching. People whose consciousness is deteriorating will be kept under close observation. If a blood clot forms inside the skull, the clot may be life-threatening and will require surgical removal; severe skull fractures may also require surgery.

OUTLOOK

Recovery from minor head injuries may take several days if there are persistent symptoms of concussion. Survival following major head injuries has been improved by advances in nursing and medical care, but permanent physical or mental disability (including changes in personality) may follow if there has been permanent damage to the brain. Epileptic seizures sometimes occur after a severe head injury (especially after a penetrating injury, severe skull fracture, or serious brain hemorrhage). Recovery from a major head injury may be very slow, but victims may continue to show signs of progressive recovery for as long as five years.

H

Head lag

The backward flopping of the head that occurs when an infant is placed in a sitting position.

Head lag is obvious in the newborn because the neck muscles are still weak, but by 4 months of age the baby can hold his or her head upright in line with the trunk. The disappearance of head lag is a measure of motor development (see *Child development*); good control of the head is essential before a baby can learn to sit.

Heaf test

A type of *tuberculin test*.

Healing

The process by which the body repairs bone, tissue, or organ damage caused by injury, infection, or disease. In popular usage, the term means simply "restoring to health."

THE HEALING PROCESS

The initial stages of healing are the same for all parts of the body. After injury, the blood forms clots in damaged areas of tissue. White blood cells, *enzymes, histamine,* other chemicals, and *proteins* from which new cells can be made accumulate at the site of damage. Fibrous tissue is laid down within the blood clot to form a supportive structure. Any dead cells are broken down and absorbed by the white blood cells. Some tissues, such as bone, are then able to regenerate by proliferation of the cells that remain around the damaged area. In such cases, the original structure and function are fully restored.

Other tissues, such as nerve tissue, may be unable to proliferate. In other cases, there may be an inadequate blood supply or persistent infection that prevents tissue regeneration. In these cases, the fibrous tissue that forms in the blood clot may develop into tough scar tissue, which keeps the tissue structure intact but may impair its function (e.g., the restriction of movement that sometimes happens after a muscle tear).

WOUND HEALING

The body repairs skin wounds by one of two processes: healing by first intention and healing by second intention.

Healing by first intention occurs when the edges of the wound are close together and there has been minimal loss of tissue. If the wound is deep, the edges of the skin may need to be held together with stitches or a butterfly bandage. The blood that seeps from the edges of the wound forms a clot which becomes the base on which scar tissue is laid down. When healing is complete, only a fine scar remains.

Healing by second intention occurs when the edges of the wound are not brought together. In this slower type of healing, pink *granulation tissue* grows from the exposed tissue. This granulation tissue is eventually covered by skin, which grows over the wound from the cut edges. By the time healing is complete, the granulation tissue has developed into tough scar tissue.

Health

At its simplest, health is the absence of physical and mental disease. However, the wider concept promoted by the World Health Organization is that all people should have the opportunity to fulfill their genetic potential. This includes the ability to grow and develop physically and mentally without the impediments of inadequate nutrition or environmental contamination, and to be protected as much as possible against infectious diseases. (See also *Diet and disease; Health hazards.*)

Health and Welfare Canada

Health and Welfare Canada is a federal department whose mandate is to promote and preserve the health, and to ensure the social security and quality of life, of all Canadians. Health and Welfare Canada directly funds and operates national income security and health protection programs and provides significant financial support for provincial and territorial health and social service programs. (See *Provincial health plans.*)

Health food

The term applied to products that are meant to promote health, including unprocessed and wholefood products, organically grown fruits and vegetables, and dietary supplements. The term is misleading because it suggests that only "health foods" are good for people. In fact, a healthy diet is based on sound *nutrition.*

Health hazards

Environmental factors that are known or suspected to cause disease. Some health hazards are obvious, such as contamination of water supplies or food with sewage or other effluents, and pollution of the air with smoke or poisonous chemicals. Others are less apparent—for example, radioactivity (which is detectable only with special instruments) and sunlight.

TYPES

For people in developing countries, in other words for the majority of the world's population, the main hazards come from lack of access to safe, pure water, from inadequate means of disposal of sewage and domestic refuse, and from insufficient or contaminated food. Foods contaminated with microorganisms, such as bacteria and molds, present far greater health hazards than those associated with the additives that are used in developed countries to combat such contamination. (See *Food additives; Food-borne infection; Food poisoning.*)

There are four other main types of health hazard, all of which are present worldwide. First, there are the numerous *infectious diseases* transmitted by contact or by insects or other animals. (See *Bacteria; Fungal infections; Insects and disease; Viruses; Zoonoses.*) The second type comprises work-related hazards, such as industrial *accidents,* and a wide variety of occupational disorders, e.g., *asbestosis, pneumoconiosis, lead poisoning,* cancers associated with exposure to chemicals. (See *Occupational disease and injury.*)

The third category includes those associated with domestic and social life, such as accidents in the home or on the road, and from recreational activities. In many developed countries, domestic and traffic accidents are the most important risks to health in early adult life. *Alcohol* and *tobaccosmoking* are other major hazards to health. Finally, there are many types of global environmental hazard, including sunlight (see *Sunlight, adverse effects of*), cosmic radiation and background radioactivity (see *Radiation, hazards*), and *pollution.*

Hearing

The sense that enables sound to be perceived. The *ear* (the organ of hearing) transforms the sound waves it receives into nerve impulses that pass to the *brain.*

MECHANISM OF HEARING

Almost all sound is heard by a mechanism known as air conduction (see illustrated box). This process is supplemented by a secondary form of hearing called bone conduction, in which sound waves set up vibrations in the skull bones that pass directly to the inner ear. This form of hearing affects the way a person hears his or her own voice.

HEARING

The ears are the organs of hearing. Each ear has three separate regions—the outer ear, middle ear, and inner ear. Sound waves are channeled through the ear canal to the middle ear, from where a complex system of membranes and tiny bones conveys the vibrations to the inner ear. A part of the auditory nerve converts the vibrations to nerve impulses, which are then transmitted to the brain.

To function properly, the eardrum must have equal air pressure on each side so that it can vibrate freely. Pressure is equalized via the eustachian tube, which runs from the back of the throat to the middle ear.

ROUTE TO THE BRAIN

Auditory sensations are picked up by nerve fibers in the cochlea and travel along the auditory nerve to the medulla. From there, they pass via the thalamus to the superior temporal gyrus—the part of the cerebral cortex involved in receiving and perceiving sound.

Thalamus

Superior temporal gyrus

Auditory nerve

Medulla

Outer ear
The pinna (the visible part of the ear) channels sound waves into the outer ear canal (auditory canal) toward the eardrum. Hairs and waxy cerumen line the canal.

Malleus (hammer) and incus (anvil)
The malleus, attached to the eardrum, transmits vibration to the incus.

Stapes (stirrup) and oval window
The incus in turn transmits vibration to the stapes and the oval window membrane.

Eardrum
The tympanic membrane (eardrum) is a taut membrane between the outer and middle ears. Sound waves of different frequencies cause the eardrum to vibrate at different speeds.

Cochlea
The cochlea consists of a hollow spiral passage in the temporal bone. The cochlear duct, a fluid-filled membranous tube, virtually divides the cochlea lengthwise; it is full of microscopic hairs that stimulate nerve cells in response to sound vibrations, transmitted through the oval window.

Function of cochlea
Inside the cochlea (shown uncoiled), the first part of the basilar membrane responds most to high-frequency vibrations; the far end registers only lower frequencies.

Cochlea

Oval window

Basilar membrane

Nerve fibers

COMPARISON OF FREQUENCY RANGES
Different animals are able to hear different ranges of sound frequencies. The diagram shows the normal ranges of sound, in hertz (cycles per second), that can be heard by a human, a bat, a dolphin, and a dog.

10 Hz   100 Hz   1,000 Hz   10,000 Hz   100,000 Hz

Lowest note on piano   Highest note on piano

Electron micrograph of inner ear
The section shows four rows of hair cells, which convert sound waves into electrical impulses to be sent to the brain.

HEARING DISORDERS

Problems with hearing (from minor sound distortions to total inability to hear) result when any part of the sound-transmitting and analyzing mechanism is damaged (see *Deafness*).

Hearing aids

Electronic devices that improve hearing in people with certain types of *deafness*. A hearing aid consists of a tiny microphone (to pick up sounds), an amplifier (to increase their volume), and a tiny speaker (to transmit sounds to the ear).

HOW IT WORKS

A tiny microphone collects sound and transforms it into electric current. The amplifier increases the strength of the current and feeds it along a tube to an earpiece, which fits into the outer ear canal (or, more rarely, onto the bone behind the ear) and converts the current back to sound (which has now been amplified).

A volume control on the aid, usually operated by turning a tiny wheel, enables the level of incoming sound to be adjusted. The aid is designed at the factory to amplify those pitches for which the user has the most loss. Further modifications of this sort may be made by the hearing aid dispenser.

TYPES

The most common types of hearing aid are inconspicuous. The mechanical parts, along with a battery to power them, are contained in a small plastic case that fits comfortably behind the ear, in the sidepiece of a pair of glasses, or entirely within the ear canal. Aids that fit entirely in the ear are most popular today.

More powerful aids that amplify sound to a greater degree are also available but are now rarely used. In these aids, the microphone, amplifier, and battery are contained in a larger case worn on the body; the current is carried to the earpiece by a thin wire.

Some people with conductive deafness, especially if there is inflammation or discharge in the ear canal, may be given a bone-conduction hearing aid. This may be fitted to a glasses frame or hair-band.

Most modern hearing aids include switches that enable normal reception to be replaced by a process known as electromagnetic induction. This process picks up transmitted speech in telephones and in public buildings that have been equipped for the purpose. The greatest advantage of electromagnetic induction is that it obscures amplified background noise.

Hearing aids

Hearing aids amplify sound waves for people who have impaired hearing. Many hearing aids include an earpiece, a microphone, an amplifier, a volume control, and a battery.

TYPES OF HEARING TEST

Tests	Function	
Tuning fork tests	These tests are used to determine whether hearing loss is conductive or sensorineural. In the Rinne test, the patient is asked whether the sound is louder with the vibrating tines held near the opening of the ear canal (air conduction) or with the base of the fork held against the mastoid bone (bone conduction). In a normal ear or in one with sensorineural loss,	air conduction is greater than bone conduction. In conductive loss, bone conduction is greater than or equal to air conduction. Weber's test, in which the base of the fork is placed on the forehead, is useful for diagnosing unilateral hearing loss. If hearing loss is conductive, the patient hears the tuning fork better in the ear with the poorer hearing.
Pure-tone audiometry	This is a test in which an audiometer is used to generate sounds of varying frequency and intensity. The audiometer is an electrical instrument that measures a person's ability to hear sounds of different frequencies and intensities. Hearing is first assessed by transmitting the sounds through one earphone while the other ear is prevented from hearing them. The sound frequencies range from 250 to 8,000 hertz (cycles per second); for each	frequency, the sound is decreased in intensity until it can no longer be heard. The person whose hearing is being tested gives a signal at the moment when he or she detects each sound, and the results are recorded on a graph called an audiogram. Bone conduction hearing is then assessed using a rubber rod connected to the audiometer (the rod is placed against the mastoid bone behind the ear and kept in place by a headband).
Auditory evoked response	In this form of testing, the brain's response to sound stimulation by the audiometer is analyzed by means of electrodes placed on the scalp. This test attempts to evaluate the presence of hearing in a person who is unable to cooperate with other tests (because of mental	handicap, for example). Auditory evoked response is commonly used to assess hearing in very young babies. The test can also help rule out acoustic neuroma (a benign tumor within the auditory canal).
Impedance audiometry	This test is used to determine the type of middle ear damage occurring in cases of conductive deafness. A probe is fitted tightly into the entrance to the outer ear canal, sealing it off from outside air pressure and sound. The probe emits a continuous sound. Air is pumped through the probe at varying pressures and, at the same time, a microphone in the probe registers the differing	reflections of sounds from the eardrum as pressure changes in the ear canal. The reflections are recorded on a graph known as a tympanogram. The pattern of differing reflections reveals the extent of elasticity in the eardrum and middle ear bones, thus indicating the type of disease that is causing the deafness. This device can also measure the air pressure in an air-filled middle ear.

H

Other devices available for the hard-of-hearing include amplified telephone receivers, flashing lights instead of doorbells and telephone bells, vibrators that respond to sound, headphones for television sets, teletypewriters, and guide dogs for the deaf. (See also *Cochlear implant*.)

Hearing loss
A deterioration in the ability to perceive sound. See *Deafness*.

Hearing tests
Tests performed to determine whether a person's hearing is impaired, the degree of impairment, and what part of the *ear* may be causing the problem. The main types of hearing test are described in the table (facing page).

WHY THEY ARE DONE
Hearing tests are performed as part of a routine assessment of *child development*. They are sometimes carried out during a general medical examination, and may be performed regularly to check the hearing of people exposed to high noise levels at work.

Hearing tests may be necessary if a person complains of impaired hearing or in cases of suspected hearing loss, such as if a child's speech development is poor or if an elderly person appears to be suffering from *dementia*. A hearing test can also help determine the cause of *tinnitus* and dizziness.

AIMS OF TESTING
The physician attempts to establish the extent and pattern of any hearing deficit by testing the person's ability to hear sounds at different frequencies and volumes. The lowest level at which a person can hear and repeat words (the speech reception threshold) is tested, as is the ability to hear words clearly (speech discrimination). The physician also tries to ascertain whether any hearing loss is conductive or sensorineural in type (see *Deafness*). Test results enable the physician and patient to decide on appropriate treatment, if necessary.

Heart
The muscular pump in the chest which, throughout life, beats continuously and rhythmically to send blood to the lungs and to the rest of the body. During an average lifetime, the heart contracts more than 2.5 billion times.

STRUCTURE
Much of the heart consists of a special type of muscle, called myocardium. The myocardium, given sufficient oxygen and nutrients, contracts rhythmically and automatically without any other stimulus.

The interior of the heart consists of four distinct chambers. A thick central muscular wall, called the septum, divides the cavity into right and left halves. Each half of the heart consists of an upper chamber, called an atrium, and a larger lower chamber, called a ventricle.

Various large blood vessels emerge from the top and sides of the heart. These vessels deliver blood to the atria or carry blood pumped out by the ventricles.

The internal surface of the heart is lined with a smooth membrane, called endocardium, and the entire heart is enclosed in a tough, membranous bag that is called the pericardium.

FUNCTION
The two sides of the heart have distinct, though interdependent, functions. The right side receives deoxygenated blood from the entire body via two large veins called the venae cavae. This blood arrives in the right atrium and, after transfer to the right ventricle, is pumped to the lungs via the pulmonary artery to be oxygenated (receive oxygen through the *alveoli*) and to lose carbon dioxide. The left side of the heart receives oxygenated blood from the lungs (via the pulmonary veins, which drain into the left atrium); this blood is first transferred to the left ventricle and then pumped to all tissues in the body. The heart can thus be viewed as a dual pump. Nonreturn (one-way) valves situated at the exits from each heart chamber guarantee that blood can flow through the circuit in only one direction (see *Heart valves*).

THE CARDIAC CYCLE
The pumping action of the heart consists of three phases, which together make up a cycle corresponding to one heartbeat. These phases are called diastole, atrial systole, and ventricular systole (see illustrated box, p. 515).

To work efficiently, the different parts of the heart must contract in a precise sequence. This sequence is brought about by electrical impulses that emanate from the sinoatrial node, the heart's own pacemaker situated at the top of the right atrium. The electrical impulses are carried partly by the heart muscle itself and partly by specialized nerve fibers.

To avoid bottlenecks developing in the blood circulation, the volume pumped at each stroke by the two sides of the heart must exactly balance each other. However, resistance to blood flow through the general circulation is much greater than resistance to blood flow through the lungs; this means that the left side of the heart must contract much more forcibly than the right side. As a result, the muscular bulk of the left side of the heart is greater than that of the right side.

FACTORS AFFECTING HEART RATE
AND OUTPUT
The rate at which the heart beats, and the amount of blood it puts out with each contraction, can vary considerably according to the demands of the body's muscles for oxygen (and thus for blood). At rest, the heart contracts at 60 to 80 beats per minute and puts out about 80 ml of blood at each stroke, thus pumping about 6 litres per minute. However, during extreme exercise, the rate may increase to 200 contractions per minute and the output may increase to almost 250 ml per beat, thereby increasing the total output to 50 litres per minute.

Such changes in heart rate and output are brought about in two ways. First, the heart muscle is able to respond automatically to any increase in the amount of blood returned to it from active muscles by increasing its output. This occurs because the more the ventricles are filled with blood during the filling phase of the heart's cycle, the more forcibly they contract during ventricular systole to expel the blood. Second, the heart rate is under external control of the *autonomic nervous system* (the part of the nervous system concerned with automatic control of body functions). The parts of the autonomic nervous system concerned with heart action are a nucleus of nerve cells called the cardiac center in the brain stem, and two sets of nerves (parasympathetic and sympathetic) whose activities, controlled by the cardiac center, exert opposing effects on the heart.

When a person is at rest, it is the parasympathetic nerves—particularly the *vagus nerve*—that are active. Signals carried along the vagus nerve act on the sinoatrial node to slow the heart rate from its inherent rate of about 140 impulses per minute to a rate closer to 70 per minute (vagal inhibition). During or in anticipation of muscular activity, the vagal inhibition lessens, the heart rate speeds up, and may speed up even more when the sympathetic nerves come into action. The nerves release *norepinephrine*, which increases the heart rate and the force of contraction.

H

THE HEART

The heart is positioned centrally in the chest, with its right margin directly underneath the right side of the sternum (breastbone). The rest of the heart points to the left, with its lowest point (the apex) located underneath the left nipple.

The heart acts as a dual pump. Deoxygenated blood from the body arrives, via the vena cava, in the right atrium (upper heart chamber), is transferred to the right ventricle (lower chamber), and is then pumped via the pulmonary artery to the lungs. There it is reoxygenated and returns, via the pulmonary veins, to the left side of the heart. It enters the left atrium, is transferred to the left ventricle, and is then pumped, via a large vessel (the aorta), to all parts of the body.

Trachea — Superior vena cava — Pulmonary artery — Right ronchus — Right atrium — Tricuspid valve — Right ventricle — Aorta — Left atrium — Pulmonary valve — Mitral valve — Left ventricle — Septum — Inferior vena cava

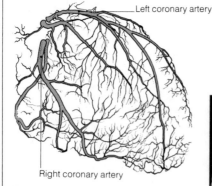

Left coronary artery

Right coronary artery

Blood supply
Although the heart muscle is continually pumping blood, it cannot obtain much oxygen from this flow, so it needs its own blood supply. This is furnished by the two coronary arteries, which arise from the aorta. With their branches, these arteries supply the entire heart muscle.

Right atrium — Left coronary artery — Circumflex branch of left coronary artery — Right coronary artery — Right ventricle

Left ventricle
Angiogram of coronary arteries
The image at left gives a view of the heart from the rear and shows clearly the coronary arteries. The image was achieved by angiography—an X ray of the heart was taken after injecting the coronary arteries with a contrast medium.

The switch from parasympathetic to sympathetic activity is triggered by any influence on the cardiac center that signals an extra need for increased blood output from the heart. Such influences may include fear or anger, low blood pressure, or a reduction of oxygen in the blood.

Heart, artificial

An implantable mechanical device that takes over the heart's action in pumping blood to maintain the circulation. First used in humans in 1985 after years of research in animals, the presently available artificial heart is now seen as a temporary measure to keep a patient alive from a few days to weeks until a *heart transplant* can be performed.

HOW IT WORKS
The type of artificial heart that has so far been used most frequently, but not exclusively, is the Jarvik 7 model. This is a metal and plastic device installed in the patient's chest in place of the diseased heart. During installation, the device is sewn to parts of the patient's own atria (upper chambers) and to the pulmonary artery and aorta (main blood vessels carrying blood out of the heart).

The device is powered by an external machine connected to the device by air lines passing through the chest wall. Pulses of pressure sent through these lines operate the device's pumping action. The patient's movements are restricted by the need to be continuously connected to the machine.

LIMITATIONS AND RISKS
As a temporary measure, the artificial heart has a place in the treatment of life-threatening heart disease, but medical opinion is, at present, strongly against attempts to employ it on a permanent basis. The complications of its use have included *kidney failure*, infection, internal bleeding, mental confusion, and *stroke*. In 1985, after all four US patients in whom an

HEART CYCLE

The pumping action of the heart has three main phases for each heartbeat. Each beat is brought about by electrical waves that emanate from the heart's own pacemaker, the sinoatrial node. The electrocardiogram tracing also shows the phases of the cycle.

Diastole
During this resting phase, the heart fills with blood. Deoxygenated blood flows into the right side of the heart; at the same time, oxygenated blood flows into the left side.

Atrial systole
In this second phase, the two atria (upper chambers of the heart) contract simultaneously, squeezing more blood into the two ventricles, which become fully filled.

Ventricular systole
The ventricles contract to pump deoxygenated blood into the pulmonary artery and oxygenated blood into the aorta. When the heart is emptied, diastole begins again.

Sinoatrial node

Atrio-ventricular node

In diastole, the heart muscle is at rest. Toward the end of this phase of the heart cycle, an electrical impulse begins to emanate from the sinoatrial node.

Atrial systole is brought about by the impulse from the sinoatrial node spreading over the atria. The impulse soon reaches another node, the atrioventricular node.

Ventricular systole is brought about by waves of electrical activity carried from the atrioventricular node to all parts of the ventricles by means of special fibers.

artificial heart had been installed on a permanent basis had died, the researchers decided to concentrate attention on assist devices.

A device known as the intra-aortic balloon pump has been in use since the middle 1970s; it has been found helpful as an alternative method of maintaining the circulation when the heart is badly diseased. The balloon is inflated automatically between each heartbeat to provide extra force to the circulation. This device has the extra advantage of increasing the pressure in the arteries that supply blood to the heart muscle and of relieving the strain on the heart.

Heart attack
A common term for the sudden death of part of the heart muscle. See *Myocardial infarction*.

Heartbeat
A contraction of the *heart* that pumps blood to the lungs and the rest of the body. The heartbeat is readily felt on the left side of the chest, where the apex of the left ventricle (lower heart chamber) lies close beneath the skin. The rate at which contractions occur is called the *heart rate*. The term *pulse* refers to the character and rate of the heartbeat when felt (at the wrist, for example).

Heart block
A common disorder of the *heartbeat* that may lead to episodes of dizziness, fainting attacks, or *stroke*. Heart block is caused by an interruption to the passage of impulses through the specialized conducting system of the heart. Consequently, although the atria beat normally, the ventricles lag behind or contract less often than the atria. This is a completely different problem from the blockage of vessels, e.g., in *atherosclerosis*.

TYPES
There are several grades of heart block. In the least severe form, the delay between the contractions of the atria and ventricles is just slightly longer than normal (called a prolonged P-R interval from its appearance on an *ECG*). Sometimes the delay lengthens with successive beats, until eventually a ventricular beat is dropped. In more severe cases, only a half, a third, or a quarter of the atrial beats is conducted to the ventricles. In complete heart block, the atria and ventricles beat independently. Thus, while the rate of atrial contraction varies according to the patient's activity, the ventricles contract at a fairly constant rate of about 40 beats per minute.

Heart block may be due to *coronary artery disease*, *myocarditis* (inflammation of heart muscle), an overdose of a *digitalis drug*, *rheumatic fever*, or syphilitic *aortitis*. In about half of all cases of heart block, the patient has no history of heart disease.

SYMPTOMS
A prolonged P-R interval causes no symptoms even though it can be detected on an *ECG*. Dropped beats may also be symptomless.

In other cases, the rate of the ventricular beat is slower than normal; in complete heart block, the rate does not increase in response to exercise. Sometimes the ventricles are able to compensate by expelling more blood with each contraction. In other cases, the blood output from the ventricles is inadequate, and the patient may become breathless due to *heart failure*, may develop the chest pains of *angina pectoris*, or may faint.

If the ventricular beat becomes very slow, or stops altogether for a few seconds, the patient may black out and have a seizure because insufficient blood reaches the brain. However, the ventricular beat usually restarts within a few seconds. If the delay is prolonged in a person whose brain is affected by atherosclerosis, a stroke may result.

H

DISORDERS OF THE HEART

Heart disorders are by far the most common cause of death in developed countries. They also impair the quality of life of millions of people, restricting activity by causing pain, breathlessness, fatigue, fainting spells, and anxiety. A wide range of conditions can affect the heart by disrupting its pumping action.

GENETIC DISORDERS

In general, inherited or genetic factors do not play a large part in causing heart disorders. However, they do contribute to the *hyperlipidemias* that predispose a person to *atherosclerosis* and *coronary artery disease.*

CONGENITAL DEFECTS

Structural abnormalities in the heart are among the most common birth defects, but are usually treatable. They result from errors of development in the fetus and include such conditions as *septal defects* ("holes in the heart") and some types of abnormal *heart valves.* (See *Heart disease, congenital.*)

INFECTION

Endocarditis is an infection of the lining of the heart and of the heart valves, usually occurring in people whose hearts have already been damaged by *rheumatic fever* or are abnormal because of some congenital or degenerative disorder. It may also affect drug addicts who inject themselves intravenously with nonsterile needles. The infection may cause damage to and malfunction of any of the heart valves, leading to, for example, *aortic insufficiency* (although heart valve disease can also have other causes). Some types of cardiomyopathy are triggered by viral infection; viruses may also cause *myocarditis* (inflammation of the heart).

TUMORS

Tumors arising from the heart tissues are rare, the most common being the benign *myxoma* (which grows inside one of the chambers of the heart and may interfere with blood flow or valve action). Occasionally a malignant *sarcoma* develops. Secondary tumors, spreading from elsewhere in the body (such as the breast or lung), are more common than primary tumors.

These *metastases* usually grow within the heart muscle or the pericardium (sac that surrounds the heart), but seldom affect the valves. The tumors may produce electrocardiographic (see *ECG*) abnormalities and, if extensive, result in congestive *heart failure.*

MUSCLE DISORDERS

Cardiomyopathy is a general term for disease of the heart muscle itself. One type of cardiomyopathy is inherited; others may be caused by vitamin deficiency or alcohol poisoning, or may be triggered by a viral infection.

Myocarditis is inflammation of the heart muscle. It may be caused by a viral infection or by toxins released during a bacterial infection. Rarely, it results from drugs or radiation therapy.

INJURY

Blunt injury to the heart most often occurs in car accidents through impact with the steering wheel. The heart is compressed between the sternum (breastbone) and the spine and may suffer injury ranging from mild bruising to complete rupture. In immediately fatal car accidents, up to two thirds of the victims have suffered rupture of a heart chamber. Seat belt use could probably prevent some of these deaths.

Stab wounds to the heart are often fatal within minutes, but, of patients who reach hospital, most survive. Bullet wounds are also very serious; only about 10 percent of people shot in the heart reach hospital alive.

NUTRITIONAL DISORDERS

The heart muscle is sensitive to severe nutritional deficiency and may become thin and flabby from simple lack of protein and calories. Thiamine (vitamin B_1) deficiency, which is common in chronic alcoholics, causes *beriberi* with congestive heart failure. *Obesity* is another important factor in causing heart disease, probably through its effect on other risk factors such as *hypertension, diabetes,* and *cholesterol.*

IMPAIRED BLOOD SUPPLY

The major cause of heart disease in developed countries is impaired blood supply. The coronary arteries (which supply blood to the heart) become narrowed due to *atherosclerosis* and parts of the heart muscle are deprived of oxygen. The result of coronary artery disease may be *angina pectoris* or, eventually, a *myocardial infarction.*

POISONING

The most common toxic substance affecting the heart is alcohol. A large intake for many years may cause a type of cardiomyopathy in which the heart becomes enlarged and heart failure develops. If alcohol intake is stopped, recovery is possible.

DRUGS

Certain drugs may disturb the heartbeat or even cause permanent damage to the heart muscle. These drugs include the anticancer drug doxorubicin, the tricyclic antidepressants, and even many drugs used to treat heart disease.

OTHER DISORDERS

Many common and serious heart disorders may be a complication of some other underlying condition, such as coronary artery disease, cardiomyopathy, or a congenital defect. Such disorders include cardiac *arrhythmia* (a disturbance in the rhythm of the heartbeat), some cases of *heart block* (in which contractions of the upper and lower parts of the heart are not synchronized), and heart failure (inability of the heart to keep up with its work load). *Cor pulmonale* is a failure of the right side of the heart; it is a consequence of lung diseases (such as *emphysema*), which increase the resistance to blood flow.

INVESTIGATION

Heart disease and disorders are investigated by such techniques as auscultation (listening to the heart sounds) and *ECG* (electrocardiography); heart *imaging techniques* such as chest X ray, echocardiography, coronary angiography, *CT scanning,* and *MRI;* cardiac catheterization; blood tests; and, in rare cases, *biopsy* of the heart muscle (removal of a small sample of tissue for analysis).

H

TYPES OF CONGENITAL HEART DISEASE

The major malformations are *septal defects*, *coarctation of the aorta*, *transposition of the great vessels*, *patent ductus arteriosus*, *tetralogy of Fallot*, *hypoplastic left heart syndrome*, *pulmonary stenosis*, and *aortic stenosis*. The bars (right) show the incidence of each type of malformation among affected babies.

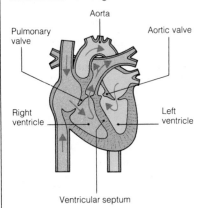

Aorta

Pulmonary valve

Aortic valve

Right ventricle

Left ventricle

Ventricular septum

How blood circulates
Deoxygenated blood (gray) is pumped from the right ventricle into the lungs, where it exchanges carbon dioxide for oxygen. The newly oxygenated blood (pink) enters the left side of the heart and is then pumped out of the left ventricle to all body tissues.

5%

Pulmonary stenosis
This is a narrowing of the pulmonary valve, or (rarely) of the upper right ventricle, which reduces blood flow to the lungs.

10%

Coarctation of the aorta
In this disorder, localized narrowing of the aorta reduces the supply of blood to the lower part of the body.

8%

Patent ductus arteriosus
The ductus arteriosus fails to close after birth and blood from the aorta continues to flow through it into the pulmonary artery.

25%

Ventricular septal defect
This is a hole in the ventricular septum, causing blood to flow from the left ventricle to the right and thence to the lungs.

7%

Tetralogy of Fallot
This is a hole in the ventricular septum, pulmonary stenosis, a displaced aorta, and a thickened right ventricle.

14%

Transposition of the great vessels
Oxygenated blood passes back to the lungs, instead of through the aorta to the body tissues.

DIAGNOSIS
Heart block may be suspected if a person has a slow, regular heartbeat (below 50 beats per minute) that does not accelerate during exercise. The diagnosis is confirmed by an ECG.

TREATMENT
Some cases of heart block do not require treatment (e.g., if there are no symptoms or if an elderly person has only minor symptoms). Heart block that is causing fainting attacks is usually treated by the fitting of an artificial *pacemaker*, which overrides the natural pacemaker and faulty electrical conducting system in the heart.

Less commonly, heart block may be treated with drugs, such as *isoproterenol*. In most cases, drug treatment is reserved for emergencies or as a temporary measure until an artificial pacemaker can be fitted.

Heartburn

A burning pain in the center of the chest which may travel from the tip of the sternum (breastbone) to the throat. Heartburn may be caused by overeating, by eating rich or spicy food, or by drinking alcohol. Recurrent heartburn is a symptom of *esophagitis* (inflammation of the esophagus), which is usually caused by *acid reflux* (backflow of stomach acid). Heartburn is often brought on by lying down or by bending forward.

Occasionally, heartburn may cause chest pain that is mistaken for the pain of heart disease.

Heart disease, congenital

Any heart abnormality that has been present from birth. Congenital heart defects are the most common major malformations compatible with life. Defects may affect the heart chambers, heart valves, or main blood vessels (see illustrated box).

CAUSES AND INCIDENCE
About 800 babies per 100,000 are born with a congenital heart defect. The errors of development leading to defects arise early in the life of the *embryo*. In most cases, there is no known cause. Of known causes, the most common is *rubella* (German measles) in the mother during the first three months of pregnancy. This can be prevented by vaccination before conception. About one third of babies with *Down's syndrome* have a congenital heart defect, and congenital heart disease often accompanies other birth defects.

Hereditary factors do not seem to play a significant role. If a couple have an affected child, there is little increased risk of a second child being affected. People born with heart defects have little increased risk of having an affected child. Prenatal diagnosis, using specialized *ultrasound scanning*, is now possible for some defects.

SYMPTOMS AND COMPLICATIONS
The symptoms of congenital heart disease arise from either insufficient or excessive circulation of blood to the lungs or to the body. The defects in heart anatomy can also mean that some deoxygenated blood is pumped

H

to the body instead of to the lungs or some oxygenated blood to the lungs instead of to the body. This is called "shunting". Heart anomalies can result in *cyanosis* (blueness caused by a reduced oxygen level in the general blood circulation), in breathlessness, or in both.

Symptoms may first appear at any time over a wide range of ages, according to the defect. Similarly, recognition of a defect may occur any time from before birth to adulthood.

Apart from cyanosis and breathlessness, an untreated heart defect can cause stunted growth and underdevelopment of the limbs and muscles. Mild respiratory infections may lead to pneumonia. With prolonged cyanosis, *clubbing* (thickening and broadening) of the ends of fingers and toes may develop. If there is insufficient capacity of the heart to increase blood flow during effort, the child may rapidly tire and be unable to take part in physical exercise. In some untreated cases, a serious complication called *Eisenmenger complex* (in which there is increased resistance of the lungs to blood flow) develops.

DIAGNOSIS
A heart defect may be diagnosed by procedures such as *chest X rays*, *ECG*, *echocardiography*, and, less commonly, cardiac *catheterization*.

TREATMENT
Rest, oxygen, and various drugs to assist the circulation and lung function may improve matters for a limited time or sometimes indefinitely. Some conditions, such as small septal defects, may get smaller or disappear on their own. Other defects are likely to worsen, and surgical correction is often a consideration.

Today, surgical correction is available for most affected children; the risk of death from unsuccessful surgery lessens every year. One condition—hypoplastic left heart syndrome (in which the left side of the heart is severely underdeveloped)—can however be treated only by performing a *heart transplant*.

Narrowed heart valves can often be treated by balloon *valvuloplasty*. In this procedure, a special catheter is introduced into the heart to widen the narrowed valve.

In other cases, *open heart surgery* is necessary. Sometimes, any of a range of *prostheses* (artificial spare parts), such as replacement heart valves or blood vessels, may be used. In some cases, a heart transplant or *heart-lung transplant* may be necessary.

OUTLOOK
Following successful heart surgery, recovery to good health with resumption of growth, increased activity, and better appetite follow rapidly, and the child usually has a near-normal life expectancy. Full activities, including sports, are generally possible after three to six months.

Children with heart defects (corrected or uncorrected) are at an increased risk of bacterial *endocarditis*, a potentially dangerous infection of the heart lining and heart valves. To protect against this possibility, children with congenital heart disease are given *antibiotic drugs* before undergoing surgical procedures.

Heart disease, ischemic
The most common form of heart disease, in which there is a reduced blood supply resulting from narrowing or obstruction of the coronary arteries. (See *Coronary artery disease*.)

Heart failure
Inability of the heart to cope with its work load of pumping blood to the lungs and to the rest of the body. Although heart failure sounds like a life-threatening disorder, the condition is usually treatable and compatible with survival for many years.

TYPES AND CAUSES
Heart failure is usually termed either left-sided or right-sided failure.

LEFT-SIDED FAILURE This may be due to *hypertension* (high blood pressure), *anemia*, or *hyperthyroidism* (overactivity of the thyroid gland), to a heart valve defect (such as *aortic stenosis, aortic insufficiency,* or *mitral insufficiency*), or to a congenital heart defect (such as *coarctation of the aorta*). In all these conditions, the left side of the heart must work harder to pump the same amount of blood. Sometimes, the extra workload can be compensated for by an increase in the size of the left side of the heart and in the thickness of its muscular walls, or by an increase in heart rate. Compensation is only temporary, however, and heart failure follows.

Other causes of left-sided heart failure include cardiac *arrhythmias* (irregularities of the heart rhythm), *coronary artery disease, myocardial infarction* (heart attack), and *cardiomyopathy* (disease of the heart muscle). In cardiomyopathy, the pumping power of the heart is reduced so it can no longer deal with its normal work load.

Whatever the cause, the left side of the heart fails to empty completely with each contraction or has difficulty accepting blood returning from the lungs. The retained blood creates a back pressure that causes the lungs to become congested with blood. This in turn leads to *pulmonary edema* (excess fluid in the lungs), of which the main symptom is shortness of breath.

RIGHT-SIDED FAILURE Right-sided failure most often results from *pulmonary hypertension* (raised pressure and resistance to blood flow through the lungs)—itself caused by left-sided failure or by lung disease (such as chronic *bronchitis* or *emphysema*). Right-sided failure can also be due to a valve defect (such as *tricuspid insufficiency*) or a congenital heart defect (such as a *septal defect, pulmonary stenosis,* or *tetralogy of Fallot*). In all types of right-sided failure, there is a back pressure in the blood circulation from the heart into the venous system, causing swollen neck veins, enlargement of the liver, and *edema* (accumulation of fluid in the tissues).

SYMPTOMS
Fatigue is an early symptom of heart failure. Breathing difficulty is the most common symptom of left-sided heart failure and is caused by fluid in the lungs. Breathlessness may first be noticed only during or after exercise, but worsens and is eventually apparent even at rest. The patient may be able to breathe easily only when well propped up in bed. Sometimes he or she may awaken at night with an attack of breathlessness, wheezing, and sweating. Attacks of acute heart failure may subside on their own or may alternatively require urgent, life-saving treatment.

Right-sided heart failure produces less breathlessness and more swelling of the ankles and legs, often with enlargement of the liver and congestion of the intestines, causing discomfort and indigestion.

TREATMENT
Immediate treatment of the heart failure is followed by treatment of its underlying cause.

Immediate treatment consists of bed rest, with the patient sitting up. The patient is given *diuretic drugs*, which increase the output of urine from the kidneys, thus ridding the body of excess fluid and reducing blood volume. In some cases, *vasodilator drugs*, which ease the work load of the heart, or *digitalis drugs*, which strengthen the contractions of the heartbeat, may also be given. *Morphine* is sometimes given as an emergency treatment in acute left-sided failure. These measures usually bring about a significant improvement within a few days.

Once the heart failure is treated, attention is directed to treating the underlying cause. If a defective heart valve is responsible, it may be treated by *heart valve surgery* (although, ideally, defective heart valves should be corrected surgically before severe heart failure develops).

Many other causes of heart failure are also treatable; hypertension and arrhythmias are treated by drug treatment, and congenital septal defects are treated by open heart surgery. However, when the cause is a long-standing cardiomyopathy or chronic lung disease, the outlook is generally not as good.

Heart imaging
Techniques that provide images of the heart and its structure. Imaging is performed to detect structural abnormality, disease, or impaired function.

TYPES
A *chest X ray* is the simplest and most widely used method of obtaining an image of the heart. An X ray can show heart size and shape, and whether or not abnormal calcification is present in the valves, major vessels, or the pericardium (membranous bag that surrounds the heart). *Pulmonary edema* (accumulation of fluid in the lungs) and engorgement (overfilling with blood) of the vessels connecting the heart and lungs are usually detectable on a chest X ray and may indicate the presence of *heart failure*. Pacemakers and artificial heart valves show up clearly on X ray and can be checked for position.

Angiography (an imaging technique in which X rays are taken after the injection of a contrast medium) may be performed to show the heart chambers. Children with complex forms of congenital heart disease, such as *tetralogy of Fallot*, may be investigated by this procedure.

Angiography is also performed to evaluate the state of the coronary arteries in patients with *coronary artery disease*. The images produced provide information affecting decisions about valve replacement.

Echocardiography (cardiac ultrasound) is most useful as the first step in investigating congenital heart abnormalities or in evaluating valvular or heart wall abnormalities. An ultrasound technique exploiting the *Doppler effect* enables the physician to measure blood flow across valves.

Radionuclide scanning is a form of imaging that shows only a limited degree of anatomical detail but that provides some information about heart function, such as how well the heart wall moves and how effectively it empties.

The development of more rapid machines for *CT scanning* has made it possible to use this technique to obtain useful information about the heart; earlier scanning machines were too slow to "freeze" a heartbeat.

High-quality images of the heart can also be obtained by *MRI* techniques. These techniques are used, for example, for assessing the results of *coronary artery bypass* surgery. In some cases, MRI techniques may eliminate the need for angiography and for other techniques used to investigate congenital heart disease.

Heart-lung machine
A machine that temporarily takes over the function of the heart and lungs to facilitate certain operations in the chest. Use of the heart-lung machine gives the surgeon more time for operations and prevents the operation site from being obscured by blood.

Operations performed using a heart-lung machine include *open heart surgery*, *heart transplants*, and *heart-lung transplants*.

A heart-lung machine consists principally of a pump (to replace the heart) and an oxygenator (to replace the lungs). The machine is sometimes called a cardiopulmonary bypass or pump oxygenator. Once the machine is connected and working, the patient's heart and lungs are effectively bypassed and the heart can be stopped.

HOW IT WORKS
Blood is taken via cannulas (tubes) inserted into the inferior and superior venae cavae (the main veins draining blood into the heart) and pumped through the oxygenator, which acts as an artificial lung, putting oxygen into the blood and removing carbon dioxide from it. The freshly oxygenated blood is then returned to the arterial circulation via a cannula inserted into the aorta (the main artery carrying blood from the heart) or the femoral artery (a large artery in the leg).

There are two main types of oxygenator. In one type, the blood is passed up a column, through which a gas mixture with a high oxygen content is bubbled. This adds oxygen and removes carbon dioxide. The blood is then treated with a defoaming agent

and held in a reservoir until it is returned to the patient. In the second type, called a membrane oxygenator, the blood and gas flow on either side of a thin, semipermeable membrane, through which oxygen passes from gas into blood; carbon dioxide passes in the opposing direction. This method more closely mimics the function of the lungs.

The heart-lung machine also contains a heat exchanger. This may be used to rewarm blood (which loses heat in the machine) before returning it to the patient. In some cases, the heat exchanger is used to cool blood intentionally to cause a drop in the patient's temperature and so give the surgeons more time for the operation (see *Hypothermia, surgical*).

LIMITATIONS
Use of a heart-lung machine tends to damage red blood cells and to cause the blood to clot; these problems are minimized by giving the patient *heparin*, an anticoagulant drug, before the machine is used.

A patient can be kept on a heart-lung machine for only a few hours. Use of the machine reduces the efficiency of the blood supply to the patient's vital organs and thus limits the time available for an operation.

Heart-lung transplant
A procedure in which both the heart and lungs of a patient are removed and replaced with organs from a donor who has been certified brain dead. (See illustrated box, p. 520, for how and why the operation is done.)

RISKS AND COMPLICATIONS
The early attempts at heart-lung transplant were unsuccessful. In the early 1980s the risk of donor organ rejection was reduced by the introduction of the drug *cyclosporine*. Some hospitals are now obtaining very good results. Nevertheless, the operation carries substantial risks. Problems may arise from airway obstruction and other lung complications (including *bronchiolitis*) in addition to the risks of organ rejection. Patients face the long-term problems associated with other forms of *transplant surgery*.

Heart rate
The rate at which the heart beats—that is, contracts to pump blood around the body.

Most people have a heart rate of between 60 and 100 beats per minute at rest. This rate remains fairly constant throughout life, although it tends to be faster in childhood and to

HEART-LUNG TRANSPLANT

In this procedure, both the heart and lungs of a patient are removed and replaced with organs taken from a brain-dead donor. The removed heart can sometimes be given to another patient.

HOW IT IS DONE

Heart and lungs must be removed from both donor and patient; the donor organs are then inserted into the patient.

1 The donor heart and lungs must be healthy, and the lungs must match the size of the patient's chest, as measured by chest X rays.

2 In both donor and patient, the heart and lungs are reached via an incision made in the sternum, and the chest is opened up.

Site of incision

3 The patient is connected to a heart-lung machine. It takes over the function of heart and lungs, oxygenating blood taken from the venae cavae and pumping it back to the body via the aorta.

— Trachea

— Aorta

— Right atrium/Vena cava

4 In both patient and donor, heart and lungs are removed through cuts in the trachea, aorta, and where the heart connects to the venae cavae. The blood vessels linking donor heart and lungs are left intact.

WHY IT IS DONE

Subject to availability of a donor, a heart-lung transplant can offer hope to someone who is dying of a terminally chronic lung disease, whether or not he or she is also suffering from heart disease. Diseases treated include *emphysema, cystic fibrosis, sarcoidosis, or interstitial pulmonary fibrosis*. The heart-lung transplant operation has a better success record than that of lung transplant alone.

These sections were taken from a healthy lung (left) and an emphysematous lung; transplantation of heart and lungs may give an emphysema patient new hope.

— Tracheal reconnection

— Aortic reconnection

— Right atrium/Vena cava reconnection

5 Insertion of the donor organs into the patient is, in some respects, easier than in the heart transplant, since fewer reconnections have to be made. The main reconnections are between the patient's and donor's tracheas and aortas and between the right atrium of the donor heart and the patient's venae cavae.

slow slightly with age. Some athletes have a resting rate below 60 beats per minute. Their hearts are very well developed and can pump blood around the body as efficiently at a slow rate as the normal heart can pump it at a faster rate.

Exercise or stress causes an increase in heart rate. In either case, the increase is due to the release of the hormones *epinephrine* and *norepinephrine* by the adrenal glands and of norepinephrine by the sympathetic nerves around the sinoatrial node, the heart's own pacemaker. A small decrease in heart rate occurs during total relaxation and sleep.

Many people have a harmless irregularity of heart rhythm in which the rate is more rapid during breathing in than breathing out.

MEASURING HEART-RATE

A doctor uses one of two methods to measure heart-rate and rhythm (the regularity of the beat). One is to feel the pulse (the expansion of an artery in response to contractions of the heart). The other method, which is sometimes more accurate, is to listen with a *stethoscope* placed just below the left nipple (see *Heart sounds*).

A more accurate record of heart rate and rhythm is provided by an *ECG* (electrocardiogram), which registers the pattern of electrical activity in the heart muscle before each beat.

DISORDERS OF HEART RATE

A resting heart rate above 100 beats per minute is termed a *tachycardia* and a rate below 60 beats per minute a *bradycardia*. Tachycardias and bradycardias are considered abnormal when the cause is a condition affecting nerve conduction pathways through the heart or the activity of the sinoatrial node, rather than a response of the heart to exercise or relaxation. (See also *Arrhythmia, cardiac*.)

Heart sounds

The sounds made by the *heart* during each heartbeat. In each heart cycle, there are two main heart sounds, known as the first heart sound and the second heart sound.

The main heart sounds can be heard simply by putting an ear to someone's chest. Using a *stethoscope*, a physician can hear the heart sounds much more clearly (and may sometimes hear additional sounds or an abnormality of one of the two main sounds). Interpretation of these sounds can be important in the diagnosis of *heart valve* disorders, as well as other heart abnormalities.

The first heart sound is often described as a "lubb." It results from closure of the tricuspid and mitral valves at the exits from the upper chambers of the heart, which occurs when the ventricles (lower chambers) begin contracting to pump blood out of the heart. The second heart sound is a higher-pitched "dupp." This sound, which is caused by closure of the pulmonary and aortic valves at the exits from the ventricles, occurs when the ventricles finish contracting. There is a pause after each lubb-dupp.

In children and young adults, there is often a normal low-pitched third heart sound after the second sound. It is thought to be caused by vibration of the muscle. In people over the age of 40, this sound is abnormal and a sign of heart failure.

Abnormal heart sounds may be a sign of various disorders of the heart. For example, an additional low-pitched sound before the first sound indicates an abnormality of the heart muscle. This sound is often present after a *myocardial infarction* (heart attack). Ejection sounds or "clicks" are high-pitched sounds caused by the abrupt halting of valve opening. These can occur in people with *hypertension* (high blood pressure) or certain heart valve defects. Heart *murmurs* are abnormal sounds caused by turbulent blood flow. They may occur as a result of any of various heart valve defects or types of congenital heart disease.

Heart surgery

Any operation performed on the heart. Heart surgery was a rare and hazardous undertaking until the early 1950s, when an operation called mitral valvotomy became a standard and successful procedure. This operation, performed to correct a narrowed mitral valve, entails passing a finger into the beating heart in order to stretch open the affected valve.

Such "closed" operations on the heart are still occasionally performed, but have largely been superseded in developed countries by *open heart surgery*, in which the heartbeat is deliberately stopped and the heart opened to make repairs. Open heart surgery was made possible by developments such as the controlled cooling of patients for surgery (see *Hypothermia, surgical*) and the introduction in the 1950s of the *heart-lung machine*, which considerably prolonged the time during which the surgeons could work. Open heart surgery allows the treatment of many previously serious or fatal con-

ditions, including most types of heart defect present at birth (see *Heart disease, congenital*) and various disorders of the *heart valves*.

Coronary artery bypass, an operation to treat obstruction of the arteries that supply the heart muscle, was first performed in 1967 and, within five years, similar surgical procedures were being carried out all over the world. Also in 1967, the first *heart transplant* was performed in South Africa; the results of heart transplant surgery are now much improved largely because of advances in preventing organ rejection.

Another significant development was the introduction in 1979 of balloon *angioplasty* to treat narrowing of the coronary arteries. The results are excellent and many lives have been saved because of it.

Angioplasty balloons are also being used to open up narrowed heart valves (see *Valvuloplasty*).

The use of *laser treatment* for stubborn cases of narrowed arteries is currently being investigated.

Heart transplant

Replacement of a person's damaged or diseased heart by a healthy human heart taken from a donor in whom *brain death* has been certified.

HISTORY

Heart transplantation in animals was first achieved in 1959. The first human heart transplant was performed by Professor Christiaan Barnard in South Africa in 1967. Early results were disappointing, however, and few patients survived more than a month or two. The team led by Professor Norman Shumway at Stanford University, California, began a program of heart transplants in 1969; by 1984 this team showed that as many as 85 percent of patients could be expected to survive for at least a year after surgery.

LIMITATIONS

Heart transplantation poses some special problems compared with the more common procedure of kidney transplantation.

First, there can be a problem of timing. Whereas the condition of a patient with kidney failure can be maintained in health by *dialysis* until a donor kidney becomes available, there is no equivalent method for maintaining the condition of someone with a nonfunctioning heart. Hence, a heart transplant is possible only when a suitable donor heart is available at the right time.

H

Second, heart transplantation has no "fallback" system; if the heart is rejected (attacked by the body's *immune system*), the only hope for the patient is another transplant.

In theory, the mechanical artificial heart (see *Heart, artificial*) is a possible solution to the problems of timing and rejection. In practice, however, the best that the artificial heart seems able to offer is a temporary respite for a patient until a donor heart becomes available.

Heart transplant operations are further limited by the fact that they are most likely to succeed if the heart is removed from the donor while it is still beating. One reason for the success of the Stanford heart transplant program was that California, often a leader in liberalized legislation, was the first North American jurisdiction to allow physicians to certify death while the heart was still beating (provided the brain was irreversibly destroyed by disease or accident). Certification of brain death in a patient connected to an artificial ventilator is now permitted in most developed countries, allowing removal of the heart in optimum condition.

WHY IT IS DONE

Heart transplantation is considered for the treatment of patients with progressive, irremediable heart disease, but who are otherwise in good health. Many such patients have advanced *coronary artery disease*; most of the others have *cardiomyopathy* (disease of the heart muscle).

If the heart disorder is associated with lung disease, a *heart-lung transplant* may be performed.

HOW IT IS DONE

Following its removal from the donor, the heart is chilled in saline to maintain its condition. If necessary, the donor heart can then be transported many miles, often by air, before being implanted into the recipient.

The actual heart transplant operation is no more or less difficult than other major heart surgery. The first step is to connect the patient's major blood vessels to a *heart-lung machine*, which pumps oxygenated blood to the brain and other vital organs while the surgeon operates. Once the blood is bypassed through the heart-lung machine, the surgeon removes the diseased heart, leaving the back walls of the atria (upper heart chambers) in place, and then inserts the donor heart. The major blood vessels are then reconnected, and the new heart can take over from the machine.

HEART VALVE REPLACEMENT

Any one of the four heart valves (aortic, pulmonary, mitral, or tricuspid) may require replacing (see diagram below right). Replacement of the aortic heart valve is described in the steps below.

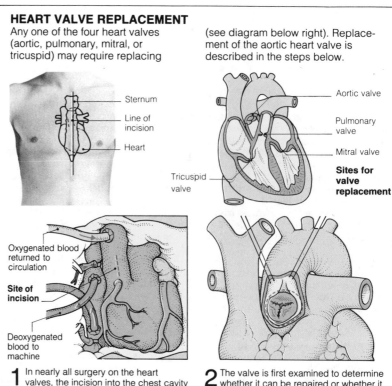

Sternum
Line of incision
Heart

Aortic valve
Pulmonary valve
Mitral valve
Tricuspid valve

Sites for valve replacement

Oxygenated blood returned to circulation
Site of incision
Deoxygenated blood to machine

1 In nearly all surgery on the heart valves, the incision into the chest cavity is made through the sternum (breastbone). The patient is put on a *heart-lung machine*, the beating of the heart is stopped, and the heart is opened.

2 The valve is first examined to determine whether it can be repaired or whether it requires replacement. If the latter is necessary (as here), the valve is excised (dotted line indicates where the incision is made).

3 A prosthesis is sutured into position and the aorta is closed. The patient is disconnected from the machine and the chest wall is sewn up. The operation takes between two and four hours.

Artificial heart valve in place
This chest X ray shows the metal components of an artificial heart valve. A ball-and-cage valve has been used to replace the patient's diseased valve.

OUTLOOK

Once the immediate postoperative period is over, the outlook is good, with more than 80 percent of patients surviving the first year in some hospitals; there is a death rate of around 5 percent per year thereafter. These results are much better than for the surgical treatment of lung or stomach cancer. The main problems are rejection, which can be countered by *immunosuppressant drugs* (such as cyclosporine, prednisone, and cyclophosphamide), and infection. Of course infection is always a hazard for people taking immunosuppressant drugs because these drugs can weaken the body's ability to fight off invading microorganisms. (See also *Transplant surgery*.)

TYPES OF REPLACEMENT HEART VALVES

The three main types

There are three main types of replacement valve—biological, mechanical, and homograft. Biological valves are taken from pigs or made from bovine tissue or the patient's own tissue; examples include the Carpentier-Edwards and Ionescu-Shiley valves. Mechanical valves are made from metal, plastic, and carbon fiber. There are two main types—ball-and-cage valves (such as the Starr-Edwards valve) and those with one or more tilting disks (such as the Bjork-Shiley and St. Jude valves). Homografts are human valves that have been removed from people who have died of a disease that does not affect the heart.

	Biological	Mechanical	Homograft
Examples	Carpentier-Edwards; Ionescu-Shiley	Starr-Edwards (ball-and-cage); Bjork-Shiley (tilting disk); St. Jude (two tilting disks)	Taken from cadaver
Availability	Readily available	Readily available	Some centers only
Ease of insertion	Routine	Routine	Specialized
Suitable age group	Over 35	All ages	All ages
Duration	About seven years	More than 12 years	More than 12 years
Postoperative drug therapy	Short-term anticoagulants	Lifelong anticoagulants	None necessary
Possible complications	Infection; stroke; damage to blood cells	Infection; stroke; calcification	Infection; calcification

H

Heart valve

A structure at the exit of a *heart* chamber that allows blood to flow out of the chamber, but which prevents backwash. There are four heart valves (one at the exit of each heart chamber). Their correct functioning is vital to the efficiency of the heart as a pump.

The opening and, more particularly, the closing of heart valves during each heart cycle are responsible for *heart sounds*.

DISORDERS

Any of the four heart valves may be affected by stenosis (narrowing), which causes the heart to work harder to force blood through the valve, or by incompetence or insufficiency (leakiness), which makes the valve unable to prevent backwash of blood. These defects cause characteristic *heart murmurs* which can be heard and identified by a physician.

Valve defects may be present at birth, either alone or with other defects (see *Heart disease, congenital*), or may be acquired later in life. The most common congenital valve defects are *aortic stenosis* and *pulmonary stenosis*.

Acquired heart valve disease is usually the result of degenerative changes or ischemia (diminished blood supply) affecting part of the heart and leading to aortic stenosis or *mitral insufficiency*.

Rheumatic fever was once the main cause of *mitral stenosis*, mitral insufficiency, aortic valve defects, and, less commonly, *tricuspid stenosis* and *tricuspid insufficiency*. Rheumatic fever is now rare in developed countries but is still prevalent in poorer countries.

Valves may also be destroyed by bacterial *endocarditis*, occurring often in intravenous drug users. Bacterial endocarditis is, however, a possible complication of any valve disorder.

The symptoms and signs of valve disorders vary but disorders commonly lead to *heart failure*, rhythm irregularities (see *Arrhythmias, cardiac*), or symptoms resulting from reduced blood supply to body tissues.

Valve defects may be diagnosed by *physical examination* (including *auscultation* to listen to the heart sounds), *chest X ray, ECG, echocardiography,* Doppler echocardiography, and cardiac *catheterization*. Valve defects may be corrected by *heart valve surgery*.

Heart valve surgery

An operation to correct a *heart valve* defect or, in many cases, to remove a diseased or damaged valve. A removed valve can be replaced by a mechanical valve (made from metal and plastic), a valve fashioned from human or bovine tissue, a pig valve, or a human valve taken from a corpse.

WHY IT IS DONE

A heart valve may have to be corrected or replaced because it is either stenotic (narrowed) or insufficient (leaky).

H

Surgery is most often performed to treat a disorder of the mitral or aortic valve (which is located on the left side of the heart).

In general, heart-valve surgery is considered only when the potential effects of the malfunctioning valve on the heart and on general health are so severe that they will soon be life-threatening. The timing of the operation is crucial and is based on an assessment of the patient's symptoms and the results of tests (such as *ECG*, *chest X rays*, *echocardiography*, and cardiac *catheterization*).

HOW IT IS DONE
The illustrated box on page 522 shows how an aortic valve is replaced.

Valvotomy is an operation in which an instrument or finger is used to widen a narrowed valve; *valvuloplasty* is a newer technique that uses a balloon catheter to widen a valve.

RECOVERY AND OUTLOOK
After the operation, the patient is usually kept in an intensive-care unit for 24 hours, followed by a few days in hospital. A longer stay may be necessary if complications develop or if the patient was suffering from severe heart failure before the operation.

Symptoms such as breathlessness may take many weeks to improve and may require continuing medication to maintain the improvement. Some people (those with a mechanical replacement valve and those with heart rhythm abnormalities, for example) require long-term treatment with *anticoagulant drugs* to prevent the formation of blood clots around the new valve, which could become detached and travel to the brain or other organs. All patients need long-term follow-up examinations to ensure that the repaired or replaced valve is working well. To reduce the risk of the valve's becoming infected, most people who have had heart-valve surgery have to take *antibiotic drugs* before any dental or certain other surgical procedures.

Most heart-valve surgery is successful; the death rate is low and is continuing to decline. If a replacement valve malfunctions, it is often possible to insert a new one.

Heat cramps
Painful contractions in muscles caused by excessive salt loss due to profuse sweating. Heat cramps are usually brought on by strenuous activity in extreme heat. The condition may occur by itself or as a symptom of *heat exhaustion* or *heatstroke*.

FIRST AID: HEAT EXHAUSTION

1 Offer plenty of salt solution to drink (about 0.25 teaspoon/0.5 litre) and seek medical help immediately.

2 Lay the victim down in a cool place and raise his or her feet by about 30 cm.

Prevention and treatment consist of taking salt tablets or drinking sufficient quantities of a weak salt solution (a quarter of a level teaspoon of salt to half a litre of cold water) to keep the urine pale. Too much salt may cause the patient to vomit.

Heat disorders
The body functions most efficiently at a temperature of 37°C; any major deviation disrupts the body processes. Malfunctioning or overloading of the body's mechanisms for keeping its temperature constant may lead to a heat disorder. For example, poor adaptation to heat may lead to *heat cramps*, *heat exhaustion*, or *heatstroke*; excessive environmental heat may result in *prickly heat*. Body functions may also be disrupted by excessive heat production in the body during a high *fever* caused by infection.

HEAT REGULATION
The mechanisms by which the body loses unwanted heat to maintain the optimum internal temperature are controlled by the *hypothalamus* (part of the brain). When the hypothalamus is disrupted (e.g., by drugs or a fever) the body may overheat progressively, which may lead to fatal heatstroke if emergency treatment is not given.

When the temperature of the blood rises, the hypothalamus sends nerve impulses to stimulate the sweat glands and dilate (widen) blood vessels in the skin. Sweating itself does not cool the body; the cooling effect is caused by the evaporation of sweat from the skin. Excessive sweating may result in an imbalance of salts and fluids in the body, which may lead to heat cramps or heat exhaustion. Dilation of the blood vessels increases the blood flow near the surface of the skin, thus increasing the amount of heat lost by convection and radiation.

ACCLIMATIZATION
Most heat disorders can be prevented by gradual acclimatization to hot conditions. Full acclimatization takes one to three weeks and involves spending gradually longer periods in the heat, alternating with rest periods in cool conditions. Strenuous exercise should be avoided. Frequent cool baths or showers should be taken and salt tablets (in moderation) or dilute salt solution used (a quarter of a level teaspoon of salt dissolved in half a litre of cold water). It is also helpful to eat a light diet, to avoid alcohol, and to wear loose, lightweight clothes.

Heat exhaustion
Fatigue, sometimes culminating in collapse, caused by overexposure to heat. It is most common in people who are unaccustomed to working in a hot environment, and, unless treated, may develop into *heatstroke*, a potentially life-threatening condition.

CAUSES
There are three main causes of heat exhaustion: insufficient water intake, insufficient salt intake, and a deficiency in the production of sweat, the evaporation of which ordinarily helps cool the body.

SYMPTOMS AND SIGNS
Heat exhaustion causes fatigue, faintness, dizziness, nausea, restlessness, headache, and, when salt loss is heavy, *heat cramps* in the legs, arms, back, or abdomen. The skin is usually pale and clammy, breathing is fast and shallow, and the pulse is rapid and weak. There may also be vomiting, and the victim may faint.

PREVENTION AND TREATMENT
Heat exhaustion can usually be prevented by appropriate acclimatization (see *Heat disorders*).

A person who develops heat exhaustion should lie down in a cool

FIRST AID: HEATSTROKE

1 Move the victim to a cool, shady place and remove clothing. Place him or her in a half-sitting position and support the head and shoulders (for example, using pillows).

2 Cover the victim with a wet sheet and keep it wet. Fan him or her with a magazine or use an electric fan until the body temperature drops to 38°C. Seek medical help immediately.

place and, if conscious, should take continual sips of a weak salt solution (made up of a quarter of a level teaspoon of salt to half a litre of cold water). If the victim is unconscious, he or she should be placed in the *recovery position* until consciousness returns. Once the patient is conscious, salt solutions can be administered.

With rest and replacement of lost water and salt, a full recovery usually takes place. Victims should, however, consult a physician because of the risk of heatstroke.

Heatstroke

A life-threatening condition, also called heat hyperpyrexia, in which overexposure to extreme heat and a consequent breakdown of the body's heat-regulating mechanisms cause the body to become dangerously overheated. In some cases, body temperature may reach 41.5°C or more. Without emergency treatment, the victim lapses into coma and death soon follows.

CAUSES
Heatstroke is most commonly brought on by prolonged, unaccustomed exposure to the sun in a hot climate. It is more likely to occur in humid conditions, which reduce the body's ability to cool itself by the evaporation of sweat. Heatstroke can also be caused by working in an extremely hot environment. Susceptibility is greater in people with a disorder of the skin or sweat glands, in people taking *anticholinergic drugs* (which reduce sweating), and in older people in poor health. Overstrenuous or unaccustomed vacation activity, un-

suitable clothing, overeating, and drinking too much alcohol are sometimes contributory factors.

SYMPTOMS AND SIGNS
Heatstroke is often preceded by *heat exhaustion*, with fatigue, weakness, faintness, and profuse sweating. With the onset of heatstroke itself, sweating diminishes markedly and often stops completely. The skin becomes hot, dry, and flushed, breathing is shallow, and the pulse is rapid and weak. As the condition progresses, body temperature rises dramatically and, without treatment, the victim may quickly lose consciousness and die.

PREVENTION AND TREATMENT
The key to preventing heatstroke is acclimatization (see *Heat disorders*).

If heatstroke develops, emergency medical help should be summoned as soon as possible. Meanwhile, the victim should be wrapped naked in a cold, wet sheet, which should then be kept continuously wet. Alternatively, the victim may be constantly sponged with cold water. Cooling should be increased by fanning. If the victim is unconscious, he or she should be placed in the *recovery position* while being cooled.

Treatment should be continued until the victim's body temperature falls to 38°C or until the body feels cool to the touch. If the victim is conscious, he or she should be given a weak salt solution to sip (a quarter of a level teaspoon of salt dissolved in half a litre of water).

If heatstroke is treated early, the victim usually makes a full recovery. Victims may, however, be at risk of a recurrence.

Heat treatment

The use of heat to treat disease or aid recovery from injury.

Moist heat may be administered by soaking the affected part in a warm bath or by applying a hot *compress* or *poultice*. Dry heat may be applied in the form of a heating pad, a hot-water bottle, or a heat lamp that produces *infrared* rays.

More precise methods of administering heat to tissues deeper in the body include *ultrasound treatment* and shortwave *diathermy*.

WHY IT IS USED
Heat is used to aid recovery from injury, such as a muscle tear or ligament sprain; by stimulating blood flow, it is thought to help tissues heal more rapidly. Heat is also useful in relieving pain and stiffness in joints and muscles caused by excessive exercise or by rheumatic disorders or *osteoarthritis*. In addition, a hot compress is effective in encouraging the formation and the drainage of pus from skin infections.

To avoid the risk of internal bleeding and swelling, heat usually should not be used within 48 hours of an injury's occurring, so as to give the blood vessels time to heal.

Heel

The part of the *foot* below the *ankle* and behind the arch. The heel consists of the *calcaneus* (heel bone), an underlying pad of fat, which acts as a protective cushion, and a layer of skin, which is usually thickened as a result of pressure from walking.

Heimlich maneuver

A first-aid treatment for *choking*, described in panel 2 of choking box.

Heliotherapy

Treatment by exposure to sunlight. Heliotherapy is a form of *phototherapy*.

Helminth infestation

Infection by any species of parasitic worm. (See *Worm infestation*.)

Hem-

A prefix indicating blood, as in *hemoglobin* (an important protein in red blood cells).

Hemangioblastoma

A rare type of *brain tumor* that consists of blood-vessel cells. Hemangioblastomas usually develop as cysts in the *cerebellum*. Slow-growing and usually benign, they most commonly affect children and young adults.

H

The principal symptoms are headache, vomiting, *ataxia* (incoordination), and *nystagmus* (abnormal jerky movements of the eyes).

A hemangioblastoma can be clearly distinguished from the surrounding brain tissue and can usually be removed surgically. In most cases, surgical removal of the tumor results in a complete cure.

Hemangioma

A birthmark caused by an abnormal distribution of blood vessels. Hemangiomas may be flat or raised.

TYPES

Port-wine stains are large, flat, purple-red marks, which are permanent and can be unsightly. In rare cases, port-wine stains are associated with abnormalities in the blood vessels of the brain (see *Sturge-Weber syndrome*).

Small, flat marks, often known as stork marks or stork bites, are common in newborn babies, particularly on the back of the neck. Most begin to fade about three weeks after birth.

Raised bright red hemangiomas, often called strawberry marks, usually enlarge rapidly during the first few weeks after birth. After the age of about 6 months, the redness gradually fades and the lump subsides. Approximately 50 percent of these marks disappear by the time the child is 5 years old; 90 percent disappear by the age of 9.

Some raised hemangiomas are tinged blue by venous blood. These hemangiomas affect deeper tissues than strawberry marks but usually disappear during childhood.

COMPLICATIONS AND TREATMENT

Hemangiomas do not usually require treatment unless they are causing a particular problem. If a hemangioma starts to bleed, medical advice should be sought; meanwhile, the bleeding can be controlled by firm pressure with a clean handkerchief.

A hemangioma that bleeds persistently may require removal, especially if it is on the lip or tongue, where it may easily be bitten, or if it is on the vulva (external female genitalia) or anus, where it is subject to repeated pressure. A hemangioma on the face may need to be removed if it is causing distress.

Removal is carried out by *laser treatment*, *cryosurgery* (destruction of tissue by extreme cold), *radiation therapy*, *embolization*, or *plastic surgery*. If removal is not possible, some hemangiomas can be disguised with cosmetics.

Hemarthrosis

Bleeding into a *joint*, causing the capsule that encloses the joint to swell. Hemarthrosis is usually the result of severe damage to a joint, such as a torn capsule, torn ligaments, or fracture of a bone forming part of the joint. The most common cause is a sports injury to the knee.

A rarer cause is a *bleeding disorder*, such as *hemophilia* (in which failure of the blood-clotting mechanism causes abnormal bleeding). Any joint may be affected and bleeding into the joint may occur spontaneously or be caused by even the slightest knock. Overuse of *anticoagulant drugs* can cause hemarthrosis.

Hemarthrosis causes a joint to swell immediately after injury; swelling that occurs 12 to 24 hours later is probably caused by *synovitis* (inflammation of the lining of the joint). In addition to swelling and pain, hemarthrosis may cause the joint to stiffen into a fixed position as a result of spasm in surrounding muscles.

DIAGNOSIS AND TREATMENT

As a first aid measure, *ice packs* may be used to reduce swelling and pain. If swelling occurs after an injury, fluid is withdrawn from the joint through a needle to relieve pain and allow analysis of the fluid to diagnose the condition. *X rays* may be necessary if a fracture is suspected. Hemophiliacs are given *factor VIII* to promote blood clotting.

To prevent further bleeding, the physician will bandage the joint and advise resting it in an elevated position; cells in the joint capsule gradually absorb any remaining blood. Surgery, such as repair of a *ligament*, is sometimes necessary.

Repeated hemarthrosis may damage the surfaces of the joint, causing *osteoarthritis*, which is characterized by persistent pain and stiffness.

Hematemesis

The medical term for *vomiting blood*.

Hematology

The study of *blood* and its formation, and the investigation and treatment of disorders affecting the blood and the *bone marrow*.

Microscopic examination and counting of blood and bone marrow cells are essential procedures in diagnosing different types of blood disorders, such as *anemia* or *leukemia*. Analysis of blood is used in the diagnosis of a wide range of disorders as well as specific blood disorders.

Hematoma

A localized collection of blood (usually clotted) caused by bleeding from a ruptured blood vessel. A hematoma may occur almost anywhere in the body and, depending on the site and amount of accumulated blood, may vary in seriousness from a minor to a potentially fatal disorder.

TYPES

Less serious types include subungual hematoma (under a fingernail or toenail), hematoma auris (in the tissues of the outer ear, better known as *cauliflower ear*), and perianal hematoma (under the skin around the anus). The accumulated blood presses on the surrounding tissues, which may cause considerable pain. In such cases, a physician may lance and drain the hematoma to relieve the pressure and thus alleviate the pain. Most hematomas disappear on their own within a few days.

Among the more serious types are those that press on the brain, notably extradural and subdural hematomas (see *Extradural hemorrhage*; *Subdural hemorrhage*). These types of hematoma are usually due to an injury that ruptures a blood vessel just under the skull and may be fatal unless they are treated promptly.

Hematoma auris

The medical term for *cauliflower ear*.

Hematuria

Red blood cells in the *urine*. Blood in the urine may be readily visible or the presence of small amounts of blood may give the urine a smoky appearance. In some cases the blood is not visible to the naked eye.

CAUSES

Hematuria can be caused by blood entering the urine at any point along the *urinary tract*, from the kidney to the urethral opening. Almost any disorder of the urinary tract can cause hematuria. *Urinary tract infection* is one of the most common causes; *prostatitis* may cause hematuria in men. Cysts, *kidney tumors*, *bladder tumors*, and stones (see *Calculus, urinary tract*) may cause blood in the sufferer's urine, as can *glomerulonephritis*, in which the glomeruli (the filtering units of the kidney) become inflamed. *Bleeding disorders* may also cause blood to appear in the urine.

INVESTIGATION

If the blood is not visible to the naked eye, it may be discovered during a urine test when the urinary sediment is examined under the microscope.

Urine dipsticks have a small patch that is impregnated with a dye at one end; when dipped in urine containing blood, the patch turns blue.

To determine the cause of blood in the urine, it may be necessary to obtain images of the urinary tract by *ultrasound scanning*, *CT scanning*, or intravenous *urography*. These tests usually detect conditions such as cysts, stones, and tumors. If bladder disease is thought to be the cause, a *cystoscopy* (direct examination of the bladder through a viewing instrument passed through the urethra) is performed. If a kidney tumor seems likely, *angiography* may be performed to show the blood vessels of the kidney, although this technique has been largely replaced by CT scanning.

Hemianopia
Loss of one half of the *visual field* in each eye. Hemianopia may be "homonymous" (in which the same side of both eyes is affected by the loss) or "heteronymous" (in which the loss is in opposite sides of the eyes). In either case the visual loss may be temporary or permanent.

Hemianopia is not due to a disorder of the eyes themselves but results from damage to the nerve tracts or brain. Transient homonymous hemianopia in young people is usually caused by *migraine*. In older people it occurs in *transient ischemic attacks* (symptoms of *stroke* lasting less than 24 hours). Permanent homonymous hemianopia is usually caused by a stroke, but in some cases results from damage to the back of the brain by a tumor, injury, or infection. Hemianopia may also be caused by pressure on the optic nerve from a tumor of the pituitary gland. In this case, the outer half of each eye's visual field is lost.

Hemiballismus
Irregular, uncontrollable, flinging movements of the arm and leg on one side of the body, caused by disease of the *basal ganglia* (part of the brain concerned with coordination). The movements are unpredictable in timing and strength, and may be severe enough to cause injury to the afflicted person or others. (See also *Athetosis*; *Chorea*.)

Hemicolectomy
Surgical removal of half or a major portion of the *colon*. The surgeon may remove either the portion between the beginning of the colon and a point two thirds of the way across the transverse

colon, or the portion between this point and the end, either including or excluding the rectum. (See also *Colectomy*.)

Hemiparesis
Muscular weakness or partial paralysis affecting only one side of the body. (See *Hemiplegia*; *Paralysis*.)

Hemiplegia
Paralysis or weakness on one side of the body, caused by damage or disease affecting the motor nerve tracts in the opposite side of the brain. If affected muscles are stiff, the disorder is known as spastic hemiplegia; if the muscles are limp and wasted, the term flaccid hemiplegia is used.

CAUSES
A common cause of hemiplegia is a *stroke*. Other causes include *head injury*, *brain tumor*, *brain hemorrhage*, *encephalitis* (inflammation of the brain), *multiple sclerosis*, or complications of *meningitis*. In *conversion disorder* (a type of psychological disorder), there may be a false paralysis or refusal to use one side of the body that is not based on brain damage.

SYMPTOMS
Paralysis or weakness occurs on only one side of the body. It may affect the arm, leg, part of the trunk, and sometimes the face; one or more sites may be involved at the same time.

TREATMENT AND OUTLOOK
Treatment is directed at the underlying cause and is carried out in conjunction with *physiotherapy* to exercise the affected muscles. The prospects for a person with hemiplegia depend mainly on the cause; in the case of stroke, the outlook depends on age, general health, and the type of stroke. Motivation plays a part, as does the treatment given, but these factors are of less importance than the extent of the brain damage.

Hemochromatosis
An inherited disease (also known as "bronze diabetes") in which too much dietary iron is absorbed. Excess iron gradually accumulates in the liver, pancreas, heart, testes, and, to a lesser extent, in other organs.

CAUSES
The disease occurs almost exclusively in men. Women are very rarely affected because they regularly lose iron in their menstrual blood. Although hemochromatosis is known to be genetic in origin, the exact method of inheritance is unclear. Male

relatives of an affected person are more likely than average to develop the disease.

SYMPTOMS AND COMPLICATIONS
Hemochromatosis rarely causes problems until middle age. A loss of sexual drive and a reduction in the size of the testes are often the first signs. Eventually, excess iron causes liver enlargement and *cirrhosis* (chronic liver damage), deficient insulin production by the pancreas leading to *diabetes mellitus*, bronzed skin coloration due to iron pigment deposition under the skin (hence the alternative name), cardiac *arrhythmia* and other heart disorders, and, during the late stages of the disease, *liver failure* and *liver cancer*.

DIAGNOSIS AND TREATMENT
The diagnosis is based on *blood tests*, which reveal a high level of iron in the blood, and a *liver biopsy* (removal of a small sample of tissue for analysis), which shows the abnormal presence of iron.

Hemochromatosis is treated by withdrawal of blood from a vein (*venesection*). Initially, the procedure is performed once or twice a week. After the iron level has returned to normal, venesection is required only three or four times a year.

In young men, treatment can prevent the development of complications; in people who have fully developed hemochromatosis, regular venesection can prolong life. Drug treatment with *chelating agents*, such as deferoxamine, has been investigated as an alternative to venesection. (See also *Hemosiderosis*.)

Hemodialysis
One of the two means of *dialysis* (removal of waste products from the blood by means of artificial filtration) used to treat *kidney failure*.

Hemoglobin
The oxygen-carrying pigment found in red *blood cells*. Hemoglobin binds with oxygen to form oxyhemoglobin, a compound that gives oxygenated blood its bright red color. There are 350 million hemoglobin molecules in the average blood cell, and each can carry four molecules of oxygen. Hemoglobin is found in many animals—from insects and worms to birds, fish, and mammals.

STRUCTURE
Hemoglobin is a large molecule made in the *bone marrow* from two components, heme and globin.

H

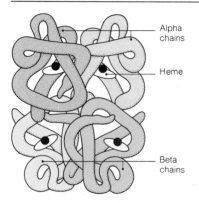

Structure of hemoglobin
Each molecule contains four globin chains—two alpha and two beta. Each chain carries a heme component capable of binding oxygen.

H

The composition of hemoglobin molecules varies, giving rise to normal and abnormal forms of hemoglobin. Hemoglobin F is the normal form in fetal life. This is replaced during infancy by the normal adult forms, hemoglobin A and A$_2$.

FUNCTION
The principal function of hemoglobin is to combine with and transport oxygen from the lungs and deliver it to all body tissues, where it is required to provide energy for the chemical reactions of all living cells. Carbon dioxide, which is produced as the waste product of these reactions, is transported to the lungs for excretion during breathing out.

DISORDERS
Some defects in hemoglobin production result from a *genetic disorder*; such defects are subdivided into errors of heme production, known as *porphyrias*, and those of globin production, known as *hemoglobinopathies*. Other defects, such as some types of *anemia*, have a nongenetic cause.

Hemoglobinopathy

A term used to describe a variety of *genetic disorders* in which there are errors in the production of globin chains (components of *hemoglobin*, the oxygen-carrying substance in the blood).

In some types of hemoglobinopathy, abnormal globin chains are produced, giving rise to abnormal hemoglobin molecules. This is the underlying defect in *sickle cell anemia*. In other types, normal globin chains are produced, but in abnormal amounts. This is the underlying defect in the *thalassemias*. Combined forms also occur.

The hemoglobinopathies cause anemia and chronic sickness in millions of people in Asia, Africa, Mediterranean countries, and the Caribbean, and in many people of these racial origins living in northern Europe and North America.

Hemoglobinuria

The presence in the *urine* of *hemoglobin* (the oxygen-carrying pigment in the blood).

Hemoglobin is mainly contained within red blood cells, although a small amount is free in the blood plasma. Excessive *hemolysis* (breakdown of red cells), which may be caused by heavy exercise, cold weather, falciparum *malaria* (blackwater fever), and hemolytic *anemia*, increases the concentration of free hemoglobin in the plasma. The excess of free hemoglobin in the plasma is excreted in the urine.

Hemolysis

The destruction of red *blood cells*. Hemolysis is the normal process by which old red blood cells that have lost their elasticity are destroyed, mainly in the *spleen*. This process releases iron for recycling in new red cells. *Bilirubin*, a waste product of hemolysis, is excreted into the *bile* by the liver.

Abnormal hemolysis in which red blood cells are destroyed prematurely may cause anemia and jaundice (see *Anemia, hemolytic*).

Hemolytic anemia

See *Anemia, hemolytic*.

Hemolytic disease of the newborn

Excessive *hemolysis* (destruction of red blood cells) in the fetus and newborn infant by *antibodies* produced by the mother. Hemolytic disease of the newborn is most often caused by *Rh incompatibility*—a blood group incompatibility between mother and baby, named after the Rhesus monkey in which the Rhesus (Rh) factor was first discovered.

A milder form of the disease may result from ABO and other blood group incompatibilities. (See *Blood groups*.)

CAUSE
Hemolytic disease may occur if the woman's blood is Rh negative, if she is carrying a baby whose blood is Rh positive, and if she has previously had a baby whose blood was Rh positive. A previous miscarriage, induced abortion, or *amniocentesis* in which the fetus's blood was Rh positive can also sensitize the woman. In each of these situations, blood has passed at some stage from the fetus to the woman. This causes the woman to produce Rh antibodies (directed against the Rh-positive blood cells) because her *immune system* recognizes the fetal blood cells as "foreign." In a first pregnancy, Rh antibodies do not form sufficiently to harm the baby. During any subsequent pregnancy, however, Rh antibodies form early on and may cross the placenta and attack the fetal blood cells.

A mismatched *blood transfusion* (giving Rh-positive blood to a woman who is Rh-negative) also sensitizes the woman to produce Rh antibodies.

DIAGNOSIS
All pregnant women have their blood types tested at the first prenatal check. If a woman is Rh negative, her husband's blood is checked. If he is positive, or if the father is unknown, the woman is checked monthly for Rh antibodies. At 28 weeks' gestation she is given an injection of *anti-D (Rh$_o$) immune globulin* to prevent her becoming sensitized to the fetal Rh antigens. If she has no antibodies throughout the rest of the monthly checks, the pregnancy proceeds normally. If the baby is Rh positive at birth, the mother is given another injection of *anti-D (Rh$_o$) immune globulin* to prevent the Rh antibodies from developing in her blood.

If a pregnant woman shows rising levels of Rh antibodies, amniocentesis is performed at intervals to measure *bilirubin* levels in the *amniotic fluid*. Bilirubin is a breakdown product of red blood cells and the level of bilirubin thus indicates the severity of hemolysis in the fetus.

SYMPTOMS AND SIGNS
In mild cases, the newborn baby becomes slightly jaundiced during the first 24 hours of life (due to excess bilirubin in the blood) and slightly anemic. In more severe cases, the level of bilirubin in the blood may increase to a dangerous level, causing a risk of *kernicterus* (a type of brain damage). The most severely affected babies have marked anemia while still in the uterus, become very swollen (hydrops fetalis), and are often stillborn. If the condition is very mild, no treatment is required. In other cases, the aim is to deliver the baby before anemia becomes severe. This usually means *induction of labor* between 35 and 39 weeks' gestation.

If the baby is severely affected before he or she is mature enough to be delivered safely (after 30 weeks' gestation), fetal blood transfusions may be necessary. Rh-negative blood is injected into the fetal umbilical vein, the fetal heart, or the fetal abdominal cavity. The procedure is monitored by *ultrasound scanning*. Transfusions of blood given in this way may need to be repeated several times until the baby has reached a size when labor may be safely induced.

After the baby is born, frequent blood tests are performed to assess jaundice and anemia. *Phototherapy* (light treatment that converts bilirubin in the skin into a water-soluble form that is more easily excreted from the body) and plenty of fluids help reduce the jaundice. If the bilirubin level becomes dangerously high, exchange transfusion (by which blood is removed from the baby and replaced by Rh-negative blood) is performed.

PREVENTION AND OUTLOOK
Hemolytic disease of the newborn is far less common since the introduction and use of *anti-D (Rh₀) immune globulin* in the early 1970s. This preparation is given by injection to any Rh-negative woman within 72 hours of childbirth, miscarriage, or elective abortion, and destroys Rh-positive blood cells from the fetus before they have had time to sensitize the woman's immune system.

Improved general obstetric and paediatric care has also resulted in a reduction in the severity of the cases that still occur.

Hemolytic-uremic syndrome

A rare disease in which red *blood cells* are destroyed prematurely and the kidneys are severely damaged, causing *kidney failure*. Hemolytic-uremic syndrome occurs mainly in infants and young children.

CAUSES
The precise cause of the disorder is unknown. It is thought that the lining of small blood vessels in the kidneys becomes damaged, causing small clots to form. These clots cause *hemolysis* (breakdown of red cells) as blood flows past them, leading to *anemia*. The resultant damage to the kidneys causes them to fail. Hemolytic-uremic syndrome often occurs in epidemics and appears to be triggered by a bacterial or viral infection.

SYMPTOMS AND SIGNS
The onset of the disease is sudden, with headache, fatigue, shortness of breath, and sometimes jaundice.

Little urine is passed and what is passed may contain blood. Severe *hypertension* (high blood pressure) is common and may cause *seizures*.

DIAGNOSIS AND TREATMENT
Blood and urine tests are performed to determine the degree of kidney damage. *Dialysis* (removal of waste products from the blood by artificial filtration) is necessary until the kidneys have recovered. *Antihypertensive drugs* are given to lower the blood pressure. Transfusions of red blood cells may be given to control the anemia. In severe cases, transfusion or exchange of plasma (the fluid in which blood cells are suspended) may prevent continual clotting of blood and excessive breakdown of red cells. Most children make a full recovery.

Hemophilia

An inherited *bleeding disorder* caused by a deficiency of a particular blood protein. Hemophiliacs (who are almost exclusively male) suffer recurrent bleeding, most often into their joints. Bleeding may occur spontaneously or after injury. Before the transmission mechanisms of *HIV* infection were understood, many hemophiliacs became infected with the virus as a direct result of treatment of their condition. Some have developed *AIDS*.

INCIDENCE AND CAUSES
About one male in 10,000 is born with hemophilia. The deficient blood protein, known as *factor VIII*, is one of a series of proteins essential to the process of *blood clotting*.

The lack of factor VIII is due to a defective gene, which shows a sex-linked pattern of inheritance (see *Genetic disorders*). Affected males pass the defective gene on to none of their sons but to all of their daughters, who are carriers of the condition. Some of the sons of carrier females may be affected, and some of the daughters of carriers may themselves be carriers. Many hemophiliacs have an uncle, brother, or grandfather also affected. About one third of cases have no family history of hemophilia.

SYMPTOMS
The severity of the disorder differs markedly among affected individuals. Most bleeding episodes involve bleeding into joints and muscles. The episodes often start when an affected child reaches weight-bearing age as a toddler. Bleeding episodes are painful and, unless treated promptly, can lead to crippling deformities of the knees, ankles, and other joints.

Injury and even minor operations such as tooth extraction may lead to profuse bleeding. Internal bleeding can give rise to symptoms such as *hematuria* (blood in the urine) or extensive bruises.

DIAGNOSIS
Hemophilia is diagnosed by *blood-clotting tests*, which reveal that factor VIII activity is abnormally low. A different type of blood test can be used to determine whether or not a woman is a carrier. *Amniocentesis* or *chorionic villus sampling* can be used to diagnose hemophilia in a fetus.

TREATMENT
Fifty years ago most hemophiliacs did not survive to adulthood; today, bleeding episodes can be controlled by infusions of concentrates of factor VIII. Regular infusions of factor VIII can be given as a preventive treatment. Alternatively, factor VIII may be given as soon as possible after the start of a bleeding episode. Patients can be shown how to administer the treatment themselves. Serious or unusual bleeding episodes may require hospitalization.

Although the use of factor VIII has considerably improved the quality of life for many hemophiliacs, the transmission of infections via factor VIII concentrates has caused problems. Factor VIII must be made from large pools of donor blood (2,000 to 5,000 individual donations) and, despite efforts to screen donors, these pools are sometimes contaminated with viruses. As a result, hemophiliacs commonly become infected with viral *hepatitis*. During the first few years of the AIDS epidemic (before its cause was recognized), large numbers of hemophiliacs became infected with HIV (the virus responsible for AIDS) through factor VIII infusions. Consequently, a percentage of hemophiliacs (and their sexual partners) have been exposed to the virus and some have died of AIDS.

Blood donations are now screened to prevent transmission of HIV by transfusion, and factor VIII is heat-treated to kill any virus that slips through the detection system. Nevertheless, there is still a risk of hepatitis transmission. Work is under way to produce a genetically engineered factor VIII, which would prevent all problems of blood-borne transmission for hemophiliacs.

OUTLOOK
A child with hemophilia should avoid activities that entail a risk of injury, including contact sports, such as

H

H

hockey and judo; activities such as swimming and walking should be encouraged.

Hemophiliacs who test positive for HIV should take the usual precautions against transmitting the virus and are advised not to have children. Hemophiliacs who do not test positive for HIV and the female relatives of hemophiliacs should obtain *genetic counseling* before starting a family.

Hemoptysis

The medical term for *coughing up blood*.

Hemorrhage

The medical term for *bleeding*.

Hemorrhoidectomy

The surgical removal of *hemorrhoids*.

WHY IT IS DONE

This operation may be carried out if simpler methods of treatment, such as banding, fail to resolve the problem. Hemorrhoidectomy tends to be reserved for people who have large, prolapsing, bleeding hemorrhoids.

HOW IT IS DONE

Stages in a hemorrhoidectomy are shown in the illustrated box.

RECOVERY PERIOD

Laxative drugs are given after the operation to soften the stools and make them easier to pass. Nonnarcotic *analgesic drugs* (painkillers) and warm baths ease discomfort. Complete healing occurs after three to six weeks. Avoidance of constipation can frequently prevent recurrences.

COMPLICATIONS

Bleeding is a possible complication. A slight loss of sensation in the anal area may impair the ability to control release of wind.

Hemorrhoids

Swollen veins in the lining of the anus. Hemorrhoids may occur close to the anal opening, in which case they are called external hemorrhoids. They may also occur higher in the anal canal, in which case they are called internal hemorrhoids. In some cases, hemorrhoids protrude outside the anus, in which case they are called prolapsing hemorrhoids.

CAUSES AND INCIDENCE

Hemorrhoids are very common, particularly during pregnancy and immediately after childbirth. Some people have a congenital weakness of the veins in the anus which makes the development of hemorrhoids more likely. Hemorrhoids are caused by increased pressure in the veins of the anus, usually due to straining to pass

REMOVING HEMORRHOIDS

In the procedures shown below, the patient is usually first given a laxative so that the lower bowel is clear of feces. Either general or epidural anesthesia is given before a hemorrhoidectomy is performed.

BANDING HEMORRHOIDS

1 This common, simple, and effective procedure is usually painless (causing no more than a mild ache afterward) and no anesthesia is required. The patient lies on one side, the proctoscope is positioned, and the hemorrhoid is grasped with the forceps.

2 Gentle traction is applied to draw the mass into the drum and the banding instrument is pressed into the anal wall.

3 The trigger mechanism of the banding instrument is fired and the bands are squeezed off onto the neck of the hemorrhoid. The proctoscope is withdrawn, leaving the hemorrhoid with its base tightly constricted by the bands. The hemorrhoid then withers and drops off painlessly within a few days.

HEMORRHOIDECTOMY

Using general or epidural anesthesia, the patient is examined with a proctosigmoidoscope to exclude a diagnosis of tumor. The patient is then placed in the *lithotomy position*. The hemorrhoid is clamped, placed under traction, secured with a suture, and then removed with a knife.

hard feces. Such feces may result from a diet containing too many refined foods and lacking sufficient fiber.

Rectal bleeding and increasing discomfort, even pain, on defecation are the most common features. Prolapsed hemorrhoids often produce a mucous discharge and itching around the anal opening. A complication of prolapse is thrombosis and strangulation (in which a clot forms in the vein, the vein does not spring back into position in the anus, and its blood supply is reduced); this can cause extreme pain. Iron-deficiency *anemia* may result from prolonged bleeding.

DIAGNOSIS

Proctoscopy (inspection of the rectum with a viewing instrument) is usually performed to exclude the possibility of cancer (see *Anus, cancer of*; *Rectum, cancer of*) and other disorders of the anus and rectum.

TREATMENT

Mild cases are controlled by drinking fluids, eating a high-fiber diet, and establishing regular toilet habits. Rectal suppositories and creams containing *corticosteroid drugs* and local anesthetics help reduce swelling and pain. More troublesome hemorrhoids may be treated on an outpatient basis by *sclerotherapy* (injection of an irritant liquid) or *cryosurgery* (application of extreme cold), which cause the swollen veins to shrivel, or by banding (see illustrated box, facing page).

Prolapsing hemorrhoids generally require a *hemorrhoidectomy*.

Hemosiderosis

A general increase in iron stores in the body, usually after repeated blood transfusions or, more rarely, as a result of excessive intake of iron. Hemosiderosis does not usually affect the function of body organs.

Hemospermia

The medical term for blood in the semen (see *Semen, blood in the*).

Hemostasis

The arrest of bleeding. There are three main natural mechanisms by which bleeding is stopped after injury. First, small blood vessels constrict (narrow) when damaged, thus lessening the "gaps" through which blood can flow. Second, blood cells called platelets aggregate (clump) and plug the bleeding points. Third, the blood plasma coagulates, forming filaments of a substance called fibrin. These filaments enmesh blood cells at the bleeding points and contract to form a solid clot that seals the damaged blood vessel (see *Blood clotting*). Defects in any of the three natural mechanisms of hemostasis can cause a *bleeding disorder*. (See also *Bleeding, treatment of*.)

Hemostatic drugs

A group of drugs used to treat *bleeding disorders* and to control bleeding.

Preparations of clotting factors are an important type of hemostatic drug. Clotting factors are present naturally in the body to aid *blood clotting* but are deficient in certain disorders. For example, preparations of factor VIII are used to treat *hemophilia*; factor IX is used to treat *Christmas disease*. The clotting factor is injected after abnormal bleeding to stimulate clotting, or before surgery to reduce the risk of excessive bleeding.

Other commonly prescribed hemostatic drugs include *vitamin K* preparations (used to treat an overdose of certain *anticoagulant drugs*) and aminocaproic acid, which disrupts *fibrinolysis* (the body's mechanism for dissolving blood clots).

Hemostatic preparations of gelatin and cellulose may be applied to the skin or gums to stop bleeding (e.g., after tooth extraction).

Hemothorax

A collection of blood in the pleural cavity (the space between the chest wall and the lung).

Hemothorax is most commonly caused by chest injury, but it may arise spontaneously in people with defects of blood coagulation or, occasionally, as a result of cancer.

Symptoms include pain in the affected side of the chest and the upper abdomen and breathlessness. The pulse rate may be raised. If extensive, hemothorax may compress the lung and cause partial lung collapse. Blood in the pleural space tends to remain fluid and can be aspirated (withdrawn through a needle).

Heparin

An *anticoagulant drug* used to prevent and treat abnormal *blood clotting*. Heparin is given by injection and is particularly useful as an immediate treatment for deep-vein *thrombosis* or *pulmonary embolism*.

POSSIBLE ADVERSE EFFECTS
Bruising around the injection site is common. Other adverse effects include rash, aching bones, and abnormal bleeding in different parts of the body. Long-term use may cause *osteoporosis* (thinning and weakening of the bones).

Hepatectomy, partial

Surgical removal of part of the *liver*. The liver has remarkable powers of regeneration; up to three quarters of the organ can be removed before it ceases to function.

WHY IT IS DONE
Severe injury to the liver sometimes occurs in road traffic accidents, causing serious bleeding in and death of the damaged area. Surgery is performed to remove the dead tissue.

Benign liver tumors and sometimes *hydatid disease* require partial hepatectomy; rarely, *liver cancer* is also treated in this way.

Hepatectomy, total

Surgical removal of the *liver*. Hepatectomy is performed as the first stage in a *liver transplant* operation.

Hepatic

Related to the *liver*. For example, the hepatic vein is the vessel that drains blood from the liver.

Hepatitis

Inflammation of the *liver*, with accompanying damage or death of liver cells. Hepatitis is most commonly caused by viral infection but may also be due to certain drugs, chemicals, or poisons. The condition may be either acute or chronic.

ACUTE HEPATITIS
This form of hepatitis is fairly common, with several thousands of cases diagnosed per year in Canada. The most frequent cause is infection with a hepatitis virus, which may be either type A, type B, or type non-A non-B (see *Hepatitis, viral*). Other causes include overdose with drugs, such as *acetaminophen*, exposure to certain chemicals, such as dry-cleaning agents, or, rarely, a reaction to certain drugs in normal dosage. Acute hepatitis may also affect heavy drinkers who have progressive liver disease (see *Liver disease, alcoholic*).

SYMPTOMS The most obvious sign of acute hepatitis is *jaundice*. In many cases, jaundice is preceded by a flu-like illness, accompanied by nausea, vomiting, loss of appetite, tenderness in the right upper abdomen, aching muscles, and sometimes joint pain.

In uncommon, severe cases, jaundice may be intense and *liver failure* may develop, with possible effects on other organs (including the brain), resulting in coma and death.

DIAGNOSIS A physician may strongly suspect acute hepatitis from the symptoms alone, particularly if the patient is in a risk group for exposure to one of the causative viruses, drugs, or chemicals. If drug or chemical poisoning is suspected, blood tests may be performed to identify the cause. *Ultrasound scanning* of the liver may help rule out *bile duct obstruction*, another cause of jaundice. *Liver-function tests* can also aid in diagnosis.

TREATMENT No specific treatment is available for most cases of acute hepatitis. In severe cases, intensive care may be required. If the disorder is caused by exposure to a chemical or drug, exposure to the causative substance should be stopped and, in some cases, detoxification using an antidote may be possible. Whatever the cause of the hepatitis, bed rest and a nourishing diet are usually recommended. Recovery usually occurs after a few weeks. Abstinence from alcohol after the illness aids in liver regeneration.

CHRONIC HEPATITIS
In some cases, a person fails to recover fully from an episode of acute hepatitis, leading to continued liver cell damage and inflammation. This usually, but not exclusively, occurs with certain types of viral hepatitis.

Chronic hepatitis may also develop insidiously over a number of years without any acute episodes. Heavy alcohol consumption may be responsible. Other possible causes are an *autoimmune disorder* (in which the body's natural defenses attack body tissues), a reaction to a medication, or a metabolic disorder which affects the liver.

Several types of chronic hepatitis are recognized. A type affecting heavy drinkers (see *Liver disease, alcoholic*) and chronic active hepatitis (see *Hepatitis, chronic active*) may both progress to liver *cirrhosis* if untreated. A third type, called chronic persistent hepatitis, is less severe and carries little risk of progression to cirrhosis.

SYMPTOMS The symptoms of chronic hepatitis are usually no worse than a vague feeling of being unwell.

DIAGNOSIS Often the disease remains undetected until the patient has a medical examination and the liver is found to be enlarged, a causative virus or specific *antibody* is found in the blood, or the results of *liver-function tests* are abnormal. A *liver biopsy* (removal of a tissue sample for microscopic analysis) helps the physician establish the type of chronic hepatitis.

TREATMENT For hepatitis caused by alcohol consumption, total abstinence is the only cure. If strictly observed, this allows complete restoration of liver function. For chronic persistent hepatitis, treatment is not usually needed. For the chronic active form, therapy depends on the precise cause of the disease.

Hepatitis A
See *Hepatitis, viral.*

Hepatitis B
See *Hepatitis, viral.*

Hepatitis, chronic active
A type of chronic *hepatitis* in which there is intense and progressive inflammation and destruction of cells surrounding certain structures within the liver. Scar tissue forms and leads to liver *cirrhosis*.

CAUSES
Chronic active hepatitis may be caused in any of four ways—as a result of an *autoimmune disorder* (in which the body's natural defenses attack body tissues), a viral infection, a reaction to a drug or chemical, or, rarely, to a *metabolic disorder*.

In the autoimmune type, antibodies (proteins with a defense role) that inappropriately attack liver cells are formed. Women are affected more often than men. Primary biliary cirrhosis may fall into this category.

Viral infection is the most common cause in Canada, most often due to viral hepatitis, caused by either hepatitis B virus or hepatitis non-A non-B virus (see *Hepatitis, viral*). Men are affected more often than women.

Drugs, including *nitrofurantoin* and *isoniazid*, are a rare cause of chronic active hepatitis. Metabolic disorders that may cause the disease include *hemochromatosis* (also known as "bronze diabetes"), a disease confined almost entirely to men, and *Wilson's disease*, a rare, inherited disorder.

SYMPTOMS AND DIAGNOSIS
The disease may cause vague feelings of tiredness, or no symptoms at all. It is diagnosed by *liver biopsy* (removal of a sample of tissue from the liver for microscopic analysis).

TREATMENT
The type caused by an autoimmune disorder is treated with *corticosteroid drugs*, which usually bring some improvement. Antiviral agents have been tried unsuccessfully against viral infections. In the drug-induced type, withdrawal of the medication can lead to recovery. For metabolic disturbances, treatment depends on the underlying disorder.

MAIN TYPES OF VIRAL HEPATITIS

	Viral hepatitis type A (infectious hepatitis)	Viral hepatitis type B (serum hepatitis)
Transmission of infection	Virus is present in feces of infected people and transmitted to others by fecal contamination of water and food (e.g., through infected people handling food). Feces are infective from two to three weeks before until eight days after the onset of jaundice. Local epidemics can occur.	Virus is present in blood and other body fluids of infected people. In Canada, virus is spread mainly sexually and by needle sharing among drug abusers. Health workers are at risk from infected blood. In Africa and Asia, spread from mother to baby is common.
Incidence	Worldwide. In Canada, about 1,500 cases are reported annually. In some parts of the world where hygiene is poor almost everyone has been exposed to this type of hepatitis.	Worldwide. In parts of Africa and Asia, up to 20 percent of the population has been carrying the virus without symptoms for years. The Canadian carrier rate is much lower. About 3,100 cases are reported annually.
Groups at particular risk	Travelers to areas where hygiene standards are poor and prevalence of the virus is high (i.e., parts of Asia, Africa, or South America).	Male homosexuals, people with multiple sexual partners, intravenous drug abusers, health care personnel, or children born to carrier mothers.
Incubation period	Three to six weeks after virus has entered the body.	A few weeks to several months after infection.
Illness	In many cases there is no illness. Otherwise, typical acute hepatitis (flulike illness with jaundice), usually mild and never progressing to chronic hepatitis.	Typical acute hepatitis, often more severe than with type A virus. Progression to chronic hepatitis and other liver disease may occur. Sometimes, no illness.
Prevention	For nonimmune travelers at risk, passive immunization with immunoglobulin plus good hygiene and care in selection of food and drink. A vaccine has also recently been developed.	Observance of safe sex with possible infected sexual partners and avoidance of blood exchange. Vaccine and/or passive immunization for groups at high risk.

Hepatitis, viral

Any type of *hepatitis* (inflammation of the liver) caused by a viral infection.

TYPES AND CAUSES

Although other viruses may infect the liver as part of a wider infection, certain viruses attack the liver as their primary target. The latter include hepatitis A virus, hepatitis B virus, and delta virus. If tests fail to find any of these viruses in a person who has obvious symptoms of viral hepatitis, the person is said to have non-A non-B hepatitis. This type of hepatitis is almost always transmitted by transfusion of infected blood and is caused by more than one virus, but in most cases the organism is a recently identified RNA virus, known as hepatitis C virus.

Hepatitis A (sometimes called infectious hepatitis) is most commonly spread by contamination of drinking water or food by infected feces. In most parts of the world, a high proportion of the population has been infected with the virus, often without symptoms, and is therefore immune to further attack.

Hepatitis B (sometimes called serum hepatitis) used to be spread mainly by transfusions of blood and blood products; this risk has now been removed by the development of screening tests for the virus.

Today, hepatitis B is mainly transmitted sexually or by the accidental inoculation of contaminated blood (for example by needle-sharing among intravenous drug abusers or by tattooing or acupuncture performed with unsterile needles).

Hepatitis B is in many respects more serious than hepatitis A. In a proportion of cases, the hepatitis B virus persists for years after the initial infection and may lead to a chronic form of hepatitis (see *Hepatitis, chronic active*) and eventually to liver *cirrhosis* or *liver cancer*. Carriers of the virus may have few or no symptoms during this time but can infect others.

Screening tests for hepatitis B and C can eliminate virtually any risk of transfusion-associated hepatitis. Hepatitis delta virus can exist only in someone who is already carrying, or has recently been infected with, hepatitis B. It seems to be spread mainly by needle-sharing among drug abusers.

SYMPTOMS

Infection with any of the causative viruses may be symptomless or may cause a typical acute *hepatitis* with a flulike illness followed by jaundice.

About 10 percent of patients infected with hepatitis B, delta, or non-A non-B viruses go on to acquire chronic hepatitis. This rarely, if ever, happens with hepatitis type A.

DIAGNOSIS AND TREATMENT

Diagnosis is usually made by identifying the virus (or antibodies to the virus) in the blood, or, in the case of non-A non-B hepatitis, by exclusion of the other types.

There is no specific treatment for any type of viral hepatitis. Bed rest, a nourishing diet, and abstinence from alcohol may speed recovery.

PREVENTION

Vaccines against hepatitis B are currently available, but are generally recommended only to people who are at high risk of infection, such as health-care workers, children born to carrier mothers, male homosexuals, and drug addicts. Vaccines against hepatitis A are being evaluated.

Passive immunization against hepatitis A and hepatitis B by means of *immunoglobulin injections* is also available and can provide some protection. Passive immunization against hepatitis A or hepatitis B may be recommended for people traveling for short periods to areas with a high incidence of the disease. The babies of carrier mothers are given hepatitis B immunoglobulin after birth in order to prevent infection while the vaccine (given at the same time) is beginning to build up immunity.

Avoidance of hepatitis A is further helped by observing good hygiene, especially food hygiene, in parts of the world where sanitary standards are low (see *Food-borne infection*). The chances of getting hepatitis B can be reduced by use of a condom during sexual intercourse, by not sharing needles, and by avoiding such activities as tattooing, unless the equipment is sterile.

Hepatoma

A type of *liver cancer*.

Hepatomegaly

Enlargement of the liver, occurring as a result of virtually any type of liver disorder. The enlargement may cause tenderness just beneath the ribs and can be detected by a physician during the course of a physical examination. (See *Liver* disorders box.)

Herbal medicine

Systems of medical treatment in which various parts of different plants are used in order to treat symptoms and to promote health.

Herbal medicine was the most common medical treatment in most cultures for many centuries.

Heredity

The transmission of traits and disorders through genetic mechanisms. Each person inherits a combination of *genes* (units of inheritance)—half paternal, half maternal—via the sperm and egg cells from which he or she is derived. The interaction of these genes determines the person's inherited characteristics, including, in some cases, disorders or susceptibility to disorders. Half of an individual's genes are passed on, in turn, to each of his or her own children. (See also *Genetic disorders; Inheritance*.)

Heritability

A measure of the extent to which a disease or disorder is the result of inherited factors—as opposed to environmental influences such as diet and climate.

Certain disorders (such as *hemophilia* or *cystic fibrosis*) are known to be caused entirely by hereditary factors. Others (such as occupational disorders) are caused entirely by environmental factors. Between these two extremes are many disorders in which both inheritance and environment probably play a part.

Pinpointing hereditary factors is notoriously difficult. A rough estimate of heritability can be obtained from the known incidence of a disorder in the first-degree relatives (i.e., parents, siblings, and offspring) of affected people and by comparing it with the incidence of the disorder in a population exposed to similar environmental influences. Other estimates of heritability are obtained from studies of identical twins who have been reared apart.

Such studies suggest a relatively high heritability for *schizophrenia*, *asthma*, *coronary artery disease*, non-insulin-dependent *diabetes mellitus*, *ankylosing spondylitis*, and some birth defects, such as *cleft lip and palate*, *pyloric stenosis*, and *talipes* (clubfoot). The heritability for congenital *heart disease* and *peptic ulcer* is low.

Estimates of heritability are useful in *genetic counseling*. (See also *Genetic disorders*.)

Hermaphroditism

A congenital disorder in which both male and female gonads (testes and ovaries) are present and the external genitalia are not clearly male or female. True hermaphroditism is extremely rare and its cause unknown. The majority of affected children are raised as males because the external genitalia usually appear more male than female.

A more common condition is pseudohermaphroditism, in which the gonads of only one sex are present, but the external genitalia may not be clearly male or female. Pseudohermaphroditism is caused by a hormonal imbalance (such as occurs in congenital *adrenal hyperplasia*, for example). Pseudohermaphroditism can usually be treated by appropriate surgery and hormone therapy.

Hernia

The protrusion of an organ or tissue through a weak area in the muscle or other tissue that normally contains it. The term is usually applied to a protrusion of the intestine through a weak area in the abdominal wall.

The main types of abdominal hernia are shown in the illustrated box. A *hiatal hernia* is a hernia in which the stomach protrudes through the diaphragm into the chest. Very rarely, other organs or tissue (e.g., the brain) may herniate.

CAUSES

Abdominal hernias are usually caused by a *congenital* weakness in the abdominal wall. They sometimes result, especially later in life, from damage caused by lifting heavy objects, substantial weight gain, persistent coughing, or straining to defecate. Hernias may also develop after surgery.

SYMPTOMS AND COMPLICATIONS

The first symptom of an abdominal hernia is usually a bulge in the abdominal wall. There may also be abdominal discomfort. In some people, the protruding intestine can be pushed back through the abdominal wall. Severe pain occurs when the hernia bulges out and cannot be replaced.

If the blood supply to a twisted, trapped intestine becomes impaired (a condition known as a strangulated hernia), gangrene (tissue death) of the bowel may develop. A strangulated hernia requires urgent treatment.

DIAGNOSIS AND TREATMENT

Hernias are diagnosed by physical examination. If the hernia is causing only slight discomfort and is readily pushed back, a supportive truss may be recommended. Hernias that are painful or that are impossible to push back are usually treated surgically (see *Hernia repair*).

MAIN TYPES OF ABDOMINAL HERNIA

Inguinal hernia

At least 2 percent of adult males suffer at some time from this kind of hernia, in which part of the intestine bulges through the inguinal canal (the passage through which the testes descend into the scrotum). The hernia is detected as a bulge in the groin or scrotum; untreated, the hernia may become stuck, so early surgery is generally recommended.

Femoral hernia

This type of hernia occurs most commonly in obese women; part of the intestine emerges where the femoral vein and artery pass from the abdomen to the thigh. A femoral hernia is noticed as a swelling of the top front of the thigh. Although the hernia itself may be large, its neck is narrow, and the condition can only be corrected by surgery.

Epigastric hernia

Also called a ventral hernia, an epigastric hernia is caused by a weakness in the muscles of the central upper abdomen; the intestine bulges out at a point between the navel and the breastbone. This form of hernia is three times more common in men than in women and is most likely to occur in people between 20 and 50 years old.

Umbilical hernia

This occurs when part of the intestine protrudes through the abdominal wall at the navel. Babies are the most common sufferers; the hernia can be repaired surgically or it may disappear naturally by about the age of 5. A similar problem, a parumbilical hernia, occurs in mostly obese, middle-aged women who have had several children.

Incisional hernia

An area of weakness may occasionally develop following a surgical incision in the wall of the abdomen. This area may then develop into an incisional hernia. The defect may become so severe that a large amount of intestine bulges through the abdominal wall; if this happens, a repair using a piece of mesh may be necessary.

Hernia repair

Surgical correction of a *hernia*. The procedure is usually performed to treat a hernia of the abdominal wall that is painful or cannot be pushed back. A strangulated hernia requires an emergency operation.

Many hernias are repaired on an outpatient basis unless an underlying medical condition necessitates hospitalization. A local, epidural, or general anesthetic may be used. The surgeon's aim is to push the protruding intestine back into place and then strengthen the weakened muscle wall (see illustrated box, facing page).

The speed of recovery depends on the underlying medical condition and on the type of hernia repaired. Lifting heavy objects should be avoided for three to six months. The risk of a recurrence of the condition varies with the type of hernia treated. Inguinal and incisional hernias both recur quite commonly; femoral and epigastric hernias, only rarely.

HERNIA REPAIR

During surgery the hernia is removed or repositioned and the weakened abdominal wall is reinforced with stitching or mesh.

1 The protruding sac of intestine is pushed back into the abdomen or, in some cases (e.g., strangulation), the sac is removed surgically.

2 The wall of the abdomen may then be repaired by overlapping the edges of the weakened area and securing them with rows of stitching.

LARGE HERNIAS

For repair of some large hernias, two mesh leaves are secured by rows of stitching, then joined at the center.

Herniated disk

See *Disk prolapse*.

Herniorrhaphy

See *Hernia repair*.

Heroin abuse

Nonmedical use of heroin, a *narcotic drug* similar to *morphine*. Heroin is a white or brownish powder that can be smoked, sniffed, or dissolved in water and injected. Medically, this drug is generally known as *diamorphine*.

Heroin abuse is a major health problem in many countries. It has many adverse effects on the user and is a sociological and economic problem of immense proportions.

EFFECTS

In addition to having an analgesic (painkilling) effect, heroin produces sensations of warmth, calmness, drowsiness, and a loss of concern for outside events.

Long-term use causes *tolerance* (the need for greater amounts of the drug to have the same effects) and psychological and physical dependence (see *Drug dependence*). Sudden withdrawal of the drug produces symptoms such as shivering, abdominal cramps, diarrhea, vomiting, sleeplessness, and restlessness. Other common problems of heroin addiction include injection scars, skin abscesses, weight loss, and impotence. Infections, such as with the viruses causing *hepatitis B* or *AIDS*, are spread by sharing needles. Death commonly occurs from accidental overdose.

Herpangina

A throat infection caused by a type of virus called coxsackievirus. Herpangina most commonly affects young children, although it also occurs in adults. The virus is usually transmitted via infected droplets coughed or sneezed into the air. Many people harbor the virus but do not experience any symptoms.

SYMPTOMS

After an incubation period of two to seven days, there is a sudden onset of fever, loss of appetite, and sore throat. There may also be headache, abdominal discomfort, and vague muscular aches and pains. The throat becomes red and a few small blisters appear, which enlarge and burst, forming shallow ulcers. The condition usually clears up within a week.

TREATMENT

Usually no treatment is required other than simple *analgesic drugs* (painkillers). There is no specific antiviral therapy available. Antibiotics are generally of no therapeutic value unless a bacterial infection develops as a complication. Recurrent attacks of herpangina may result from infection with different strains of the virus.

Herpes

Any of a variety of conditions, which are characterized by an eruption of small, and usually painful, blisters on the patient's skin.

When a person is said to be suffering from herpes, the term usually refers to an infection with the *herpes simplex* virus. Forms of the virus are responsible for *cold sores* (painful blisters around the lips) and for the sexually transmitted infection genital herpes, which is characterized by blisters on the sex organs (see *Herpes, genital*). The virus can also cause a number of other conditions affecting the skin, mouth, eyes, brain, or, in rare cases, the whole body.

A closely related virus, the varicella-zoster virus, is responsible for two more conditions in which skin blisters are a feature—*chickenpox* (also known as varicella) and *herpes zoster* (also known as shingles). Like herpes simplex virus, varicella-zoster virus can also affect the eyes or, rarely, may infect the brain or cause a generalized infection throughout the body.

Herpes gestationis and *dermatitis herpetiformis* are among various other conditions in which "herpetiform" (herpeslike) groups of blisters may appear on the skin, but neither is related to herpes simplex or varicella-zoster virus infections.

Herpes, genital

A sexually transmitted disease that produces a painful rash on the genitals. Caused by the *herpes simplex* virus, genital herpes is transmitted by sexual intercourse with an infected person.

SYMPTOMS AND SIGNS

After an incubation period of about a week, the virus produces itching, burning, soreness, and small blisters in the genital area. The blisters burst to leave small, painful ulcers, which heal within 10 to 21 days. The lymph nodes in the groin may become enlarged and painful, and the affected person may feel unwell, with headache and fever. Women may find urination very painful if the urine comes into contact with the sores.

TREATMENT

Genital herpes cannot be cured, but the earlier treatment is given, the more likely the treatment will prevent or reduce the severity of an attack. Antiviral drugs, such as *acyclovir*, help make the ulcers less painful and encourage faster healing. Other soothing measures include taking *analgesic drugs* (painkillers) and bathing the area with a salt solution by adding a heaped teaspoon of salt to a half-litre of water.

Subsequent attacks tend to occur when the patient is anxious or

H

depressed, before menstrual periods, after sexual intercourse, after sunbathing, or when the affected person is run down; these recurrent attacks often clear up quickly with or without treatment. Sexual activity should be avoided until the symptoms have disappeared. If a pregnant woman has an attack of genital herpes when the baby is due, a cesarean section is performed to prevent the baby from being infected during delivery.

OUTLOOK
Once the virus enters the body, it stays there for the rest of the person's life. About 12 to 20 percent of those affected never have another attack after the first. Others, however, suffer four or five attacks annually for several years. Gradually, the attacks become less severe and the intervals between recurrences become longer.

The herpes virus may have a role in the development of cervical cancer (see *Cervix, cancer of*); women who have had herpes should have a *cervical smear test* every year.

Herpes gestationis
A rare skin disorder of pregnant women, characterized by crops of blisters on the legs and abdomen. The cause is not known and, despite its name, herpes gestationis is not related to any of the disorders caused by the *herpes simplex* viruses.

Severe herpes gestationis is treated with *corticosteroid drugs* in tablet form and may require hospital admission because of the risk of *miscarriage*. The disorder usually clears up completely after the birth of the baby, but tends to recur in subsequent pregnancies.

Herpes simplex
A common and troublesome viral infection, characterized by the appearance of small, fluid-filled blisters. Although most herpes simplex infections are symptomless, mild, or merely irritating, others can be extremely distressing (notably infections affecting the genitals) or, in rare cases, even life-threatening. Herpes simplex infections are *contagious* and usually spread by direct contact with the blisters or the fluid they contain.

TYPES
The virus exists in two forms, known as HSV1 (herpes simplex virus, type 1) and HSV2 (herpes simplex virus, type 2). HSV1 is usually associated with infections of the lips, mouth, and face, whereas HSV2 is often associated with infections of the genitals and infections acquired by babies at birth.

However, there is a considerable amount of overlap. Some conditions usually caused by HSV1 are sometimes caused by HSV2 and vice versa.

TYPE 1 VIRUS Most people have been infected with HSV1 by the time they reach adulthood; most of the remainder are infected during adulthood. The initial infection may cause no symptoms or may cause a sometimes severe flulike illness with mouth ulcers. Thereafter, the virus remains in the nerve cells within the facial area. In many people, the virus is periodically reactivated, causing recurrent *cold sores* that always erupt in the same site (usually around the lips). Cold sores often recur when the temperature at the affected site is raised, such as in a fever or during prolonged exposure to the sun.

Rarely, the virus may infect the fingers, causing an eruption of very painful blisters known as a herpetic *whitlow*. Sometimes the virus may cause an extensive rash of blisters (known as eczema herpeticum) in a person with a preexisting skin condition such as one of the forms of dermatitis.

If a person with an *immunodeficiency disorder*, such as *AIDS*, or someone who is taking *immunosuppressant drugs* is infected with the virus, it may cause a severe generalized infection that is occasionally fatal.

If the virus gets into an eye, it may cause *conjunctivitis*, which usually lasts only a few days, or, more seriously, a *corneal ulcer*. Very rarely, the type 1 virus may spread to the brain, leading to serious *encephalitis* (inflammation of the brain).

TYPE 2 VIRUS This form of the virus is the usual cause of sexually transmitted genital herpes, in which painful blisters erupt on the sex organs (see *Herpes, genital*). As with cold sores, the blisters recur in some people.

TREATMENT
Treatment of herpes simplex depends on its type, site, and severity. *Antiviral drugs*, such as *acyclovir*, are sometimes helpful. If sores become infected with bacteria, *antibiotic drugs* and bathing in tepid water may be helpful.

Herpes zoster
The medical term for shingles. Herpes zoster is an infection of the nerves that supply certain areas of the skin. This disorder causes a painful rash of small, crusting blisters. After the rash heals, pain may persist for months or, rarely, years.

Herpes zoster often affects a strip of skin over the ribs on one side. Less

Example of herpes zoster
An extensive rash of crusting blisters over one side of the neck spreads over the shoulder and onto the front of the chest.

commonly, it affects a strip on one side of the neck and arm, or on one side of the lower part of the body. Sometimes, herpes zoster involves one side of the upper half of the face, and the eye may also be affected. Shingles in this area is known as herpes zoster ophthalmicus.

CAUSES
Herpes zoster is caused by the varicella-zoster virus, which also causes *chickenpox*. During an attack of chickenpox, most of the viral organisms are destroyed, but some survive and lie dormant in certain sensory nerves, remaining there for many years. In some people, a decline in the efficiency of the *immune system* (the body's defenses against infection) allows the viruses to reemerge and cause shingles.

The efficiency of the immune system declines with age; this decline is probably accelerated by stress and by the use of *corticosteroid drugs*. Herpes zoster commonly follows a stressful episode.

INCIDENCE
The disorder mainly affects people over 50 and the incidence rises with age. Herpes zoster is very common in people whose immune systems have been weakened either by diseases, such as *lymphoma* or *AIDS*, or by treatment with *immunosuppressant drugs* or *anticancer drugs*.

SYMPTOMS AND SIGNS
The first indication is excessive sensitivity in the area of skin to be affected; this is soon followed by pain, which is sometimes severe and which may, until the rash appears, be mistaken for pleurisy or appendicitis.

After about five days, the rash appears, starting as small, slightly raised red spots that quickly turn to tense blisters, teeming with viruses. Within three days the blisters have turned yellowish and soon dry, flatten, and crust over. During the next two weeks or so these crusts drop off, often leaving small pitted scars.

The most serious feature of herpes zoster is pain following the attack, a condition known as postherpetic pain. This pain is a consequence of damage to the nerves, causing strong nerve impulses to be constantly produced and passed upward to the brain. The pain, which affects about one third of sufferers, may be severe and last for months or years. The older the patient and the more pronounced the rash, the more likely it is that the pain will be severe and persistent.

Ophthalmic herpes zoster may be confined to the eyelids and forehead and need not affect the eye itself. But if it does affect the eye, it may cause a *corneal ulcer* or *uveitis*, both of which are potentially serious.

TREATMENT

Provided that treatment is begun soon after the rash appears, *antiviral drugs* (such as *acyclovir*) will reduce the severity of the active stage and minimize nerve damage. If treatment is delayed beyond the early stage of the disease, little can be done to influence the course of the disease or the likelihood of postherpetic pain.

Some relief from pain may be obtained by taking *analgesic drugs*. Many other measures have been advocated for the relief of postherpetic pain, but none has been shown to be consistently effective. Such measures include stimulation of the skin by intermittent rubbing, the passage of alternating electric currents through the skin, local heat, cold spraying, the injection of local anesthetics, and even surgical cutting of the nerves.

Heterosexuality

Sexual attraction to members of the opposite sex. (See also *Bisexuality*; *Homosexuality, male*; *Lesbianism*.)

Heterozygote

A term used to describe a person whose cells contain two different *genes* controlling a specified inherited trait, in contrast to a *homozygote* who has identical genes controlling that trait. (See also *Genetic disorders* and *Inheritance*.)

Hiatal hernia

A condition in which the upper part of the stomach protrudes through the hiatus (opening) in the *diaphragm* through which the esophagus passes from the chest into the abdominal cavity.

CAUSES AND INCIDENCE

The underlying cause of hiatal hernia is unknown, but this common condition tends to occur more commonly in obese people (and especially in women in later middle age) and in those who smoke. In some cases, it is present at birth.

SYMPTOMS

Many people have no symptoms, but in some people hiatal hernia affects the efficiency of the muscle at the junction between the *esophagus* and stomach, permitting *acid reflux* (backflow of acidic juices from the stomach into the esophagus). This reflux may in turn cause *heartburn*, which is often made worse by bending over or lying down, or *esophagitis* (inflammation of the esophagus). The pain of esophagitis may mimic the pain of *coronary artery disease*.

DIAGNOSIS

Esophagoscopy (a type of *endoscopy* in which a viewing instrument is passed down the throat into the esophagus) may be performed, and a *biopsy* sample of esophageal tissue taken for microscopic analysis. A *barium X-ray examination* is usually performed, with the patient tilted head-down; incompetence at the junction between the esophagus and stomach is indicated if the X ray shows reflux of the barium into the esophagus. *Manometry* (the taking of pressure measurements) can

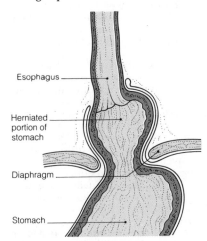

Common type of hiatal hernia
The stomach slides into the chest through the esophageal hiatus (opening).

confirm the reduced pressure at the junction between the esophagus and the stomach.

TREATMENT

To alleviate symptoms, the patient should avoid eating large, heavy meals and should never lie down or bend over immediately after a meal. The head end of the bed should be raised to prevent reflux during the night. People who are obese should lose weight and smokers should stop smoking. *Antacid drugs* may be given to reduce stomach acidity and to protect the esophagus against acid juices. In severe cases, an operation may be required to return the protruding part of the stomach to the abdomen and to prevent the further reflux of acid stomach contents into the esophagus.

Hiccup

A sudden, involuntary contraction of the *diaphragm* followed by rapid closure of the *vocal cords* (which causes the characteristic sound). Hiccups, which are also spelled hiccoughs, are extremely common. Most attacks last only a few minutes, consisting of individual hiccups usually with a brief interval between.

CAUSES

In almost all cases, hiccups occur without obvious cause and are not medically significant. Rarely, hiccups may be due to a condition that causes irritation of the diaphragm or of the *phrenic nerves* that supply it. Known causes include *pleurisy*, *pneumonia*, certain disorders of the stomach or esophagus, *pancreatitis*, *alcohol dependence*, and *hepatitis*. Frequent, prolonged attacks of hiccups, which are extremely rare, may lead to severe exhaustion.

TREATMENT

Most minor attacks clear up without treatment. Numerous popular remedies, such as drinking cold water or provoking a sneeze, have been tried with varying success in different people. Drugs, such as *chlorpromazine*, *haloperidol*, and *diazepam* are sometimes prescribed in severe cases. If medication fails to cure severe hiccups, surgery on the phrenic nerve to paralyse half of the diaphragm may be performed but this may affect breathing and may not succeed.

Hip

The joint between the *pelvis* and the upper end of the *femur* (thighbone). The hip is an extremely stable ball-and-socket joint; the smooth, rounded head of the femur fits securely into the acetabulum, a deep, cuplike cavity in the pelvis. Tough ligaments attach the femur to the pelvis, further stabilizing the joint and providing it with the necessary strength to support the weight of the upper body and to take the strain of running, jumping, and other vigorous leg movements. In addition, the ball-and-socket structure of the joint allows the leg a considerable range of movement that is available only because of the unique design of this joint.

DISORDERS

ARTHRITIS *Osteoarthritis* of the hip, one of the most common of all disorders, causes stiffness and pain in the joint, particularly during movement. Occasionally, *ankylosing spondylitis* and rheumatoid arthritis of the hip cause similar problems.

FRACTURE What is commonly called fracture of the hip (most common in elderly people as a result of a fall) is in fact fracture of the head or neck of the femur (see *Femur, fracture of*).

DISLOCATION Congenital dislocation of the hip is remediable (see *Hip, congenital dislocation of*).

Dislocation of the hip by injury is rare and usually results only from extreme force, such as may occur in a road traffic accident.

Dislocation may cut off the blood supply to the head of the femur, causing avascular necrosis (a condition in which the bone dies because of impaired blood supply). It may also injure the sciatic nerve, leading to weakness in the leg.

Hip, congenital dislocation of

A disorder present at birth in which the ball-like head of the femur (thighbone) fails to fit into the cuplike socket in the pelvis to form a joint but instead lies outside. One or both of the hips may be affected.

CAUSES AND INCIDENCE

The cause of congenital dislocation of the hip is not known, but it is more common in babies born by *breech delivery* and following pregnancies in which there was *oligohydramnios* (an abnormally small amount of amniotic fluid surrounding the fetus).

About 400 in every 100,000 babies born are affected by instability of the hip joint. In most cases the condition soon corrects itself, but true dislocation does not correct itself. The disorder affects approximately five times as many girls as boys and sometimes runs in families.

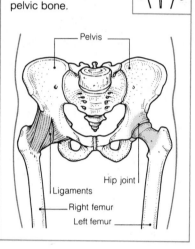

LOCATION OF HIP
The hip is a ball-and-socket joint comprising the dome at the top of the femur (thighbone) and the cup-shaped depression in the pelvic bone.

Pelvis

Hip joint

Ligaments

Right femur

Left femur

DIAGNOSIS

Shortly after birth and at intervals until walking starts, all babies are given a routine physical examination of the hip to check its stability and range of motion. *Ultrasound scanning* is currently being evaluated as a screening test. If the condition is not detected in infancy, dislocation may cause a limp when the child is learning to walk.

TREATMENT

If the condition is found in early infancy, light *splints* are applied to the thigh to maneuver the ball of the joint into the socket and keep it in position. The splints are worn for two to four months and usually help to correct the problem.

If the condition is not discovered until later in infancy, *traction* is used. The head of the femur is moved into the correct position and kept there by a system of weights and pulleys attached to the leg or by being nursed with the legs raised on a "gallows."

If detection of dislocation is delayed, surgery under a general anesthetic may be required to correct it. The child must usually stay in hospital for several weeks and wear a plaster *cast* for a few months.

OUTLOOK

Provided the disorder is treated in infancy, the child usually walks normally and there are no aftereffects. When treatment is delayed,

however, there may be lifelong problems with walking. Without treatment, the dislocation often leads to shortening of the leg, limping, and early *osteoarthritis* in the joint.

Hippocratic oath

A set of ethical principles derived from the writings of the ancient Greek physician Hippocrates. The Hippocratic oath is concerned with a physician's duty to work for the good of his or her patients and to cause no harm, whether by deliberate intent, by prescribing deadly drugs, or by giving advice that might cause death. The oath also covers the principle of confidentiality and condemns abuse of the physician-patient relationship for sexual purposes.

Hip replacement

A surgical procedure to replace all or part of a diseased hip joint with an artificial substitute.

WHY IT IS DONE

Hip replacement is most often carried out in older people whose joints are stiff and painful as a result of *osteoarthritis*. It may also be needed if *rheumatoid arthritis* has spread to the hip joint, making walking difficult, or if the top end of the femur is badly fractured (see *Femur, fracture of*).

The operation is not usually advised for young patients, since their greater activity puts more strain on the joints and it is not known how long an artificial replacement is likely to last.

HOW IT IS DONE

A procedure for hip replacement is shown in the illustrated box on the facing page.

RECOVERY PERIOD

The joint remains unstable for a week or two after the operation, and patients must take care not to dislocate the new joint during this time. Patients are advised to sleep on their backs and not to cross their legs, and are taught how to get in and out of the bath without disturbing the joint.

OUTLOOK

Hip replacement is a remarkably successful operation that has transformed the lives of many people who, before undergoing this procedure, suffered from severe pain and stiffness. However, with time, a substantial proportion of artificial joints show signs on X ray of loosening at the cemented union between the bone and the metal. Surgeons and engineers are continuing to develop newer joint designs that do not rely on cement to hold them in place.

PERFORMING A HIP REPLACEMENT

In this operation, the surgeon pushes aside or cuts through the surrounding muscles to expose the hip joint. The femur (thighbone) is cut and the pelvis is drilled to make room for the two components of the artificial joint. These parts are secured in place, the femur is repaired, and the muscles and tendons are replaced and repaired.

Sites of incision

Pelvis

Trochanter

Femur

1 The trochanter at the top of the femur is detached, and the hip joint is dislocated to separate the femur and the pelvis. The ball at the top of the femur is then cut away.

2 An instrument known as a reamer is used to make the hollow in the pelvis large enough to make room for the cup-shaped socket formed by the two components of the artificial hip joint.

3 A coarse file is used to cut a shaft in the femur, and the ball part of the artificial joint is inserted. The components are fixed in place with a special cement, which binds them to the bone.

4 The ball is placed in the socket and the trochanter is reattached to the femur with wires. The muscles and tendons are replaced and repaired, and the incision is then closed.

Before
This X ray shows a hip joint that has been badly damaged by arthritis.

Ball

Socket

Shaft

Components
An artificial hip joint has two parts. The ball and shaft are metal; the socket may be metal or plastic.

After
This X ray shows the artificial hip joint in position after surgery.

Hip, snapping

A fairly common condition in adults in which a characteristic clicking is heard and felt during certain movements of the joint.

Snapping hip is generally harmless and does not indicate that the patient is suffering from a disease of the hip joint. In fact, the noise and sensation are simply caused by a tendon slipping over the bony prominence on the outside of the femur when the hip is bent upward.

A snapping hip is different from the clicking that can be heard during examination of the hip of a newborn baby suffering from dislocation of the hip (see *Hip, congenital dislocation of*).

Hirschsprung's disease

A congenital disorder in which a segment of intestine lacks the ganglion cells that control the intestine's rhythmic contractions. The segment without ganglion cells extends up from the lower end of the rectum, usually also involving the last part of the colon. This segment becomes narrowed and blocks the movement of fecal material. As a result, the area of intestine above the narrowed segment becomes widened and convoluted.

Hirschsprung's disease is uncommon and tends to run in families. It occurs about four times more often in boys than in girls.

SYMPTOMS

Symptoms usually appear in infancy or early childhood; they include constipation and bloating. The child usually has a poor appetite and may fail to grow properly.

DIAGNOSIS

A barium enema (see *Barium X-ray examinations*) can show the narrowed segment of the intestine. A *biopsy* (removal of a sample of tissue for microscopic analysis) may be performed during *proctoscopy* (inspection of the rectum with a viewing instrument) or during a surgical procedure. Examination of the biopsy sample will show whether ganglion cells are lacking and thus confirm the diagnosis.

Treatment involves removing the narrowed intestinal segment and rejoining the normal areas of intestine. Before surgery, a temporary *colostomy* (creation of an artificial outlet for the colon through the abdominal wall) may be necessary if the child is considerably underweight.

Hirsutism

Excessive hairiness, particularly in women. The additional hair is coarse, like a man's, and grows in a male pattern on the face, trunk, and limbs.

CAUSES AND INCIDENCE

Hirsutism occurs in some conditions, such as polycystic ovary syndrome (see *Ovary, polycystic*) and congenital *adrenal hyperplasia*, in which the level of male hormones in the blood is abnormally high. Hirsutism can also be caused by taking anabolic steroids (see *Steroids, anabolic*).

Much more commonly, hirsutism is not a sign of any underlying disorder; it occurs in many normal women, especially after the *menopause*. The condition tends to run in families. Women with dark hair, particularly those of Indian or Hispanic extraction, are particularly likely to be hirsute.

H

H

TREATMENT

Hair can be bleached or removed in various ways (see *Hair removal*); the only method of permanent removal is by *electrolysis*. (See also *Hypertrichosis*.)

Histamine

A chemical present in cells (mainly *mast cells*) throughout the body that is released during an allergic reaction (see *Allergy*). Histamine is one of the substances responsible for the swelling and redness that occur in *inflammation*. Histamine also narrows the bronchi (airways) in the lungs, causes itching, and stimulates production of acid by the stomach.

The effects of histamine can be counteracted by *antihistamine drugs*; its action on the acid-forming glands in the stomach is blocked by a group of *Histamine₂-receptor antagonists*.

Histamine₂-receptor antagonists

A group of *ulcer-healing drugs* related to the *antihistamine drug* group. These drugs work by blocking the action of the chemical *histamine* at specific *receptors* (sites on a cell's surface), preventing release of acid in the stomach. Acid reduction promotes the healing of *peptic ulcers* and relieves symptoms of *esophagitis*. (See also *Cimetidine*; *Famotidine*; *Ranitidine*.)

Histiocytosis X

A rare childhood disease in which there is an overgrowth of a type of tissue cell called a histiocyte. The cause is unknown, but histiocytosis X probably results from a disturbance of the *immune system*.

In the mildest form of the disease, rapid cell growth occurs in one bone only, usually affecting the skull, a clavicle, a rib, or a vertebra, causing swelling and pain. The chances of recovery are good in these cases.

The most severe, and least common, form of the disease affects infants. This form causes a skin rash and enlargement of the liver, spleen, and lymph nodes. The chance of recovery in these cases is poor.

Histocompatibility antigens

A group of proteins that are naturally present within tissues and that have a role in the *immune system* (body's natural defenses). The main group of histocompatibility antigens is known as the HLA (human leukocyte antigen) system. A person's tissue type (i.e., the particular set of HLAs in the body tissues) is inherited half from the father and half from the mother. The main role of HLAs is their defense role against infections and tumors, but they also influence the outcome of organ transplantation (see *Transplant surgery*) and seem to have an effect on individuals' susceptibility to certain diseases.

TYPES AND STRUCTURE

Synthesis of histocompatibility antigens takes place within cells and is under the control of genes. These genes, which are known as the major histocompatibility complex, give rise to several series of antigens, called HLA-A, HLA-B, HLA-C, and HLA-D.

Each histocompatibility antigen is composed of two parts, a constant region (which is the same for all people) and a variable region (which differs among people). The structure of this region is genetically determined (inherited from one of the parents) and can take any of several forms, which have been given numbers. Thus, a particular antigen has a letter (the series it belongs to) and a number corresponding to the form within the series—for example, HLA-A3, HLA-B13, or HLA-C5 types. The number of possible combinations of antigens from the different series is vast, but unrelated people with identical combinations occur at a rate of one in 50,000. By a technique called *tissue typing* every person can be immunologically "fingerprinted."

IMMUNOLOGICAL FUNCTION

Histocompatibility antigens within the series HLA-A, B, and C are present on virtually all living cells in the body. They are essential for the function of certain *lymphocytes* (white blood cells with an immunological function) called killer T cells. The antigens act as a guide for killer T cells to recognize and kill abnormal cells.

Histocompatibility antigens within the HLA-D series are present on the surfaces of various other cells with a defense role; they influence the interactions of these cells in fighting infection and tumors.

EFFECT IN TRANSPLANTATION

When an organ is transplanted from one person to another, the histocompatibility antigens in the donor organ are generally recognized as foreign and are attacked by the recipient's immune system, leading to rejection. However, if a donor can be found whose HLA types are very similar to those of the recipient (often a blood relative and ideally an identical twin), the chances of rejection occurring are minimized.

DISEASE ASSOCIATION

Certain HLA types occur more frequently in patients with particular diseases than in the rest of the population. For example, *multiple sclerosis* is associated with HLA-A3, *celiac disease* with HLA-B8, and *ankylosing spondylitis* with HLA-B27.

It is suspected that susceptibility to these diseases is influenced by the HLA types, presumably as a result of their immunological actions. The associations are of interest because they allow identification of individuals at risk and can help in the confirmation of disease.

PATERNITY TESTING

Comparison of HLA types can sometimes show that two people are likely to be related and HLA analysis has therefore sometimes been used in *paternity testing*. This use is now being superseded by modern techniques of *genetic fingerprinting*, which can show relationship with greater certainty.

Histology

The study of tissues, including their cellular structure and function. The main practical use of histology in medicine is in the diagnosis of disease. This often involves obtaining a tissue sample by *biopsy* and examining it under a microscope for abnormalities. The histologist's skill lies in his or her familiarity with the range of normal appearances of tissues and the recognition of the abnormal appearances that occur in different diseases.

Histopathology

The branch of *histology* concerned with the effects of disease on the microscopic structure of tissues.

Histoplasmosis

An infection caused by inhaling the spores of *HISTOPLASMA CAPSULATUM*, a fungus found in soil, particularly in soil contaminated with droppings from birds or bats. Histoplasmosis is very rare in Canada, but there are known *endemic* areas in the central and southern parts of the US.

History-taking

The process by which a physician learns from patients the symptoms of their illnesses and any previous disorders. (See *Diagnosis*.)

HIV

Human immunodeficiency virus. HIV belongs to the class of retroviruses (see *Viruses*) and is the cause of *AIDS* and *AIDS-related complex*.

HOW HUMAN IMMUNODEFICIENCY VIRUS (HIV) MULTIPLIES

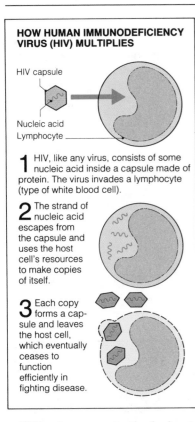

HIV capsule

Nucleic acid
Lymphocyte

1 HIV, like any virus, consists of some nucleic acid inside a capsule made of protein. The virus invades a lymphocyte (type of white blood cell).

2 The strand of nucleic acid escapes from the capsule and uses the host cell's resources to make copies of itself.

3 Each copy forms a capsule and leaves the host cell, which eventually ceases to function efficiently in fighting disease.

HIV gains access to the body via contaminated blood transfusions, nonsterile needles, or sexual intercourse. A fetus may be infected via the placenta. HIV has an affinity for the T-*lymphocytes*, in which the virus multiplies and, in some cases, destroys function. HIV also attacks the brain and may cause severe damage with *dementia*, although most infected people succumb to AIDS before this.

HIV is an organism of low infectivity; infected people present no threat to the health of their contacts at work or home, except for sexual partners and needle sharers.

The virus that causes AIDS was discovered at the Institut Pasteur in Paris and named the lymphadenopathy associated virus (LAV). In 1984, research workers in the US identified an AIDS virus which they classed as a retrovirus similar to viruses already linked with a rare type of human leukemia. They named their virus human T cell lymphotropic virus III or HTLV III. The LAV virus and the HTLV virus subsequently proved to be identical and the name now generally agreed for the organism that causes AIDS is the human immunodeficiency virus or HIV.

More recent research has shown that some AIDS patients in Africa have been infected with a virus that is very similar to HIV. This variant is known as HIV II. A third related virus causes an AIDS-like disease in monkeys. At present, these rarer viruses seem to be found only in Africa.

Hives
An alternative name for *urticaria*.

HLA types
See *Histocompatibility antigens*.

Hoarseness
A rough, husky, or croaking voice, usually caused by interference with the normal working of the vocal cords in the *larynx* (voice box). Most attacks do not last long and clear up of their own accord, but persistent hoarseness requires investigation to exclude the possibility of serious disease.

CAUSES
Hoarseness of limited duration is often due to overuse of the voice (for example, in teachers or singers), which strains small muscles in the larynx. It is also commonly caused by inflammation of the vocal cords as part of acute *laryngitis*, which is usually due to an upper respiratory tract infection such as a cold or sore throat. (See pp. 542-543.)

Persistent hoarseness has many possible causes. It may be due to chronic irritation of the larynx (which can be caused by smoking or excessive consumption of alcohol) or to chronic *bronchitis*. Irritation can also be caused by mucus dripping onto the larynx, which may occur in people with nasal *polyps* (harmless growths in the nose), allergic *rhinitis* (hay fever), *sinusitis*, or a deviated *nasal septum* (displacement of the cartilage that separates the two nasal passages).

Polyps on the vocal cords may also cause hoarseness, as may any accidental damage to them during surgery on the thyroid gland. In people with *hypothyroidism* (underactivity of the thyroid gland), hoarseness can result from formation of tissue on the vocal cords.

In young children, hoarseness is a symptom of *croup* (inflammation and narrowing of the airways).

Occasionally, persistent hoarseness in adults has a more serious cause—including cancer of the larynx (see *Larynx, cancer of*). Less commonly, persistent hoarseness is caused by *thyroid cancer* or by *lung cancer*.

SELF-HELP
Anyone suffering from hoarseness believed to be brought on by straining the voice should rest his or her voice until it has returned to normal; otherwise, permanent damage may eventually occur in the vocal cords. Voice training may reduce the likelihood of the hoarseness recurring. Resting the voice, along with not smoking or drinking alcohol, also helps recovery from laryngitis.

INVESTIGATION
It is essential to consult a physician if hoarseness persists for more than two weeks. In such cases, a *laryngoscopy* (examination of the larynx with a mirror or viewing tube) will be performed to exclude the possibility of cancer (which can be completely cured if diagnosed early).

Hodgkin's disease
Also known as Hodgkin's lymphoma, a malignant disorder in which there is proliferation of cells in the lymphoid tissue (found mainly in the *lymph nodes* and *spleen*) and a resultant enlargement of the lymph nodes. Lymphoid tissue is an important part of the *immune system*. The cause of Hodgkin's disease is unknown.

INCIDENCE
Hodgkin's disease is an uncommon cancer; about 800 new cases are diagnosed annually in Canada. This disorder is more common in men than in women, and most commonly develops between the ages of 20 and 30, and between 55 and 70.

SYMPTOMS AND SIGNS
The most common sign is painless enlargement of a group of lymph nodes, typically those in the neck or armpits. Most symptoms are caused by the presence of the enlarged nodes, invasion of other organs by proliferating lymphoid tissue, or impairment of the body's immune system. Thus, a Hodgkin's disease victim may suffer from a general feeling of illness, with fever, loss of appetite, weight loss, and night sweats. There may also be such discomforts as generalized itching and, rarely, pain after drinking alcohol.

Invasion of other organs by this disease may cause a diverse range of symptoms (such as breathlessness if the lungs are involved or paralysis if the spine is affected). As the disease progresses, the immune system becomes increasingly impaired and the patient may suffer life-threatening complications from an infection that would normally be trivial.

H

H

HOARSENESS OR LOSS OF VOICE
Any abnormal huskiness in the voice that may be so severe that you can make little or no sound.

Has the hoarseness started within the past three days?

YES → **Do you have or have you just had a cold, cough, or sore throat?**

YES → You probably have inflammation of the vocal cords.
See • *Laryngitis*

NO ↓

Had you been using your voice more than usual just before the hoarseness or loss of voice developed?

YES → Overuse can irritate the vocal cords.
See • *Laryngitis*

NO ↓

Have you recently become tense, nervous, or depressed?

YES → Anxiety can sometimes cause a sudden loss of voice.
See • *Anxiety*

NO

NO ↓

Are you over 40 years old and has your voice deepened?

YES → **Have you noticed two or more of the following symptoms?**
• feeling the cold more than you used to
• dry skin or hair
• weight increase without overeating
• unexplained tiredness

YES → An underactive thyroid gland is a possibility. This is an uncommon problem that is most likely to occur in middle-aged women. Consult your physician.
See • *Hypothyroidism*

NO

NO ↓

Do you smoke?

YES → Smoking can lead to inflammation of the vocal cords.
See • *Laryngitis*

NO ↓

Have you been drinking alcohol recently?

YES → Drinking alcohol can lead to inflammation of the vocal cords.
See • *Laryngitis*

NO ↓

Self-help
Hoarseness usually clears up after a few days with simple measures such as resting the voice and abstaining from smoking and alcohol.

Continued on next page

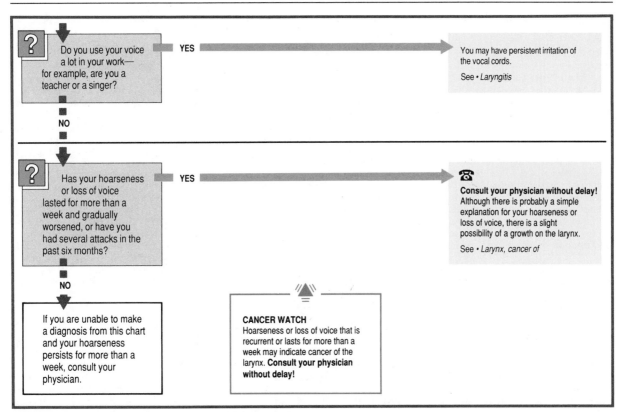

Do you use your voice a lot in your work—for example, are you a teacher or a singer?

YES → You may have persistent irritation of the vocal cords.

See • *Laryngitis*

NO

Has your hoarseness or loss of voice lasted for more than a week and gradually worsened, or have you had several attacks in the past six months?

YES → ☎ **Consult your physician without delay!** Although there is probably a simple explanation for your hoarseness or loss of voice, there is a slight possibility of a growth on the larynx.

See • *Larynx, cancer of*

NO

If you are unable to make a diagnosis from this chart and your hoarseness persists for more than a week, consult your physician.

CANCER WATCH
Hoarseness or loss of voice that is recurrent or lasts for more than a week may indicate cancer of the larynx. **Consult your physician without delay!**

H

DIAGNOSIS

Diagnosis of Hodgkin's disease depends on the identification of characteristic cells, called Reed-Sternberg cells, in a *biopsy* specimen (sample of tissue removed for microscopic analysis) from an enlarged lymph node or other affected organ.

Analysis is also made of the relative proportions of other cells in the specimen—including plasma cells, eosinophils, lymphocytes, and granulocytes (all types of white blood cell). This enables the disease to be classified according to its histological type, which is one factor that affects the chances of a cure.

The extent of the disease (known as its *stage*) is also assessed in terms of the number of groups of lymph nodes affected and in terms of any other organs that are involved. This process, called staging, is important for the planning of treatment. Typically, staging includes a *chest X ray*, *CT scanning* of the abdomen, and a *bone marrow biopsy*.

Other tests may include *laparotomy* (surgical exploration of the abdomen), *liver biopsy*, *splenectomy*, or *lymphangiography* (X-ray imaging of the lymphatic system) of the abdomen.

TREATMENT AND OUTLOOK

Treatment varies according to the stage of the disease. In an early stage, *radiation therapy* is usually curative. If the disease has progressed to involve many organs, however, treatment with *anticancer drugs* is usually recommended and may have to be continued for several months. In some cases, both radiation therapy and drug treatment are used.

The outlook depends on the stage to which the disease has progressed and on the histological type. However, after treatment, some 70 to 80 percent of patients survive for at least five years. The condition is apparently cured in most people who receive treatment at an early stage. (See also *Lymphoma, non-Hodgkin's*.)

Hole in the heart

The common name for a *septal defect*.

Holistic medicine

A form of therapy aimed at treating the whole person—body and mind—not just the part in which symptoms occur. This approach is emphasized by many practitioners of *alternative medicine*, such as homeopathists, acupuncturists, and herbalists.

Homatropine

An *anticholinergic drug* that is similar to, but less powerful than, *atropine*. Homatropine is used mainly to enlarge the pupils.

Homeopathy

A system of *alternative medicine* that seeks to treat patients by administering small doses of medicines that in a healthy person would bring on symptoms similar to that the medicine is prescribed to treat.

For example, the homeopathic treatment for diarrhea would be a very dilute laxative preparation.

Homeostasis

The dynamic processes by which an organism maintains a constant internal environment despite external changes. Homeostasis is a major function of most body organs. Examples of homeostatic mechanisms include the regulation of blood pressure, body temperature, and blood sugar levels.

Homeostasis plays a vital role in the body because tissues and organs can function efficiently only within a narrow range of conditions such as temperature and acidity. The homeostatic mechanisms regulate such conditions

H

by negative feedback. When a certain factor varies from its optimum set point, automatic regulatory mechanisms act to counterbalance the disturbance and reestablish the internal equilibrium. For example, when the body overheats, sweating is stimulated until the temperature returns to normal. Similarly, when the level of oxygen in the blood is low, breathing is stimulated; when blood pressure falls, the heart rate increases.

Homeostatic mechanisms sometimes malfunction. For example, in malignant *hyperthermia*, the body's thermostat is somehow reset to a higher temperature than normal. In *diabetes mellitus*, blood sugar levels can no longer be regulated because of a malfunction in insulin production.

Homocystinuria

A rare, inherited condition caused by an *enzyme* deficiency. Homocystinuria is a type of inborn error of metabolism (see *Metabolism, inborn errors of*) in which there is an abnormal presence of homocystine (an *amino acid*) in the blood and urine. Affected people are very tall, with long limbs and long, spindly fingers. Some have skeletal deformities, such as curvature of the spine, and abnormalities of the lens of the eye.

Homocystinuria cannot be cured, but some cases may be improved by vitamin B$_6$ and a special diet.

Homosexuality, female

See *Lesbianism*.

Homosexuality, male

Sexual attraction to other men. According to Alfred Kinsey's studies of sexuality carried out in the 1940s, about 5 to 10 percent of men are completely homosexual; up to one third of men have had sexual contact with another man at some time.

People who are homosexual achieve orgasm in various ways, including oral sex, mutual masturbation, and anal penetration.

Each partner may adopt a particular role in the relationship (either active or passive) but more often the roles are interchangeable.

CAUSES

Various theories have been put forward to explain homosexuality. Some studies have shown an increased incidence of homosexuality among men who had absent or weak fathers and who formed close emotional relationships with their mothers. Evidence for either a genetic tendency or a hor-

mone imbalance is lacking. The prevalence of homosexuality appears to be much the same in all cultures, with no change over thousands of years—suggesting that homosexuality is a consistent variation in behavior.

PROBLEMS

Homosexuality is more openly considered than it once was, but some homosexuals feel guilty about their sexual orientation. This may cause them to mask their feelings behind a cloak of apparent heterosexuality or to seek medical help.

The fact that some homosexuals have multiple partners and high rates of sexual activity has placed them at high risk of *sexually transmitted diseases*; it was in homosexual males that the virus responsible for *AIDS* was first identified. (See also *Bisexuality*.)

Homozygote

A term used to describe a person whose cells contain two identical *genes* controlling a specified inherited trait, in contrast to a *heterozygote*, whose cells contain two different genes controlling that trait. (See also *Genetic disorders; Inheritance*.)

Hookworm infestation

An infestation of the small intestine by small, round, blood-sucking worms of the species NECATOR AMERICANUS or ANCYLOSTOMA DUODENALE. The worms are about 12 mm long and have hooklike teeth.

INCIDENCE AND CAUSES

Hookworms infest about 1 billion people worldwide, primarily in tropical and subtropical regions. Hookworms cannot be acquired or transmitted in Canada. Persons originating from, or visiting, endemic areas may be at risk.

The accompanying illustration shows how hookworms can enter and multiply in the body. In a heavy infestation, there may be several hundred worms in the intestine, consuming up to 50 ml of blood every day.

SYMPTOMS AND COMPLICATIONS

When the larvae penetrate the skin, a red and intensely itchy rash may develop on the feet. This is called ground itch and may last for several days. In light infestations, there may be no further symptoms. In heavier infestations, migration of the larvae through the lungs may produce cough and pneumonia; adult worms in the intestines may cause vague abdominal discomfort.

By far the most important problem caused by a heavy infestation of hookworms is iron-deficiency *anemia* due to loss of blood.

DIAGNOSIS AND TREATMENT

Diagnosis is made by microscopic examination of feces, which can reveal hookworm eggs. *Anthelmintic drugs*, such as *mebendazole*, kill the worms. Treatment also involves improving nutrition with a high-protein diet and correcting anemia with iron tablets or blood transfusions, if necessary. Elimination of the disease from a community depends on efficient sanitation. (See also *Larva migrans*.)

Hormonal disorders

Conditions that are caused by malfunction of an endocrine gland. See *Endocrine system* and disorders of the *adrenal glands; ovaries; pancreas; parathyroid glands; pituitary gland; testes; thyroid gland*.

Hormonal methods of contraception

See *Contraception, hormonal methods of*.

Hormone

A chemical released into the bloodstream by a particular gland or tissue that has a specific effect on tissues elsewhere in the body.

Many hormones are produced by the glands of the *endocrine system* (the *adrenal glands, ovaries* or *testes, pancreas, parathyroid glands, pituitary gland*, and *thyroid gland*). Hormones are also secreted by other organs, including the kidneys, intestines, brain, and, in women who are pregnant, the *placenta*.

Hormones control numerous body functions, including the *metabolism* (chemical activity) of cells, growth, sexual development, and the body's response to stress or illness. (See the table, p. 546.)

Hormone antagonist

A drug that blocks the action of a *hormone* (chemical messenger released by a gland). *Tamoxifen*, for example, blocks the effects of *estrogen hormones* and is used in the treatment of some types of breast cancer.

Hormone replacement therapy

The use of a synthetic or natural *hormone* (chemical messenger released by a gland) to treat a hormone deficiency. In its broadest sense, the term describes the replacement of any deficient hormone, such as giving *thyroid*

HOOKWORM LIFE CYCLE

Infestation begins with larvae that penetrate the skin or are ingested and enter the bloodstream. They migrate throughout the body, particularly to the small intestine. Adult worms develop and lay eggs, which leave the body in feces and eventually hatch into larvae.

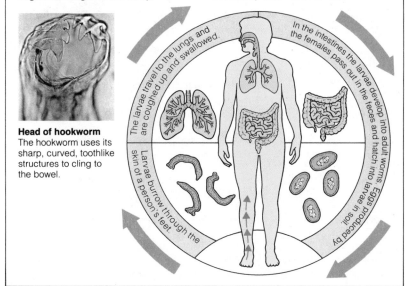

Head of hookworm
The hookworm uses its sharp, curved, toothlike structures to cling to the bowel.

hormones to treat *hypothyroidism* or *insulin* to treat *diabetes mellitus*. More commonly, hormone replacement therapy refers to the use of *estrogen hormones* to treat symptoms afflicting some women when their estrogen levels fall after the *menopause*.

Estrogen replacement therapy is given to relieve menopausal symptoms such as hot flashes and excessive sweating at night. Estrogen hormones help prevent atrophic *vaginitis* (thinning and dryness of the vagina), which may make sexual intercourse painful and difficult. Estrogen hormone, replacement also delays, or helps prevent, some of the long-term consequences of reduced estrogen levels in old age, including the development of *osteoporosis* (reduction in bone density) and *atherosclerosis* (narrowing of the arteries by deposits of fatty material).

HOW IT IS DONE
In hormone replacement therapy, estrogen drugs are usually prescribed in combination with a *progesterone drug* because estrogen drugs given alone may increase a woman's susceptibility to cancer of the uterus.

The drugs are usually taken orally in a three-stage cycle repeated each month—estrogen for the first 11 to 14 days, estrogen and a progesterone for the next seven to 10 days, and no drugs for the last seven days, during which there is often a light menstrual period. Alternatively, estrogen may be released slowly into the bloodstream from an adhesive patch placed on the skin of the lower trunk. The progesterone is still taken in tablet form.

Therapy is usually continued for between two and five years. Regular tests, including weight and blood pressure checks, breast and pelvic examinations, and *cervical smear tests*, are carried out to monitor the effects of the therapy. Occasionally, a *biopsy* (removal of a sample of tissue for microscopic analysis) of the lining of the uterus may be carried out to test for cancer.

POSSIBLE ADVERSE EFFECTS
Minor adverse effects include nausea, breast tenderness, fluid retention, and leg cramps. In some women, estrogen replacement therapy may increase the risk of abnormal blood clotting. Estrogen replacement therapy is therefore not usually given to women who smoke heavily or have suffered from *thrombosis*, *stroke*, liver disease, or severe *hypertension* (raised blood pressure). Women who have had cancer of the breast or uterus are not usually given estrogen replacement therapy because such therapy may increase the risk of a recurrence of the cancer.

Horn, cutaneous

A hard, noncancerous protrusion occasionally found on the skin (usually the face) of elderly people. Horns are slow-growing and vary in color from yellow to brown to black. They may develop where there was previously a wart on normal skin.

Left untreated, they can grow to a considerable size and may protrude as much as 2 cm. Surgical removal is usually recommended.

Horner's syndrome

A group of physical signs that affects one side of the face and indicates damage to part of the sympathetic nervous system (see *Autonomic nervous system*). The signs of Horner's syndrome are narrowing of the pupil of the eye, drooping of the lid, and absence of sweating. They are caused by damage to or destruction of sympathetic nerve fibers, usually in the lower part of the neck, and may be the first indication of disease in the area.

Hornet stings

See *Insect stings*.

Horseshoe kidney

A congenital abnormality in which the two kidneys are fused or joined at the base, forming a horseshoe shape. The condition may be diagnosed prenatally by *ultrasound scanning*.

The joined kidneys usually function normally but they may be associated with other congenital abnormalites of the kidneys.

Hospice

A hospital or part of a hospital devoted to the care of patients who are dying (usually of cancer). (See *Dying, care of the*.)

Hospitals, types of

With very few exceptions, Canadian hospitals are public institutions offering a full range of diagnostic and medical care services (both inpatient and outpatient) at little or no direct cost to the patient. (See *Medicare*.)

There are more than 1,200 general, teaching, pediatric, and allied specialty hospitals. These provide more than 176,000 beds, or about seven beds per 1,000 population. More than half of Canadian hospitals are small, having 100 beds or less. Nearly one half are short-term medical and surgical beds; about one quarter are for extended and chronic care.

Many of these are organized to provide special services to residents of remote areas. A person to be hospitalized may choose any hospital to which the physician has admitting privileges. As well, there are about 5,600 special care facilities such as nursing homes and homes for the elderly.

Hot flashes

Reddening of the face, neck, and upper trunk usually caused by decreased *estrogen hormone* production by the ovaries during or after the *menopause*. Hot flashes may also occur after removal of the ovaries (see *Oophorectomy*). Occasionally, men experience hot flashes after removal of the testes (see *Orchiectomy*), which causes a reduction in testosterone levels.

THE SOURCES AND MAIN EFFECTS OF SELECTED HORMONES

Section of body	Hormone secreted	Effects
Hypothalamus	Releasing hormones	Stimulate hormone secretion by pituitary gland
Pituitary gland	Growth hormone	Stimulates growth and metabolism
	Prolactin	Stimulates milk production after childbirth
	ACTH (adrenocorticotropic hormone)	Stimulates hormone production by adrenal glands
	TSH (thyroid-stimulating hormone)	Stimulates hormone production by thyroid gland
	FSH (follicle-stimulating hormone); LH (luteinizing hormone)	Stimulate gonads (ovaries or testes)
	ADH (antidiuretic hormone)	Acts on kidneys to reduce urine production
	Oxytocin	Stimulates contractions of uterus during labor and ejection of milk during breast-feeding
	MSH (melanocyte-stimulating hormone)	Acts on the skin to promote production of skin pigment (melanin)
Brain	Endorphins; enkephalins	Alleviate pain
Thyroid gland	Thyroid hormone	Increases metabolic rate; affects growth
	Calcitonin	Controls level of calcium in blood
Parathyroid glands	Parathyroid hormone	Controls level of calcium in blood
Thymus	Thymic hormone	Stimulates lymphocyte development
Adrenal glands	Epinephrine; norepinephrine	Prepare body for stress
	Hydrocortisone	Affects metabolism
	Aldosterone	Regulates sodium and potassium excretion by kidneys
	Androgens	Affect growth and sex drive
Kidneys	Renin	Regulates blood pressure
	Erythropoietin	Stimulates erythrocyte production
	Vitamin D	Controls calcium and phosphate metabolism
Pancreas	Insulin; glucagon	Regulate blood sugar level
Placenta	Chorionic gonadotropin; estrogens; progesterone	Maintain pregnancy
Gastrointestinal tract	Gastrin; secretin; cholecystokinin	Regulate secretion of some digestive enzymes
Testes	Testosterone	Affects development of male secondary sexual characteristics and genital organs
Ovaries	Estrogens; progesterone	Affect development of female secondary sexual characteristics and genital organs; control menstrual cycle; maintain pregnancy

The various glands that make up the hormonal system constitute a control and communications network that is complementary to the nervous system. The glands secrete chemical messengers (hormones) to affect other glands and tissues in various parts of the body. Hormones are carried in the bloodstream to their targets. This table lists the hormones secreted by different parts of the body and gives a description of their wide-ranging actions.

Hot flashes typically last one to two minutes. They are accompanied by a sensation of heat, are often followed by sweating, and are aggravated by stress. If hot flashes are severe, they can usually be alleviated by *hormone replacement therapy*.

Housemaid's knee
Inflammation of the *bursa* (fluid-filled sac) that acts as a cushion over the kneecap. The inflammation is usually caused by prolonged kneeling, but may develop after a blow to the front of the knee. (See also *Bursitis*.)

House staff
A term for an *intern* or *resident* who is assigned to, and takes care of, patients in a specific hospital.

HTLV III
An old name for *HIV*.

Human chorionic gonadotropin
See *Gonadotropin, human chorionic*.

Humerus
The bone of the upper arm. The smooth, dome-shaped head of the bone lies at an angle to the shaft and fits into a shallow socket in the scapula (shoulder blade) to form the shoulder joint. Below its head, the bone narrows to form a cylindrical shaft. It flattens and widens at its lower end, forming a prominence on each side called an epicondyle. At its base, the humerus articulates with the *ulna* and *radius* (the bones of the lower arm) to form the elbow.

A spiral groove in the shaft of the humerus carries the *radial nerve*, one of the main nerves of the arm.

Humerus, fracture of
Fractures of the *humerus* (the bone of the upper arm) may affect the upper end, the shaft, or the lower end of the bone. The part of the humerus most commonly fractured is the neck of the bone (at the upper end of the humerus, just below the bone's head). This type of fracture most often occurs in elderly people.

Fractures of the shaft of the humerus usually affect the middle third of the bone. Such fractures occur in adults of all ages but are uncommon in children. Supracondylar fractures (at the lower end of the bone) occur most commonly in children.

DIAGNOSIS AND TREATMENT
An *X ray* is performed if any fracture of the humerus is suspected.

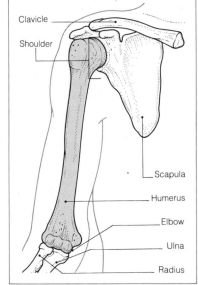

LOCATION OF HUMERUS
The humerus is the bone of the upper arm, located between the shoulder and elbow joints.

Clavicle
Shoulder
Scapula
Humerus
Elbow
Ulna
Radius

A fracture of the neck of the bone usually requires only a *sling* to keep the bone immobilized; a fracture of the shaft or of the lower end of the bone usually needs to be put in a plaster *cast*. Most fractures of the humerus heal in six to eight weeks.

COMPLICATIONS
Damage to the radial nerve may occur when the shaft of the humerus is fractured. In severe cases, this may result in *wristdrop*. Fracture of the humerus may be accompanied by damage to the brachial artery. If such damage is undetected, circulation to the arm may be impaired, resulting in *Volkmann's contracture* (a deformity of the forearm and hand). Some supracondylar fractures fail to mend properly—despite all remedial efforts and traction—resulting in elbow deformity and an increased risk that *osteoarthritis* will eventually develop.

Humors
Liquid or jellylike substances in the body. The term usually refers to the aqueous humor (the watery fluid in the front chamber of the *eye*) and the *vitreous humor* (the jellylike substance in the rear chamber of the eye).

According to early medical theory, four humors—blood, phlegm, black bile, and yellow bile—permeated the entire body, the balance between them determining its state of health.

Hunchback
See *Kyphosis*.

Hunger
A disagreeable feeling caused by the need for food (as opposed to *appetite*, a pleasant sensation felt in anticipation of a meal).

Hunger occurs when the stomach is empty and when the blood sugar level is low. In response to these stimuli, messages from the hypothalamus in the brain cause the muscular wall of the stomach to contract rhythmically, signaling the need for food; if pronounced, these contractions produce hunger pains.

Hunger caused by a low blood sugar level usually results from strenuous exercise. It can also occur in certain diseases, notably in *thyrotoxicosis*, a disorder of the thyroid gland that causes marked speeding-up of body processes, and in insulin-dependent *diabetes mellitus*, in cases where an incorrect balance between insulin and carbohydrate intake causes *hypoglycemia* (low blood sugar level).

Huntington's chorea
An uncommon disease in which degeneration of the *basal ganglia* (paired nerve cell clusters in the brain) results in *chorea* (rapid, jerky, involuntary movements) and *dementia* (progressive mental impairment). Symptoms do not usually appear until the age of 35 to 50; in rare cases the condition is apparent in childhood.

Huntington's chorea is a *genetic disorder* with an autosomal dominant pattern of inheritance. Because the age of onset of symptoms is generally so late, an affected person may bear children before realizing that he or she has the disease. Each child has a 50 percent chance of the condition developing. The disease is present in five to eight persons per 100,000.

SYMPTOMS
The chorea usually affects the face, arms, and trunk, resulting in random grimaces and twitches and general clumsiness. Dementia takes the form of personality and behavior changes, irritability, difficulty making decisions, memory loss, and apathy.

When the disease starts in childhood, it may be marked by loss of movement and muscle rigidity.

DIAGNOSIS
Until recently there was no way of detecting whether a child of a person with Huntington's chorea had inherited the abnormal gene responsible for the condition. As a result of recent

H

H

advances in genetics, young adults with parents who have the condition can now learn, with 95 percent accuracy, whether or not they have the abnormal gene and thus have the disorder. This may affect decisions about having children of their own (see *Genetic counseling*). In addition, *chorionic villus sampling* during pregnancy can now determine whether a fetus is at high or low risk of inheriting the disorder.

TREATMENT AND OUTLOOK

There is no known cure. Treatment is aimed at lessening the chorea with drugs, such as tetrabenazine, and alleviating the effects of dementia with good nursing care.

Most sufferers survive for about 15 years after the onset of symptoms; some live for up to 30 years.

Hurler's syndrome

A rare, inherited condition caused by an *enzyme* defect. Hurler's syndrome is a type of inborn error of metabolism (see *Metabolism, inborn errors of*) in which there is an abnormal accumulation of substances known as mucopolysaccharides in the tissues.

Affected children may appear normal at birth, but, between 6 and 12 months of age develop cardiac abnormalities, umbilical hernia, skeletal deformities, and enlargement of the tongue, liver, and spleen. Physical growth is limited and mental development slows, leaving the child mentally retarded.

The strange physical features of affected children gave the condition its former name of gargoylism.

Hydatid disease

A rare infestation caused by the larval stage of the small tapeworm *ECHINO-COCCUS GRANULOSUS*. Larvae most often settle in the liver, lungs, or muscle, causing the development of slowly growing cysts. In rare cases, the brain or other organs are affected.

The illustration above shows how tapeworm eggs or larvae can enter the human body, migrating to the liver, lungs, or other organs, which they sometimes inhabit for years.

Hydatid disease is prevalent only in areas of the world, such as Australia and New Zealand, where sheep are managed with the aid of dogs. About 200 cases of the disease are diagnosed in the US each year; a few occur in Canada.

Although the infestation is usually

ORIGINS OF HYDATID DISEASE

The infestation is generally confined to dogs and sheep, but occasionally a child swallows eggs from dog feces. These hatch into larvae, which migrate through the body, especially to the liver or lungs, to form slow-growing cysts. Symptoms may not appear until years later.

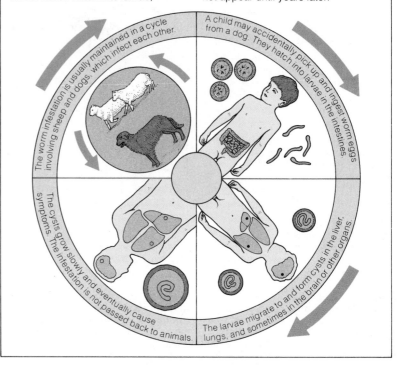

The worm infestation is usually maintained in a cycle involving sheep and dogs, which infect each other.

A child may accidentally pick up and ingest worm eggs from a dog. They hatch into larvae in the intestines.

The cysts grow slowly and eventually cause symptoms. The infestation is not passed back to animals.

The larvae migrate to and form cysts in the liver, lungs, and sometimes in the brain or other organs.

acquired in childhood, the cysts grow very slowly, so symptoms, if any, occur mainly in adults. In many cases there are no symptoms.

Cysts in the liver may cause a tender, localized lump or lead to *bile duct obstruction* and jaundice. Cysts in the lungs may press on an airway, causing inflammation; rupture of a lung cyst may cause chest pain, coughing up blood, and wheezing. Cysts in the brain can cause seizures or other symptoms similar to those of a brain tumor. Ruptured cysts may rarely cause *anaphylactic shock*.

DIAGNOSIS AND TREATMENT

Hydatid cysts are diagnosed by *CT scanning*. Cysts may be removed surgically. Alternatively, they may be sterilized and then drained. Drug treatments are being investigated.

Hydatidiform mole

An uncommon benign tumor that develops from placental tissue early in a pregnancy in which the embryo has failed to develop normally. A hydatidiform mole, which resembles a bunch of small grapes, is caused by degeneration of the chorionic villi, minute fingerlike projections in the placenta. The cause of the degeneration is unknown.

INCIDENCE

A hydatidiform mole is the most common form of trophoblastic tumor. It occurs in about one in 2,000 pregnancies in developed countries; the incidence is much higher in some developing countries. In about 3 percent of affected pregnancies the growth develops into a *choriocarcinoma*, a malignant tumor that can invade the walls of the uterus if it is left untreated.

SYMPTOMS, DIAGNOSIS, AND TREATMENT

Vaginal bleeding and excessive morning sickness usually occur.

A hydatidiform tumor shows up on *ultrasound scanning*. Urine and blood tests detect excessive amounts of human chorionic gonadotropin (see *Gonadotropin, human chorionic*), which are produced by the tumor.

The tumor can be removed either by suctioning out the contents of the uterus or by a *D and C*. A *hysterectomy* may be considered.

OUTLOOK

There is a small risk that a malignant tumor may develop later; for this reason, tests are performed regularly for several years to determine the levels of human chorionic gonadotropin in the blood and urine.

A woman should not become pregnant again until her human chorionic gonadotropin levels have returned to normal for at least a year. There is a one in 75 risk of a recurrence of the condition in a future pregnancy.

Hydralazine

An *antihypertensive drug* which is particularly useful as an emergency treatment for *hypertension*. Hydralazine is also often used when the combination of *diuretic drugs* and *beta-blocker drugs* fails to control high blood pressure.

Hydralazine may cause nausea, vomiting, headache, dizziness, and irregular heartbeat. Less common adverse effects include loss of appetite, rash, and joint pain. When prescribed in high doses over a prolonged period, hydralazine may cause *lupus erythematosus*.

Hydramnios

See *Polyhydramnios*.

Hydrocele

A soft, painless swelling in the *scrotum* caused by the space around a *testis* filling with fluid. A hydrocele is sometimes caused by inflammation, infection, or injury to the testis; occasionally, the cause is a tumor. In most cases, however, there is no apparent cause.

Treatment is rarely necessary. If the swelling is large enough to be uncomfortable or painful, the fluid may be aspirated (drawn off through a hollow needle) under a local anesthetic. Recurrent swelling may be treated by surgery.

Hydrocephalus

An excessive amount of *cerebrospinal fluid*, usually under increased pressure, within the skull. The term "water on the brain" is a nonmedical phrase which is sometimes used to describe this condition.

Hydrocephalus is often associated with other congenital abnormalities, particularly *spina bifida*.

CAUSES

The condition may be *congenital* (present at birth) or may develop as a result of major head injury, brain hemorrhage, infection (*meningitis*, for example), or a tumor. Hydrocephalus

Infant with hydrocephalus
Skull enlargement is due to pressure from excess fluid within the cavities of the brain. To prevent brain damage, the fluid must be drained by means of a tube inserted through a hole made in the skull.

is caused by excessive formation of cerebrospinal fluid, by a block in the circulation of this fluid, or both.

SYMPTOMS

When the condition is congenital, the main feature is an enlarged head that continues to grow at an abnormally fast rate because the bones are not rigid and expand to accommodate the fluid. Other features are rigidity of the legs, *epilepsy*, irritability, lethargy, vomiting, and the absence of normal reflex actions. If the condition is not treated, it progresses to extreme drowsiness, severe brain damage, and seizures, which may lead to the baby's death within a matter of weeks.

When the condition occurs later in childhood or in adulthood, the skull is no longer flexible and symptoms are caused by raised pressure within the skull. Symptoms include headache, vomiting, loss of coordination, and deterioration of mental function.

DIAGNOSIS AND TREATMENT

CT scanning or *MRI* show the location and nature of any obstruction.

In most cases, treatment aims to drain excess fluid away from the brain to another part of the body, such as the peritoneal cavity (lining of the abdomen), where it can be absorbed. Drainage is achieved by means of a valve and *shunt* (tube), which is inserted into the brain through a hole made in the skull. In some cases, the shunt must be left in position for an indefinite period.

In older children and adults, treatment is sometimes only for the underlying cause.

Hydrochloric acid

A strong acid released by the stomach lining. It forms part of the stomach juices and is important in the diges-

tion of proteins. Excessive acid production, which may be stimulated by stress or tobacco smoking, is an important factor in the development of *peptic ulcers*. In *acid reflux* (backflow of stomach acid into the esophagus), hydrochloric acid may cause *esophagitis* and heartburn. (See also *Digestive system*.)

Hydrochlorothiazide

A thiazide *diuretic drug* used to reduce *edema* (fluid retention) in people with *heart failure* (reduced pumping efficiency), *nephrotic syndrome* (a kidney disorder), *cirrhosis* of the liver, and breast tenderness before menstruation. Hydrochlorothiazide is also given to treat *hypertension* (high blood pressure), and is occasionally used to prevent the recurrence of certain types of kidney stones (see *Calculus, urinary tract*).

POSSIBLE ADVERSE EFFECTS

Adverse effects include leg cramps, lethargy, dizziness, rash, and impotence. Hydrochlorothiazide may rarely cause *gout* and may aggravate *diabetes mellitus*.

Hydrocortisone

CORTICOSTEROID
Tablet Injection Rectal suppository Cream Eye drops
Prescription sometimes needed

A *corticosteroid drug* used in creams, sprays, and other *topical* preparations for the treatment of inflammatory or allergic conditions, such as *ulcerative colitis* or *dermatitis*. Hydrocortisone, also called cortisol, is a hormone produced by the *adrenal gland*.

POSSIBLE ADVERSE EFFECTS

Hydrocortisone creams used in excess may cause thinning of the skin. However, if the preparation is dilute, the risk of this is slight.

Hydrogen peroxide

An *antiseptic* solution used to treat infections of the skin or mouth and to bleach hair. Hydrogen peroxide combines with catalase, an enzyme present in the skin and mouth, to release oxygen. This effect kills bacteria and cleanses infected areas. Hydrogen peroxide occasionally causes soreness.

Hydronephrosis

A condition in which a *kidney* becomes distended (swollen) with urine due to an obstruction in the *urinary tract*.

H

Untreated hydronephrosis can severely damage a kidney and, if both kidneys are affected, it can lead to *kidney failure*.

CAUSES
Many people with hydronephrosis have a *congenital* constriction (narrowing) of the ureter. Obstruction of a ureter may be due to a stone (see *Calculus, urinary tract*), a *kidney tumor*, or, less commonly, a blood clot. In some cases, the kidney becomes distended because of obstruction to the outflow of urine from the bladder due to an enlarged *prostate gland*.

SYMPTOMS AND SIGNS
Acute hydronephrosis, with sudden blockage of the ureter, results in severe pain in the loin. Chronic hydronephrosis, in which the obstruction develops slowly, may cause no symptoms until the ureter has become completely blocked and kidney failure occurs. The kidney may also become infected, resulting in pyonephrosis (pus-filled kidney).

DIAGNOSIS AND TREATMENT
Ultrasound scanning can provide an image of the kidneys and ureter. If the scan reveals an obstruction and if the kidney is still relatively healthy, the blockage is removed or relieved by surgery; the kidney usually resumes normal, or near normal, function. Occasionally, however, a kidney is so badly damaged that it requires removal (see *Nephrectomy*); the remaining kidney, provided it is healthy, will compensate for the loss of the other.

Hydrophobia
A once popular term—now almost obsolete—for *rabies*. Meaning "fear of water," hydrophobia refers to the inability to drink that is one of the characteristic symptoms of rabies.

Hydrops
An abnormal accumulation of fluid in body tissues or in a sac (baglike organ or body structure). Hydrops fetalis, which may be caused by severe *Rh incompatibility*, is marked by generalized *edema* (fluid collection causing tissue swelling) of the fetus.

Hydrotherapy

The external use of water to treat patients recovering from injury or suffering from lack of mobility. Hydrotherapy includes the use of exercise pools, whirlpool baths, and showers.

People who are unable to bear full weight on a limb (because of arthritis

or after a fracture, for example) can often exercise more fully and effectively in a hydrotherapy pool. The buoyant effect of the water allows a greater range of movement and permits fuller use of the limb with little discomfort. Warm whirlpool baths provide a gentle massage to stimulate areas of the body and relieve stiffness. Cold baths or showers after an injury can reduce blood flow, swelling, and bruising and can help to minimize tissue damage. (See also *Heat treatment; Ice packs*).

Hydroxocobalamin
A long-acting synthetic preparation of *vitamin B$_{12}$* given by injection.

Hydroxyzine
Hydroxyzine is an *antihistamine* drug that has three uses: it helps control hives and itching, it reduces nausea and vomiting, and it is a mild tranquilizer. It commonly causes drowsiness.

Hygiene
The science and practice of preserving health. Today the word is commonly equated with cleanliness, particularly in the sense of personal hygiene. However, in the last century and early years of this century, the term hygiene was widely used as an equivalent to *public health*—the scientific study of environmental influences on health (with particular regard to the provision of pure water supplies, safe sanitation, good housing, and safe conditions in the workplace).

The terms industrial hygiene and occupational hygiene refer to the science of measuring, assessing, and controlling the environment to prevent *occupational disease*.

Hygiene, oral
See *Oral hygiene*.

Hygroma, cystic
A type of *lymphangioma* which may be present around the head and neck, armpits, or groin. Cystic hygromas contain clear fluid. They increase during infancy, usually reaching their maximum size by the age of 2, and then gradually disappear. Most are left to disappear naturally, but surgical removal is performed if a cystic hygroma is very unsightly or if it obstructs the airway.

Hymen
The thin fold of membrane surrounding the vaginal opening. The hymen has a central perforation which is

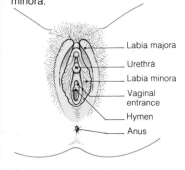

LOCATION OF HYMEN
The membrane that forms the hymen surrounds the opening to the vagina, inside a woman's labia minora.

Labia majora
Urethra
Labia minora
Vaginal entrance
Hymen
Anus

usually stretched or torn by the use of tampons or during first sexual intercourse. Once torn, the hymen becomes an irregular ring of tissue around the vaginal opening.

Imperforate hymen is a rare condition in which the hymen has no perforation; at the onset of menstruation, menstrual blood collects in the vagina, causing lower abdominal pain. The condition is easily corrected by a minor operation.

Hyoid
A small, U-shaped bone situated centrally in the upper part of the neck. The hyoid is not joined to any other bone but is suspended by ligaments from the base of the skull. Its function is to provide an anchor point for the muscles of the tongue and for those in the upper part of the front of the neck.

LOCATION OF HYOID BONE
The U-shaped hyoid bone provides an anchor for the muscles at the back of the tongue.

Muscles of tongue

Hyoid bone

Hyoscyamine
An *anticholinergic* drug used in treating irritable bladder and *irritable bowel syndrome*.

Hyper-
A prefix meaning above, excessive, or greater than normal, as in *hypertension* (high blood pressure) and *hyperthyroidism* (overactivity of the thyroid gland).

Hyperacidity
A condition in which an excessive amount of acid is produced by the stomach. Hyperacidity is commonly confused with *acid reflux* (which causes a burning sensation in the upper abdomen or lower chest) or *water brash* (sudden filling of the person's mouth with a watery fluid). Most people with a duodenal ulcer (see *Peptic ulcer*) produce more acid than normal, and those with *Zollinger-Ellison syndrome* produce vast amounts.

Hyperactivity
A behavior pattern of childhood in which the child is continually overactive and has difficulty concentrating on a single activity or task. It is four times more common in boys than in girls. The incidence is uncertain because various diagnostic criteria are used, but in some estimates it may be as high as 5 percent of children in the susceptible age group.
CAUSES
It has been suggested that some hyperactive children, especially those who are clumsy, may have a subtle form of "minimal" brain damage. However, there is no definite, conclusive evidence.

Hyperactive children seem more likely to have fathers who were hyperactive, suggesting that the condition may be partly inherited. Children with *mental retardation, cerebral palsy,* or *temporal lobe epilepsy* may also be hyperactive. Although food allergy is widely believed to be a common cause, research studies suggest that it is involved only rarely.
SYMPTOMS
The main feature of hyperactivity is continual overactivity. Such children are always on the go, full of energy, fidgety, and seem to sleep less than their peers. They also tend to be impulsive and reckless, with no sense of danger, and are usually irritable, emotionally immature, and aggressive. Their attention span is short and, as a result, they do not conform to orderly routine.

In those afflicted with the condition, hyperactivity can lead to antisocial acts and to learning difficulty, although IQ is normal. It is not known whether this behavior is a part of the disorder or simply a result of an affected child's poor attention span and disruptive activity.
DIAGNOSIS
Overactivity in itself does not indicate that a child is hyperactive. A stressful home environment or physical illness may also cause overactivity. It is also true that many of the behavioral problems mentioned are, to some degree, common to all young children. However, when other causes have been eliminated and the behavior continues past the age of 4 years, is intense, and is different from that of "normal" children, then it seems reasonable to regard the child as being hyperactive.
TREATMENT
Paradoxically, *stimulant drugs* (such as amphetamines) seem to be the most effective treatment for those suffering from this condition. This suggests that hyperactivity results from "underarousal" of the midbrain, which causes no damping down or control of movements and sensations. Stimulant drugs seem to work by stimulating the midbrain enough to suppress the extra activity. Behavior therapy and counseling of the child and parents are also useful.

Diets that exclude certain artificial food colorings, additives, or foods benefit very few children.

Hyperactive children should have formal educational and psychological assessment; many need help with reading and spelling.
OUTLOOK
In many cases, hyperactivity disappears completely at puberty. In others, the overactivity subsides and is replaced by sluggishness, depression, and moodiness; these teenagers often fail at school and resort to antisocial behavior. Sometimes all the symptoms of hyperactivity continue into adult life.

Hyperacusis
An exceptionally developed sense of hearing. Hyperacusis may cause the sensation of pain or discomfort in the ears on exposure to loud noises.

Hyperaldosteronism
A metabolic disorder that is caused by an overproduction of the hormone *aldosterone* by the adrenal glands. See *Aldosteronism*.

Hyperalimentation
Administration of excess amounts of calories, usually intravenously or by stomach tube. (See *Feeding, artificial*.)

Hyperbaric oxygen treatment
A method of increasing the amount of oxygen in the tissues by exposing a person to oxygen at a much higher than normal atmospheric pressure.
WHY IT IS DONE
This technique is occasionally used to treat poisoning from *carbon monoxide*, in which the tissues are starved of oxygen because *hemoglobin* (the oxygen-carrying component of red blood cells) is prevented from taking up oxygen. Hyperbaric oxygen treatment is also used in cases of gas *gangrene*; the bacteria that infect gangrenous tissue cannot survive if they are oxygenated.
HOW IT IS DONE
The patient is placed in a chamber into which oxygen is pumped at up to three times normal atmospheric pressure for no more than three hours. The inhaled oxygen dissolves in the patient's blood.

Hyperbilirubinemia
A raised blood level of *bilirubin* (a waste product formed from the destruction of red blood cells). Hyperbilirubinemia may be undetectable except by a blood test, but *jaundice* becomes apparent if the blood bilirubin rises to twice the normal level.

Hypercalcemia
An abnormally high level of *calcium* in the blood. Minor degrees of hypercalcemia are quite common in healthy people and probably not significant.
CAUSES
Hypercalcemia is commonly caused by *hyperparathyroidism* (overproduction of parathyroid hormone, which helps control the blood calcium level).

Cancer may cause hypercalcemia, either by spreading to bone or by producing abnormal hormones which cause bone to soften, releasing calcium from bone into the blood.

Less commonly, hypercalcemia is due to excessive intake of *vitamin D*, which helps regulate the absorption of calcium, or to certain inflammatory disorders, such as *sarcoidosis*.
SYMPTOMS
Hypercalcemia causes nausea, vomiting, lethargy, depression, thirst, and excessive urination. Higher levels of calcium in the blood produce confusion, extreme fatigue, and muscle weakness. If the disorder is untreated and the blood calcium level continues

H

to increase, cardiac arrhythmias (irregularities of the heartbeat), kidney failure, coma, and even death may result. Long-standing hypercalcemia may cause *nephrocalcinosis* (calcification of the kidney) or kidney stones (see *Calculus, urinary tract*).

DIAGNOSIS AND TREATMENT

The condition is diagnosed by measuring the level of calcium in the blood. If the diagnosis is confirmed, more tests are performed to discover the underlying cause. Any treatment is of the underlying cause.

Hypercapnia

Excessive carbon dioxide in the blood. Carbon dioxide is a waste product of the metabolic processes that produce energy in body cells and is eliminated from the body during *breathing* out. Normally, the amount of carbon dioxide in the blood is maintained within narrow limits. Hypercapnia is caused by failure of mechanisms, such as breathing rate, that normally control blood carbon dioxide levels; it usually leads to respiratory *acidosis*.

Hyperemesis

The medical term for excessive *vomiting*, which may cause dehydration and weight loss. When the condition occurs in pregnancy, it is known as hyperemesis gravidarum.

Hyperglycemia

An abnormally high level of glucose (sugar) in the blood, occurring in people suffering from untreated or inadequately controlled *diabetes mellitus*. It may also occur in diabetics as a result of an infection, stress, or surgery.

The symptoms of hyperglycemia are the same as those of diabetes: thirst, the passing of large amounts of urine, *glycosuria* (glucose in the urine), and *ketosis* (an accumulation of ketones in the body). In severe cases, hyperglycemia may lead to confusion and coma, which require emergency medical treatment with *insulin* and an intravenous infusion of fluids.

Hypergonadism

Overactivity of the gonads (*testes* or *ovaries*) resulting in overproduction of *androgen hormones* or *estrogen hormones*. Hypergonadism may be caused by disorders of the gonads or by a disorder of the *pituitary gland* that results in overproduction of *gonadotropin hormone*. During childhood, the condition causes precocious sexual development and excessive growth in its victims.

Hyperhidrosis

A term meaning excessive sweating. Hyperhidrosis may be localized, affecting only the armpits, feet, palms, or face. Alternatively, it may be generalized, affecting all areas supplied by *sweat glands*.

CAUSES

Excessive sweating may be caused by hot weather, exercise, or anxiety. In some cases, the condition is due to a disorder, such as an infection, *thyrotoxicosis, hypoglycemia*, or a disorder of the nervous system. More commonly, hyperhydrosis is idiopathic (of unknown cause), usually beginning at puberty and disappearing by the mid-20s or early 30s.

TREATMENT

Sufferers should pay special attention to personal hygiene. Clothing and shoes made of natural materials, such as cotton and leather, tend to be more comfortable than less absorbent materials. Regular use of *antiperspirants* may help; potent preparations of aluminum chloride and aluminum hydroxychloride may be prescribed by a physician. Some cases may respond to treatment with *anticholinergic drugs*.

Hyperkeratosis

Thickening of the outer layer of the skin due to an increased amount of *keratin* (a tough protein that is the major component of the outer layer of skin). The most common forms of hyperkeratosis are *corns* and *calluses*, caused by prolonged pressure or friction. Hyperkeratosis is a feature of warts on the soles of the feet (see *Wart, plantar*). It is also a feature of *lichen planus*.

The term hyperkeratosis is sometimes used to describe abnormal thickening of the *nails*.

Hyperkinetic syndrome

Another name for *hyperactivity*.

Hyperlipidemias

A group of *metabolic disorders* characterized by high levels of *lipids* (fats) in the blood.

TYPES

Hyperlipidemias may be classified into six types. These six types are differentiated by the extent to which the blood levels of different forms of lipids are higher than normal (see the table on facing page).

Lipids are carried in the blood in several forms, chiefly *cholesterol*, triglycerides, and lipoproteins. Lipoproteins consist of fat and cholesterol

molecules linked to protein molecules. Lipoproteins are classified according to their density, which depends on their relative proportions of cholesterol and protein; the higher the proportion of cholesterol, the lower the density of the lipoprotein. According to this classification, lipoproteins are divided into: very low-density lipoproteins (VLDLs), low-density lipoproteins (LDLs), and intermediate-density lipoproteins (IDLs). There are also high-density lipoproteins (HDLs), but these are not involved in the hyperlipidemias. Chylomicrons (microscopic fat droplets in the blood) are usually also classed as lipoproteins.

CAUSES

Hyperlipidemias may be inherited or may be a consequence of another disorder, such as *hypothyroidism, alcohol dependence, diabetes mellitus, kidney failure,* and *Cushing's syndrome.* Hyperlipidemias may also result from treatment with *corticosteroid drugs* or *estrogen drugs*.

RISKS

Hyperlipidemias are associated with a number of serious disorders, notably *atherosclerosis* (narrowing of arteries by deposits of fatty material) and *coronary artery disease*. For this reason, if a close relative has, or has had, either of these disorders, particularly if he or she has had a heart attack while still under 50 years of age, other members of the family should be tested.

SYMPTOMS, DIAGNOSIS, AND TREATMENT

The symptoms and treatments for the different types of hyperlipidemia are shown in the table on page 553. Because many of the types produce similar symptoms, diagnosis usually depends on blood tests to measure the levels of the different lipids.

Treatment depends to some extent on the type of hyperlidemia, but in all cases is aimed at reducing blood lipid levels and thus lowering the risk of atherosclerosis.

Hypernephroma

An alternative and older name for renal cell carcinoma, which is a type of *kidney cancer*.

Hyperopia

Commonly called farsightedness, an error of *refraction* that initially causes difficulty in seeing near objects and then affects distance vision. Hyperopia tends to run in families.

Hyperopia is caused by the eye being too short from front to back, so that images are not clearly focused on

TYPES OF HYPERLIPIDEMIA

Type	Lipoprotein elevated	Blood cholesterol level	Blood triglyceride level	Symptoms and signs in addition to risk of heart disease	Treatment
I	Chylomicrons	Small elevation	Large elevation	Fatty nodules in skin; abdominal pain; inflammation of pancreas	Diet very low in fats.
IIa	Low-density lipoproteins	Small to medium elevation	Normal	Fatty nodules around tendons (especially Achilles tendon and hand tendons) and over joints; white line around rim of cornea	Diet low in saturated fats and cholesterol; cholestyramine, colestipol, or clofibrate may be prescribed.
IIb	Low-density and very low-density lipoproteins	Small to medium elevation	Small elevation	Fatty nodules on eyelids; white line around rim of cornea	Diet low in saturated fats, cholesterol, and carbohydrates; cholestyramine or colestipol may be prescribed.
III	Intermediate-density lipoproteins	Small to medium elevation	Small to medium elevation	Fat deposits in palms and sometimes over joints	Diet low in fats and carbohydrates; clofibrate, nicotinic acid or gemfibrozil may be prescribed.
IV	Very low-density lipoproteins	Normal	Small to medium elevation	Fatty nodules in skin; patient is often obese	Diet low in carbohydrates; weight reduction; clofibrate and sometimes nicotinic acid and gemfibrozil may be prescribed.
V	Chylomicrons and very low-density lipoproteins	Small elevation	Small to medium elevation	Fatty nodules in skin; abdominal pain; inflammation of pancreas; patient may be obese	Diet low in fats and carbohydrates; weight reduction; gemfibrozil and nicotinic acid may be prescribed.

the retina. Mild or moderate hyperopia in the young is overcome by *accommodation* (the action of the ciliary muscles to change the shape of the lens), which brings the point of focus forward to produce a clear image.

SYMPTOMS AND SIGNS
The error is present from birth, but symptoms generally do not appear until later life. The more severe the hyperopia, the lower the age at which people experience difficulty viewing close objects, because the power of accommodation declines with age. In time, distant objects also become blurred.

TREATMENT
If necessary, an ophthalmologist may prescribe *glasses* or *contact lenses* with convex lenses which will reinforce focusing power.

Hyperparathyroidism
Overactivity of the *parathyroid glands*. These pea-sized glands are embedded in the thyroid gland in the neck and produce parathyroid hormone. This hormone, together with *vitamin D* and *calcitonin* (a hormone produced by the thyroid gland), controls the level of calcium in the body. Overproduction of parathyroid hormone raises the level of calcium in the blood (a condition called *hypercalcemia*) by removing the calcium from bones. This condition may lead to bone disorders, for example *osteoporosis*.

In an attempt to normalize the high blood calcium level, the kidneys excrete large amounts of calcium in the urine, which can result in the formation of kidney stones (see *Calculus, urinary tract*).

CAUSES AND INCIDENCE
Hyperparathyroidism is most often caused by a small benign tumor of one or more of the parathyroid glands. In other cases, it occurs when the patient's glands become enlarged for no known reason.

About 35 people per 100,000 suffer from the disorder, which usually develops after the age of 40 and is twice as common in women as in men.

SYMPTOMS
Hyperparathyroidism may cause generalized aches and pains, depression, and abdominal pain. Often, the only symptoms are those caused by kidney stones.

If hypercalcemia is severe, there may be nausea, vomiting, tiredness, excessive urination, confusion, and muscle weakness.

DIAGNOSIS AND TREATMENT
The condition is diagnosed by X rays of the hands and skull and by tests to measure the level of calcium, phosphorus, and parathyroid hormone in the blood.

Surgical removal of all abnormal parathyroid tissue usually cures the condition. In some cases, the amount of parathyroid tissue remaining after the operation may be insufficient to meet the body's needs. The affected person may then require treatment for *hypoparathyroidism* (underactivity of the parathyroid glands).

Hyperplasia
Enlargement of an organ or tissue due to an increase in the number of its constituent cells. The new cells are normal, unlike those of a tumor.

Hyperplasia is usually the result of hormonal stimulation. It may be a normal occurrence (such as in the enlargement of breast tissue and uterine muscle that occurs during pregnancy)

HYPERPARATHYROIDISM

In this disorder, the parathyroid glands produce too much parathyroid hormone. Symptoms, signs, and complications of the disorder occur as a result of an increased calcium level in the blood and urine, the loss of calcium from bones, and calcinosis (the formation of calcium deposits in different tissues). Surgical removal of abnormal parathyroid tissue is carried out to prevent complications.

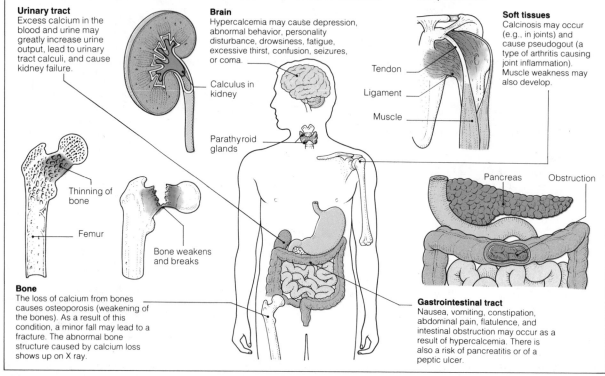

Urinary tract
Excess calcium in the blood and urine may greatly increase urine output, lead to urinary tract calculi, and cause kidney failure.

Calculus in kidney

Parathyroid glands

Brain
Hypercalcemia may cause depression, abnormal behavior, personality disturbance, drowsiness, fatigue, excessive thirst, confusion, seizures, or coma.

Tendon

Ligament

Muscle

Pancreas   Obstruction

Soft tissues
Calcinosis may occur (e.g., in joints) and cause pseudogout (a type of arthritis causing joint inflammation). Muscle weakness may also develop.

Thinning of bone

Femur

Bone weakens and breaks

Bone
The loss of calcium from bones causes osteoporosis (weakening of the bones). As a result of this condition, a minor fall may lead to a fracture. The abnormal bone structure caused by calcium loss shows up on X ray.

Gastrointestinal tract
Nausea, vomiting, constipation, abdominal pain, flatulence, and intestinal obstruction may occur as a result of hypercalcemia. There is also a risk of pancreatitis or of a peptic ulcer.

or it may indicate a disorder (such as in hyperplasia of the thyroid or adrenal glands, which may be due to oversecretion of certain pituitary hormones). Hyperplasia of the prostate gland is a common benign condition of men after middle age. (See also *Hypertrophy*.)

Hyperplasia, gingival

Abnormal enlargement of the gums. The condition may be a feature of *gingivitis* (inflammation of the gums), especially when it occurs during pregnancy. Gingival hyperplasia can also develop around the front teeth as a result of persistent breathing through the mouth. The condition can also be caused by *phenytoin*, an anticonvulsant drug used to treat *epilepsy*. Gums may be enlarged for other reasons too. For example, ill-fitting dentures may cause rolls of fibrous gum tissue to form beyond the edges of the dentures.

Enlarged gums should be examined by a dentist whether or not one wears dentures; surgical removal of surplus tissue may be necessary.

Hyperpyrexia

A medical term for extremely high body temperature; it is synonymous with hyperthermia. Heat hyperpyrexia is another name for *heatstroke*.

Hypersensitivity

Overreaction of the *immune system* (defense against infection) to an *antigen* (protein recognized as foreign). Hypersensitivity reactions occur only on second or subsequent exposures to particular antigens, after the first exposure has sensitized the immune system. Such reactions have the same mechanisms as those of protective *immunity*. However, while the latter protect against disease, hypersensitivity reactions lead to tissue damage and disease.

Hypersensitivity is closely related to *allergy*, except that only one of the four main types of hypersensitivity reaction (type I) is closely associated with allergic illnesses.

TYPES
The four main types of hypersensitivity reaction are as follows.

TYPE I This type is also called immediate or anaphylactic hypersensitivity. After a first exposure to an antigen (which may be a harmless substance such as grass pollen), *antibodies* (substances that can recognize and bind to the antigen) are formed; these antibodies coat cells called mast cells in various tissues. On second exposure, the antigen and antibodies combine, causing the mast cells to disintegrate and release various chemicals that cause the symptoms of *asthma*, allergic *rhinitis* (hay fever), *urticaria* (hives), *anaphylactic shock*, or other illnesses of an allergic nature.

TYPE II In this type, antibodies that bind to antigens on cell surfaces are formed, leading to possible destruction of the cells. Type II reactions may be responsible for certain *autoimmune disorders* (in which antibodies attack the body's own tissues) and for some cases of *hemolysis* (red blood cell destruction) triggered by certain drugs.

TYPE III Antibodies combine with antigens to form particles called immune complexes, which can lodge in various tissues and activate further immune system responses, leading to tissue damage. This type of hypersensitivity reaction is responsible for *serum sickness*, for allergic *alveolitis* (a lung disease caused by exposure to the spores of certain fungi), and for the large swellings that sometimes form after booster vaccinations.

TYPE IV This type is also called delayed hypersensitivity. In type IV, sensitized *T-lymphocytes* (a class of white blood cell and an important component of the immune system) bind to antigens and subsequently release chemicals called lymphokines, which promote an inflammatory reaction. Type IV reactions are responsible for contact *dermatitis* and the rash of *measles*; they are important in the body's defense against *tuberculosis* and may also play a part in some "allergic" reactions to drugs.

TREATMENT
Effective treatment of a hypersensitivity reaction depends on its type, cause, and severity. When possible, exposure to the offending antigen should be avoided.

Hypersplenism
Overactivity of the *spleen*, resulting in and associated with blood disease. One of the functions of the spleen is to break down blood cells as they age and wear out. An overactive spleen may begin to destroy cells indiscriminately, causing a deficiency of any of the types of blood cell. In most cases, the spleen will also be enlarged.

Hypersplenism may be primary, occurring for no known reason, but more commonly it is secondary to another disorder in which the spleen has become enlarged, such as *Hodgkin's disease* or *malaria*.

SYMPTOMS AND TREATMENT
A person with hypersplenism is likely to have the symptoms of *anemia* (due to destruction of red blood cells) or of *thrombocytopenia* (platelet deficiency), and there is sometimes a decrease in resistance to infection due to lack of white cells. There may also be symptoms of an underlying disorder, such as malaria.

Treatment of secondary hypersplenism is aimed at controlling the underlying cause. Primary hypersplenism requires *splenectomy* (removal of the spleen).

Hypertension
Abnormally high *blood pressure* (the pressure of blood in the main arteries). Blood pressure goes up as a normal response to stress and physical activity. However, a person with hypertension has a high blood pressure even at rest. A large number of people have hypertension without even realizing it; because the condition increases the chances of having a *stroke* or of developing heart disease, regular medical checks are advised in order to detect hypertension as early as possible.

Blood pressure is measured by two values, each expressed as millimetres (mm) of mercury (chemical symbol Hg) or mm Hg. The systolic value (the higher value) is the pressure when blood surges into the aorta from the heart; the diastolic value is the pressure when the ventricles (larger heart chambers) relax between beats.

There is no clear dividing line between "normal" and "high" blood pressure, but in Canada mild hypertension is considered to begin at levels of 140 systolic and 90 diastolic. Although average blood pressures rise with age in developed countries, a person over 65 who has a blood pressure at these levels has a significantly increased risk of having the cardiovascular complications described above. A diastolic pressure of 105 or above is considered to indicate severe hypertension.

INCIDENCE AND CAUSES
Hypertension is an extremely common condition, affecting 12 percent of the Canadian adult population. The condition is more common in men than in women and its incidence is highest in the middle-aged and elderly, although significant numbers of young adults are also hypertensive.

Blood pressure rises as a result of an increase in resistance to the flow of blood in both large and small blood vessels. Resistance increases in the large vessels as they become more rigid with age. Resistance in the smaller vessels depends on the extent to which they are constricted, which is under nerve and chemical control.

About 95 percent of people with hypertension have no obvious underlying cause for their elevated blood pressure; in such cases it is called essential hypertension. Apart from age and male gender, factors associated with an increased risk of essential hypertension include: obesity, excess alcohol intake, a family history of hypertension, a sedentary lifestyle, and a high degree of social and occupational stress. In the other 10 percent of patients with hypertension, a definite cause is found; it is then called secondary hypertension. Specific causes include various disorders of the *kidneys*, certain disorders of the *adrenal glands*, *preeclampsia* (a complication of pregnancy), *coarctation of the aorta* (a type of congenital heart defect), and use of certain drugs. Taking the combined (estrogen-containing) contraceptive pill appears to increase the risk of hypertension.

SYMPTOMS AND COMPLICATIONS
Hypertension usually causes no symptoms and generally goes undiscovered until detected by a physician during the course of a routine physical examination. Severe hypertension may sometimes cause headaches, shortness of breath, giddiness and visual disturbances.

Hypertension puts a considerable strain on the heart and blood vessels. Apart from increasing the risk of having a stroke or developing *heart failure* or *coronary artery disease*, high blood pressure may eventually cause kidney damage and *retinopathy* (damage to the retina at the back of the eye). Severe hypertension may cause confusion and seizures.

All these risks increase with the degree of hypertension. For example, for a man in his 40s, each rise of 10 mm Hg in the systolic blood pressure increases the risk of heart disease by about 20 percent.

DIAGNOSIS
Because of the health risks associated with hypertension, everyone should have his or her blood pressure checked at least once every five years, and if previous readings have shown borderline or raised blood pressure, more frequently than this. Many family physicians now check the blood pressure of their middle-aged and elderly patients at virtually every consultation.

A diagnosis of hypertension is usually not confirmed until the patient's blood pressure at rest is found to be raised on three separate occasions. However, hypertension is sometimes diagnosed on the first reading if the blood pressure is exceptionally high and accompanied by one of the complications of hypertension, such as retinopathy.

TREATMENT
Occasionally, in the most severe cases of hypertension, immediate admission to hospital for emergency treatment, investigation of the cause, and bed rest, is required.

With mild to moderate hypertension, if no underlying cause (such as a kidney disorder) is found, the first line

H

HYPERTENSION

Hypertension affects about 12 percent of adults in Canada. It is diagnosed if a person's resting blood pressure is persistently raised.

Blood pressure is expressed by two values—the systolic and diastolic pressures—and measured in millimetres of mercury.

Although hypertension rarely causes symptoms, it is a serious condition. Left untreated, it increases the risk of stroke and other disorders. In many cases, there is no obvious cause, but, in some, there is a specific cause, such as a kidney disorder, pregnancy, or use of oral contraceptives. Hypertension is linked to obesity and, in some people, to a high salt intake. Smoking appears to aggravate the effects of hypertension.

Stress and hypertension
Stress acts on the nervous system, causing blood vessels to constrict and the heart to work harder. Both lead to a temporary rise in blood pressure. Hence, pressure should be measured when a person is relaxed. It is possible (but unproven) that frequent stress may eventually cause hypertension.

Atheroma
Hypertension and atherosclerosis, in which arteries are narrowed (left), are closely linked.

Fatty deposits
Contracted muscle

Constriction
Factors such as nicotine in tobacco cause artery constriction (left) and a short-term rise in blood pressure that may worsen hypertension.

Artery wall

Variation in blood pressure
In any population, blood pressure varies over a wide range in the same way as height. Many people are considered to be hypertensive because they are at the top end of this range (see above). In obese people, the range is similarly wide but shifted toward the top end; hence, more obese people are hypertensive.

COMMON FACTORS AND PREVENTIVE MEASURES

Factors associated with essential hypertension	Age (incidence higher in the elderly)	Family history of the condition	Gender (incidence higher in men than in women)	
Factors that may aggravate hypertension	Smoking Obesity	Excess alcohol intake	Diabetes mellitus	Stress
Self-help and treatment	1. Regular screening of blood pressure is important for early diagnosis and can help to prevent complications 2. Sufferers from essential hypertension should: Reduce weight Not smoke Reduce or stop alcohol intake Reduce salt intake Learn relaxation methods to combat stress 3. Antihypertensive drugs, prescribed by a physician, can usually keep high blood pressure under control			

of attack is alteration of life-style. Smokers should stop smoking and drinkers should reduce their consumption of alcohol. Any overweight person with hypertension should make an attempt to reduce weight through restriction of food intake and gradually increased exercise. A restricted intake of salt is also sometimes recommended. All these general health measures may also help to prevent hypertension from developing in the first place.

A number of stress management techniques have been tried for mild hypertension. These include relaxation and *biofeedback training* techniques. So far, controlled trials of these techniques have yielded inconsistent results, and they are still under investigation.

If these non-drug measures have no effect, or in the case of more severe hypertension, *antihypertensive drugs* may be prescribed. A large number of different types of antihypertensive drug are available, including diuretics, beta-blockers, vasodilators, and calcium antagonists, which work in different ways on the heart, blood vessels, and nervous system to reduce blood pressure. One or a combination of drugs may be prescribed, leading to satisfactory control of the hypertension in the majority of cases. Usually, the physician will wish to monitor the effects of treatment through measurement of blood pressure every two to four weeks, so that adjustment to the drug dosages or regimen can be made if necessary. If any side effects develop, the physician should be told, as a more suitable alternative therapy may be available.

Most people who have a sustained elevation of blood pressure will have to take drugs for several years or even for the rest of their lives.

Hyperthermia
A medical term for extremely high body temperature. (See also *Heatstroke*.)

Hyperthermia, malignant
A rapid rise in body temperature to a dangerously high level brought on by general *anesthesia*. The condition is rare, occurring in only about one in 50,000 operations. In most cases, susceptibility to the condition is inherited; people suffering from certain muscle disorders may also be at risk.

The patient's temperature rises soon after the anesthetic is given. At the same time, large amounts of *lactic acid* pass from the muscles into the blood, causing *acidosis*. The muscles then stiffen and the patient turns blue; without emergency treatment, seizures and death may follow rapidly.

Malignant hyperthermia may be suspected if the patient does not relax normally during the early, induction stage of anesthesia, or if he or she shows signs of abnormal muscle contractions after administration of succinylcholine (a chemical used to relax muscles during operations).

If malignant hyperthermia occurs, the anesthetic is stopped immediately and the patient is cooled with ice packs. Pure oxygen and intravenous injections of sodium bicarbonate may be given to counteract acidosis. Injections of dantrolene sodium are given intravenously at 5- to 10-minute intervals as required.

Hyperthyroidism

Overproduction of *thyroid hormones* by an overactive *thyroid gland*.

CAUSES AND INCIDENCE

The most common form of hyperthyroidism is *Graves' disease*, an *auto-immune disorder* in which the body develops antibodies that stimulate the production of excessive amounts of thyroid hormones. This condition affects about 1 percent of the adult population and is most common in young to middle-aged women. More rarely, hyperthyroidism may be associated with the development of enlarged nodules in the thyroid.

SYMPTOMS AND SIGNS

Symptoms and signs are described in the illustrated box below.

DIAGNOSIS AND TREATMENT

The diagnosis of hyperthyroidism is confirmed by tests to measure the level of thyroid hormones in the blood. The condition may be treated with drugs that inhibit the production of thyroid hormones or by surgical removal of part of the thyroid gland. In older patients, an alternative is a single dose of radioactive iodine, which is taken up by the thyroid and destroys some of its tissue.

Hypertonia

Increased rigidity in a muscle. Hypertonia may be caused by damage to its nerve supply or by cell changes within the muscle itself. Hypertonia causes episodes of continuous muscle spasm (as may occur in the bladder wall, for example, when the outflow of urine is being obstructed by an enlarged prostate gland).

Persistent hypertonia in limb muscles following a *stroke* or major *head injury* causes *spasticity* (increased rigidity). A variable increase in muscle tension associated with abnormal patterns of movement and posture is referred to as *dystonia*.

Hypertrichosis

Growth of excessive hair, often in places that are not normally hairy. Hypertrichosis is often a result of taking certain drugs (including *cyclosporine*, *minoxidil*, and *diazoxide*). The term hypertrichosis is also used to describe hair growth in a colored, fleshy mole.

Hypertrichosis is not the same as *hirsutism*, which is excessive hairiness, particularly in women, due to abnormally high levels of male hormones in the blood.

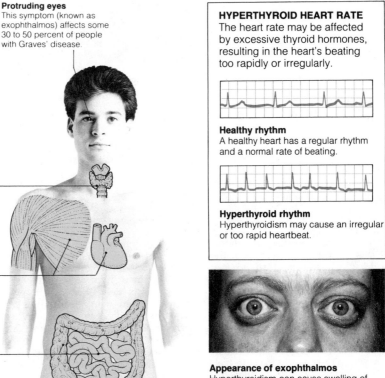

SYMPTOMS AND SIGNS OF HYPERTHYROIDISM

Oversecretion of thyroid hormones produces symptoms associated with overactivity of the body's metabolism. Weight loss, increased appetite, intolerance to heat, and increased sweating are early signs; there may also be tremors and a rapid heart rate. In more severe cases, the thyroid gland is often enlarged and there tends to be physical and mental hyperactivity and wasting of the muscles.

Thyroid gland enlargement
This symptom (known as goiter) may be due to hyperthyroidism. However, it may also be associated with hypothyroidism (underactivity of the thyroid).

Muscle wasting
Severe hyperthyroidism may cause wasting of both skeletal and heart muscle; it may also lead to irregularities of heart rhythm.

Increased appetite
This symptom is a result of the metabolic overactivity that hyperthyroidism causes. Despite increased appetite, there is often weight loss.

Protruding eyes
This symptom (known as exophthalmos) affects some 30 to 50 percent of people with Graves' disease.

HYPERTHYROID HEART RATE
The heart rate may be affected by excessive thyroid hormones, resulting in the heart's beating too rapidly or irregularly.

Healthy rhythm
A healthy heart has a regular rhythm and a normal rate of beating.

Hyperthyroid rhythm
Hyperthyroidism may cause an irregular or too rapid heartbeat.

Appearance of exophthalmos
Hyperthyroidism can cause swelling of tissues around the eyes, resulting in a staring appearance.

Hypertrophy

Enlargement of an organ or tissue due to an increase in the size, rather than the number, of its constituent cells. For example, skeletal muscles increase in size in response to increased physical demands. (See also *Hyperplasia*.)

Hyperuricemia

An abnormally high level of *uric acid* in the blood. Hyperuricemia may lead to the development of *gout* due to the deposition of uric acid crystals in the joints; it may also cause kidney stones (see *Calculus, urinary tract*) and the deposition of crystals elsewhere in the body, especially around joints (see *Tophus*).

CAUSES

Hyperuricemia may be caused by an inborn error of metabolism (see *Metabolism, inborn error of*), by rapid destruction of cells as part of a disease such as *leukemia*, or by medication (such as *diuretic drugs*) that reduces the excretion of uric acid by the kidneys. Increased amounts of *purine* (a nitrogen-containing substance) in the diet may raise the level of uric acid in the blood, precipitating gout.

TREATMENT

Drugs, such as *allopurinol* (which reduces uric acid production in cells) and *probenecid* or *sulfinpyrazone* (which increase the excretion of uric acid by the kidneys), may be prescribed for the rest of the patient's life to prevent complications. Foods that are high in purine (such as liver, poultry, and dried peas and beans) should be avoided.

Hyperventilation

Abnormally deep or rapid breathing, usually caused by *anxiety*. Hyperventilation may also occur as a result of uncontrolled *diabetes mellitus*, oxygen deficiency, *kidney failure*, and some lung disorders (such as *pulmonary edema* and *emphysema*).

Hyperventilation causes an abnormal loss of carbon dioxide from the blood, which can lead to *alkalosis* (increase in blood alkalinity). Symptoms include numbness of the extremities, faintness, *tetany* (painful spasms and twitches of the muscles, especially in the hands and feet), and a sensation of not being able to take a full breath. The effects of alkalosis often add to the already existing feelings of anxiety, and may give rise to "hyperventilation syndrome," in which the sufferer experiences a feeling of impending doom.

Breathing into a plastic or paper bag during an attack may help reduce the loss of carbon dioxide and avoid the risk of alkalosis.

Hyperventilation associated with uncontrolled diabetes or with kidney failure represents the body's efforts to eliminate excess carbon dioxide in dealing with *acidosis*.

Hyphema

Blood in the front chamber of the *eye*, almost always caused by an injury that ruptures a small blood vessel in the iris or the ciliary body.

Vision is blurred while the blood remains mixed with the aqueous humor, but clears as the red cells sink. In most cases, the blood disappears completely within a few days and vision is fully restored. There is, however, a risk of delayed bleeding three to five days after the injury.

Appearance of hyphema
Blood that has collected in the front chamber of the eye is clearly visible in front of the iris; hyphema is usually caused by injury.

Hypnosis

A trancelike state of altered awareness characterized by extreme suggestibility. Although it was once believed to be a form of sleep, the *EEG* (electrical tracing of brain-wave activity) of a hypnotized person does not show any normal sleep patterns.

HISTORY

A form of hypnotism was first practiced by the Austrian physician Franz Mesmer in the 18th century. Mesmerism (renamed hypnotism after the Greek god of sleep) began to receive attention from many leading members of the medical community in the 19th century. The celebrated Parisian physician Charcot gave public demonstrations, and Freud used hypnosis in his early treatment of hysteria.

In some provinces, hypnosis is regulated and its use limited to specified practitioners, such as physicians, den-

tists, and psychologists. Most provincial health plans pay for hypnotherapy. Hypnosis is not a medical specialty, but a means of treating certain conditions.

HOW IT IS DONE

For hypnosis to succeed, the subject must first want to be hypnotized. The second requirement is relaxation, so a comfortable chair and a quiet, dimly lit room are usually necessary. The subject is usually asked to fix his or her attention on a particular object while the therapist quietly repeats phrases such as "Be still and listen to my voice" or "Empty your mind of all thoughts." The subject gradually becomes more and more relaxed, eventually losing touch with the environment and hearing only the therapist's voice. At the end of the session, the subject "wakes up" when told to do so.

With training, it is possible for people to practice autohypnosis (self-hypnosis) by repeating certain phrases to themselves or imagining relaxing scenes.

Some people are more easily hypnotized than others, usually those with an intense imaginative life. The ability seems to be related to early childhood experiences and may be partly inherited.

CHARACTERISTICS

Hypnotized subjects wait passively to be told what to do by the therapist and are very suggestible—they touch or hold imaginary objects and act out suggested roles. They do not, however, obey commands to behave in a manner they would normally regard as dangerous or improper.

Attention usually becomes highly selective, so that only one person at a time is heard. Subjects frequently will obey orders to forget everything that has happened during hypnosis, or, alternatively, to remember or repeat behavior learned while hypnotized (a phenomenon known as posthypnotic suggestion).

THERAPEUTIC USES

Physicians probably use hypnosis most frequently as a way to help patients relax. It is also used in the treatment of phobias, anxiety states, multiple personality syndromes, and sexual dysfunction. It has been used in smoking cessation, but it is no more successful than other antismoking programs.

Hypnotic drugs

Drugs that induce sleep. (See *Sleeping drugs*.)

Hypo-

A prefix meaning under, below, or less than normal, as in hypodermic (under the skin), *hypoglycemia* (abnormally low blood sugar level), and *hypotension* (lower than normal blood pressure).

Hypoaldosteronism

A rare deficiency of the hormone *aldosterone*, which is produced by the adrenal glands. Hypoaldosteronism may be caused by damage or disease affecting the adrenal glands. The disorder may produce weakness and is treated by the drug fludrocortisone.

Hypocalcemia

An abnormally low level of *calcium* in the blood. The most common cause is *vitamin D* deficiency, due to a poor diet or, occasionally, to lack of sunshine. Rarer causes include chronic *kidney failure*, which leads to poor absorption of calcium from the diet, and *hypoparathyroidism* (underactivity of the parathyroid glands), resulting in insufficient production of parathyroid hormone, which helps control the level of calcium in the blood.

In mild cases, hypocalcemia is symptomless. In severe cases, it causes *tetany* (painful spasms and twitches of the muscles, especially in the hands and feet) due to the effect of low blood calcium on muscle activity. Hypocalcemia may lead to softening of the bones. In children, such softening takes the form of *rickets*; in adults, it takes the form of *osteomalacia*.

Hypochondriasis

The unrealistic belief or fear that one is suffering from a serious illness, despite medical reassurance.

SYMPTOMS

Hypochondriacs worry constantly about their bodily health and interpret any physical symptom, however trivial, as evidence of a serious disorder. The feared disease may involve many parts of the body or may center on a particular organ or a single disease, as in *cardiac neurosis* (fear of heart disease). People with hypochondriasis constantly seek medical advice and are likely to undergo numerous tests.

Hypochondriasis may be a complication of other psychological disorders, including *obsessive-compulsive disorder*, *phobia*, *generalized anxiety disorder*, *schizophrenia*, *depression*, and brain diseases, such as *dementia*.

The cause of hypochondriasis in the absence of an underlying disorder is uncertain. However, it seems to be more common in people who suffered from a true organic illness during childhood or were constantly exposed to sick relatives. The reason for this may be that the hypochondriac becomes programmed to overreact to every bodily feeling. In some cases, however, there may be an inherited sensitivity to pain. Other factors responsible for hypochondriasis include social stresses and personality type (typically orderly and obstinate).

TREATMENT

Any underlying mental disorder is treated as required. Hypochondriasis without an underlying cause is more difficult to treat, although an understanding and sympathetic physician may help relieve distress.

Hypochondrium

The region on each side of the upper abdomen below the lower ribs.

Hypoglossal nerve

The 12th *cranial nerve*, which controls movements of the *tongue*. The hypoglossal nerve is rarely damaged. If damage does occur (as a result of a stroke, for example), one side of the tongue becomes paralyzed.

LOCATION OF HYPOGLOSSAL NERVE

The hypoglossal nerve arises in the medulla oblongata (part of the brain stem), passes through the base of the skull, and runs around the throat to the tongue.

Skull

Brain stem

Tongue muscles

Hypoglossal nerve

Hypoglycemia

An abnormally low level of glucose (sugar) in the blood. Almost all cases of hypoglycemia occur in people with insulin-dependent *diabetes mellitus*. In this disease, the pancreas fails to produce enough *insulin* (a hormone that regulates the level of glucose in the blood), resulting in an abnormally high level of glucose. To lower the blood glucose level, diabetics take hypoglycemic drugs by mouth (see *Hypoglycemics, oral*) or insulin by injection. Too high a dose of either can reduce the blood glucose to too low a level, thus starving the body cells of energy. Hypoglycemia can also occur if a person with diabetes misses a meal, fails to eat enough carbohydrates, or takes too much exercise.

Rarely, hypoglycemia can result from drinking a large amount of alcohol or from an *insulinoma*. Some children suffer from hypoglycemia for no known reason, but in most cases the condition is temporary.

Hypoglycemia is a serious condition. Failure of the brain to receive sufficient glucose may lead to permanent intellectual impairment.

SYMPTOMS

The principal symptoms include sweating, weakness, hunger, dizziness, trembling, headache, palpitations, confusion, and sometimes double vision. Behavior is often irrational and aggressive and movements are uncoordinated; this state may be mistaken for drunkenness. The victim may lapse into coma.

TREATMENT

Insulin-dependent diabetics should always carry sugar with them (in a convenient form such as sugar lumps or glucose tablets) to take at the first sign of an attack of hypoglycemia. If it is suspected that an unconscious person has suffered a hypoglycemic attack, medical help should be summoned immediately. The physician will give an injection of either glucose solution or the hormone glucagon; the latter counteracts the effects of insulin and raises the blood glucose level by stimulating the conversion of glycogen to glucose.

Hypoglycemics, oral

COMMON DRUGS
Chlorpropamide Glibenclamide Gliclazide Glipizide Tolazamide Tolbutamide

WARNING
Consult your physician if you regularly experience symptoms, such as dizziness, nausea, and sweating, that are relieved only by food or a sugary drink. You might be taking too large a dose.

H

H

A group of drugs used in the treatment of non-insulin-dependent *diabetes mellitus* when *hyperglycemia* (raised blood glucose level) cannot be controlled simply by diet.

Oral hypoglycemics lower blood glucose levels by increasing the production by the pancreas of *insulin*, a hormone that increases the amount of glucose that is absorbed from the bloodstream into body cells. Insulin rather than oral hypoglycemics may need to be prescribed temporarily to control the blood glucose level (e.g., during surgery, pregnancy, or a severe illness). Oral hypoglycemics are of no use in treating insulin-dependent diabetes, in which the pancreas is unable to produce any insulin.

POSSIBLE ADVERSE EFFECTS

Oral hypoglycemic drugs may cause *hypoglycemia* (abnormally low blood glucose) if the dosage is too high or if the person has not had enough to eat.

Hypogonadism

Underactivity of the gonads (*testes* or *ovaries*). Hypogonadism may be caused by disorders of the gonads or by a disorder of the *pituitary gland* that results in deficient production of *gonadotropin hormone*. In men, hypogonadism causes the symptoms and signs of *androgen hormone* deficiency. In women, it causes those of *estrogen hormone* deficiency.

Hypohidrosis

Reduced activity of the *sweat glands*. It is a feature of hypohidrotic ectodermal dysplasia, a rare, inherited, incurable condition characterized by reduced production of sweat and usually accompanied by dry, wrinkled skin, sparse, dry hair, small, brittle nails, and conical teeth.

Other causes include *exfoliative dermatitis* and some *anticholinergic drugs*.

Hypomania

A mild form of *mania*.

Hypoparathyroidism

Insufficient production of parathyroid hormone by the *parathyroid glands*, which lie behind the *thyroid gland* in the neck. Parathyroid hormone, along with *vitamin D* and *calcitonin* (a hormone produced by the thyroid gland), regulates the level of *calcium* in the body. A deficiency of the hormone results in *hypocalcemia* (low levels of calcium in the blood).

The most common cause of hypoparathyroidism is accidental removal of the parathyroid glands during surgery on the thyroid gland. The condition may also result from surgery to remove a portion of the parathyroid glands themselves in the treatment of *hyperparathyroidism* (overactivity of the parathyroid glands). Occasionally the parathyroid glands are absent from birth, or they may cease to function for no apparent reason.

SYMPTOMS

The main effect of a low level of calcium in the body is *tetany*, an increased excitability of the nerves that causes uncontrollable, painful, cramplike spasms of the hands, feet, and sometimes other parts of the body. Very occasionally, general seizures similar to those of an epileptic attack may occur.

DIAGNOSIS AND TREATMENT

The condition is diagnosed by tests to measure the level of calcium and parathyroid hormone in the blood.

If the patient is suffering from an attack of tetany, calcium may be injected slowly into a vein to provide quick relief. To maintain the blood calcium at a normal level, a lifelong course of calcium and vitamin D tablets is necessary (the vitamin D is needed to increase absorption of calcium from the diet). Regular checkups are necessary to monitor the blood calcium level.

Hypophysectomy

The removal or destruction of the *pituitary gland*.

Hypophysectomy is sometimes performed to remove *pituitary tumors*, which can cause various endocrine disorders, such as *acromegaly* and *Cushing's syndrome*.

The operation may also be performed to treat some cancers of the breast, ovary, or prostate gland, the growth of which is stimulated by hormones secreted by the pituitary gland.

HOW IT IS DONE

In some cases, the pituitary gland is removed surgically. The patient is given a general anesthetic and the gland is removed, usually through the nose. Very large tumors may be removed through an incision into the skull (see *Craniotomy*).

In other cases, the gland may be destroyed by a radioactive implant which can be inserted into the gland by *stereotaxic surgery*.

Hypopituitarism

Underactivity of the *pituitary gland*, resulting in inadequate production of pituitary hormones. Hypopituitarism may lead to deficiency of one or more of the pituitary hormones and thus may produce a variety of effects on the body depending on which hormones are affected. Possible causes of hypopituitarism are a *pituitary tumor*, an abnormality affecting the *hypothalamus* (part of the brain), or injury to the pituitary gland. Hypopituitarism may also follow surgical treatment or *radiation therapy* of the pituitary gland.

The condition is treated by replacing the deficient hormones.

Hypoplasia

Failure of an organ or a tissue to develop fully and reach its normal adult size.

Hypoplasia, enamel

A defect in tooth enamel. It is usually due to *amelogenesis imperfecta* (a hereditary condition), but may also be caused by vitamin deficiency, injury, or infection of a primary tooth that interferes with maturation of enamel.

Hypoplastic left heart syndrome

A serious and usually fatal form of congenital *heart disease* that affects about one to two newborn babies in every 10,000 live births. The baby is born with a poorly formed ventricle (pumping chamber) on the left side of the heart and with other heart defects. The aorta (main artery carrying blood from the heart to the body) is malformed and blood can reach it only via a duct (the ductus arteriosus) that links the aorta to the pulmonary artery, which transports blood to the lungs.

At birth the baby may seem healthy, but within a day or two the ductus arteriosus closes off and the baby collapses, becoming pale and breathless. Surgical correction of the defects is very difficult, and only about 20 percent of children survive a two-stage operation. Heart transplantation has also been used, but the supply of infant hearts is erratic. Untreated, affected babies die within a week. The risk of parents having another affected child is small.

Hyposensitization

A preventive treatment of *allergy* to substances such as grass pollens, house-dust mites, and wasp and bee venom. Hyposensitization involves giving gradually increasing doses of an allergen (substance to which the person is allergic). This works by making the *immune system* less sensitive to that substance, probably by causing production of a particular "blocking" *antibody*, which reduces the symptoms of allergy when the substance is encountered.

Skin tests or sometimes blood tests are performed to confirm the specific allergens to which the person has antibodies. Hyposensitization is usually recommended only if the person seems to be selectively sensitive to a specific allergen.

HOW IT IS DONE
A purified extract of a small amount of the allergen is injected into the skin of the arm in a course of injections. The course may need to be repeated annually for a few years.

RISKS
There is a danger of *anaphylactic shock* (a severe allergic reaction) shortly after an injection. Hyposensitization must therefore be performed under close medical supervision.

Hypospadias
A *congenital* defect of the *penis*, occurring in about one in 300 male babies, in which the opening of the *urethra* is situated on the underside of the penis. The urethral opening may be on the glans (head) or the shaft of the penis. In some cases, the penis curves downward, a condition known as *chordee*, and the foreskin is limited to the front of the penis.

In severe forms of hypospadias the urethral opening lies well back along the penis toward the scrotum. The scrotum may be small, and the testes are undescended (see *Testis, undescended*). In such cases, the true sex of the child may be in doubt.

TREATMENT
Hypospadias can be corrected by a single operation in which the penis is straightened and a tube of skin (or occasionally bladder lining) is used to create a new urethra that extends to the tip of the penis. The operation is normally performed before the child is 2 years old; circumcision should not be performed prior to a hypospadias repair because the foreskin may be needed at the operation.

Surgery is usually successful, allowing the child to pass urine normally and, in later years, to have satisfactory sexual intercourse.

Hypotension
The medical term for low *blood pressure*. Some healthy people with a normal heart and blood vessels have blood pressure well below average for their age. The term hypotension is usually used only when blood pressure has fallen to the extent that blood flow to the brain is reduced, causing dizziness and fainting.

In the most common type of hypotension, known as postural hypotension, symptoms occur after abruptly standing or sitting up. Usually, blood pressure increases slightly with these changes in posture; in people with postural hypotension, this normal increase fails to occur. Postural hypotension is sometimes an adverse effect of *antidepressant drugs* or of *antihypertensive drugs* (drugs used to treat high blood pressure). Postural hypotension may also occur in people with *diabetes mellitus*.

Another type of hypotension develops suddenly as a result of serious burns or injuries that lead to a reduction in blood volume and to *shock*. Acute hypotension may also develop when a disease, such as *myocardial infarction* (heart attack) or *adrenal failure*, leads to shock.

Treatment of hypotension depends on the underlying cause.

Hypothalamus
A region of the *brain*, roughly the size of a cherry, situated behind the eyes and beneath another brain region called the thalamus. The hypothalamus has nerve connections to most other regions of the nervous system.

FUNCTION
The hypothalamus exerts overall control over the sympathetic nervous system (part of the *autonomic nervous system*). In response to sudden alarm or excitement, signals are sent from higher regions of the brain to the hypothalamus, which initiates sympathetic nervous system activity. This causes a faster heartbeat, increased breathing, widening of the pupils of the eye, and increased blood flow to muscles (all together known as the "fight or flight" response).

Other groups of nerve cells in the hypothalamus are concerned with the control of body temperature. Some are sensitive to heat and cold so that, when blood flowing to the brain is hotter or cooler than normal, the hypothalamus switches on temperature-regulating mechanisms (among them sweating or shivering). The hypothalamus receives information from internal sense organs regarding the body's water content and the level of glucose in the blood; if these are too low, the hypothalamus stimulates thirst and appetite for food. The hypothalamus is also involved in regulating sleep, in motivating sexual behavior, and in determining mood and the experience of emotions.

Another role is to coordinate the function of the nervous and endocrine (hormonal) systems. The hypothalamus connects with the *pituitary gland* through a short stalk of nerve fibers and controls hormonal secretions from this gland. It does this in two ways—through direct nerve connections and through specialized nerve cells, which secrete hormones called releasing factors into the blood to travel to the pituitary gland. In this way, the hypothalamus can convert nerve signals into hormonal signals. Thus, the hypothalamus indirectly

H

HYPOPLASTIC LEFT HEART SYNDROME
The heart defects associated with this syndrome are shown (at right) and compared with those of the normal heart (at left). Neither the left ventricle (pumping chamber) nor the aorta is properly formed.

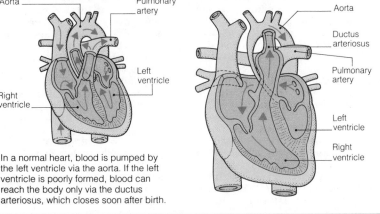

In a normal heart, blood is pumped by the left ventricle via the aorta. If the left ventricle is poorly formed, blood can reach the body only via the ductus arteriosus, which closes soon after birth.

Aorta — Pulmonary artery
Left ventricle
Right ventricle

Aorta
Ductus arteriosus
Pulmonary artery
Left ventricle
Right ventricle

H

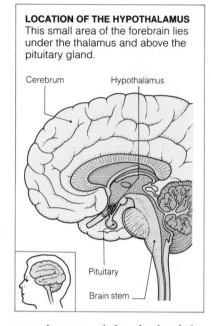

LOCATION OF THE HYPOTHALAMUS
This small area of the forebrain lies under the thalamus and above the pituitary gland.

Cerebrum   Hypothalamus

Pituitary

Brain stem

controls many of the glands of the *endocrine system*, including the pituitary gland, *thyroid gland*, cortex of the *adrenal glands*, *ovaries*, and *testes*.

Disorders of the hypothalamus are usually caused by a hemorrhage within the hypothalamic region (see *Intracerebral hemorrhage*) or by an expanding *pituitary tumor*. Loss of hypothalamic function can have effects ranging from hormonal disorders to disturbances in temperature regulation, and increased or decreased appetite for food, sex, and sleep.

Hypothermia
A fall in body temperature to below 35°C. Hypothermia causes drowsiness, lowers breathing and heart rates, and may lead to unconsciousness or death. Many victims are elderly people who are unable to keep sufficiently warm in winter.

Hypothermia also includes the deliberate lowering of body temperature during some forms of surgery (see *Hypothermia, surgical*).

CAUSES
Most cases of serious hypothermia in Canada occur after exposure outdoors to cold and wind. Alcohol intoxication, inadequate clothing and a cold winter night can be a fatal combination. Alcohol consumption reduces resistance to cold, dulls the sense of discomfort, and may disorient a person walking home. Hypothermia is also a hazard for travelers trapped in a car in a snowstorm.

Hypothermia may develop at above-freezing temperatures if exposure to wind and cold rain is prolonged and clothing is damp. It is now thought that some deaths attributed to drowning in cold water are actually due to hypothermia. Except in July and August, all bodies of water in or surrounding Canada are cold enough to induce severe hypothermia in a few minutes.

Elderly people are particularly at risk, especially if they live in poorly heated buildings or if they have conditions such as *hypothyroidism*, impaired mental function (*dementia*) or poor mobility (*arthritis*) that reduce the body's heat production. Babies also are at increased risk because they lose heat rapidly and cannot easily reverse a fall in temperature.

Certain drugs may also contribute to the onset of hypothermia. For example, *tranquilizer drugs* (such as chlorpromazine) may lower the level of consciousness and reduce the ability to shiver, which helps protect the body against cold.

SIGNS
A person suffering from hypothermia is usually pale, puffy-faced, and listless, and shows changes in behavior, such as withdrawal and apathy. The heart rate is slow and the victim is often drowsy and confused. Areas of the body that are normally warm (e.g., the armpits, the groin) are cold.

In severe hypothermia, breathing becomes slow and shallow, the muscles are often stiff, the victim may become unconscious, and the heart may beat only faintly and irregularly or—especially if the body temperature falls below 32.2°C—it may stop beating altogether.

DIAGNOSIS
The condition is usually obvious from the above signs and the victim's circumstances. To determine how cold the body has become, the rectal temperature is taken with a special low-reading thermometer. Household rectal thermometers do not read below 33°C, but hospital emergency departments have low-reading thermometers. Alternatively, the temperature of the urine may be measured.

TREATMENT
A person with impaired consciousness or abnormalities of heartbeat or respiration due to hypothermia requires immediate medical attention. Even if heartbeat and respiration are undetectable, it is possible that proper emergency treatment can save the person's life.

If the person is unconscious and has no heartbeat or respiration, start *cardiopulmonary resuscitation*.

If there is a heartbeat but no respiration, start *artificial respiration*.

If the victim has a heartbeat and respiration, but is unconscious, place in the *recovery position*.

All unconscious victims should be warmed by raising the room temperature to at least 25°C, and by wrapping in a heat-reflective (thermal) blanket. Victims of severe hypothermia may be admitted to an intensive care unit for controlled warming and warm fluids may be given either intravenously or by introduction into the abdominal cavity.

If the person is conscious, he or she may be warmed in a bath heated to about 40°C (warm to the touch). This is not recommended for elderly victims because rapid warming of the skin and muscles may cause a rush of blood to the surface of the body with consequent reduction in blood supply to the brain and other organs. Elderly people should be warmed gradually by being placed in a very warm room (25°C), covered with blankets or heat-reflecting material, and their rectal temperature monitored every half hour. The temperature should rise at least 0.6°C per hour.

In mild cases, changing into dry warm clothes and drinking warm drinks (never give alcohol) may be sufficient. Do not attempt to warm the victim by rubbing the skin.

PREVENTION
The best protection against hypothermia is clothing that blocks wind and completely covers the body with heavy insulation. A hooded parka (more than 20 percent of the body's heat is lost through the head) is the best protection against cold and windy weather, especially when traveling any distance at night. People driving long distances in winter should equip their cars with candles and matches, reflective blanket, extra clothing, and emergency rations.

For elderly infirm people, care should be taken to ensure that their living quarters are kept at a temperature of at least 20°C, and that hot drinks and meals are available.

Hypothermia, surgical
The deliberate reduction of body temperature to prolong the period for which the vital organs can safely be deprived (partly or totally) of their normal blood supply during *open heart surgery*.

Cold reduces the rate of metabolism in cells and tissues and thus increases their tolerance to lack of oxygen.

In the early days of heart surgery, induced hypothermia allowed surgeons to perform quick (eight to 10 minutes) operations on the heart while blood circulation throughout the body was completely stopped.

Today, open heart surgery is usually performed with the general blood circulation maintained by means of a *heart-lung machine*. Nevertheless, mild hypothermia—with the body temperature reduced from 37°C to about 28 to 31°C—is still generally induced as a safety measure. It can allow heart operations to proceed for several hours. A heat exchanger, installed into the machine circuit, can be used to cool the blood before it is returned to the body, thus inducing hypothermia.

During open heart surgery, because the blood supply to the heart is interrupted, the heart muscle itself must also be vigorously cooled. Cooling can be achieved by continuously instilling cold saline at a temperature of about 4°C into the open chest cavity. As a result, damage to the heart muscle from lack of oxygen is minimal, even if an operation lasts several hours.

Rewarming of the patient afterward is carefully synchronized with restarting the heart and stopping use of the heart-lung machine.

Hypothyroidism

Underproduction of *thyroid hormones* by an underactive *thyroid gland*.

CAUSES AND INCIDENCE

Most cases of hypothyroidism are caused by the body developing *antibodies* against its own thyroid gland (an example of an *autoimmune disorder*) with a resultant reduction in thyroid hormone production. *Hashimoto's thyroiditis* is an example of this phenomenon. More rarely, hypothyroidism may result from surgery to remove part of the thyroid gland or the giving of radioactive iodine as a treatment for *hyperthyroidism*.

About 1 percent of the adult population suffer from hypothyroidism. It is most common in elderly women, although it occurs at all ages and in both sexes.

SYMPTOMS AND SIGNS

Thyroid hormones stimulate energy production, so a deficiency of them causes generalized tiredness and lethargy. There may also be muscle weakness, cramps, a slow heart rate, dry and flaky skin, hair loss, a deep and husky voice, and weight gain. A syndrome known as *myxedema*, in which the skin and other body tissues thicken, may develop. In some cases, a *goiter* (enlargement of the thyroid gland) develops, although not all goiters are due to hypothyroidism.

The severity of the symptoms depends on the degree of thyroid deficiency. Mild deficiency may cause no symptoms; severe deficiency may produce all of the above symptoms.

If hypothyroidism occurs in childhood and remains untreated, it may retard growth, delay sexual maturation, and inhibit normal development of the brain.

DIAGNOSIS AND TREATMENT

The disorder is diagnosed by tests to measure the level of thyroid hormones in the blood.

Treatment consists of replacement therapy with the thyroid hormone thyroxine; in most cases, hormone therapy must be continued for life. If this treatment does not cure a goiter, surgery may be required.

Hypotonia

Abnormal muscle slackness. Normally, a muscle that is not being used has a certain inbuilt tension, but in a number of disorders affecting the nervous system (such as *Huntington's chorea*) this natural tension or tone is moderately or markedly reduced.

Hypotonia in infants

Excessive limpness in infants. Hypotonia is sometimes known as the floppy infant syndrome.

FEATURES

Hypotonic babies cannot hold their limbs up against gravity and thus tend to lie flat with their arms and legs splayed. Their limbs and joints seem slack when moved by someone else. Floppy babies move around less than normal babies and their mothers may not have felt the baby move much during pregnancy. When held horizontally by the trunk, face downward, floppy babies hang limply.

CAUSES

Premature infants are naturally more floppy than full-term infants, but normal muscle tension will develop as they mature.

Hypotonia may be caused by a general disorder, such as *hypothyroidism* or *Down's syndrome*. It may also be an early feature of *cerebral palsy* as a result of brain damage, and occurs in disorders of the spinal cord, such as *Werdnig-Hoffman disease*, and in some children with *muscular dystrophy*.

Hypovolemia

An abnormally low volume of blood in the circulation. Hypovolemia usually follows severe blood loss, which may occur as a result of injury, internal bleeding, or surgery. It also occurs in other conditions, such as serious burns and severe dehydration.

Hypovolemia, untreated, can lead to *shock*, which is potentially fatal.

Hypoxia

An inadequate supply of oxygen to the tissues.

CAUSES

Temporary hypoxia may occur as a result of strenuous exercise in which the normal supply of oxygen cannot meet the additional requirements of the tissues. In such cases, the condition disappears once exercise has stopped and breathing has reoxygenated the tissues.

More serious causes include impaired breathing (see *Respiratory failure*), usually as a result of a lung disorder; *ischemia* (reduced blood flow to a tissue), which may be due to an artery disorder or a heart disorder; and severe *anemia*, in which the oxygen-carrying capacity of the blood is reduced. Another, rare, cause is *carbon monoxide* poisoning, which prevents the blood from being adequately oxygenated. In severe cases, any of these more serious causes may lead to *anoxia* (complete absence of oxygen in a tissue), which, if prolonged, may cause tissue death.

SYMPTOMS AND SIGNS

Hypoxia in muscles forces the muscle cells to produce energy by *anaerobic* metabolism, which produces lactic acid as a by-product. The accumulation of lactic acid causes cramps. Hypoxia in heart muscle may cause the chest pain of *angina pectoris*. Hypoxia of the brain initially causes confusion, dizziness, and incoordination, progressing to unconsciousness and death if the condition persists.

TREATMENT

Severe, potentially life-threatening hypoxia may require treatment by *oxygen therapy* or artificial *ventilation*. Otherwise, the treatment depends on the underlying cause.

Hysterectomy

Removal of the uterus. Hysterectomy is the most frequently performed major operation in Canada.

Hysterectomy is often performed to treat *fibroids* (benign tumors of the uterus) that are causing symptoms. It is also performed to treat cancer of the

H

uterus (see *Uterus, cancer of*) or of the cervix (see *Cervix, cancer of*). Hysterectomy may be performed to relieve *menorrhagia* (heavy menstrual bleeding) or *endometriosis* (a condition in which fragments of the uterine lining occur elsewhere in the pelvis) that have not responded to treatment. A hysterectomy may also be performed to remove a severely prolapsed uterus (see *Uterus, prolapse of*).

TYPES

The most common type of hysterectomy is a total hysterectomy, in which the uterus and cervix are removed. Sometimes, the fallopian tubes and ovaries are removed in addition to the uterus. The operation known as a subtotal hysterectomy, in which the cervix is not removed, is now obsolete. For cervical cancer, a radical hysterectomy (in which the pelvic lymph nodes are also removed) is necessary.

RECOVERY PERIOD

After the operation, a drainage tube may be inserted at the site of the incision. For a few days there may be some vaginal bleeding and discharge and considerable tenderness and pain. The stay in hospital depends on the age and health of the woman and whether there are postoperative problems. Full recovery requires another three to six weeks; sexual intercourse can be resumed about a month after the surgery.

After hysterectomy, the woman is unable to bear children; she does not menstruate and needs no contraception. If the ovaries have also been removed from a woman before or around the *menopause, hormone replacement therapy* should be considered.

Many women worry that their sex lives will be affected, but there should be no noticeable change. Early counseling can help dispel fears. Depression is not uncommon if women are inadequately counseled.

Hysteria

A term encompassing a wide range of physical or mental symptoms that are attributed to mental stress.

Derived from the Greek word for uterus, hysteria was once thought to be a physical disorder confined to women. By the 19th century, it was believed to have a psychological origin and was used to describe many seemingly bizarre states (e.g., hallucination, trances, and sleepwalking).

Today, many psychiatrists feel that the term hysteria is no longer helpful in diagnosis. In modern classifications, therefore, the symptoms for-

---

PERFORMING A HYSTERECTOMY

Hysterectomy may be performed through the abdomen or the vagina. For an abdominal hysterectomy, the incision is made in the lower abdomen (see below). In vaginal hysterectomy, the uterus is removed through an incision at the top of the vagina.

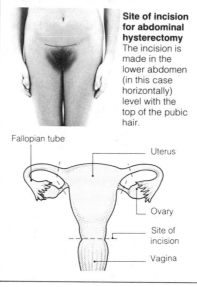

Site of incision for abdominal hysterectomy
The incision is made in the lower abdomen (in this case horizontally) level with the top of the pubic hair.

Fallopian tube

Uterus

Ovary

Site of incision

Vagina

Abdominal hysterectomy
The uterine vessels are clamped. Traction is placed on the top of the uterus and the vessels are tied and then divided. In some cases, the fallopian tubes are cut and the tubes and ovaries left in place.

Vaginal hysterectomy
After a vaginal incision is made, the uterus and cervix are removed. The upper end of the vagina is repaired by stitching.

---

merly grouped under this term are now included in the more specific diagnostic categories of *conversion disorder; dissociative disorders; factitious disorders;* and *somatization disorder*.

The term is still sometimes used loosely to describe any difficult or unusual behavior that does not seem consistent with the symptoms or situation of the patient. Mass hysteria describes the spread of psychologically produced symptoms (such as fainting) from person to person. It usually occurs in schools or institutions of young women in response to group tensions or worries and is often triggered by a charismatic personality.

Hysterosalpingography

An *X-ray* procedure performed to examine the inside of the uterus and fallopian tubes.

WHY IT IS DONE

The examination is performed as part of the investigation of *infertility*. *Laparoscopy* can indicate whether the tubes are blocked, but hysterosalpingography may be needed to determine the site of the blockage, which is most often due to scar tissue caused by a

previous infection. Hysterosalpingography also outlines any distortion in the uterus, such as a congenital abnormality or a *fibroid*.

HOW IT IS DONE

The test is an outpatient procedure performed by a radiologist and/or a gynecologist. It may cause discomfort or a cramplike pain, so the patient may be mildly sedated.

A plastic or metal *cannula* (tube) is inserted into the cervix (neck of the uterus), a radiopaque contrast medium (one that shows up on X-ray film) is passed through it into the uterus and the fallopian tubes; X-ray pictures are taken to reveal any abnormalities. The procedure takes 10 to 30 minutes.

Hysterotomy

A method of late abortion in which the abdomen and uterus are surgically opened to remove the fetus. Hysterotomy is the most complicated method of abortion and carries the highest risk. It is rarely used today; instead, most late abortions are performed by giving *prostaglandin drugs* to induce labor. (See also *Abortion, induced*.)

SEE END OF VOLUME 2 FOR